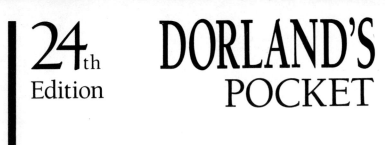

24th Edition

DORLAND'S POCKET

Medical Dictionary

**ABRIDGED FROM DORLAND'S ILLUSTRATED
MEDICAL DICTIONARY**

with a series of 16 color plates:
The Human Body – Highlights of Structure and Function

W. B. SAUNDERS COMPANY
Harcourt Brace Jovanovich, Inc.

Philadelphia   London   Toronto   Montreal   Sydney   Tokyo

W.B. SAUNDERS COMPANY
Harcourt Brace Jovanovich, Inc.

The Curtis Center
Independence Square West
Philadelphia, PA 19106

Dorland's pocket medical dictionary.
Philadelphia, W.B. Saunders Co.

v. ill. 17 cm.

"Abridged from Dorland's illustrated medical dictionary."
Continues: American pocket medical dictionary.

1. Medicine—Dictionaries.
R121.A5   610'.3—dc19   98-578
Library of Congress   [8701r85]rev2   MARC-S

Print No.:   9 8 7 6 5

PREFACE

Ninety years have passed since the publication of the first edition of *Dorland's Pocket Medical Dictionary* (then titled *The American Pocket Medical Dictionary*). The twenty-fourth edition stands in the tradition of the previous twenty-three and has been governed by the same purpose: to provide in a compact and convenient form a comprehensive and authoritative guide to the spelling, pronunciation, and meaning of the vocabulary of medicine. Like its predecessors, this new edition draws extensively on *Dorland's Illustrated Medical Dictionary*, now in its twenty-seventh edition. The care and effort put forth in the preparation of the larger volume are thus passed on to the smaller.

It is an often-stated truth that medical and scientific knowledge is increasing at a prodigious rate. To keep up with the corresponding growth in terminology, thousands of new and up-to-date terms have been added in this edition. The entire Dictionary has been subjected to a thorough examination to ensure that the terminology and definitions are in accord with current usage. In addition to the revisions in the vocabulary, a number of other changes have been made with the aim of increasing the book's usefulness. Several of the color plates have been redrawn to make them clearer and more modern in appearance. The tables have been examined thoroughly and revised as necessary and have been reset in their entirety to make them easier to read. The temperature conversion tables have been moved from *thermometry* to their logical place at *temperature*. A table of SI units has been added, and the table "Multiples and Submultiples of the Metric System" has been moved to appear on the same page with it. Names of specific acids have been removed as subentries of the *acid* entry and added to the vocabulary as main entries alphabetized by the first word of the name; this was done to eliminate the extremely dense look of the former arrangement, with its sometimes long boldface entry words, fairly short definitions, and long chemical formulas. A change that will make an entire section of the Dictionary accessible to those who may have despaired of using it is the transliteration of the Greek characters in the section "Combining Forms in Medical Etymology." It is now possible to consult this

convenient guide to the formation of medical terms and the disentanglement of their parts without either knowing Greek or having constant recourse to a table of the Greek alphabet (two strong deterrents to the use of this section).

In order to make room for this new material, while keeping the book within the limits required by a compact dictionary, all terms, both new and old, were subjected to severe scrutiny and those considered obsolete or too specialized for inclusion were discarded. Additional space was gained by eliminating elements that are properly included in a large dictionary but are beyond what is necessary in a small one; these include rarely used or archaic variant spellings and entries for some of the grammatical forms (as the participles of a verb) related to an entry at which a definition appears, when these additional entries add nothing to the user's understanding. To give an extreme but illustrative possibility, there could be three or four variant spellings of a noun, sometimes with an adjectival form for each, the corresponding verb for the defined form, and present and past participles of the verb. Although such a list is appropriate to a larger dictionary, it is excessive in a smaller one when there are thousands of new terms to be added and the volume is approaching the limit of what could be called pocket-sized. All of the deleted forms can be deduced easily by means of the user's knowledge of English; anything odd or irregular has been retained. In addition, some of the long definitions that seemed more at home in the larger *Dorland's* than in a shorter dictionary have been rewritten. In all of these decisions, the compilers have been guided by the principle that was set forth in the first edition, that this dictionary is not intended "to take the place of the larger dictionaries indispensible to a thorough understanding of the language of medicine" but "to make the selection of words as complete as possible."

The result of all this care and effort is, we believe, a dictionary that upholds the tradition of its predecessors in providing a current, comprehensive yet compact, authoritative guide to medical vocabulary. We hope that you, the user, will find that this new edition of *Dorland's Pocket Medical Dictionary* remains as helpful today as its predecessors have been to countless others in the past.

Douglas M. Anderson
Editor

CONTENTS

NOTES ON THE USE
OF THIS BOOK

ARRANGEMENT OF ENTRIES

All terms in this Dictionary are listed in one alphabetical sequence except the open compound terms, which are listed as subentries under the principal word (the *noun*). Thus, Addison's disease, collagen disease, Raynaud's disease, etc., are subentries under *disease*. Interstitial pneumonia, primary atypical pneumonia, lobar pneumonia, etc., are subentries under *pneumonia*, and so on.

Chemical compounds embodying the name of the element are given as subentries under the element, so that sodium chloride is a subentry under *sodium;* compounds with names that indicate the oxidation state of the element, e.g., *cupric, cuprous,* will be found as subentries under the salt or ester, so that cupric sulfate appears as a subentry under *sulfate*. Names of specific acids form an exception to the general rule of arrangement and will be found as main entries alphabetized on the first word of the name rather than subentries under *acid*.

In all subentries, the noun (main entry) is repeated in abbreviated form (e.g., *a.* for acid, *d.* for disease). Subentries that are plural in form are indicated by adding an apostrophe and *s* to the abbreviation of the noun. Thus, under *body,* the subentry *Aschoff's b's* is read Aschoff's bodies, *ketone b's* is read ketone bodies, etc. Irregular and Latin plurals in subentries are spelled out, as *esophageal varices* under *varix*.

Adjectival forms of many words are given on the noun entries in many instances (e.g., **allele . . . allel'ic,** adj.; **allergen . . . allergen'ic,** adj.). In similar fashion, irregular plural forms are given on the singular forms (e.g., **epiphysis . . .** pl. *epiphyses*). When, however, such forms may not be readily recognizable they are also given as separate entries (e.g., **viscera . . .** plural of *viscus*).

PRONUNCIATION

The pronunciation of words is indicated by a phonetic respelling which appears in parentheses immediately following each main entry. These phonetic respellings, devised for ease of interpretation, are presented with a minimum of diacritical markings. The basic rule is this: An unmarked vowel ending a syllable is long; an unmarked vowel in a syllable ending with a consonant is short. By the same token, a long vowel in a syllable ending with a consonant is indicated by a macron (ā, ē, ī, ō, and ū): for example, ah-bāt′ (abate), lēd (lead), bīl (bile), hor′mōn (hormone), and am′pūl (ampule). A short vowel that constitutes or ends a syllable is indicated by a breve (ĕ, ĭ, ŏ, or ŭ): for example, ĕ-fu′zhun (effusion), ĭ-mu′nĭ-te (immunity), and ŏ-fish′al (official).

The syllable *ah* is used to represent the sound of *a* in open unaccented syllables (ah-pof′ĭ-sis, ah-tak′se-ah) and to indicate a broader *a* sound in syllables ending with a consonant, as in fahr′mah-se (pharmacy).

The primary accent in a word is indicated by a boldface, single accent, the secondary accent by a light face, double accent.

When, on successive words, the first syllables are pronounced in the same way, these syllables are given in the phonetic respelling of only the first of the sequence of terms. If the accent varies or other change occurs in the pronunciation of these syllables, even when they involve the same letters, the entire pronunciation is indicated in the phonetic respelling. For example:

> **ichthyophagous** (ik″the-of′ah-gus)
> **ichthyosarcotoxin** (ik″the-o-sar″ko-tok′sin)
> **ichthyosarcotoxism** (-sar″ko-tok′sizm)
> **ichthyosis** (ik″the-o′sis)
> **ichthyotoxin** (ik″the-o-tok′sin)

ABBREVIATIONS USED IN THIS DICTIONARY

a.	artery (L. *arteria*)
aa.	arteries (L. *arteriae*)
adj.	adjective
ant.	anterior
b.	bone
cf.	compare (L. *confer*)
e.g.	for example (L. *exempli gratia*)
ext.	external
Fr.	French
Ger.	German
Gr.	Greek
i.e.	that is (L. *id est*)
inf.	inferior
int.	interior
L.	Latin
lat.	lateral
m.	muscle (L. *musculus*)
mm.	muscles (L. *musculi*)
n.	nerve (L. *nervus*)
nn.	nerves (L. *nervi*)
o.	os (bone)
oss.	ossa (bones)
pl.	plural
post.	posterior
pr.	process
q.v.	which see (L. *quod vide*)
sing.	singular
sup.	superior
v.	vein (L. *vena*)
vv.	veins (L. *venae*)

COMBINING FORMS IN
MEDICAL TERMINOLOGY*

The following is a list of combining forms encountered frequently in the vocabulary of medicine. A dash or dashes are appended to indicate whether the form usually precedes (as *ante-*) or follows (as *-agra*) the other elements of the compound or usually appears between the other elements (as *-em-*). Following each combining form, the first item of information is the Greek or Latin word, or both a Greek and a Latin word, from which it is derived. Greek words have been transliterated into Roman characters. Latin words are identified by [L.], Greek words by [Gr.]. Information necessary to an understanding of the form appears next in parentheses. Then the meaning or meanings of the words are given, followed where appropriate by reference to a synonymous combining form. Finally, an example is given to illustrate the use of the combining form in a compound English derivative.

a-	*a*-[L.] (*n* is added before words beginning with a vowel) negative prefix. Cf. in-³. a*metria*
ab-	*ab* [L.] away from. Cf. apo-. *ab*ducent
abdomin-	*abdomen, abdominis* [L.] abdomen. *abdomino*scopy
ac-	See ad-. *ac*cretion
acet-	*acetum* [L.] vinegar. *aceto*meter
acid-	*acidus* [L.] sour. *acid*uric
acou-	*akouō* [Gr.] hear. *acou*ethesia. (Also spelled acu-)
acr-	*akron* [Gr.] extremity, peak. *acro*megaly
act-	*ago, actus* [L.] do, drive, act. re*action*
actin-	*aktis, aktinos* [Gr.] ray, radius. Cf. radi-. *actino*genesis
acu-	See acou-. osteo*acusis*
ad-	*ad* [L.] (*d* changes to *c, f, g, p, s,* or *t* before words beginning with those consonants) to. *ad*renal
aden-	*adēn* [Gr.] gland. Cf. gland-. *adeno*ma
adip-	*adeps, adipis* [L.] fat. Cf. lip- and stear-. *adipo*cellular
aer-	*aēr* [Gr.] air. an*aero*biosis
aesthe-	See esthe-. *aesthe*sioneurosis
af-	See ad-. *af*ferent
ag-	See ad-. *ag*glutinant
-agogue	*agōgos* [Gr.] leading, inducing. galact*agogue*
-agra	*agra* [Gr.] catching, seizure. pod*agra*
alb-	*albus* [L.] white. Cf. leuk-. *albo*cinereous
alg-	*algos* [Gr.] pain. neur*algia*
all-	*allos* [Gr.] other, different, *all*ergy
alve-	*alveus* [L.] trough, channel, cavity. *alve*olar
amph-	See amphi-. *amph*eclexis
amphi-	*amphi* [Gr.] (*i* is dropped before words beginning with a vowel) both, doubly. *amphi*celous
amyl-	*amylon* [Gr.] starch. *amylo*synthesis
an-¹	See ana-. *an*agogic
an-²	See a-. *an*omalous
ana-	*ana* [Gr.] (final *a* is dropped before words beginning with a vowel) up, positive. *ana*phoresis
ancyl-	See ankyl-. *ancylo*stomiasis
andr-	*anēr, andros* [Gr.] man. gyn*andro*id
angi-	*angeion* [Gr.] vessel. Cf. vas-. *angiem*phraxis
ankyl-	*ankylos* [Gr.] crooked, looped. *ankylo*dactylia. (Also spelled ancyl-)
ant-	See anti-. *ant*ophthalmic
ante-	*ante* [L.] before. *ante*flexion
anti-	*anti* [Gr.] (*i* is dropped before words beginning with a vowel) against, counter. Cf. contra-. *anti*pyogenic
antr-	*antron* [Gr.] cavern. *antro*dynia
ap-¹	See apo-. *ap*heter
ap-²	See ad-. *ap*pend
-aph-	*haptō, haph-* [Gr.] touch. dys*aph*ia. (See also hapt-)
apo-	*apo* [Gr.] (*o* is dropped before words beginning with a vowel) away from, detached. Cf. ab-. *apo*physis
arachn-	*arachnē* [Gr.] spider. *arachno*dactyly
arch-	*archē* [Gr.] beginning, origin. *arch*enteron
arter(i)-	*arteria* [Gr.] windpipe, artery. *arteri*osclerosis, peri*arter*itis
arthr-	*arthron* [Gr.] joint. Cf. articul-. syn*arthr*osis
articul-	*articulus* [L.] joint. Cf. arthr-. dis*articul*ation
as-	See ad-. *as*similation

*Compiled by Lloyd W. Daly, A.M., Ph.D., Litt. D., Allen Memorial Professor of Greek Emeritus, University of Pennsylvania.

at-   See ad-. *attrition*
aur-   *auris* [L.] ear. Cf. ot-. *auri*nasal
aux-   *auxō* [Gr.] increase. enter*auxe*
ax-   *axōn* [Gr.] or *axis* [L.] axis. *axo*fugal
axon-   *axōn* [Gr.] axis. *axono*meter
ba-   *bainō, ba-* [Gr.] go, walk, stand. hyp-
               no*batia*
bacill-   *bacillus* [L.] small staff, rod. Cf. bac-
               ter-. actino*bacill*osis
bacter-   *bactērion* [Gr.] small staff, rod. Cf. ba-
               cill-. *bacter*iophage
ball-   *ballō, bol-* [Gr.] throw. *ball*istics. (See
               also bol-)
bar-   *baros* [Gr.] weight. pedo*baro*meter
bi-1   *bios* [Gr.] life. Cf. vit-. aero*bic*
bi-2   *bi-* [L.] two (see also di-1). *bi*lobate
bil-   *bilis* [L.] bile. Cf. chol-. *bili*ary
blast-   *blastos* [Gr.] bud, child, a growing
               thing in its early stages. Cf. germ-.
               *blast*oma, zygoto*blast*
blep-   *blepō* [Gr.] look, see. hemia*blep*sia
blephar-   *blepharon* [Gr.] (from *blepō;* see blep-)
               eyelid. Cf. cili-. *blephar*oncus
bol-   See ball-. em*bol*ism
brachi-   *brachiōn* [Gr.] arm. *brachi*ocephalic
brachy-   *brachys* [Gr.] short. *brachy*cephalic
brady-   *bradys* [Gr.] slow. *brady*cardia
brom-   *brōmos* [Gr.] stench. podo*brom*idrosis
bronch-   *bronchos* [Gr.] windpipe. *bronch*oscopy
bry-   *bryō* [Gr.] be full of life. em*bry*onic
bucc-   *bucca* [L.] cheek. disto*bucc*al
cac-   *kakos* [Gr.] bad, abnormal. Cf. mal*ca*-
               codontia, arthro*cace*. (See also dys-)
calc-1   *calx, calcis* [L.] stone (cf. lith-), lime-
               stone, lime. *calc*ipexy
calc-2   *calx, calcis* [L.] heel. *calc*aneotibial
calor-   *calor* [L.] heat. Cf. therm-. *calor*imeter
cancr-   *cancer, cancri* [L.] crab, cancer. Cf.
               carcin-. *cancr*ology. (Also spelled
               chancr-)
capit-   *caput, capitis* [L.] head. Cf. cephal-.
               de*capit*ator
caps-   *capsa* [L.] (from *capio;* see cept-) con-
               tainer. en*caps*ulation
carbo(n)-   *carbo, carbonis* [L.] coal, charcoal. *car*-
               *bo*hydrate, *carbon*uria
carcin-   *karkinos* [Gr.] crab, cancer. Cf. cancr-.
               *carcin*oma
cardi-   *kardia* [Gr.] heart. lipo*cardi*ac
cary-   See kary-. *cary*okinesis
cat-   See cata-. *cat*hode
cata-   *kata* [Gr.] (final *a* is dropped before
               words beginning with a vowel)
               down, negative. *cata*batic
caud-   *cauda* [L.] tail. *caud*ad
cav-   *cavus* [L.] hollow. Cf. coel-. con*cav*e
cec-   *caecus* [L.] blind. Cf. typhl-. *cec*opexy
cel-1   See coel-. amphi*cel*ous
cel-2   See -cele. *cel*ectome
-cele   *kēlē* [Gr.] tumor, hernia. gastro*cele*
cell-   *cella* [L.] room, cell. Cf. cyt-. *cell*iferous
cen-   *koinos* [Gr.] common. *cen*esthesia
cent-   *centum* [L.] hundred. Cf. hect-. Indi-
               cates fraction in metric system.

[This exemplifies the custom in the
metric system of identifying frac-
tions of units by stems from the
Latin, as centimeter, decimeter, millimeter, and multiples of units by the
similar stems from the Greek, as
hectometer, decameter, and kilometer.] *centi*meter, *centi*pede
cente-   *kenteō* [Gr.] to puncture. Cf. punct-.
               entero*cente*sis
centr-   *kentron* [Gr.] or *centrum* [L.] point,
               center. neuro*centr*al
cephal-   *kephalē* [Gr.] head. Cf. capit-. en*cephal*-
               itis
cept-   *capio, -cipientis, -ceptus* [L.] take, re-
               ceive, re*ceptor*
cer-   *kēros* [Gr.] or *cera* [L.] wax. *cer*oplasty,
               *cer*omel
cerat-   See kerat-. *acerat*osis
cerebr-   *cerebrum* [L.] brain. *cerebr*ospinal
cervic-   *cervix, cervicis* [L.] neck. Cf. trachel-.
               *cervic*itis
chancr-   See cancr-. *chancr*iform
cheil-   *cheilos* [Gr.] lip. Cf. labi-. *cheil*oschisis
cheir-   *cheir* [Gr.] hand. Cf. man-. macro-
               *cheir*ia. (Also spelled chir-)
chir-   See cheir-. *chir*omegaly
chlor-   *chlōros* [Gr.] green. a*chlor*opsia
chol-   *cholē* [Gr.] bile. Cf. bil-. hepato*chol*-
               angeitis
chondr-   *chondros* [Gr.] cartilage. *chondro*-
               malacia
chord-   *chordē* [Gr.] string, cord. peri*chord*al
chori-   *chorion* [Gr.] protective fetal mem-
               brane. endo*chori*on
chro-   *chrōs* [Gr.] color. poly*chro*matic
chron-   *chronos* [Gr.] time. syn*chron*ous
chy-   *cheō, chy-* [Gr.] pour. ec*chy*mosis
-cid(e)   *caedo, -cisus* [L.] cut, kill. infanti*cide*,
               germi*cid*al
cili-   *cilium* [L.] eyelid. Cf. blephar-. super-
               *cili*ary
cine-   See kine-. auto*cine*sis
-cipient   See cept-. in*cipient*
circum-   *circum* [L.] around. Cf. peri-. *circum*-
               ferential
-cis-   *caedo, -cisus* [L.] cut, kill. ex*cis*ion
clas-   *klaō* [Gr.] break, cranio*clas*t
clin-   *klinō* [Gr.] bend, incline, make lie
               down. *clin*ometer
clus-   *claudo, -clusus* [L.] shut. Malo*cclus*ion
co-   See con-. *co*hesion
cocc-   *kokkos* [Gr.] seed, pill. gono*cocc*us
coel-   *koilos* [Gr.] hollow. Cf. cav-. *coel*en-
               teron. (Also spelled cel-)
col-1   See colon-. *col*ic
col-2   See con-. *col*lapse
colon-   *kolon* [Gr.] lower intestine, *colon*ic
colp-   *kolpos* [Gr.] hollow, vagina. Cf. sin-. en-
               do*colp*itis
com-   See con-. *com*masculation
con-   *con-* [L.] (becomes co- before vowels
               or *h;* col- before *l;* com- before *b, m,*

or *p;* cor- before *r*) with, together. Cf. syn-. contraction

contra-   *contra* [L.] against, counter. Cf. anti-. contraindication

copr-   *kopros* [Gr.] dung. Cf. sterco-. coproma

cor-[1]   *korē* [Gr.] doll, little image, pupil. isocoria

cor-[2]   See con-. corrugator

corpor-   *corpus, corporis* [L.] body. Cf. somat-. intracorporal

cortic-   *cortex, corticis* [L.] bark, rind. corticosterone

cost-   *costa* [L.] rib. Cf. pleur-. intercostal

crani-   *kranion* [Gr.] or *cranium* [L.] skull. pericranium

creat-   *kreas, kreato-* [Gr.] meat, flesh. creatorrhea

-crescent   *cresco, crescentis, cretus* [L.] grow. excrescent

cret-[1]   *cerno, cretus* [L.] distinguish, separate off. Cf. crin-. discrete

cret-[2]   See -crescent. accretion

crin-   *krinō* [Gr.] distinguish, separate off. Cf. cret-[1]. endocrinology

crur-   *crus, cruris* [L.] shin, leg. brachiocrural

cry-   *kryos* [Gr.] cold. cryesthesia

crypt-   *kryptō* [Gr.] hide, conceal. cryptorchism

cult-   *colo, cultus* [L.] tend, cultivate. culture

cune-   *cuneus* [L.] wedge. Cf. sphen-. cuneiform

cut-   *cutis* [L.] skin. Cf. derm(at)-. subcutaneous

cyan-   *kyanos* [Gr.] blue, anthocyanin

cycl-   *kyklos* [Gr.] circle, cycle. cyclophoria

cyst-   *kystis* [Gr.] bladder. Cf. vesic-. nephrocystitis

cyt-   *kytos* [Gr.] cell. Cf. cell-. plasmocytoma

dacry-   *dakry* [Gr.] tear. dacryocyst

dactyl-   *daktylos* [Gr.] finger, toe. Cf. digit-. hexadactylism

de-   *de* [L.] down from. decomposition

dec-[1]   *deka* [Gr.] ten. Indicates multiple in metric system. Cf. dec-[2]. decagram

dec-[2]   *decem* [L.] ten. Indicates fraction in metric system. Cf. dec-[1]. decipara, decimeter

dendr-   *dendron* [Gr.] tree. neurodendrite

dent-   *dens, dentis* [L.] tooth. Cf. odont-. interdental

derm(at)-   *derma, dermatos* [Gr.] skin. Cf. cut-. endoderm, dermatitis

desm-   *desmos* [Gr.] band, ligament. syndesmopexy

dextr-   *dexter, dextr-* [L.] right-hand. ambidextrous

di-[1]   *di-* [Gr.] two. dimorphic. (See also bi-[2])

di-[2]   See dia-. diuresis

di-[3]   See dis-. divergent

dia-   *dia* [Gr.] (*a* is dropped before words beginning with a vowel) through, apart. Cf. per-. diagnosis

didym-   *didymos* [Gr.] twin. Cf. gemin-. epididymal

digit-   *digitus* [L.] finger, toe. Cf. dactyl-. digitigrade

diplo-   *diploos* [Gr.] double. diplomyelia

dis-   *dis-* [L.] (*s* may be dropped before a word beginning with a consonant) apart, away from. dislocation

disc-   *diskos* [Gr.] or *discus* [L.] disk. discoplacenta

dors-   *dorsum* [L.] back. ventrodorsal

drom-   *dromos* [Gr.] course, hemodromometer

-ducent   See duct-. adducent

-duct   *duco, ducentis, ductus* [L.] lead, conduct. oviduct

dur-   *durus* [L.] hard. Cf. scler-. induration

dynam(i)-   *dynamis* [Gr.] power. dynamoneure, neurodynamic

dys-   *dys-* [Gr.] bad, improper. Cf. mal-. dystrophic. (See also cac-)

e-   *e* [L.] out from. Cf. ec- and ex-. emission

ec-   *ek* [Gr.] out of. Cf. e-. eccentric

-ech-   *echō* [Gr.] have, hold, be. synechotomy

ect-   *ektos* [Gr.] outside. Cf. extra-. ectoplasm

ede-   *oideō* [Gr.] swell. edematous

ef-   See ex-. efflorescent

-elc-   *helkos* [Gr.] sore, ulcer. enterelcosis. (See also helc-)

electr-   *ēlectron* [Gr.] amber. electrotherapy

em-   See en-. embolism, empathy, emphlysis

-em-   *haima* [Gr.] blood. anemia. (See also hem(at)-)

en-   *en* [Gr.] (*n* changes to *m* before *b, p* or *ph*) in, on. Cf. in-[2]. encelitis

end-   *endon* [Gr.] inside. Cf. intra-. endangium

enter-   *enteron* [Gr.] intestine. dysentery

ep-   See epi-. epaxial

epi-   *epi* [Gr.] (*i* is dropped before words beginning with a vowel) upon, after, in addition. epiglottis

erg-   *ergon* [Gr.] work, deed. energy

erythr-   *erythros* [Gr.] red. Cf. rub(r)-. erythrochromia

eso-   *esō* [Gr.] inside. Cf. intra-. esophylactic

esthe-   *aisthanomai, aisthē-* [Gr.] perceive, feel. Cf. sens-. anesthesia

eu-   *eu* [Gr.] good, normal. eupepsia

ex-   *ex* [Gr.] or *ex* [L.] out of. Cf. e-. excretion

exo-   *exō* [Gr.] outside. Cf. extra-. exopathic

extra-   *extra* [L.] outside of, beyond. Cf. ect- and exo-. extracellular

faci-   *facies* [L.] face. Cf. prosop-. brachiofaciolingual

-facient   *facio, facientis, factus, -fectus* [L.] make. Cf. poie-. calefacient

-fact-   See facient-. artefact

fasci-   *fascia* [L.] band. fasciorrhaphy

febr-   *febris* [L.] fever. Cf. pyr-. febricide

-fect-   See -facient. defective

-ferent   *fero, ferentis, latus* [L.] bear, carry. Cf. phor-. ef*ferent*

ferr-   *ferrum* [L.] iron. *ferro*protein

fibr-   *fibra* [L.] fiber. Cf. in-¹. chondro*fibroma*

fil-   *filum* [L.] thread. *fili*form

fiss-   *findo, fissus* [L.] split. Cf. schis-. *fission*

flagell-   *flagellum* [L.] whip. *flagell*ation

flav-   *flavus* [L.] yellow. Cf. xanth-. ribo*flavin*

-flect-   *flecto, flexus* [L.] bend, divert. de*flection*

-flex-   See -flect-. re*flex*ometer

flu-   *fluo, fluxus* [L.] flow. Cf. rhe-. *flu*id

flux-   See flu-. af*flux*ion

for-   *foris* [L.] door, opening. per*for*ated

-form   *forma* [L.] shape. Cf. -oid. ossi*form*

fract-   *frango, fractus* [L.] break. re*fract*ive

front-   *frons, frontis* [L.] forehead, front. naso*front*al

-fug(e)   *fugio* [L.] flee, avoid. vermi*fuge*, centri*fug*al

funct-   *fungor, functus* [L.] perform, serve, function. mal*function*

fund-   *fundo, fusus* [L.] pour. in*fund*ibulum

fus-   See fund-. dif*fus*ible

galact-   *gala, galactos* [Gr.] milk. Cf. lact-. dys*galact*ia

gam-   *gamos* [Gr.] marriage, reproductive union. a*gam*ont

gangli-   *ganglion* [Gr.] swelling, plexus. neuro*gangli*itis

gastr-   *gastēr, gastros* [Gr.] stomach. cholangio*gastr*ostomy

gelat-   *gelo, gelatus* [L.] freeze, congeal. *gelat*in

gemin-   *geminus* [L.] twin, double. Cf. didym-. quadri*gemin*al

gen-   *gignomai, gen-, gon-* [Gr.] become, be produced, originate, or *gennaō* [Gr.] produce, originate. cyto*gen*ic

germ-   *germen, germinis* [L.] bud, a growing thing in its early stages. Cf. blast-. *germin*al, ovi*germ*

gest-   *gero, gerentis, gestus* [L.] bear, carry. con*gest*ion

gland-   *glans, glandis* [L.] acorn. Cf. aden-. intra*gland*ular

-glia   *glia* [Gr.] glue. neuro*glia*

gloss-   *glōssa* [Gr.] tongue. Cf. lingu-. tricho*gloss*ia

glott-   *glōtta* [Gr.] tongue, language. *glott*ic

gluc-   See glyc(y)-. *gluc*ophenetidin

glutin-   *gluten, glutinis* [L.] glue. ag*glutin*ation

glyc(y)-   *glykys* [Gr.] sweet. *glyc*emia, *glyc*yrrhizin. (Also spelled gluc-)

gnath-   *gnathos* [Gr.] jaw. ortho*gnath*ous

gno-   *gignōsiō, gnō-* [Gr.] know, discern. di*agno*sis

gon-   See gen-. anphi*gon*y

grad-   *gradior* [L.] walk, take steps. retro*grad*e

-gram   *gramma* [Gr.] letter, drawing. cardio*gram*

gran-   *granum* [L.] grain, particle. lipo*gran*uloma

graph-   *graphō* [Gr.] scratch, write, record. histo*graphy*

grav-   *gravis* [L.] heavy. multi*grav*ida

gyn(ec)-   *gynē, gynaikos* [Gr.] woman, wife. androgyny, *gynec*ologic

gyr-   *gyros* [Gr.] ring, circle. *gyr*ospasm

haem(at)-   See hem(at)-. *haem*orrhagia, *haemat*oxylon

hapt-   *haptō* [Gr.] touch. *hapt*ometer

hect-   *hekt-* [Gr.] hundred. Cf. cent-. Indicates multiple in metric system. *hect*ometer

helc-   *helkos* [Gr.] sore, ulcer. *helc*osis

hem(at)-   *haima, haimatos* [Gr.] blood. Cf. sanguin-. *hem*angioma, *hemat*ocyturia. (See also -em-)

hemi-   *hēmi-* [Gr.] half. Cf. semi-. *hemi*ageusia

hen-   *heis, henos* [Gr.] one. Cf. un-. *heno*genesis

hepat-   *hēpar, hēpatos* [Gr.] liver. gastro*hepat*ic

hept(a)-   *hepta* [Gr.] seven. Cf. sept-². *hept*atomic, *hepta*valent

hered-   *heres, heredis* [L.] heir. *heredo*immunity

hex-¹   *hex* [Gr.] six. Cf. sex-. *hex*yl-. An *a* is added in some combinations

hex-²   *echō, hex-* [Gr.] (added to *s* becomes *hex-*) have, hold, be. cac*hex*ia

hexa-   See hex-¹. *hexa*chromic

hidr-   *hidros* [Gr.] sweat. hyper*hidr*osis

hist-   *histos* [Gr.] web, tissue. *histo*dialysis

hod-   *hodos* [Gr.] road, path. *hodo*neuromere. (See also od- and -ode¹)

hom-   *homos* [Gr.] common, same. *homo*morphic

horm-   *ormē* [Gr.] impetus, impulse. *hormo*ne

hydat-   *hydōr, hydatos* [Gr.] water. *hydat*ism

hydr-   *hydōr, hydr-* [Gr.] water. Cf. lymph-. anchlor*hydr*ia

hyp-   See hypo-. *hyp*axial

hyper-   *hyper* [Gr.] above, beyond, extreme. Cf. super-. *hyper*trophy

hypn-   *hypnos* [Gr.] sleep. *hypn*otic

hypo-   *hypo* [Gr.] (*o* is dropped before words beginning with a vowel) under, below. Cf. sub-. *hypo*metabolism

hyster-   *hystera* [Gr.] womb. colpo*hyster*opexy

iatr-   *iatros* [Gr.] physician. pedi*atr*ics

idi-   *idios* [Gr.] peculiar, separate, distinct. *idi*osyncrasy

il-   See in-²,³. *il*linition (in, on), *il*legible (negative prefix)

ile-   See ili- [ile- is commonly used to refer to the portion of the intestines known as the ileum]. *ile*ostomy

ili-   *ilium (ileum)* [L.] lower abdomen, intestines [ili- is commonly used to refer to the flaring part of the hip bone known as the ilium]. *ili*osacral

im-
: See in-[2,3]. *immersion* (in, on), *imper*foration (negative prefix)

in-[1]
: *is, inos* [Gr.] fiber. Cf. fibr-. *ino*steatoma

in-[2]
: *in* [L.] (*n* changes to *l, m,* or *r* before words beginning with those consonants) in, on. Cf. en-. *in*sertion

in-[3]
: *in-* [L.] (*n* changes to *l, m,* or *r* before words beginning with those consonants) negative prefix. Cf. a-. *in*valid

infra-
: *infra* [L.] beneath. *infra*orbital

insul-
: *insula* [L.] island. *insul*in

inter-
: *inter* [L.] among, between. *inter*carpal

intra-
: *intra* [L.] inside. Cf. end- and eso-. *in*travenous

ir-
: See in-[2,3]. *irradiation* (in, on), *irre*ducible (negative prefix)

irid-
: *iris, iridos* [Gr.] rainbow, colored circle. *kerato*irid*o*cyclitis

is-
: *isos* [Gr.] equal. *iso*tope

ischi-
: *ischion* [Gr.] hip, haunch, *ischi*opubic

jact-
: *iacio, iactus* [L.] throw. *jact*itation

-ject
: *iacio, -iectus* [L.] throw. *in*jection

jejun-
: *ieiunus* [L.] hungry, not partaking of food. *gastroje*junostomy

jug-
: *iugum* [L.] yoke. *con*jugation

junct-
: *iungo, iunctus* [L.] yoke, join. *conjunct*iva

kary-
: *karyon* [Gr.] nut, kernel, nucleus. Cf. nucle-. *mega*karyocyte. (Also spelled cary-)

kerat-
: *keras, keratos* [Gr.] horn. *kerat*olysis. (Also spelled cerat-)

kil-
: *chilioi* [Gr.] one thousand. Cf. mill-. Indicates multiple in metric system. *kilo*gram

kine-
: *kineō* [Gr.] move. *kine*matograph. (Also spelled cine-)

labi-
: *labium* [L.] lip. Cf. cheil-. *gingivo*labial

lact-
: *lac, lactis* [L.] milk. Cf. galact-. *glucolact*one

lal-
: *laleō* [Gr.] talk, babble. *glossolal*ia

lapar-
: *lapara* [Gr.] flank. *lapar*otomy

laryng-
: *larynx, laryngos* [Gr.] windpipe. *laryng*endoscope

lat-
: *fero, latus* [L.] bear, carry. See -ferent. *trans*lation

later-
: *latus, lateris* [L.] side. *ventro*lateral

lent-
: *lens, lentis* [L.] lentil. Cf. phac-. *lent*iconus

lep-
: *lambanō, lēp-* [Gr.] take, seize. *cat*aleptic

leuc-
: See leuk-. *leuc*inuria

leuk-
: *leukos* [Gr.] white. Cf. alb-. *leuk*orrhea. (Also spelled leuc-)

lien-
: *lien* [L.] spleen. Cf. splen-. *lien*ocele

lig-
: *ligo* [L.] tie, bind. *lig*ate

lingu-
: *lingua* [L.] tongue. Cf. gloss-. *sublin*gual

lip-
: *lipos* [Gr.] fat. Cf. adip-. *glycolip*in

lith-
: *lithos* [Gr.] stone. Cf. calc-[1]. *nephrolith*otomy

loc-
: *locus* [L.] place. Cf. top-. *loc*omotion

log-
: *legō, log-* [Gr.] speak, give an account. *logo*rrhea, embry*olog*y

lumb-
: *lumbus* [L.] loin. *dorsolumb*ar

lute-
: *luteus* [L.] yellow. Cf. xanth-. *lute*oma

ly-
: *lyō* [Gr.] loose, dissolve. Cf. solut-. ker*atolys*is

lymph-
: *lympha* [Gr.] water. Cf. hydr-. *lymphadenosis

macr-
: *makros* [Gr.] long, large. *macr*omyeloblast

mal-
: *malus* [L.] bad, abnormal. Cf. cac- and dys-. *malfunction

malac-
: *malakos* [Gr.] soft. *osteomalac*ia

mamm-
: *mamma* [L.] breast. Cf. mast-. *submammary

man-
: *manus* [L.] hand. Cf. cheir-. *mani*phalanx

mani-
: *mania* [Gr.] mental aberration. *man*igraphy, klepto*mani*a

mast-
: *mastos* [Gr.] breast. Cf. mamm-. hy*permast*ia

medi-
: *medius* [L.] middle. Cf. mes-. *medi*frontal

mega-
: *megas* [Gr.] great, large. Also indicates multiple (1,000,000) in metric system. *mega*colon, *mega*dyne. (See also megal-)

megal-
: *megas, megalou* [Gr.] great, large. *acromegal*y

mel-
: *melos* [Gr.] limb, member. *symmel*ia

melan-
: *melas, melanos* [Gr.] black. *hippomelan*in

men-
: *mēn* [Gr.] month. *dysmen*orrhea

mening-
: *mēninx, mēningos* [Gr.] membrane. *encephalomening*itis

ment-
: *mens, mentis* [L.] mind. Cf. phren-, psych- and thym-. *dementia

mer-
: *meros* [Gr.] part. *polymer*ic

mes-
: *mesos* [Gr.] middle. Cf. medi-. *meso*derm

met-
: See meta-. *met*allergy

meta-
: *meta* [Gr.] (*a* is dropped before words beginning with a vowel) after, beyond, accompanying. *meta*carpal

metr-[1]
: *metron* [Gr.] measure. *stereometr*y

metr-[2]
: *metra* [Gr.] womb. *endometr*itis

micr-
: *mikros* [Gr.] small. *photomicr*ograph

mill-
: *mille* [L.] one thousand. Cf. kil-. Indicates fraction in metric system. *milli*gram, *milli*pede

miss-
: See -mittent. *intromiss*ion

-mittent
: *mitto, mittentis, missus* [L.] send. *intermittent

mne-
: *mimnērcō, mnē-* [Gr.] remember. *pseudomne*domnesia

mon-
: *monos* [Gr.] only, sole. *mono*plegia

morph-
: *morphē* [Gr.] form, shape. *polymorpho*nuclear

mot-
: *moveo, motus* [L.] move. *vasomot*or

my-
: *mys* [Gr.] muscle. *inoleiomy*oma

-myces
: *mykēs, mykētos* [Gr.] fungus. *myelomyces

myc(et)-
: See -myces. *ascomycetes, *streptomyc*in

myel-	*myelos* [Gr.] marrow. polio*myel*itis
myx-	*myxa* [Gr.] mucus. *myx*edema
narc-	*narkē* [Gr.] numbness. topo*narc*osis
nas-	*nasus* [L.] nose. Cf. rhin-. palato*nas*al
ne-	*neos* [Gr.] new, young. *ne*ocyte
necr-	*nekros* [Gr.] corpse. *necr*ocytosis
nephr-	*nephros* [Gr.] kidney. Cf. ren-. para-*nephr*ic
neur-	*neuron* [Gr.] nerve. esthesio*neur*e
nod-	*nodus* [L.] knot. *nod*osity
nom-	*nomos* [Gr.] (from *nemō* deal out, distribute) law, custom. taxo*nom*y
non-	*nona* [L.] nine. *non*acosane
nos-	*nosos* [Gr.] disease. *nos*ology
nucle-	*nucleus* [L.] (from *nux, nucis* nut) kernel. Cf. kary-. *nucle*ide
nutri-	*nutrio* [L.] nourish. mal*nutri*tion
ob-	*ob* [L.] (*b* changes to *c* before words beginning with that consonant) against, toward, etc. *ob*tuse
oc-	See ob-. *oc*clude
ocul-	*oculus* [L.] eye. Cf. ophthalm-. *ocul*omotor
-od-	See -ode¹. peri*od*ic
-ode¹	*hodos* [Gr.] road, path. cath*ode*. (See also hod-)
-ode²	See -oid. nemat*ode*
odont-	*odous, odontos* [Gr.] tooth. Cf. dent-. orth*odont*ia
-odyn-	*odynē* [Gr.] pain, distress. gastr*odyn*ia
-oid	*eidos* [Gr.] form. Cf. -form. hy*oid*
-ol	See ole-. cholester*ol*
ole-	*oleum* [L.] oil. *ole*oresin
olig-	*oligos* [Gr.] few, small. *olig*ospermia
omphal-	*omphalos* [Gr.] navel. peri*omphal*ic
onc-	*onkos* [Gr.] bulk, mass. hemat*onc*ometry
onych-	*onyx, onychos* [Gr.] claw, nail. an*onych*ia
oo-	*ōon* [Gr.] egg. Cf. ov-. *oo*theocitis
op-	*horaō, op-* [Gr.] see. erythr*op*sia
ophthalm-	*ophthalmos* [Gr.] eye. Cf. ocul-. ex*ophthalm*ic
or-	*os, oris* [L.] mouth. Cf. stom(at)-. intra*or*al
orb-	*orbis* [L.] circle. sub*orb*ital
orchi-	*orchis* [Gr.] testicle. Cf. test-. *orchi*opathy
organ-	*organon* [Gr.] implement, instrument. *organ*oleptic
orth-	*orthos* [Gr.] straight, right, normal. *orth*opedics
oss-	*os, ossis* [L.] bone. Cf. ost(e)-. *oss*iphone
ost(e)-	*osteon* [Gr.] bone. Cf. oss-. en*ost*osis, *oste*anaphysis
ot-	*ous, ōtos* [Gr.] ear. Cf. aur-. par*ot*id
ov-	*ovum* [L.] egg. Cf. oo-. syn*ov*ia
oxy-	*oxys* [Gr.] sharp. *oxy*cephalic
pachy(n)-	*pachynō* [Gr.] thicken. *pachy*derma, myo*pachyn*sis
pag-	*pēgnymi, pag-* [Gr.] fix, make fast. thoraco*pag*us

par-¹	*pario* [L.] bear, give birth to. primip*ar*ous
par-²	See para-. *par*epigastric
para-	*para* [Gr.] (final *a* is dropped before words beginning with a vowel) beside, beyond. *para*mastoid
part-	*pario, partus* [L.] bear, give birth to. *part*urition
path-	*pathos* [Gr.] that which one undergoes, sickness. psycho*path*ic
pec-	*pēgnymi, pēg-* [Gr.] (*pēk-* before *t*) fix, make fast. sym*pec*tothiene. (See also pex-)
ped-	*pais, paidos* [Gr.] child. ortho*ped*ic
pell-	*pellis* [L.] skin, hide. *pell*agra
-pellent	*pello, pellentis, pulsus* [L.] drive. re*pellent*
pen-	*penomai* [Gr.] need, lack. erythrocyto*pen*ia
pend-	*pendeo* [L.] hang down. ap*pend*ix
pent(a)-	*pente* [Gr.] five. Cf. quinque-. *pent*ose, *penta*ploid
peps-	*peptō, peps-* [Gr.] digest. brady*peps*ia
pept-	*peptō* [Gr.] digest. dys*pept*ic
per-	*per* [L.] through. Cf. dia-. *per*nasal
peri-	*peri* [Gr.] around. Cf. circum-. *peri*phery
pet-	*peto* [L.] seek, tend toward. centri*pet*al
pex-	*pēgnumi, pēg-* [Gr.] (added to *s* becomes *pēx*) fix, make fast. hepato*pex*y
pha-	*phēmi, pha-* [Gr.] say, speak. dys*pha*sia
phac-	*phakos* [Gr.] lentil, lens. Cf. lent-. *phac*osclerosis. (Also spelled phak-)
phag-	*phagein* [Gr.] eat. lipo*phag*ic
phak-	See phac-. *phak*itis
phan-	See phen-. dia*phan*oscopy
pharmac-	*pharmakon* [Gr.] drug. *pharmac*ognosy
pharyng-	*pharynx, pharyng-* [Gr.] throat. glosso*pharyng*eal
phen-	*phainō, phan-* [Gr.] show, be seen. phos*phen*e
pher-	*pherō, phor-* [Gr.] bear, support. peri*pher*y
phil-	*phileō* [Gr.] like, have affinity for. eosino*phil*ia
phleb-	*phleps, phlebos* [Gr.] vein. peri*phleb*itis
phleg-	*phlogō, phlog-* [Gr.] burn, inflame. adeno*phleg*mon
phlog-	See phleg-. anti*phlog*istic
phob-	*phobos* [Gr.] fear, dread. claustro*phob*ia
phon-	*phōne* [Gr.] sound. echo*phon*y
phor-	See pher-. Cf. -ferent. exo*phor*ia
phos-	See phot-. *phos*phorus
phot-	*phōs, phōtos* [Gr.] light. *phot*erythrous
phrag-	*phrassō, phrag-* [Gr.] fence, wall off, stop up. Cf. sept-¹. dia*phrag*m
phrax-	*phrassō, phrag-* [Gr.] (added to *s* becomes *phrax-*) fence, wall off, stop up. em*phrax*is
phren-	*phrēn* [Gr.] mind, midriff. Cf. ment-. meta*phren*ia, meta*phren*on

phthi-   *phthinō* [Gr.] decay, waste away. *phthi*sis

phy-   *phyō* [Gr.] beget, bring forth, produce, be by nature. *nosophyte*

phyl-   *phylon* [Gr.] tribe, kind. *phylogeny*

-phyll   *phyllon* [Gr.] leaf. *xanthophyll*

phylac-   *phylax* [Gr.] guard. *prophylactic*

phys(a)-   *physaō* [Gr.] blow, inflate. *physocele, physalis*

physe-   *physaō, physē-* [Gr.] blow, inflate. *emphysema*

pil-   *pilus* [L.] hair. *epilation*

pituit-   *pituita* [L.] phlegm, rheum. *pituitous*

placent-   *placenta* [L.] (from *plakous* [Gr.]) cake. *extraplacental*

plas-   *plassō* [Gr.] mold, shape. *cineplasty*

platy-   *platys* [Gr.] broad, flat. *platyrrhine*

pleg-   *plēssō* [Gr.] strike. *diplegia*

plet-   *pleo, -pletus* [L.] fill. *depletion*

pleur-   *pleura* [Gr.] rib, side. Cf. *cost-*. *peripleural*

plex-   *plēssō, plēg-* (added to s becomes *plēx-*) strike. *apoplexy*

plic-   *plico* [L.] fold. *complication*

pne-   *pneuma, pneumatos* [Gr.] breathing. *traumatopnea*

pneum(at)-   *pneuma, pneumatos* [Gr.] breath, air. *pneumodynamics, pneumatothorax*

pneumo(n)-   *pneumōn* [Gr.] lung. Cf. *pulmo(n)-*. *pneumocentesis, pneumonotomy*

pod-   *pous, podos* [Gr.] foot. *podiatry*

poie-   *poieō* [Gr.] make, produce. Cf. *-facient*. *sarcopoietic*

pol-   *polos* [Gr.] axis of a sphere. *peripolar*

poly-   *polys* [Gr.] much, many. *polyspermia*

pont-   *pons, pontis* [L.] bridge. *pontocerebellar*

por-[1]   *poros* [Gr.] passage. *myelopore*

por-[2]   *pōros* [Gr.] callus. *porocele*

posit-   *pono, positus* [L.] put, place. *repositor*

post-   *post* [L.] after, behind in time or place. *postnatal, postoral*

pre-   *prae* [L.] before in time or place. *prenatal, prevesical*

press-   *premo, pressus* [L.] press. *pressoreceptive*

pro-   *pro* [Gr.] or *pro* [L.] before in time or place. *progamous, procheilon, prolapse*

proct-   *prōktos* [Gr.] anus. *enteroproctia*

prosop-   *prosōpon* [Gr.] face. Cf. *faci-*. *diprosopus*

pseud-   *pseudēs* [Gr.] false. *pseudoparaplegia*

psych-   *psychē* [Gr.] soul, mind. Cf. *ment-*. *psychosomatic*

pto-   *piptō, ptō* [Gr.] fall. *nephroptosis*

pub-   *pubes* and *puber, puberis* [L.] adult. *ischiopubic.* (See also *puber-*)

puber-   *puber* [L.] adult. *puberty*

pulmo(n)-   *pulmo, pulmonis* [L.] lung. Cf. *pneumo(n)-*. *pulmolith, cardiopulmonary*

puls-   *pello, pellentis, pulsus* [L.] drive, propulsion

punct-   *pungo, punctus* [L.] prick, pierce. Cf. *cente-*. *punctiform*

pur-   *pus, puris* [L.] pus. Cf. *py-*. *suppuration*

py-   *pyon* [Gr.] pus. Cf. *pur-*. *nephropyosis*

pyel-   *pyelos* [Gr.] trough, basin, pelvis. *nephropyelitis*

pyl-   *pylē* [Gr.] door, orifice. *pylephlebitis*

pyr-   *pyr* [Gr.] fire. Cf. *febr-*. *galactopyra*

quadr-   *quadr-* [L.] four. Cf. *tetra-*. *quadrigeminal*

quinque-   *quinque* [L.] five. Cf. *pent(a)-*. *quinquecuspid*

rachi-   *rachis* [Gr.] spine. Cf. *spin-*. *encephalorachidian*

radi-   *radius* [L.] ray. Cf. *actin-*. *irradiation*

re-   *re-* [L.] back, again. *retraction*

ren-   *renes* [L.] kidneys. Cf. *nephr-*. *adrenal*

ret-   *rete* [L.] net. *retothelium*

retro-   *retro* [L.] backwards. *retrodeviation*

rhag-   *rhēgnymi, rhag-* [Gr.] break, burst. *hemorrhagic*

rhaph-   *rhaphē* [Gr.] suture. *gastrorrhaphy*

rhe-   *rhaphē* [Gr.] flow. Cf. *flu-*. *diarrheal*

rhex-   *rhēgnymi, rhēg-* [Gr.] (added to s becomes *rhēx*) break, burst. *metrorrhexis*

rhin-   *rhis, rhinos* [Gr.] nose. Cf. *nas-*. *basirhinal*

rot-   *rota* [L.] wheel. *rotator*

rub(r)-   *ruber, rubri* [L.] red. Cf. *erythr-*. *bilirubin, rubrospinal*

salping-   *salpinx, salpingos* [Gr.] tube, trumpet. *salpingitis*

sanguin-   *sanguis, sanguinis* [L.] blood. Cf. *hem(at)-*. *sanguineous*

sarc-   *sarx, sarkos* [Gr.] flesh. *sarcoma*

schis-   *schizō, schid-* [Gr.] (before *t* or added to s becomes *schis-*) split. Cf. *fiss-*. *schistorachis, rachischisis*

scler-   *sklēros* [Gr.] hard. Cf. *dur-*. *sclerosis*

scop-   *skopeō* [Gr.] look at, observe. *endoscope*

sect-   *seco, sectus* [L.] cut. Cf. *tom-*. *sectile*

semi-   *semi* [L.] half. Cf. *hemi-*. *semiflexion*

sens-   *sentio, sensus* [L.] perceive, feel. Cf. *esthe-*. *sensory*

sep-   *sepō* [Gr.] rot, decay. *sepsis*

sept-[1]   *saepio, saeptus* [L.] fence, wall off, stop up. Cf. *phrag-*. *nasoseptal*

sept-[2]   *septem* [L.] seven. Cf. *hept(a)-*. *septan*

ser-   *serum* [L.] whey, watery substance, serum. *serosynovitis*

sex-   *sex* [L.] six. Cf. *hex-*[1]. *sexdigitate*

sial-   *sialon* [Gr.] saliva. *polysialia*

sin-   *sinus* [L.] hollow, fold. Cf. *colp-*. *sinobronchitis*

sit-   *sitos* [Gr.] food. *parasitic*

solut-   *solvo, solventis, solutus* [L.] loose, dissolve, set free. Cf. *ly-*. *dissolution*

-solvent   See *solut-*. *dissolvent*

somat-   *sōma, somatos* [Gr.] body. Cf. *corpor-*. *psychosomatic*

-some   See *somat-*. *dictyosome*

spas- *spaō, spas-* [Gr.] draw, pull. *spasm,* *spastic*

spectr- *spectrum* [L.] appearance, what is seen. micro*spectr*oscope

sperm(at)- *sperma, spermatos* [Gr.] seed. *sperm*acrasia, *spermat*ozoon

spers- *spargo, -spersus* [L.] scatter. di*spers*ion

sphen- *sphēn* [Gr.] wedge. Cf. cune-. *sphen*oid

spher- *sphaira* [Gr.] ball. hemi*spher*e

sphygm- *sphygmos* [Gr.] pulsation. *sphygm*omanometer

spin- *spina* [L.] spine. Cf. rachi-. cerebro*spin*al

spirat- *spiro, spiratus* [L.] breathe. in*spira*tory

splanchn- *splanchna* [Gr.] entrails, viscera. neuro*splanchn*ic

splen- *splēn* [Gr.] spleen. Cf. lien-. *splen*omegaly

spor- *sporos* [Gr.] seed. *sporo*phyte, zygo*spore*

squam- *squama* [L.] scale. de*squam*ation

sta- *histēmi, sta-* [Gr.] make stand, stop. genesi*sta*sis

stal- *stellō, stal-* [Gr.] send. peri*stal*sis. (See also stol-)

staphyl- *staphylē* [Gr.] bunch of grapes, uvula. *staphyl*ococcus, *staphyl*ectomy

stear- *stear, steatos* [Gr.] fat. Cf. adip-. *stear*odermia

steat- See stear-. *steat*opygous

sten- *stenos* [Gr.] narrow, compressed. *sten*ocardia

ster- *stereos* [Gr.] solid. chole*ster*ol

sterc- *stercus* [L.] dung. Cf. copr-. *sterc*oporphyrin

sthen- *sthenos* [Gr.] strength. a*sthen*ia

stol- *stellō, stol-* [Gr.] send. dia*stol*e

stom(at)- *stoma, stomatos* [Gr.] mouth, orifice. Cf. or-. ana*stom*osis, *stomat*ogastric

strep(h)- *strephō, strep-* (before *t*) [Gr.] twist. Cf. tors-. *strep*hosymbolia, *strep*tomycin. (See also stroph-)

strict- *stringo, stringentis, strictus* [L.] draw tight, compress, cause pain. con*strict*ion

-stringent See strict-. a*stringent*

stroph- *strephō, stroph-* [Gr.] twist. ana*stroph*ic. (See also strep[h]-)

struct- *struo, structus* [L.] pile up (against). ob*struct*ion

sub- *sub* [L.] (*b* changes to *f* or *p* before words beginning with those consonants) under, below. Cf. hypo-. *sub*lumbar

suf- See sub-. *suf*fusion

sup- See sub-. *sup*pository

super- *super* [L.] above, beyond, extreme. Cf. hyper-. *super*motility

sy- See syn-. *sy*stole

syl- See syn-. *syl*lepsiology

sym- See syn-. *sym*biosis, *sym*metry, *sym*pathetic, *sym*physis

syn- *syn* [Gr.] (*n* disappears before *s*, changes to *l* before *l*, and changes to *m* before *b, m, p,* and *ph*) with, together. Cf. con-. myo*syn*izesis

ta- See ton-. ec*ta*sis

tac- *tassō, tag-* [Gr.] (*tak-* before *t*) order, arrange. a*tac*tic

tact- *tango, tactus* [L.] touch. con*tact*

tax- *tassō, tag-* [Gr.] (added to *s* becomes *tax-*) order, arrange. a*tax*ia

tect- See teg-. pro*tect*ive

teg- *tego, tectus* [L.] cover. in*teg*ument

tel- *telos* [Gr.] end. *tel*osynapsis

tele- *tēle* [Gr.] at a distance. *tele*ceptor

tempor- *tempus, temporis* [L.] time, timely or fatal spot, temple. *tempor*omalar

ten(ont)- *tenōn, tenontos* [Gr.] (from *teinō* stretch) tight stretched band. *teno*dynia, *ten*onitis, *tenont*agra

tens- *tendo, tensus* [L.] stretch. Cf. ton-. ex*tens*or

test- *testis* [L.] testicle. Cf. orchi-. *test*itis

tetra- *tetra-* [Gr.] four. Cf. quadr-. *tetra*genous

the- *tithēmi, thē-* [Gr.] put, place. syn*the*sis

thec- *thēkē* [Gr.] repository, case. *theco*stegnosis

thel- *thēlē* [Gr.] teat, nipple. *thel*erethism

therap- *therapeia* [Gr.] treatment. hydro*therap*y

therm- *thermē* [Gr.] heat. Cf. calor-. dia*therm*y

thi- *theion* [Gr.] sulfur. *thi*ogenic

thorac- *thōrax, thōrakos* [Gr.] chest. *thorac*oplasty

thromb- *thrombos* [Gr.] lump, clot. *thromb*openia

thym- *thymos* [Gr.] spirit. Cf. ment-. dys*thym*ia

thyr- *thyreos* [Gr.] shield (shaped like a door *thyra*). *thyr*oid

tme- *temnō, tmē-* [Gr.] cut. axono*tme*sis

toc- *tokos* [Gr.] childbirth, dys*toc*ia

tom- *temnō, tom-* [Gr.] cut. Cf. sect-. appendec*tom*y

ton- *teino, ton-* [Gr.] stretch, put under tension. Cf. tens-. peri*ton*eum

top- *topos* [Gr.] place. Cf. loc-. *top*esthesia

tors- *torqueo, torsus* [L.] twist. Cf. strep-. ec*tors*ion

tox- *toxicon* [Gr.] (from *toxon* bow) arrow poison, poison. *tox*emia

trache- *tracheia* [Gr.] windpipe. *trache*otomy

trachel- *trachēlos* [Gr.] neck. Cf. cervic-. *trachel*opexy

tract- *traho, tractus* [L.] draw, drag. pro*tract*ion

traumat- *trauma, traumatos* [Gr.] wound. *traumat*ic

tri- *treis, tria* [Gr.] or *tri-* [L.] three. *tri*gonid

trich- *thrix, trichos* [Gr.] hair. *trich*oid

trip- *tribō* [Gr.] rub. en*trip*sis

trop- *trepō, trop-* [Gr.] turn, react. sito*trop*ism

troph-   *trepō, troph-* [Gr.] nurture. a*troph*y

tuber-   *tuber* [L.] swelling, node. *tuber*cle

typ-   *typos* [Gr.] (from *typto* strike) type. a*typ*ical

typh-   *typhos* [Gr.] fog, stupor. adeno*typh*us

typhl-   *typhlos* [Gr.] blind. Cf. cec-. *typh*lectasis

un-   *unus* [L.] one. Cf. hen-. *uni*oval

ur-   *ouron* [Gr.] urine. poly*ur*ia

vacc-   *vacca* [L.] cow. *vacc*ine

vagin-   *vagina* [L.] sheath. in*vagin*ated

vas-   *vas* [L.] vessel. Cf. angi-. *vas*cular

vers-   See vert-. in*vers*ion

vert-   *verto, versus* [L.] turn. di*vert*iculum

vesic-   *vesica* [L.] bladder. Cf. cyst-. *vesic*ovaginal

vit-   *vita* [L.] life. Cf. bi-[1]. de*vit*alize

vuls-   *vello, vulsus* [L.] pull, twitch. con*vuls*ion

xanth-   *xanthos* [Gr.] yellow, blond. Cf. flav- and lute-. *xanth*ophyll

-yl-   *hyte* [Gr.] substance. cacod*yl*

zo-   *zoē* [Gr.] life, *zōon* [Gr.] animal. micro*zo*aria

zyg-   *zygon* [Gr.] yoke, union. *zyg*odactyly

zym-   *zymē* [Gr.] ferment, en*zym*e

A

Å symbol, *angstrom* or *Angström unit.*

A absorbance; accommodation; ampere; anterior; axial; total acidity.

A₂ aortic second sound.

a. [L.] *arteria* (artery); atto-.

a- word element [Gr.], *without; not.*

A.A. achievement age; Alcoholics Anonymous.

aa. [L. pl.] *arteriae* (arteries).

āā ana (*of each*).

A.A.A. American Association of Anatomists.

A.A.A.S. American Association for the Advancement of Science.

A.A.B.B. American Association of Blood Banks.

A.A.C.P. American Academy for Child Psychiatry.

A.A.D. American Academy of Dermatology.

A.A.D.P. American Academy of Denture Prosthetics.

A.A.D.R. American Academy of Dental Radiology.

A.A.D.S. American Association of Dental Schools.

A.A.E. American Association of Endodontists.

A.A.F.P. American Academy of Family Physicians.

A.A.I. American Association of Immunologists.

A.A.I.D. American Academy of Implant Dentistry.

A.A.I.N. American Association of Industrial Nurses.

A.A.M.A. American Association of Medical Assistants.

A.A.O. American Association of Orthodontists; American Academy of Ophthalmology; American Academy of Otolaryngology.

A.A.O.P. American Academy of Oral Pathology.

A.A.O.S. American Academy of Orthopaedic Surgeons.

A.A.P. American Academy of Pediatrics; American Academy of Pedodontics; American Academy of Periodontology; American Association of Pathologists.

A.A.P.A. American Academy of Physician Assistants.

A.A.P.M.R. American Academy of Physical Medicine and Rehabilitation.

A.B. [L.] *Artium Baccalaureus* (Bachelor of Arts).

Ab antibody.

ab [L.] *from.*

ab- word element [L.], *from; off; away from.*

abarognosis (ah-bar″og-no′sis) loss of sense of weight.

abarthrosis (ab″ar-thro′sis) abarticulation.

abarticulation (-ar-tik″u-la′shin) 1. synovial joint. 2. dislocation of a joint.

abasia (ah-ba′ze-ah) inability to walk. aba′sic, abat′ic, adj. a.-asta′sia, astasia-abasia. a. atac′tica, abasia with uncertain movements, due to a defect of coordination. choreic a., abasia due to chorea of the legs. paralytic a., aba-sia due to paralysis of leg muscles. paroxysmal trepidant a., abasia due to spastic stiffening of the legs on attempting to stand. spastic a., paroxysmal trepidant a. trembling a., a. tre′pidans, abasia due to trembling of the legs.

abatement (ah-bāt′mint) decrease in severity of a pain or symptom.

ABC aspiration biopsy cytology.

abdomen (ab-do′min) that part of the body lying between the thorax and the pelvis, and containing the abdominal cavity and viscera. abdom′inal, adj. acute a., an acute intra-abdominal condition of abrupt onset, usually associated with pain due to inflammation, perforation, obstruction, infarction, or rupture of abdominal organs, and usually requiring emergency surgical intervention. carinate a., navicular a., scaphoid a. a. obsti′pum, congenital shortness of the rectus abdominis muscle. scaphoid a., one whose anterior wall is hollowed, occurring in children with cerebral disease. surgical a., acute a.

abdomin(o)- word element [L.], *abdomen.*

abdominocentesis (ab-dom″ĭ-no-sen-te′sis) surgical puncture of the abdomen.

abdominocystic (-sis′tik) pertaining to the abdomen and gallbladder.

abdominohysterectomy (-his″ter-ek′tah-me) hysterectomy through an abdominal incision.

abdominoscopy (ab-dom″ĭ-nos′kah-pe) examination of the abdominal cavity.

abdominovaginal (ab-dom″ĭ-no-vaj′ĭ-nil) pertaining to the abdomen and vagina.

abducens (ab-doo′senz) [L.] drawing away.

abduct (-dukt′) to draw away from the median plane, or (the digits) from the axial line of a limb. abdu′cent, adj.

aberrant (ab″er-a′she-o) [L.] aberration.

aberration (ab-er-a′shin) 1. deviation from the normal or usual. 2. unequal refraction or focalization of a lens. chromatic a., unequal refraction of light rays of different wavelength, producing a blurred image with fringes of color. chromosomal a., loss, gain, or exchange of genetic material in the chromosomes of a cell, resulting in a deletion, duplication, inversion, or translocation of genes. mental a., unsoundness of mind of mild degree, not affecting intelligence.

abetalipoproteinemia (a-ba″tah-lip″o-pro″te-in-e′me-ah) a hereditary syndrome marked by a lack of β-lipoproteins in the blood and by acanthocytosis, hypocholesterolemia, progressive ataxic neuropathy, atypical retinitis pigmentosa, and malabsorption.

abiosis (ah-be-o′sis) absence or deficiency of life. abiot′ic, adj.

abiotrophy (ah-be-ah′trah-fe) progressive loss of vitality of certain tissues leading to disorders applied to degenerative hereditary diseases of late onset, e.g., Huntington's chorea.

1

abirritant (ab-ir′ĭ-tint) 1. diminishing irritation; soothing. 2. an agent that relieves irritation.

ablactation (ab″lak-ta′shin) weaning or cessation of milk secretion.

ablatio (ab-la′she-o) [L.] ablation.

ablation (ab-la′shin) 1. separation or detachment; extirpation; eradication. 2. removal, especially by cutting.

ablepharia (a″blef-a′re-ah) cryptophthalmos. **ablephʹarous,** adj.

ablepsia (a-blep′se-ah) blindness.

abluent (ab′loo-ent) 1. detergent; cleansing. 2. a cleansing agent.

abnormality (ab″nor-mal′it-e) 1. the state of being abnormal. 2. a malformation.

abomasum (-o-ma′sum) the fourth stomach of ruminants.

aborad (ab-o′rad) moving away from the mouth.

aboral (-o′ril) opposite to, or remote from, the mouth.

abort (ah-bort′) to arrest prematurely a disease or developmental process; to expel the products of conception before the fetus is viable.

abortifacient (ah-bort″ĭ-fa′shint) 1. causing abortion. 2. an agent that induces abortion.

abortion (ah-bor′shin) 1. expulsion from the uterus of the products of conception before the fetus is viable. 2. premature arrest of a natural or morbid process. **artificial a.,** induced a. **complete a.,** one in which all the products of conception are expelled from the uterus and identified. **contagious a.,** infectious a. **enzootic a.,** an infectious abortion of cattle (*foothill a.*) and ewes caused by organisms of the genus *Chlamydia.* **equine virus a.,** see under *rhinopneumonitis.* **foothill a.,** enzootic a. of cattle. **habitual a.,** spontaneous abortion occurring in three or more successive pregnancies, at about the same level of development. **incomplete a.,** that with retention of parts of the products of conception. **induced a.,** that brought on intentionally by medication or instrumentation. **inevitable a.,** a condition in which vaginal bleeding has been profuse and the cervix has become dilated, and abortion will invariably occur. **infected a.,** that associated with infection of the genital tract. **infectious a.,** 1. a disease of cattle due to *Brucella abortus,* causing premature loss of the developing calf. 2. an infectious disease of horses due to *Salmonella abortusequi* and of sheep due to *S. abortusovis.* **missed a.,** retention in the uterus of an abortus that has been dead for at least eight weeks. **septic a.,** that associated with serious infection of the uterus leading to generalized infection. **spontaneous a.,** that occurring naturally. **therapeutic a.,** interruption of pregnancy by artificial means for medical considerations. **threatened a.,** a condition in which vaginal bleeding is less than in inevitable abortion and the cervix is not dilated, and abortion may or may not occur.

abortionist (ah-bor′shin-ist) one who makes a business of inducing illegal abortions.

abortus (ah-bor′tus) a dead or nonviable fetus (weighing less than 500 gm. at birth).

abrasio (ah-bra′se-o) [L.] abrasion. **a. cor′neae,** the scraping off of corneal excrescences.

abrasion (ah-bra′zhun) 1. a rubbing or scraping off; see also *planing.* 2. a rubbed or scraped area on skin or mucous membrane. **dental a.,** the wearing away of tooth structure due to mechanical action other than mastication.

abreaction (ab″re-ak′shin) the reliving of an experience in such a way that previously repressed emotions associated with it are released.

abruptio (ah-brup′she-o) [L.] separation. **a. placen′tae,** premature detachment of the placenta.

abscess (ab′ses) a localized collection of pus in a cavity formed by disintegration of tissues. **amebic a.,** one caused by *Entamoeba histolytica,* usually occurring in the liver but also in the lungs, brain, and spleen. **apical a.,** a suppurative inflammatory reaction involving the tissues surrounding the apical portion of a tooth, occurring in acute and chronic forms. **appendiceal a., appendicular a.,** one resulting from perforation of an acutely inflamed appendix. **Bezold's a.,** one deep in the neck resulting from a complication of acute mastoiditis. **brain a.,** one affecting the brain as a result of extension of an infection (e.g., otitis media) from an adjacent area, or through bloodborne infection. **Brodie's a.,** a roughly spherical region of bone destruction, filled with pus or connective tissue, usually in the metaphyseal region of long bones and caused by *Staphylococcus aureus* or *S. albus.* **cold a.,** one of slow development and with little inflammation, usually tuberculous. **diffuse a.,** a collection of pus not enclosed by a capsule. **gas a.,** one containing gas, caused by gas-forming bacteria such as *Clostridium perfringens.* **miliary a.,** one of a set of small multiple abscesses. **pancreatic a.,** one that occurs as a complication of acute pancreatitis or postoperative pancreatitis caused by secondary bacterial contamination. **Pautrier's a.,** focal collections of reticular cells in the epidermis. **peritonsillar a.,** an abscess in the connective tissue of the tonsil capsule, resulting from suppuration of the tonsil. **phlegmonous a.,** one associated with acute inflammation of the subcutaneous connective tissue. **ring a.,** a ring-shaped purulent infiltration at the periphery of the cornea. **shirt-stud a.,** one separated into two cavities connected by a narrow channel. **stitch a.,** one developed about a stitch or suture. **strumous a.,** tuberculous a. **thecal a.,** one arising in a sheath, as in a tendon sheath. **tuberculous a.,** one due to infection with tubercle bacilli. **vitreous a.,** an abscess of the vitreous humor of the eye due to infection, trauma, or foreign body. **wandering a.,** one that burrows into tissues and finally points at a distance from the site of origin. **Welch's a.,** gas a.

abscise (ab′sīz) to cut off or remove.

abscissa (ab-sis′ah) the horizontal line in a graph along which are plotted the units of one of the factors considered in the study, as time in a time-temperature study.

abscission (-sish′in) removal by cutting.

abscopal (-sko′p′l) pertaining to the effect on nonirradiated tissue resulting from irradiation of other tissue of the organism.

Absidia (-sid′ĭ-ah) a genus of fungi (order Mucorales), including *A. corymbif′era*, which may cause mycosis in man, and *A. ramo′sa*, which grows on bread and decaying vegetation and causes otomycosis and sometimes mucormycosis.

absorb (ab-sorb′) 1. to take in or assimilate, as to take up substances into or across tissues, e.g., the skin or intestine. 2. to stop particles of radiation so that their energy is totally transferred to the absorbing material.

absorbance (-sor′bins) in radiology, a measure of the ability of a medium to absorb radiation, expressed as the logarithm of the quotient of the intensity of the radiation entering the medium divided by that leaving it.

absorbent (-sorb′int) 1. able to take in, or suck up and incorporate. 2. a tissue structure involved in absorption. 3. a substance that absorbs or promotes absorption.

absorption (-sorp′shin) 1. the uptake of substances into or across tissues. 2. in psychology, devotion of thought to one object or activity only. 3. in radiology, uptake of energy by matter with which the radiation interacts. **intestinal a.**, the uptake from the intestinal lumen of fluids, solutes, proteins, fats, and other nutrients into the intestinal epithelial cells, blood, lymph, or interstitial fluids.

abstergent (ab-ster′jint) 1. cleansing or detergent. 2. a cleansing agent.

abstinence (ab′stĭ-nins) a refraining from the use of or indulgence in food, stimulants, or sex.

abstraction (ab-strak′shin) 1. the withdrawal of any ingredient from a compound. 2. malocclusion in which the occlusal plane is further from the eye-ear plane, causing lengthening of the face; cf. *attraction* (2).

abtropfung (ahp′tropf-oong) the proliferative transition of theques of nevus cells from the epidermis down into the dermis.

abulia (ah-bu′le-ah) loss or deficiency of will power, initiative, or drive. **abu′lic,** adj.

abuse (ah-būs′) misuse, maltreatment, or excessive use. **child a.,** see *battered-child syndrome.* **drug a.,** use of illegal drugs or misuse of prescribed drugs. See also *dependence.* **substance a., psychoactive,** use of a substance that modifies mood or behavior in a manner characterized by a maladaptive pattern of use. See also *dependence.*

abutment (ah-but′mint) a supporting structure to sustain lateral or horizontal pressure, as the anchorage tooth for a fixed or removable partial denture.

A.C. acromioclavicular; air conduction; alternating current; anodal closure; aortic closure; axiocervical.

Ac chemical symbol, *actinium.*

a.c. [L.] *an′te ci′bum* (before meals).

A.C.A. American College of Angiology; American College of Apothecaries.

acacia (ah-ka′shah) the dried gummy exudate from stems and branches of species of *Acacia,* prepared as a mucilage or syrup, and used as a pharmaceutical aid.

acalcicosis (ah-kal″sĭ-ko′sis) a condition due to deficiency of calcium in the diet.

acampsia (a-kamp′se-ah) rigidity of a part or limb.

acanth(o)- word element [Gr.], *sharp spine; thorn.*

acantha (ah-kan′tha) 1. the spine. 2. a spinous process of a vertebra.

acanthamebiasis (ah-kan″thah-me-bi′ah-sis) infection with *Acanthamoeba castellani.*

Acanthamoeba (-me′bah) a genus of amebas of the order Amoebida, including *A. castella′ni,* which ordinarily inhabits moist soil or water, but has been found as an opportunistic parasite of man, causing a fatal meningoencephalitis.

acanthesthesia (a-kan″thes-the′ze-ah) perverted sensation of a sharp point pricking the body.

acanthion (ah-kan′the-on) a point at the base of the anterior nasal spine.

Acanthocephala (ah-kan″tho-sef′ah-lah) a phylum of elongate, mostly cylindrical organisms (thorny-headed worms) parasitic in the intestines of all classes of vertebrates; in some classifications, considered to be a class of the phylum Nemathelminthes.

Acanthocephalus (-sef′ah-lus) a genus of parasitic worms (phylum Acanthocephala).

Acanthocheilonema (-ki″lo-ne′mah) a genus of long, threadlike worms. **A. per′stans,** *Dipetalonema perstans.*

acanthocyte (ah-kan′tho-sīt) a distorted erythrocyte with protoplasmic projections giving it a "thorny" appearance; seen in abetalipoproteinemia.

acanthocytosis (ah-kan″tho-si-to′sis) the presence in the blood of acanthocytes.

acantholysis (ah″kan-thol′ĭ-sis) dissolution of the intercellular bridges of the prickle-cell layer of the epidermis. **acantholyt′ic,** adj.

acanthoma (ak″an-tho′mah) a tumor composed of epidermal or squamous cells.

acanthosis (ak″an-tho′sis) diffuse hyperplasia and thickening of the prickle-cell layer of the epidermis. **acanthot′ic,** adj. **a. ni′gricans,** diffuse velvety acanthosis with gray, brown, or black pigmentation, chiefly in the axillae and other body folds; it occurs in an adult form, often associated with an internal carcinoma (*malignant acanthosis nigricans*), and in a benign, nevoid form, more or less generalized. A benign juvenile form associated with obesity, which is sometimes due to endocrine disturbance, is called *pseudoacanthosis nigricans.*

acanthrocytosis (ah-kan″thro-si-to′sis) acanthocytosis.

acapnia (a-kap′ne-ah) decrease of carbon dioxide in the blood; hypocapnia. **acap′nic,** adj.

acarbia (ah-kar′be-ah) decrease of bicarbonate in the blood.

acardia (ah-kar′de-ah) congenital absence of the heart.

acariasis (ak″ah-ri′ah-sis) infestation with mites.

acaricide (ah-kar′ĭ-sīd) 1. destructive to mites. 2. an agent that destroys mites.

acarid (ak'ah-rid) a tick or mite of the order Acarina.

acaridiasis (ah-kar''ĭ-di'ah-sis) acariasis.

Acarina (ak''ah-ri'nah) an order of arthropods (class Arachnida), including mites and ticks.

acarinosis (ah-kar''ĭ-no'sis) any disease caused by mites; acariasis.

acarodermatitis (ak''ah-ro-der''mah-ti'tis) any skin inflammation caused by mites (acarids). **a. urticarioi'des,** grain itch.

acarology (ak''ah-rol'ah-je) the scientific study of mites and ticks.

Acarus (ak'ah-rus) a genus of small mites. **A. folliculo'rum,** Demodex folliculorum. **A. scabie'i,** Sarcoptes scabiei. **A. si'ro,** a mite that causes vanillism in vanilla pod handlers.

acaryote (ah-kăr'e-ōt) akaryote.

acatalasemia (a''kat-ah-la-se'me-ah) acatalasia.

acatalasia (-la'ze-ah) a rare hereditary disease seen mostly in Japan and Switzerland, marked by absence of catalase; it may be associated with infections of oral structures.

acatamathesia (ah-kat''ah-mah-the'ze-ah) 1. loss or impairment of the power to understand speech. 2. impairment of any one of the perceptive faculties, due to a central lesion.

acataphasia (-fa''ze-ah) speech disorder, with inability to express one's thoughts in a connected manner, due to a central lesion.

acathexia (ak''ah-thek'se-ah) inability to retain bodily secretions. **acathec'tic,** adj.

acathexis (-sis) a mental disturbance in which certain things, such as objects, ideas, and memories, that ordinarily have great significance to an individual arouse no emotional response.

acaudate (a-kaw'dāt) lacking a tail.

A.C.C. American College of Cardiology.

ACC anodal closure contraction.

accelerator (ak-sel''er-a'tor) [L.] 1. an agent or apparatus that increases the rate at which something occurs or progresses. 2. any nerve or muscle that hastens the performance of a function. **serum prothrombin conversion a. (SPCA),** coagulation Factor VII. **serum thrombotic a.,** a factor in serum which has procoagulant properties and the ability to induce blood coagulation.

acceptor (ak-sep'ter) a substance which unites with another substance; specifically, one that unites with hydrogen or oxygen in an oxidoreduction reaction and so enables the reaction to proceed.

accessory (ak-ses'o-re) supplementary; affording aid to another similar and generally more important thing.

accident prone specially susceptible to accidents owing to psychological factors.

acclimation (ă-kli-ma'shin) the process of becoming accustomed to a new environment.

accommodation (ah-kom''ah-da'shin) adjustment, especially of the eye for seeing objects at various distances. **negative a.,** adjustment of the eye for long distances by relaxation of the ciliary muscles. **positive a.,** adjustment of the eye for short distances by contraction of the ciliary muscles.

accommodometer (ah-kom''ah-dom'it-er) an instrument for measuring accommodative capacity of the eye.

accouchement (ah-kōōsh-maw') [Fr.] delivery; labor. **a. forcé,** rapid forcible delivery by one of several methods; originally, rapid dilatation of the cervix with the hands, followed by version and extraction of the fetus.

accrementition (ă''kri-men-tish'in) growth by addition of similar tissue.

accretion (ah-kre'shin) 1. growth by addition of material. 2. accumulation. 3. adherence of parts normally separated.

acedapsone (as''ah-dap'sōn) a dapsone derivative, $C_{16}H_{16}N_2O_4S$, having antimalarial and leprostatic activities.

acellular (a-sel'u-ler) not cellular in structure.

acelomate (ah-se'lo-māt) having no coelom or body cavity.

acentric (a-sen'tric) 1. not central; not located in the center. 2. lacking a centromere, so that the chromosome will not survive cell divisions.

ACEP American College of Emergency Physicians.

acephalocyst (ah-sef'ah-lo-sist'') a sterile cyst.

acephalous (ah-sef'ah-lus) headless.

acephalus (ah-sef'ah-lus) a headless monster.

acepromazine (ah-se-pro'mah-zēn) a phenothiazine tranquilizer, $C_{19}H_{22}N_2OS$, used in veterinary medicine to immobilize large animals.

acervuline (ah-ser'vu-līn) aggregated; heaped up; said of certain glands.

acervulus (ah-ser'vu-lus), pl. acer'vuli [L.] gritty matter in or near the pineal body, the choroid plexus, and other parts of the brain. **a. ce'rebri,** acervulus.

acetabulectomy (as''ah-tab''u-lek'tah-me) excision of the acetabulum.

acetabuloplasty (as''ah-tab'u-lo-plas''te) plastic repair of the acetabulum.

acetabulum (as''ah-tab'u-lum) the cup-shaped cavity on the lateral surface of the hip bone, receiving the head of the femur. **acetab'ular,** adj. **sunken a.,** Otto pelvis.

acetal (as'ah-tal) an organic compound formed by a combination of an aldehyde with an alcohol.

acetaldehyde (as''it-al'de-hīd) a colorless, volatile, flammable liquid, CH_3CHO, used in the manufacture of acetic acid, perfumes, and flavors. It is also an intermediate in the metabolism of alcohol.

acetaminophen (as''it-am'ĭ-no-fen'') an analgesic and antipyretic, $C_8H_9NO_2$.

acetanilid (as''ah-tan'ĭ-lid) a colorless crystalline powder, C_8H_9NO; analgesic and antipyretic.

acetate (as'ah-tāt) any salt of acetic acid.

acetazolamide (as''it-ah-zol'ah-mīd) a renal carbonic anhydrase inhibitor, $C_4H_6N_4O_3S_2$, used as a diuretic in the treatment of carbon dioxide retention in chronic lung disease and to reduce intraocular pressure in glaucoma. **sodium a.,** a form suitable for parenteral use.

Acetest (ah'sah-test) trademark for reagent tablets containing sodium nitroprusside, aminoacetic acid, disodium phosphate, and lactose. A drop of urine is placed on a tablet on a sheet of white paper; if significant quantities of acetone are present the tablet changes from a purple tint (1+), to lavender (2+), to moderate purple (3+), or to deep purple (4+).

acetic (ah-se′tik, ah-set′ik) pertaining to vinegar or its acid; sour.

acetic acid (ah-se′tik) a saturated fatty acid, CH_3COOH, the characteristic component of vinegar; used in solutions of various strengths, as *dilute acetic acid* (6%) and *glacial acetic acid* (99.4%). Its salts (*potassium* and *sodium acetate*) are useful as urinary and systemic alkalizers.

acetoacetic acid (ah′se″to-ah-se′tik) CH_3-$COCH_2COOH$, one of the ketone bodies produced in diabetic ketoacidosis.

Acetobacter (ah-se″to-bak′ter) a genus of schizomycetes (family Pseudomonadaceae) important in completion of the carbon cycle and in production of vinegar.

acetohexamide (as″ah-to-heks′ah-mīd) an oral hypoglycemic, $C_{15}H_{20}O_4S$.

acetone (as′ah-tōn) a compound, CH_3COCH_3, with solvent properties and characteristic odor, obtained by fermentation or produced synthetically; one of the ketone bodies produced in abnormal amounts in diabetes mellitus. It is used as a solvent for fats, resins, rubber, and plastic and to cleanse the skin before injections and vaccinations.

acetonemia (as″it-ōn-ēm′e-ah) ketonemia.

acetonitrile (-ni′trīl) methyl cyanide, CH_3CN, a poisonous colorless acid.

acetonuria (-nu′re-ah) ketonuria.

acetophenazine (-fen′ah-zēn) a mildly sedative substance, $C_{23}H_{29}N_3O_2S$, whose maleate salt is used as a tranquilizer.

acetous (as′ah-tis) pertaining to, producing, or resembling acetic acid.

aceturate (ah-set′u-rāt) USAN contraction for *N*-acetylglycinate.

acetyl (as′ah-til) the monovalent radical, CH_3-CO, a combining form of acetic acid. **a. sulfisoxazole**, a sulfanilamide used as an antimicrobial.

acetylation (ah-set″ĭ-la′shin) introduction of an acetyl radical into an organic molecule.

acetylator (ah-set″ĭ-la′ter) an organism capable of metabolic acetylation. Individuals that differ in their inherited ability to metabolize certain drugs, e.g., isoniazid, are termed fast or slow acetylators.

acetylcholine (as″ah-til-ko′lēn) the acetic acid ester of choline, $CH_3COOCH_2CH_2N(CH_3)_3{}^+$, which is a neurotransmitter at cholinergic synapses in the central, sympathetic, and parasympathetic nervous systems; used in medicine as a miotic. Abbreviated ACh.

acetylcholinesterase (-ko″lin-es′ter-ās) an enzyme present in nervous tissue, muscle, and red cells that catalyzes the hydrolysis of acetylcholine to choline and acetic acid.

acetyl-CoA acetylcoenzyme A.

acetyl-CoA carboxylase (as′ah-til ko′a′ kar-

bok′sil-ās) an enzyme that catalyzes the conversion of ATP, acetyl-CoA, CO_2, and water to ADP, orthophosphate, and malonyl-CoA.

acetyl coenzyme A (as″ah-til ko-en′zīm) an important intermediate in the citric acid (Krebs) cycle and the chief precursor of lipids; it is formed by the attachment to coenzyme A of an acetyl group during the oxidation of pyruvate, fatty acids, or amino acids.

acetylcysteine (-sis′te-in) a compound, C_5H_9-NO_3S, with mucolytic properties, used as an adjuvant in various bronchopulmonary disorders.

acetylene (ah-set′ĭ-lēn) a colorless, volatile, explosive gas, C_2H_2; it is the simplest alkyne (unsaturated, triple-bonded hydrocarbon).

acetylsalicylic acid (ASA) (ah-se″til-sal″ah-sil′ik) aspirin.

acetyltransferase (as″ah-til-trans′fer-ās) any of a group of enzymes that catalyze the transfer of an acetyl group from one substance to another.

A.C.G. American College of Gastroenterology.

AcG accelerator globulin (coagulation Factor V).

ACh acetylcholine.

A.C.H.A. American College of Hospital Administrators.

achalasia (ak″ah-la′ze-ah) failure to relax of smooth muscle fibers at any junction of one part of the gastrointestinal tract with another, especially failure of the esophagogastric sphincter to relax with swallowing, due to degeneration of ganglion cells in the wall of the organ.

Achatina (ak″ah-ti′nah) a genus of very large land snails, including *A. fuli′ca*, which serves as an intermediate host of *Angiostrongylus cantonensis*.

AChE acetylcholinesterase.

acheiria (ah-ki′re-ah) sense as of the loss of the hands, seen in hysteria.

achillobursitis (ah-kil″o-ber-sīt′is) inflammation of the bursae about the Achilles tendon.

achillodynia (-din′e-ah) pain in the Achilles tendon or its bursa.

achillorrhaphy (ak″il-lor′ah-fe) suturing of the Achilles tendon.

achillotenotomy (ah-kil″o-ten-ot′ah-me) surgical division of the Achilles tendon.

achlorhydria (a″klōr-hi′dre-ah) absence of hydrochloric acid from gastric secretions. **achlorhy′dric,** adj.

acholia (a-ko′le-ah) lack or absence of bile secretion. **acho′lic,** adj.

acholuria (ah″ko-lu′re-ah) lack of bile pigments in the urine.

achondrogenesis (a-kon″dro-jen′ĭ-sis) a hereditary disorder characterized by hypoplasia of bone, resulting in markedly shortened limbs; the head and trunk are normal.

achondroplasia (-pla′ze-ah) a hereditary, congenital disorder of cartilage formation, leading to a type of dwarfism. **achondroplas′tic,** adj.

Achorion (ah-ko′re-on) *Trichophyton.*

achromasia (ak″ro-ma′se-ah) 1. lack of normal skin pigmentation. 2. the inability of tissues or cells to be stained.

achromat (ak′ro-mat) 1. an achromatic objective. 2. monochromat.

Achromatiaceae (ah-kro''mah-ti-a'se-e) a family of schizomycetes (order Beggiatoales) whose cells lack photosynthetic pigments.

achromatic (ak''ro-mat'ik) 1. producing no discoloration. 2. staining with difficulty. 3. pertaining to achromatin. 4. refracting light without decomposing it into its component colors. 5. monochromatic (2).

achromatin (ah-kro'mah-tin) the faintly staining groundwork of a cell nucleus.

Achromatium (ah''kro-ma'te-um) a genus of schizomycetes (family Achromatiaceae).

achromatolysis (ak''ro-mah-tol'ĭ-sis) disorganization of cell achromatin.

achromatophil (ak''ro-mat'ah-fil, a''kro-mat'ah-fil) 1. not easily stainable. 2. an organism or tissue that does not stain easily.

achromatopsia (ah-kro''mah-top'se-ah) monochromatism.

achromatosis (-to'sis) 1. deficiency of pigmentation in the tissues. 2. lack of staining power in a cell or tissue.

achromatous (a-kro'mah-tis) colorless.

achromaturia (a-kro''mah-tu're-ah) colorless state of the urine.

achromia (ah-kro'me-ah) the lack or absence of normal color or pigmentation, as of the skin. **achro'mic,** adj.

achromocyte (ah-kro'mah-sīt) a red cell artifact in the shape of a quarter moon which stains more faintly than intact red cells.

Achromycin (ak''ro-mi'sin) trademark for preparations of tetracycline.

achylia (ah-ki'le-ah) absence of hydrochloric acid and pepsinogens (pepsin) in the gastric juice (gastric a.).

achylous (ah-ki'lis) deficient in chyle.

achymia (ah-ki'me-ah) imperfect, insufficient, or absence of chyme formation.

acicular (ah-sik'u-ler) needle-shaped.

aciculum (ah-sik'u-lum) a bent, finger-like structure observed in certain flagellates.

acid (as'id) 1. sour. 2. a chemical compound that dissociates in solution, releasing hydrogen ions (a proton donor). An acidic solution has a pH below 7.0. Cf. base (3). **amino a.,** see under amino. **amino a., essential,** see under amino. **bile a's,** see under bile. **fatty a.,** see under fatty. **a. fuchsin,** see under fuchsin. **haloid a.,** see under haloid. **inorganic a.,** see under inorganic. **keto a's,** see under keto. **nucleic a's,** see under nucleic. **organic a.,** see under organic. **phosphatidic a.,** see under phosphatidic. **polyunsaturated fatty a's,** see under polyunsaturated.

acidemia (as''id-e'me-ah) abnormal acidity of the blood. **argininosuccinic a.,** the presence in the blood of argininosuccinic acid. **isovaleric a.,** an inborn error of leucine metabolism characterized by high levels of isovaleric acid in the blood, periodic acidosis with coma, objectionable body odor, and psychomotor retardation. **methylmalonic a.,** an inborn error of metabolism characterized by excretion of excessive amounts of methylmalonic acid in the urine, developmental retardation, hepatomegaly, intermittent neutropenia, thrombocytopenia, and severe metabolic acidosis. It is due to an inability to convert D- to L-methylmalonyl-CoA or of the latter to succinyl-CoA or to a defect in the metabolism of vitamin B_{12}. **propionic a.,** an excess of propionic acid in the blood, due to failure of activity of propionyl-CoA carboxylase and characterized by ketosis, acidosis, and hyperglycinemia and, in the absence of dietary controls, by developmental retardation, ECG abnormalities, and osteoporosis.

acid-fast not readily decolorized by acids after staining.

acidifiable (ah-sid''ĭ-fi'ah-b'l) capable of being made acid.

acidifier (ah-sid'ĭ-fi-er) an agent that causes acidity; a substance used to increase gastric acidity.

acidity (ah-sid'it-e) the quality of being acid; the power to unite with positively charged ions or with basic substances.

acidology (as''id-ol'ah-je) the science of surgical appliances.

acidophil (as'id-ah-fil'') 1. a histologic structure, cell, or other element staining readily with acid dyes. 2. an alpha cell of the adenohypophysis or the pancreatic islets. 3. an organism that grows well in highly acid media. 4. acidophilic.

acidophilic (as''id-ah-fil'ik) 1. easily stained with acid dyes. 2. growing best on acid media.

acidosis (as''id-o'sis) a pathologic condition resulting from accumulation of acid in, or loss of base from, the body. Cf. alkalosis. **acidot'ic,** adj. **compensated a.,** a condition in which the compensatory mechanisms have returned the pH toward normal. **diabetic a.,** metabolic acidosis produced by accumulation of ketones in uncontrolled diabetes mellitus. **hypercapnic a.,** respiratory a. **hyperchloremic a.,** metabolic acidosis accompanied by elevated plasma chloride. **metabolic a.,** a disturbance in which the acid-base status shifts toward the acid because of loss of base or retention of noncarbonic, or fixed (nonvolatile), acids. **nonrespiratory a.,** metabolic a. **renal hyperchloremia a.,** renal tubular a. **renal tubular a.,** metabolic acidosis resulting from impairment of renal function. **respiratory a.,** a state due to excess retention of carbon dioxide in the body. **starvation a.,** metabolic acidosis due to accumulation of ketone bodies which may accompany a caloric deficit. **uremic a.,** the condition in chronic renal disease in which the ability to excrete acid is decreased, causing acidosis.

acidulous (ah-sid'u-lis) somewhat acid.

acidum (as'id-um) [L.] acid.

aciduria (as''id-ūr'e-ah) the presence of acid in the urine. **beta-aminoisobutyric a.,** excessive excretion of β-aminoisobutyric acid in the urine; it occurs as a benign genetic metabolic variant and in certain illnesses. **methylmalonic a.,** excretion of excessive amounts of methylmalonic acid in the urine; a characteristic symptom of methylmalonic acidemia. **orotic a.,** a hereditary disorder in which a defect in the metabolism of pyrimidines is associated with excessive excretion of orotic acid in the urine, with megaloblastic anemia, crystalluria, and frequently physical and mental retardation.

aciduric (as″id-ūr′ik) capable of growing in extremely acid media; said of bacteria.

aciniform (ah-sin′ĭ-form) shaped like an acinus, or grape.

acinitis (as″ĭ-nīt′is) inflammation of the acini of a gland.

acinose (as′ĭ-nōs) made up of acini.

acinous (as′ĭ-nis) shaped like a grape.

acinus (as′ĭ-nus), pl. *ac′ini* [L.] a small saclike dilatation, particularly one found in various glands; see also *alveolus*. **liver a.**, the smallest functional unit of the liver, a mass of liver parenchyma that is supplied by terminal branches of the portal vein and hepatic artery and drained by a terminal branch of the bile duct.

acladiosis (ah-klad″e-o′sis) an ulcerative dermatomycosis caused by *Acladium castellani*.

Acladium (ah-kla′de-um) a genus of fungi sometimes infecting man.

aclasis (ak′lah-sis) pathologic continuity of structure, as in enchondromatosis. **diaphyseal a.**, enchondromatosis.

acleistocardia (ah-klīs″to-kar′de-ah) an open state of the foramen ovale of the fetal heart.

acme (ak′me) the critical stage or crisis of a disease.

acne (ak′ne) an inflammatory disease of the skin with the formation of an eruption of papules or pustules; more particularly, acne vulgaris. **bromide a.**, an acneiform eruption without comedones, one of the most constant symptoms of brominism. **common a.**, a. vulgaris. **a. conglobata'ta, conglobate a.**, severe acne with many comedones, marked by suppuration, cysts, sinuses, and scarring. **a. cosme′tica,** a persistent, low-grade acne usually affecting the chin and cheeks of a woman who uses cosmetics. **a. deter′gicans,** aggravation of existing acne lesions by too frequent and too severe washing with comedogenic soaps and rough cloths or pads. **a. ful′minans,** a rare form affecting teenage males, marked by sudden onset of fever and eruption of highly inflammatory, tender, ulcerative, and crusted lesions on the back, chest, and face. **halogen a.,** an acneiform eruption from ingestion of the simple salts of bromine and iodine present in cold remedies, sedatives, analgesics, and vitamins. **a. indura′ta,** a progression of papular acne, with deep-seated and destructive lesions that may produce severe scarring. **keloid a.,** keloid folliculitis. **a. mecha′nica, mechanical a.,** aggravation of existing acne lesions by mechanical factors (rubbing, stretching, pressing, pinching, pulling) caused by chin straps, clothing, back packs, casts, and seats. **a. necrot′ica milia′ris,** a rare and chronic form of folliculitis of the scalp, occurring principally in adults, with formation of tiny superficial pustules which are destroyed by scratching; see also *a. variolifor-mis*. **a. papulo′sa,** acne vulgaris with the formation of papules. **pomade a.,** acne vulgaris in blacks who groom their scalp and facial hair with greasy lubricants, marked by closed come-

dones on the forehead, temples, cheeks, and chin. **premenstrual a.,** acne of a cyclic nature, appearing shortly before (rarely after) the onset of menses. **a. rosa′cea,** rosacea. **tropical a., a. tropica′lis,** a severe and extensive form of acne occurring in hot, humid climates, with nodular, cystic, and pustular lesions chiefly on the back, buttocks, and thighs; conglobate abscesses frequently form, especially on the back. **a. variolifor′mis,** a rare condition with reddish-brown, papulopustular umbilicated lesions, usually on the brow and scalp; probably a deep variant of acne necrotica miliaris. **a. venena′ta,** acne produced by contact with a great variety of acnegenic chemicals, including those used in cosmetics and grooming agents and in industry. **a. vulga′ris,** chronic acne, usually occurring in adolescence, with comedones, papules, nodules, and pustules on the face, neck, and upper part of the trunk. Many factors, including certain foods, stress, hereditary factors, hormones, drugs, and the bacteria *Corynebacterium acnes, Staphylococcus albus,* and *Pityrosporon ovale* have been suggested as causative agents.

acnegenic (ak″nĕ-jen′ik) producing acne.

acnitis (ak-nīt′is) papulonecrotic tuberculid.

A.C.N.M. American College of Nurse-Midwives; see *nurse-midwife* and *nurse-midwifery.*

acoelomate (a-se′lah-māt) without a coelom or body cavity; an animal lacking a body cavity.

A.C.O.G. American College of Obstetricians and Gynecologists.

aconite (ak′o-nīt) a poisonous drug from the dried tuberous root of *Aconitum napellus,* containing several closely related alkaloids, the principal one being aconitine.

aconitine (ah-kon′ĭ-tin) a poisonous alkaloid, $C_{34}H_{47}O_{11}N$, the active principle of aconite.

acorea (ah″ko-re′ah) absence of the pupil.

acoria (ah-ko′re-ah) excessive ingestion of food, not from hunger but due to loss of the sensation of satiety.

A.C.O.S. American College of Osteopathic Surgeons.

acoustic (ah-koos′tik) relating to sound or hearing.

acoustics (-tiks) the science of sound or of hearing.

acoustogram (-tah-gram) the graphic tracing of the curves of sounds produced by motion of a joint.

A.C.P. American College of Physicians.

acquired (ah-kwi′erd) incurred as a result of factors acting from or originating outside the organism; not inherited.

acquisition (ak″wĭ-zish′in) in psychology, the period in learning during which progressive increments in response strength can be measured. Also, the process involved in such learning.

A.C.R. American College of Radiology.

acral (a′kral) pertaining to or affecting the extremities.

acridine (ak′rĭ-dēn) an alkaloid of anthracene,

$CH:(C_6H_4)_2:N$, used in the synthesis of dyes and drugs.

acriflavine (ak″rĭ-fla′vin) a deep orange, granular powder, used as a topical and urinary antiseptic. **a. hydrochloride,** a brownish red crystalline acridine dye; used as an antiseptic and germicide.

acrisorcin (ak″rĭ-sor′sin) a topical antifungal agent, $C_{13}H_{10}N_2 \cdot C_{12}H_{18}O_2$, used in the treatment of tinea versicolor.

acro- word element [Gr.], *extreme; top; extremity.*

acroagnosis (ak″ro-ag-no′sis) lack of sensory recognition of a limb; lack of acrognosis.

acroanesthesia (-an″es-the′ze-ah) anesthesia of the extremities.

acroarthritis (-ar-thrĭt′is) arthritis of the extremities.

acroblast (ak′ro-blast) Golgi material in the spermatid from which the acrosome arises.

acrobrachycephaly (ak″ro-brak″ĕ-sef′ah-le) abnormal height of the skull, with shortness of its anteroposterior dimension. **acrobrachycephal′ic,** adj.

acrocentric (-sen′trik) having the centromere toward one end of the replicating chromosome so that one arm is much longer than the other.

acrocephalia (-sĕ-fa′le-ah) oxycephaly.

acrocephalic (-sĕ-fal′ik) oxycephalic.

acrocephalopolysyndactyly (ACPS) (-sef″ ah-lo-pol″e-sin-dak′tĭ-le) acrocephalosyndactyly with polydactyly as an additional feature. Four types are known: *type I* (Noack syndrome), *type II* (Carpenter syndrome), *type III* (Sakati-Nyhan syndrome), and *type IV* (Goodman syndrome).

acrocephalosyndactyly (-sin-dak′tĭ-le) any of a group of autosomal dominant syndromes, in which craniostenosis is associated with acrocephaly and syndactyly. Called also *a. type I, Apert Syndrome, Apert-Crouzon disease, Chotzen syndrome* (a. type III), or *Pfeiffer syndrome* (a. type V).

acrochordon (-kor′don) a pedunculated skin tag, occurring principally on the neck, eyelids, upper chest, and axillae in older women.

acrocontracture (-kon-trak′cher) contracture of the muscles of the hand or foot.

acrocyanosis (-si″ah-no′sis) cyanosis of the extremities with mottled discoloration of the skin of the digits, wrists, and ankles, and with profuse sweating and coldness of the digits.

acrodermatitis (-der″mah-tīt′is) inflammation of the skin of the hands or feet. **chronic atrophic a., a. chro′nica atro′phicans,** chronic, idiopathic inflammation of the skin, usually of the extremities, leading to atrophy of the skin. **a. contin′ua** chronic inflammation of the extremities, in some cases becoming generalized. **a. enteropa′thica,** a hereditary disorder associated with a defect in zinc uptake, with a vesiculopustulous dermatitis preferentially located periorificially and on the head, elbows, knees, hands, and feet, associated with gastrointestinal disturbances, chiefly manifested by diarrhea, and total alopecia. **Hallopeau's a.,** a. continua. **infantile lichenoid a., infantile**

papular a., a. papulo′sa infan′tum, Gianotti-Crosti syndrome. **a. per′stans,** a. continua.

acrodermatosis (-der″mah-to′sis) any disease of the skin of the hands and feet.

acrodolichomelia (-dol″ĭ-ko-me′le-ah) abnormal length of hands and feet.

acrodynia (-din′e-ah) a disease of infancy and early childhood marked by pain and swelling in, and pink coloration of, the fingers and toes and by listlessness, irritability, failure to thrive, profuse perspiration, and sometimes scarlet coloration of the cheeks and tip of the nose.

acroesthesia (-es-the′ze-ah) 1. exaggerated sensitiveness. 2. pain in the extremities.

acrohypothermy (ak″ro-hi′po-ther″me) abnormal coldness of the hands and feet.

acrokeratosis (-kĕ″rah-to′sis) a condition involving the skin of the extremities, with the appearance of horny growths.

acrokinesia (-ki-ne′se-ah) abnormal motility or movement of the extremities. **acrokinet′ic,** adj.

acrolein (ak-ro′le-in) a volatile liquid, C_3H_4O, from decomposition of glycerin.

acromegaly (-meg′ah-le) abnormal enlargement of the extremities of the skeleton caused by hypersecretion of the pituitary growth hormone after maturity.

acrometagenesis (-met″ah-jen′ĭ-sis) undue growth of the extremities.

acromicria (-mi′kre-ah) abnormal hypoplasia of the extremities of the skeleton—nose, jaws, fingers, and toes.

acromio- word element [Gr.], *acromion.*

acromioclavicular (ah-kro″me-o-klah-vik′u-ler) pertaining to the acromion and clavicle.

acromion (ah-kro′me-on) the lateral extension of the spine of the scapula, forming the highest point of the shoulder. **acro′mial,** adj.

acromionectomy (ah-kro″me-on-ek′tah-me) resection of the acromion.

acromphalus (ah-krom′fah-lus) 1. bulging of the navel; sometimes a sign of umbilical hernia. 2. the center of the navel.

acromyotonia (ak″ro-mi″o-to′ne-ah) myotonia of the extremities.

acroneurosis (-noo-ro′sis) any neuropathy of the extremities.

acronym (ak′rah-nim) a word formed by the initial letters of the principal components of a compound term, as *rad* from *radiation ab-* sorbed dose.

acro-osteolysis (ak″ro-os″te-ol′ĭ-sis) osteolysis involving the distal phalanges of the fingers and toes.

acropachy (ak′ro-pak″e) clubbing of the fingers and toes.

acropachyderma (ak″ro-pak″e-der′mah) thickening of the skin over the face, scalp, and extremities, clubbing of the extremities, and deformities of the long bones; usually associated with acromegaly.

acroparalysis (-pah-ral′ĭ-sis) paralysis of the extremities.

acroparesthesia (-par″es-the′ze-ah) 1. paresthesia of the digits. 2. a disease marked by attacks of tingling, numbness, and stiffness chiefly in the fingers, hands, and forearms, sometimes with pain, skin pallor, or slight cyanosis.

acropathology (-pah-thol′ah-je) pathology of diseases of the extremities.

acrophobia (ak″ro-fo′be-ah) morbid fear of heights.

acroposthitis (-pos-thīt′is) inflammation of the prepuce.

acropurpura (-pur′pu-rah) purpura affecting the extremities, especially the digits.

acroscleroderma (-sklĕ″ro-der′mah) acrosclerosis.

acrosclerosis (-skler-o′sis) a combination of Raynaud's disease and scleroderma of the distal parts of the extremities, especially of the digits, and of the neck and face, particularly the nose.

acrosome (ak′rah-sōm) the caplike, membrane-bound structure covering the anterior portion of the head of a spermatozoon; it contains enzymes for penetrating the ovum.

acrotism (ak′rah-tizm) absence or imperceptibility of the pulse. **acrot′ic,** adj.

acrotrophoneurosis (ak″ro-trof″o-noo-ro′sis) trophoneurotic disturbance of the extremities.

acrylamide (ah-kril′ah-mīd) a highly toxic crystalline solid, $CH_2=CHCONH_2$, that readily polymerizes. Polymerized acrylamide gel is used as a medium for electrophoresis and thin-layer chromatography.

A.C.S. American Cancer Society; American Chemical Society; American College of Surgeons.

A.C.S.M. American College of Sports Medicine.

ACTH adrenocorticotropic hormone; see *corticotropin.*

Actifed (ak′tĭ-fed) trademark for a fixed combination preparation of triprolidine hydrochloride and pseudoephedrine hydrochloride.

actin (ak′tin) a muscle protein localized in the I band of the myofibrils; acting along with myosin, it is responsible for contraction and relaxation of muscle.

acting out the behavioral expression of hidden emotional conflicts, such as hostile feelings, in various kinds of neurotic behavior, as a defense pattern analogous to somatic conversion.

actinic (ak-tin′ik) producing chemical action; said of rays of light beyond the violet end of the spectrum.

actinium (ak-tin′e-im) a chemical element (*see table*), at. no. 89, symbol Ac.

actino- word element [Gr.], *ray; radiation.*

actinobacillosis (ak″tĭ-no-bas″ĭ-lo′sis) an actinomycosis-like disease of domestic animals caused by *Actinobacillus ligniere'sii,* in which the bacilli form radiating structures in the tissues; sometimes seen in man.

Actinobacillus (-bah-sil′us) a genus of schizomycetes (family Brucellaceae) capable of infecting cattle, but rarely man. **A. ligniere′sii,** the causative agent of actinobacillosis. **A. mal′lei,** *Pseudomonas mallei.*

actinodermatitis (-der″mah-tīt′is) radiodermatitis.

Actinomadura (ak″tĭ-no-mad′ŭ-rah) a genus of schizomycetes (family Actinomycetaceae), including A. *madu′rae,* the cause of maduromycosis in which the granules in the discharged pus are white, and A. *pelletie′rii,* the cause of maduromycosis in which the granules are red.

Actinomyces (ak″tĭ-no-mi′sēz) a genus of schizomycetes (family Actinomycetaceae). **A. bo′ vis,** a gram-positive microorganism causing actinomycosis in cattle. **A. israe′lii,** a species parasitic in the mouth, proliferating in necrotic tissue; it is the cause of some cases of human actinomycosis. **A. naeslun′dii,** an anaerobic species that is a normal inhabitant of the oral cavity and a cause of human actinomycosis and periodontal disease.

Actinomycetaceae (-mi″sah-ta′se-e) a family of schizomycetes (order Actinomycetales).

Actinomycetales (-mi″sah-ta′lēz) an order of schizomycetes made up of elongated cells having a definite tendency to branch.

actinomycin (-mi′sin) a family of antibiotics from various species of *Streptomyces,* which are active against bacteria and fungi; it includes the antineoplastic agents cactinomycin (actinomycin C) and dactinomycin (actinomycin D).

actinomycosis (-mi-ko′sis) an infectious disease caused by *Actinomyces,* marked by indolent inflammatory lesions of the lymph nodes draining the mouth, by intraperitoneal abscesses, or by lung abscesses due to aspiration. **actinomycot′ic,** adj.

actinotherapy (ak″tĭ-no-thĕ′rah-pe) treatment of disease with ultraviolet rays.

action (ak′shin) the accomplishment of an effect, whether mechanical or chemical, or the effect so produced. **ac′tive,** adj. **cumulative a.,** the sudden and markedly increased action of a drug after administration of several doses. **reflex a.,** involuntary response to a stimulus conveyed to the nervous system by passage of excitation potential from a receptor to a muscle or gland, over a system of neurons without the necessity of volition.

activator (ak′ti-vāt-er) a substance that makes another substance active or that renders an inactive enzyme capable of exerting its proper effect.

activity (ak-tiv′it-e) the quality or process of exerting energy or of accomplishing an effect. **enzyme a.,** the catalytic effect exerted by an enzyme, expressed as units per milligram of enzyme (*specific a.*) or as molecules of substrate transformed per minute per molecule of enzyme (*molecular a.*). **optical a.,** the ability of a chemical compound to rotate the plane of polarization of plane-polarized light.

actomyosin (ak″to-mi′o-sin) the complex of actin and myosin occurring in muscle fibers.

acuity (ah-ku′it-e) clarity or clearness, especially of vision.

acuminate (ah-ku′mĭ-nāt) sharp-pointed.

acupuncture (-punk′cher) the Chinese practice of piercing specific areas of the body along peripheral nerves with fine needles to relieve pain, to induce surgical anesthesia, and for therapeutic purposes.

acus (a′kus) a needle or needle-like process.

acute (ah-kūt′) 1. sharp. 2. having severe symptoms and a short course.

acutorsion (ak″u-tor′shin) twisting of a blood vessel with a needle to control bleeding.

acyanotic (ah-si″ah-not′ik) characterized by absence of cyanosis.

acyclovir (a-si′klo-vir) a synthetic purine nucleoside with selective activity against herpes simplex virus; used in the treatment of genital and mucocutaneous herpesvirus infections.

acylase (as′ĭ-lās) any enzyme that catalyzes the hydrolysis of acylated amino acids.

acyltransferase (-trans′fer-ās) any of a group of enzymes that catalyze the transfer of an acyl group from one substance to another.

acystinervia (ah-sis″tĭ-ner′ve-ah) paralysis of the bladder.

A.D. [L.] *au′ris dex′tra* (right ear).

ad [L.] preposition, *to*.

ad. [L.] *adde* (add).

A.D.A. American Dental Association; American Diabetes Association; American Dietetic Association.

adactyly (a″dak′tĭ-le) congenital absence of fingers or toes. **adac′tylous,** adj.

Adam's apple a subcutaneous prominence on the front of the neck produced by the thyroid cartilage of the larynx.

adamantine (ad″ah-man′tin) pertaining to the enamel of the teeth.

adamantoblast (ad″ah-man′to-blast) ameloblast.

adamantoma (ad″ah-man-to′mah) ameloblastoma.

adaptation (ad″ap-ta′shin) 1. the adjustment of an organism to its environment, or the process by which it enhances such fitness. 2. the normal ability of the eye to adjust itself to variations in the intensity of light; the adjustment to such variations. 3. the decline in the frequency of firing of a neuron, particularly of a receptor, under conditions of constant stimulation. 4. in dentistry, (*a*) the proper fitting of a denture, (*b*) the degree of proximity and interlocking of restorative material to a tooth preparation, (*c*) the exact adjustment of bands to teeth. 5. in microbiology, the adjustment of bacterial physiology to a new environment. **color a.,** 1. changes in visual perception of color with prolonged stimulation. 2. adjustment of vision to degree of brightness or color tone of illumination. **dark a.,** adaptation of the eye to vision in the dark or in reduced illumination. **enzymatic a.,** inducible enzyme synthesis. **genetic a.,** the natural selection of the progeny of a mutant better adapted to a new environment; especially seen in the development of microbes resistant to chemotherapeutic agents or to other inhibitors of growth (drug resistance). **light a.,** adaptation of the eye to vision in the sunlight or in bright illumination (photopia), with reduction in the concentration of the photosensitive pigments of the eye. **phenotypic a.,** a change in the properties of an organism, without any change in genotype, in response to a change in the environment. In microbiology, especially the formation of specific enzymes required for the utilization

of new foodstuffs (induced enzyme formation), or a change in cell size and composition with variation in growth rate.

adaptometer (ad″ap-tom′ĭt-er) an instrument for measuring the time required for retinal adaptation, i.e., for regeneration of the visual purple; used in detecting night blindness, vitamin A deficiency, and retinitis pigmentosa. **color a.,** an instrument to demonstrate adaptation of the eye to color or light.

adder (ad′er) 1. *Vipera berus.* 2. any of many venomous snakes of the family Viperidae, such as the puff adder and European viper.

addiction (ah-dik′shin) physiologic or psychologic dependence on some agent (e.g., alcohol, drug), with a tendency to increase its use.

addisonism (ad′ĭ-son-izm″) symptoms seen in pulmonary tuberculosis, consisting of debility and pigmentation, resembling Addison's disease.

adduct (ad-dukt′) to draw toward the median plane or (in the digits) toward the axial line of a limb.

adduction (ad-duk′shin) the act of adducting; the state of being adducted.

adelomorphous (ah-del″o-mor′fis) of indefinite form.

adenalgia (ad″in-al′je-ah) pain in a gland.

adenase (ad′in-ās) a deaminizing enzyme of the spleen, liver, and pancreas that converts adenine into hypoxanthine and ammonia.

adenasthenia (ad″in-as-the′ne-ah) deficient glandular activity.

adendritic (ah″den-drit′ik) lacking dendrites.

adenectomy (ad″in-ek′tah-me) excision of a gland.

adenectopia (ad″in-ek-to′pe-ah) malposition or displacement of a gland.

adenia (ah-de′ne-ah) chronic enlargement of the lymphatic glands; see also *lymphoma.*

adenine (ad′in-ēn) a white crystalline base, $C_5H_5N_5$, found in plant and animal tissues as one of the purine base constituents of DNA and RNA; it is one of the decomposition products of nuclein. **a. arabinoside (ara-A),** vidarabine.

adenitis (ad″in-īt′is) inflammation of a gland. **cervical a.,** a condition characterized by enlarged, inflamed, and tender lymph nodes of the neck; seen in certain infectious diseases of children, such as acute throat infections. **mesenteric a.,** mesenteric lymphadenitis.

adenization (ad″in-ĭ-za′shin) assumption by other tissue of an abnormal glandlike appearance.

adeno- word element [Gr.], *gland.*

adenoacanthoma (ad″in-o-ak″an-tho′mah) adenocarcinoma in which some of the cells exhibit squamous differentiation.

adenoameloblastoma (-ah-mel″o-blas-to′mah) an odontogenic tumor with formation of ductlike structures in place of or in addition to a typical ameloblastic pattern.

adenoblast (ad′in-o-blast″) embryonic forerunner of gland tissue.

adenocarcinoma (ad″in-o-kar″sĭ-no′mah) carcinoma derived from glandular tissue or in which the tumor cells form recognizable glandular structures.

adenocele (ad'in-o-sēl″) a cystic adenomatous tumor.

adenocellulitis (ad″in-o-sel″u-līt'is) inflammation of a gland and the tissue around it.

adenochondroma (-kon-dro'mah) a tumor containing both glandular and cartilaginous elements.

adenocystoma (ad″in-o-sis-to'mah) adenoma in which there is cyst formation. **papillary a. lymphomato'sum**, a cystic tumor containing epithelial and lymphoid tissue, found in the regions of the submaxillary and parotid glands.

adenocyte (ad'in-o-sīt″) a mature secretory cell of a gland.

adenoepithelioma (-ep″ĭ-the″le-o'mah) a tumor composed of glandular and epithelial elements.

adenogenous (ad″in-ah'jĭ-nus) originating from glandular tissue.

adenography (ad″in-ah'grah-fe) roentgenography of the glands.

adenohypophysectomy (ad″in-o-hi-pof″ĭ-sek'tah-me) excision of the glandular portion (the adenohypophysis) of the pituitary gland.

adenohypophysis (-hi-pof'ĭ-sis) the anterior (or glandular) lobe of the pituitary gland. **adenohypophys'eal**, adj.

adenoid (ad'in-oid) 1. resembling a gland. 2. (pl.) hypertrophy of the adenoid tissue (pharyngeal tonsil) that normally exists in the nasopharynx of children.

adenoiditis (-īt'is) inflammation of the adenoids.

adenolipoma (ad″in-o-lĭ-po'mah) a tumor composed of both glandular and fatty tissue elements.

adenolipomatosis (-lip″o-mah-to'sis) the formation of numerous adenolipomas in the neck, axilla, and groin.

adenolymphitis (-lim-fīt'is) lymphadenitis.

adenolymphoma (-lim-fo'mah) papillary adenocystoma lymphomatosum.

adenoma (ad″in-o'mah) a benign epithelial tumor in which the cells form recognizable glandular structures or in which the cells are derived from glandular epithelium. **acidophilic a.**, a tumor of the alpha cells of the anterior lobe of the pituitary gland, which may secrete an excess of growth hormone causing gigantism or acromegaly. **basophilic a.**, a tumor of the beta cells of the anterior lobe of the pituitary gland, which may secrete an excess of corticotropin (ACTH) resulting in Cushing's syndrome. **bronchial a's**, adenomas situated in the submucosal tissues of large bronchi; sometimes composed of well differentiated cells and usually circumscribed, these tumors have two histologic types: carcinoid and cylindroma. Although termed "adenomas," these tumors are now recognized as being of low grade malignancy. **chromophobe a., chromophobic a.**, a tumor of the anterior lobe of the pituitary gland whose cells do not readily stain with either acid or basic dyes. **malignant a.**, adenocarcinoma. **pituitary a.**, a benign neoplasm of the pituitary

gland; see *acidophilic a., basophilic a.*, and *chromophobe a.*

adenomalacia (ad″in-o-mah-la'she-ah) undue softness of a gland.

adenomatoid (ad″in-o'mah-toid) resembling adenoma.

adenomatosis (ad″in-o″mah-to'sis) the development of numerous adenomatous growths. **polyendocrine a.**, a rare syndrome in which there are adenomas or hyperplasia of more than one endocrine tissue; common sites are the anterior pituitary gland, the islets of Langerhans, and the parathyroid. The Zollinger-Ellison syndrome may occur in affected families.

adenomere (ad'in-o-mēr″) the blind terminal portion of the glandular cavity of a developing gland, becoming the functional portion of the organ.

adenomyofibroma (ad″in-o-mi″o-fi-bro'mah) a fibroma containing both glandular and muscular elements.

adenomyoma (-mi-o'mah) see *adenomyosis*.

adenomyomatosis (-mi″o-mah-to'sis) the formation of multiple adenomyomatous nodules in the tissues around or in the uterus.

adenomyometritis (-mi″o-mĕ-trīt'is) adenomyosis.

adenomyosarcoma (-sar-ko'mah) a mixed mesodermal tumor containing striated muscle cells.

adenomyosis (-mi-o'sis) benign ingrowth of the endometrium into the uterine musculature, sometimes with overgrowth of the latter; if the lesion forms a circumscribed tumor-like nodule, it is called *adenomyoma*. **a. subbasa'lis**, a bandlike, usually diffuse and superficial invasion of the myometrium by epithelial elements, accompanied by small clusters of endometrial stromal cells.

adenoncus (ad″in-ong'kus) enlargement of a gland.

adenopathy (ad″in-op'ah-the) enlargement of glands, especially of the lymph nodes.

adenopharyngitis (ad″in-o-far″in-jīt'is) inflammation of the adenoids and pharynx, usually involving the tonsils.

adenosarcoma (-sar-ko'mah) a mixed tumor composed of both glandular and sarcomatous elements.

adenosclerosis (-skler-o'sis) hardening of a gland.

adenosine (ah-den'ah-sēn) a nucleoside consisting of adenine and the pentose sugar D-ribose. **cyclic a. monophosphate (cyclic AMP, cAMP, 3′,5′AMP)**, a cyclic nucleotide, adenosine 3′,5′-cyclic monophosphate, involved in the action of many hormones, including catecholamines, ACTH, and vasopressin. The hormone binds to a specific receptor on the cell membrane of target cells. This activates an enzyme, adenylate cyclase, which produces cyclic AMP from ATP. Cyclic AMP acts as a second messenger activating other enzymes within the cell. **a. diphosphate (ADP)**, a nucleotide, adenosine 5′-pyrophosphate produced by the hydrolysis of adenosine triphosphate (ATP). It is then converted back to ATP by the metabolic process oxidative phosphorylation, glycolysis, and the tricarboxylic acid cycle. **a. monophosphate (AMP),** a nucleotide, adenosine 5'-phosphate, involved in energy metabolism and nucleotide synthesis. Called also *adenylic acid.* **a. triphosphate (ATP),** a nucleotide, adenosine 5'-triphosphate, occurring in all cells, where it stores energy in the form of high-energy phosphate bonds. Free energy is supplied to drive metabolic reactions or to transport molecules against concentration gradients, when ATP is hydrolyzed to ADP and inorganic phosphate or to AMP and inorganic pyrophosphate. ATP is also used to produce high-energy phosphorylated intermediary metabolites, such as glucose 6-phosphate.

adenosis (ad''in-o'sis) 1. any disease of a gland. 2. the abnormal development of a gland.

adenotome (ad'in-o-tōm'') an instrument for excision of adenoids.

adenovirus (-vi'rus) any of a large group of viruses causing disease of the upper respiratory tract and conjunctiva, and also present in latent infections in normal persons; many induce malignancy. **adenovi'ral,** adj.

adenyl (ad'in-il) the chemical radical produced by removal of a hydroxy group from the phosphorus of adenosine monophosphate (adenylic acid).

adenylate (ah-den'ĭ-lāt) adenylic acid, or any salt of adenylic acid.

adenylate kinase (ki'nās) ATP: AMP phosphotransferase; an enzyme occurring in muscle, heart, brain, and liver that converts AMP and ATP to two molecules of ADP.

adenyl cyclase (ad'in-il si'klās) an enzyme that catalyzes the conversion of adenosine triphosphate (ATP) to cyclic adenosine monophosphate (cAMP) and inorganic pyrophosphate (PP_i). It is activated by the attachment of a hormone or neurotransmitter to a specific membrane-bound receptor.

adenylic acid (ad''in-il'ik) adenosine monophosphate.

adenylyl (ad'in-il-il) the radical of adenylic acid with one H ion removed.

adequacy (ad'ĭ-kwah-se) the state of being sufficient for a specific purpose. **velopharyngeal a.,** sufficient functional closure of the velum against the postpharyngeal wall so that air and hence sound cannot enter the nasopharyngeal and nasal cavities.

adermogenesis (ah-der''mo-jen'ĭ-sis) imperfect development of skin.

ADH antidiuretic hormone.

adherence (ad-hēr'ĭns) the act or quality of sticking to something. **immune a.,** a complement-dependent phenomenon in which antigen-antibody complexes or particulate antigens coated with antibody (e.g., antibody-coated bacteria) adhere to red blood cells when complement component C3 is bound. It is a sensitive detector of complement-fixing antibody.

adhesion (ad-he'zhin) 1. the property of remaining in close proximity. 2. the stable joining of parts to one another, which may occur abnormally. 3. a fibrous band or structure by which parts abnormally adhere. **primary a.,** healing by first intention. **secondary a.,** healing by second intention.

adhesiotomy (ad-he''ze-ot'ah-me) surgical division of adhesions.

adiadochokinesia (ah-di''ah-do''ko-ki-ne'ze-ah) inability to perform fine, rapidly repeated, coordinated movements.

adiaphoria (-fo're-ah) nonresponse to stimuli as a result of previous exposure to similar stimuli; see also *refractory period.*

adiaspiromycosis (ad''ĭ-ah-spi''ro-mi-ko'sis) a pulmonary disease of many species of rodents throughout the world and rarely of man, due to inhalation of spores produced by the fungi, *Emmonsia parva* and *E. crescens,* and marked by the presence of huge spherules (adiaspores) without endospores in the lungs.

adiaspore (ad'ĭ-ah-spōr'') a spore produced by the soil fungi *Emmonsia parva* and *E. crescens;* see *adiospiromycosis.*

adip(o)- word element [L.], *fat.*

adipocele (ad'ĭ-pah-sēl'') a hernia containing fat.

adipocellular (ad''ĭ-pah-sel'u-ler) composed of fat and connective tissue.

adipocere (ad'ĭ-pah-sēr'') a waxy substance formed during decomposition of dead animal bodies, consisting mainly of insoluble salts of fatty acids.

adipocyte (-sīt) fat cell.

adipofibroma (ad''ĭ-po-fi-bro'mah) a lipoma with fibrous elements.

adipogenic (-jen'ik) producing fat or fatness.

adipokinesis (ad''ĭ-po-ki-ne'sis) the mobilization of fat in the body. **adipokinet'ic,** adj.

adipokinin (-ki'nin) a hormone from the anterior pituitary which accelerates mobilization of stored fat.

adipolysis (ad''ĭ-pol'ĭ-sis) the digestion of fats. **adipolyt'ic,** adj.

adiponecrosis (ad''ĭ-po-nah-kro'sis) necrosis of fatty tissue.

adipopexis (-pek'sis) the fixation or storing of fats. **adipopec'tic,** adj.

adiposis (ad''ĭ-po'sis) 1. obesity; excessive accumulation of fat. 2. fatty change in an organ or tissue. **a. cerebra'lis,** cerebral adiposity. **a. doloro'sa,** a disease, usually of women, marked by painful localized fatty swellings and by various nerve lesions; death may result from pulmonary complications. **a. hepa'tica,** fatty change in the liver.

adipositis (ad''ĭ-po-sīt'is) panniculitis.

adiposity (ad''ĭ-pos'it-e) the state of being fat; obesity. **cerebral a.,** fatness due to cerebral disease, especially of the hypothalamus.

adiposuria (ad''ĭ-pōs-ūr'e-ah) the occurrence of fat in the urine.

adipsia (a-dip'se-ah) absence of thirst, or abnormal avoidance of drinking.

aditus (ad'ĭ-tus), pl. *ad'itus* [L.] in anatomic nomenclature, an approach or entrance to an organ or part.

adjuvant (ă''jĭ-vint, ad'joo-vint) 1. assisting or aiding. 2. a substance which, administered with a drug or antigen, enhances its pharmacologic effect or its antigenicity. **Freund's a.,** a water-in-oil emulsion incorporating antigen, in the aqueous phase, into light-weight paraffin oil with the aid of an emulsifying agent. On injection, this mixture (*Freund's incomplete a.*) induces strong persistent antibody formation. The addition of killed, dried mycobacteria, e.g., *Mycobacterium tuberyicum,* to the oil phase (*Freund's complete a.*) elicits cell-mediated immunity (delayed hypersensitivity), as well as humoral antibody formation.

adjuvanticity (ad″joo-vin-tǐ′sit-e) the ability to modify the immune response.

adnerval (ad-ner′vil) 1. situated near a nerve. 2. toward a nerve, said of electric current that passes through muscle toward the entrance point of a nerve.

adneural (ad-noo′ril) adnerval.

adnexa (ad-nek′sah) [L., pl.] appendages or accessory structures of an organ, as the appendages of the eye (*a. o′culi*), including the eyelids and lacrimal apparatus, or of the uterus (*a. u′teri*), including the uterine tubes and ligaments and ovaries. **adnex′al,** adj.

adolescence (ad″o-les′ins) the period between puberty and the completion of physical growth, roughly from 11 to 19 years of age. **adoles′cent,** adj.

adoral (ad-o′ral) toward or near the mouth.

ADP adenosine diphosphate.

adren(o)- word element [L.], *adrenal gland.*

adrenal (ah-dre′nil) 1. near the kidney. 2. an adrenal gland.

Adrenalin (ah-dren′ah-lin) trademark for epinephrine.

adrenaline (-ah-lēn) official British Pharmacopoeia name for epinephrine.

adrenalinuria (-u′re-ah) the presence of epinephrine in the urine.

adrenalism (ah-dren′ah-lizm) ill health due to adrenal dysfunction.

adrenalitis (ah-dre″nal-īt′is) inflammation of the adrenal glands.

adrenergic (ă″dren-er′jik) sympathomimetic: activated or transmitted by epinephrine; said of those nerve fibers that liberate epinephrine (sympathin) at a synapse when a nerve impulse passes, i.e., the sympathetic fibers. Also, any agent that produces such an effect. See also under *receptor.*

adrenoceptor (ah-dren″no-sep′ter) adrenergic receptor. **adrenocep′tive,** adj.

adrenocorticohyperplasia (-kor″tǐ-ko-hi″perpla′ze-ah) adrenal cortical hyperplasia.

adrenocorticomimetic (-mi-met′ik) having effects similar to those of hormones of the adrenal cortex.

adrenocorticotrophic (-trof′ik) corticotropic.

adrenocorticotrophin (-trof′in) corticotropin.

adrenocorticotropin (-trōp′in) corticotropin.

adrenodoxin (-dok′sin) an iron-sulfide protein of the adrenal cortex that serves as an electron carrier in the biosynthesis of adrenal steroids.

adrenoglomerulotropin (-glo-mer″u-lo-tro′-pin) a hormone alleged to stimulate production of aldosterone by the adrenal cortex.

adrenoleukodystrophy (-loo″ko-dis′tro-fe) an X-linked disorder characterized by diffuse abnormality of the cerebral white matter and adrenal atrophy.

adrenolytic (-lit′ik) inhibiting the action of the adrenergic nerves or the response to epinephrine.

adrenomegaly (-meg′ah-le) enlargement of one or both of the adrenal glands.

adrenomimetic (-mi-met′ik) having actions similar to those of adrenergic compounds; sympathomimetic.

adrenoreceptor (ah-dre″no-re-sep′tor) adrenergic receptor.

adrenotoxin (-tok′sin) any substance that is toxic to the adrenal glands.

Adriamycin (a″dre-ah-mi′sin) trademark for preparations of doxorubicin hydrochloride.

adsorb (ad-sorb′) to attract and retain other material on the surface.

adsorbent (-int) 1. pertaining to or characterized by adsorption. 2. a substance that attracts other materials or particles to its surface.

adsorption (ad-sorp′shin) the action of a substance in attracting and holding other materials or particles on its surface.

adtorsion (ad-tor′shin) intorsion.

adult (ah-dult′) having attained full growth or maturity, or an organism that has done so.

adulteration (ah-dul″ter-a′shin) addition of an impure, cheap, or unnecessary ingredient to cheat, cheapen, or falsify a preparation; in legal terminology, incorrect labeling, including dosage not in accordance with the label.

advancement (ad-vans′mint) surgical detachment, as of a muscle or tendon, followed by reattachment at an advanced point; chiefly done with an eye muscle for correction of strabismus.

adventitia (ad″ven-tish′e-ah) the outer coat of an organ or structure, especially the outer coat of an artery.

adventitious (ad″ven-tish′is) 1. accidental or acquired; not natural or hereditary. 2. found out of the normal or usual place.

adynamia (ad″ǐ-na′me-ah) lack or loss of normal or vital powers; asthenia. **adynam′ic,** adj.

Aedes (a-e′dēz) a genus of mosquitoes, including approximately 600 species; some are vectors of disease, others are pests. It includes *A. aegyp′ti,* a vector of yellow fever and dengue.

aeg- for words beginning thus, see those beginning *eg-.*

aer(o)- word element [Gr.], *air; gas.*

aeration (a″er-a′shin) 1. the exchange of carbon dioxide for oxygen by the blood in the lungs. 2. the charging of a liquid with air or gas.

Aerobacter (a″er-o-bak′ter) a former name for a genus of bacteria now of the family Enterobacteriaceae; individual species are assigned to the genera *Enterobacter* and *Klebsiella.*

aerobe (a′er-ōb) a microorganism that lives and grows in the presence of free oxygen. **aero′bic,** adj. **facultative a.,** one that can live in the presence of oxygen, but does not require it. **obligate a.,** one that cannot live without oxygen.

aerobiology (a″er-o-bi-ol′o-je) the study of the distribution of living organisms (microorganisms) by the air.

aerobiosis (-bi-o′sis) life requiring free oxygen.

aerocele (a′er-o-sēl″) a tumor formed by air filling an adventitious pouch. **epidural a.,** a collection of air between the dura mater and the wall of the spinal column.

aerodermectasia (-der″mek-ta′ze-ah) subcutaneous emphysema, which may be spontaneous, traumatic, or surgical in origin.

aerodontalgia (-don-tal′je-ah) pain in the teeth due to lowered atmospheric pressure at high altitudes.

aeroembolism (-em′bo-lizm) obstruction of a blood vessel by air or gas.

aeroemphysema (-em″fi-ze′mah) pulmonary emphysema and edema with collection of nitrogen bubbles in the lung tissues; due to excessively rapid atmospheric decompression.

aerogen (a′er-o-jen″) a gas-producing bacterium.

Aeromonas (a″er-o-mo′nas) a genus of schizomycetes (family Pseudomonadaceae), usually found in water, some being pathogenic for fish, amphibians, reptiles, and humans.

aeroneurosis (-noo-ro′sis) a functional nervous disorder occurring in pilots.

aero-otitis (-o-tīt′is) barotitis.

aeropathy (a″er-op′ah-the) any disease due to change in atmospheric pressure, e.g., decompression sickness.

aeroperitonia (a″er-o-per″ĭ-to-ne′ah) pneumoperitoneum.

aerophilic (-fil′ik) requiring air for proper growth.

aerophyte (a′er-ah-fīt″) any plant organism that lives upon air.

aeropiesotherapy (a″er-o-pi-e″so-ther′ah-pe) treatment by compressed or rarefied air.

aeroplethysmograph (a″er-o-plĕ-thiz′mo-graf) an apparatus for measuring respiratory volumes by recording changes in body volume.

aerosinusitis (-si″nus-īt′is) barosinusitis.

aerosol (ār′o-sol) a colloid system in which solid or liquid particles are suspended in a gas, especially a suspension of a drug or other substance to be dispensed in a fine spray or mist.

aerotaxis (-tak′sis) movement of an organism in response to the presence of molecular oxygen.

aerotitis (-tīt′is) barotitis.

aerotolerant (-tol′er-int) surviving and growing in small amounts of air; said of anaerobic microorganisms.

aes-, aet- for words beginning thus, see also those beginning *es-, et-*.

Aesculapius (es″cu-la′pe-us) the god of healing in Roman mythology; see also *caduceus*, and under *staff*.

afebrile (a-feb′ril) without fever.

affect (af′ekt) the external expression of emotion attached to ideas or mental representations of objects.

affection (ah-fek′shin) 1. a state of emotion or feeling. 2. a morbid condition or diseased state.

affective (ah-fek′tiv) pertaining to affect.

afferent (af′er-int) conducting toward a center or specific site of reference.

affinity (ah-fin′it-e) 1. attraction; a tendency to seek out or unite with another object or substance. 2. in chemistry, the tendency of two substances to form strong or weak chemical bonds forming molecules or complexes. 3. in immunology, the thermodynamic bond strength of an antigen-antibody complex. Cf. *avidity*.

afibrinogenemia (a-fi″brin-o-jĭ-ne′me-ah) deficiency or absence of fibrinogen in the blood. **congenital a.,** an uncommon hemorrhagic coagulation disorder, probably autosomal recessive, and characterized by complete incoagulability of the blood.

aflatoxin (-tok′sin) a toxin, $C_{17}H_{12}O_6$, produced by *Aspergillus flavus* and *A. parasiticus,* molds which contaminate ground nut seedlings; it produces aflatoxicosis (x disease), with high mortality rates in fowl and other farm animals fed with infected ground nut meal and has been implicated as a cause of hepatic carcinoma in humans.

AFP alpha-fetoprotein.

afterbirth the placenta and membranes delivered from the uterus after childbirth.

afterbrain metencephalon.

afterimage a retinal impression remaining after cessation of the stimulus causing it.

afterpains cramplike pains that follow expulsion of the placenta, due to uterine contractions.

aftertaste a taste continuing after the substance producing it has been removed.

AG atrial gallop.

Ag chemical symbol, *silver* [L. *argentum*]; antigen.

A.G.A. American Gastroenterological Association.

agalactia (ag″ah-lak′she-ah) absence or failure of secretion of milk.

agammaglobulinemia (a″gam-ah-glob″u-line′me-ah) absence of all classes of immunoglobulins in the blood. **Swiss type a.,** a lethal form with associated alymphocytosis and aplasia of the thymus, first recognized in Switzerland.

aganglionosis (a-gang″gle-on-o′sis) congenital absence of parasympathetic ganglion cells.

agar (ag′ar) a dried hydrophilic, colloidal substance extracted from various species of red algae; used in solid culture media for bacteria and other microorganisms, as a bulk laxative, in making emulsions, and as a supporting medium for immunodiffusion and immunoelectrophoresis.

agaric (ah-gar′ik) 1. any mushroom, more especially any species of *Agaricus*. 2. the tinder or punk prepared from dried mushrooms.

agastric (ah-gas′trik) having no alimentary canal.

age (āj) 1. the duration, or the measure of time, of the existence of a person or object. 2. to undergo change as a result of passage of time.

achievement a., the age of a person expressed as the chronologic age of a normal person showing the same proficiency in study. **chronologic a.**, the actual measure of time elapsed since a person's birth. **mental a.**, the age level of mental ability of a person as gauged by standard intelligence tests.

agenesia (ah″jĭ-ne′ze-ah) 1. imperfect development. 2. sterility or impotence.

agenesis (a-jen′ĭ-sis) absence of an organ due to nonappearance of its primordium in the embryo; imperfect development of a part. **gonadal a.**, complete failure of gonadal development; see *Turner's syndrome*. **nuclear a.**, Möbius' syndrome. **ovarian a.**, failure of development of the ovaries; see *Turner's syndrome*.

agenitalism (a-jen′ĭ-til-izm″) absence of the genitals, or a condition due to lack of secretion of the testes or ovaries.

agenosomia (ah-jen″ah-so′me-ah) congenital absence or imperfect development of the genitals and eventration of the lower part of the abdomen.

agent (a′jint) something capable of producing an effect. **adrenergic blocking a.**, one that inhibits response to sympathetic impulses by blocking the alpha or beta receptor sites of effector organs. **adrenergic neuron blocking a.**, one that inhibits the release of norepinephrine from postganglionic adrenergic nerve endings. **alkylating a.**, a cytotoxic agent, e.g., a nitrogen mustard, which is highly reactive and can donate an alkyl group to another compound. Alkylating agents inhibit cell division by reacting with DNA and are used as antineoplastic agents. **blocking a.**, an agent that inhibits the response of effector organs to neural impulses of the autonomic nervous system; it may be an adrenergic or anticholinergic blocking agent. **chelating a.**, a compound which combines with metals to form weakly dissociated complexes in which the metal is part of a ring; used to extract certain elements from a system. **cholinergic blocking a.**, one that blocks the action of acetylcholine at nicotinic or muscarinic receptors of nerves or effector organs. **ganglionic blocking a.**, one that blocks cholinergic transmission at autonomic ganglionic synapses. **A. Orange**, a herbicide containing 2,4,5-T, 2,4-D, and the contaminant dioxin and which is suspected of being carcinogenic and teratogenic. **oxidizing a.**, a substance that acts as an electron acceptor in a chemical oxidation-reduction reaction. **progestational a's**, a group of hormones secreted by the corpus luteum and placenta and, in small amounts, by the adrenal cortex, including progesterone, Δ⁴-3-ketopregnene-20(α)-ol, and Δ⁴-3-ketopregnene-20(β)-ol; agents having progestational activity are also produced synthetically. **reducing a.**, a substance that acts as an electron donor in a chemical oxidation-reduction reaction.

ageusia (ah-gu′ze-ah) lack or impairment of the sense of taste. **ageu′sic**, adj.

agger (aj′er), pl. **ag′geres** [L.] an eminence or elevation.

agglutinant (ah-glōōt′in-int) 1. promoting union by adhesion. 2. a tenacious or gluey substance that holds parts together during the healing process.

agglutination (ah-glōōt′in-a″shin) 1. aggregation of suspended cells into clumps or masses, especially the clumping together of bacteria exposed to specific immune serum. 2. the process of union in wound healing. **agglutina′tive**, adj. **group a.**, agglutination of members of a group of biologically related organisms or corpuscles by an agglutinin specific for that group. **intravascular a.**, clumping of particulate elements within the blood vessels; used conventionally to denote red blood cell aggregation.

agglutinator (ah-glōōt′in-āt″er) an agglutinin.

agglutinin (ah-glōōt′in-in) an antibody in serum, which when combined with its homologous antigen, causes the antigen elements to adhere to one another in clumps. Also, any other substance, e.g., a lectin, capable of causing agglutination. **anti-Rh a.**, an agglutinin not normally present in human plasma, which may be produced in Rh-negative mothers carrying an Rh-positive fetus or after transfusion of Rh-positive blood into an Rh-negative patient. **chief a.**, the specific immune agglutinin in the blood of an animal immunized against an infectious disease agent. **cold a.**, one that acts only at relatively low temperatures (0°–20° C.). **group a.**, one that has a specific action on a particular group of microorganisms. **H a.**, one that is specific for flagellar antigens of the motile strain of a microorganism. **immune a.**, a specific agglutinin found in the blood after recovery from the disease or injection with the microorganism causing the disease. **incomplete a.**, one that at appropriate concentrations fails to agglutinate the homologous antigen. **leukocyte a.**, one that is directed against neutrophilic and other leukocytes. **major a.**, chief a. **minor a.**, partial a. **partial a.**, one present in agglutinative serum which acts on organisms and cells that are closely related to the specific antigen, but in a lower dilution.

agglutinogen (ag″loo-tin′o-jen) any substance that stimulates the production of agglutinin.

agglutinophilic (ah-glōōt′in-o-fil′ik) agglutinating easily.

aggregation (ag-re-ga′shin) 1. massing or clumping of materials together. 2. a clumped mass of material. **familial a.**, the occurrence of more cases of a given disorder in close relatives of a person with the disorder than in control families. **platelet a.**, a clumping together of platelets induced by various agents (e.g., thrombin) as part of the mechanism leading to thrombus formation.

aggression (ah-gresh′in) behavior leading to self-assertion, which may arise from innate drives and/or a response to frustration, and may be manifested by destructive and attacking behavior, by hostility and obstructionism, or by self-expressive drive to mastery.

aging (āj′ing) the gradual structural changes that occur with the passage of time, that are not due to disease or accident, and that eventually lead to death.

agitated (aj′ĭ-tāt″id) marked by restlessness and increased activity intermingled with anxiety, fear, and tension.

aglutition (ag″loo-tish′in) inability to swallow.

aglycemia (a″gli-se′me-ah) absence of sugar from the blood.

aglycone (a-gli′kōn) the noncarbohydrate portion of a glycoside molecule.

agnogenic (ag-no-jen′ik) of unknown origin.

agnosia (ag-no′ze-ah) inability to recognize the import of sensory impressions; the varieties correspond with several senses and are distinguished as *auditory* (*acoustic*), *gustatory*, *olfactory*, *tactile*, and *visual*. **finger a.**, loss of ability to indicate one's own or another's fingers. **time a.**, loss of comprehension of the succession and duration of events.

-agogue word element [Gr.], *something which leads or induces*.

agonadism (ah-go′nah-dizm) the condition of being without sex glands.

agonal (ag′ŏ-n′l) 1. pertaining to the death agony; occurring at the moment of or just before death. 2. pertaining to terminal infection.

agonist (ag′o-nist) 1. in anatomy, a prime mover. 2. in pharmacology, a drug that has an affinity for and stimulates physiologic activity at cell receptors normally stimulated by naturally occurring substances.

agony (ag′o-ne) 1. death struggle. 2. extreme suffering.

agoraphobia (ag″o-rah-fo′be-ah) morbid dread of open spaces.

-agra word element [Gr.], *attack; seizure*.

agranulocyte (ah-gran′u-lah-sīt″) a nongranular leukocyte.

agranulocytosis (a-gran″u-lo-si-to′sis) a symptom complex characterized by a marked decrease in the number of granulocytes and by lesions of the throat and other mucous membranes, of the gastrointestinal tract, and of the skin.

agranuloplastic (-plas′tik) forming nongranular cells only; not forming granular cells.

agraphia (a-graf′e-ah) inability to express thoughts in writing, due to a lesion of the cerebral cortex. **agraph′ic**, adj.

A.G.S. American Geriatrics Society.

ague (a′gu) 1. malarial fever, or any other severe recurrent symptom of malarial origin. 2. a chill.

agyria (ah-ji′re-ah) a malformation in which the gyri of the cerebral cortex are not normally developed and the brain is usually small.

A.H.A. American Heart Association; American Hospital Association.

AHF antihemophilic factor (coagulation Factor VIII; see under *factor*).

AHG antihemophilic globulin (coagulation Factor VIII; see under *factor*).

A.H.P. Assistant House Physician.

A.H.S. Assistant House Surgeon.

A.I. aortic incompetence; aortic insufficiency; apical impulse; artificial insemination.

A.I.C. Association des Infirmières Canadiennes.

A.I.D. donor insemination.

aid (ād) help or assistance; by extension, applied to any device by which a function can be improved or augmented, as a hearing aid. **first a.**, emergency assistance and treatment of an injured or ill person before regular surgical or medical therapy can be obtained. **pharmaceutic a., pharmaceutical a.**, see under *necessity*.

AIDS acquired immunodeficiency syndrome.

A.I.H. American Institute of Homeopathy; homologous insemination.

A.I.H.A. American Industrial Hygiene Association.

ailurophobia (i-loo″ro-fo′be-ah) morbid fear of cats.

A.I.N. American Institute of Nutrition.

air (ār) the gaseous mixture which makes up the atmosphere. **alveolar a.**, air in the lungs, varying in volume (during normal respiration) from the functional residual capacity at the end of expiration to the functional residual capacity plus tidal volume at the end of inspiration. **reserve a.**, see *expiratory* and *inspiratory reserve volume*. **residual a.**, see under *volume*. **tidal a.**, see under *volume*.

airborne (ār′born) suspended in, transported by, or spread by air.

airway (ār′wa) 1. the passage by which air enters and leaves the lungs. 2. a tube for securing unobstructed respiration. **esophageal obturator a.**, a hollow tube inserted into the esophagus to maintain airway patency in unconscious persons and to permit positive-pressure ventilation through the face mask connected to the tube. **nasopharyngeal a.**, a hollow tube inserted into a nostril and directed along the floor of the nose to the nasopharynx to prevent the tongue from blocking off passage of air in unconscious persons. **oropharyngeal a.**, a hollow tube inserted into the mouth and back of the throat to prevent the tongue from blocking off passage of air in unconscious persons.

A.I.U.M. American Institute of Ultrasound in Medicine.

akaryocyte (ah-kar′e-o-sīt″) a non-nucleated cell, e.g., an erythrocyte.

akaryote (ah-kar′e-ōt) akaryocyte.

akatamathesia (ah-kat″ah-mah-the′ze-ah) inability to understand.

akathisia (ak″ah-the′ze-ah) a condition marked by motor restlessness, ranging from anxiety to inability to lie or sit quietly or to sleep, as seen in toxic reactions to phenothiazines.

akinesia (a″ki-ne′ze-ah) absence or poverty of movements. **akinet′ic**, adj. **a. al′gera**, Möbius' syndrome.

akinesthesia (ah-kin″es-the′ze-ah) absence of movement sense.

Al chemical symbol, *aluminum*.

Ala alanine.

ala (a′lah), pl. *a′lae* [L.] a winglike process. **a′late**, adj.

alacrima (a-lak′rĭ-mah) a deficiency or absence of secretion of tears.

alactasia (ah-lak-ta′se-ah) a genetically determined condition marked by malabsorption of lactose due to deficiency of lactase; it is very rare in infants of any race, but is common in nonwhite adults.

alanine (al'ah-nēn) a natural amino acid occurring in two forms: alpha-alanine, CH_3CH-$(NH_2)\cdot COOH$, and beta-alanine, CH_2-$NH_2 \cdot CH_2COOH$.

alanine aminotransferase (ALT) (ah-me''no-trans'fer-ās) an enzyme normally present in serum and body tissues, especially in the liver; it is released into the serum as a result of tissue injury, hence the concentration in the serum may be increased in patients with acute damage to hepatic cells.

alar (a'lar) pertaining to an ala, or wing.

alba (al'bah) [L.] white.

albedo (al-be'do) [L.] whiteness. **a. re'tinae,** paleness of the retina due to edema caused by transudation of fluid from the retinal capillaries.

albicans (al'bĭ-kans) [L.] white.

albiduria (al''bid-ūr'e-ah) the discharge of white or pale urine.

albinism (al'bĭ-nizm) congenital absence, either total or partial, of normal pigmentation in the body (hair, skin, eyes) due to a defect in melanin synthesis.

albino (al-bi'no) a person affected with albinism.

albinoidism (al-bĭ-noid'izm) deficiency of pigment in the hair, skin, and eyes, but not to the degree seen in albinism.

albinuria (al''bin-u're-ah) albiduria.

albuginea (al''bu-jin'e-ah) 1. a tough, whitish layer of fibrous tissue investing a part or organ. 2. the tunica albuginea. **a. oc'uli,** sclera. **a. ova'rii,** the outer layer of the ovarian stroma. **a. pe'nis,** the outer envelope of the corpora cavernosa.

albumin (al-bu'min) 1. any protein that is soluble in water and also in moderately concentrated salt solutions. 2. serum a. **egg a.,** albumin of egg whites. **iodinated I-125 serum a.,** a radiopharmaceutical used in plasma volume determinations, consisting of albumin human labeled with iodine-125. **iodinated I-131 serum a.,** a radiopharmaceutical used in blood pool imaging and plasma volume determinations, consisting of albumin human labeled with iodine-131. **a. human,** a sterile, nonpyrogenic preparation of human serum albumin tested for absence of hepatitis B surface antigen, used in the treatment of shock and hypoproteinemia.

albuminocholia (-no-ko'le-ah) presence of protein in the bile.

albuminoid (al-bu'mĭ-noid) 1. resembling albumin. 2. a scleroprotein.

albuminoptysis (-nop'tĭ-sis) albumin in the sputum.

albuminuretic (al-bu''min-u-ret'ik) pertaining to, characterized by, or promoting albuminuria; also, an agent that promotes albuminuria.

albuminuria (al-bu''min-u're-ah) presence in the urine of serum albumin; see *proteinuria.* **albuminu'ric,** adj.

Alcaligenes (al''kah-lij'ĭ-nēz) a genus of schizomycetes (family Achromobacteraceae) found in the intestinal tract of vertebrates or in dairy products. **A. faeca'lis,** a species that is a cause of nosocomial septicemia, which arises from contaminated hemodialysis or intravenous fluid, in immunocompromised patients.

alcapton (al-kap'ton) see *alkapton bodies,* under *body.*

alcohol (al'kah-hol) 1. any organic compound containing the hydroxy (—OH) functional group except those in which the OH group is attached to an aromatic ring, which are called *phenols.* Alcohols are classified as *primary, secondary,* or *tertiary* according to whether the carbon atom to which the OH group is attached is bonded to one, two, or three other carbon atoms and as *monohydric, dihydric,* or *trihydric* according to whether they contain one, two, or three OH groups; the latter two are called *diols* and *triols,* respectively. 2. common name for ethyl alcohol (see *ethanol*). **absolute a.,** dehydrated a. **benzyl a.,** a colorless liquid, $C_6H_5\cdot$-$CH_2\cdot OH$, used as a bacteriostatic in solutions for injection; also applied topically as a local anesthetic. **cetyl a.,** a solid alcohol, $C_{16}H_{34}O$, used as an emulsifying and stiffening agent. **dehydrated a.,** an extremely hygroscopic, transparent, colorless, volatile liquid, containing 99.5% by volume of C_2H_5OH. **denatured a.,** alcohol rendered unfit for human consumption. **ethyl a.,** ethanol, CH_3CH_2OH. **isopropyl a.,** transparent, colorless, volatile liquid, CH_3-$CHOH\cdot CH_3$, used as a solvent. **isopropyl rubbing a.,** a preparation containing between 68% and 72% isopropyl alcohol in water, used as a rubefacient. **methyl a.,** methanol. **nicotinyl a.,** an alcohol, C_6H_7NO, used as a peripheral vasodilator in vasospastic conditions. **phenylethyl a.,** a colorless liquid, $C_8H_{10}O$, used as a bacteriostatic and preservative. **polyvinyl a.,** a water-soluble synthetic polymer used as a viscosity-increasing agent in pharmaceuticals. **propyl a.,** a colorless fluid of alcoholic taste and fruity odor; used as a solvent. **rubbing a.,** a preparation of acetone, methyl isobutyl ketone, and 68.5% to 71.5% ethyl alcohol; used as a rubefacient. **stearyl a.,** a mixture of solid alcohols, consisting chiefly of $CH_3(CH_2)_{16}CH_2OH$; used as an ingredient of various pharmaceutic or cosmetic preparations. **wood a.,** methanol.

alcoholism (al'kah-hol-izm) a disorder marked by a pathological pattern of alcohol use that causes serious impairment in social or occupational functioning (alcohol abuse). If tolerance or withdrawal is present, it is called alcohol dependence.

alcoholysis (al''kah-hol'ĭ-sis) decomposition of a compound due to the incorporation and splitting of alcohol.

Aldactazide (al-dak'tah-zīd) trademark for a preparation of spironolactone with hydrochlorothiazide.

Aldactone (al-dak'tōn) trademark for a preparation of spironolactone.

aldehyde (al'dĕ-hīd) an organic compound containing the aldehyde functional group (—CHO), i.e., one with a carbonyl group (C=O) located at one end of the carbon chain.

aldehyde-lyase (-li'ās) a group of lyases that catalyze the removal of an aldehyde group.

aldolase (al'do-lās) an enzyme in muscle extract that acts as a catalyst in the production of dihydroxyacetone phosphate and glyceraldehyde phosphate from fructose 1,6-diphosphate.

Aldomet (-met) trademark for a preparation of methyldopa.

aldopentose (al″do-pen'tōs) any of a class of sugars containing five carbon atoms and an aldehyde group (—CHO).

Aldoril (-ril) trademark for a fixed combination preparation of methyldopa and hydrochlorothiazide.

aldose (al'dōs) a sugar containing an aldehyde group (—CHO).

aldosterone (al'do-ster-ōn″, al-dos'ter-ōn) the main mineralocorticoid hormone secreted by the adrenal cortex, the principal biological activity of which is the regulation of electrolyte and water balance by promoting the retention of sodium and the excretion of potassium.

aldosteronism (-izm″) hyperaldosteronism; an abnormality of electrolyte balance caused by excessive secretion of aldosterone. **primary a.,** that arising from oversecretion of aldosterone by an adrenal adenoma, characterized typically by hypokalemia, alkalosis, muscular weakness, polyuria, polydipsia, and hypertension. Called also *Conn's syndrome.* **pseudoprimary a.,** that caused by bilateral adrenal hyperplasia and having the same signs and symptoms as primary aldosteronism. **secondary a.,** that due to extra-adrenal stimulation of aldosterone secretion; it is commonly associated with edematous states, as in nephrotic syndrome, hepatic cirrhosis, heart failure, and accelerated phase hypertension.

alecithal (ah-les'ĭ-thal) without yolk; applied to eggs with very little yolk; see under *ovum.*

aleukemia (ah″loo-ke'me-ah) 1. absence or deficiency of leukocytes in the blood. 2. aleukemic leukemia.

aleukia (ah-loo'ke-ah) leukopenia; absence of leukocytes from the blood. **alimentary toxic a.,** a form of mycotoxicosis associated with the ingestion of grain that has overwintered in the field; abbreviated ATA.

aleukocytosis (-si-to'sis) deficiency in the proportion of white cells in the blood; leukopenia.

alexia (ah-lek'se-ah) inability to read; see *word blindness.* **cortical a.,** a form of sensory aphasia due to lesions of the left gyrus angularis. **motor a.,** alexia in which the patient understands what he sees written or printed, but cannot read it aloud. **musical a.,** loss of the ability to read music. **optical a.,** word blindness.

alexic (ah-lek'sik) 1. pertaining to alexia. 2. having the properties of an alexin.

aleydigism (ah-lid'ig-izm) absence of secretion of the interstitial cells of Leydig.

ALG antilymphocyte globulin.

alga (al'gah), pl. *al'gae* [L.] an individual organism of the algae.

algae (al'je) a group of plants, including the seaweeds and many unicellular marine and fresh-water plants, most of which contain chlorophyll and account for about 90% of the earth's photosynthetic activity. **al'gal,** adj.

algefacient (al″jĕ-fa'shint) cooling or refrigerant.

algesia (al-je'ze-ah) sensitiveness to pain; hyperesthesia. **alge'sic, alget'ic,** adj.

algesimeter (al″jĕ-sim'it-er) an instrument used in measuring the sensitiveness to pain as produced by pricking with a sharp point.

algesthesis (-sis) the perception of pain; a painful sensation.

-algia word element [Gr.], *pain.*

algicide (al'jĭ-sīd) 1. destructive to algae. 2. an agent which destroys algae.

algid (al'jid) chilly; cold.

alginate (al'jĭ-nāt) a salt of alginic acid; certain alginates have been used as foam, clot, or gauze for absorbable surgical dressings, and others are useful as materials for dental impressions.

alginic acid (al-jin'ik) an acid polysaccharide obtained from seaweed, used for thickening, emulsifying, and stabilizing foods and drugs.

algo- word element [Gr.], *pain; cold.*

algodystrophy (al″go-dis'tro-fe) a combination of pain and dystrophic changes in bone.

algogenic (-jen'ik) 1. causing pain. 2. lowering the temperature.

algology (al-gol'o-je) 1. the scientific study of pain. 2. phycology.

algometry (-ĭ-tre) measurement of the sensitivity to painful stimuli.

algor (al'gor) chill or rigor; coldness. **a. mor'tis,** the gradual decrease of body temperature after death.

algorithm (al'go-rith'm) a mechanical procedure for solving a certain type of mathematical problem; a step-by-step method of solving a problem, as making a diagnosis.

alienia (ah″li-e'ne-ah) absence of the spleen.

aliform (al'ĭ-form) shaped like a wing.

alimentation (-min-ta'shin) giving or receiving of nourishment. **rectal a.,** feeding by injection of nutriment into the rectum. **total parenteral a.,** parenteral hyperalimentation.

alimentotherapy (-men″to-thĕ'rah-pe) treatment by systematic feeding.

alinasal (-na'z'l) pertaining to either ala of the nose.

aliphatic (-fat'ik) 1. fatty or oily. 2. pertaining to a hydrocarbon that does not contain an aromatic ring.

alisphenoid (al-ĭ-sfe'noid) 1. pertaining to the great wing of the sphenoid. 2. a cartilage of the fetal chondrocranium on either side of the basisphenoid; later in development it forms the greater part of the great wing of the sphenoid.

alizarin (ah-liz'ah-rin) a red crystalline dye, $C_{14}H_8O_4$, prepared synthetically or obtained from madder; its compounds are used as indicators.

alkalemia (al″kah-le'me-ah) increased pH (abnormal alkalinity) of the blood.

alkali (al'kah-li) a strong, caustic base, e.g., sodium or potassium hydroxide.

alkaline (al'kah-līn) having the reactions of an alkali.

alkalinuria (-lin-ūr′e-ah) an alkaline condition of the urine.

alkalizer (-līz′er) an agent that causes alkalization.

alkaloid (al′kah-loid) any of a group of organic basic substances found in plants, many of which are pharmacologically active, e.g., atropine, caffeine, morphine, nicotine, quinine, and strychnine. **vinca a's,** alkaloids produced by the common periwinkle plant (*Vinca rosea*); two, vincristine and vinblastine, are used as antineoplastic agents.

alkalosis (al″kah-lo′sis) a pathologic condition due to accumulation of base in, or loss of acid from, the body. Cf. *acidosis*. **alkalot′ic,** adj. **altitude a.,** increased alkalinity in blood and tissues due to exposure to high altitudes. **compensated a.,** a condition in which compensatory mechanisms have returned the pH toward normal. **hypokalemic a.,** metabolic alkalosis associated with a low serum potassium level. **metabolic a.,** a disturbance in which the acid-base status shifts toward the alkaline side because of retention of base or loss of noncarbonic, or fixed (nonvolatile), acids.

alkane (al′kān) a saturated hydrocarbon, i.e., one that has no carbon-carbon multiple bonds; formerly called *paraffin*.

alkapton (al-kap′tŏn) see under *body*.

alkaptonuria (al-kap″tŏn-ūr′e-ah) excretion in the urine of alkapton bodies (most commonly homogentisic acid) as a result of a genetic disorder of phenylalanine-tyrosine metabolism, characterized by darkening of the urine when left standing or on addition of alkali; it is the precursor of ochronosis. **alkap′tonuric,** adj.

alkavervir (al″kah-verv′er) a yellow powdery mixture of alkaloids extracted from *Veratrum viride;* used to lower blood pressure.

alkyl (al′k'l) a monovalent radical of the general formula C_nH_{2n+1}, formed when an aliphatic hydrocarbon loses one hydrogen atom.

alkylation (al″kĭ-la′shin) the substitution of an alkyl group for an active hydrogen atom in an organic compound.

all(o)- word element [Gr.], *other; deviating from normal.*

allachesthesia (al″ah-kes-the′ze-ah) allesthesia. **optical a.,** visual allesthesia.

allantiasis (al″an-ti′ah-sis) sausage poisoning; botulism from improperly prepared sausages.

allantochorion (ah-lan″to-kor′e-on) the allantois and chorion as one structure.

allantoid (ah-lan′toid) 1. resembling the allantois. 2. sausage-shaped.

allantoin (ah-lan′to-in) a crystalline substance, $C_4H_6N_4O_3$, found in allantoic fluid, fetal urine, and many plants, and as a urinary excretion product of purine metabolism in most mammals but not in man or the higher apes; used topically to promote wound healing.

allantois (ah-lan′to-is) a ventral outgrowth of the embryos of reptiles, birds, and mammals. In man, it is vestigial except that its blood vessels give rise to those of the umbilical cord. **allanto′ic,** adj.

allele (ah-lēl′) one of two or more alternative forms of a gene at corresponding sites (loci) on homologous chromosomes, which determine alternative characters in inheritance. **allel′ic,** adj. **multiple a's,** alleles of which there are more than two alternative forms possible at any one locus.

allelochemics (al-le″lo-kem′iks) chemical interactions between species, involving release of active chemical substances, such as scents, pheromones, and toxins.

allelotaxis (ah-le″lo-tak′sĭs) development of an organ from several embryonic structures.

allergen (al′er-jen) an antigenic substance capable of producing immediate hypersensitivity (allergy). **allergen′ic,** adj. **pollen a.,** any protein antigen of weed, tree, or grass pollens capable of causing allergic asthma or rhinitis; pollen antigen extracts are used in skin testing for pollen sensitivity and in immunotherapy (desensitization) for pollen allergy.

allergy (al′er-je) a hypersensitive state acquired through exposure to a particular allergen, reexposure bringing to light an altered capacity to react. See *hypersensitivity*. **aller′gic,** adj. **atopic a.,** atopy. **bacterial a.,** specific hypersensitivity to a particular bacterial antigen. **bronchial a.,** see *asthma*. **cold a.,** a condition manifested by local and systemic reactions, mediated by histamine, which is released from mast cells and basophils as a result of exposure to cold. **contact a.,** hypersensitiveness marked by an eczematous reaction to contact between the epidermis and the allergen. **delayed a.,** see under *hypersensitivity*. **drug a.,** an allergic reaction occurring as the result of unusual sensitivity to a drug. **food a., gastrointestinal a.,** allergy, usually manifested by a skin reaction, in which the ingested antigens include food as well as drugs. **hereditary a.,** atopy. **immediate a.,** see under *hypersensitivity*. **latent a.,** that not manifested by symptoms but which may be detected by tests. **physical a.,** a condition in which the patient is sensitive to the effects of physical agents, such as heat, cold, light, etc. **pollen a.,** hay fever. **polyvalent a.,** see *pathergy* (2). **spontaneous a.,** atopy.

allesthesia (al″es-the′ze-ah) the experiencing of a sensation, e.g., pain or touch, as occurring at a point remote from where the stimulus actually is applied.

alloantibody (al″o-an′tĭ-bod-e) isoantibody.

alloantigen (-an′tĭ-jen) isoantigen.

allobarbital (-bar′bĭ-tal) a hypnotic and sedative, $(C_3H_5)_2C(CO\cdot NH)_2CO$.

allocheiria (-ki′re-ah) allesthesia.

allochroism (-kro′izm) change or variation in color, as in certain minerals.

allochromasia (-kro-ma′ze-ah) change in color of hair or skin.

allodynia (-din′e-ah) pain produced by a non-noxious stimulus.

alloeroticism (-ĕ-rot′ĭ-sizm) sexuality directed to another.

allogeneic (-ji-ne′ik) 1. having cell types that are antigenically distinct. 2. in transplantation biology, denoting individuals (or tissues) that are of the same species but antigenically distinct.

NOTE: In contrast, *syngeneic* (or *isogeneic*) refers to individuals having identical genotypes, and *xenogeneic* to individuals of different species, which by definition have different genotypes.

allogenic (-jen'ik) allogeneic.

allograft (al'o-graft) a graft between animals of the same species, but of different genotype.

allogroup (-grōōp) an allotype linkage group, especially of allotypes for the four IgG subclasses, which are closely linked and inherited as a unit.

alloimmune (al″o-im-ūn') specifically immune to an allogeneic antigen.

alloimmunization (-im″u-ni-za'shin) isoimmunization.

allomerism (ah-lom'er-izm) change in chemical constitution without change in crystalline form.

allomorphism (al″o-mor'fizm) change in crystalline form without change in chemical constitution.

alloplasia (al″o-pla'ze-ah) heteroplasia.

alloplast (al'o-plast) an inert foreign body used for implantation into tissue. **alloplas'tic,** adj.

alloplasty (-plas″te) adaptation by alteration of the environment.

allopsychic (-si'kik) pertaining to the mind in its relation to the external world.

allopurinol (-pūr'in-ol) an isomer of hypoxanthine, capable of inhibiting xanthine oxidase and thus of reducing serum and urinary levels of uric acid; used in the treatment of gout.

allorhythmia (-rith'me-ah) irregularity of the heart beat or pulse that recurs regularly.

all-or-none the heart muscle, under whatever stimulation, will contract to the fullest extent or not at all; in other muscles and in nerves, stimulation of a fiber causes an action potential to travel over the entire fiber, or not to travel at all.

allosensitization (al″o-sen″sĭ-ti-za'shin) sensitization to alloantigens (isoantigens), as to Rh antigens during pregnancy.

allosome (al'o-sōm) a foreign constituent of the cytoplasm which has entered from outside the cell.

allosteric (al″o-stĕ'rik) pertaining to an effect on the biological function of a protein produced by a compound not directly involved in that function (an allosteric effector) or to regulation of an enzyme involving cooperativity between multiple binding sites (allosteric sites).

allotherm (al'ah-therm) 1. poikilotherm. 2. heterotherm.

allotope (-tōp) a site on the constant or nonvarying portion of an antibody molecule that can be recognized by a combining site of other antibodies.

allotropic (al″ah-trop'ik) 1. exhibiting allotropism. 2. concerned with others; said of a type of personality that is more preoccupied with others than with oneself.

allotropism (ah-lah'trah-pizm) existence of an element in two or more distinct forms.

allotype (al'ah-tīp) any of several allelic variants of a protein that are characterized by antigenic differences. **allotyp'ic,** adj.

alloxan (ah-lok'san) an oxidized product of uric acid, $C_4H_2N_2O_4$, which tends to destroy the islet cells of the pancreas, thus producing diabetes. It has been obtained from intestinal mucus in diarrhea and has been used in nutrition experiments and as an antineoplastic.

alloxuria (al″ok-su're-ah) presence of purine bases in the urine. **alloxu'ric,** adj.

alloy (al'oi) a solid mixture of two or more metals or metalloids that are mutually soluble in the molten condition.

allyl (al″l) a univalent radical, $CH_2{:}CH{\cdot}CH_2$.

aloe (al'o) the dried juice of leaves of various species of *Aloe,* used in pharmaceutical preparations.

alopecia (al″o-pe'she-ah) baldness; absence of hair from skin areas where it is normally present. **a. area'ta,** hair loss, usually reversible, in sharply defined areas, usually involving the beard or scalp. **cicatricial a., a. cicatrisa'ta,** irreversible loss of hair associated with scarring, usually on the scalp. **male pattern a.,** loss of scalp hair genetically determined and androgen-dependent, beginning with frontal recession and progressing symmetrically to leave ultimately only a sparse peripheral rim of hair. **a. symptomat'ica,** loss of hair due to systemic or psychogenic causes, or to other stress. **a. tota'lis,** loss of hair from the entire scalp. **a. universa'lis,** loss of hair from the entire body.

alpha (al'fah) first letter of the Greek alphabet, α; used in names of chemical compounds to distinguish the first in a series of isomers, or to indicate position of substituting atoms or groups.

alpha₁-antitrypsin (al″fah-an″tĭ-trip'sin) a plasma protein (an α_1-globulin) produced in the liver, which inhibits the activity of trypsin and other proteolytic enzymes. Deficiency of this protein is associated with development of emphysema. Also written α_1-*antitrypsin.*

alpha-fetoprotein (AFP) (-fēt″to-pro'tēn) a protein with alpha electrophoretic mobility produced by the fetal liver, yolk sac, and gastrointestinal tract and also by hepatocellular carcinoma, germ cell neoplasms, and other cancers in adults. The serum AFP level is used to monitor the effectiveness of cancer treatment, and the amniotic fluid AFP level is used in the prenatal diagnosis of neural tube defects.

alphalytic (-lit'ik) blocking the α-adrenergic receptors of the sympathetic nervous system; also, an agent that so acts.

alphamimetic (-mi-met'ik) stimulating or mimicking the stimulation of the α-adrenergic receptors of the sympathetic nervous system; also, an agent that so acts.

alphaprodine (-pro'dēn) a narcotic analgesic, $C_{16}H_{23}NO_2$; used as the hydrochloride salt.

ALS antilymphocyte serum.

alseroxylon (al″sĕ-rok'sĭ-lon) a purified extract of *Rauwolfia serpentina,* containing reserpine and other amorphous alkaloids; used as a tranquilizer and sedative.

alternans (awl-ter'nanz) [L.] alternating or alternation, as in pulsus alternans (alternating strength of the pulse). **electrical a.,** alternating variations in the amplitude of electrocardiographic waves. **a. of the heart,** alternating strength in the heart beat or pulse. **pul′sus a.,** the presence of alteration of intensity of heart sounds, indicating left ventricular failure.

alternation (awl″ter-na′shin) the regular succession of two opposing or different events in turn. **a. of generations,** alternate sexual and asexual reproduction, one generation reproducing sexually, the next asexually.

alum (al′um) a crystalline substance, ammonium alum, $AlNH_4(SO_4)_2 \cdot 12H_2O$, or potassium alum, $AlK(SO_4)_2 \cdot 12H_2O$; used topically as an astringent and styptic.

alumina (ah-loo′mĭ-nah) aluminum oxide, Al_2O_3.

aluminosis (ah-loo″mĭ-no′sis) pneumoconiosis due to the presence of aluminum-bearing dust in the lungs.

aluminum (ah-loo′mĭ-num) a chemical element (*see table*), at. no. 13, symbol Al. **a. chloride,** $AlCl_3 \cdot 6H_2O$, used topically as an astringent solution, and as an antiperspirant. **a. hydroxide,** $AL(OH)_3$, used as a gastric antacid. **a. nicotinate,** a complex of aluminum nicotinate, aluminum hydroxide, and nicotinic acid used as an anticholesterolemic, antilipoproteinemic, and peripheral vasodilator. **a. phosphate,** $AlPO_4$, used with calcium sulfate and sodium silicate in dental cements, and in pharmacy as the gel. **a. subacetate,** a compound used as an astringent when diluted with water.

alveolitis (-lit′is) inflammation of an alveolus. **allergic a., extrinsic allergic a.,** hypersensitivity pneumonitis caused by repeated exposure to an allergen; e.g., farmer's lung, bagassosis, and pigeon breeder's lung.

alveoloclasia (-lo-kla′ze-ah) disintegration or resorption of the inner wall of a tooth alveolus.

alveoloplasty (al-ve′ah-lo-plas″te) surgical alteration of the shape and condition of the alveolar process, in preparation for denture construction.

alveolus (al-ve′o-lus), pl. *alve′oli* [L.] a small saclike dilatation; see also *acinus.* **alve′olar,** adj. **dental alveoli,** the cavities or sockets of either jaw, in which the roots of the teeth are embedded. **pulmonary alveoli,** small outpocketings of the alveolar ducts and sacs and terminal bronchioles through whose walls the exchange of carbon dioxide and oxygen takes place between alveolar air and capillary blood; see Plate VII.

alveus (al′ve-us), pl. *al′vei* [L.] a canal or trough.

alymphocytosis (a-lim″fo-si-to′sis) deficiency or absence of lymphocytes from the blood; lymphopenia.

alymphoplasia (-pla′ze-ah) failure of development of lymphoid tissue.

A.M. amperemeter; [L.] ante meridiem (*before noon*); meter angle.

Am chemical symbol, *americium.*

A.M.A. Aerospace Medical Association; American Medical Association; Australian Medical Association.

amacrine (am′ah-krīn) 1. without long processes. 2. any of a group of branched retinal structures regarded as modified nerve cells.

amalgam (ah-mal′gam) an alloy of two or more metals, one of which is mercury.

Amanita (am″ah-nīt′ah) a genus of mushrooms, some of which are poisonous and others edible; ingestion of *A. phalloi′des, A. musca′ria, A. pantheri′na, A. ver′na,* and others, is manifested by vomiting, abdominal pain, and diarrhea, followed by a period of improvement, and culminating in signs of severe hepatic, renal, and central nervous system damage.

amantadine (ah-man′tah-dēn) an antiviral agent used against the influenza A virus, also used as an antidyskinetic in the treatment of Parkinson's disease.

amastia (ah-mas′te-ah) congenital absence of one or both mammary glands.

amastigote (ah-mas′tĭ-gōt) the nonflagellate, intracellular, morphologic stage in the development of certain hemoflagellates, resembling the typical adult form of *Leishmania.*

amaurosis (am″aw-ro′sis) blindness, especially that occurring without apparent lesion of the eye. **amaurot′ic,** adj. **a. congen′ita of Leber, Leber's congenital a.,** hereditary blindness, occurring at or shortly after birth, associated with an atypical form of diffuse pigmentation and commonly with optic atrophy and attenuation of the retinal vessels.

ambenonium (am″bĭ-no′ne-um) a cholinergic, $C_{28}H_{42}N_4O_2$; the chloride salt is used to treat symptoms of muscular weakness and fatigue in myasthenia gravis.

ambidextrous (am″bĭ-deks′tris) able to use either hand with equal dexterity.

ambilateral (-lat′er-il) pertaining to or affecting both sides.

ambilevous (-le′vus) unable to use either hand with dexterity.

ambiopia (am″be-o′pe-ah) diplopia.

ambisexual (am″bĭ-sek′shoo-il) denoting sexual characteristics common to both sexes, e.g., pubic hair.

ambivalence (am-biv′ah-lins) simultaneous existence of conflicting emotional attitudes toward a goal, object, or person. **ambiv′alent,** adj.

Amblyomma (-om′ah) a genus of hard-bodied ticks of worldwide distribution. **A. america′num,** the Lone Star tick, found in southern and southwestern United States, Central America, and Brazil; a vector of Rocky Mountain spotted fever. **A. cajennen′se,** a common pest of domestic animals and man in the southern United States, Central and South America, and the West Indies; a vector of Rocky Mountain spotted fever. **A. macula′tum,** the Gulf Coast tick, infesting cattle in southwestern United States and Central and South America; its bite causes painful sores that serve as sites of screwworm infections and secondary bacterial and fungal infections.

amblyopia (-o′pe-ah) dimness of vision without detectable organic lesion of the eye. **amblyop′ic,** adj. **alcoholic a.,** nutritional a.; toxic a. **a. ex anop′sia,** that resulting from long disuse. **color a.,** dimness of color vision due to toxic or other influences. **nocturnal a.,** abnormal dimness of vision at night. **nutritional a.,** scotomata due to poor nutrition; seen in alcoholics, the malnourished, and those with vitamin B_{12} deficiency or pernicious anemia. **tobacco a.,** nutritional a., toxic a. **toxic a.,** that due to poisoning, as from alcohol or tobacco.

amblyoscope (am'blĕ-o-skōp''), p''. an instrument for training an amblyopic eye to take part in vision and for increasing fusion of the eyes.

ambo (am'bo) ambon.

amboceptor (am'bo-sep''ter) hemolysin, particularly its double receptors, the one combining with the blood cell, the other with complement.

ambon (am'bon) the fibrocartilaginous ring forming the edge of the socket in which the head of a long bone is lodged.

ambulatory (am'bu-lah-tor''e) walking or able to walk; not confined to bed.

amdinocillin (am-de'no-sil''in) a semisynthetic penicillin effective against many gram-negative bacteria and used in the treatment of urinary tract infections.

ameba (ah-me'bah), pl. *ame'bae, ame'bas* [L.] a minute protozoon (class Rhizopoda, subphylum Sarcodina), occurring as a single-celled nucleated mass of protoplasm that changes shape by extending cytoplasmic processes (pseudopodia), by means of which it moves about and absorbs food; most amebae are free-living but some parasitize man. **ame'bic,** adj.

amebiasis (am''ĕ-bi'ah-sis) infection with amebae, especially with *Entamoeba histolytica,* the causative agent of amebic dysentery. **a. cu'tis,** painful ulcers with distinct borders and erythematous rims, seen in those with active intestinal or hepatic disease. **hepatic a.,** amebic hepatitis. **intestinal a.,** amebic dysentery. **pulmonary a.,** infection of the thoracic space secondary to intestinal amebiasis and associated with amebic liver abscesses.

amebicide (ah-me'bĭ-sīd) an agent that is destructive to amebae.

amebocyte (ah-me'bo-sīt) any cell showing ameboid movement.

ameboid (ah-me'boid) resembling an ameba in form or movement.

ameboma (am''ĭ-bo'mah) a tumor-like mass caused by granulomatous reaction in the intestines in amebiasis.

amebula (ah-meb'u-lah) the motile ameboid stage of spores of certain sporozoa.

amelia (ah-me'le-ah) congenital absence of a limb or limbs.

amelification (ah-mel'ĭ-fĭ-ka'shin) the development of enamel cells into enamel.

ameloblast (ah-mel'o-blast) a cell which takes part in forming dental enamel.

ameloblastoma (ah-mel''o-blas-to'mah) a true neoplasm of tissue of the type characteristic of the enamel organ, but which does not differentiate to the point of enamel formation. **melanotic a.,** melanotic neuroectodermal tumor. **pituitary a.,** craniopharyngioma.

amelogenesis (ah-mel''o-jen'ĭ-sis) the formation of dental enamel. **a. imperfec'ta,** a hereditary

condition resulting in defective development of dental enamel, marked by a brown color of the teeth; due to improper differentiation of the ameloblasts.

amelogenin (-jen''in) any of several proteins secreted by ameloblasts and forming the organic matrix of tooth enamel.

amelus (am'ĭ-lus) an individual exhibiting amelia.

amenorrhea (a-men''o-re'ah) absence or abnormal stoppage of the menses. **amenorrhe'al,** adj. **dietary a., nutritional a.,** cessation of menstruation accompanying loss of weight due to dietary restriction, the loss of weight and of appetite being less extreme than in anorexia nervosa and unassociated with psychological problems. **primary a.,** failure of menstruation to occur at puberty. **secondary a.,** cessation of menstruation after it has once been established at puberty.

amensalism (a-men'sil-izm) symbiosis in which one population (or individual) is adversely affected and the other is unaffected.

amentia (a-men'she-ah) 1. (obs.) profound mental retardation. 2. the terminal stage of degenerative dementia.

americium (am''er-ish'e-um) chemical element (*see table*), at. no. 95, symbol Am.

ametria (ah-me'tre-ah) congenital absence of the uterus.

ametropia (am''ĭ-tro'pe-ah) a condition of the eye in which images fail to come to a proper focus on the retina, due to a discrepancy between the size and refractive powers of the eye. **ametrop'ic,** adj.

AMI acute myocardial infarction.

amicrobic (ah''mi-kro'bik) not produced by microbes.

amiculum (ah-mik'u-lum) a dense surrounding coat of white fibers, as the sheath of the inferior olive and of the dentate nucleus.

amidase (am'ĭ-dās) a deamidizing enzyme.

amide (am'ĭd) any compound derived from ammonia by substitution of an acid radical for hydrogen, or from an acid by replacing the —OH group by —NH₂.

amidine-lyase (am'ĭ-dēn-li'ās) an enzyme that catalyzes the removal of an amindino group, as from L-argininosuccinate to form fumarate and L-arginine.

amido-ligase (am''ĭ-do-li'gās) any enzyme that catalyzes the coupling of two molecules, with glutamine acting as an ammonia donor.

amikacin (am''ĭ-ka'sin) a semisynthetic aminoglycoside antibiotic derived from kanamycin, $C_{22}H_{43}N_5O_{13}$, used in the treatment of a wide range of infections due to susceptible organisms.

amimia (a-mim'e-ah) loss of the power of expression by the use of signs or gestures.

aminacrine (am''in-ak'rin) an amino derivative of acridine, $C_{13}H_{10}N_2$, effective against many gram-negative and gram-positive bacteria; used as a topical anti-infective.

amine (am'in, ah-mēn') an organic compound containing nitrogen; any of a group of compounds formed from ammonia by replacement of one or more hydrogen atoms by organic radicals. **biogenic a's,** amine neurotransmitters, e.g., epinephrine, norepinephrine, serotonin, and dopamine.

amino (am′ĭ-no, ah-me′no) the monovalent radical NH_2, when not united with an acid radical.

aminoacetic acid (-ah-se′tik) glycine.

amino acid one of a class of organic compounds containing the amino (NH_2) and the carboxyl (COOH) groups occurring naturally in plant and animal tissue and forming the chief constituents of protein. **essential a., a.,** one of nine α-amino acids that cannot be synthesized by humans but must be obtained from the diet. **nonessential a., a.,** one of eleven α-amino acids that can be synthesized by humans and are not specifically required in the diet.

aminoacidemia (-as″id-e′me-ah, ah-me″no-) an excess of amino acids in the blood.

aminoacidopathy (-as″id-op′ah-the) any of a group of disorders due to a defect in an enzymatic step in the metabolic pathway of one or more amino acids or in a protein mediator necessary for transport of certain amino acids into or out of cells.

aminoaciduria (-as″ĭd-ūr′e-ah) an excess of amino acids in the urine.

aminoacylase (-as′ĭ-lās) an enzyme in the kidney that catalyzes the hydrolysis of hippuric acid to benzoic acid and glycine.

aminobenzoic acid, p-aminobenzoic acid (-ben-zo′ik) para-aminobenzoic acid.

γ-aminobutyrate (-būt′ĭ-rāt) the anion of gamma-aminobutyric acid.

γ-aminobutyric acid, 4-aminobutyric acid (-bu-tir′ik) gamma-aminobutyric acid.

ε-aminocaproic acid (-kah-pro′ik) a nonessential amino acid that is an inhibitor of plasmin and of plasminogen and, indirectly, of fibrinolysis; used as a hemostatic.

aminoglycoside (-gli-ko′sīd) any of a group of antibacterial antibiotics (e.g., streptomycin and gentamicin), derived from various species of *Streptomyces*, which interfere with the function of bacterial ribosomes. Aminoglycosides contain an inositol substituted with two amino or guanidino groups and with one or more sugars and aminosugars.

aminohippurate (-hip′ūr-āt) any salt of aminohippuric acid.

aminohippuric acid (hĭ-pūr′ik) para-aminohippuric acid (PAH), the glycine conjugate of para-aminobenzoic acid; the sodium salt (aminohippurate sodium) is used as a diagnostic aid in the determination of effective renal plasma flow.

δ-aminolevulinate (-lev″u-lin′āt) the anion of δ-aminolevulinic acid.

δ-aminolevulinic acid (-lev″u-lin′ik) a precursor of porphyrins and hemoglobin, H_2NCH_2-$COCH_2CH_2COOH$, produced from succinyl coenzyme A and glycine by the enzyme δ-aminolevulinate synthase.

aminolysis (am″ĭ-nol′ĭ-sis) reaction with an amine, resulting in the addition of (or substitution by) an imino group —NH—.

aminophylline (am″ĭ-no-fil′in) a bronchial smooth muscle relaxant, respiratory stimulant, and diuretic, $C_{16}H_{25}N_{10}O_4$.

aminopterin (am″in-op′ter-in) a folic acid antagonist, $C_{19}H_{20}N_8O_5$, used in the treatment of leukemia, and as a rodenticide.

aminosalicylate (am″ĭ-no-sal″ĭ-sil′āt, ah-me″no-) any salt of aminosalicylic acid.

aminosalicylic acid (-sal-ĭ-sil′ik) para-aminosalicylic acid (PAS); an analogue of p-aminobenzoic acid (PABA), $NH_2 \cdot C_6H_3 \cdot OH \cdot COOH$, with antibacterial properties, whose salts (*calcium, potassium,* and *sodium aminosalicylate*) are used as tuberculostatics.

aminotransferase (-trans′fer-ās) an enzyme that catalyzes the reversible transfer of an amino group from an α-amino acid to an α-keto acid using the coenzyme pyridoxal phosphate.

aminuria (am″ĭn-ūr′e-ah) an excess of amines in the urine.

amitosis (am″ĭ-to′sis) direct cell division, i.e., the cell divides by simple cleavage of the nucleus without formation of spireme spindle figures or chromosomes. **amitot′ic,** adj.

amitriptyline (am″ĭ-trip′tĭ-lēn) an antidepressant, $C_{20}H_{23}N$, used as the hydrochloride salt.

ammeter (am′mēt-er) an instrument for measuring in amperes or subdivisions of amperes the strength of a current flowing in a circuit.

ammoaciduria (am″o-as″id-ūr′e-ah) an excess of ammonia and amino acids in the urine.

ammonia (ah-mo′ne-ah) a colorless alkaline gas with a pungent odor and acrid taste, NH_3.

ammonia-lyase (-li′ās) any of a group of lyases that catalyze the removal of ammonia by cleaving a C—N bond.

ammonium (ah-mo′ne-um) the hypothetical radical, NH_4, forming salts analogous to those of the alkaline metals. **a. carbonate,** a mixture of NH_4HCO_3 (ammonium bicarbonate) and NH_4COONH_4 (ammonium carbamate), used as a stimulant, as in smelling salts, and as an expectorant. **a. chloride,** crystalline compound, NH_4Cl, used as a systemic acidifier.

ammoniuria (ah-mo″ne-ūr′e-ah) excess of ammonia in the urine.

ammonolysis (am″o-nol′ĭ-sis) a process analogous to hydrolysis, but in which ammonia takes the place of water.

amnalgesia (am″nal-je′ze-ah) abolition of pain and memory of a painful procedure by the use of drugs or hypnosis.

amnesia (am-ne′zhe-ah) pathologic impairment of memory. **amnes′tic,** adj. **anterograde a.,** amnesia for events occurring subsequent to the episode precipitating the disorder. **auditory a.,** auditory aphasia. **psychogenic a.,** a dissociative disorder characterized by a sudden loss of memory for important personal information, not due to any organic mental disorder. **retrograde a.,** amnesia for events occurring prior to the episode precipitating the disorder. **transient global a.,** a temporary episode of short-term memory loss without other neurological impairment. **visual a.,** alexia.

amniocele (am′ne-o-sēl″) omphalocele.

amniocentesis (am″ne-o-sen-te′sis) surgical transabdominal or transcervical penetration of the uterus for aspiration of amniotic fluid.

amniogenesis (-jen′ĭ-sis) the development of the amnion.

amnion (am′ne-on) the extraembryonic membrane of birds, reptiles, and mammals, which lines the chorion and contains the fetus and the amniotic fluid. **amnion′ic, amniot′ic,** adj. **a. nodo′sum,** a nodular condition of the fetal surface of the amnion, observed in oligohydramnios associated with absence of the kidneys of the fetus.

amniorrhexis (-rek′sis) rupture of the amnion.

amnioscope (am′ne-ah-skōp″) an endoscope that, by passage through the maternal abdominal wall into the amniotic cavity, permits direct visualization of the fetus and amniotic fluid.

amniotomy (am″ne-ot′ah-me) surgical rupture of the fetal membranes to induce labor.

amobarbital (am″o-bar′bĭ-tal) a hypnotic and sedative, $C_{11}H_{18}N_2O_3$, having a short to intermediate action; also used as the sodium salt.

amodiaquine (-di′ah-kwin) a drug, $C_{20}H_{22}Cl-N_3O$, used as the hydrochloride salt in treatment of malaria, especially falciparum malaria, and of amebic abscess.

Amoeba (ah-me′ba) a genus of amebae.

amorph (a′morf) a mutant gene that produces no detectable phenotypic effect.

amorphia (ah-mor′fe-ah) the fact or quality of being amorphous.

amorphous (ah-mor′fis) having no definite form; shapeless; having no specific orientation of atoms; in pharmacy, not crystallized.

amotio (ah-mo′she-o) [L.] a removing. **a. re′tinae,** detachment of the retina.

amoxapine (ah-mok′sah-pēn) a drug, $C_{17}H_{16}Cl-N_3O$, chemically related to the dibenzoxazepine antipsychotic agents but having uses and activities similar to those of the tricyclic antidepressants.

amoxicillin (ah-moks″ĭ-sil′in) a semisynthetic derivative of ampicillin, $C_{16}H_{19}N_3O_5S$, effective against a broad spectrum of gram-positive and gram-negative bacteria.

Amoxil (ah-moks′il) trademark for a preparation of amoxicillin.

AMP adenosine monophosphate. **cyclic AMP,** cyclic adenosine monophosphate.

amp. ampere.

ampere (am′pēr) unit of electric current strength, the current yielded by one volt of electromotive force against one ohm of resistance.

amphetamine (am-fet′ah-mēn) 1. a synthetic, powerful central nervous system stimulant, $C_6H_5CH_2CHNH_2CH_3$, most commonly used as the sulfate salt. Abuse may lead to dependence. 2. any drug closely related to amphetamine and having similar actions, e.g., methamphetamine.

amphi- word element [Gr.], *both; on both sides.*

amphiarthrosis (am″fi-ar-thro′sis) a joint permitting little motion, the opposed surfaces being connected by fibrocartilage, as between vertebrae.

Amphibia (am-fib′e-ah) a class of vertebrates,

including frogs, toads, newts, and salamanders, capable of living both on land and in water.

amphibolic (am″fi-bol′ik) 1. uncertain. 2. having both an anabolic and a catabolic function.

amphicelous (-se′lis) concave at both ends.

amphicentric (-sen′trik) beginning and ending in the same vessel.

amphidiarthrosis (-di″ar-thro′sis) a joint having the nature of both ginglymus and arthrodia, as that of the lower jaw.

amphigonadism (-gon′ah-dizm) possession of both ovarian and testicular tissue.

amphistome (am-fis′tōm) a fluke having the ventral sucker near the posterior end, usually found in the rumen or intestine of herbivorous mammals.

amphitrichous (am-fi′trĭ-kis) having flagella at each end.

amphocyte (am′fo-sīt) a cell staining with either acid or basic dyes.

ampholyte (-līt) an organic or inorganic substance capable of acting as either an acid or a base.

amphophilic (am″fo-fil′ik) staining with either acid or basic dyes.

amphoric (am-for′ik) pertaining to a bottle; resembling the sound made by blowing across the neck of a bottle.

amphoteric (am″fo-tě′rik) having opposite characters; capable of acting as both an acid and a base; capable of neutralizing either bases or acids.

amphotericin B (-tě′rĭ-sin) an antibiotic derived from strains of *Streptomyces nodosus;* used in cryptococcal meningitis and systemic fungal infections, and applied topically for treatment of candidiasis.

amphotony (am-fot′o-ne) tonicity of the sympathetic and parasympathetic nervous systems.

ampicillin (amp″ĭ-sil′in) a semisynthetic, acid-resistant penicillin, $C_{16}H_{19}N_3O_4S$, used as an antibacterial against gram-negative bacteria and nonpenicillinase-producing strains of *Escherichia coli.*

amplification (am″plĭ-fĭ-ka′shin) the process of making larger, as the increase of an auditory stimulus, as a means of improving its perception.

amplitude (am′plĭ-tōōd) largeness, fullness; wideness in range or extent. **a. of accommodation,** amount of accommodative power of the eye.

ampule (am′pūl) a small, hermetically sealed glass flask, e.g., one containing medication for parenteral administration.

ampulla (am-pul′ah), pl. *ampul′lae* [L.] a flask-like dilatation of a tubular structure, especially of the expanded ends of the semicircular canals of the ear. **ampul′lar,** adj. **a. chy′li,** cisterna chyli. **a. duc′tus defe′rentis,** the enlarged and tortuous distal end of the ductus deferens. **hepatopancreatic a., a. hepatopancreat′ica,** the dilatation formed by junction of the common bile duct and the pancreatic duct proximal to their opening into the lumen of the duodenum. **ampul′lae lacti′ferae,** lactiferous sinuses. **Lieberkühn's a.**, the blind termination of lacteals in the villi of the intestines. **ampul′lae membrana′ceae**, the dilatations at one end of each of the three semicircular ducts. **ampul′lae os′seae**, the dilatations at one of the ends of the semicircular canals. **phrenic a.**, the dilatation at the lower end of the esophagus. **rectal a.**, **a. rec′ti**, the dilated portion of the rectum just proximal to the anal canal. **a. of Thoma**, one of the small terminal expansions of an interlobar artery in the pulp of the spleen. **a. of uterine tube**, the thin-walled, almost muscle-free, midregion of the uterine tube; its mucosa is greatly plicated. **a. of vas deferens**, a. ductus deferentis.

amputation (am″pu-ta′shin) removal of a limb or other appendage of the body. **above-knee (A-K) a.**, that in which the femur is divided in the supracondylar region, at midthigh, or high on the thigh. **below-knee (B-K) a.**, that in which the bone division is done a few centimeters distal to the tibial tuberosity. **Chopart's a.**, amputation of the foot by a midtarsal disarticulation. **closed a.**, one in which flaps are made from the skin and subcutaneous tissue and sutured over the end of the bone. **congenital a.**, absence of a limb at birth, attributed to constriction of the part by an encircling band during intrauterine development. **consecutive a.**, an amputation during or after the period of suppuration. **a. in contiguity**, amputation at a joint. **a. in continuity**, amputation of a limb elsewhere than at a joint. **double-flap a.**, one in which two flaps are formed. **Dupuytren's a.**, amputation of the arm at the shoulder joint. **elliptical a.**, one in which the cut has an elliptical outline. **flap a.**, closed a. **flapless a.**, guillotine a. **Gritti-Stokes a.**, amputation of the leg through the knee, using an oval anterior flap. **guillotine a.**, one performed rapidly by a circular sweep of the knife and a cut of the saw, the entire cross-section being left open for dressing. **Hey's a.**, amputation of the foot between the tarsus and metatarsus. **interpleviabdominal a.**, amputation of the thigh with excision of the lateral portion of the pelvic girdle. **interscapulothoracic a.**, amputation of the arm with excision of the lateral portion of the shoulder girdle. **intrauterine a.**, congenital a. **Larrey's a.**, amputation at the shoulder joint. **Lisfranc's a.**, 1. Dupuytren's a. 2. amputation of the foot between the metatarsus and tarsus. **oblique a.**, oval a. **open a.**, guillotine a. **oval a.**, one in which the incision consists of two reversed spirals. **Pirigoff's a.**, amputation of the foot at the ankle, through the malleoli of the tibia and fibula. **pulp a.**, pulpotomy. **racket a.**, one in which there is a single longitudinal incision continuous below with a spiral incision on either side of the limb. **root a.**, removal of one or more roots from a multirooted tooth, leaving at least one root to support the crown; when only the apex of a root is involved, it is called *apicoectomy*. **spontaneous a.**, loss of a part without surgical intervention, as in diabetes mellitus, etc. **Stokes' a.**, Gritti-Stokes a. **subperiosteal a.**, one in which the cut end of the bone is covered by periosteal flaps. **Syme's a.**, disarticulation of the foot with removal of both malleoli. **Teale's a.**, amputation with short and long rectangular flaps.

A.M.R.L. Aerospace Medical Research Laboratories.

A.M.S. American Meteorological Society.

amu atomic mass unit.

A.M.W.A. American Medical Women's Association; American Medical Writers' Association.

amyelinic (ah-mi″il-in′ik) without myelin.

amyelonic (-on′ik) 1. having no spinal cord. 2. having no marrow.

amyelotrophy (-ah′trah-fe) atrophy of spinal cord.

amygdala (ah-mig′dah-lah) an almond-shaped structure; often used to refer to the corpus amygdaloideum.

amygdalin (-lin) a glycoside, $C_{20}H_{27}NO_{11}$, found in almonds and other members of the same family.

amygdaline (-lin) 1. like an almond. 2. pertaining to a tonsil; tonsillar.

amyl (am′il) the radical C_5H_{11}. **a. nitrite**, a volatile, inflammable liquid, $C_5H_{11}NO_2$, with a pungent ethereal odor. It is administered by inhalation for the treatment of angina pectoris (acting as a coronary vasodilator) or cyanide poisoning (producing methemoglobin, which binds cyanide).

amyl(o)- word element [Gr.], *starch.*

amylaceous (am″ï-la′shis) composed of or resembling starch.

amylase (am′ï-las) an enzyme that catalyzes the hydrolysis of starch into simpler compounds. The *α-amylases* occur in animals and include pancreatic and salivary amylase; the *β-amylases* occur in higher plants.

amyloid (am′ï-loid) 1. starchlike; amylaceous. 2. an optically homogeneous, waxy, translucent material, probably a glycoprotein, bearing a superficial resemblance to starch and deposited intercellularly in a variety of pathologic conditions; see *amyloidosis.*

amyloidosis (am″ï-loi-do′sis) extracellular deposition of amyloid in tissues; when sufficiently advanced, the accumulations obliterate the parenchyma of affected organs. The disease may be primary (of unknown cause), secondary to chronic diseases (e.g., tuberculosis and rheumatoid arthritis), hereditary, as in familial Mediterranean fever, associated with multiple myeloma, associated with aging, or local amyloidosis (tumor-like deposits).

amylopectin (am″ï-lo-pek′tin) the insoluble constituent of starch; the soluble constituent is amylose.

amylopectinosis (-pek′tï-no″sis) glycogenosis (type IV) in which deficiency of the brancher enzyme amylo-1:4,1:6-transglucosidase results in cirrhosis of the liver, hepatosplenomegaly, and progressive hepatic failure and death.

amylorrhea (am″ï-lo-re′ah) presence of excessive starch in the stools.

amylorrhexis (-reks′is) the enzymatic splitting of starch.

amylose (am′ï-los) 1. any carbohydrate other

than a glucose or saccharose. 2. the soluble constituent of starch, as opposed to amylopectin.

amyluria (am″ĭ-lūr′e-ah) an excess of starch in the urine.

amyoplasia (ah-mi″o-pla′ze-ah) lack of muscle formation or development. **a. conge′nita,** generalized lack in the newborn of muscular development and growth, with contracture and deformity at most joints.

amyostasia (-sta′ze-ah) a tremor of the muscles.

amyosthenia (ah-mi″os-the′ne-ah) deficient muscular strength.

amyotaxy (ah-mi′o-tak″se) ataxia.

amyotonia (a-mi″o-to′ne-ah) atonic condition of the muscles. **a. conge′nita,** any of several rare congenital diseases marked by general hypotonia of the muscles.

amyotrophy (ah″mi-ah′trah-fe) muscular atrophy. **amyotroph′ic,** adj. **diabetic a.,** a painful condition, associated with diabetes, with progressive wasting and weakening of muscles, usually limited to the muscles of the pelvic girdle and thigh. **neuralgic a.,** atrophy and paralysis of the muscles of the shoulder girdle, with pain across the shoulder and upper arm.

amyxia (ah-mik′se-ah) absence of mucus.

amyxorrhea (a-mik″sah-re′ah) absence of mucous secretion.

An. anode.

ANA antinuclear antibody.

A.N.A. American Nurses' Association.

ana (an′ah) [Gr.] of each.

ana- word element [Gr.], *upward; again; backward; excessively.*

anabasis (ah-nab′ah-sis) the stage of increase in a disease. **anabat′ic,** adj.

anabiosis (an″ah-bi-o′sis) restoration of the vital processes after their apparent cessation; bringing back to consciousness. **anabiot′ic,** adj.

anabolism (-lizm) the constructive process by which living cells convert simple substances into more complex compounds, especially into living matter. **anabol′ic,** adj.

anabolite (-līt″) any product of anabolism.

anachoresis (an″ah-kah-re′sis) preferential collection or deposit of particles at a site, as of bacteria or metals that have localized out of the blood stream in areas of inflammation. **anachoret′ic,** adj.

anacidity (-sid′it-e) lack of normal acidity. **gastric a.,** achlorhydria.

anaclisis (-kli′sis) the state of leaning against or depending on something; in psychoanalysis, the development of the infant's love for his mother from his original dependence on her care. **anaclit′ic,** adj.

anacrotism (ah-nak′rah-tizm) a pulse anomaly evidenced by the presence of a prominent notch on the ascending limb of the pulse tracing. **anacrot′ic,** adj.

anadipsia (an″ah-dip′se-ah) intense thirst.

anadrenalism (-dre′nil-izm) absence or failure of adrenal function.

anaerobe (an-a′er-ōb) an organism that lives and grows in the absence of molecular oxygen. **anaero′bic,** adj. **facultative a.,** a microorganism that can live and grow with or without molecular oxygen. **obligate a.,** a microorganism that can grow only in the complete absence of molecular oxygen; some are killed by oxygen.

anaerobiosis (an-a″er-o-bi-o′sis) life cnly in the absence of molecular oxygen. **anaerobiot′ic,** adj.

anaerogenic (-jen′ik) 1. producing little or no gas. 2. suppressing the formation of gas by gas-producing bacteria.

anaerosis (an″a-er-o′sis) interruption of respiratory function.

anagen (an′ah-jen) the first phase of the hair cycle, during which synthesis of hair takes place.

anakusis (-ku′sis) total deafness.

anal (a′n′l) relating to the anus.

analbuminemia (an″al-bu″min-e′me-ah) absence or deficiency of serum albumins.

analeptic (an″ah-lep′tik) a drug that acts as a restorative, such as caffeine, etc.

analgesia (an″al-je′ze-ah) absence of sensibility to pain, particularly the relief of pain without loss of consciousness; absence of pain or noxious stimulation. **a. al′gera,** spontaneous pain in a denervated part; pain in an area or region which is anesthetic. **audio a.,** audioanalgesia. **continuous caudal a.,** continuous injection of an anesthetic solution into the sacral and lumbar plexuses within the epidural space to relieve the pain of childbirth; also used in general surgery to block the pain pathways below the navel. **a. doloro′sa,** a. algera. **epidural a.,** analgesia induced by introduction of the analgesic agent into the epidural space of the vertebral canal. **infiltration a.,** paralysis of the nerve endings at the site of operation by subcutaneous injection of an anesthetic. **paretic a.,** loss of the sense of pain accompanied by partial paralysis. **relative a.,** in dental anesthesia, a maintained level of conscious-sedation, short of general anesthesia, in which the pain threshold is elevated; usually induced by inhalation of nitrous oxide and oxygen. **surface a.,** local analgesia produced by an anesthetic applied to the surface of such mucous membranes as those of the eye, nose, urethra, etc.

analgesic (-je′sik) 1. relieving pain. 2. pertaining to analgesia. 3. an agent that relieves pain without causing loss of consciousness.

analgia (an-al′je-ah) painlessness. **anal′gic,** adj.

analogous (ah-nal′ah-gus) resembling or similar in some respects, as in function or appearance, but not in origin or development.

analogue (an′ah-log) 1. a part or organ having the same function, but of different evolutionary origin. 2. a chemical compound having a structure similar to that of another but differing from it in respect to a certain component; it may have similar or opposite action metabolically.

analogy (ah-nal′o-je) the quality of being analogous; resemblance or similarity in function or appearance, but not in origin or development.

analysand (ah-nal′ĭ-sand) a person undergoing psychoanalysis.

analysis (ah-nal′ĭ-sis) 1. separation into component parts; the act of determining the component parts of a substance. 2. psychoanalysis. **analyt′ic,** adj. **bite a.,** occlusal a. **blood gas a.,** the determination of oxygen and carbon dioxide concentrations and the pH of the blood by laboratory tests; the following measurements may be made: PO_2, partial pressure of oxygen in arterial blood; PCO_2, partial pressure of carbon dioxide in arterial blood; SO_2, percent saturation of hemoglobin with oxygen in arterial blood; the total CO_2 content of (venous) plasma; and the pH. **gasometric a.,** analysis by measurement of the gas evolved. **gravimetric a.,** quantitative analysis in which the analyte or a derivative is determined by weighing after purification. **occlusal a.,** study of the relations of the occlusal surfaces of opposing teeth. **qualitative a.,** chemical analysis in which the presence or absence of certain compounds in a specimen is determined. **quantitative a.,** chemical analysis in which the concentration of a specific compound in a specimen is determined. **spectroscopic a., spectrum a.,** that done by determining the wave length(s) at which electromagnetic energy is absorbed by the sample. **transactional a.,** a type of psychotherapy involving an understanding of the interpersonal interchanges between the components of the personalities of the participants (individuals or members of a group). **vector a.,** analysis of a moving force to determine both its magnitude and its direction, e.g., analysis of the scalar electrocardiogram to determine the magnitude and direction of the electromotive force for one complete cycle of the heart.

analyzer (an″ah-līz′er) 1. a Nicol prism attached to a polarizing apparatus which extinguishes the ray of light polarized by the polarizer. 2. Pavlov's name for a specialized part of the nervous system which controls the reactions of the organism to changing external conditions. 3. a nervous receptor together with its central connections, by means of which sensitivity to stimulations is differentiated.

anamnesis (an″am-ne′sis) 1. the faculty of memory. 2. the past history of a patient and his family.

anaphase (an′ah-fāz) the third stage of division of the nucleus in either meiosis or mitosis.

anaphia (an-a′fe-ah) lack or loss of the sense of touch.

anaphoria (an″ah-for′e-ah) the tendency to tilt the head downward, with the visual axes deviating upward, on looking straight ahead.

anaphrodisiac (-diz′e-ak) 1. repressing sexual desire. 2. a drug that represses sexual desire.

anaphylactin (an″ah-fĭ-lak′tin) the antibody in anaphylaxis, now identified as IgE.

anaphylactogenesis (-fĭ-lak″tah-jen′ĭ-sis) the production of anaphylaxis. **anaphylactogen′ic,** adj.

anaphylatoxin (-fil″ah-tok′sin) a substance produced in blood serum during complement fixation which serves as a mediator of inflammation by inducing mast cell degranulation and histamine release; on injection into animals, it causes anaphylactic shock.

anaphylaxis (-fĭ-lak′sis) 1. exaggerated reaction of an organism to a foreign protein or other sustance to which it has previously become sensitized; resulting from the release of histamine, serotonin, and other vasoactive substances. Cf. *allergy.* 2. anaphylactic shock. **anaphylac′tic,** adj. **active a.,** that produced by injection of a foreign protein. **antiserum a.,** passive a. **local a.,** that confined to a limited area, e.g., cutaneous anaphylaxis. **passive a.,** that resulting in a normal person from injection of serum of a sensitized person. **passive cutaneous a.,** localized anaphylaxis passively transferred by intradermal injection of an antibody and, after a latent period (about 24 to 72 hours), intravenous injection of the homologous antigen and Evans blue dye; blueing of the skin at the site of the intradermal injection is evidence of the permeability reaction. Used in studies of antibodies causing immediate hypersensitivity reaction. **reverse a.,** that following injection of antigen, succeeded by injection of antiserum.

anaplasia (-pla′ze-ah) loss of differentiation of cells (dedifferentiation) and of their orientation to one another and to their axial framework and blood vessels, a characteristic of tumor tissue. **anaplas′tic,** adj.

Anaplasma (-plaz′mah) a genus of microorganisms (family Anaplasmataceae), including *A. margina′le,* the etiologic agent of anaplasmosis.

Anaplasmataceae (-plaz″mah-ta′se-e) a family of microorganisms (order Rickettsiales).

anaplasmodastat (-plaz-mōd′ah-stat″) any of a group of chemical agents used to control anaplasmosis in animals.

anaplasmosis (-plaz-mo′sis) a disease of cattle and related ruminants, marked by high temperature, anemia, and icterus, and caused by infection with *Anaplasma marginale.* Called also *gallsickness.*

anapophysis (-pof′ĭ-sis) an accessory vertebral process.

anaptic (an-ap′tik) marked by anaphia.

anarthria (an-ar′thre-ah) severe dysarthria resulting in speechlessness.

anastalsis (-stal′sis) reversed peristalsis.

anastaltic (-stal′tik) styptic; astringent.

anastole (ah-nas′tah-le) retraction, as of the edges of a wound.

anastomosis (ah-nas″tah-mo′sis) 1. communication between vessels by collateral channels. 2. surgical, traumatic, or pathological formation of an opening between two normally distinct spaces or organs. **anastomot′ic,** adj. **arteriovenous a.,** one between an artery and a vein. **crucial a.,** an arterial anastomosis in the upper part of the thigh. **heterocladic a.,** one between branches of different arteries. **ileorectal a.,** surgical anastomosis of the ileum and rectum after total colectomy, as is sometimes performed in the treatment of ulcerative colitis. **intestinal a.,** establishment of a communication between two formerly distant portions of the intestine. **a. of Riolan,** anastomosis of the superior and inferior mesenteric arteries. **Roux-en-Y a.,** any Y-shaped anastomosis in which the small intestine is included.

anat. anatomy.

anatomy (ah-me) the science of the structure of living organisms. **applied a.**, anatomy as applied to diagnosis and treatment. **comparative a.**, comparison of the structure of different animals and plants, one with another. **developmental a.**, structural embryology. **gross a.**, that dealing with structures visible with the unaided eye. **histologic a.**, histology. **homologic a.**, the study of the related parts of the body in different animals. **macroscopic a.**, gross a. **microscopic a.**, histology. **morbid a.**, **pathologic a.**, that of diseased tissues. **physiological a.**, the study of the organs with respect to their normal functions. **radiological a.**, the study of the anatomy of tissues based on their visualization on x-ray films. **special a.**, the study of particular organs or parts. **topographic a.**, the study of parts in their relation to surrounding parts. **veterinary a.**, the anatomy of domestic animals. **x-ray a.**, radiological a.

anatropia (an″ah-tro′pe-ah) upward deviation of the visual axis of one eye when the other eye is fixing. **anatrop′ic**, adj.

anchorage (ang′ker-ij) fixation, e.g., surgical fixation of a displaced viscus or, in operative dentistry, fixation of fillings or of artificial crowns or bridges. In orthodontics, the support used for a regulating apparatus.

anchylo- for words beginning thus, see those beginning *ankylo-*.

ancipital (an-sip′it′l) two-edged or two-headed.

anconad (ang′kon-ad) toward the elbow or olecranon.

anconagra (ang″kon-ag′rah) gout of the elbow.

anconeal (ang-ko′ne-il) pertaining to the elbow.

anconitis (an″kon-īt′is) inflammation of the elbow joint.

ancrod (an′krod) a proteinase obtained from the venom of the Malayan pit viper *Agkistrodon rhodostoma*, acting specifically on fibrinogen; used as an anticoagulant in the treatment of retinal vein occlusion and deep vein thrombosis and to prevent postoperative rethrombosis.

ancylo- for words beginning thus, see also those beginning *ankylo-*.

Ancylostoma (an″sĭ-los′tah-mah, an″kĭ-) a genus of hookworms (family Ancylostomidae). **A. america′num,** *Necator americanus.* **A. brazilien′se,** a species parasitizing dogs and cats in tropical areas; its larvae may cause creeping eruption in man. **A. cani′num,** the common hookworm of dogs and cats; its larvae may cause creeping eruption in man. **A. ceylo′nicum,** A. *brazilien'se.* **A. duodena′le,** the common European or Old World hookworm, parasitic in the small intestine, producing the condition known as *hookworm disease.*

ancylostomiasis (an″sĭ-los″tah-mi′ah-sis, an″ki-) infection with hookworms; see *hookworm disease.* **a. brazilien′sis,** larva migrans.

Ancylostomidae (an″sĭ-los-to′mĭ-de, an″kĭ-los-) a family of nematode parasites having two ventrolateral cutting plates at the entrance to a large buccal capsule and small teeth at its base; the hookworms.

ancyroid (an′sĭ-roid) anchor-shaped.

andr(o)- word element [Gr.], *male; masculine.*

androblastoma (an″dro-blas-to′mah) 1. a rare benign tumor of the testis histologically resembling the fetal testis; there are three varieties: diffuse stromal, mixed (stromal and epithelial), and tubular (epithelial). The epithelial elements contain Sertoli cells, which may produce estrogen and thus cause feminization. 2. arrhenoblastoma.

androgen (an′dro-jen) any substance, e.g., androsterone and testosterone, that stimulates male characteristics. **androgen′ic**, adj.

androstane (an′dro-stān) the hydrocarbon nucleus, $C_{19}H_{32}$, from which androgens are derived.

androstanediol (an″dro-stān′de-ol) an androgen, $C_{19}H_{32}O_2$.

androstanedione (-stān′de-ōn) an androgen, $C_{19}H_{28}O_2$, formed in the testes.

androstene (an′dro-stēn) cyclic hydrocarbon, $C_{19}H_{30}$, forming the nucleus of testosterone and certain other androgens.

androstenediol (an″dro-stēn′de-ol) a crystalline androgenic steroid, $C_{19}H_{30}O_2$.

androstenedione (-stēn′di-ōn) an androgen, $C_{19}H_{26}O_2$, less potent than testosterone, secreted by the testis, ovary, and adrenal cortex.

androsterone (an-dros′ter-ōn) an androgenic hormone, $C_{19}H_{30}O_2$, occurring in urine or prepared synthetically.

-ane word termination denoting a saturated open-chain hydrocarbon (C_nH_{2n+2}).

anecdotal (an″ek-dōt′l) based on case histories rather than on controlled clinical trials.

anechoic (an-ĕ-ko′ik) without echoes; said of a chamber for measuring the effects of sound.

anectasis (an-ek′tah-sis) congenital atelectasis due to developmental immaturity.

anemia (ah-ne′me-ah) reduction below normal of the number of erythrocytes, quantity of hemoglobin, or the volume of packed red cells in the blood; a symptom of various diseases and disorders. **ane′mic**, adj. **achrestic a.**, megaloblastic anemia morphologically resembling pernicious anemia, but with multiple other causes. **aplastic a.**, that resistant to therapy and characterized by absence of regeneration of red blood cells. **autoimmune hemolytic a.**, a general term covering a large group of anemias involving antoantibodies against red cell antigens; they may be idiopathic or may have any of a number of causes, including autoimmune disease, hematologic neoplasms, viral infections, or immunodeficiency disorders. **Cooley's a.,** see *β-thalassemia,* under *thalassemia.* **drug-induced hemolytic a.,** immune hemolytic anemia produced by drugs, classified as *penicillin type,* in which the drug induces the formation of specific antibodies, the *methyldopa* type, in which the drug induces the formation of anti-Rh antibodies, and the *stibophen type,* in which circulating drug-antibody complexes bind to red cells. **equine infectious a.,** a viral disease of equines, with recurring malaise and abrupt temperature rises, weight loss, edema, and anemia; transmission to man has been suggested, in whom it causes anemia, neutropenia, and relative lymphocytosis. **hemolytic a.,** see *autoimmune hemolytic a.* and *drug-induced hemolytic a.* **hypoplastic a.,** that due to varying degrees of erythrocytic hypoplasia without leukopenia or thrombocytopenia. **hypoplastic a., congenital,** 1. idiopathic progressive anemia occurring in the first year of life, without leukopenia and thrombocytopenia; it is unresponsive to hematinics and requires multiple blood transfusions to sustain life. 2. Fanconi's syndrome (1). **iron deficiency a.,** a form characterized by low or absent iron stores, low serum iron concentration, low transferrin saturation, elevated transferrin, low hemoglobin concentration or hematocrit, and hypochromic, microcytic red blood cells. **macrocytic a.,** a group of anemias, of varying etiologies, marked by larger than normal red cells, absence of the customary central area of pallor, and an increased mean corpuscular volume and mean corpuscular hemoglobin. **Mediterranean a.,** see *β-thalassemia,* under *thalassemia.* **megaloblastic a.,** that marked by the presence of megaloblasts in the bone marrow. **microcytic a.,** that marked by decrease in size of the red cells. **miner's a.,** hookworm disease. **myelopathic a., myelophthisic a.,** leukoerythroblastosis. **normocytic a.,** that marked by a proportionate decrease in the hemoglobin content, the packed red cell volume, and the number of erythrocytes per cubic millimeter of blood. **pernicious a.,** megaloblastic anemia, most commonly affecting adults, due to failure of the gastric mucosa to secrete adequate and potent intrinsic factor, resulting in malabsorption of vitamin B_{12}. **a. pseudoleuke'mica infan'tum,** a syndrome caused by many factors, e.g., malnutrition, chronic infection, malabsorption, etc., with anisocytosis, poikilocytosis, peripheral red cell immaturity, leukocytosis, lymphadenopathy, and hepatosplenomegaly; once considered to be a specific entity in children under age 3. **sickle cell a.,** a genetically determined defect of hemoglobin synthesis, occurring almost exclusively in blacks, characterized by the presence of sickle-shaped erythrocytes in the blood, arthralgia, acute adominal pain, ulcerations of the legs, and homozygosity for S hemoglobin. **sideroblastic a.,** a heterogeneous group of anemias with diverse clinical manifestations and with multiple causes each involving a derangement in the final pathway of heme synthesis, in which iron stores of the reticuloendothelial tissues are almost always increased and bone marrow normoblasts contain iron (sideroblasts). **sideropenic a.,** a group of anemias marked by low levels of iron in the plasma; it includes iron deficiency anemia and the anemia of chronic disorders. **spur-cell a.,** anemia in which the red cells have a bizarre spiculated shape and are destroyed prematurely, primarily in the spleen; it is an acquired form occurring in severe liver disease, and represents an abnormality in the cholesterol content of the red cell membrane.

anencephaly (an″en-sef′ah-le) congenital absence of the cranial vault, with the cerebral hemispheres completely missing or reduced to small masses. **anancephal′ic,** adj.

anergy (an′er-je) diminished reactivity to specific antigen(s). **aner′gic,** adj.

anerythroplasia (an″ĕ-rith″ro-pla′ze-ah) absence of erythrocyte formation. **anerythroplas′tic,** adj.

anerythropoiesis (-poi-e′sis) deficient production of erythrocytes.

anesthesia (an″es-the′ze-ah) loss of feeling or sensation, especially the loss of pain sensation induced to permit the performance of surgery or other painful procedures. **basal a.,** narcosis produced by preliminary medication so that the inhalation of anesthetic necessary to produce surgical anesthesia is greatly reduced. **block a.,** see *regional a.,* and see *block.* **bulbar a.,** that due to a lesion of the pons. **caudal a.,** anesthesia produced by injection of a local anesthetic into the caudal or sacral canal. **central a.,** that due to disease of the nerve centers. **closed a.,** that produced by continuous rebreathing of a small amount of anesthetic gas in a closed system with an apparatus for removing carbon dioxide. **crossed a.,** see under *hemianesthesia.* **doll's head a.,** anesthesia of the head, neck, and upper part of the chest. **a. doloro′sa,** pain in an area or region that is anesthetic. **electric a.,** that induced by passage of an electric current. **endotracheal a.,** that produced by introduction of a gaseous mixture through a tube inserted into the trachea. **epidural a.,** that produced by injection of the anesthetic between the vertebral spines and beneath the ligamentum flavum into the extradural space. **frost a.,** abolition of feeling or sensation as a result of topical refrigeration produced by a jet of a highly volatile liquid. **general a.,** a state of unconsciousness and insusceptibility to pain, produced by administration of anesthetic agents by inhalation, intravenously, intramuscularly, rectally, or via the gastrointestinal tract. **infiltration a.,** local anesthesia produced by injection of the anesthetic solution in the area of terminal nerve endings. **inhalation a.,** that produced by the inhalation of vapors of a volatile liquid or gaseous anesthetic agent. **insufflation a.,** that produced by blowing a mixture of gases or vapors into the respiratory tract through a tube. **intraoral a.,** that within the oral cavity produced by injection, spray, pressure, etc. **local a.,** that produced in a limited area, as by injection of a local anesthetic or by freezing with ethyl chloride. **lumbar epidural a.,** that produced by injection of the anesthetic into the epidural space at the second or third lumbar interspace. **open a.,** general inhalation anesthesia utilizing a cone; there is no significant rebreathing of expired gases. **partial a.,** that with retention of some degree of sensibility. **peripheral a.,** that due to changes in the peripheral nerves. **refrigeration a.,** local anesthesia produced by applying a tourniquet and chilling the part to near freezing temperature. **regional a.,** insensibility of a part induced by interrupting the sensory nerve conductivity of that region of the body; it may be produced by (1) *field block,* encircling the operative field by means of injections of a local anesthetic; or (2) *nerve block,* making injections in close proximity to the nerves supplying the area. **saddle-block a.,** that produced in a region corresponding roughly with the areas of the buttocks, perineum, and inner aspects of the thighs which impinge on the saddle in riding, by introducing the anesthetic low in the dural sac. **spinal a.,** 1. that produced by injection of a local anesthetic into the subarachnoid space around the spinal cord. 2. loss of sensation due to a spinal lesion. **splanchnic a.,** regional anesthesia for visceral operation by injection of anesthetic agent into the region of the semilunar ganglia. **surgical a.,** that degree of anesthesia at which operation may safely be performed. **tactile a.,** loss or impairment of the sense of touch. **topical a.,** that produced by application of a local anesthetic directly to the area involved, as to the oral mucosa or the cornea. **transsacral a.,** spinal anesthesia produced by injection of the anesthetic into the sacral canal and about the sacral nerves through each of the posterior sacral foramina. **twilight a.,** twilight sleep.

anesthesimeter (an″es-thĕ-sim′it-er) 1. an instrument for testing degree of anesthesia. 2. a device for regulating the amount of anesthetic given.

anesthesiology (-ol′ah-je) that branch of medicine which studies anesthesia and anesthetics.

anesthetic (an″es-thet′ik) 1. pertaining to, characterized by, or producing anesthesia. 2. an agent that produces anesthesia. **local a.,** an agent, e.g., lidocaine, procaine, or tetracaine, that produces anesthesia by paralyzing sensory nerve endings or nerve fibers at the site of application. The conduction of nerve impulses is blocked by stopping the entry of sodium into nerve cells. **topical a.,** a local anesthesia applied directly to the area to be anesthetized, usually the mucous membranes or the skin.

anesthetist (ah-nes′thĕ-tist) a person not an anesthesiologist trained in administering anesthetics.

anetoderma (ah-ne″to-der′mah) looseness and atrophy of the skin. **perifollicular a.,** anetoderma occurring around hair follicles not preceded by folliculitis; it may be caused by elastase-producing staphylococci, by drugs, or by endocrine factors. **postinflammatory a.,** a condition occurring usually during infancy, marked by the development of erythematous papules that enlarge to form plaques, followed by laxity of the skin resembling cutis laxa.

aneuploidy (an″u-ploid′e) any deviation from an exact multiple of the haploid number of chromosomes, whether fewer or more.

aneurysm (an′ūr-izm) a sac formed by localized dilatation of an artery or vein. **aneurys′mal,** adj. **aortic a.,** aneurysm of the aorta. **arteriovenous a.,** abnormal communication between an artery and a vein in which the blood flows directly into a neighboring vein or is carried into the vein by a connecting sac. **atherosclerotic a.,** one arising as a result of weakening of the tunica media in severe atherosclerosis. **berry a.,** a small saccular aneurysm of a cerebral artery, usually at the junction of vessels in the circle of Willis, having a narrow opening into the artery. **compound a.,** one in which some of the layers of the wall of the vessel are ruptured and some merely dilated. **dissecting a.,** one in which rupture of the inner coat has permitted blood to escape between layers of the vessel wall. **false a.,** one in which the entire wall is injured and the blood is retained in the surrounding tissues; a sac communicating with the artery (or heart) is eventually formed. **infected a.,** one produced by growth of microorganisms (bacteria or fungi) in the vessel wall, or infection arising within a preexisting arteriosclerotic aneurysm. **mixed a.,** compound a. **mycotic a.,** an infected aneurysm caused by fungi. **racemose a.,** dilatation and tortuous lengthening of the blood vessels. **saccular a., sacculated a.,** a distended sac affecting only part of the arterial circumference. **varicose a.,** one in which an intervening sac connects the artery with contiguous veins.

aneurysmoplasty (an″ūr-iz′mo-plas″te) plastic repair of the affected artery in the treatment of aneurysm.

aneurysmorrhaphy (an″ūr-iz-mor′ah-fe) suture of an aneurysm.

angi(o)- word element [Gr.], *vessel (channel).*

angiasthenia (an″je-as-the′ne-ah) loss of tone in the vascular system.

angiectasis (-ek′tah-sis) gross dilatation and, often, lengthening of a blood vessel. **angiectat′ic,** adj.

angiectomy (-ek′tah-me) excision or resection of a vessel.

angiectopia (-ek-to′pe-ah) abnormal position or course of a vessel.

angiitis (-īt′is) inflammation of the coats of a vessel, chiefly blood or lymph vessels; vasculitis.

angina (an-ji′nah, an′jĭ-nah) spasmodic, choking, or suffocating pain; used almost exclusively to denote angina pectoris. **an′ginal,** adj. **agranulocytic a.,** agranulocytosis. **intestinal a.,** generalized cramping abdominal pain occurring shortly after a meal and persisting for one to three hours, due to ischemia of the smooth muscle of the bowel. **a. inver′sa,** a variant form of angina pectoris in which there is elevation, rather than depression, of the RS-T interval of the electrocardiogram. **a. ludovi′ci,** a. ludwig′ii, Ludwig's a.,** diffuse purulent inflammation of the floor of the mouth, usually due to streptococcal infection. **a. pec′toris,** paroxysmal pain in the chest, usually due to interference with the supply of oxygen to the heart muscle, and precipitated by excitement or effort. **Plaut's a.,** necrotizing ulcerative gingivostomatitis. **Prinzmetal's a.,** a variant of angina pectoris in which the attacks occur during rest, exercise capacity is well preserved, and attacks are associated electrocardiographically with elevation of the ST-segment. **streptococcus a.,** that due to streptococci. **a. tonsilla′ris,** peritonsillar abscess. **a. trachea′lis,** croup. **variant a. pectoris,** Prinzmetal's a.

anginose (an′jĭ-nōs) characterized by angina.

angioblast (an′je-o-blast″) 1. the earliest formative tissue from which blood cells and blood vessels arise. 2. an individual vessel-forming cell. **angioblast′ic,** adj.

angioblastoma (an″je-o-blas-to′mah) a term applied to certain blood-vessel tumors of the brain: those arising in the cerebellum (*cerebellar a.*) may be cystic and associated with von Hippel-Lindau disease; also, a blood-vessel tumor arising from the meninges of the brain or spinal cord (angioblastic meningioma).

angiocardiography (-kar″de-og′rah-fe) radiography of the heart and great vessels after introduction of an opaque contrast medium into a blood vessel or a cardiac chamber.

angiocardiokinetic (-kar″de-o-ki-net′ik) affecting the movements of the heart and blood vessels; also, an agent that affects such movements.

angiocarditis (-kar-dīt′is) inflammation of the heart and blood vessels.

angiochondroma (-kon-dro′mah) chondroma with excessive development of blood vessels.

angiodysplasia (-dis-pla′ze-ah) small vascular abnormalities, especially of the intestinal tract.

angioedema (-e-de′mah) a vascular reaction involving the deep dermis or subcutaneous or submucosal tissues, representing localized edema caused by dilatation and increased permeability of the capillaries, and characterized by the development of giant wheals. *Hereditary angioedema,* transmitted as an autosomal dominant trait, tends to involve more visceral lesions than the sporadic form.

angioendothelioma (-en″do-the″le-o′mah) hemangioendothelioma.

angiofibroma (-fi-bro′mah) an angioma containing fibrous tissue. **nasopharyngeal a.,** a relatively benign tumor of the nasopharynx composed of fibrous connective tissue with abundant endothelium-lined vascular spaces, usually occurring during puberty, most commonly in boys. It is marked by nasal obstruction which may become total, adenoid speech, discomfort in swallowing, and auditory tube obstruction.

angiofollicular (-fol-lik′u-ler) pertaining to a lymphoid follicle and its blood vessels.

angiogenesis (-jen′ĭ-sis) development of blood vessels in the embryo.

angiogenic (-jen′ik) 1. pertaining to angiogenesis. 2. of vascular origin.

angiography (an″je-og′rah-fe) roentgenography of the blood vessels after introduction of a contrast medium. **intravenous digital subtraction a.,** a fluoroscopic imaging technique in which electronic circuitry is used to subtract the background of bone and soft tissue and provide a useful image of vessels following the injection of contrast medium.

angiohemophilia (an″je-o-he″mah-fil′e-ah) von Willebrand's disease.

angiohyalinosis (-hi″ah-lin-o′sis) hyaline degeneration of the walls of blood vessels.

angioid (an′je-oid) resembling blood vessels.

angiokeratoma (an″je-o-kĕ″rah-to′mah) a skin disease in which telangiectasis or warty growths occur in groups, together with epidermal thickening. **a. circumscrip′tum,** a rare form with discrete papules and nodules usually localized to a small area on the leg or trunk.

angiokinetic (-ki-net′ik) vasomotor.

angioleiomyoma (-li″o-mi-o′mah) a leiomyoma arising from vascular smooth muscle, usually occurring as a solitary nodular, sometimes painful, tumor on the lower extremity in middle-aged women.

angiolipoleiomyoma (-lip″o-li″o-mi-o′mah) see *angiomyolipoma.*

angiolipoma (-lĭ-po′mah) a tumor composed of adipose tissue and blood vessels.

angiolith (an′je-o-lith″) a calcareous deposit in the wall of a blood vessel. **angiolith′ic,** adj.

angiology (an″je-ol′ah-je) the scientific study of the vessels of the body; also, the sum of knowledge relating to the blood and lymph vessels.

angiolupoid (an″je-o-loo′poid) a granuloma occurring chiefly on the side of the nose, consisting of small, oval red plaques with telangiectases over the surface.

angiolysis (an″je-ol′ĭ-sis) retrogression or obliteration of blood vessels, as in embryologic development.

angioma (an″je-o′mah) a tumor whose cells tend to form blood vessels (hemangioma) or lymph vessels (lymphangioma); a tumor made up of blood vessels or lymph vessels. **angiom′atous,** adj. **a. caverno′sum, cavernous a.,** see under *hemangioma.* **cherry a's,** bright red, circumscribed, round or oval angiomas, 2 to 6 mm. in diameter, containing many vascular loops, due to a telangiectatic vascular disturbance, usually seen on the trunk but may appear on other areas of the body, as in angioma serpiginosum, and occurring in most of the middle-aged and elderly. **senile a's,** cherry a's. **a. serpigino′sum,** a skin disease marked by minute vascular points arranged in rings on the skin.

angiomatosis (an″je-o-mah-to′sis) a diseased state of the vessels with formation of multiple angiomas. **cerebroretinal a.,** von Hippel-Lindau disease. **encephalofacial a., encephalotrigeminal a.,** Sturge-Weber syndrome. **hemorrhagic familial a.,** hereditary hemorrhagic telangiectasia. **a. of retina,** von Hippel's disease. **retinocerebral a.,** von Hippel-Lindau disease.

angiomyolipoma (-mi″o-lĭ-po′mah) a benign tumor containing vascular, adipose, and muscle elements, occurring most often in the kidney with smooth muscle elements (angiolipoleiomyoma) in association with tuberous sclerosis, and considered to be a hamartoma.

angiomyoma (-mi-o′mah) angioleiomyoma.

angiomyosarcoma (-mi″o-sar-ko′mah) a tumor composed of elements of angioma, myoma, and sarcoma.

angioneuroma (-noo-ro′mah) glomangioma.

angioneuromyoma (-noo″ro-mi-o′mah) glomangioma.

angioneuropathy (-noo-rop′ah-the) any neuropathy affecting the blood vessels; a disorder of the vasomotor system, as angiospasm or vasomotor paralysis. **angioneuropath′ic,** adj.

angionoma (-no′mah) ulceration of blood vessels.

angioparalysis (-pah-ral′ĭ-sis) vasomotor paralysis.

angioparesis (-pah-re′-sis) vasomotor paralysis.

angioplasty (an′je-o-plas″te) surgical reconstruction of blood vessels. **percutaneous transluminal a.**, dilatation of a blood vessel by means of a balloon catheter inserted through the skin and into the chosen vessel and then passed through the lumen of the vessel to the site of the lesion, where the balloon is inflated to flatten plaque against the artery wall.

angiopoiesis (an″je-o-poi-e′sis) the formation of blood vessels. **angiopoiet′ic,** adj.

angiopressure (-presh′er) the application of pressure to a blood vessel to control hemorrhage.

angiorrhaphy (an″je-or′ah-fe) suture of a vessel or vessels.

angiosarcoma (an″je-o-sar-ko′mah) hemangiosarcoma.

angiosclerosis (-skler-o′sis) hardening of the walls of blood vessels. **angiosclerot′ic** adj.

angioscope (an′je-o-skōp″) a microscope for observing the capillaries.

angioscotoma (an″je-o-sko-to′mah) a cecocentral scotoma caused by shadows of the retinal blood vessels.

angioscotometry (-sko-tom′ĭ-tre) the plotting or mapping of an angioscotoma; done particularly in diagnosing glaucoma.

angiospasm (an′je-o-spazm″) spasmodic contraction of the walls of a blood vessel. **angiospas′tic,** adj.

angiostaxis (an″je-o-stak′sis) hemorrhagic diathesis.

angiostenosis (-stah-no′sis) narrowing of the caliber of a vessel.

angiosteosis (an″je-os″te-o′sis) ossification or calcification of a vessel.

angiostrongyliasis (an″je-o-stron″jĭ-li′ah-sis) infection with *Angiostrongylus cantonensis*.

Angiostrongylus (-stron′jĭ-lus) a genus of nematode parasites. **A. cantonen′sis,** the rat lungworm of Australia and many Pacific islands, including Hawaii; human infection—thought to be due to ingestion of larvae in intermediate hosts, e.g., freshwater crabs—results in migration of the larval worms to the central nervous system, where they provoke eosinophilic meningoencephalitis. **A. vaso′rum,** a species parasitic in the pulmonary arteries of dogs.

angiostrophe, angiostrophy (an″je-os′trah-fe) twisting of a vessel to arrest hemorrhage.

angiotelectasis (an″je-o-tel-ek′tah-sis) dilatation of the minute arteries and veins.

angiotensin (-ten′sin) a decapeptide hormone (a. I) formed from the plasma glycoprotein angiotensinogen by renin secreted by the juxtaglomerular apparatus. It is in turn hydrolyzed by a peptidase in the lungs to form an octapeptide (a. II), which is a powerful vasopressor and stimulator of aldosterone secretion by the adrenal cortex. This is in turn hydrolyzed to form a heptapeptide (a. III), which has less vasopressor activity but more adrenal cortex–stimulating activity. **a. amide,** $C_{49}H_{70}N_{14}O_{11}$, used as a vasopressor.

angiotensinase (-ten′sin-ās) any of a group of peptidases in plasma and tissues that inactivate angiotensin.

angiotensinogen (-ten′sin-o-jin) a serum α_2-globulin secreted in the liver which, on hydrolysis by renin, gives rise to angiotensin.

angiotitis (-ti′is) inflammation of the vessels of the ear.

angiotome (an′je-o-tōm″) one of the segments of the vascular system of the embryo.

angiotonic (an″je-o-ton′ik) increasing vascular tension.

angiotribe (an′je-o-trīb″) a strong forceps in which pressure is applied by means of a screw; used to crush tissue containing an artery in order to check hemorrhage from the vessel.

angiotrophic (an″je-o-trof′ik) pertaining to nutrition of vessels.

angle (ang′g′l) 1. the space or figure formed by two diverging lines, measured as the number of degrees one would have to be moved to coincide with the other. 2. the point at which two intersecting borders or surfaces converge. **acromial a.,** the subcutaneous bony point at which the lateral border becomes continuous with the spine of the scapula. **axial a.,** any line angle parallel with the long axis of a tooth. **cardiodiaphragmatic a.,** that formed by the junction of the shadows of the heart and diaphragm in posteroanterior roentgenograms of the chest. **costovertebral a.,** that formed on either side of the vertebral column between the last rib and the lumbar vertebrae. **filtration a.,** a narrow recess between the sclerocorneal junction and the attached margin of the iris, at the periphery of the anterior chamber of the eye; it is the principal exit site for the aqueous fluid. **iridocorneal a., a. of iris,** filtration a. **line a.,** an angle formed by the junction of two planes; in dentistry, the junction of two surfaces of a tooth or of two walls of a tooth cavity. **Louis' a., Ludwig's a.,** that between manubrium and gladiolus. **point a.,** one formed by the junction of three planes; in dentistry, the junction of three surfaces of a tooth, or of three walls of a tooth cavity. **a. of pubis,** that formed by the conjoined rami of the ischial and pubic bones. **subpubic a.,** a. of pubis. **tooth a's,** those formed by two or more tooth surfaces. **Y a.,** that between the radius fixus and the line joining the lambda and inion.

angstrom (ang′strom) an unsystematic unit of length equal to 10^{-10} meter or 0.1 nanometer; symbol Å.

angulation (ang″gu-la′shun) 1. formation of a sharp obstructive bend, as in the intestine, ureter, or similar tubes. 2. deviation from a straight line, as in a badly set bone.

angulus (ang′gu-lus) [L.] angle; used in names of anatomic structures or landmarks. **a. infectio′sus,** perlèche. **a. i′ridis,** filtration angle. **a. Ludovi′ci,** Louis' angle. **a. o′culi,** the canthus of the eye. **a. pu′bis,** angle of pubis. **a. ster′ni,** Louis' angle. **a. veno′sus,** the angle at the junction of the internal jugular vein and the subclavian vein.

anhedonia (an″he-do′ne-ah) inability to experience pleasure in normally pleasurable acts.

anhidrotic (an″hǐ-drot′ik) 1. checking the flow of sweat. 2. an agent which suppresses perspiration.

anhydrase (an-hi′drās) an enzyme that catalyzes the removal of water from a compound.

anhydremia (an″hi-dre′me-ah) deficiency of water in the blood.

anhydride (an-hi′drīd) any compound derived from a substance, especially an acid, by abstraction of a molecule of water. **chromic a.,** chromic acid (2).

anileridine (an″ĭ-lĕr′ĭ-dēn) a narcotic analgesic, $C_{22}H_{28}N_2O_2$.

anilide (an′ĭ-lĭd) any compound formed from aniline by substituting a radical for the hydrogen of NH_2.

aniline (an′ĭ-lēn) an oily liquid, $C_6H_5NH_2$, from coal tar and indigo or prepared by reducing nitrobenzene; the parent substance of colors or dyes derived from coal tar. It is an important cause of serious industrial poisoning associated with bone marrow depression as well as methemoglobinemia.

anilinism, anilism (an′ĭ-lin-izm; an′ĭ-lizm) poisoning by exposure to aniline.

anility (ah-nil′it-e) 1. the state of being like an old woman. 2. imbecility.

anima (an′ĭ-mah) 1. the soul. 2. Jung's term for the unconscious, or inner being, of the individual, as opposed to the personality he presents to the world (persona). In jungian psychoanalysis, the more feminine soul or feminine component of a man's personality; cf. *animus.*

animal (an′ĭ-m′l) 1. a living organism having sensation and the power of voluntary movement and requiring for its existence oxygen and organic food. 2. of or pertaining to such an organism. **control a.,** an untreated animal otherwise identical in all respects to one that is used for purposes of experimentation, used for checking results of treatment. **hyperphagic a.,** an experimental animal in which the cells of the ventromedial nucleus of the hypothalamus have been destroyed, abolishing its awareness of the point at which it should stop eating; excessive eating and savageness characterize such an animal. **spinal a.,** one whose spinal cord has been severed, cutting off communication with the brain.

animus (an′ĭ-mis) in jungian psychoanalysis, the more male soul or masculine component of a woman's personality; cf. *anima* (2).

anion (an′i-on) a negatively charged ion. In an electrolytic cell anions are attracted to the positive electrode (anode).

aniridia (an″ĭ-rid′e-ah) congenital absence of the iris.

anisakiasis (an″is-ah-ki′ah-sis) infection with the third-stage larvae of the roundworm *Anisakis marina,* which burrow into the stomach wall, producing an eosinophilic granulomatous mass. Infection is acquired by eating undercooked marine fish.

Anisakis (an″ĭ-sa′kis) a genus of nematodes that parasitize the stomachs of marine mammals and birds.

aniseikonia (an″ĭ-si-ko′ne-ah) inequality of the retinal images of the two eyes.

anisindione (an″is-in-di′ōn) an anticoagulant, $C_{16}H_{12}O_3$.

aniso- word element [Gr.], *unequal.*

anisochromatic (an-i″so-kro-mat′ik) not of the same color throughout.

anisocoria (-kor′e-ah) inequality in size of the pupils of the eyes.

anisocytosis (-si-to′sis) presence in the blood of erythrocytes showing excessive variations in size.

anisogamete (-gam′ēt) a gamete differing in size and structure from the one with which it unites. **anisogamet′ic,** adj.

anisokaryosis (an-i″so-kar″e-o′sis) inequality in the size of the nuclei of cells.

anisometropia (-mah-tro′pe-ah) inequality in refractive power of the two eyes. **anisometrop′ic,** adj.

anisopiesis (-pi-e′sis) variation or inequality in the blood pressure as registered in different parts of the body.

anisopoikilocytosis (-poi″kĭ-lo-si-to′sis) the presence in the blood of erythrocytes of varying sizes and abnormal shapes.

anisospore (an-i′so-spor) 1. an anisogamete of organisms reproducing by spores. 2. an asexual spore produced by heterosporous organisms.

anisosthenic (an-i″sos-then′ik) not having equal power; said of muscles.

anisotonic (an-i″so-ton′ik) 1. varying in tonicity or tension. 2. having different osmotic pressure; not isotonic.

anisotropic (-trop′ik) 1. having unlike properties in different directions. 2. doubly refracting, or having a double polarizing power.

anisotropine (-tro′pēn) an anticholinergic, C_{17}-$H_{32}BrNO_2$, which produces relaxation of visceral smooth muscle; used as a spasmolytic in various gastrointestinal disorders.

anisotropy (an″i-ah′tro-pe) the quality of being anisotropic.

anisuria (an″ĭs-u′re-ah) alternating oliguria and polyuria.

ankle (ang′k′l) the region of the joint between leg and foot; the tarsus. Also, the ankle joint.

ankylo- word element [Gr.], *bent; crooked; in the form of a loop; adhesion.*

ankyloblepharon (ang″kĭ-lo-blef′ah-ron) adhesion of the ciliary edges of the eyelids to each other.

ankyloglossia (-glos′e-ah) tongue-tie. **a. superior,** extensive adhesion of the tongue to the palate, associated with deformities of hands and feet.

ankylosed (ang′kĭ-lōst, -lōzd) fused or obliterated, as an ankylosed joint.

ankylosis (ang″kĭ-lo′sis) immobility and consolidation of a joint due to disease, injury, or surgical procedure. **ankylot′ic,** adj. **artificial a.,** arthrodesis. **bony a.,** union of the bones of a joint by proliferation of bone cells, resulting in complete immobility; true a. **extracapsular a.,** that due to rigidity of structures outside the joint capsule. **false a.,** fibrous a. **fibrous a.,** reduced joint mobility due to proliferation of fibrous tissue. **intracapsular a.,** that due to disease, injury, or surgery within the joint capsule.

ankyroid (ang'kĭ-roid) hook-shaped.

anlage (ahn'lah-gah), pl. *anla'gen* [Ger.] primordium.

anneal (ah-nēl') to soften a material, as a metal, by controlled heating and cooling, to make its manipulation easier.

annectent (ah-nek'tint) connecting; joining together.

annelid (an'el-id) any member of Annelida.

Annelida (ah-nel'ĭ-dah) a phylum of metazoan invertebrates, the segmented worms, including leeches.

annular (an'u-ler) ring-shaped.

annuloplasty (an"u-lo-plas'te) plastic repair of a cardiac valve.

annulorrhaphy (an"u-lor'ah-fe) closure of a hernial ring or defect by sutures.

annulus (an'u-lus), pl. *an'nuli* [L.] [NA] a small ring or encircling structure; spelled also *anulus.* **a. of nuclear pore,** a circular filamentous structure surrounding a nuclear pore in the nuclear membrane of a cell. **a. of spermatozoon,** an electron-dense body at the caudal end of the neck of a spermatozoon.

anode (an'ōd) the positive electrode or pole to which negative ions are attracted. **ano'dal,** adj.

anodontia (an"ah-don'she-ah) congenital absence of some or all of the teeth.

anodyne (an'ah-dīn) 1. relieving pain. 2. a medicine that eases pain.

anodynia (an"o-din'e-ah) freedom from pain.

anomalad (ah-nom'ah-lad) a single, localized anomaly occurring during morphogenesis, together with the pattern of subsequent morphologic defects that stem from it.

anomaly (ah-nom'ah-le) marked deviation from normal, especially as a result of congenital or hereditary defects. **anom'alous,** adj. **Alder's a.,** a hereditary condition in which all leukocytes, but mainly those of the myelocytic series, contain coarse, azurophilic granules. **Chédiak-Higashi a.,** see under *syndrome.* **developmental a.,** a defect resulting from imperfect embryonic development. **Ebstein's a.,** a malformation of the tricuspid valve, usually associated with an atrial septal defect. **May-Hegglin a.,** a rare dominantly inherited disorder of blood cell morphology, characterized by RNA-containing cytoplasmic inclusions (similar to Döhle bodies) in granulocytes, by large, poorly granulated platelets, and by thrombocytopenia. **Pelger's nuclear a., Pelger-Huët nuclear a.,** a hereditary or acquired defect in which the nuclei of neutrophils and eosinophils appear rodlike, spherical, or dumbbell-shaped; the nuclear structure is coarse and lumpy.

anomer (an'o-mer) one of two stereoisomers (designated α or β) of the furanose or pyranose form of a sugar, e.g., α-D-glucose. **anomer'ic,** adj.

anonychia (an"on-ik'e-ah) congenital absence of a nail or nails.

Anopheles (ah-nof'ĭl-ēz) a widely distributed genus of mosquitoes, comprising over 300 species, many of which are vectors of malaria; some are vectors of *Wuchereria bancrofti.*

anophthalmia (an"of-thal'me-ah) a developmental anomaly characterized by complete absence of the eyes (rare) or by the presence of vestigial eyes.

anoplasty (a'no-plas"te) plastic or reparative surgery of the anus.

anorchid (an-or'kid) a person with no testes or with undescended testes.

anorchism (an-or'kizm) congenital absence of one or both testes.

anorectic (an"o-rek'tik) 1. pertaining to anorexia. 2. an agent that diminishes the appetite.

anorexia (-rek'se-ah) lack or loss of appetite for food. **a. nervo'sa,** a psychophysiologic condition in girls and young women, characterized by prolonged inability or refusal to eat, sometimes accompanied by vomiting, extreme emaciation, amenorrhea, and other biological changes.

anorexigenic (-rek"sĭ-jen'ik) 1. producing anorexia. 2. an agent that diminishes or controls the appetite.

anorthography (an"or-thog'rah-fe) loss of the ability to write correctly.

anorthopia (-tho'pe-ah) asymmetrical or distorted vision.

anosigmoidoscopy (a"no-sig"moid-os'kah-pe) endoscopic examination of the anus, rectum, and sigmoid colon. **anosigmoidoscop'ic,** adj.

anosmia (an-oz'me-ah) absence of the sense of smell. **anos'mic, anosmat'ic,** adj.

anosognosia (an"o-sog-no'zhe-ah) unawareness or denial of a neurological deficit, such as hemiplegia. **anosogno'sic,** adj.

anostosis (an"os-to'sis) defective formation of bone.

anotia (an-o'she-ah) congenital absence of the external ears.

anovarism (an-o'var-izm) absence of the ovaries.

anovular (an-ov'u-ler) not associated with ovulation.

anovulatory (an-ov'u-lah-tor"e) anovular.

anoxemia (an"ok-se'me-ah) reduction in oxygen content of the blood below normal levels. **anoxe'mic,** adj.

anoxia (an-ok'se-ah) absence of oxygen supply to tissues despite adequate perfusion of the tissue by blood; the term is often used interchangeably with *hypoxia* to indicate a reduced oxygen supply. **anox'ic,** adj. **altitude a.,** that due to reduced oxygen pressure at high altitudes. **anemic a.,** that due to decrease in amount of hemoglobin or number of erythrocytes in the blood. **anoxic a.,** that due to interference with the oxygen supply. **histotoxic a.,** that resulting from diminished ability of cells to utilize available oxygen.

ansa (an'sah), pl. *an'sae* [L.] a looplike structure. **a. cervica'lis,** a nerve loop in the neck that supplies the infrahyoid muscles. **a. hypo-**

glos′si, a. cervicalis. **a. lenticula′ris**, a small nerve fiber tract arising in the globus pallidus and joining the anterior part of the ventral thalamic nucleus. **an′sae nervo′rum spina′lium**, loops of spinal nerves joining the ventral roots of the spinal nerves. **a. peduncula′ris**, a complex grouping of nerve fibers connecting the amygdaloid nucleus, piriform area, and anterior hypothalamus, and various thalamic nuclei. **a. subcla′via, a. of Vieussens**, nerve filaments passing around the subclavian artery to form a loop connecting the middle and inferior cervical ganglia. **a. vitelli′na**, an embryonic vein from the yolk sac to the umbilical vein.

Antabuse (an′tah-būs) trademark for a preparation of disulfiram.

antacid (ant-as′id) counteracting acidity; an agent that so acts.

antagonism (an-tag′o-nizm) opposition or contrariety between similar things, as between muscles, medicines, or organisms; cf. *antibiosis*.

antagonist (an-tag′o-nist) 1. a muscle that counteracts the action of another muscle, its agonist. 2. a drug that binds to a cell receptor for a hormone, a neurotransmitter, or another drug, and thus blocks the action of the other substance without producing any physiological effect itself. 3. a tooth in one jaw that articulates with one in the other jaw. **folic acid a.**, an antimetabolite, e.g., methotrexate, that interferes with DNA replication and cell division by inhibiting the enzyme dihydrofolate reductase; used in cancer chemotherapy.

antarthritic (ant″ar-thrit′ik) alleviating arthritis; an agent that so acts.

antalgic (ant-al′jik) 1. counteracting or avoiding pain, as a posture or gait assumed so as to lessen pain. 2. analgesic.

ante (an′te) [L.] *before*.

ante- word element [L.], *before* (in time or space).

antebrachium (an″te-bra′ke-um) the forearm. **antebra′chial**, adj.

antecedent (-sēd′int) a precursor. **plasma thromboplastin a. (PTA)**, coagulation Factor XI.

anteflexion (-flek′shin) 1. abnormal forward bending of an organ or part. 2. the normal forward curvature of the uterus.

ante mortem (an′te mort′em) [L.] before death.

antenna (an-ten′ah) either of the two lateral appendages on the anterior segment of the head of arthropods.

antepartal (an″te-part′′l) occurring before childbirth, with reference to the mother.

ante partum (an′te part′um) [L.] before parturition.

antepartum (an″te-part′um) antepartal.

antepyretic (an″te-pi-ret′ik) occurring before the stage of fever.

anterior (an-te′re-or) situated at or directed toward the front; opposite of posterior.

antero- word element [L.], *anterior; in front of*.

anteroclusion (an″ter-o-kloo′zhin) mesioclusion.

anterograde (an′ter-o-grād″) extending or moving forward.

anterolateral (-lat′er-il) situated in front and to one side.

anteroposterior (-pos-tēr′e-er) directed from the front toward the back.

anteversion (an″te-ver′zhin) the tipping forward of an entire organ.

anthelix (ant′he-liks) the semicircular ridge on the flap of the ear, anteroinferior to the helix.

anthelmintic (ant″hel-min′tik) 1. destructive to worms. 2. an agent destructive to worms.

anthocyanin (an″tho-si′ah-nin) any of a class of glycoside pigments of blue, red, and violet flowers.

anthracene (an′thrah-sēn) 1. a crystalline hydrocarbon, $C_{14}H_{10}$, from coal tar. 2. a ptomaine from *Bacillus anthracis*.

anthracoid (an′thrah-koid) resembling anthrax or a carbuncle.

anthraconecrosis (an″thrah-ko-nah-kro′sis) degeneration of tissue into a black mass.

anthracosilicosis (-sil″ĭ-ko′sis) a combination of anthracosis and silicosis.

anthracosis (an″thrah-ko′sis) pneumoconiosis, usually asymptomatic, due to deposition of coal dust in the lungs.

anthracycline (an″thrah-si′klēn) a class of antibiotics isolated from cultures of *Streptomyces peucetius*; it includes the antineoplastic agents daunomycin and doxorubicin.

anthralin (an′thrah-lin) a compound, $C_{14}H_{10}O_3$, used topically in eczema and psoriasis.

anthraquinone (an″thrah-kwin′ōn) a yellow substance, $C_{14}H_8O_2$, from anthracene.

anthrax (an′thraks) an often fatal, infectious disease of ruminants due to ingestion of spores of *Bacillus anthracis* in soil; acquired by man through contact with contaminated wool or other animal products or by inhalation of airborne spores. **cutaneous a.**, that due to inoculation of *Bacillus anthracis* into superficial wounds or abrasions of the skin, producing a black crusted pustule on a broad zone of edema. **gastrointestinal a., intestinal a.**, anthrax involving the gastrointestinal tract, caused by ingestion of poorly cooked meat contaminated by *Bacillus anthracis* spores; bowel obstruction, hemorrhage, and necrosis may result. **inhalational a.**, a highly fatal form of anthrax due to inhalation of dust containing anthrax spores, which are transported by the alveolar pneumocytes to the regional lymph nodes, where they germinate; it is primarily an occupational disease affecting those who handle and sort wools and fleeces. **localized a.**, cutaneous a. **pulmonary a.**, inhalation a. **symptomatic a.**, blackleg; a disease of sheep, cattle, and goats marked by emphysematous and subcutaneous swellings and nodules, due to *Clostridium chauvoei* and sometimes *C. septicum*.

anthropo- word element [Gr.], *man (human being)*.

anthropocentric (an″thrah-po-sen′trik) with a human bias; considering man the center of the universe.

anthropoid (an′thrah-poid) resembling man; the anthropoid apes are tailless apes, including the chimpanzee, gibbon, gorilla, and orangutan.

Anthropoidea (an″thro-poi′de-ah) a suborder of Primates, including monkeys, apes, and man.

anthropology (an″thrah-pol′o-je) the science that treats of man, his origins, historical and cultural development, and races.

anthropometry (-pom′ĭ-tre) the science dealing with measurement of the size, weight, and proportions of the human body. **anthropomet′ric**, adj.

anthropomorphism (an″thrah-po-mor′fizm) the attribution of human characteristics to nonhuman objects.

anthropophilic (-fil′ik) preferring man to animals; said of mosquitoes.

anthropozoonosis (-zo″o-no′sis) a disease of either animals or man that may be transmitted from one to the other.

anti- word element [Gr.], *counteracting; effective against.*

antiabortifacient (an″tĭ-ah-bor″tĭ-fa′shint) 1. preventing abortion or promoting gestation. 2. an antiabortifacient agent.

antiadrenergic (-ah-dren-er″jik) 1. sympatholytic: opposing the effects of impulses conveyed by adrenergic postganglionic fibers of the sympathetic nervous system. 2. an antiadrenergic agent.

antiagglutinin (-ah-glōōt′in-in) a substance that opposes the action of an agglutinin.

antiamebic (-ah-me′bik) 1. destroying or suppressing the growth of amebas. 2. an agent having such properties.

antianaphylactin (-an″ah-fi-lak′tin) an antibody which counteracts anaphylactin.

antianaphylaxis (-an″ah-fi-lak′sis) a condition in which the anaphylaxis reaction does not occur because of free antigens in the blood; the state of desensitization to antigens.

antiandrogen (-an′drah-jen) any substance capable of inhibiting the biological effects of androgenic hormones.

antianemic (-ah-ne′mik) 1. counteracting anemia. 2. an agent that so acts.

antiantibody (-an′tĭ-bod-e) an immunoglobulin formed in the body after administration of antibody acting as immunogen, and which interacts with the latter.

antianxiety (-ang-zi′it-e) dispelling anxiety; relating to an agent (anxiolytic, minor tranquilizer) that so acts. There are two types: sedative-hypnotic (benzodiazepines, barbiturates, meprobamate) and sedative-autonomic (diphenhydramine-type antihistamines and the more sedating phenothiazines and tricyclic antidepressants).

antiarrhythmic (-ah-rith′mik) 1. preventing or alleviating cardiac arrhythmias. 2. an agent that so acts.

antibacterial (-bak-te′re-il) destroying or suppressing growth or reproduction of bacteria; also, an agent having such properties.

antibiosis (-bi-o′sis) an association between two organisms that is detrimental to one of them, or between one organism and an antibiotic produced by another.

antibiotic (-bi-ot′ik) a chemical substance produced by a microorganism, which has the capacity to inhibit the growth of or to kill other microorganisms; antibiotics sufficiently nontoxic to the host are used in the treatment of infectious diseases. **broad-spectrum a.**, one effective against a wide range of bacteria.

antibody (an″tĭ-bod-e) an immunoglobulin molecule that reacts with a specific antigen that induced its synthesis and with similar molecules; classified according to mode of action as agglutinin, bacteriolysin, hemolysin, opsonin, or precipitin. Antibodies are synthesized by B lymphocytes that have been activated by the binding of an antigen to a cell surface receptor. Abbreviated Ab. See *immunoglobulin.* **anaphylactic a.**, anaphylactin. **antimitochondrial a's**, circulating antibodies directed against inner mitochondrial antigens seen in almost all patients with primary biliary cirrhosis. **antinuclear a's (ANA)**, autoantibodies directed against components of the cell nucleus, e.g., DNA, RNA, and histones. **antireceptor a's**, autoantibodies against cell-surface receptors, e.g., those directed against β_2-adrenergic receptors in some patients with allergic disorders. **antithyroglobulin a's**, those directed against thyroglobulin, demonstrable in about one-third of patients with thyroiditis, Graves' disease, and thyroid carcinoma. **blocking a.**, 1. one (usually IgG) that reacts preferentially with an antigen, preventing it from reacting with a cytotropic antibody (IgE), and producing a hypersensitivity reaction. 2. incomplete a. **complement-fixing a.**, one that activates complement when reacted with antigen: IgM and IgG fix complement by the classic pathway; IgA, by the alternative pathway. **complete a.**, one that reacts with the antigen in saline, producing an agglutination or precipitation reaction. **cytophilic a.**, cytotropic a. **cytotoxic a.**, any specific antibody directed against cellular antigens, which when bound to the antigen, activates the complement pathway or activates killer cells, resulting in cell lysis. **cytotropic a.**, any of a class of antibodies that attach to tissue cells through their Fc segments to induce the release of histamine and other vasoconstrictive amines important in immediate hypersensitivity reactions. **Forssman a.**, heterophile antibody directed against the Forssman antigen. **heteroclitic a.**, antibody produced in response to immunization with one antigen but having a higher affinity for a second antigen that was not present during immunization. **heterogenetic a.**, **heterophil a.**, **heterophile a.**, antibody directed against heterophile antigens. Heterophile sheep erythrocyte agglutinins appear in the serum of patients with infectious mononucleosis. **immune a.**, one induced by immunization or by transfusion incompatibility, in contrast to natural antibodies. **incomplete a.**, 1. antibody that binds to erythrocytes or bacteria but does not produce agglutination. 2. a univalent antibody fragment, e.g., Fab fragment. **isophil a's**, antibodies against red blood cell antigens produced in members of the species from which the red cells originated. **monoclonal a's**, chemically and immunologically homogeneous antibodies produced by hybridomas, used as laboratory reagents in radioimmunoassays, ELISA, and immunofluorescence assays. **natural a's**, ones that react with antigens to which the individual has had no known exposure. **neutralizing a.**, one which, on mixture with the homologous infectious agent, reduces the infectious titer. **Prausnitz-Küstner (P-K) a's**, homocytotropic antibodies of the immunoglobulin class IgE responsible for cutaneous anaphylaxis. See *reagin*. **protective a.**, one responsible for immunity to an infectious agent observed in passive immunity. **reaginic a.**, reagin. **saline a.**, complete a. **sensitizing a.**, anaphylactic a.

anticalculous (-kal′ku-lis) suppressing the formation of calculi.

anticariogenic (-kăr″e-o-jen′ik) effective in suppressing caries production.

anticheirotonus (-ki-rot′in-us) spasmodic flexion of the thumb.

anticholelithogenic (-ko″lĭ-lith″o-jen′ik) 1. preventing the formation of gallstones. 2. an agent that so acts.

anticholesteremic (-kah-les″ter-e′mik) promoting a reduction of cholesterol levels in the blood; also, any agent that so acts, e.g., the sitosterols and clofibrate.

anticholinergic (-ko″lin-er′jik) parasympatholytic: blocking the passage of impulses through the parasympathetic nerves; also, an agent that so acts.

anticholinesterase (-ko″lin-es′ter-ās) a drug that inhibits the enzyme acetylcholinesterase, thereby potentiating the action of acetylcholine at postsynaptic membrane receptors in the parasympathetic nervous system.

anticlinal (-kli′n′l) sloping or inclined in opposite directions.

anticoagulant (-ko-ag′u-lint) 1. acting to prevent clotting of blood. 2. any substance which suppresses, delays, or nullifies blood coagulation. **circulating a.**, a substance in the blood which inhibits normal blood clotting and may cause a hemorrhagic syndrome.

anticoagulin (-ko-ag′u-lin) a substance that suppresses, delays, or nullifies coagulation of the blood.

anticodon (-ko′don) a triplet of nucleotides in transfer RNA that is complementary to the codon in messenger RNA which specifies the amino acid.

anticomplement (-kom′plĭ-ment) a substance that counteracts a complement.

anticonvulsant, anticonvulsive (-kon-vul′sint; -kon-vulsiv) 1. inhibiting convulsions. 2. an agent that suppresses convulsions.

anticus (an-ti′kus) [L.] anterior.

anti-D antibody against D antigen, the most immunogenic of the Rh antigens. Commercial preparations of anti-D, Rh₀(D) immune globulin, are administered to Rh-negative women following the birth of an Rh-positive baby in order to prevent maternal alloimmunization against the D-antigen, which may cause hemolytic disease of the newborn in a subsequent pregnancy. Called also anti-Rh₀.

antidepressant (an″tĭ-de-pres′int) preventing or relieving depression; also, an agent that so acts. **tricyclic a's**, a class of drugs, including imipramine, amitriptyline, nortriptyline, protriptyline, desipramine, and doxepin, used for the treatment of depression.

antidinic (-din′ik) relieving giddiness or vertigo.

antidiuretic (-di″u-ret′ik) 1. pertaining to or causing suppression of urine. 2. an agent that causes suppression of urine.

antidote (an′tĭ-dōt) an agent that counteracts a poison. **antido′tal,** adj. **chemical a.**, one that neutralizes the poison by changing its chemical nature. **mechanical a.**, one that prevents absorption of the poison. **physiologic a.**, one that counteracts the effects of the poison by producing opposing physiologic effects.

antidromic (an″tĭ-drom′ik) conducting impulses in a direction opposite to the normal; said of neurons in the posterior roots of the spinal cord.

antiemetic (-e-met′ik) preventing or alleviating nausea and vomiting; also, an agent that so acts.

antifebrile (-feb′ril) antipyretic.

antifibrinolysin (-fi″brĭ-no-li′sin) an inhibitor of fibrinolysin.

antifibrinolytic (-fi″brĭ-no-lit′ik) inhibiting fibrinolysis.

antiflatulent (-flă′choo-lint) relieving or preventing flatulence; also, an agent that so acts.

antifungal (-fung′g′l) 1. destructive to fungi; suppressing the growth or reproduction of fungi; effective against fungal infections. 2. an agent that so acts.

antigalactic (-gah-lak′tik) 1. diminishing secretion of milk. 2. an agent that tends to suppress milk secretion.

antigen (an′tĭ-jen) any substance capable of inducing a specific immune response and of reacting with the products of that response, i.e., with specific antibody or specifically sensitized T-lymphocytes, or both. Abbreviated Ag. **antigen′ic,** adj. **Au a., Australia a.**, hepatitis B surface a. **B a.**, an antigenic component of the K antigen complex. **blood group a's,** erythrocyte surface antigens whose antigenic differences determine blood groups. **capsular a.**, specific capsular substance. **carcinoembryonic a. (CEA),** a cancer-specific glycoprotein antigen of colon carcinoma, also present in many adenocarcinomas of endodermal origin and in normal gastrointestinal tissues of human embryos. **class I a's,** major histocompatibility antigens found on every cell except erythrocytes, recognized during graft rejection, and involved in MHC restriction. **class II a's,** major histocompatibility antigens found only on immunocompetent cells, primarily B lymphocytes and macrophages. **common acute lymphoblastic leukemia a. (CALLA),** a tumor-associated antigen occurring on lymphoblasts in about 80 per cent of patients with acute lymphoblastic leukemia (ALL) and in 40–50 per cent of patients with blastic phase chronic myelogenous leukemia (CML). **complete a.**, one which both stimulates an immune response and reacts with the products of that response. **conjugated a.**, one produced by coupling a hapten to a protein carrier molecule through covalent bonds; when it induces immunization, the resultant immune response is directed against both the hapten and the carrier. **D a.,** a red cell antigen of the Rh blood group system, important in the development of isoimmunization in Rh-negative persons exposed to the blood of Rh-positive persons. **E a.,** a red cell antigen of the Rh blood group system. **flagellar a.,** H antigen. **Forssman a.,** a heterogenetic antigen inducing the production of antisheep hemolysin, occurring in various unrelated species, mainly in the organs but not in the erythrocytes (guinea pig, horse), but sometimes only in the erythrocytes (sheep), and occasionally in both (chicken). **H a.** the antigen which occurs in the flagella of motile bacteria. **hepatitis a., hepatitis-associated a. (HAA),** hepatitis B surface a. **hepatitis B core a. (HB₍c₎Ag),** the antigen of the DNA core of the hepatitis B virus. **hepatitis B e a. (HB₍e₎Ag),** one contained on the outer lipoprotein coat of the hepatitis B virus. **hepatitis B surface a. (HB₍s₎Ag),** one present in the serum of those infected with hepatitis B, consisting of the surface coat lipoprotein of the hepatitis B virus. Tests for serum Hb₍s₎Ag are used in the diagnosis of hepatitis B and in testing blood products for infectivity. **heterogenetic a., heterologous a., heterophil a.,** an antigen common to more than one species and whose species distribution is unrelated to its phylogenetic distribution (viz., Forssman's antigen, lens protein, certain caseins, etc.). **histocompatibility a's,** genetically determined isoantigens found on the surface of nucleated cells of most tissues, which incite an immune response when grafted onto a genetically different individual and thus determine compatibility of tissues in transplantation. **HLA a's** (*human leukocyte antigen*), histocompatibility antigens (glycoproteins) on the surface of nucleated cells (including circulating and tissue cells) determined by a region on chromosome 6 bearing several genetic loci, designated HLA-A, -B, -C, -DP, -DQ, -DR, -MB, -MT, and -Te. They are important in cross-matching procedures and are partially responsible for the rejection of transplanted tissues when donor and recipient HLA antigens do not match. **homologous a.,** 1. the antigen inducing antibody formation. 2. isoantigen. **H-Y a.,** a histocompatibility antigen of the cell membrane, determined by a locus on the Y chromosome; it is a mediator of testicular organization (hence, sexual differentiation) in the male. **Ia a's,** histocompatibility antigens governed by the I region of the major histocompatibility complex (MHC), located principally on B cells, although T cells, skin, and certain macrophages may also contain Ia antigens. **Inv group a.,** Km a. **isogeneic a.,** an antigen carried by an individual which is capable of eliciting an immune response in genetically different individuals of the same species, but not in an individual bearing it. **isophil a.,** isoantigen. **K a's,** antigens that function as blocking antigens in that their presence interferes with agglutination with O antisera. **Km a.,** one of the three alloantigens found in the constant region of the κ light chains of immunoglobulins.

Ly a's, Lyt a's, antigenic cell-surface markers of subpopulations of T lymphocytes, classified as Ly 1, 2, and 3; they are associated with helper and suppressor activities of T lymphocytes. **lymphogranuloma venereum a.,** a sterile suspension of *Chlamydia lymphogranulomatis;* used as a dermal reactivity indicator. **mumps skin test a.,** a sterile suspension of mumps virus; used as a dermal reactivity indicator. **O a.** one occurring in the lipopolysaccharide layer of the wall of gram-negative bacteria. **oncofetal a.,** carcinoembryonic a. **organ-specific a.,** any antigen occurring only in a particular organ and serving to distinguish it from other organs; it may be limited to an organ of a single species or be characteristic of the same organ in many species. **partial a.,** hapten. **private a's,** antigens of the low frequency blood groups, probably differing from ordinary blood group systems only in their incidence. **public a's,** antigens of the high frequency blood groups, so called because they are found in almost all persons tested. **self a.,** an autoantigen, a normal constituent of the body against which antibodies are formed in autoimmune disease. **T a.,** 1. a tumor antigen, coded for by the viral genome, and associated with transformation of infected cells by certain DNA tumor viruses. 2. any of a series, T_1 through T_{10}, of human T lymphocyte cell-surface markers. 3. an antigen present on human erythrocytes that is exposed by treatment with neuraminidase or contact with certain bacteria. **T-dependent a.,** one requiring the presence of helper T cells to stimulate antibody production by B cells. **T-independent a.,** one able to trigger B cells to produce antibodies without the presence of T cells. **tumor-specific a. (TSA),** cell-surface antigens of tumors that elicit a specific immune response in the host. **Vi a.,** a K antigen of *Salmonella typhi* originally thought responsible for virulence.

antigenemia (an″tĭ-jin-e′me-ah) the presence of antigen (e.g., hepatitis B surface antigen) in the blood. **antigene′mic,** adj.

antigenicity (-jĭ-nis′ĭt-e) the capacity to stimulate the production of antibodies or the capacity to react with an antibody.

antiglobulin (-glob′u-lin) an antibody directed against gamma globulin, as used in the Coombs' test.

antihemolysin (-he-mol′ĭ-sin) any agent that opposes the action of a hemolysin.

antihemorrhagic (-hem″o-raj′ik) 1. exerting a hemostatic effect; counteracting hemorrhage. 2. an agent that so acts.

antihistamine (-his′tah-min) a drug that counteracts the effect of histamine. There are two types: H_1-receptor blockers, which inhibit the effects of histamine released from mast cells and are used in the treatment of allergic disorders, and H_2-receptor blockers, e.g., cimetidine, which inhibit the secretion of gastric acid stimulated by histamine, pentagastrin, food, and insulin, and are used in the treatment of peptic ulcer.

antihypercholesterolemic (-hi″per-kah-les′ter-ol-e″mik) 1. effective against hypercholesterolemia. 2. an agent that prevents or relieves hypercholesterolemia.

antihyperlipoproteinemic (-lip″o-pro″te-in-e′mik) 1. promoting a reduction of lipoprotein levels in the blood. 2. an agent that so acts.

anti-immune (-ĭ-mūn′) preventing immunity.

anti-infective (-in-fek′tiv) 1. counteracting infection. 2. a substance that so acts.

anti-inflammatory (-in-flam′ah-tor″e) counteracting or suppressing inflammation; also, an agent that so acts.

antileukocytic (-loo″ko-sit′ik) destructive to white blood corpuscles (leukocytes).

antilipemic (-li-pe′mik) counteracting high levels of lipids in the blood; also an agent that so acts.

antilithic (-lith′ik) preventing calculus formation; also, an agent that so acts.

antilysis (-li′sis) inhibition of lysis.

antilytic (-lit′ik) 1. pertaining to antilysis. 2. inhibiting or preventing lysis.

antimere (an′tĭ-mēr) one of the opposite corresponding parts of an organism that are symmetrical with respect to the longitudinal axis of its body.

antimetabolite (an″tĭ-mĕ-tab′ol-īt) a substance bearing a close structural resemblance to one required for normal physiological functioning, and exerting its effect by interfering with the utilization of the essential metabolite.

antimethemoglobinemic (-met″he-mah-glo″-bin-e′mik) 1. promoting reduction of methemoglobin levels in the blood. 2. an agent that so acts.

antimetropia (-mah-tro′pe-ah) hyperopia of one eye, with myopia in the other.

antimicrobial (an″tĭ-mi-kro′be-il) 1. killing microorganisms or suppressing their multiplication or growth. 2. an agent with such effects.

antimongolism (-mong′gul-izm) a term applied to syndromes associated with certain chromosomal abnormalities, in which some of the clinical signs, e.g., downward-slanting palpebral fissures, are variations of those seen in Down's syndrome.

antimony (an′tĭ-mo″ne) chemical element (*see table*), at. no. 51, symbol Sb, forming various medicinal and poisonous salts; ingestion of antimony compounds, and rarely industrial exposure to them, may produce symptoms similar to acute arsenic poisoning, with vomiting a prominent symptom. **antimo′nial,** adj. **a. potassium tartrate,** a compound used in treatment of parasitic infections, e.g., schistosomiasis or leishmaniasis. **a. sodium thioglycollate,** a compound used in treatment of schistosomiasis.

antimycotic (an″tĭ-mi-kot′ik) suppressing the growth of fungi; antifungal.

antineoplastic (-ne″o-plas′tik) 1. inhibiting or preventing development of neoplasms; checking maturation and proliferation of malignant cells. 2. an agent having such properties.

antineoplaston (-ne″o-plas′ton) any of a number of peptides isolated from human urine that inhibit cell division in certain cancer cells but not in normal cells.

antinion (an-tin′e-on) the frontal pole of the head; the median frontal point farthest from the inion.

antioxidant (-ok′sid-int) a substance added to a product to prevent or delay its deterioration by the oxygen in air.

antiparallel (an″te-par′ah-lel) denoting molecules arranged side by side but in opposite directions.

antiparkinsonian (-par″kin-so′ne-in) 1. effective in the treatment of parkinsonism. 2. an agent effective in the treatment of parkinsonism.

antipediculotic (-pĕ-dik″u-lot′ik) 1. effective against lice. 2. an agent effective against lice.

antiperistalsis (-pĕ″ri-stal′sis) reversed peristalsis. **antiperistal′tic,** adj.

antiplasmin (-plaz′min) a substance in the blood that inhibits plasmin.

antiplastic (-plas′tik) 1. unfavorable to healing. 2. an agent that suppresses formation of blood or other cells.

antiport (an′tĭ-port) a cell membrane structure that transports two molecules at once through the membrane in opposite directions.

antiprothrombin (an″tĭ-pro-throm′bin) an anticoagulant that retards the conversion of prothrombin into thrombin.

antiprotozoal (-pro″tah-zo′l) lethal to protozoa, or checking their growth or reproduction; also, an agent that so acts.

antipruritic (-proo-rit′ik) 1. preventing or relieving itching. 2. an agent that counteracts itching.

antipsychotic (-si-kot′ik) effective in the management of manifestations of psychotic disorders; also an agent that so acts. There are several classes of antipsychotic drugs (phenothiazines, thioxanthines, dibenzazepines, and butyrophenones), of which all may act by the same mechanism, i.e., blockade of dopaminergic receptors in the central nervous system. Called also *neuroleptic* and *major tranquilizer.*

antipyretic (-pi-ret′ik) relieving or reducing fever; also, an agent that so acts.

antipyrotic (-pi-rot′ik) 1. effective in the treatment of burns. 2. an agent used in the treatment of burns.

antiscorbutic (-skor-būt′ik) effective in the prevention or relief of scurvy.

antisecretory (-se-krēt′ah-re) 1. inhibiting or diminishing secretion; secretoinhibitory. 2. an agent that so acts, as certain drugs that inhibit or diminish gastric secretions.

antiseptic (-sep′tik) 1. preventing sepsis. 2. a substance that inhibits the growth and development of microorganisms but does not necessarily kill them.

antiserum (-sēr′um) a serum containing antibody(ies), obtained from an animal immunized either by injection of antigen or by infection with microorganisms containing antigen.

antisialagogue (-si-al′ah-gog) counteracting saliva formation; also, an agent that inhibits flow of saliva. **antisialagog′ic,** adj.

antisialic (-si-al′ik) checking the flow of saliva; also, an agent that so acts.

antisocial (-so′sh′l) denoting (1) behavior that violates the rights of others or is criminal or (2) a specific syndrome of personality traits, *antisocial personality disorder* (under *personality*).

antispasmodic (an″tĭ-spaz-mod′ik) 1. preventing or relieving spasms. 2. an agent that so acts.

antisudoral, antisudorific (-soo′der-′l; -soo″ der-if′ik) inhibiting perspiration; also an agent that so acts.

antisympathetic (-sim″pah-thet′ik) 1. producing effects resembling those of interruption of the sympathetic nerve supply. 2. an agent that produces such effects.

antithenar (-the′nar) placed opposite to the palm or sole.

antithrombin (-throm′bin) any naturally occurring or therapeutically administered substance that neutralizes the action of thrombin and thus limits or restricts blood coagulation. **a. I,** the capacity of fibrin to adsorb thrombin and thus neutralize it. **a. III,** a plasma protein (alpha₂-globulin) that inactivates thrombin; it is also a heparin cofactor and an inhibitor of certain coagulation factors.

antithromboplastin (-throm″bo-plas′tin) any agent or substance that prevents or interferes with the interaction of blood coagulation factors as they generate prothrombinase (thromboplastin).

antithyroid (-thi′roid) counteracting thyroid functioning, especially in its synthesis of thyroid hormones.

antitoxin (-tok′sin) antibody produced in response to a toxin of bacterial (usually an exotoxin), animal (zootoxin), or plant (phytotoxin) origin, which neutralizes the effects of the toxin. **antitox′ic,** adj. **botulism a.,** a sterile solution of antitoxic substances from blood serum or plasma of healthy horses immunized against toxins of both types of *Clostridium botulinum.* **diphtheria a.,** a sterile solution of refined and concentrated antibody globulins from the blood serum or plasma of a healthy animal (usually the horse) immunized against diphtheria toxin. **gas gangrene a.,** a sterile solution of antibody globulins from the serum of horses immunized against toxins of certain species of pathogenic clostridia. **scarlet fever streptococcus a.,** a sterile solution of antitoxic substances (i.e., immunoglobulins) from the serum of healthy animals immunized against toxin from the streptococci causing scarlet fever. **tetanus a.,** a sterile solution of refined and concentrated antibody globulins from blood serum or plasma of a healthy animal (usually the horse) immunized against tetanus toxin or toxoid. **tetanus and gas gangrene a's,** a sterile solution of antitoxic substances (immunoglobulins) from the blood of healthy animals immunized against the toxins of *Clostridium tetani, C. perfringens,* and *C. septicum.*

antitragus (-tra′gus) a projection on the ear opposite the tragus.

antitrichomonal (-trich″ah-mo′n′l) effective against *Trichomonas;* also, an agent having such effects.

antitrope (an′tĭ-trōp) one of two symmetrical but oppositely oriented structures. **antitrop′ic,** adj.

α₁-antitrypsin (-trip′sin) alpha₁-antitrypsin.

antituberculin (-too-ber′ku-lin) an antibody developed after injection of tuberculin into the body.

antitussive (-tus′iv) 1. effective against cough. 2. an agent that suppresses coughing.

antivenin (-ven′in) a material used in treatment of poisoning by animal venom. **black widow spider (Latrodectus mactans) a.,** an antitoxic serum prepared by immunizing horses against venom of the black widow spider. **a. (Crotalidae) polyvalent, crotaline a., polyvalent,** a serum containing specific venom-neutralizing globulin, produced by hyperimmunization of horses with venoms of the fer-de-lance and the Florida, Texas, and tropical rattlesnakes, used for treatment of envenomation by most pit vipers throughout the world. **a. (Micrurus fulvius),** a serum containing specific venom-neutralizing globulin, produced by immunization of horses with venom of the eastern coral snake.

antixerotic (-ze-rot′ik) counteracting or preventing dryness.

antr(o)- word element [L.], *chamber; cavity;* often used with specific reference to the maxillary antrum or sinus.

antritis (an-trīt′is) inflammation of an antrum, chiefly of the maxillary antrum (sinus).

antrocele (an′tro-sēl) cystic accumulation of fluid in the maxillary antrum.

antronasal (an″tro-na′z′l) pertaining to the maxillary antrum and nasal fossa.

antroscope (an′tro-skōp) an instrument for inspecting the maxillary antrum (sinus).

antrotomy (an-trot′ah-me) incision of an antrum.

antrotympanitis (-tim″pah-nīt′is) inflammation of the tympanic (mastoid) antrum and tympanum.

antrum (an′trum) pl. *an′tra* [L.] a cavity or chamber. **an′tral,** adj. **a. of Highmore,** maxillary sinus. **mastoid a., a. mastoi′deum,** an air space in the mastoid portion of the temporal bone communicating with the tympanic cavity and the mastoid cells. **a. maxilla′re, maxillary a.,** maxillary sinus. **pyloric a., a. pylo′ricum,** the dilated portion of the pyloric part of the stomach, between the body of the stomach and pyloric canal. **tympanic a., a tympa′nicum,** mastoid a.

anulus (an′u-lus), pl. *an′uli* [L.] NA alternative for *annulus;* used in names of certain ringlike or encircling structures of the body.

anuresis (an″ūr-e′sis) 1. retention of urine in the bladder. 2. anuria. **anuret′ic,** adj.

anuria (an-ūr′e-ah) complete suppression of urine formation by the kidney. **anu′ric,** adj.

anus (a′nus) the opening of the rectum on the body surface; the distal orifice of the alimentary canal. **imperforate a.,** congenital absence of the anal canal or persistence of the anal membrane so that the anus is closed, either completely or partially.

Anusol (an′u-sol) trademark for a fixed combination preparation of bismuth subgallate, bismuth resorcin compound, benzyl benzoate, Peruvian balsam, zinc oxide, and either pramoxine hydrochloride or (in Anusol-HC) hydrocortisone acetate; used for relief of anorectal pain and itching.

anvil (an′vil) incus.

anxiety (ang-zi′it-e) a feeling of apprehension, uncertainty, and fear without apparent stimulus, associated with physiological changes (tachycardia, sweating, tremor, etc.). **separation a.,** apprehension due to removal of significant persons or familiar surroundings, common in infants six to 10 months old.

anxiolytic (ang″zĭ-o-lit′ik) an antianxiety agent; see *antianxiety.*

A.O.A. American Optometric Association; American Orthopsychiatric Association; American Osteopathic Association.

aorta (a-ort′ah), pl. *aor′tae, aor′tas* [Gr.] the great artery arising from the left ventricle, being the main trunk from which the systemic arterial system proceeds; see *Table of Arteries* for parts of aorta, and see Plate VIII. **overriding a.,** a congenital anomaly occurring in tetralogy of Fallot, in which the aorta is displaced to the right so that it appears to arise from both ventricles and straddles the ventricular septal defect.

aortitis (a″or-tīt′is) inflammation of the aorta.

aortography (a″or-tog′rah-fe) radiography of the aorta after introduction into it of a contrast material.

aortopathy (a″or-top′ah-the) any disease of the aorta.

aortorrhaphy (a″or-tor′ah-fe) suture of the aorta.

aortosclerosis (a-ort″o-skler-o′sis) sclerosis of the aorta.

aortotomy (a″or-tot′ah-me) incision of the aorta.

A.O.T.A. American Occupational Therapy Association.

AP angina pectoris; anteroposterior; arterial pressure.

A.P.A. American Pharmaceutical Association; American Podiatric Association; American Psychiatric Association; American Psychological Association.

apallesthesia (ah-pal″es-the′ze-ah) pallanesthesia.

apancrea (ah-pan′kre-ah) absence of the pancreas.

apathism (ap′ah-thizm) slowness of response to stimuli.

apathy (ap′ah-the) lack of feeling or emotion; indifference. **apathet′ic,** adj.

APC 1. abbreviation for aspirin, phenacetin, and caffeine, used as an analgesic or antipyretic. 2. atrial premature contraction.

APE anterior pituitary extract.

apellous (ah-pel′is) 1. skinless; not covered with skin; not cicatrized (said of a wound). 2. having no prepuce.

aperient (ah-pēr′e-ent) a mild laxative or gentle purgative.

aperistalsis (ah″per-ĭ-stal′sis) absence of peristaltic action.

apertognathia (ah-pert″og-na′the-ah) open bite.

apertura (ap″er-tu′rah), pl. *apertu′rae* [L.] aperture.

aperture (ap′er-cher) an opening or orifice. **numerical a.,** an expression of the measure of efficiency of a microscope objective.

apex (a′peks), pl. *a′pices* [L.] tip; the pointed end of a conical part; the top of a body, organ, or part. **ap′ical,** adj. **root a.,** the terminal end of the root of the tooth.

A.P.H.A. American Public Health Association.

A.Ph.A. American Pharmaceutical Association.

aphagia (ah-fa′je-ah) abstention from eating.

aphakia (ah-fa′ke-ah) absence of the lens of an eye, occurring congenitally or as a result of trauma or surgery. **apha′kic,** adj.

aphalangia (ah″fah-lan′je-ah) absence of fingers or toes.

aphasia (ah-fa′zhe-ah) defect or loss of the power of expression by speech, writing, or signs, or of comprehending spoken or written language, due to injury or disease of the brain centers. For types of aphasia not given below, see *agrammatism, anomia, paragrammatism,* and *paraphasia.* **apha′sic,** adj. **amnesic a., amnestic a.,** anomic a. **anomic a.,** fluent aphasia in which comprehension and repetition are preserved. **ataxic a.,** expressive a. **auditory a.,** word deafness; loss of the ability to comprehend spoken language. **Broca's a.,** expressive a. **conduction a.,** aphasia due to lesion of the path between sensory and motor speech centers. **expressive a.,** that in which the patient understands written and spoken words and knows what he wishes to say, but cannot utter the words. **fluent a.,** that in which speech is well articulated and grammatically correct but is lacking in content. **gibberish a.,** jargon a. **global a.,** total aphasia involving all the functions which go to make up speech or communication. **jargon a.,** that with utterance of meaningless phrases. **mixed a.,** global a. **motor a.,** expressive a. **nominal a.,** that marked by defective use of names (L. *nomina*) of objects. **nonfluent a.,** that in which little speech is produced and is uttered slowly, with great effort and poor articulation, due to a lesion in Broca's area. **receptive a.,** inability to understand written, spoken, or tactile speech symbols. **sensory a.,** receptive a. **total a.,** global a. **visual a.,** alexia. **Wernicke's a.,** receptive a.

aphasiology (-ol′ah-je) the scientific study of aphasia and the specific neurologic lesions producing it.

aphemia (ah-fe′me-ah) expressive aphasia.

apheresis (ah-fē′ris-is) any procedure in which blood is withdrawn from a donor, a portion (plasma, leukocytes, platelets, etc.) is separated and retained, and the remainder is retransfused into the donor. It includes leukapheresis, thrombocytapheresis, etc. Called also *pheresis*.

aphonia (a-fo′ne-ah) loss of voice; inability to produce vocal sounds. **a. clerico′rum,** see under *dysphonia.*

aphotic (a-fōt′ik) without light; totally dark.

aphrasia (ah-fra′zhe-ah) inability to speak.

aphrenia (ah-fre′ne-ah) dementia.

aphrodisiac (af″ro-diz′e-ak) 1. arousing sexual desire. 2. a drug that arouses sexual desire.

aphtha (af′thah), pl. *aph′thae* [L.] (usually plural) small ulcers, especially the whitish or reddish spots in the mouth characteristic of aphthous stomatitis. **aph′thous,** adj. **Bednar's a.,** an infected traumatic ulcer on the posterior hard palate in infants. **contagious aphthae, epizootic aphthae,** foot-and-mouth disease.

aphthosis (af-tho′sis) a condition marked by the presence of aphthae.

aphylaxis (a″fi-lak′sis) absence of phylaxis or immunity. **aphylac′tic,** adj.

apical (ap′ĭ-k'l) pertaining to an apex.

apicectomy (a″pĭ-sek′to-me) excision of the apex of the petrous portion of the temporal bone.

apicitis (-sīt′is) inflammation of an apex, as of the lung or the root of a tooth.

apicoectomy (-ko-ek′tah-me) excision of the apical portion of the root of a tooth through an opening in overlying tissues of the jaw.

apicolysis (a″pĭ-kol′ĭ-sis) surgical collapse of the apex of the lung to obliterate the apical cavity.

aplanatic (ap″lah-nat′ik) correcting spherical aberration, as an aplanatic lens.

aplasia (ah-pla′ze-ah) lack of development of an organ or tissue, or of the cellular products from an organ or tissue. **aplas′tic,** adj. **a. axia′lis extracortica′lis conge′nita,** familial centrolobar sclerosis. **a. cu′tis conge′nita,** localized failure of development of skin, most commonly of the scalp; the defects are usually covered by a thin translucent membrane or scar tissue, or may be raw, ulcerated, or covered by granulation tissue.

apnea (ap′ne-ah) 1. cessation of breathing. 2. asphyxia. **apne′ic,** adj. **sleep a.,** transient attacks of failure of autonomic control of respiration, becoming more pronounced during sleep and resulting in acidosis and pulmonary arteriolar vasoconstriction and hypertension.

apneusis (ap-noo′sis) sustained inspiratory effort unrelieved by expiration. **apneu′stic,** adj.

apo- word element [Gr.], *away from; separated; derived from.*

apochromat (ap″o-kro′mat) an apochromatic objective.

apochromatic (-kro-mat′ik) free from chromatic and spherical aberrations.

apocope (ah-pok′ah-pe) a cutting off; amputation. **apocop′tic,** adj.

apocrine (ap′o-krīn) exhibiting that type of glandular secretion in which the free end of the secreting cell is cast off along with the secretory products accumulated therein (e.g., mammary and sweat glands).

apoenzyme (ap″o-en′zīm) the protein compo-

nent of an enzyme separable from the prosthetic group (coenzyme) but requiring the presence of the prosthetic group to form the functioning compound (holoenzyme).

apoferritin (-fĕ′rĭ-tin) an apoprotein that can bind many atoms of iron per molecule, forming ferritin, the intracellular storage form of iron.

apogee (ap′ah-je) the state of greatest severity of a disease.

apolar (a-po′ler) having neither poles nor processes; without polarity.

apolipoprotein (ap″o-lip″o-pro′tēn) a protein moiety occurring in plasma lipoproteins; there are five families of apolipoproteins, designated A–E.

apomorphine (ap″o-mor′fēn) a morphine derivative, $C_{17}H_{17}NO_2$, used as a potent and prompt emetic; also used as the hydrochloride salt.

aponeurorrhaphy (-noo-ror′ah-fe) suture of an aponeurosis.

aponeurosis (-noo-ro′sis), pl. *aponeuro′ses* [Gr.] a sheetlike tendinous expansion, mainly serving to connect a muscle with the parts it moves. **aponeurot′ic,** adj.

apophysis (ah-pof′ĭ-sis), pl. *apoph′yses* [Gr.] any outgrowth or swelling, especially a bony outgrowth that has never been entirely separated from the bone of which it forms a part, such as a process, tubercle, or tuberosity. **apophys′eal,** adj.

apophysitis (ah-pof″ĭ-zīt′is) inflammation of an apophysis.

apoplectiform (ap″ah-plek″tĭ-form) resembling apoplexy.

apoplexy (ap′ah-plek″se) 1. sudden neurologic impairment due to a cerebrovascular disorder, limited classically to intracranial hemorrhage, but extended by some to include occlusive cerebrovascular lesions; see *stroke syndrome.* 2. copious extravasation of blood within any organ. **apoplec′tic,** adj. **adrenal a.,** sudden massive hemorrhage into the adrenal gland, occurring in Waterhouse-Friderichsen syndrome. **pancreatic a.,** extensive hemorrhage of the pancreas; seen in cardiac failure and portal hypertension.

apoprotein (ap″ah-pro′tēn) the protein moiety of a molecule or complex, as of a lipoprotein.

aporepressor (-re-pres′er) in genetic theory, a product of regulator genes that combines with the corepressor to form the complete repressor.

apothecary (ah-poth′ĭ-kĕ-re) pharmacist.

apotripsis (ap″ah-trip′sis) removal of a corneal opacity.

apparatus (ap″ah-rāt′is) an arrangement of a number of parts acting together to perform a special function. **Golgi a.,** see under *complex.* **juxtaglomerular a.,** see under *cell.* **Kirschner's a.,** a wire and stirrup apparatus for applying skeletal traction in leg fractures. **lacrimal a., a. lacrima′lis,** the lacrimal gland and ducts and associated structures. **subneural a.,** an infolding of the sarcolemma, forming a series of grooves beneath the terminal branches of motor nerve fibers at neuromuscular junctions.

appendage (ah-pen′dij) a subordinate portion of

a structure, or an outgrowth, such as a tail. **epiploic a's,** appendices epiploicae.

appendectomy (ap″en-dek′tah-me) excision of the vermiform appendix.

appendicitis (-sīt′is) inflammation of the vermiform appendix. **acute a.,** appendicitis of acute onset, requiring prompt surgery, and usually marked by pain in the right lower abdominal quadrant, referred rebound tenderness, overlying muscle spasm, and cutaneous hyperesthesia. **chronic a.,** 1. that characterized by fibrotic thickening of the organ wall due to previous acute inflammation. 2. formerly, chronic or recurrent pain in the appendiceal area, evidence of acute inflammation being absent. **fulminating a.,** that marked by sudden onset and death. **gangrenous a.,** that complicated by gangrene of the organ, due to interference of blood supply. **obstructive a.,** a common form with obstruction of the lumen, usually by a fecalith.

appendicostomy (ah-pen″dĭ-kos′tah-me) surgical creation of an opening into the vermiform appendix to irrigate or drain the large bowel.

appendix (ah-pen′diks), pl. *appen′dices* [L.] 1. a supplementary, accessory, or dependent part attached to a main structure. 2. vermiform a. **appen′dices epiplo′icae,** small peritoneum-covered tabs of fat attached in rows along the taeniae coli. **vermiform a., a. vermifor′mis,** a wormlike diverticulum of the cecum. **xiphoid a.,** see under *process.*

apperception (ap″er-sep′shin) the process of receiving, appreciating, and interpreting sensory impressions.

appestat (ap′ĭ-stat) the brain center (probably in the hypothalamus) concerned in controlling the appetite.

applanometer (ap″lah-nom′it-er) an instrument for determining intraocular pressure in the detection of glaucoma; see *tonometer.*

appliance (ah-pli′ins) a device used for performing or for facilitating the performance of a particular function.

apposition (ap″o-zish′in) juxtaposition; the placing of things in proximity; specifically, the deposition of successive layers upon those already present, as in cell walls.

apprehension (ap″re-hen′shin) 1. perception and understanding. 2. anticipatory fear or anxiety.

approach (ah-prōch′) 1. in surgery, the specific procedures by which an organ or part is exposed. 2. in psychiatry, the manner in which personal conflicts are dealt with.

approximation (ah-prok″sĭ-ma′shin) 1. the act or process of bringing into proximity or apposition. 2. a numerical value of limited accuracy.

apraxia (ah-prak′se-ah) loss of ability to carry out familiar purposeful movements in the absence of motor or sensory impairment, especially inability to use objects correctly. **amnestic a.,** loss of ability to carry out a movement on command due to inability to remember the command. **Bruns' a. of gait,** a common disorder of the elderly in which the patient walks with a broad-based gait, taking short steps and placing the feet flat on the ground. **cortical a.,**

motor a. **ideational a.,** sensory a. **innervation a., motor a.,** loss of ability to make proper use of an object, although its proper nature is recognized. **sensory a.,** loss of ability to use an object due to lack of perception of its purpose.

aprobarbital (ap″ro-bar′bĭ-tal) a hypnotic and sedative, $C_{10}H_{14}N_2O_3$.

A.P.S. American Physiological Society.

apsychia (ah-si′ke-ah) loss of consciousness.

A.P.T.A. American Physical Therapy Association.

aptyalism (ap-ti′ah-lizm) xerostomia; deficiency or absence of saliva.

APUD (*amine precursor uptake and decarboxylation*) see *APUD cells.*

apudoma (ah-pu-do′mah) a tumor derived from APUD cells.

apyretic (a″pi-ret′ik) without fever; afebrile.

apyrexia (ah″pi-rek′se-ah) absence of fever.

A.Q. achievement quotient.

aq. [L.] *a′qua* (water). **aq. dest.,** *a′qua destilla′ta* (distilled water).

aqua (ak′wah) [L.] 1. water, H_2O. 2. a saturated solution of a volatile oil or other aromatic or volatile substance in purified water.

aquaphobia (ak″wah-fo′be-ah) morbid fear of water.

aqueduct (ak′wĭ-dukt″) any canal or passage. **cerebral a.,** a narrow channel in the midbrain connecting the third and fourth ventricles. **a. of cochlea, cochlear a.,** cochlear canaliculus; a small canal in the petrous portion of the temporal bone that interconnects the scala tympani with the subarachnoid cavity. **sylvian a., a. of Sylvius, ventricular a.,** cerebral a.

aqueous (a′kwe-is) 1. watery; prepared with water. 2. see under *humor.*

AR alarm reaction; aortic regurgitation; artificial respiration.

Ar chemical symbol, *argon.*

ara-A adenine arabinoside; see *vidarabine.*

ara-C cytosine arabinoside; see *cytarabine.*

arachic acid, arachidic acid (ah-rak′ik, ar″ah-kid′ik) a saturated fatty acid, $C_{19}H_{39}COOH$, occurring in peanut oil.

arachidonic acid (ah-rah-kĭ-don′ik) a polyunsaturated essential fatty acid, $C_{19}H_{39}COOH$; a constituent of lecithin and a source of some prostaglandins.

Arachnida (ah-rak′nĭ-dah) a class of the Arthropoda, including the spiders, scorpions, ticks, and mites.

arachnodactyly (ah-rak″no-dak′tĭ-le) extreme length and slenderness of fingers and toes.

arachnoid (ah-rak′noid) 1. resembling a spider's web. 2. the delicate membrane interposed between the dura mater and the pia mater, and with them constituting the meninges.

arachnophobia (ah-rak″no-fo′be-ah) morbid fear of spiders.

araphia (ah-ra′fe-ah) dysraphia. **ara′phic,** adj.

arbor (ar′bor), pl. *arbo′res* [L.] a treelike structure or part. **a. vi′tae,** 1. treelike outlines seen in a median section of the cerebellum. 2. palmate folds.

arborization (ar″ber-ĭ-za′shin) a collection of branches, as the branching terminus of a nerve-cell process.

arborvirus (-vi′ris) arbovirus.

arbovirus (ar″bo-vi′ris) any of a group of viruses, including the causative agents of yellow fever, viral encephalitides, and certain febrile infections, transmitted to man by various mosquitoes and ticks; those transmitted by ticks are often considered in a separate category (tick-borne viruses). **arbovi′ral,** adj.

ARC AIDS-related complex.

A.R.C. American Red Cross; anomalous retinal correspondence.

arc (ark) a structure or projected path having a curved outline; by extension, a visible electrical discharge taking the outline of an arc. In neurophysiology, the pathway of neural reactions. **reflex a.,** the neural arc utilized in a reflex action; an impulse travels centrally over afferent fibers to a nerve center, and the response outward to an effector organ or part over efferent fibers; see Plate XIV.

arch (arch) a structure of bowlike or curved outline. **a. of aorta,** the curving portion between the ascending aorta and the descending aorta, giving rise to the brachiocephalic trunk and the left common carotid and the left subclavian artery. **aortic a's,** paired vessels arching from the ventral to the dorsal aorta through the branchial clefts of fishes and amniote embryos. In mammalian development, arches 1 and 2 disappear; 3 joins the common to the internal carotid artery; 4 becomes the arch of the aorta and joins the aorta and subclavian artery; 5 disappears; 6 forms the pulmonary arteries and, until birth, the ductus arteriosus. **branchial a's,** paired arched columns that bear the gills in lower aquatic vertebrates and which, in embryos of higher vertebrates, become modified into structures of the head and neck. **dental a.,** the curving structure formed by the teeth in their normal position; the *inferior dental a.* is formed by the mandibular teeth, the *superior dental a.* by the maxillary teeth. **double aortic a.,** a congenital anomaly in which the aorta divides into two branches which embrace the trachea and esophagus and reunite to form the descending aorta. **a's of foot,** the longitudinal and transverse arches of the foot. **lingual a.,** a wire appliance that conforms to the lingual aspect of the dental arch, used to promote or prevent movement of the teeth in orthodontic work. **mandibular a.,** 1. the first branchial arch, from which are developed the bone of the lower jaw, malleus, and incus. 2. inferior dental a. **maxillary a.,** 1. the palatal arch. 2. superior dental a. 3. residual dental a. **open pubic a.,** a congenital anomaly in which the pubic arch is not fused, the bodies of the pubic bones being spread apart. **oral a., palatal a.,** one formed by the roof of the mouth from the teeth (or residual dental arch) on one side to those on the other. **palmar a's,** two arches in the palm, one (*deep palmar a.*) formed by anastomosis of the terminal part of the radial artery with the deep branch of the ulnar, and the other (*superficial palmar a.*) by anastomosis of the terminal part

of the ulnar artery with the superficial palmar branch of the radial. **passive lingual a.,** an orthodontic appliance for maintaining space and preserving arch length when bilateral primary molars are prematurely lost. **plantar a.,** the arch in the foot formed by anastomosis of the lateral plantar artery with the deep plantar branch of the dorsal artery. **pubic a., a. of pubis,** the arch formed by the conjoined rami of the ischial and pubic bones on two sides of the body. **pulmonary a.,** the most caudal of the aortic arches, which become the pulmonary arteries. **right aortic a.,** a congenital anomaly in which the aorta is displaced to the right and passes behind the esophagus, thus forming a vascular ring that may cause compression of the trachea and esophagus. **supraorbital a.,** curved margin of frontal bone forming upper boundary of orbit. **tarsal a's,** two arches of the median palpebral artery, one of which supplies the upper eyelid, the other the lower. **tendinous a.,** a linear thickening of fascia over some part of a muscle. **zygomatic a.,** one formed by processes of zygomatic and temporal bones.

archaeocerebellum (ar″ke-o-sĕ-rĕ-bel′um) the phylogenetically old part of the cerebellum, viz., the flocculonodular node and the lingula.

archaeocortex (ar″ke-o-kor′teks) that part of the cerebral cortex (pallium) that with the palaeocortex develops in association with the olfactory system and is phylogenetically older than the neocortex (neopallium) and lacks its layered structure.

arch(i)-, archae(o)-, arche(o)- word element [Gr.], *ancient; beginning; original; first; chief; leading.*

archencephalon (ark″en-sef′ah-lon) the primitive brain from which the midbrain and forebrain develop.

archenteron (ark-en′ter-on) the primitive digestive cavity of those embryonic forms whose blastula become a gastrula by invagination.

archeokinetic (ar″ke-o-ki-net′ik) relating to the primitive motor nerve mechanism seen in the peripheral and ganglionic nervous systems.

archetype (-tīp) an ideal, original, or standard type or form.

archinephron (ar″kĭ-nef′ron) a unit of the pronephros.

archipallium (-pal′e-um) archaeocortex.

arciform (ar′sĭ-form) arcuate.

arcuation (ar″ku-a′shin) a curvature, especially an abnormal curvature.

arcus (ar′kus), pl. *ar′cus* [L.] arch; bow. **a. adipo′sus,** a. corneae. **a. cor′neae,** a gray opaque line surrounding the margin of the cornea, but separated from the margin by an area of clear cornea, sometimes present at birth, but usually occurring bilaterally in persons of 50 years or older as a result of lipoid degeneration. **a. juveni′lis,** a corneae.

area (ār′e-ah), pl. *a′reae, areas* [L.] a limited space; in anatomy, a specific surface or functional region. **association a's,** areas of the cerebral cortex (excluding primary areas) connected with each other and with the neothalamus; they are responsible for higher mental and emotional processes, including memory, learning, etc. **Broca's motor speech a.**, an area comprising parts of the opercular and triangular portions of the inferior frontal gyrus; injury to this area may result in motor aphasia. **Brodmann's a's**, areas of the cerebral cortex distinguished by differences in arrangement of their six cellular layers; identified by numbering each area. **embryonic a.**, see under *disk*. **Kiesselbach's a.**, one on the anterior part of the nasal septum above the intermaxillary bone, richly supplied with capillaries, and a common site of nosebleed. **motor a.**, that area of the cerebral cortex which, on brief electrical stimulation, shows the lowest threshold and shortest latency for the production of muscle movement. **a. perfora'ta**, perforated space. **prefrontal a.**, the cortex of the frontal lobe immediately in front of the premotor cortex, concerned chiefly with associative functions. **premotor a.**, the motor cortex of the frontal lobe immediately in front of the precentral gyrus. **primary a's**, areas of the cerebral cortex comprising the motor and sensory regions; cf. *association a's*. **a. subcallo'sa, subcallosal a.**, an area of the cortex on the medial surface of each cerebral hemisphere, immediately in front of the gyrus subcallosus. **thymus-dependent a's**, those areas of the peripheral lymphoid organs populated by the thymus-dependent lymphocytes, e.g., the pericortical areas of the lymph nodes, the centers of the malpighian corpuscle of the spleen, and the internodular zone of Peyer's patches. **thymus-independent a's**, those areas of the peripheral lymphoid organs populated by thymus-independent lymphocytes, e.g., the medullary and outer cortical regions of the lymph node. **vocal a.**, the part of the glottis between the vocal cords. **Wernicke's a.**, originally a term denoting a speech center on the posterior part of the superior temporal gyrus, but not including the supramarginal and angular gyri.

Arenaviridae (ah″re-nah-vi′ri-de) a family of viruses comprising the arenaviruses.

arenavirus (ah″re-nah-vi′ris) any of a group of spherical or pleomorphic RNA viruses containing host cell–derived ribonucleoproteins, including Lassa virus, lymphocytic choriomeningitis (LCM) virus, and Tacaribe viruses. The natural hosts are rodents.

areola (ah-re′ah-lah), pl. *are'olae* [L.] 1. any minute space or interstice in a tissue. 2. a circular area of different color surrounding a central point, as that surrounding the nipple of the breast. **are'olar**, adj.

Arg arginine.

Argas (ar′gas) a genus of ticks (family Argasidae), parasitic in poultry and other birds and sometimes man. **A. per'sicus**, the fowl tick, parasitic in chickens and turkeys, the vector of fowl spirochetosis.

Argasidae (ar-gas′ĭ-de) a family of arthropods (superfamily Ixodidea) made up of the soft-bodied ticks.

argentaffin (ar-jen′tah-fin) staining with silver and chromium salts; see also under *cell*.

argentaffinoma (ar″jen-taf″ĭ-no′mah) carci-

noid, a tumor of the gastrointestinal tract formed from the argentaffin cells of the enteric canal and producing carcinoid syndrome.

argentum (-tum) [L.] silver (symbol Ag).

arginase (ar′jĭ-nās) an enzyme existing primarily in the liver, which splits arginine into urea and ornithine.

arginine (-nēn) an amino acid occurring in proteins; it is also involved in the urea cycle, which converts ammonia to urea.

argininosuccinate (ar″jĭ-nĭ″no-suk′sĭ-nāt) a compound formed by the condensation of aspartic acid and citrulline; an intermediate in the urea cycle.

argininosuccinic acid (-suk-sin′ik) an amino acid normally formed in the ornithine cycle of urea formation in the liver, but not normally present in the urine.

argininosuccinicaciduria (-suk-sin″ik-as″id-ūr′e-ah) excretion in the urine of argininosuccinic acid, a feature of an inborn error of metabolism marked also by mental retardation.

argon (ar′gon) chemical element (*see table*), at. no. 18, symbol Ar.

argyria (ar-ji′re-ah) poisoning by silver or its salts; chronic argyria is marked by a permanent ashen-gray discoloration of the skin, conjunctivae, and internal organs.

argyrophil (ar-ji′ro-fil) capable of binding silver salts.

ariboflavinosis (a-ri″bo-fla″vĭ-no′sis) deficiency of riboflavin in the diet, marked by angular cheilosis, nasolabial lesions, optic changes, and seborrheic dermatitis.

Aristocort (ah-ris′tah-cort) trademark for a preparation of triamcinolone.

arm (arm) 1. brachium: the upper extremity from shoulder to elbow; popularly, the entire extremity, from shoulder to hand. 2. an armlike part, e.g., the portion of the chromatid extending in either direction from the centromere of a mitotic chromosome. **chromosome a.**, either of two segments of a chromosome separated by the centromere.

Armillifer (ar-mil′ĭ-fer) a genus of wormlike endoparasites of reptiles; the larvae of *A. armilla'tus* and *A. monilifor'mis* are occasionally found in man.

aromatase (ah-ro′mah-tās) an enzyme that catalyzes the aromatization of its substrate, e.g., the conversion of testosterone to estradiol.

aromatic (ar″o-mat′ik) 1. having a spicy odor. 2. in chemistry, denoting a compound (an arene) containing a resonance-stabilized ring, e.g., benzene or naphthalene.

arrector (ah-rek′tor), pl. *arrecto'res* [L.] raising, or that which raises; an arrector muscle.

arrest (ah-rest′) cessation or stoppage, as of a function or a disease process. **cardiac a.**, sudden cessation of cardiac function. **developmental a.**, a temporary or permanent cessation of development. **epiphyseal a.**, premature interruption of longitudinal growth of bone by fusion of the epiphysis and diaphysis. **maturation a.**, interruption of the process of development, as of blood cells, before the final stage is reached. **sinus a.**, a pause in cardiac rhythm due to a momentary failure of the sinus node to initiate an impulse.

arrheno- word element [Gr.], *male; masculine.*

arrhenoblastoma (ah-re″no-blas-to′mah) a neoplasm of the ovary, sometimes causing virilization.

arrhinia (ah-rin′e-ah) arhinia.

arrhythmia (ah-rith′me-ah) variation from the normal rhythm of the heart beat. **arrhyth′mic,** adj. **sinus a.,** the physiologic cyclic variation in heart rate related to vagal impulses to the sinoatrial node; it occurs commonly in children and in the aged.

arrhythmogenic (ah-rith″mah-jen′ik) producing or promoting arrhythmia.

A.R.R.S. American Roentgen Ray Society.

arsenate (ar′sah-nāt) any salt of arsenic acid.

arseniasis (ar″sah-ni′ah-sis) chronic arsenic poisoning; see *arsenic* (1).

arsenic (ar′sah-nik) 1. a medicinal and poisonous element (*see table*), at. no. 33, symbol As. Acute arsenic poisoning may result in shock and death, with skin rashes, vomiting, diarrhea, abdominal pain, muscular cramps, and swelling of eyelids, feet, and hands; the chronic form, due to ingestion of small amounts of arsenic over long periods, is marked by skin pigmentation accompanied by scaling, hyperkeratosis of palms and soles, transverse lines on the fingernails, headache, peripheral neuropathy, and confusion. 2. pertaining to or containing arsenic in a pentavalent state.

arsenoblast (ar-sen′ah-blast) the male element of a zygote; a male pronucleus.

arsine (ar′sēn) a very poisonous gas, AsH₃; some of its compounds have been used in warfare.

A.R.T. Accredited Record Technicians.

Artane (ar′tān) trademark for preparations of trihexyphenidyl hydrochloride.

artefact (art′ah-fakt) artifact.

arteralgia (art″er-al′je-ah) pain emanating from an artery, such as headache from an inflamed temporal artery.

arteria (ar-tēr′e-ah), pl. *arte′riae* [L.] artery. **a. luso′ria,** an abnormally situated retroesophageal vessel, usually the subclavian artery from the aortic arch.

arteriectasis (ar-tēr″e-ek′tah-sis) dilatation and, usually, lengthening of an artery.

arterio- word element [L., Gr.], *artery.*

arteriography (ar-tēr″e-og′rah-fe) radiography of an artery or arterial system after injection of a contrast medium into the blood stream. **catheter a.,** radiography of vessels after introduction of contrast material through a catheter inserted into an artery. **selective a.,** radiography of a specific vessel which is opacified by a medium introduced directly into it, usually via a catheter.

arteriol(o)- word element [L.], *arteriole.*

arteriola (ar-tēr″e-o′lah), pl. *arteriolae* [L.] arteriole.

arteriole (ar-tēr′e-ōl) a minute arterial branch. **arterio′lar,** adj. **glomerular a., afferent,** a branch of an interlobar artery that goes to a renal artery. **glomerular a., efferent,** one aris-

ing from a renal glomerulus, breaking up into capillaries to supply renal tubules. **postglomerular a.,** efferent glomerular a. **precapillary a's,** arterial capillaries. **preglomerular a.,** afferent glomerular a.

arteriolith (ar-tēr′e-ah-lith″) a chalky concretion in an artery.

arteriolonecrosis (ar-tēr″e-o″lo-nĭ-kro′sis) necrosis or destruction of arterioles.

arteriolosclerosis (-skler-o′sis) sclerosis and thickening of the walls of arterioles. The hyaline form may be associated with nephrosclerosis, the hyperplastic with malignant hypertension, nephrosclerosis, and scleroderma. **arteriolosclerot′ic,** adj.

arteriomotor (ar-tēr″e-o-mōt′er) involving or causing dilation or constriction of arteries.

arteriomyomatosis (-mi″o-mah-to′sis) growth of muscular fibers in the walls of an artery, causing thickening.

arteriopathy (ar-tēr″e-op′ah-the) any disease of an artery. **hypertensive a.,** widespread involvement of arterioles and small arteries, associated with arterial hypertension, and characterized by hypertrophy of the tunica media.

arterioplasty (ar-tēr′e-o-plas″te) surgical repair or reconstruction of an artery; applied especially to Matas' operation for aneurysm.

arteriorrhaphy (ar-tēr″e-or′ah-fe) suture of an artery.

arteriorrhexis (ar-tēr″e-o-rek′sis) rupture of an artery.

arteriosclerosis (-skler-o′sis) a group of diseases characterized by thickening and loss of elasticity of the arterial walls occurring in three forms, atherosclerosis, Mönckeberg's arteriosclerosis, and arteriolosclerosis. **arteriosclerot′ic,** adj. **Mönckeberg's a.,** arteriosclerosis with extensive deposits of calcium in the middle coat of the artery. **a. obli′terans,** that in which proliferation of the intima of the small vessels has caused complete obliteration of the lumen of the artery. **peripheral a.,** arteriosclerosis of the extremities.

arteriostenosis (ar-tēr″e-o-stĭ-no′sis) constriction of an artery.

arteriosympathectomy (-sim″pah-thek′tah-me) periarterial sympathectomy.

arteriotony (ar-ter″e-ot′ah-ne) blood pressure.

arteritis (art″er-īt′is) inflammation of an artery. **brachiocephalic a., a. brachiocephal′ica,** pulseless disease. **coronary a.,** inflammation of the coronary arteries. **cranial a.,** temporal a. **giant-cell a.,** temporal a. **a. oblit′erans,** endarteritis obliterans. **rheumatic a.,** generalized inflammation of arterioles and arterial capillaries occurring in rheumatic fever. **Takayasu's a.,** pulseless disease. **temporal a.,** a chronic vascular disease of unknown origin, occurring in the elderly, characterized by severe headache, fever, and accumulation of giant cells in the walls of medium-sized arteries, especially the temporal arteries. Ocular involvement may cause blindness.

artery (art′er-e) a vessel in which blood flows away from the heart, in the systemic circulation carrying oxygenated blood. **arte′rial,** adj.

For named arteries of the body, see Table of Arteries and see Plates VIII and IX.

arthr(o)- word element [Gr.], *joint; articulation.*

arthragra (ar-thrag'rah) gouty pain in a joint.

arthralgia (ar-thral'je-ah) pain in a joint.

arthritide (ar'thrĭ-tīd) a skin eruption of gouty origin.

arthritis (ar-thrīt'is) inflammation of a joint. **arthrit'ic,** adj. **acute a.,** arthritis marked by pain, heat, redness, and swelling. **atrophic a.,** rheumatoid a. **chronic inflammatory a.,** rheumatoid a. **a. defor'mans,** rheumatoid a. **degenerative a.,** osteoarthritis. **hypertrophic a.,** osteoarthritis. **infectious a.,** arthritis caused by bacteria, rickettsiae, mycoplasmas, viruses, fungi or parasites. **Lyme a.,** a recurrent, tickborne form of arthritis affecting a few large joints, especially the knees, shoulders, and elbows, and associated with erythema chronicum migrans, malaise, and myalgia. **menopausal a.,** that seen in some menopausal women, due to ovarian hormonal deficiency, and marked by pain in the small joints, shoulders, elbows, or knees. **a. mu'tilans,** severe deforming polyarthritis with gross bone and cartilage destruction an atypical variant of rheumatoid arthritis. **rheumatoid a.,** a chronic systemic disease primarily of the joints, usually polyarticular, marked by inflammatory changes in the synovial membranes and articular structures and by atrophy and rarefaction of the bones. In late stages, deformity and ankylosis develop. The cause is unknown, but autoimmune mechanisms and viral infection have been postulated. **rheumatoid a., juvenile,** rheumatoid arthritis in children, with swelling, tenderness, and pain involving one or more joints, leading to impaired growth and development, limitation of movement, and ankylosis and flexion contractures of the joints; often accompanied by systemic manifestations. **suppurative a.,** a form marked by purulent joint infiltration, chiefly due to bacterial infection but also seen in Reiter's disease. **tuberculous a.,** that due to tuberculous infection, usually affecting a single joint, marked by chronic inflammation with effusion and destruction of contiguous bone.

arthrocentesis (ar''thro-sen-te'sis) puncture of a joint cavity with aspiration of fluid.

arthrochondritis (-kon-drīt'is) inflammation of the cartilage of a joint.

arthroclasia (-kla'ze-ah) surgical breaking of an ankylosis to permit a joint to move.

arthrodia (ar-thro'de-ah) a synovial joint which allows a gliding motion.

arthrodysplasia (-dis-pla'ze-ah) hereditary deformity of various joints.

arthroempyesis (-em''pi-e'sis) suppuration within a joint.

arthrography (ar-throg'rah-fe) radiography of a joint after injection of opaque contrast material. **air a.,** pneumarthrography.

arthrogryposis (ar''thro-grĭ-po'sis) 1. persistent flexure of a joint. 2. tetanoid spasm.

arthrolith (ar'thro-lith) calculous deposit within a joint.

arthroneuralgia (ar''thro-noo-ral'je-ah) pain in or around a joint.

arthro-ophthalmopathy (-of''thal-mop'ah-the) an association of degenerative joint disease and eye disease.

arthropathy (ar-throp'ah-the) any joint disease. **arthropath'ic,** adj. **Charcot's a., neuropathic a.,** chronic progressive degeneration of the stress-bearing portion of a joint, with hypertrophic changes at the periphery; it is associated with neurologic disorders involving loss of sensation in the joint. **chondrocalcific a.,** progressive polyarthritis with joint swelling and bony enlargement, most commonly in the small joints of the hand but also affecting other joints, characterized roentgenographically by narrowing of the joint space with subchondral erosions and sclerosis and frequently chondrocalcinosis. **osteopulmonary a.,** clubbing of fingers and toes and enlargement of ends of the long bones, in cardiac or pulmonary disease.

arthroplasty (-plas''te) plastic repair of a joint.

Arthropoda (ar-throp'ah-dah) the largest phylum of animals, composed of bilaterally symmetrical organisms with hard, segmented bodies bearing jointed legs, including, among other related forms, arachnids, crustaceans, and insects, many species of which are parasites or are vectors of disease-causing organisms.

arthropyosis (ar''thro-pi-o'sis) formation of pus in a joint cavity.

arthrosclerosis (-skler-o'sis) stiffening or hardening of the joints.

arthroscintigram (ar''thro-sin'tĭ-gram) a scintiscan of a joint.

arthrosis (ar-thro'sis) 1. a joint or articulation. 2. disease of a joint.

arthrostomy (ar-thros'tah-me) surgical creation of an opening into a joint, as for drainage.

arthrosynovitis (ar''thro-sin''o-vi'tis) inflammation of the synovial membrane of a joint.

articular (ar-tik'u-ler) pertaining to a joint.

articulare (ar-tĭ''ku-la're) the point of intersection of the dorsal contours of the articular process of the mandible and the temporal bone.

articulate (ar-tik'u-lit, -lāt) 1. divided into or united by joints. 2. enunciated in words and sentences. 3. to divide into or to unite so as to form a joint. 4. in dentistry, to adjust or place the teeth in their proper relation to each other in making an artificial denture.

articulatio (-la'she-o), pl. *articulatio'nes* [L.] an articulation or joint.

articulation (-la'shin) 1. a joint; the place of union or junction between two or more bones of the skeleton. 2. enunciation of words and sentences. 3. in dentistry: (a) the contact relationship of the occlusal surfaces of the teeth while in action; (b) the arrangement of artificial teeth so as to accommodate the various positions of the mouth and to serve the purpose of the natural teeth which they are to replace.

articulo (-lo) [L.] at the moment, or crisis. **a. mor'tis,** at the point or moment of death.

artifact (art'ĭ-fakt) any artificial (man-made) product; anything not naturally present, but introduced by some external source.

TABLE OF ARTERIES

COMMON NAME*	NA EQUIVALENT†	ORIGIN*	BRANCHES*	DISTRIBUTION
accompanying a. of ischiadic nerve. See sciatic a.				
alveolar a's, anterior superior	aa. alveolares superiores anteriores	infraorbital a.	dental and peridental branches	incisor and canine regions of upper jaw, maxillary sinus
alveolar a., inferior	a. alveolaris inferior	maxillary a.	dental, peridental, mental, mylohyoid branches	lower jaw, lower lip, chin
alveolar a., posterior superior	a. alveolaris superior posterior	maxillary a.	dental and peridental branches	molar and premolar regions of upper jaw, maxillary sinus
angular a.	a. angularis	facial a.		lacrimal sac, lower eyelid, nose
a. of angular gyrus	a. gyri angularis	terminal part of middle cerebral a.		temporal, parietal, occipital lobes
aorta	aorta	left ventricle		
abdominal aorta	pars abdominalis aortae	lower portion of descending aorta, from aortic hiatus of diaphragm to bifurcation into common iliac a's	inferior phrenic, lumbar, median sacral, superior and inferior mesenteric, middle suprarenal, renal, and testicular or ovarian a's, celiac trunk	
arch of aorta	arcus aortae	continuation of ascending aorta	brachiocephalic trunk, left common carotid and left subclavian a's; continues as descending (thoracic) aorta	
ascending aorta	pars ascendens aortae	proximal portion of aorta, arising from left ventricle	right and left coronary a's; continues as arch of aorta	
descending aorta. See thoracic aorta and abdominal aorta	pars descendens aortae	continuation of aorta from arch of aorta to division into common iliac arteries		
thoracic aorta	pars thoracica aortae	proximal portion of descending aorta, continuing from arch of aorta to aortic hiatus of diaphragm	bronchial, esophageal, pericardiac, and mediastinal branches, superior phrenic a's, posterior intercostal a's [III–XI], subcostal a's, continues as abdominal aorta	
appendicular a.	a. appendicularis	ileocolic a.		vermiform appendix
arcuate a. of foot	a. arcuata pedis	dorsalis pedis a.	deep plantar branch, dorsal metatarsal a's	foot, toes
arcuate a's of kidney	aa. arcuatae renis	interlobar a.	interlobular a's, straight arterioles of kidney	parenchyma of kidney
auditory a., internal. See a. of labyrinth				
auricular a., deep	a. auricularis profunda	maxillary a.		skin of auditory canal, tympanic membrane, temporomandibular joint

48

49

auricular a., posterior	a. auricularis posterior	external carotid a.	auricular and occipital branches, stylomastoid a.	middle ear, mastoid cells, auricle, parotid gland, digastric and other muscles
axillary a.	a. axillaris	continuation of subclavian a.	subscapular branches, highest thoracic, thoracoacromial, lateral thoracic, subscapular, and anterior and posterior circumflex humeral a's	upper limb, axilla, chest, shoulder
basilar a.	a. basilaris	from junction of right and left vertebral a's	pontine branches, anterior inferior cerebellar, labyrinthine, superior cerebellar, posterior cerebral a's	brain stem, internal ear, cerebellum, posterior cerebrum
brachial a.	a. brachialis	continuation of axillary a.	superficial and deep brachial, nutrient of humerus, superior and inferior ulnar collateral, radial, ulnar a's	shoulder, arm, forearm, hand
brachial a., deep	a. profunda brachii	brachial a.	nutrient to humerus, deltoid branch, middle and radial collateral a's	humerus, muscles and skin of arm
brachial a., superficial	a. brachialis superficialis	variant brachial a., taking a more superficial course than usual	see *brachial a.*	see *brachial a.*
brachiocephalic trunk	truncus brachiocephalicus	arch of aorta	right common carotid, right subclavian a's	right side of head and neck, right arm
buccal a.	a. buccalis	maxillary a.		buccinator muscle, oral mucous membrane
a. of bulb of penis	a. bulbi penis	internal pudendal a.		bulbourethral gland, bulb of penis
bulbourethral a. *See* a. of bulb of penis				
a. of bulb of vestibule of vagina	a. bulbi vestibuli vaginae	internal pudendal a.		bulb of vestibule of vagina, Bartholin glands
callosomarginal a.	a. callosomarginalis	anterior cerebral a.	anteromedial frontal, intermediomedial frontal, posteromedial frontal, cingular branches	medial and upper lateral surfaces of cerebral hemisphere
caroticotympanic a's	aa. caroticotympanicae	internal carotid a.		tympanic cavity
carotid a., common	a. carotis communis	brachiocephalic trunk (right), arch of aorta (left)	external and internal carotid a's	see *carotid a., external* and *carotid a., internal*
carotid a., external	a. carotis externa	common carotid a.	superior thyroid, ascending pharyngeal, lingual, facial, sternocleidomastoid, occipital, posterior auricular, superficial temporal, maxillary a's	neck, face, skull

*a. = artery; a's = (pl.) arteries.
†a. = [L.] arteria; aa. = [L. (pl.)] arteriae.

COMMON NAME*	NA EQUIVALENT†	ORIGIN*	BRANCHES*	DISTRIBUTION
carotid a., internal	a. carotis interna	common carotid a.	caroticotympanic, ophthalmic, posterior communicating, anterior choroid, anterior cerebral, middle cerebral a's	middle ear, brain, hypophysis, orbit, choroid plexus
caudal a. See sacral a., median				
cecal a., anterior	a. caecalis anterior	ileocolic a.		cecum
cecal a., inferior	a. caecalis inferior	ileocolic a.		cecum
celiac trunk	truncus celiacus	abdominal aorta	left gastric, common hepatic, splenic a's	esophagus, stomach, duodenum, spleen, pancreas, liver, gallbladder
central a's, anterolateral	aa. centrales laterales	middle cerebral a.	medial and lateral branches	anterior lenticular and caudate nuclei and internal capsule of brain
central a's, anteromedial	aa. centrales anteromediales	anterior cerebral a.		anterior and medial corpus striatum
central a's, posterolateral	aa. centrales posterolaterales	posterior cerebral a.		cerebral peduncle, posterior thalamus, colliculi, pineal and medial geniculate bodies
central a's, posteromedial	aa. centrales posteromediales	posterior cerebral a.		anterior thalamus, lateral wall of third ventricle, globus pallidus
central a., long	a. centralis longa	anterior cerebral a.		
central a. of retina	a. centralis retinae	ophthalmic a.		retina
central a., short	a. centralis brevis	anterior cerebral a.		
a. of central sulcus	a. sulci centralis	middle cerebral a.		cortex on either side of central sulcus
cerebellar a., anterior, inferior	a. inferior anterior cerebelli	basilar a.	posterior, spinal (usually), and labyrinthine (usually) a's	lower anterior cerebellum, lower and lateral parts of pons, (sometimes) upper part of medulla oblongata
cerebellar a., posterior inferior	a. inferior posterior cerebelli	vertebral a.		lower part of cerebellum, medulla, choroid plexus of fourth ventricle
cerebellar a., superior	a. cerebelli superior	basilar a.		upper part of cerebellum, midbrain, pineal body, choroid plexus of third ventricle
cerebral a., anterior	a. cerebri anterior	internal carotid a.	*precommunical part:* anteromedial central, long and short central, anterior communicating a's, anteromedial central branch; *precommunical part:* medial frontobasal, callosomarginal, paracentral, precuneal, parietooccipital a's	orbital, frontal, and parietal cortex, corpus callosum, diencephalon, corpus striatum, internal capsule, choroid plexus of lateral ventricle

cerebral a., middle	a. cerebri media	internal carotid a.	*sphenoidal part:* anterolateral central a; *insular part:* insular lateral frontobasilar, temporal a's; *terminal* or *cortical part:* a's of sulcus, parietal a's, a. of angular gyri	orbital, frontal, parietal, and temporal cortex, corpus striatum, internal capsule
cerebral a., posterior	a. cerebri posterior	terminal bifurcation of basilar a.	*precommunical part:* posteromedial central a's; *postcommunical part:* posterolateral central a's, medial and lateral posterior choroidal, peduncular branches; *terminal* or *cortical part:* lateral and medial occipital a's	occipital and temporal lobes, basal ganglia, choroid plexus of lateral ventricle, thalamus, midbrain
cervical a., ascending	a. cervicalis ascendens	inferior thyroid a.		muscles of neck, vertebrae, vertebral canal
cervical a., deep	a. cervicalis profunda	costocervical trunk subclavian a.	deep and superficial branches	deep neck muscles root of neck, muscles of scapula
cervical a., transverse	a. transversa cervicis			
choroidal a., anterior	a. choroidea anterior	internal carotid or middle cerebral a.	many small branches	interior of brain, choroid plexus of lateral ventricle and related parts
ciliary a's, anterior	aa. ciliares anteriores	ophthalmic and lacrimal a's	episcleral and anterior conjunctival a's	iris, conjunctiva
ciliary a's, posterior, long	aa. ciliares posteriores longae	ophthalmic a.		iris, ciliary process
ciliary a's, posterior, short	aa. ciliares posteriores breves	ophthalmic a.		choroid coat of eye
circumflex femoral a., lateral	a. circumflexa femoris lateralis	deep femoral a.	ascending, descending, and transverse branches	hip joint, thigh muscles
circumflex femoral a., medial	a. circumflexa femoris medialis	deep femoral a.	deep, ascending, transverse, and acetabular branches	hip joint, thigh muscles
circumflex humeral a., anterior	a. circumflexa anterior humeri	axillary a.		shoulder joint and head of humerus, long tendon of biceps, tendon of greater pectoral muscle
circumflex humeral a., posterior	a. circumflexa posterior humeri	axillary a.		deltoid, shoulder joint, teres minor and triceps muscles
circumflex iliac a., deep	a. circumflexa ilium profunda	external iliac a.	ascending branches	iliac region, abdominal wall, groin
circumflex iliac a., superficial	a. circumflexa ilium superficialis	femoral a.		groin, abdominal wall
circumflex a. of scapula	a. circumflexa scapulae	subscapular a.		inferolateral muscles of scapula
coccygeal a. *See* sacral a., median				
colic a., left	a. colica sinistra	inferior mesenteric a.		descending colon
colic a., middle	a. colica media	superior mesenteric a.		transverse colon

TABLE OF ARTERIES—*Continued*

COMMON NAME*	NA EQUIVALENT†	ORIGIN*	BRANCHES*	DISTRIBUTION
colic a., right	a. colica dextra	superior mesenteric a.		ascending colon
colic a., right, inferior. *See* ileocolic a.				
colic a., superior accessory. *See* colic a., middle				
collateral a., inferior ulnar	a. collateralis ulnaris inferior	brachial a.		arm muscles at back of elbow
collateral a., middle	a. collateralis media	deep brachial a.		triceps muscle, elbow joint
collateral a., radial	a. collateralis radialis	deep brachial a.		brachioradial and brachial muscles
collateral a., superior ulnar	a. collateralis ulnaris superior	brachial a.		elbow joint, triceps muscle
communicating a., anterior	a. communicans anterior cerebri	precommunical part of anterior cerebral a.		interconnects anterior cerebral a's
communicating a., posterior	a. communicans posterior cerebri	interconnects internal carotid and posterior cerebral a's	branches to optic chiasm, oculomotor nerve, thalamus, hypothalamus, and tail of caudate nucleus	
conjunctival a's, anterior	aa. conjunctivales anteriores	anterior ciliary a's		conjunctiva
conjunctival a's, posterior	aa. conjunctivales posteriores	medial palpebral a.		lacrimal caruncle, conjunctiva
coronary a., left	a. coronaria sinistra	left aortic sinus	anterior interventricular and circumflex branches	left ventricle, left atrium
coronary a., right	a. coronaria dextra	right aortic sinus	posterior interventricular branch	right ventricle, right atrium
costocervical trunk	truncus costocervicalis	subclavian a.	deep cervical and highest intercostal a's	deep neck muscles, first two intercostal spaces, vertebral column, back muscles
cremasteric a.	a. cremasterica	inferior epigastric a.		cremaster muscle, coverings of spermatic cord
cystic a.	a. cystica	right branch of proper hepatic a.		gallbladder
deep brachial a. *See* brachial a., deep				
deep a. of clitoris	a. profunda clitoridis	internal pudendal a.		clitoris
deep femoral a. *See* femoral a., deep.				
deep lingual a. *See* profunda linguae a.				
deep a. of penis	a. profunda penis	internal pudendal a.		corpus cavernosum penis
deferential a. *See* a. of ductus deferens				
dental a's. *See* alveolar a's				
diaphragmatic a's. *See* phrenic a's				

52

Common Name	NA Term	Origin	Branches	Distribution
digital a's, palmar, proper / digital a's of foot, common. *See* metatarsal a's, plantar				
digital a's of foot, dorsal	aa. digitales dorsales pedis	dorsal metatarsal a's		dorsum of toes
digital a's of hand, dorsal	aa. digitales dorsales manus	dorsal metacarpal a's		dorsum of fingers
digital a's, palmar, common	aa. digitales palmares communes	superficial volar arch	proper palmar digital a's	fingers
digital a's, palmar, proper	aa. digitales palmares propriae	common palmar digital a's		fingers
digital a's, plantar, common	aa. digitales plantares communes	plantar metatarsal a's	proper plantar digital a's	toes
digital a's, plantar, proper	aa. digitales plantares propriae	common plantar digital a's		toes
dorsal a. of clitoris	a. dorsalis clitoridis	internal pudendal a.		clitoris
dorsal a. of foot. *See* dorsalis pedis a.				
dorsal a. of nose	a. dorsalis nasi	ophthalmic a.	lacrimal branch	dorsum of nose
dorsal a. of penis	a. dorsalis penis	internal pudendal a.		glans, corona, and prepuce of penis
dorsalis pedis a.	a. dorsalis pedis	continuation of anterior tibial a.	lateral and medial tarsal, arcuate, deep plantar a's	foot, toes
a. of ductus deferens	a. ductus deferentis	umbilical a.	ureteral artery	ureter, ductus deferens, seminal vesicles, testes
duodenal a's. *See* pancreaticoduodenal a's, inferior				
epigastric a., external. *See* circumflex iliac a., deep				
epigastric a., inferior	a. epigastrica inferior	external iliac a.	pubic branch, cremasteric a., a. of round ligament of uterus	abdominal wall
epigastric a., superficial	a. epigastrica superficialis	femoral a.		abdominal wall, groin
epigastric a., superior	a. epigastrica superior	internal thoracic a.		abdominal wall, diaphragm
episcleral a's	aa. episclerales	anterior ciliary a.		iris, ciliary process
ethmoidal a., anterior	a. ethmoidalis anterior	ophthalmic a.	anterior meningeal, anterior septal, anterior lateral nasal branches	dura mater, nose, frontal sinus, anterior ethmoidal cells
ethmoidal a., posterior	a. ethmoidalis posterior	ophthalmic a.		conjunctival ethmoidal cells, dura mater, nose
facial a.	a. facialis	external carotid a.	ascending palatine, submental, inferior and superior labial, septal, lateral nasal, and angular a's, tonsillar and glandular branches	face, tonsil, palate, submandibular gland
facial a., deep. *See* maxillary a.				
facial a., transverse	a. transversa faciei	superficial temporal a.		parotid region

COMMON NAME*	NA EQUIVALENT†	ORIGIN*	BRANCHES*	DISTRIBUTION
fallopian a. See uterine a.				
femoral a.	a. femoralis	continuation of external iliac a.	superficial epigastric, superficial circumflex iliac, external pudendal, profunda femoris, descending genicular a's	lower abdominal wall, external genitalia, lower limb
femoral a., deep	a. profunda femoris	femoral a.	medial and lateral circumflex femoral a's, perforating a's	thigh muscles, hip joint, gluteal muscle, femur
fibular a. See peroneal a.				
frontal a. See supratrochlear a.				
frontobasal a., lateral	a. frontobasalis lateralis	middle cerebral a.		cortex of frontal lobe
frontobasal a., medial	a. frontobasalis medialis	anterior cerebral a.		cortex of frontal lobe
funicular a. See testicular a.				
gastric a., left	a. gastrica sinistra	celiac trunk	esophageal branches	esophagus, lesser curvature of stomach
gastric a., posterior	a. gastrica posterior	splenic a.		posterior gastric wall
gastric a., right	a. gastrica dextra	common hepatic a.		lesser curvature of stomach
gastric a's, short	aa. gastricae breves	splenic a.		upper part of stomach
gastroduodenal a.	a. gastroduodenalis	common hepatic a.	superior pancreaticoduodenal and right gastro-omental a's	stomach, duodenum, pancreas, greater omentum
gastroepiploic a., left. See gastro-omental a., left				
gastroepiploic a., right. See gastro-omental a., right				
gastro-omental a., left	a. gastro-omentalis sinistra	splenic a.	gastric and omental branches	stomach and greater omentum
gastro-omental a., right	a. gastro-omentalis sinistra	gastroduodenal a.	gastric and omental branches	stomach and greater omentum
genicular a., descending	a. descendens genicularis	femoral a.	saphenous, articular branches	knee joint, upper and medial part of leg
genicular a., lateral inferior	a. inferior lateralis genus	popliteal a.		knee joint
genicular a., lateral superior	a. superior lateralis genus	popliteal a.		knee joint, femur, patella, contiguous muscles
genicular a., medial inferior	a. inferior medialis genus	popliteal a.		knee joint
genicular a., medial superior	a. superior medialis genus	popliteal a.		knee joint, femur, patella, contiguous muscles
genicular a., middle	a. media genus	popliteal a.		knee joint, cruciate ligaments, patellar synovial and alar folds
gluteal a., inferior	a. glutea inferior	internal iliac a.	sciatic a.	buttock, back of thigh
gluteal a., superior	a. glutea superior	internal iliac a.	superficial and deep branches	buttocks
helicine a's of penis	aa. helicinae penis	deep and dorsal a's of penis	superficial and deep branches	erectile tissue of penis
hemorrhoidal a's. See rectal a's				

54

hepatic a., common	a. hepatica communis	celiac trunk	right gastric, gastroduodenal, proper hepatic a's	stomach, pancreas, duodenum, liver, gallbladder, greater omentum
hepatic a., proper	a. hepatica propria	common hepatic a.	right and left branches	liver, gallbladder
hypogastric a. See iliac a., internal				
hypophyseal a., inferior	a. hypophysialis inferior	internal carotid a.		pituitary gland
hypophyseal a., superior	a. hypophysialis superior	internal carotid a.		pituitary gland
ileal a's	aa. ilei	superior mesenteric a.		ileum
ileocolic a.	a. ileocolica	superior mesenteric a.	anterior and posterior cecal and appendicular a's, colic (ascending) and ileal branches	ileum, cecum, vermiform appendix, ascending colon
iliac a., common	a. iliaca communis	abdominal aorta	internal and external iliac a's	pelvis, abdominal wall, lower limb
iliac a., external	a. iliaca externa	common iliac a.	inferior epigastric, deep circumflex iliac a's	abdominal wall, external genitalia, lower limb
iliac a., internal	a. iliaca interna	continuation of common iliac a.	iliolumbar, obturator, superior and inferior gluteal, umbilical, inferior vesical, uterine, middle rectal, internal pudendal a's	wall and viscera of pelvis, buttock, reproductive organs, medial aspect of thigh
iliolumbar a.	a. iliolumbalis	internal iliac a.	iliac and lumbar branches, lateral sacral a's	pelvic muscles and bones, fifth lumbar vertebra, sacrum
infraorbital a.	a. infraorbitalis	maxillary a.	anterior superior alveolar a's	maxilla, maxillary sinus, upper teeth, lower eyelid, cheek, nose
innominate a. See brachiocephalic trunk				
insular a's	aa. insulares	insular part of cerebral a.		cortex of insula
intercostal a's, highest	a. intercostalis suprema	costocervical trunk	posterior intercostal a's I and II	upper thoracic wall
intercostal a's, posterior, I and II	aa. intercostales posteriores I et II	highest intercostal a.	dorsal and spinal branches	upper thoracic wall
intercostal a's, posterior (III–XI)	aa. intercostales posteriores (III–XI)	thoracic aorta	dorsal, spinal, lateral and medial cutaneous collateral, lateral mammary branches	thoracic wall
interlobar a's of kidney	aa. interlobares renis	renal a.	arcuate a's of kidney	lobes of kidney
interlobular a's of kidney	aa. interlobulares renis	arcuate a's of kidney		renal glomeruli
interlobular a's of liver	aa. interlobulares hepatis	right or left branch of proper hepatic a.		between lobules of liver
interosseous a., anterior	a. interossea anterior	posterior or common interosseous a.	median a.	deep parts of front of forearm
interosseous a., common	a. interossea communis	ulnar a.	anterior and posterior interosseous a's	antecubital fossa
interosseous a., posterior	a. interossea posterior	common interosseous a.	recurrent interosseous a's	deep parts of back of forearm
interosseous a., recurrent	a. interossea recurrens	posterior or common interosseous a.		back of elbow joint

TABLE OF ARTERIES—*Continued*

COMMON NAME*	NA EQUIVALENT†	ORIGIN*	BRANCHES*	DISTRIBUTION
intestinal a's		vessels arising from superior mesenteric a. and supplying intestines; they include pancreaticoduodenal, jejunal, ileal, ileocolic, and colic a's		
jejunal a's	aa. jejunales	superior mesenteric a.		jejunum
labial a., inferior	a. labialis inferior	facial a.		lower lip
labial a., superior	a. labialis superior	facial a.	septal and alar branches	upper lip and nose
a. of labyrinth	a. labyrinthi	basilar or anterior inferior cerebellar a.	vestibular and cochlear branches	internal ear
lacrimal a.	a. lacrimalis	ophthalmic a.	lateral palpebral a., recurrent meningeal branch	lacrimal gland, eyelids, conjunctiva
laryngeal a., inferior	a. laryngea inferior	inferior thyroid a.		larynx, trachea, esophagus
laryngeal a., superior	a. laryngea superior	superior thyroid a.		larynx
lingual a.	a. lingualis	external carotid a.	suprahyoid, sublingual, dorsal lingual, profunda linguae branches	tongue, sublingual gland, tonsil, epiglottis
lingual a., deep. *See* profunda linguae a.				
lumbar a's	aa. lumbales	abdominal aorta	dorsal and spinal branches	posterior abdominal wall, renal capsule
lumbar a., lowest	a. lumbalis ima	median sacral a.		sacrum, gluteus maximus muscle
malleolar a., anterior, lateral	a. malleolaris anterior lateralis	anterior tibial a.		ankle joint
malleolar a., anterior, medial	a. malleolaris anterior medialis	anterior tibial a.		ankle joint
mammary a., external. *See* lateral thoracic a., lateral mammary a., internal. *See* internal thoracic a., internal mandibular a. *See* alveolar a., inferior				
masseteric a.	a. masseterica	maxillary a.		masseter muscle
maxillary a.	a. maxillaris	external carotid a.	pterygoid branches, deep auricular, anterior tympanic, inferior alveolar, middle meningeal, masseteric, deep temporal, buccal, posterior superior alveolar, infraorbital, descending palatine, and sphenopalatine a's, and a. of pterygoid canal	both jaws, teeth, muscles of mastication, ear, meninges, nose, paranasal sinuses, palate
maxillary a., external. *See* facial a.				

Common Name	Latin	Origin	Branches	Distribution
maxillary a., internal. see maxillary a.				
median a.	a. comitans nervi mediani	anterior interosseous a.		median nerve, muscles of front of forearm
meningeal a., middle	a. meningea media	maxillary a.	frontal, parietal, lacrimal anastomotic, accessory meningeal, petrous branches, superior tympanic a.	cranial bones, dura mater
meningeal a., posterior	a. meningea posterior	ascending pharyngeal a.		bones and dura mater of posterior cranial fossa
mesencephalic a's	aa. mesencephalicae	basilar a.		cerebral peduncle
mesenteric a., inferior	a. mesenterica inferior	abdominal aorta	left colic, sigmoid, superior rectal a's	descending colon, rectum
mesenteric a., superior	a. mesenterica superior	abdominal aorta	inferior pancreaticoduodenal, jejunal, ileal, ileocolic, right and middle colic a's	small intestine, proximal half of colon
metacarpal a's, dorsal	aa. metacarpales dorsales	dorsal carpal rete and radial a.	dorsal digital a's	dorsum of fingers
metacarpal a's, palmar	aa. metacarpales palmares	deep palmar arch		deep parts of metacarpus
metatarsal a's, dorsal	aa. metatarsales dorsales	arcuate a. of foot	dorsal digital a's	foot, toes
metatarsal a's, plantar	aa. metatarsales plantares	plantar arch	perforating branches, common and proper plantar digital a's	toes
musculophrenic a.	a. musculophrenica	internal thoracic a.		diaphragm, abdominal and thoracic walls
nasal a's, posterior lateral	aa. nasales posteriores laterales	sphenopalatine a.		frontal, maxillary, ethmoidal and sphenoidal sinuses
nutrient a's of femur	aa. nutriciae femoris	third perforating a.		femur
nutrient a's of fibula	aa. nutriciae fibulae	fibular a.		fibula
nutrient a's of humerus	aa. nutriciae humeri	brachial and deep brachial a's		humerus
nutrient a's of tibia	aa. nutriciae tibiae	posterior tibial a.		tibia
obturator a.	a. obturatoria	internal iliac a.	pubic, acetabular, anterior, posterior branches	pelvic muscles, hip joint
obturator a., accessory	a. obturatoria accessoria	variant obturator a. arising from inferior epigastric instead of internal iliac a.		
occipital a.	a. occipitalis	external carotid a.	auricular, meningeal, mastoid, descending, occipital, sternocleidomastoid branches	muscles of neck and scalp, meninges, mastoid cells
occipital a., lateral	a. occipitalis lateralis	posterior cerebral a.	anterior temporal, middle intermediate temporal, posterior temporal branches	anterior, medial, intermediate, and posterior parts of temporal lobe
occipital a., middle	a. occipitalis medialis	posterior cerebral a.	dorsal corpus callosum, parietal, parieto-occipital, calcarine, occipital, occipitotemporal branches	dorsum of corpus callosum, precuneus, cuneus, lingual gyrus, posterior part of lateral surface of occipital lobe

COMMON NAME*	NA EQUIVALENT†	ORIGIN*	BRANCHES*	DISTRIBUTION
ophthalmic a.	a. ophthalmica	internal carotid a.	lacrimal and supraorbital a's, central a. of retina, ciliary, posterior and anterior ethmoidal, palpebral, supratrochlear, dorsal nasal a's	eye, orbit, adjacent facial structures
ovarian a.	a. ovarica	abdominal aorta	ureteral and tubal branches	ureter, ovary, uterine tube
palatine a., ascending	a. palatina ascendens	facial a.		soft palate, wall of pharynx, tonsil, auditory tube
palatine a., descending	a. palatina descendens	maxillary a.	greater and lesser palatine a's	soft and hard palates, tonsil
palatine a's, greater	a. palatina major	descending palatine a.		hard palate
palatine a's, lesser	aa. palatinae minores	descending palatine a.		soft palate, tonsil
palpebral a's, lateral	aa. palpebrales laterales	lacrimal a.		eyelids, conjunctiva
palpebral a's, medial	aa. palpebrales mediales	ophthalmic a.	posterior conjunctival a's	eyelids
pancreatic a., dorsal	a. pancreatica dorsalis	splenic a.	inferior pancreatic a.	neck and body of pancreas
pancreatic a., great	a. pancreatica magna	splenic a.	right and left branches anastomose with other pancreatic a's	body and tail of pancreas
pancreatic a., inferior	a. pancreatica	dorsal pancreatic		body and tail of pancreas
pancreaticoduodenal a., anterior superior	a. pancreaticoduodenalis superior anterior	gastroduodenal a.	pancreatic and duodenal branches	pancreas, duodenum
pancreaticoduodenal a's, inferior	aa. pancreaticoduodenales inferiores	superior mesenteric a.	anterior and posterior branches	pancreas, duodenum
pancreaticoduodenal a., posterior superior	a. pancreaticoduodenalis posterior	gastroduodenal a.	pancreatic and duodenal branches	pancreas, duodenum
paracentral a.	a. paracentralis	anterior cerebral a.		cerebral cortex and medial central sulcus
parietal arteries, anterior and posterior	aa. parietales anterior et posterior	middle cerebral a.	anterior and posterior branches	anterior parietal lobe and posterior temporal lobe
parieto-occipital a.	a. parieto-occipitalis	anterior cerebral a.		parietal lobe and sometimes occipital lobe
perforating a's	aa. perforantes	deep femoral a.	nutrient a's	adductor, hamstring, and gluteal muscles, femur
pericardiacophrenic a.	a. pericardiacophrenica	internal thoracic a.		pericardium, diaphragm, pleura
perineal a.	a. perinealis	internal pudendal a.		perineum, skin of external genitalia
peroneal a.	a. fibularis	posterior tibial a.	perforating, communicating, calcaneal, and lateral and medial malleolar branches, calcaneal rete	outside and back of ankle, deep calf muscles
pharyngeal a., ascending	a. pharyngea ascendens	external carotid a.	posterior meningeal, pharyngeal, inferior tympanic branches	pharynx, soft palate, ear, meninges
phrenic a's, great. See phrenic a's, inferior				
phrenic a's, inferior	aa. phrenicae inferiores	abdominal aorta	superior suprarenal a's	diaphragm, suprarenal gland
phrenic a's, superior	aa. phrenicae superiores	thoracic aorta		upper surface of vertebral portion of diaphragm

58

plantar a., lateral	a. plantaris lateralis	posterior tibial a.	plantar arch, plantar metatarsal a's	sole of foot, toes
plantar a., medial	a. plantaris medialis	posterior tibial a.	deep and superficial branches	sole of foot, toes
pontine a's	aa. pontis	basilar a.		pons and adjacent areas of the brain
popliteal a.	a. poplitea	continuation of femoral a.	lateral and medial superior genicular, middle genicular, sural, lateral and medial inferior genicular, anterior and posterior tibial a's, articular rete of knee, patellar rete	knee, calf
a. of postcentral sulcus	a. sulci postcentralis	middle cerebral a.		cortex of either side of postcentral sulcus
a. of precentral sulcus	a. sulci precentralis	middle cerebral a.		cortex on either side of precentral sulcus
precuneal a.	a. precunealis	anterior cerebral a.		inferior precuneus
princeps pollicis a.	a. princeps pollicis	radial a.	radialis indicis a.	sides and palmar aspect of thumb
principal a. of thumb. See princeps pollicis a.				
profunda linguae a.	a. profunda linguae	lingual a.		tongue
a. of pterygoid canal	a. canalis pterygoidei	maxillary a.		roof of pharynx, auditory tube
pudendal a's, external	aa. pudendae externae	femoral a.	anterior scrotal or anterior labial branches, inguinal branches	external genitalia, upper medial thigh
pudendal a., internal	a. pudenda interna	internal iliac a.	posterior scrotal or posterior labial branches, inferior rectal, perineal, urethral a's, a. of bulb of penis or vestibule, deep a. of penis or clitoris, dorsal a. of penis or clitoris	external genitalia, anal canal, perineum
pulmonary a., left	a. pulmonalis sinistra	pulmonary trunk	numerous branches named according to segments of lung to which they distribute unaerated blood	left lung
pulmonary a., right	a. pulmonalis dextra	pulmonary trunk	numerous branches named according to segments of lung to which they distribute unaerated blood	right lung
pulmonary trunk	truncus pulmonalis	right ventricle	right and left pulmonary a's	conveys unaerated blood toward lungs
radial a.	a. radial	brachial a.	palmar carpal, superficial palmar and dorsal carpal branches; recurrent radial a., princeps pollicis a., deep palmar arch	forearm, wrist, hand
radial a., collateral. See collateral a., radial				
radial a. of index finger. See radialis indicis a.				

TABLE OF ARTERIES—*Continued*

COMMON NAME*	NA EQUIVALENT†	ORIGIN*	BRANCHES*	DISTRIBUTION
radialis indicis a.	a. radialis indicis	princeps pollicis a.		index finger
radiate a's of kidney. *See* interlobular a's of kidney				
ranine a. *See* profunda linguae a.				
rectal a., inferior	a. rectalis inferior	internal pudendal a.		rectum, anal canal
rectal a., middle	a. rectalis media	internal iliac a.		rectum, prostate, seminal vesicles, vagina
rectal a., superior	a. rectalis superior	inferior mesenteric a.		rectum
recurrent a., radial	a. recurrens radialis	radial a.		brachioradial and brachial muscles, elbow region
recurrent a., tibial, anterior	a. recurrens tibialis anterior	anterior tibial a.		anterior tibial muscle and long extensor muscle of toes, knee joint, contiguous fascia and skin
recurrent a., tibial, posterior	a. recurrens tibialis posterior	anterior tibial a.		knee
recurrent a., ulnar	a. recurrens ulnaris	ulnar a.		elbow region
renal a.	a. renalis	abdominal aorta	anterior and posterior branches ureteral branches, inferior suprarenal a.	kidney, adrenal gland, ureter
renal a's. *See* arcuate, interlobar, *and* interlobular a's, *and* straight arterioles of kidney	aa. renis			
a. of round ligament of uterus	a. ligamenti teretis uteri	inferior epigastric a.		round ligament of uterus
sacral a's, lateral	aa. sacrales laterales	iliolumbar a.	spinal branches	structures about coccyx and sacrum
sacral a., median	a. sacralis mediana	central continuation of abdominal aorta, beyond origin of common iliac a's	lowest lumbar a.	sacrum, coccyx, rectum
scapular a., dorsal	a. dorsalis scapularis	subclavian (deep) branch of transverse cervical a.		rhomboid, latissimus dorsi, trapezius muscles
scapular a., transverse. *See* suprascapular a.				
sciatic a.	a. comitans nervi ischiadici	inferior gluteal a.		accompanies sciatic nerve
segmental a., anterior	a. segmenti anterioris	right hepatic		anterior segment of right lobe of liver
segmental a., anterior inferior	a. segmenti anterior inferior	anterior branch of renal a.		anterior inferior segment of kidney
segmental a., anterior superior	a. segmenti anterioris superioris	anterior branch of renal a.		anterior superior segment of kidney
segmental a., inferior	a. segmenti inferioris	anterior branch of renal a.		inferior segment of kidney

segmental a., lateral	a. segmenti lateralis	left branch of common hepatic a.		lateral segment of left lobe of liver
segmental a., medial	a. segmenti medialis	left branch of common hepatic a.		medial segment of left lobe of liver
segmental a., posterior	a. segmenti posterioris	1. right hepatic a. 2. posterior branch of renal a.		1. posterior segment of right lobe of liver 2. posterior segment of kidney
segmental a., superior	a. segmenti superioris	anterior branch of renal a.		superior segment of kidney
sigmoid a's	aa. sigmoideae	inferior mesenteric a.		sigmoid colon
spermatic a., external. See cremasteric a.				
sphenopalatine a.	a. sphenopalatina	maxillary a.	posterior lateral nasal a. and posterior septal branches	structures adjoining nasal cavity, nasopharynx
spinal a., anterior	a. spinalis anterior	intracranial part of vertebral a.		spinal cord
spinal a., posterior	a. spinalis posterior	vertebral a.		spinal cord
splenic a.	a. splenica	celiac trunk	pancreatic and splenic branches, left gastro-omental, short gastric a's	spleen, pancreas, stomach, greater omentum
straight arterioles of kidney	arteriolae rectae renis	arcuate a's of kidney		renal pyramids
stylomastoid a.	a. stylomastoidea	posterior auricular a.	mastoid and stapedial branches, posterior tympanica	tympanic cavity walls, mastoid cells, stapedius muscle
subclavian a.	a. subclavia	brachiocephalic trunk (right), arch of aorta (left)	vertebral, internal thoracic a's, thyrocervical and costocervical trunks	neck, thoracic wall, spinal cord, brain, meninges, upper limb
subcostal a.	a. subcostalis	thoracic aorta	dorsal and spinal branches	upper posterior abdominal wall
sublingual a.	a. sublingualis	lingual a.		sublingual gland
submental a.	a. submentalis	facial a.		tissue under chin
subscapular a.	a. subscapularis	axillary a.	thoracodorsal and circumflex scapular a's	scapular and shoulder region
supraduodenal a.	a. supraduodenalis	gastroduodenal a.	duodenal branch	superior part of duodenum
supraorbital a.	a. supraorbitalis	ophthalmic a.		forehead, superior muscles of orbit, upper eyelid, frontal sinus
suprarenal a., inferior	a. suprarenalis inferior	renal a.		adrenal gland
suprarenal a., middle	a. suprarenalis media	abdominal aorta		adrenal gland
suprarenal a's, superior	aa. suprarenales superiores	inferior phrenic a.		adrenal gland
suprascapular a.	a. suprascapularis	thyrocervical trunk	acromial branch	clavicular, deltoid, and scapular regions
supratrochlear a.	a. supratrochlearis	ophthalmic a.		anterior scalp
sural a's	aa. surales	popliteal a.		popliteal space, calf
sylvian a. See cerebral a., middle				
tarsal a., lateral	a. tarsalis lateralis	dorsalis pedis a.		tarsus

TABLE OF ARTERIES—Continued

COMMON NAME*	NA EQUIVALENT†	ORIGIN*	BRANCHES*	DISTRIBUTION
tarsal a's, medial	aa. tarsales mediales	dorsalis pedis a.		side of foot
temporal a., anterior	a. temporalis anterior	middle cerebral a.		cortex of anterior temporal lobe
temporal a., anterior deep	a. temporalis profunda anterior	maxillary a.	to zygomatic bone and greater wing of sphenoid bone	temporal muscle
temporal a., middle	a. temporalis media	1. superficial temporal a. 2. middle cerebral a.		1. temporal region 2. cortex of temporal lobe
temporal a., posterior	a. temporalis posterior	middle cerebral a.		cortex of posterior temporal lobe
temporal a., posterior deep	a. temporalis profunda posterior	maxillary a.		temporal muscle
temporal a., superficial	a. temporalis superficialis	external carotid a.	parotid, auricular, occipital branches, transverse facial, zygomatico-orbital, middle temporal a's	parotid and temporal regions
testicular a.	a. testicularis	abdominal aorta	ureteral and epididymal branches	ureter, epididymis, testis
thalamostriate a's, anterolateral. See central a's, anterolateral				
thalamostriate a's, anteromedial. See central a's, anteromedial				
thoracic a., highest	a. thoracica suprema	axillary a.		axillary aspect of chest wall
thoracic a., internal	a. thoracica interna	subclavian a.	mediastinal, thymic, bronchial, tracheal, sternal, perforating, medial mammary, lateral costal, anterior intercostal branches, pericardiacophrenic, musculophrenic, superior epigastric a's	anterior thoracic wall, mediastinal structures, diaphragm
thoracic a., lateral	a. thoracica lateralis	axillary a.	mammary branches	pectoral muscles, mammary gland
thoracoacromial a.	a. thoracoacromialis	axillary a.	clavicular, pectoral, deltoid, acromial branches	deltoid, clavicular, thoracic regions
thoracodorsal a.	a. thoracodorsalis	subscapular a.		subscapular and teres major and minor muscles
thyrocervical trunk	truncus thyrocervicalis	subclavian a.	inferior thyroid, suprascapular and transverse cervical a's	deep neck, including thyroid gland, scapular region
thyroid a., inferior	a. thyroidea inferior	thyrocervical trunk	pharyngeal, esophageal, tracheal branches, inferior laryngeal, ascending cervical a's	thyroid gland and adjacent structures
thyroid a., lowest. See thyroidea ima a.				
thyroid a., superior	a. thyroidea superior	external carotid a.	hyoid, sternocleidomastoid, superior laryngeal, cricothyroid, muscular, glandular branches	thyroid gland and adjacent structures

thyroidea ima a.	a. thyroidea ima	arch of aorta, brachiocephalic trunk or right common carotid a.		thyroid gland
tibial a., anterior	a. tibialis anterior	popliteal a.	posterior and anterior tibial recurrent a's, lateral and medial anterior malleolar a's, lateral and medial malleolar retia	leg, ankle, foot
tibial a., posterior	a. tibialis posterior	popliteal a.	fibular circumflex branch, peroneal, medial plantar, lateral plantar a's	leg, foot
transverse a. of face. See facial a., transverse / transverse a. of neck. See cervical a., transverse / transverse a. of scapula. See suprascapular a.				
tympanic a., anterior	a. tympanica anterior	maxillary a.		tympanic cavity
tympanic a., inferior	a. tympanica inferior	ascending pharyngeal a.		tympanic cavity
tympanic a., posterior	a. tympanica posterior	stylomastoid a.		tympanic cavity
tympanic a., superior	a. tympanica superior	middle meningeal a.		tympanic cavity
ulnar a.	a. ulnaris	brachial a.	palmar carpal, dorsal carpal, deep palmar branches, ulnar recurrent and common interosseous a's, superficial palmar arch	forearm, wrist, hand
ulnar a., collateral. See collateral a., inferior ulnar and collateral a., superior ulnar				
umbilical a.	a. umbilicalis	internal iliac a.	a. of ductus deferens, superior vesical a's	ductus deferens, seminal vesicles, testes, urinary bladder, ureter
urethral a.	a. urethralis	internal pudendal a.		urethra
uterine a.	a. uterina	internal iliac a.	ovarian and tubal branches, vaginal a.	uterus, vagina, round ligament of uterus, uterine tube, ovary
vaginal a.	a. vaginalis	uterine a.		vagina, fundus of bladder
vertebral a.	a. vertebralis	subclavian a.	transverse part: spinal and muscular branches; intracranial part: anterior spinal a., posterior inferior cerebellar a. and its branches	muscles of neck, vertebrae, spinal cord, cerebellum, interior of cerebrum
vesical a., inferior	a. vesicalis inferior	internal iliac a.	prostatic	bladder, prostate, seminal vesicles, lower ureter
vesical a's, superior	aa. vesicales superiores	umbilical a.		bladder, urachus, ureter
zygomatico-orbital a.	a. zygomatico-orbitalis	superficial temporal a.		lateral side of orbit

A.R.V.O. Association for Research in Vision and Ophthalmology.

aryl- in organic chemistry, a prefix denoting any radical having the free valence on a carbon atom in an aromatic ring.

arytenoid (ar″ĭ-te′noid) shaped like a jug or pitcher as arytenoid cartilage.

arytenoidopexy (ar″ĭ-te-noid′ah-pek″se) surgical fixation of arytenoid cartilage or muscle.

AS aortic stenosis; arteriosclerosis.

A.S. [L.] *au′ris sinis′tra* (left ear).

As chemical symbol, *arsenic.*

As. astigmatism.

ASA acetylsalicylic acid; arginosuccinic acid.

A.S.A. American Society of Anesthesiologists; American Standards Association; American Surgical Association.

A.S.B. American Society of Bacteriologists.

asbestos (as-bes′tis) a fibrous incombustible magnesium and calcium silicate.

asbestosis (as″bes-to′sis) a pneumoconiosis caused by inhaled asbestos fibers, characterized by interstitial fibrosis and associated with pleural mesothelioma and bronchogenic carcinoma.

ascariasis (as″kah-ri′ah-sis) infection with the roundworm *Ascaris lumbricoides.* After ingestion, the larvae migrate first to the lungs then to the intestine.

ascaricide (as-kar′ĭ-sīd) an agent that destroys ascarids. **ascarici′dal,** adj.

ascarid (as′kah-rid) any of the phasmid nematodes of the Ascaridoidea, which includes the genera *Ascaridia, Ascaris, Toxocara,* and *Toxascaris.*

Ascaris (-ris) a genus of large intestinal nematode parasites. **A. lumbricoi′des,** a species causing ascariasis. **A. su′is,** a name given to *A. lumbricoides* found in swine.

Ascarops (-rops) a genus of parasitic nematodes. **A. strongyli′na,** a blood-sucking species found in the stomach of pigs.

ascertainment (as-er-tān′mint) in genetics, the method by which persons with a trait are selected or discovered by an investigator.

A.S.C.H. American Society of Clinical Hypnosis.

Aschelminthes (ask″hel-minth′ēz) a phylum of unsegmented, bilaterally symmetrical, pseudocoelomate, mostly vermiform animals whose bodies are almost entirely covered with a cuticle, and which possess a complete digestive tract lacking definite muscular walls.

A.S.C.I. American Society for Clinical Investigation.

ascites (ah-sīt′ēz) effusion and accumulation of serous fluid in the abdominal cavity. **ascit′ic,** adj. **chylous a.,** the presence of chyle in the peritoneal cavity owing to anomalies, injuries, or obstruction of the thoracic duct.

A.S.C.L.T. American Society of Clinical Laboratory Technicians.

Ascomycetes (as″ko-mi-sēt′ēz) a class of perfect fungi which form ascospores, including yeasts, mildew, and molds.

ascorbic acid (ah-skor′bik) vitamin C, $C_6H_8O_6$, found in many vegetables and fruits, and an essential element in the diet of man and many other animals; deficiency produces scurvy and poor wound repair. Its sodium salt *(sodium ascorbate)* is used in solution for parenteral administration.

A.S.C.P. American Society of Clinical Pathologists.

-ase suffix used in enzyme names, affixed to a stem indicating the substrate (luciferase), the general nature of the substrate (proteinase), the reaction catalyzed (hydrolase), or a combination of these (transaminase).

asemasia (as″ĭ-ma′ze-ah) aphasia in which there is lack or loss of ability to communicate by words or by signals.

asepsis (a-sep′sis) 1. freedom from infection. 2. the prevention of contact with microorganisms. **asep′tic,** adj.

asexualization (a-sek″shoo-il-ĭ-za′shin) sterilization of an individual, as by castration or vasectomy.

A.S.G. American Society for Genetics.

A.S.H. American Society of Hematology.

A.S.H.A. American School Health Association; American Speech and Hearing Association.

A.S.H.P. American Society of Hospital Pharmacists.

asialia (ah″si-a′le-ah) aptyalism.

asiderosis (ah″sid-er-o′sis) deficiency of iron reserve of the body.

A.S.I.I. American Science Information Institute.

A.S.I.M. American Society of Internal Medicine.

-asis word element, *state; condition.*

Asn asparagine.

ASO arteriosclerosis obliterans.

A.S.P. American Society of Parasitologists.

Asp aspartic acid.

asparaginase (as-par′ah-jin-ās″) an enzyme that catalyzes the deamination of asparagine; used as an antineoplastic agent against cancers, e.g., acute lymphocytic leukemia, in which the malignant cells require exogenous asparagine for protein synthesis.

asparagine (as-par′ah-jēn) the β-amide of aspartic acid, a nonessential amino acid occurring in proteins; used in bacterial culture media.

aspartase (as′par-tās) an enzyme that splits aspartic acid into fumaric acid and ammonia.

aspartate (ah-spar′tāt) a salt of aspartic acid, or aspartic acid in dissociated form.

aspartate aminotransferase (AST) (ah-me″no-trans′fer-ās) an enzyme normally present in serum and in various body tissues, especially in the heart and liver; it is released into the serum as the result of tissue injury, hence the concentration in the serum may be increased in myocardial infarction or acute damage to hepatic cells.

aspartic acid (ah-spar′tik) a nonessential, natural dibasic amino acid, $COOH \cdot CH(NH_2 \cdot CH_2 \cdot \cdot COOH$, involved in transamination reactions, the ornithine cycle, and the formation of carnosine, anserine, purines, and pyrimidines.

aspect (as′pekt) that part of a surface facing in any designated direction. **dorsal a.,** that surface of a body viewed from the back (human anatomy) or from above (veterinary anatomy).

ventral a., that surface of a body viewed from the front (human anatomy) or from below (veterinary anatomy).

aspergilloma (as″per-jil-o′mah) a tumor-like granulomatous mass formed by colonization of *Aspergillus* in a bronchus or pulmonary cavity; the organism may disseminate through the blood stream to the brain, heart, and kidneys.

aspergillosis (-o′sis) a disease caused by species of *Aspergillus*, marked by inflammatory granulomatous lesions in the skin, ear, orbit, nasal sinuses, lungs, bones, and meninges.

Aspergillus (as″per-jil′is) a genus of fungi (molds), several species of which are endoparasitic and opportunistic pathogens. **A. fumiga′tus,** a species growing in soil and manure, which has been found in infections of the ear, lungs, and other organs of humans and animals, and is considered a primary pathogen of birds. Its cultures produce various antibiotics, e.g., fumagillin and helvolic acid.

aspergillustoxicosis (as″per-jil″is-tok″sĭ-ko′sis) mycotoxicosis caused by *Aspergillus*.

aspermia (ah-sper′me-ah) failure of formation or emission of semen.

asphyxia (as-fik′se-ah) apparent or actual cessation of life due to interruption of effective gaseous exchange in the lungs. **asphyx′ial,** adj. **a. carbo′nica,** suffocation from the inhalation of coal gas, water gas, or carbon monoxide. **fetal a.,** asphyxia *in utero* due to anoxia caused by abruptio placentae, injudicious use of anesthetics, etc. **a. li′vida,** that in which the skin is cyanotic. **local a.,** acroasphyxia. **a. neonato′rum,** respiratory failure in the newborn; see also *respiratory distress syndrome of newborn.* **traumatic a.,** that due to sudden or severe compression of the thorax or upper abdomen, or both.

aspidium (as-pid′e-um) the rhizome and stipes of the male fern, the source of an oleoresin used as an anthelmintic in intestinal tapeworm infestations.

aspiration (as″pĭ-ra′shin) 1. the act of inhaling. 2. removal of fluids or gases from a cavity by suction. **vacuum a.,** removal of the uterine contents by application of a vacuum through a hollow curet or a cannula introduced into the uterus.

aspirin (as′pĭ-rin) acetylsalicylic acid, $C_9H_8O_4$, an analgesic, antipyretic, and antirheumatic.

asplenia (ah-sple′ne-ah) absence of the spleen. **functional a.,** impaired reticuloendothelial function of the spleen, as seen in children with sickle-cell anemia.

A.S.R.T. American Society of Radiologic Technologists.

assay (as′a) determination of the amount of a particular constituent of a mixture, or of the potency of a drug. **biological a.,** bioassay. **microbiological a.,** the assay of nutrient or other substances by their effect on living microorganisms. **stem cell a.,** a measurement of the potency of antineoplastic drugs, based on their ability to retard the growth of cultures of human tumor cells.

assimilation (ah-sim″ĭ-la′shin) 1. conversion of

nutritive material into living tissue; anabolism. 2. psychologically, absorption of new experiences into existing psychologic make-up.

assistant (ah-sis′tint) one who aids or helps another; an auxiliary. **physician a.,** see under *physician.*

association (ah-so″se-a′shin) close relation in time or space. In neurology, correlation involving a high degree of modifiability and also consciousness; see *association areas.* In genetics, the occurrence together of two characteristics (e.g., blood group O and peptic ulcers) at a frequency greater than would be predicted on the basis of chance. **free a.,** oral expression of one's ideas as they arrive spontaneously; a method used in psychoanalysis.

assortment (ah-sort′mint) the random distribution of nonhomologous chromosomes to daughter cells in metaphase of the first meiotic division.

AST aspartate aminotransferase.

astasia (as-ta′zhe-ah) motor incoordination with inability to stand. **astat′ic,** adj. **a.-aba′sia,** inability to stand or walk although the legs are otherwise under control.

astatine (as′tah-tēn) chemical element (*see table*), at. no. 85, symbol At.

asteatosis (as″te-ah-to′sis) any disease in which persistent dry scaling of the skin suggests scantiness or absence of sebum.

asterion (as-tēr′e-on) the point on the skull at the junction of occipital, parietal, and temporal bones.

asterixis (as″ter-ik′sis) a motor disturbance marked by intermittent lapses of an assumed posture as a result of intermittency of sustained contraction of groups of muscles; called *liver flap* because of its occurrence in hepatic coma, but observed also in other conditions.

asteroid (as′ter-oid) star-shaped.

asthen(o)- word element [Gr.], *weak; weakness.*

asthenia (as-the′ne-ah) lack or loss of strength and energy; weakness. **asthen′ic,** adj. **neurocirculatory a.,** a syndrome of breathlessness, giddiness, a sense of fatigue, precordial pain, and palpitation, seen chiefly in soldiers in active war service. **tropical anhidrotic a.,** a condition due to generalized anhidrosis in conditions of high temperature, characterized by a tendency to overfatigability, irritability, anorexia, inability to concentrate, and drowsiness, with headache and vertigo.

asthenocoria (as″thĭ-no-kor′e-ah) sluggishness of the pupillary light reflex; seen in hypoadrenalism.

asthenometer (as″thĭ-nom′ĭt-er) a device used in measuring the degree of muscular asthenia or of asthenopia.

asthenopia (as″thĭ-no′pe-ah) weakness or easy fatigue of the eye, with pain in the eyes, headache, dimness of vision, etc. **asthenop′ic,** adj. **accommodative a.,** asthenopia due to strain of ciliary muscle. **muscular a.,** asthenopia due to weakness of external ocular muscles.

asthma (az′mah) a condition marked by recurrent attacks of paroxysmal dyspnea, with wheezing due to spasmodic contraction of the bronchi. In some cases, it is an allergic manifestation in sensitized persons; in others it may be induced by vigorous exercise, irritant particles, or physiologic stress. **asthmat′ic,** adj. **bronchial a.,** see *asthma.*

astigmatism (ah-stig′mah-tizm) ametropia caused by differences in curvature in different meridians of the refractive surfaces of the eye so that light rays are not sharply focused on the retina. **astigmat′ic,** adj. **compound a.,** that complicated with hypermetropia or myopia in all meridians. **corneal a.,** that due to irregularity in the curvature or refracting power of the cornea. **irregular a.,** that in which the curvature varies in different parts of the same meridian or in which refraction in successive meridians differs irregularly. **mixed a.,** that in which one principal meridian is myopic and the other hyperopic. **myopic a.,** that in which the light rays are brought to a focus in front of the retina. **regular a.,** that in which the refractive power of the eye shows a uniform increase or decrease from one meridian to another.

astragalus (ah-strag′ah-lus) talus (see *Table of Bones).* **astrag′alar,** adj.

astral (as′tril) of or relating to an aster.

astringent (ah-strin′jint) causing contraction, usually locally after topical application.

astroblast (as′trah-blast) a cell that develops into an astrocyte.

astroblastoma (as″tro-blas-to′mah) an astrocytoma of Grade II, composed of cells with abundant cytoplasm and two or three nuclei.

astrocyte (as′tro-sīt) a neuroglial cell of ectodermal origin. Based on differences in stained appearance, astrocytes are divided into *fibrous a.'s,* those found in the white matter, and *protoplasmic a.'s;* however, these are modifications of a single cell type. Collectively called *astroglia.*

astrocytoma (-si-to′mah) a tumor composed of astrocytes; classified in order of malignancy as: *Grade I,* consisting of fibrillary or protoplasmic astrocytes; *Grade II* (see *astroblastoma); Grades III* and *IV* (see *glioblastoma multiforme).*

asymmetry (a-sim′ĭ-tre) lack or absence of symmetry; dissimilarity in corresponding parts or organs on opposite sides of the body which are normally alike. In chemistry, lack of symmetry in the special arrangements of the atoms and radicals within the molecule or crystal. **asymmet′rical,** adj.

asynchronism (a-sing′krah-nizm) lack of synchronism; disturbance of coordination.

asynclitism (a-sing′klĭ-tizm) 1. oblique presentation of the fetal head in labor, called *anterior a.* when the anterior parietal bone is designated the point of presentation, and *posterior a.* when the posterior parietal bone is so designated. 2. maturation at different times of the nucleus and cytoplasm of blood cells.

asyndesis (ah-sin′dis-is) a language disorder in which related elements of a sentence cannot be welded together as a whole.

asynechia (ah″sĭ-nek′e-ah) absence of continuity of structure.

asynergy (a″sin′er-je) lack of coordination among parts or organs normally acting in unison; in neurology, failure of cooperation among muscle groups that is necessary for movement.

asystole (a-sis′tah-le) cardiac standstill or arrest—absence of heartbeat. **asystol′ic,** adj.

At chemical symbol, *astatine.*

at. atmosphere; atomic.

atactiform (-tĭ-form) resembling ataxia.

ataractic (at″ah-rak′tik) 1. pertaining to ataraxia. 2. a tranquilizer.

ataralgesia (at″er-al-je′ze-ah) combined sedation and analgesia intended to abolish mental distress and pain from surgical procedures, with the patient remaining conscious and alert.

ataraxia (at″ah-rak′se-ah) a state of detached serenity without depression of mental faculties.

atavism (at′ah-vizm) apparent inheritance of a characteristic from remote rather than immediate ancestors. **atavis′tic,** adj.

ataxia (ah-tak′se-ah) failure of muscular coordination; irregularity of muscular action. **atac′tic, atax′ic,** adj. **alcoholic a.,** a condition resembling tabes dorsalis, due to loss of proprioception in chronic alcoholism. **Friedreich's a.,** hereditary sclerosis of the dorsal and lateral columns of the spine, usually beginning in childhood or youth; it is attended with ataxia, speech impairment, scoliosis, peculiar movements, paralysis, and often hypertrophic cardiomyopathy. **locomotor a.,** tabes dorsalis. **motor a.,** inability to control the coordinate movements of the muscles. **sensory a.,** ataxia due to loss of proprioception (joint position sensation) between the motor cortex and peripheral nerves, resulting in poorly judged movements, the incoordination becoming aggravated when the eyes are closed. **a.-telangiectasia,** a severe hereditary progressive cerebellar ataxia, transmitted as an autosomal recessive trait, and associated with oculocutaneous telangiectasia, abnormal eye movements, sinopulmonary disease, and immunodeficiency.

atel(o)- word element [Gr.], *incomplete; imperfectly developed.*

atelectasis (at″′l-ek′tah-sis) incomplete expansion of the lungs at birth, or collapse of the adult lung. **atelectat′ic,** adj. **congenital a.,** that present at birth (*primary a.*) or immediately thereafter (*secondary a.*). **lobar a.,** that affecting only a lobe of the lung. **lobular a.,** that affecting only a lobule of the lung.

atelia (ah-tēl′e-ah) imperfect or incomplete development. **ateliot′ic,** adj.

ateliosis (ah-tēl″e-o′sis) hypophyseal infantilism.

atelocardia (at″′l-o-kar′de-ah) imperfect development of the heart.

athelia (ah-thēl′e-ah) congenital absence of the nipples.

athermic (ah-ther′mik) without rise of temperature; afebrile; apyretic.

athermosystaltic (ah-ther″mo-sis-tal′tik) not contracting under the action of cold or heat; said of skeletal muscle.

atheroembolus (-em′bah-lus), pl. *atheroemboli.* an embolus composed of cholesterol or its esters (typically lodging in small arteries) or of fragments of atheromatous plaques.

atherogenesis (-jen″ĭ-sis) formation of atheromatous lesions in arterial walls. **atherogen′ic,** adj.

atheroma (ath″er-o′mah) a mass or plaque of degenerated thickened arterial intima, occurring in atherosclerosis.

atheromatosis (ath″er-o-mah-to′sis) diffuse atheromatous arterial disease.

atherosclerosis (ath″er-o-skler-o′sis) a form of arteriosclerosis in which atheromas containing cholesterol, lipoid material, and lipophages are formed within the intima and inner media of large and medium-sized arteries.

athetosis (ath″ĭ-to′sis) repetitive involuntary, slow, sinuous, writhing movements, especially severe in the hands.

athrepsia (ah-threp′se-ah) marasmus. **athrep′-tic,** adj.

athymia (ah-thi′me-ah) 1. dementia. 2. absence of functioning thymus tissue.

athyreosis (ah-thi″re-o′sis) hypothyroidism. **athyreot′ic,** adj.

athyria (ah-thi′re-ah) 1. a condition resulting from absence of the thyroid gland. 2. hypothyroidism.

atlantad (at-lan′tad) toward the atlas.

atlantal (at-lan′t'l) pertaining to the atlas.

atlantoaxial (at-lan″to-ak′se-'l) pertaining to the atlas and the axis.

atlas (at′lis) the first cervical vertebra; see *Table of Bones.*

atloaxoid (at″lo-ak′soid) pertaining to the atlas and axis.

atmosphere (at′mis-fēr) 1. the gaseous envelope around the earth, including the troposphere, tropopause, and stratosphere. 2. the unit of pressure equal to 101325 pascals, the pressure exerted by the earth's atmosphere at sea level, about 760 mm Hg. **atmospher′ic,** adj.

at. no. atomic number.

atocia (ah-to′se-ah) sterility in the female.

atom (at′'m) the smallest particle of an element with all the properties of the element; it consists of a positively charged nucleus (made up of protons and neutrons) and negatively charged electrons, which move in orbits about the nucleus. **atom′ic,** adj.

atomization (at′″m-ĭ-za′shin) the act or process of breaking up a liquid into a fine spray.

atony (at′ah-ne) lack of normal tone or strength. **aton′ic,** adj.

atopic (ah-top′ik) 1. ectopic. 2. pertaining to atopy; allergic.

atopognosia (ah-top″ahg-no′ze-ah) inability to correctly locate a sensation.

atopy (at′ah-pe) a clinical hypersensitivity state with a hereditary predisposition; i.e., the tendency to develop an allergy is inherited, but not the specific clinical form (hay fever, asthma, etc.) The antibody reagin is involved.

atoxic (ah-tok′sik) not poisonous; not due to a poison.

ATP adenosine triphosphate.

ATPase adenosinetriphosphatase.

atransferrinemia (a-trans″fer-in-e′me-ah) ab-

sence of circulating iron-binding protein (transferrin).

atraumatic (a″traw-mat′ik) not producing injury or damage.

atresia (ah-tre′ze-ah) congenital absence or closure of a normal body opening or tubular structure. **atret′ic,** adj. **anal a., a. a′ni,** imperforate anus. **aortic a.,** congenital absence of the opening from the left ventricle of the heart into the aorta. **biliary a.,** obliteration or hypoplasia of one or more components of the bile ducts due to arrested fetal development, resulting in persistent jaundice and liver damage ranging from biliary stasis to biliary cirrhosis, with splenomegaly as portal hypertension progresses. **follicular a., a. follic′uli,** degeneration and resorption of an ovarian follicle before it reaches maturity and ruptures. **mitral a.,** congenital obliteration of the mitral valve orifice; it is associated with hyperplastic left-heart syndrome or transposition of the great vessels. **prepyloric a.,** congenital membranous obstruction of the gastric outlet, characterized by vomiting of gastric contents only. **pulmonary a.,** congenital severe narrowing of the opening between the pulmonary artery and the right ventricle, with cardiomegaly, reduced pulmonary vascularity, and right ventricular atrophy. It is usually associated with tetralogy of Fallot, transposition of the great vessels, or other cardiovascular anomalies. **tricuspid a.,** congenital absence of the opening between the right atrium and right ventricle, circulation being made possible by the presence of an atrial septal defect.

atrichia (ah-trik′e-ah) 1. absence of hair; alopecia. 2. absence of flagella or cilia.

atriomegaly (a″tre-o-meg′ah-le) abnormal enlargement of an atrium of the heart.

atrioseptopexy (-sep′tah-pek″se) surgical correction of a defect in the interatrial septum.

atrioseptoplasty (-sep′tah-plas″te) plastic repair of the interatrial septum.

atrioventricularis communis (-ven-trik″u-la′-ris kŏ-mu′nis) a congenital cardiac anomaly in which the endocardial cushions fail to fuse, the ostium primum persists, the atrioventricular canal is undivided, a single atrioventricular valve has anterior and posterior cusps, and there is a defect of the membranous interventricular septum.

atrium (a′tre-um) pl. *a′tria* [L.] a chamber; in anatomy, a chamber affording entrance to another structure or organ, especially the upper, smaller cavity (*a. cordis*) on either side of the heart, which receives blood from the pulmonary veins (*left a.*) or venae cavae (*right a.*) and delivers it to the ventricle on the same side. **a′trial,** adj. **common a.,** the single atrium found in a form of three-chambered heart.

Atromid-S (ă′tro-mid) trademark for a preparation of clofibrate.

atrophoderma (ă″trah-fo-der′mah) atrophy of the skin.

atrophy (ă′trah-fe) 1. a wasting away; a diminution in the size of a cell, tissue, organ, or part. 2. to undergo or cause atrophy. **atro′phic,** adj. **acute yellow a.,** the shrunken, yellow liver which is a complication, usually fatal, of fulminant hepatitis with massive hepatic necrosis. **Aran-Duchenne a.**, spinal muscular a. **bone a.**, resorption of bone evident in both external form and internal density. **Duchenne-Aran a.**, spinal muscular a. **healed yellow a.**, postnecrotic cirrhosis. **Leber's optic a.**, an X-linked bilateral progressive optic atrophy seen in males. **lobar a.**, progressive atrophy of the cerebral convolutions in a limited area (lobe) of the brain. **myelopathic muscular a.**, muscular atrophy due to lesion of the spinal cord, as in spinal muscular atrophy. **optic a.**, atrophy of the optic disk due to degeneration of the nerve fibers of the optic nerve and optic tract. **physiologic a.**, that affecting certain organs in all individuals as part of the normal aging process. **progressive neuropathic (peroneal) muscular a.** hereditary muscular atrophy, beginning in the muscles supplied by the peroneal nerves, progressing slowly to involve the muscles of the hands and arms. **senile a. of the skin,** the mild atrophic changes in the dermis and epidermis that occur naturally with aging. **spinal muscular a.**, progressive degeneration of the motor cells of the spinal cord, beginning usually in the small muscles of the hands, but in some cases (scapulohumeral type) in the upper arm and shoulder muscles, and progressing slowly to the leg muscles. **subacute yellow a.**, hepatic necrosis with broad zones of necrosis, due to viral, toxic, or drug-induced hepatitis; it may have an acute course with death occurring after several weeks of liver failure, or clinical recovery may be associated with regeneration of the parenchymal cells.

atropine (ă′trah-pēn) an anticholinergic alkaloid, $C_{17}H_{23}NO_3$, occurring in belladonna. It acts as a competitive antagonist of acetylcholine at muscarinic receptors, blocking stimulation of muscles and glands by parasympathetic and cholinergic sympathetic nerves; used as a smooth muscle relaxant, as a preanesthetic to reduce secretions, and as an antidote to organophosphate poisoning.

A.T.S. American Thoracic Society; antitetanic serum.

attack (ah-tak′) an episode or onset of illness. **panic a.**, an episode of acute intense anxiety, the essential feature of panic disorder. **transient ischemic a's,** brief attacks (a few hours or less) of cerebral dysfunction of vascular origin, without lasting effect. **vagal a., vasovagal a.**, a transient vascular and neurogenic reaction marked by pallor, nausea, sweating, bradycardia, and rapid fall in arterial blood pressure, which may result in syncope.

attenuation (ah-ten″u-a′shin) 1. the act of thinning or weakening, as (a) the alteration of virulence of a pathogenic microorganism by passage through another host species, decreasing the virulence of the organism for the native host and increasing it for the new host, or (b) the process by which a beam of radiation is reduced in energy when passed through tissue or other material.

attic (at′ik) the upper portion of the tympanic cavity, extending above the level of the tympanic membrane and containing the greater part of the incus and the head of the malleus.

atticoantrotomy (at″ĭ-ko-an-trot′ah-me) surgical exposure of the attic and mastoid antrum.

attitude (at′ĭ-tood) 1. a position of the body; in obstetrics, the relation of the various parts of the fetal body. 2. a pattern of mental views established by cumulative prior experience.

atto- a prefix signifying one quintillionth, or 10^{-18}; symbol a.

attraction (ah-trak′shin) 1. the force, act, or process that draws one body toward another. 2. malocclusion in which the occlusal plane is closer than normal to the eye-ear plane, causing shortening of the face; cf. *abstraction* (3). **capillary a.**, the force which causes a liquid to rise in a fine-caliber tube.

at. wt. atomic weight.

atypia (a-tip′e-ah) deviation from the normal.

atypical (-ĭ-k'l) irregular; not conformable to the type; in microbiology, applied specifically to strains of unusual type.

A.U. [L.] *aures unitas,* both ears together or *auris uterque,* each ear.

Au chemical symbol, *gold* (L. *aurum*).

audi(o)- word element [L.], *hearing.*

audiogenic (-jen′ik) produced by sound.

audiology (-ol′ah-je) the study of impaired hearing that cannot be improved by medication or surgical therapy.

audiometry (aw″de-om′ĭ-tre) measurement of the acuity of hearing for the various frequencies of sound waves. **audiomet′ric,** adj. **Békésy a.,** that in which the patient, by pressing a signal button, traces his monaural thresholds for pure tones: the intensity of the tone decreases as long as the button is depressed and increases when it is released; both continuous and interrupted tones are used. **cortical a.,** an objective method of determining auditory acuity by recording and averaging electric potentials evoked from the cortex of the brain in response to stimulation by pure tones. **electrocochleographic a.,** measurement of electrical potentials from the middle ear or external auditory canal (cochlear microphonics and eighth nerve action potentials) in response to acoustic stimuli. **electrodermal a.,** audiometry in which the subject is conditioned by harmless electric shock to pure tones; thereafter he anticipates a shock when he hears a pure tone, the anticipation resulting in a brief electrodermal response, which is recorded; the lowest intensity at which the response is elicited is taken to be his hearing threshold. **localization a.,** a technique for measuring the capacity to locate the source of a pure tone received binaurally in a sound field. **pure tone a.,** audiometry utilizing pure tones that are relatively free of noise and overtones.

audition (aw-dish′in) perception of sound; hearing. **chromatic a.,** chromesthesia in which a sensation of color is produced by sound.

aula (aw′lah) the red areola formed around a vaccination vesicle.

aura (aw′rah) a subjective sensation or motor phenomenon that precedes and marks the onset of a paroxysmal attack, as of an epileptic attack.

aural (aw′r′l) 1. pertaining to or perceived by the ear. 2. pertaining to an aura.

auric (aw′rik) pertaining to or containing gold.

auricle (aw′rĭ-k'l) 1. the flap of the ear. 2. the ear-shaped appendage of either atrium of the heart.

auricula (aw-rik′u-lah), pl. *auri′culae* [L.] auricle.

auriculare (aw-rik″u-lār′e) a point at the top of the opening of the external auditory meatus.

auricularis (-ris) [L.] pertaining to the ear; auricular.

auripuncture (aw′rĭ-punk″cher) surgical puncture of the tympanic membrane.

auris (aw′ris), pl. *au′res* [L.] ear.

auriscope (aw′rĭ-skōp) otoscope.

aurothioglucose (-thi″o-gloo′kōs) a gold preparation, $C_6H_{11}Au_5S$, used in treating rheumatoid arthritis.

aurum (aw′rum) [L.] gold (symbol Au).

auscultation (aws″kul-ta′shin) listening for sounds within the body, chiefly to ascertain the condition of the thoracic or abdominal viscera and to detect pregnancy; it may be performed with the unaided ear (*direct* or *immediate a.*) or with a stethoscope (*mediate a.*).

aut(o)- word element [Gr.], self.

autecic, autecious (aw-te′sik; aw-te′shis) autoecious.

autism (aw′tizm) the condition of being dominated by subjective, self-centered trends of thought or behavior which are not subject to correction by external information. **autis′tic,** adj. **early infantile a., infantile a.,** a severe disorder of communication and behavior, usually beginning at birth, invariably present by age 3; it is characterized by self-absorption, profound withdrawal from contact with people, including the mother figure, a desire for sameness, preoccupation with inanimate objects, and developmental language disorders.

autoagglutination (awt″o-ah-gloot″in-a′shin) 1. clumping or agglutination of an individual's cells by his own serum, as in autohemagglutination. Autoagglutination occurring at low temperatures is called *cold agglutination.* 2. agglutination of particulate antigens, e.g., bacteria, in the absence of specific antigens.

autoagglutinin (-ah-gloot′in-in) a factor in serum capable of causing clumping together of the subject's own cellular elements.

autoamputation (-am″pu-ta′shin) spontaneous detachment from the body and elimination of an appendage or an abnormal growth, such as a polyp.

autoantibody (-an′tĭ-bod-e) an antibody formed in response to, and reacting against, an antigenic constituent of the one's own tissues.

autoantigen (-an′tĭ-jen) a tissue constituent immunogenic in the organism, and stimulating the production of autoantibodies.

autocatalysis (-kah-tal′ĭ-sis) catalysis in which a product of the reaction hastens the catalysis.

autochthonous (aw-tok′thah-nus) 1. originat-

ing in the same area in which it is found. 2. denoting a tissue graft to a new site on the same individual.

autoclasis (aw-tok′lah-sis) destruction of a part by influences within itself, as by autoimmune processes.

autoclave (awt′o-klāv) a self-locking apparatus for the sterilization of materials by steam under pressure.

Autoclip (awt′o-klip″) trademark for a stainless steel surgical clip inserted by means of a mechanical applier that automatically feeds a series of clips for wound closing.

autodigestion (-dĭ-jes′chin) self-digestion; autolysis; especially, digestion of the stomach wall and contiguous structures after death.

autoecious (aw-te′shis) pertaining to parasitic fungi that pass through their life cycle in the same host.

autoeczematization (awt″o-ek-zem″ah-tĭ-za′-shin) the spread, at first locally and later more generally, of lesions from an orginally circumscribed focus of eczema.

autoerotism (-ĕ′ro-tizm) erotic behavior directed toward one's self. **autoerot′ic,** adj.

autogamy (aw-tog′ah-me) 1. self-fertilization; fertilization by union of two chromatin masses derived from the same primary nucleus within a cell. 2. reproduction in which the two gametes are derived from division of a single mother cell.

autogenesis (-jen′ĭ-sis) self-generation; origination within the organism. **autogenet′ic, autog′enous,** adj.

autograft (awt′o-graft) a tissue graft transferred from one part of the patient's body to another part.

autohemagglutination (awt″o-hem″ah-gloot″in-a′shin) agglutination of erythrocytes by a factor produced in the subject's own body.

autohemagglutinin (-hem″ah-gloot′in-in) a substance produced in a person's body that causes agglutination of his own erythrocytes.

autohemolysin (-he-mol′ĭ-sin) a hemolysin produced in the body of an animal which lyses its own erythrocytes.

autohemolysis (-he-mol′ĭ-sis) hemolysis of an individual's blood cells by his own serum. **autohemolyt′ic,** adj.

autohemotherapy (-he″mo-thĕ′rah-pe) treatment by reinjection of the patient's own blood.

autohypnosis (-hip-no′sis) a self-induced hypnotic state; the act or process of hypnotizing oneself. **autohypnot′ic,** adj.

autoimmune (-ĭ-mūn′) directed against the body's own tissue; see under *disease* and *response.*

autoimmunity (-ĭ-mu′nit-e) a condition characterized by a specific humoral or cell-mediated immune response against the constituents of the body's own tissues (autoantigens); it may result in hypersensitivity reactions or, if severe, in autoimmune disease.

autoimmunization (-ĭ″mu-nĭ-za′shin) induction in an organism of an immune response to its own tissue constituents.

autoinoculation (-in-ok″u-la′shin) inoculation with microorganisms from one's own body.

autoisolysin (-i-sol′ĭ-sin) a substance that lyses cells (e.g., blood cells) of the individual in which it is formed, as well as those of other members of the same species.

autokeratoplasty (-kĕ′rah-to-plas″te) grafting of corneal tissue from one eye to the other.

autolesion (-le′zhin) a self-inflicted injury.

autologous (aw-tol′ah-gis) related to self; belonging to the same organism.

autolysin (aw-tol′ĭ-sin) a lysin originating in an organism and capable of destroying its own cells and tissues.

autolysis (aw-tol′ĭ-sis) 1. spontaneous disintegration of cells or tissues by autologous enzymes, as occurs after death and in some pathologic conditions. 2. destruction of cells of the body by its own serum. **autolyt′ic,** adj.

automatism (aw-tom′ah-tizm) performance of nonreflex acts without conscious volition. **command a.,** abnormal responsiveness to commands, as in hypnosis.

autonomic (awt″o-nom′ik) not subject to voluntary control. See under *system.*

autonomotropic (-nom″ah-trop′ik) having an affinity for the autonomic nervous system.

autopathy (aw-top′ah-the) idiopathic disease; one without apparent external causation.

autophagia (awt″o-fa′je-ah) 1. eating one's own flesh. 2. nutrition of the body by consumption of its own tissues. 3. autophagy.

autophagosome (-fag′ah-sōm) a secondary lysosome in which elements of a cell's own cytoplasm are digested.

autophagy (aw-tof′ah-je) 1. lysosomal digestion of a cell's own cytoplasmic material. 2. autophagia.

autopharmacologic (awt″o-far″mah-ko-lah′jik) pertaining to substances (e.g., hormones) produced in the body that have pharmacologic activities.

autophilia (-fil′e-ah) pathologic self-esteem; narcissism.

autoplasmotherapy (-plaz″mo-thě′rah-pe) therapeutic injection of one's own blood plasma.

autoplasty (awt′o-plas″te) 1. replacement or reconstruction of diseased or injured parts with tissues taken from another region of the patient's own body. 2. in psychoanalysis, instinctive modification within the psychic systems in adaptation to reality. **autoplas′tic,** adj.

autopsy (aw′top-se) postmortem examination of a body to determine the cause of death or the nature of pathological changes; necropsy.

autoradiography (-ra″de-og′rah-fe) the making of a radiograph of an object or tissue by recording on a photographic plate the radiation emitted by radioactive material within the object.

autoreactive (-re-ak′tiv) pertaining to an immune response directed against the body's own tissues.

autoregulation (-reg″u-la′shin) control of certain phenomena by factors inherent in a situation; specifically, (1) maintenance by an organ

or tissue of a constant blood flow despite changes in arterial pressure, and (2) adjustment of blood flow through an organ in accordance with its metabolic needs. **heterometric a.,** intrinsic mechanisms controlling the strength of ventricular contractions that depend on the length of myocardial fibers at the end of diastole. **homeometric a.,** intrinsic mechanisms controlling the strength of ventricular contractions that are independent of the length of myocardial fibers at the end of diastole.

autosensitization (-sen″sĭ-ti-za′shin) autoimmunization. **erythrocyte a.,** autoerythrocyte sensitization; see under *syndrome.*

autosepticemia (-sep″tĭ-se′me-ah) septicemia from poisons developed within the body.

autosite (awt′o-sīt) the larger, more normal member of asymmetrical conjoined twin fetuses, to which the parasite is attached.

autosome (-sōm) any non–sex-determining chromosome; in man there are 22 pairs of autosomes. **autoso′mal,** adj.

autosplenectomy (awt″o-sple-nek″tah-me) almost complete disappearance of the spleen through progressive fibrosis and shrinkage.

autosuggestion (-sug-jes′chin) suggestion arising in one's self, as opposed to heterosuggestion.

autotomography (-tah-mog′rah-fe) a method of body section roentgenography involving movement of the patient instead of the x-ray tube. **autotomograph′ic,** adj.

autotoxin (-tok′sin) a toxin which acts against the body in which it is formed.

autotransfusion (-trans-fu′zhin) reinfusion of a patient's own blood.

autotransplantation (-trans″plan-ta′shin) transfer of tissue from one part of the body to another part.

autotroph (awt′o-trōf) an autotrophic organism.

autotrophic (awt″o-trof′ik) self-nourishing; able to build organic constituents from carbon dioxide and inorganic salts.

autovaccine (-vak′sēn) a vaccine prepared from cultures of organisms isolated from the patient's own tissues or secretions.

autoxidation (aw-tok″sĭ-da′shin) spontaneous oxidation of a substance that is in direct contact with oxygen.

auxanography (awk″sah-nog′rah-fe) a method used for determining the most suitable medium for the cultivation of microorganisms. **auxanograph′ic,** adj.

auxesis (awk-se′sis) increase in size of an organism, especially that due to growth of its individual cells rather than an increase in their number. **auxet′ic,** adj.

auxilytic (awk″sĭ-lit′ik) increasing the lytic or destructive power.

auxocyte (-sīt) an oocyte, spermatocyte, or sporocyte in the early stages of development.

auxotrophic (awk″sah-trof′ik) 1. requiring a growth factor not required by the parental or prototype strain; said of microbial mutants. 2. requiring specific organic growth factors in addition to the carbon source present in a minimal medium.

AV, A-V atrioventricular; arteriovenous.

av., avoir. avoirdupois.

avascular (ah-vas'ku-ler) not vascular; bloodless.

avascularization (ah-vas"ku-ler-i-za'shin) diversion of blood from tissues, as by ligation of vessels or tight bandaging.

aversive (ah-ver'siv) characterized by or giving rise to avoidance; noxious; cf. *appetitive*.

avian (a've-in) of or pertaining to birds.

avidity (ah-vid'it-e) in immunology, an imprecise measure of the strength of antigen-antibody binding based on the rate at which the complex is formed. Cf. *affinity* (3).

avirulence (a-vir'u-lins) lack of virulence; lack of competence of an infectious agent to produce pathologic effects. **avir'ulent,** adj.

avoidance (ah-void'ins) a conscious or unconscious defensive reaction intended to escape anxiety, conflict, danger, fear, or pain.

avoirdupois (av"er-dĭ-poiz') a system of weight used in English-speaking countries; see *Table of Weights and Measures.*

avulsion (ah-vul'shin) the tearing away of a structure or part. **phrenic a.,** extraction of a portion of the phrenic nerve, producing one-sided paralysis of the diaphragm and partial collapse of the lung.

ax. axis.

axenic (a-zen'ik) not contaminated by or associated with any foreign organisms; used in reference to pure cultures of microorganisms or to germ-free animals. Cf. *gnotobiotic.*

axiation (ak"se-a'shin) establishment of an axis; development of polarity in an ovum, embryo, organ, or other body structure.

axilla (ak-sil'ah) the armpit. **ax'illary,** adj.

axio- word element [L., Gr.], *axis;* in dentistry, the *long axis of a* tooth.

axipetal (ak-sip'it'l) directed toward an axis or axon.

axis (ak'sis) 1. a line through the center of a body, or about which a structure revolves; a line around which body parts are arranged. 2. see *Table of Bones.* **ax'ial,** adj. **basibregmatic a.,** the vertical line from the basion to the bregma. **basicranial a.,** a line from basion to gonion. **basifacial a.,** a line from gonion to subnasal point. **binauricular a.,** a line joining the two auricular points. **celiac a.,** see under *trunk.* **dorsoventral a.,** one passing from the back to the belly surface of the body. **electrical a. of heart,** the resultant of the electromotive forces within the heart at any instant. **frontal a.,** an imaginary line running from right to left through the center of the eyeball. **a. of heart,** a line passing through the center of the base of the heart and the apex. **optic a.,** 1. visual a. 2. the hypothetical straight line passing through the centers of curvature of the front and back surfaces of a simple lens. **visual a.,** an imaginary line passing from the midpoint of the visual field to the fovea centralis.

axis cylinder (ak"sis sil'in-der) axon.

axoaxonic (ak"so-ak-son'ik) referring to a synapse between the axon of one neuron and the axon of another.

axodendritic (-den-drit'ik) referring to a synapse between the axon of one neuron and dendrites of another.

axolemma (ak"so-lem'ah) the surface membrane of an axon.

axolysis (ak-sol'ĭ-sis) degeneration of an axon.

axon (ak'son) 1. the process of a nerve cell along which impulses travel away from the cell body. It branches at its termination, forming synapses at other nerve cells or effector organs. Many axons are covered by a myelin sheath formed from the cell membrane of a glial cell. 2. the axis of the body.

axoneme (ak'son-ēm) the central core of a cilium or flagellum, consisting of two central fibrils surrounded by nine peripheral fibrils.

axonotmesis (ak"son-ot-me'sis) nerve injury characterized by disruption of the axon and myelin sheath but with preservation of the connective tissue fragments, resulting in degeneration of the axon distal to the injury site; regeneration of the axon is spontaneous and of good quality. Cf. *neurapraxia* and *neurotmesis.*

axophage (ak'so-fāj) a glia cell occurring in excavations in the myelin in myelitis.

axoplasm (-plazm) cytoplasm of an axon. **axoplas'mic,** adj.

axopodium (ak"so-po'de-um) a more or less permanent type of pseudopodium, long and needle-like, characterized by an axial rod, composed of a bundle of fibrils inserted near the center of the cell body.

axosomatic (-so-mat'ik) referring to a synapse between the axon of one neuron and the cell body of another.

axostyle (ak'sah-stīl) 1. the central supporting structure of an axopodium. 2. a supporting rod running through the body of a trichomonad and protruding posteriorly.

azatadine (ah-zat'ah-dēn) an antihistaminic, $C_{20}H_{22}N_2$, used in the treatment of allergic rhinitis and chronic urticaria.

azathioprine (a"zah-thi'ah-prēn) a mercaptopurine derivative used as a cytotoxic and immunosuppressive agent in the treatment of leukemia and autoimmune diseases and in transplantation therapy.

azeotrope (a'ze-o-trōp") a mixture of two substances that has a constant boiling point and cannot be separated by fractional distillation.

azidothymidine (az"ĭ-do-thi'mĭ-dēn) zidovudine.

azoospermia (a"zo-o-sper'me-ah) absence of spermatozoa in the semen, or failure of formation of spermatozoa.

azote (a'zōt) nitrogen.

azoturia (-ūr'e-ah) excess of urea or other nitrogenous compounds in the urine. **azotu'ric,** adj.

azure (azh'er) one of three metachromatic basic dyes (A, B, and C).

azuresin (azh"er-ez'in) a complex combination of azure A dye and carbacrylic cationic exchange resin used as a diagnostic aid in detection of gastric secretion.

azurophil (azh-ōōr'ah-fil) a tissue constituent staining with azure or a similar metachromatic thiazin dye.

azurophilia (azh''er-ah-fil'e-ah) a condition in which the blood contains cells having azurophilic granules.

azygography (az''ĭ-gog'rah-fe) radiography of the azygous venous system. **azygograph'ic,** adj.

azygos (az'ĭ-gis) 1. unpaired. 2. any unpaired part, as the azygos vein.

B

B chemical symbol, *boron;* symbol for *bel.*

B.A. Bachelor of Arts.

Ba chemical symbol, *barium.*

Babesia (bah-be'ze-ah) a genus of protozoa found as parasites in red blood cells and transmitted by ticks; its numerous species cause disease in both wild and domestic animals and a malarialike illness in humans.

babesiasis (ba''be-si'ah-sis) 1. chronic, asymptomatic infection with protozoa of the genus *Babesia.* 2. babesiosis.

babesiosis (bah-be''ze-o'sis) a group of tickborne diseases due to infection with *Babesia* species, occurring in both wild and domestic animals and usually associated with anemia, hemoglobinuria, and hemoglobemia; human illness resembles malaria.

baby (ba'be) an infant; a child not yet able to walk. **blue b.,** an infant born with cyanosis due to a congenital heart lesion or atelectasis. **collodion b.,** an infant born completely covered by a collodion- or parchment-like membrane; see *lamellar exfoliation of the newborn,* under *exfoliation.*

bacca (bak'ah) [L.] a berry.

baccate (-āt) resembling a berry.

Bacillaceae (bas''il-la'se-e) a family of mostly saprophytic bacteria (order Eubacteriales), commonly found in soil; a few are insect or animal parasites and many cause disease.

bacillary (bas'ĭ-lĕ-re) pertaining to bacilli or to rodlike structures.

bacilli (bah-sil'i) plural of *bacillus.*

bacillin (bah-sil'in) an antibiotic substance isolated from strains of *Bacillus subtilis,* highly active on both gram-positive and gram-negative bacteria.

bacillosis (bas''il-o'sis) infection with bacilli.

bacilluria (bas''il-ür'e-ah) bacilli in the urine.

Bacillus (bah-sil'us) a genus of bacteria (family Bacillaceae), including gram-positive, spore-forming bacteria, separated into 33 species, three of which are pathogenic, or potentially so, the remainder being saprophytic soil forms. **B. an'thracis,** the causative agent of anthrax. **B. co'li,** *Escherichia coli.* **B. dysente'riae,** *Shigella dysenteriae.* **B. enteri'tidis,** *Salmonella enteritidis.* **B. le'prae,** *Mycobacterium leprae.* **B. mal'lei,** *Pseudomonas mallei.* **B. pneumo'-niae,** *Klebsiella pneumoniae.* **B. pseudomal'-lei,** *Pseudomonas pseudomallei.* **B. pyocya'-neus,** *Pseudomonas aeruginosa.* **B. sub'tilis,** a common saprophytic soil and water form, often occurring as a laboratory contaminant, and, rarely, in apparently causal relation to pathologic processes, such as conjunctivitis. **B. te'tani,** *Clostridium tetani.* **B. ty'phi,** **B. ty-pho'sus,** *Salmonella typhosa.* **B. welch'ii,** *Clostridium perfringens.*

bacillus (bah-sil'us), pl. *bacil'li* [L.] 1. an organism of the genus *Bacillus.* 2. a rod-shaped bacterium; any spore-forming, rod-shaped microorganism of the order Eubacteriales. **Bang's b.,** *Brucella abortus.* **Battey bacilli,** *Mycobacterium intracellulare.* **Bordet-Gengou b.,** *Bordetella pertussis.* **Calmette-Guerin b.,** *Mycobacterium bovis* rendered completely avirulent by cultivation over a long period on bile-glycerol-potato medium; see *BCG vaccine.* **coliform b.,** gram-negative bacilli resembling *Escherichia coli* that are found in the intestinal tract; the term generally refers to the genera *Citrobacter, Escherichia, Edwardiella, Enterobacter, Klebsiella,* and *Serratia.* **colon b.,** *Escherichia coli.* **Ducrey's b.,** *Haemophilus ducreyi.* **dysentery bacilli,** see *Shigella.* **enteric b.,** any bacillus belonging to the family Enterobacteriaceae. **Flexner's b.,** *Shigella flexneri.* **Friedländer's b.,** *Klebsiella pneumoniae.* **Gärtner's b.,** *Salmonella enteritidis.* **glanders b.,** *Pseudomonas mallei.* **Hansen's b.,** *Mycobacterium leprae.* **Johne's b.,** *Mycobacterium paratuberculosis.* **Klebs-Löffler b.,** *Corynebacterium diphtheriae.* **Koch-Weeks b.,** *Haemophilus aegyptius.* **legionnaire's b.,** *Legionella pneumophila.* **Morax-Axenfeld b.,** *Haemophilus duplex.* **Morgan's b.,** *Proteus morgani.* **Pfeiffer's b.,** *Haemophilus influenzae.* **Sonne-Duval b.,** *Shigella sonnei.* **tubercle b.,** *Mycobacterium tuberculosis.* **typhoid b.,** *Salmonella typhosa.*

bacitracin (bas''ĭ-tra'sin) an antibacterial polypeptide elaborated by the licheniformis group of *Bacillus subtilis,* effective against a wide range of infections; usually applied topically, but also given intramuscularly.

back-cross (-kros) a mating between a heterozygote and a homozygote.

backflow (-flo) abnormal backward flow of fluids; regurgitation. **pyelovenous b.,** drainage from the renal pelvis into the venous system occurring under certain conditions of back pressure.

baclofen (bak'lo-fen) an analogue of gamma-aminobutyric acid, $C_{10}H_{12}ClNO_2$, used as a muscle relaxant.

bacter(io)- word element [Gr.], *bacteria.*

Bacteria (bak-tēr'e-ah) in some former systems

of classification, a division of the kingdom Procaryotae including all prokaryotic organisms that are not blue-green algae (*Cyanophyceae*).

bacteria (bak-tēr′e-ah) plural of *bacterium*. **bacte′rial,** adj.

bactericidal (bak-tēr″ĭ-si′d′l) destructive to bacteria.

bactericidin (bak″ter-ĭ-sīd′in) bactericidal antibody.

bacterid (bak′ter-id) a skin eruption caused by bacterial infection elsewhere in the body.

bacteriochlorophyll (bak-tēr″e-o-klōr′ah-fil) a form of chlorophyll produced by certain bacteria and capable of carrying out photosynthesis.

bacteriocidin (-si′d′n) a bactericidal antibody.

bacteriocin (-sin) any of a group of substances, e.g., colicin, released by certain bacteria that kill other strains of bacteria by inducing metabolic block.

bacteriocinogenic (-sin″ah-jen′ik) giving rise to bacteriocin; denoting bacterial plasmids that synthesize bacteriocin.

bacteriology (-ol′ah-je) the scientific study of bacteria. **bacteriolog′ic,** adj.

bacteriolysin (-ol′ĭ-sin) an antibacterial antibody that lyses bacteria.

bacteriopexy (bak-tēr″e-ah-pek′se) the fixation of bacteria by histiocytes.

bacteriophage (bak-tēr′e-ah-fāj″) a virus that lyses bacteria; see *bacterial virus*. **bacteriopha′gic,** adj. **temperate b.,** one whose genetic material (prophage) becomes an intimate part of the bacterial genome, persisting and being reproduced through many cell division cycles; the affected bacterial cell is known as a *lysogenic bacterium* (q.v.).

bacteriopsonin (bak-tēr″e-op′so-nin) an antibody that acts on bacteria.

bacteriostatic (-stat′ik) inhibiting growth or multiplication of bacteria; an agent that so acts.

Bacterium (bak-tēr′e-um) former name for a genus of schizomycetes the species of which are now assigned to other genera, e.g., *Aerobacter, Pseudomonas, Salmonella,* etc.

bacterium (bak-tēr′e-um), pl. *bacte′ria* [L., Gr.] any prokaryotic organism. Bacteria are single-celled microorganisms about 1 μm in diameter; most species have a rigid cell wall. They differ from other organisms (eukaryotes) in lacking a nucleus and membrane-bound organelles and also in much of their biochemistry. **acid- fast b.,** one not readily decolorized by acids after staining. **coliform bacteria,** see *Escherichia, Aerobacter* and *Paracolobactrum.* **coryneform bacteria,** a group of bacteria that are morphologically similiar to organisms of the genus *Corynebacterium.* **hemophilic bacteria,** microorganisms of the genera *Haemophilus* and *Bordetella,* which have a nutritional affinity for constituents of fresh blood or whose growth is significantly stimulated on blood-containing media. **lactic acid bacteria,** those producing fermentation of carbohydrate materials to form lactic acid. **lysogenic b.,** a bacterial cell that harbors in its genome the genetic material (prophage) of a temperate bacteriophage and thus reproduces the bacteriophage in cell division; occasionally the prophage develop into the mature form, replicates, lyses the bacterial cell, and is free to infect other cells.

Bacteroidaceae (bak″tĕ-roi-da′se-e) a family of schizomycetes (order Eubacteriales).

Bacteroides (bak″tĕ-roi′des) a genus of gram-negative, anaerobic, rod-shaped bacteria, which are normal inhabitants of the oral, respiratory, intestinal, and urogenital cavities of humans and animals; some species are potential pathogens and cause possibly fatal abscesses and bacteremias.

bacteroides (-roid′ēz) 1. any highly pleomorphic rod-shaped bacteria. 2. an organism of the genus *Bacteroides.*

Bactrim (bak-trim) trademark for preparations of trimethoprim and sulfamethoxazole.

bag (bag) a sac or pouch. **Barnes' b.,** a water-filled rubber bag for dilating the uterine cervix. **colostomy b.,** a receptacle worn over the stoma to receive the fecal discharge after colostomy. **ileostomy b.,** any of various plastic or latex bags attached to the body for the collection of urine or fecal material following ileostomy or the establishment of an ileal bladder. **Politzer b.,** a soft bag of rubber for inflating the auditory tube. **b. of waters,** the membranes enclosing the liquor amnii and the developing fetus *in utero.*

bagassosis (bag″ah-so′sis) a lung disease due to inhalation of dust from the residue of cane after extraction of sugar (bagasse).

BAL dimercaprol (British anti-lewisite).

balance (bal′ins) 1. an instrument for weighing. 2. harmonious adjustment of parts; harmonious performance of functions. **acid-base b.,** a normal balance between production and excretion of acid or alkali by the body, resulting in a stable concentration of H^+ in body fluids. **analytical b.,** a laboratory balance sensitive to variations of the order of 0.05 to 0.1 mg. **fluid b.,** the state of the body in relation to ingestion and excretion of water and electrolytes. **nitrogen b.,** the state of the body in regard to ingestion and excretion of nitrogen. In *negative nitrogen b.* the amount excreted is greater than the quantity ingested; in *positive nitrogen b.* the amount excreted is smaller than the quantity ingested. **water b.,** fluid b.

balanitis (bal″ah-nīt′is) inflammation of the glans penis. **gangrenous b.,** erosion of the glans penis leading to rapid destruction, believed to be due to continually unhygienic conditions together with secondary spirochetal infection.

balanoposthitis (bal″ah-no-pos-thīt′is) inflammation of the glans penis and prepuce.

balanorrhagia (-ra′je-ah) balanitis with free discharge of pus.

balantidiasis (bal″in-tĭ-di′ah-sis) infection by protozoa of the genus *Balantidium;* in man, *B. coli* may cause diarrhea and dysentery with ulceration of the colonic mucosa.

Balantidium (bal″in-tid′e-um) a genus of ciliated protozoa, including many species found in

ballismus

the intestine in vertebrates and invertebrates, including *B. co'li,* a common parasite of swine, rarely in man, in whom it may cause dysentery, and *B. su'is,* found in pigs, often considered the same as *B. coli.*

ballismus (bah-liz'mus) violent movements of the limbs, as in chorea, sometimes affecting only one side of the body (hemiballismus).

ballottement (bah-lot'maw) [Fr.] a palpatory maneuver to test for a floating object, especially a maneuver for detecting pregnancy by inserting two fingers into the vagina and pushing the fetal head or breech, causing the fetus to leave and quickly return to the fingers.

balm (bahm) 1. a balsam. 2. a soothing or healing medicine.

balsam (bawl'sim) a semifluid, fragrant, resinous vegetable juice; balsams are resins combined with oils. **balsam'ic,** adj. **Canada b.,** an oleoresin from the balsam fir, used as a microscopic mounting medium. **b. of Peru, peruvian b.,** a dark brown viscid liquid from the tree *Myroxylon pereirae,* used as a local protectant and as a rubefacient. **tolu b.,** a brown or yellowish brown, plastic solid from the tree *Myroxylon balsamum,* used as an ingredient of compound benzoin tincture and as an expectorant.

bambermycins (bam''ber-mi'sinz) a complex of antibiotics produced by *Streptomyces* strains, used as a feed additive for livestock.

band (band) 1. a part, structure, or appliance that binds. 2. in dentistry, a thin metal strip fitted around a tooth or its roots. 3. in histology, a zone of a myofibril of striated muscle. 4. in cytogenetics, a segment of a chromosome stained brighter or darker than the adjacent bands; used in identifying the chromosomes and in determining the exact extent of chromosomal abnormalities. Called *Q-bands, G-bands, C-bands, T-bands,* etc., according to the staining method used. **A b.,** the dark-staining zone of a sarcomere, whose center is traversed by the H band. **H b.,** a pale zone sometimes seen traversing the center of the A band of a striated muscle fibril. **I b.,** the band within a striated muscle fibril, seen as a light region under the light microscope and as a dark region under polarized light. **iliotibial b.,** see under *tract.* **M b.,** the narrow dark band in the center of the H band. **matrix b.,** a thin piece of metal fitted around a tooth to supply a missing wall of a multisurface cavity to allow adequate condensation of amalgam into the cavity. **Z b.,** a thin membrane seen on longitudinal section as a dark line in the center of the I band; the distance between Z bands delimits the sarcomeres of striated muscle.

bandage 1. a strip or roll of gauze or other material for wrapping or binding a body part. 2. to cover by wrapping with such material. **Ace b.,** trademark for a bandage of woven elastic material. **Barton's b.,** a double figure-of-8 bandage for fracture of the lower jaw. **demigauntlet b.,** one that covers the hand but leaves the fingers exposed. **Desault's b.,** one binding the elbow to the side, with a pad in the axilla, for fractured clavicle. **Esmarch's b.,** an India rubber bandage applied upward around (from the distal

part to the proximal) a part in order to expel blood from it; the part is often elevated as the elastic pressure is applied. **gauntlet b.,** one which covers the hand and fingers like a glove. **Gibney b.,** strips of ½-inch adhesive overlapped along the sides and back of the foot and leg to hold the foot in slight varus position and leave the dorsum of foot and anterior aspect of leg exposed. **plaster b.,** one stiffened with a paste of plaster of Paris. **pressure b.,** one for applying pressure. **roller b.,** a tightly rolled, circular bandage of varying width and materials, often commercially prepared. **scultetus b.,** a many-tailed bandage applied with the tails overlapping each other and held in position by safety pins. **spica b.,** a figure-of-8 bandage with turns that cross one another regularly like the letter V, usually applied to anatomical areas whose dimensions vary, as the pelvis and thigh. **Velpeau b.,** one used in immobilization of certain fractures about the upper end of the humerus and shoulder joint, binding the arm and shoulder to the chest.

banding (band'ing) 1. the act of encircling and binding with a thin strip of material. 2. in genetics, any of several techniques of staining chromosomes so that a characteristic pattern of transverse dark and light bands becomes visible, permitting identification of individual chromosome pairs.

bar (bar) 1. a unit of pressure, being the pressure exerted by 1 megadyne per square cm. 2. a heavy wire or wrought or cast metal segment, longer than its width, used to connect parts of a removable partial denture. **chromatoidal b.,** chromatoid body. **median b.,** a fibrotic formation across the neck of the prostate gland, producing obstruction of the urethra. **Mercier's b.,** interureteric ridge. **terminal b.,** the beltlike seal between epithelial cells at the luminal surface as visualized by the light microscope. The electron microscope shows that it is composed of elements of the junctional complex.

barbital (bar'bit-ahl) the first of the barbiturates, being a long-acting hypnotic and sedative.

barbiturate (bar-bit'choor-āt) a salt or derivative of barbituric acid; barbiturates are used for their hypnotic and sedative effects.

barbituric acid (bar-bǐ-tōōr'ik) $C_4H_4N_2O_3$, the parent substance of barbiturates.

barbotage (bar''bo-tahzh') [Fr.] repeated alternate injection and withdrawal of fluid with a syringe, as in gastric lavage or administration of an anesthetic agent into the subarachnoid space by alternate injection of part of the anesthetic and withdrawal of cerebrospinal fluid into the syringe.

baresthesiometer (bar''es-the''ze-om'it-er) instrument for estimating sense of weight or pressure.

bariatrics (bar''e-ă'triks) a field of medicine encompassing the study of overweight, its causes, prevention, and treatment.

barium (bar'e-um) chemical element (*see table*), at. no. 56, symbol Ba. **b. sulfate,** a water-insoluble salt, $BaSO_4$, used as an opaque contrast medium in roentgenography of the digestive tract.

baroceptor (bar″ah-sep′ter) baroreceptor.

barophilic (-fil′ik) growing best under high atmospheric pressure; said of bacteria.

baroreceptor (-re-sep′ter) a sensory nerve ending that is stimulated by pressure changes, as those in blood vessel walls.

barosinusitis (-si″nis-īt′tis) a symptom complex due to differences in environmental atmospheric pressure and the air pressure in the paranasal sinuses.

barotaxis (-tak′sis) stimulation of living matter by change of atmospheric pressure.

barotitis (-tīt′is) a morbid condition of the ear due to exposure to differing atmospheric pressures. **b. me′dia**, a symptom complex due to difference between atmospheric pressure of the environment and air pressure in the middle ear.

barotrauma (-traw′mah) injury due to pressure, as to structures of the ear, in high-altitude flyers, owing to differences between atmospheric and intratympanic pressures; see *barosinusitis* and *barotitis*.

barrier (bă′re-er) an obstruction. **blood-air b.**, alveolocapillary membrane. **blood-aqueous b.**, the physiologic mechanism that prevents exchange of materials between the chambers of the eye and the blood. **blood-brain b.**, **blood-cerebral b.**, the selective barrier separating the blood from the parenchyma of the central nervous system. Abbreviated *BBB*. **blood-gas b.**, alveolocapillary membrane. **blood-testis b.**, a barrier separating the blood from the seminiferous tubules, consisting of special junctional complexes between adjacent Sertoli cells near the base of the seminiferous epithelium. **placental b.**, the tissue layers of the placenta which regulate the exchange of substances between the fetal and maternal blood.

Bartonella (bar″to-nel′ah) a genus of the family Bartonellaceae, including *B. bacillifor′mis*, the etiologic agent of Carrión's disease.

Bartonellaceae (-nel-a′se-e) a family of the order Rickettsiales, occurring as pathogenic parasites in the erythrocytes of man and other animals.

bartonelliasis, bartonellosis (-nel-i′ah-sis; -nel-o′sis) Carrión's disease.

baryphonia (-fo′ne-ah) deepness and hoarseness of the voice.

basad (ba′sad) toward a base or basal aspect.

basal (ba′s′l, ba′z′l) pertaining to or situated near a base; in physiology, pertaining to the lowest possible level.

base (bās) 1. the lowest part or foundation of anything; see also *basis*. 2. the main ingredient of a compound. 3. in chemistry, a substance that combines with acids to form salts; a substance that dissociates to give hydroxide ions in aqueous solutions; a substance whose molecule or ion can combine with a proton (hydrogen ion); a substance capable of donating a pair of electrons (to an acid) for the formation of a coordinate covalent bond. **denture b.**, the material in which the teeth of a denture are set and which rests on the supporting tissues when the denture is in place in the mouth. **nitrogenous b.**, an aromatic, nitrogen-containing molecule that serves as a proton acceptor, e.g., purine or pyrimidine. **ointment b.**, a vehicle for medicinal substances intended for external application to the body. **purine b's**, a group of chemical compounds of which purine is the base, including adenine, theobromine, uric acid, and xanthine. **pyrimidine b's**, a group of chemical compounds of which pyrimidine is the base, including uracil, thymine, and cytosine, which are common constituents of nucleic acids. **record b.**, baseplate. **b. of stapes**, footplate. **temporary b.**, trial b., baseplate.

baseline (bās′līn) a known value or quantity used to measure or assess an unknown, as a baseline urine sample.

baseplate (-plāt) a sheet of plastic material used in making trial plates for artificial dentures.

basial (ba′se-il) pertaining to the basion.

basic (ba′sik) 1. pertaining to or having properties of a base. 2. capable of neutralizing acids.

basicity (ba-sis′it-e) 1. the quality of being a base, or basic. 2. the combining power of an acid.

Basidiobolus (bah-sid″ī-ob′ah-lus) a genus of phycomycetous fungi (family Entomophthoraceae, order Entomophthorales), including *B. haptospo′rus*, the cause of subcutaneous phycomycosis.

basidium (-um), pl. *basi′dia* [L.] the clublike organ bearing basidiospores.

basihyoid (ba″se-hi′oid) the body of the hyoid bone; in certain lower animals, either of two lateral bones that are its homologues.

basilad (bas′ī-lad) toward the base.

basilemma (-lem′ah) basement membrane.

basiloma (bas-ī-lo′mah) basal cell carcinoma.

basion (ba′se-on) the midpoint of the anterior border of the foramen magnum.

basipetal (ba-sip′it′l) descending toward the base; developing in the direction of the base, as a spore.

basis (ba′sis) the lower, basic, or fundamental part of an object, organ, or substance.

basisphenoid (ba″sah-sfe′noid) an embryonic bone which becomes the back part of the body of the sphenoid.

basoerythrocyte (ba″so-ĕ-rith′rah-sīt) an erythrocyte containing basophil granules.

basophil (ba′sah-fil) 1. any structure, cell, or histologic element staining readily with basic dyes. 2. a granular leukocyte with an irregularly shaped, relatively pale-staining nucleus that is partially constricted into two lobes, and with cytoplasm containing coarse bluish black granules of variable size. 3. a beta cell of the adenohypophysis. 4. basophilic.

basophilia (ba″sah-fil′e-ah) 1. reaction of relatively immature erythrocytes to basic dyes whereby the stained cells appear blue, gray, or grayish-blue, or bluish granules appear. 2. abnormal increase of basophilic leukocytes in the blood. 3. basophilic leukocytosis.

basophilism (ba-sof′ī-lizm) abnormal increase

of basophilic cells. **Cushing's b., pituitary b.,** see under *syndrome* (1).

bath (bath) 1. a medium, e.g., water, vapor, sand, or mud, with which the body is washed or in which the body is wholly or partially immersed for therapeutic or cleansing purposes; application of such a medium to the body. 2. the equipment or apparatus in which a body or object may be immersed. **colloid b.,** one containing gelatin, starch, bran, or similar substances. **contrast b.,** alternate immersion of a body part in hot and cold water. **cool b.,** one in water from 65° to 75° F. **douche b.,** application of water to the body from a jet spray. **emollient b.,** one in an emollient liquid, e.g., a decoction of bran. **graduated b.,** one in which the temperature of the water is gradually lowered. **half b.,** a bath of the hips and lower part of the body. **hip b.,** sitz b. **hot b.,** one in water from 98° to 104° F. **mud b.,** application of wet sticky earth to the body, or immersion of the body in such material. **needle b.,** a shower bath in which the water is projected in a fine, needle-like spray. **sitz b.,** immersion of only the hips and buttocks. **sponge b.,** one in which the body is not immersed but is rubbed with a wet cloth or sponge. **tepid b.,** one in water 75° to 92° F. **warm b.,** one in water 92° to 97° F. **whirlpool b.,** one in which the water is kept in constant motion by mechanical means.

bathrocephaly (bath″ro-sef′ah-le) a developmental anomaly marked by a steplike posterior projection of the skull, caused by excessive growth of the lambdoid suture.

bathy- word element [Gr.], *deep.*

bathypnea (-ne′ah) deep breathing.

battery (bat′er-e) 1. a set or series of cells affording an electric current. 2. any set, series, or grouping of similar things, as a battery of tests.

B.C. bone conduction.

BCG bacille Calmette-Guérin (see under *vaccine*).

BCNU carmustine.

Bdellovibrio (del″o-vib′re-o) a genus of small, rod-shaped or curved, actively motile bacteria that are obligate parasites on certain gram-negative bacteria, including *Pseudomonas, Salmonella,* and coliform bacteria.

bdellovibrio (del″o-vib′re-o) any microorganism of the genus *Bdellovibrio.*

Be chemical symbol, *beryllium.*

beaker (bēk′er) a glass cup, usually with a lip for pouring, used by chemists and pharmacists.

beat (bēt) a throb or pulsation, as of the heart or of an artery. **apex b.,** the beat felt over the apex of the heart, normally in the fifth left intercostal space. **capture b's,** occasional ventricular responses to a sinus impulse that reaches the atrioventricular node in a nonrefractory phase. **ectopic b.,** a heart beat originating at some point other than the sinus node. **escaped b's,** heart beats that follow an abnormally long pause. **forced b.,** an extrasystole produced by artificial stimulation of the heart. **fusion b.,** in electrocardiography, the complex resulting when an ectopic ventricular beat coincides with normal conduction to the ventricle. **premature b.,** extrasystole.

bechic (bek′ik) pertaining to cough.

beclomethasone dipropionate (bek″lo-meth′-ah-sōn) a glucocorticoid, $C_{28}H_{37}ClO_7$; administered by aerosol inhalation to patients who require chronic treatment with corticosteroids for control of bronchial asthma symptoms.

becquerel (bek-rel′) the proposed SI unit of radioactivity defined as the quantity of a radionuclide that undergoes one decay per second (s^{-1}). One curie equals 3.7×10^{10} becquerels. Abbreviated Bq.

bed (bed) 1. a supporting structure or tissue. 2. a couch or support for the body during sleep. **capillary b.,** the capillaries, collectively, and their volume capacity; see Plate IX. **fracture b.,** one for the use of patients with broken bones. **Klondike b.,** one arranged to protect the patient from drafts in outdoor sleeping. **nail b.,** matrix unguis; the area of modified epithelium beneath the nail, over which the nail plate slides forward as it grows.

bedbug (bed′bug) a bug of the genus *Cimex.*

Bedsonia (bed-so′ne-ah) *Chlamydia.*

bedsore (bed′sōr) decubitus ulcer.

behavior (be-hāv′yer) deportment or conduct; any or all of a person's total activity, especially that which is externally observable.

behaviorism (-izm) the psychologic theory based upon objectively observable, tangible, and measurable data, rather than subjective phenomena, such as ideas and emotions.

bel (bel) a unit used to express the ratio of two powers, usually electric or acoustic powers; an increase of 1 bel in intensity approximately doubles loudness of most sounds. See also *decibel.*

belemnoid (bel′im-noid, bah-lem′-noid) 1. dart-shaped. 2. the styloid process.

belladonna (bel″ah-don′ah) 1. *Atropa belladonna* (deadly nightshade), a plant that is the source of various alkaloids, e.g., atropine, hyoscyamine, etc. 2. belladonna leaf; the dried leaves and fruiting flowering tops of *Atropa belladonna,* used as an anticholinergic.

belly (bel′e) 1. the abdomen. 2. the fleshy, contractile part of a muscle.

belonoid (bel′ah-noid) needle-shaped; styloid.

benactyzine (ben-ak′tĭ-zēn) an ataraxic, $C_{20}H_{25}$-NO_3, used as the hydrochloride salt.

Benadryl (ben′ah-dril) trademark for a preparation of diphenhydramine.

bend (bend) a flexure or curve; a flexed or curved part. **varolian b.,** the third cerebral flexure in the developing fetus.

bendroflumethiazide (ben″dro-floo″mĭ-thi′-ah-zīd) a diuretic and antihypertensive, $C_{15}H_{14}$-$F_3N_3O_4S_2$.

bends (bendz) pain in the limbs and abdomen due to rapid reduction of air pressure; see *decompression sickness.*

benign (bĭ-nīn′) not malignant; not recurrent; favorable for recovery.

benoxinate (bah-nok′sĭ-nāt) a surface anesthetic for the eye, $C_{17}H_{28}N_2O_3$, used as the hydrochloride salt.

bentonite (ben′tah-nīt) a native colloidal hydrated aluminum silicate that swells in water; used as a suspending agent and as a bulk laxative.

Bentyl (ben′til) trademark for preparations of dicyclomine hydrochloride.

Benylin (ben′ĭ-lin) trademark for a preparation of diphenhydramine hydrochloride and alcohol.

benzaldehyde (ben-zal′dĕ-hīd) artificial essential oil of almond; used as a flavoring agent.

benzalkonium chloride (ben″zal-ko′ne-um) a quaternary ammonium compound, used as a surface disinfectant and detergent and as a topical antiseptic and antimicrobial preservative.

Benzedrex (ben′zah-dreks) trademark for a propylhexedrine inhaler.

Benzedrine (-drēn) trademark for a preparation of amphetamine.

benzene (ben′zēn) a liquid hydrocarbon, C_6H_6, from coal tar; used as a solvent. **b. hexachloride,** a compound, $C_6H_6Cl_6$, having five isomers, the gamma isomer being a powerful insecticide.

benzethonium chloride (ben″zah-tho′ne-um) a quaternary ammonium compound, $C_{27}H_{42}Cl$-NO_2; used as a local anti-infective, as a preservative in pharmaceutical preparations, and as a detergent and disinfectant.

benzidine (ben′zĭ-dēn) a compound, $NH_2 \cdot C_6$-$H_4 \cdot C_6H_4NH_2$, used as a test for blood.

benzin, benzine (ben′zin; ben′zēn) petroleum b. **petroleum b.,** a purified distillate from petroleum, a solvent for organic compounds.

benzoate (ben′zo-āt) a salt of benzoic acid.

benzocaine (-kān) a local anesthetic, $C_9H_{11}NO_2$, used topically.

benzodiazepine (ben″zo-di-az′ah-pēn) any of a group of minor tranquilizers, including chlordiazepoxide, clorazepate, diazepam, flurazepam, and oxazepam, having a common molecular structure and similar pharmacological activities, such as antianxiety, muscle relaxing, and sedative and hypnotic effects.

benzoic acid (ben-zo′ik) a crystalline acid, C_6H_5-COOH, from benzoin and other resins and from coal tar; used as an antifungal agent and as a germicide. Its sodium salt (sodium benzoate) is also used as an antifungal agent, and may be used as a test for liver function.

benzoin (ben′zo-in, -zoin) a balsamic resin from *Styrax benzoin* and other *Styrax* species, used as a topical protectant and antiseptic and as an expectorant.

benzonatate (ben-zo′nah-tāt) an antitussive, $C_{30}H_{53}NO_{11}$.

benzothiadiazide, benzothiadiazine (ben″zo-thi″ah-di′ah-zīd; -zēn) thiazide.

benzoyl (ben′zo-il) the acyl radical formed from benzoic acid, C_6H_5CO—. **b. peroxide,** dibenzoyl peroxide, used as a topical keratolytic in the treatment of acne vulgaris.

benzphetamine (benz-fet′ah-mēn) a sympathomimetic amine, $C_{17}H_{21}N$, used as an anorexiant in the form of the hydrochloride salt.

benzquinamide (-kwin′ah-mīd) a compound,

$C_{22}H_{32}N_2O_5$, used intramuscularly or intravenously as an antiemetic; it also has antihistaminic and mild anticholinergic and sedative action.

benzthiazide (-thi′ah-zīd) a diuretic and antihypertensive, $C_{15}H_{14}ClN_3O_4S_3$.

benztropine (benz′trah-pēn) a parasympatholytic, $C_{21}H_{25}NO$, used as the mesylate salt in parkinsonism.

benzyl (ben′zil) the hydrocarbon radical, C_7H_7. **b. benzoate,** a clear, colorless, oily liquid, C_{14}-$H_{12}O_2$, used as a pharmaceutic necessity in the preparation of dimercaprol for injection and applied topically as a scabicide.

benzylpenicillin (ben″zil-pen″ĭ-sil′in) penicillin G.

beriberi (bĕ′re-bĕ′re) a disease due to thiamine (vitamin B_1) deficiency, marked by polyneuritis, cardiac pathology, and edema; the epidemic form occurs primarily in areas in which white (polished) rice is the staple food.

berkelium (ber-kēl′e-um, berk′le-um) chemical element (*see table*), at. no. 97, symbol Bk.

berylliosis (bah-ril″e-o′sis) a morbid condition due to exposure to fumes or finely divided dust of beryllium salts, marked by formation of granulomas, usually involving the lungs and, rarely, the skin, subcutaneous tissue, lymph nodes, liver, and other organs.

beryllium (bah-ril′le-um) chemical element (*see table*), at. no. 4, symbol Be.

Besnoitia (bes-noit′e-ah) a genus of sporozoa, including *B. bennetti* and *B. besnoiti*, which cause benoitiosis in horses and cattle, respectively.

besnoitiosis (bes-noit″e-o′sis) a disease of cattle, horses, sheep, goats, and other herbivorous animals, due to sporozoan parasites of the genus *Besnoitia*, in which the organisms localize in the skin, blood vessels, mucous membranes, and other tissues, where they eventually form characteristic thick-walled cysts.

besylate (bes′ĭ-lāt) USAN contraction for benzenesulfonate.

beta (bāt′ah) second letter of the Greek alphabet, β; used in names of chemical compounds to distinguish one of two or more isomers or to indicate position of substituting atoms or groups.

Betadine (-dēn) trademark for preparations of povidone-iodine.

beta-hydroxybutyric acid, beta-oxybutyric acid (bāt′ah-hi-drok″se-bu-tir′ik) CH_3CHOH--CH_2COOH, one of the ketone bodies, occurring in the urine in diabetic ketoacidosis and starvation due to incomplete fatty acid oxidation.

beta-ketobutyric acid (kēt″o-bu-tir′ik) acetoacetic acid.

betaine (bēt′ah-ēn) the carboxylic acid derived by oxidation of choline; it acts as a transmethylating metabolic intermediate. The hydrochloride salt is used as a gastric acidifier.

betamethasone (bāt-ah-meth′ah-sōn) a synthetic glucocorticoid, $C_{22}H_{29}FO_5$, the most active of the anti-inflammatory steroids; available as a cream or tablet for topical or oral use.

betazole (bat′ah-zōl) a pyrazole derivative, C_5-H_9N_3; its hydrochloride salt is used in gastric function tests to stimulate gastric secretion.

bethanechol (bĕ-than′ĕ-kol) a cholinergic antagonist, $C_7H_{17}N_2O_2$, used to stimulate smooth muscle contraction of the gastrointestinal tract and urinary bladder in cases of postoperative or neurognic atony and retention; used as the chloride salt.

BF blastogenic factor.

Bi chemical symbol, *bismuth.*

bi- word element [L.], *two.*

bicameral (bi-kam′er-il) having two chambers or cavities.

bicarbonate (-kar′bi-nāt) any salt containing the HCO_3^- anion. **blood b., plasma b.,** the bicarbonate of the blood plasma, an index of alkali reserve. **b. of soda,** sodium bicarbonate.

biceps (bi′seps) a muscle having two heads.

bicipital (bi-sip′it′l) having two heads; pertaining to a biceps muscle.

biconcave (-kon-kāv′) having two concave surfaces.

biconvex (-kon-veks′) having two convex surfaces.

bicornate, bicornuate (-kor′nāt; -kor′nu-āt, -it) having two horns or cornua.

bicuspid (-kus′pid) 1. having two cusps. 2. a bicuspid (mitral) valve. 3. a premolar tooth.

b.i.d. [L.] *bis in di′e* (twice a day).

bidermoma (bid″er-mo′mah) a teratoma composed of cells and tissues from two germ layers.

biduous (bĭ′du-us) lasting two days.

bifid (bi′fid) cleft into two parts or branches.

Bifidobacterium (bi″fid-o-bak-te′re-um) a genus of obligate anaerobic lactobacilli commonly occurring in the feces.

biforate (bi-for′āt) having two perforations or foramina.

bifurcation (bi″fer-ka′shin) 1. a division into two branches. 2. the point at which division into two branches occurs.

bighead (big′hed) 1. a condition of young rams characterized by edematous swelling of the head and neck, due to *Clostridium novyi.* 2. thickening of face and ears in white sheep, due to photosensitivity after ingestion of certain plants. 3. hydrocephalus in mink.

bile (bīl) a fluid secreted by the liver, concentrated in the gallbladder, and poured into the small intestine via the bile ducts, which helps in alkalinizing the intestinal contents and plays a role in emulsification, absorption, and digestion of fat; its chief constituents are conjugated bile salts, cholesterol, phospholipid, bilirubin, and electrolytes.

bile acids steroid acids derived from cholesterol; classified as primary, those synthesized in the liver, e.g., cholic and chendeoxycholic acid, or secondary, produced from primary bile acids by intestinal bacteria and returned to the liver by enterohepatic circulation, e.g., deoxycholic and lithocholic acid. Cf. *bile salt* under *salt.*

Bilharzia (bil-har′ze-ah) *Schistosoma.*

bilharziasis (bil″har-zi′ah-sis) schistosomiasis.

bili- word element [L.], *bile.*

biliousness (-nis) a symptom complex comprising nausea, abdominal discomfort, headache,

and constipation, formerly attributed to excessive bile secretion.

bilirachia (bil″i-ra′ke-ah) presence of bile pigments in spinal fluid.

bilirubin (-roo′bin) a bile pigment produced by breakdown of heme and reduction of biliverdin; it normally circulates in plasma and is taken up by liver cells and conjugated to form bilirubin diglucuronide, the water-soluble pigment excreted in bile. High concentrations of bilirubin may result in jaundice. **conjugated b., direct b.,** bilirubin that has been taken up by the liver cells and conjugated to form the water-soluble bilirubin diglucuronide. **indirect b., unconjugated b.,** bilirubin.

biliverdin (bil″i-ver′d′n) a green bile pigment formed by catabolism of hemoglobin and converted to bilirubin in the liver; it may also arise from oxidation of bilirubin.

bilocular (-lok′u-ler) having two compartments.

biloma (bi′lo-mah) an encapsulated collection of bile in the peritoneal cavity.

binary (bi′nah-re) made up of two elements or of two equal parts; denoting a number system with a base of two.

binaural (bi-naw′r′l, bin-aw′r′l) pertaining to both ears.

binauricular (bin″aw-rik′u-ler) pertaining to both auricles of the ears.

binder (bīnd′er) a girdle or large bandage for support of the abdomen or breasts. **abdominal b.,** one applied to the abdomen after childbirth to support relaxed abdominal walls. **obstetric b.,** an abdominal girdle or bandage chiefly for women in labor who have pendulous abdomen.

binocular (bin-ok′u-ler) 1. pertaining to both eyes. 2. having two eyepieces, as in a microscope.

binomial (bi-no′me-il) composed of two terms, e.g., names of organisms formed by combination of genus and species names.

binovular (bin-ov′u-ler) pertaining to or derived from two distinct ova.

binucleation (bi″noo-kle-a′shin) formation of two nuclei within a cell through division of the nucleus without division of the cytoplasm.

bio- word element [Gr.], *life; living.*

bioaminergic (-am″in-er′jik) of or pertaining to neurons that secrete biogenic amines.

bioassay (-as′a) determination of the active power of a drug sample by comparing its effects on a live animal or an isolated organ preparation with those of a reference standard.

bioavailability (-ah-val″ah-bil′it-e) the degree to which a drug or other substance becomes available to the target tissue after administration.

biochemistry (-kem′is-tre) the chemistry of living organisms and of vital processes.

biocompatibility (-kom-pat″i-bil′it-e) the quality of not having toxic or injurious effects on biological systems. **biocompat′ible,** adj.

biodegradable (-de-grād′ah-b′l) susceptible of degradation by biological processes, as by bacterial or other enzymatic action.

biodegradation (-deg″rah-da′shin) the series of

processes by which living systems render chemicals less noxious to the environment.

bioequivalence (-ĕ-kwiv′ah-lins) the relationship between two preparations of the same drug in the same dosage form that have a similar bioavailability. **bioequiv′alent,** adj.

biofeedback (-fēd′bak) the process of furnishing an individual with information on the state of one or more physiologic variables, such as heart rate, blood pressure, or skin temperature; this often enables the individual to gain some voluntary control over them. **alpha b.,** the visual presentation of his own brain wave patterns to a subject who is instructed to try to produce alpha brain wave activity to achieve the alpha state of relaxation and peaceful wakefulness. An acoustic tone is used to indicate nonproduction of alpha waves.

biogenesis (-jen′ĭ-sis) 1. origin of life, or of living organisms. 2. the theory that living organisms originate only from other living organisms.

bioimplant (-im′plant) a prosthesis made of biosynthetic material.

biokinetics (-ki-net′iks) the study of the movements of tissue and other changes that occur in the development of organisms.

biological (-lah′jĭ-k′l) 1. pertaining to biology. 2. a medicinal preparation made from living organisms and their products, including serums, vaccines, etc.

biology (bi-ol′ah-je) scientific study of living organisms. **molecular b.,** study of molecular structures and events underlying biological processes, including relation between genes and the functional characteristics they determine. **radiation b.,** scientific study of effects of ionizing radiation on living organisms.

bioluminescence (bi″o-loo″mĭ-nes′ins) chemoluminescence occurring in living cells.

biomass (bi′o-mas) the entire assemblage of living organisms of a particular region, considered collectively.

biomaterial (bi″o-mah-tēr′e-il) a synthetic dressing with selective barrier properties, used in the treatment of burns; it consists of a liquid solvent (polyethylene glycol-400) and a powdered polymer.

biome (bi′ōm) a large, distinct, easily differentiated community of organisms arising as a result of complex interactions of climatic factors, biota, and substrate; usually designated, according to kind of vegetation present, as tundra, coniferous or deciduous forest, grassland, etc.

biomedicine (-med′ĭ-sin) clinical medicine based on the principles of the natural sciences (biology, biochemistry, etc.) **biomed′ical,** adj.

biomembrane (-mem′brān) any membrane, e.g., the cell membrane, of an organism. **biomem′-branous,** adj.

biometry (bi-om′ĭ-tre) the application of statistical methods to biological facts.

biomicroscope (bi″o-mi′krah-skōp) a microscope for examining living tissue in the body.

biomolecule (-mol′ĭ-kūl) a molecule produced by living cells, e.g., a protein, carbohydrate, lipid, or nucleic acid.

bionics (bi-on′-iks) scientific study of functions, characteristics, and phenomena observed in the living world, and the application of knowledge gained therefrom to nonliving systems.

biophysics (bi″o-fiz′iks) the science dealing with the application of physical methods and theories to biological problems. **biophys′ical,** adj.

biophysiology (-fiz″e-ol′ah-je) that portion of biology including organogeny, morphology, and physiology.

biopsy (bi′op-se) removal and examination, usually microscopic, of tissue from the living body, performed to establish precise diagnosis. **aspiration b.,** biopsy in which tissue is obtained by application of suction through a needle attached to a syringe. **brush b.,** biopsy in which cells or tissue are obtained by manipulating tiny brushes against the tissue or lesion in question (e.g., through a bronchoscope) at the desired site. **cone b.,** biopsy in which an inverted cone of tissue is excised, as from the uterine cervix. **endoscopic b.,** removal of tissue by appropriate instruments through an endoscope. **excisional b.,** biopsy of tissue removed by surgical cutting. **incisional b.,** biopsy of a selected portion of a lesion. **needle b.,** biopsy in which tissue is obtained by puncture of a tumor, the tissue within the lumen of the needle being detached by rotation, and the needle withdrawn. **percutaneous b.,** biopsy in which tissue is obtained by a needle inserted through the skin. **punch b.,** biopsy in which tissue is obtained by a punch. **sternal b.,** biopsy of bone marrow of the sternum removed by puncture or trephining.

bioptome (bi′op-tōm″) a cutting instrument for taking biopsy specimens.

bioreversible (bi″o-re-ver′sĭ-b′l) capable of being changed back to the original biologically active chemical form by processes within the organism; said of drugs.

bioscience (-si′ins) the study of biology wherein all the applicable sciences (physics, chemistry, etc.) are applied.

biosphere (bi′o-sfēr) 1. that part of the universe in which living organisms are known to exist, comprising the atmosphere, hydrosphere, and lithosphere. 2. the sphere of action between an organism and its environment.

biostatistics (bi″o-stah-tis′tiks) vital statistics.

biostereometrics (-stĕr″e-o-mĕ′triks) analysis of the spatial and spatial-temporal characteristics of biological form and function by means of three-dimensional mapping of the body.

biosynthesis (-sin′thĭ-sis) creation of a compound by physiologic processes in a living organism. **biosynthet′ic,** adj.

biota (bi-ōt′ah) all the living organisms of a particular area; the combined flora and fauna of a region.

biotelemetry (bi″o-tel-em′ĭ-tre) the recording and measuring of certain vital phenomena of living organisms that are situated at a distance from the measuring device.

biotin (bi′o-tin) a member of the vitamin B complex, $C_{10}H_{16}O_3N_2S$, required by or occurring in all forms of life tested.

biotoxicology (bi″o-tok″sĭ-kol′ah-je) scientific

study of poisons produced by living organisms, and treatment of conditions produced by them.

biotransformation (-trans″for-ma′shin) the series of chemical alterations of a compound (e.g., a drug) occurring within the body, as by enzymatic activity.

biotype (bi′o-tīp) 1. a group of individuals having the same genotype. 2. any of a number of strains of a species of microorganisms having differentiable physiologic characteristics.

biovular (bi-ov′u-ler) binovular.

biparous (bip′ah-ris) producing two ova or offspring at one time.

bipenniform (bi-pen′ĭ-form) doubly feather-shaped; said of muscles whose fibers are arranged on each side of a tendon like barbs on a feather shaft.

biperiden (-pĕ′rĭ-den) a synthetic anticholinergic, $C_{21}H_{29}NO$, used to reduce tremors of parkinsonism and in the treatment of drug-induced extrapyramidal reactions.

biphenyl (-fen′il) diphenyl, $(C_6H_5)_2$. **polychlorinated b's (PCBs),** chlorinated derivatives of biphenyl, used as heat-transfer agents and as electrical insulators; they are toxic and not biodegradable.

bipotentiality (bi″pah-ten″she-al′it-e) ability to develop or act in either of two possible ways.

biramous (bi-ra′mis) having two branches.

birefringence (-re-frin′jens) the quality of transmitting light unequally in different directions. **birefrin′gent,** adj.

birth (berth) a coming into being; act or process of being born. **complete b.,** entire separation of the infant from the maternal body (after cutting of the umbilical cord). **multiple b.,** the birth of two or more offspring produced in the same gestation period. **premature b.,** birth of a premature infant.

birthmark (berth′mark) nevus; a circumscribed blemish or spot on the skin of congenital origin.

bisacodyl (bis-ah-kōd′'l) a cathartic, $C_{22}H_{19}NO_4$.

bisacromial (bis″ah-kro′me-il) pertaining to the two acromial processes.

bisalbuminemia (-al-bu″min-e′me-ah) a congenital abnormality marked by the presence of two distinct serum albumins that differ in mobility on electrophoresis.

bisection (bi-sek′shin) division into two parts by cutting.

bisexual (-sek′shoo-il) 1. having gonads of both sexes. 2. hermaphrodite. 3. having both active and passive sexual interests or characteristics. 4. capable of the function of both sexes. 5. both heterosexual and homosexual. 6. an individual who is both heterosexual and homosexual. 7. of, relating to, or involving both sexes, as bisexual reproduction.

bisferious (bis-fe′re-us) dicrotic; having two beats.

bisiliac (bis-il″e-ak) pertaining to the two iliac bones or to any two corresponding points on them.

bis in die (bis in de′a) [L.] twice a day.

bismuth (biz′muth) chemical element (*see table*), at. no. 83, symbol Bi. Its salts have been used in

inflammatory diseases of the stomach and intestines and in syphilis.

bismuthosis (biz″muth-o′sis) chronic bismuth poisoning, with anuria, stomatitis, dermatitis, and diarrhea.

2,3-bisphosphoglycerate (bis-fos″fo-glis′er-āt) an intermediate in the conversion of 3-phosphoglycerate to 2-phosphoglycerate; it also acts as an allosteric effector in the regulation of oxygen binding by hemoglobin.

bistoury (bis′too-re) a long, narrow, straight or curved, surgical knife.

bisulfate (bi-sul′fāt) an acid sulfate.

bite 1. seizure with the teeth. 2. a wound or puncture made by a living organism. 3. an impression made by closure of the teeth upon some plastic material, e.g., wax. 4. occlusion (2). **closed b.,** malocclusion in which the incisal edges of the mandibular anterior teeth protrude past those of the maxillary teeth. **cross b.,** crossbite. **edge-to-edge b., end-to-end b.,** occlusion in which the incisors of both jaws are closed. **open b.,** occlusion in which certain opposing teeth fail to come together when the jaws are closed; usually confined to anterior teeth. **over-b.,** overbite.

bite-block (bīt′blok) occlusion rim.

bitelock (-lok) a dental device for retaining occlusion rims in the same relation outside the mouth which they occupied in the mouth.

biteplate (bīt′plāt) an appliance, usually plastic and wire, worn in the palate as a diagnostic or therapeutic adjunct in orthodontics or prosthodontics.

bite-wing (-wing) a wing or fin attached along the center of the tooth side of a dental x-ray film and bitten on by the patient, permitting production of images of the corona of the teeth in both dental arches and their contiguous periodontal tissues.

Bitis (bit′is) a genus of venomous, brightly colored, thick-bodied, viperine snakes, possessing heart-shaped heads; including the puff adder (*B. arientans*), Gaboon viper (*B. gabonica*), and rhinoceros viper (*B. nasicornis*).

bitrochanteric (bi-tro″kan-tĕ′tik) pertaining to both trochanters on one femur or to both greater trochanters.

bituminosis (bĭ-too″min-o′sis) a form of pneumoconiosis due to dust from soft coal.

biuret (bi′ūr-it) a urea derivative, $C_2O_3N_3H_5$; its presence is detected after addition of sodium hydroxide and copper sulfate solutions by a pinkish-violet color (protein test) or a pink and finally a bluish color (urea test).

bivalent (bi-va′lent) 1. having a valence of two. 2. denoting homologous chromosomes associated in pairs during the first meiotic prophase.

biventricular (bi″ven-trik′u-ler) pertaining to or affecting both ventricles of the heart.

bizygomatic (bi-zi″go-mat′ik) pertaining to the two most prominent points on the two zygomatic arches.

Bk chemical symbol, *berkelium.*

black (blak) reflecting no light or true color; of the darkest hue.

blackhead (blak′hed) 1. comedo. 2. histomoniasis of turkeys.

blackleg (-leg) symptomatic anthrax.

blackout (-owt) loss of vision and momentary lapse of consciousness due to diminished circulation to the brain and retina.

bladder (blad′er) a membranous sac, such as one serving as receptacle for a secretion, especially the urinary bladder. **automatic b.,** neurogenic bladder due to complete transection of the spinal cord above the sacral segments, with loss of micturition reflexes and bladder sensation, involuntary voiding, and an abnormal amount of residual urine. **autonomic b., autonomous b.,** neurogenic bladder due to a lesion in the sacral portion of the spinal cord that interrupts the reflex arc controlling the bladder, with loss of normal bladder sensation and reflexes, inability to initiate urination normally, and incontinence. **irritable b.,** a condition of the bladder marked by increased frequency of contraction with associated desire to urinate. **motor paralytic b.,** neurogenic bladder due to impairment of the motor neurons or nerves controlling the bladder; the *acute* form is marked by painful distention and inability to initiate micturition, and the *chronic* form by difficulty in initiating micturition, straining, decreased size and force of stream, interrupted stream, and recurrent urinary tract infection. **neurogenic b., atonic,** neurogenic bladder due to destruction of the sensory nerve fibers from the bladder to the spinal cord, with absence of control of bladder functions and of desire to void, overdistention of the bladder, and an abnormal amount of residual urine; most frequently associated with tabes dorsalis (*tabetic b.*) and pernicious anemia. **neurogenic b., uninhibited,** neurogenic bladder due to a lesion in the region of the upper motor neurons with subtotal interruption of corticospinal pathways, with urgency, frequent involuntary voiding, and small-volume threshold of activity. **urinary b.,** the musculomembranous sac in the anterior part of the pelvic cavity that serves as a reservoir for urine, which it receives through the ureters and discharges through the urethra.

blast (blast) 1. an immature stage in cellular development before appearance of the definitive characteristics of the cell; used also as a word termination, as in adamantoblast, etc. 2. the wave of air pressure produced by the detonation of high-explosive bombs or shells or by other explosions; it causes pulmonary concussion and hemorrhage (*lung blast, blast chest*), laceration of other thoracic and abdominal viscera, ruptured ear drums, and minor effects in the central nervous system. 3. see *blasto-.*

blastema (blas-te′mah) 1. the primitive substance from which cells are formed. 2. a group of cells giving rise to a new individual (in asexual reproduction) or to an organ or part (in either normal development or in regeneration). **blastem′ic,** adj.

blasto- word element [Gr.], *a bud; budding.*

blastocoele (blas′tah-sēl) the fluid-filled central segmentation cavity of the blastula. **blastocoe′lic,** adj.

blastocyst (-sist) the mammalian conceptus in the post-morula stage, consisting of the trophoblast and an inner cell mass.

blastocyte (-sīt) an undifferentiated embryonic cell.

blastoderm (blas′tah-derm) the single layer of cells forming the wall of the blastula, or the cellular cap above the floor of segmented yolk in the discoblastula of telolecithal ova.

blastodisc (-disk) the convex structure formed by the blastomeres at the animal pole of an ovum undergoing incomplete cleavage.

blastogenesis (blas″to-jen′ĭ-sis) 1. development of an individual from a blastema, i.e., by asexual reproduction. 2. transmission of inherited characters by the germ plasm. 3. morphological transformation of small lymphocytes into larger cells resembling blast cells on exposure to phytohemagglutinin or to antigens to which the donor is immunized. **blastogenet′ic, blastogen′ic,** adj.

blastoma (blas-to′mah) a neoplasm composed of embryonic cells derived from the blastema of an organ or tissue. **blasto′matous,** adj.

blastomere (blas′to-mēr) one of the cells produced by cleavage of a fertilized ovum.

Blastomyces (blas″to-mi′sēz) a genus of pathogenic fungi growing as mycelial forms at room temperature and as yeastlike forms at body temperature; applied to the yeasts pathogenic for man and animals. **B. brasilien′sis,** *Paracoccidioides brasiliensis.* **B. dermati′tidis,** the agent of North American blastomycosis.

blastomycosis (-mi-ko′sis) 1. infection with *Blastomyces.* 2. any infection caused by a yeast-like organism. **North American b.,** a chronic infection due to *Blastomyces dermatitidis,* predominately involving the skin, lungs, and bones. **South American b.,** paracoccidioidomycosis.

blastopore (blas′to-por) the opening of the archenteron to the exterior of the embryo, at the gastrula stage.

blastula (blas′tu-lah), pl. *blas′tulae.* The usually spherical body produced by cleavage of a fertilized ovum, consisting of a single layer of cells (blastoderm) surrounding a fluid-filled cavity (blastocoele).

bleb (bleb) a large flaccid vesicle, usually at least 1 cm. in diameter.

bleeder (blēd′er) 1. one who bleeds freely; a hemophiliac. 2. any large blood vessel cut during surgery.

bleeding (-ing) 1. the escape of blood, as from an injured vessel. 2. the letting of blood. **functional b.,** bleeding from the uterus when no organic lesions are present. **implantation b.,** that occurring at the time of implantation of the fertilized ovum in the decidua. **occult b.,** escape of blood in such small quantity that it can be detected only by chemical test or by microscopic or spectroscopic examination. **placentation b.,** bleeding from the uterus during the early weeks of pregnancy, when the maternal blood vessels are being eroded.

blenn(o)- word element [Gr.], *mucus.*

blennadenitis (blen″ad-in-īt′is) inflammation of mucous glands.

blennoid (blen′oid) resembling mucus.

blennorrhagia (blen″ah-ra′je-ah) 1. any excessive discharge of mucus; blennorrhea. 2. gonorrhea.

blennorrhea (-re′ah) any free discharge of mucus, especially a gonorrheal discharge from the urethra or vagina; gonorrhea. **blennorrhe′al,** adj. **inclusion b.,** see under *conjunctivitis.*

blennostasis (blen-os′tah-sis) suppression of an abnormal mucous discharge, or correction of an excessive one. **blennostat′ic,** adj.

blennothorax (blen″o-thor′aks) an accumulation of mucus in the chest.

bleomycin (ble-o-mi′sin) a polypeptide antibiotic mixture having antineoplastic properties, obtained from cultures of *Streptomyces verticellus.* Evidence indicates that bleomycin inhibits cell division, thymidine incorporation into DNA, and DNA synthesis.

blephar(o)- word element [Gr.], *eyelid; eyelash.*

blepharadenitis (blef″ar-ad″in-īt′is) inflammation of the meibomian glands.

blepharitis (blef″ah-rīt′is) inflammation of the eyelids. **angular b.,** inflammation involving the angles of the eyelids. **squamous b.,** blepharitis in which the edge of the eyelid is covered with small, white or gray scales. **ulcerative b.,** that marked by small ulcerated areas along the eyelid margin, multiple, suppurative lesions, and loss of lashes.

blepharoatheroma (-ath″er-o′mah) an encysted tumor or sebaceous cyst of an eyelid.

blepharochalasis (-kal′ah-sis) hypertrophy and loss of elasticity of the skin of the upper eyelid.

blepharoncus (blef″er-ong′kus) a tumor on the eyelid.

blepharophimosis (blef″ah-ro-fī-mo′sis) abnormal narrowness of the palpebral fissures.

blepharoplasty (blef″ah-ro-plas′te) plastic surgery of the eyelids.

blepharoplegia (blef″ah-ro-ple′je-ah) paralysis of an eyelid.

blepharoptosis (blef′er-op-to′sis) drooping of an upper eyelid; ptosis.

blepharopyorrhea (blef″ah-ro-pi″ah-re′ah) purulent ophthalmia.

blepharorrhaphy (blef″ah-ror′ah-fe) 1. suture of an eyelid. 2. tarsorrhaphy.

blepharostenosis (blef″ah-ro-stah-no′sis) blepharophimosis.

blepharosynechia (-sin-ek′e-ah) a growing together or adhesion of the eyelids.

blight (blīt) any fungal disease of plants.

blindness (blīnd′nis) lack or loss of ability to see; lack of perception of visual stimuli. **blue b.,** tritanopia. **blue-yellow b.,** 1. tritanopia. 2. tetartanopia. **color b.,** popular term for any deviation from normal perception of color. **day b.,** defective vision in bright light. **epidemic b.,** a form of avian leukosis with blindness and misshapen pupil or irregular depigmentation of the iris in one or both eyes. **flight b.,** amaurosis fugax due to high centrifugal forces encountered in aviation. **green b.,** deuteranopia.

legal b., that defined by law, usually, maximal visual acuity in the better eye after correction of 20/200 with a total diameter of the visual field in that eye of 20 degrees. **letter b.,** inability to recognize individual letters. **mind b.,** psychic b. **moon b.,** periodic ophthalmia. **night b.,** failure or imperfection of vision at night or in dim light. **note b.,** inability to read musical notes because of a brain lesion. **object b.,** inability to recognize the nature and purpose of objects seen. **psychic b.,** failure of proper interpretation of visual stimuli due to a brain lesion. **red b.,** protanopia. **snow b.,** dimness of vision, usually temporary, due to glare of sun upon snow. **text b., word b.,** alexia.

blister (blis′ter) a vesicle, especially a bulla. **blood b.,** a vesicle having bloody contents, as may be caused by a pinch or bruise. **fever b.,** see *herpes simplex.* **water b.,** one with clear watery contents.

bloat (blōt) 1. tympany of the stomach or cecum. 2. enteritis in young rabbits, accompanied by gaseous distention of the abdomen.

block (blok) 1. an obstruction or stoppage. 2. regional anesthesia. **bundle-branch b.,** see under *heart block.* **caudal b.,** anesthesia produced by injection of a local anesthetic into the caudal or sacral canal. **epidural b.,** anesthesia produced by injection of the anesthetic between the vertebral spines and beneath the ligamentum flavum into the extradural space. **heart b.,** see *heart block.* **mental b.,** obstruction to thought or memory, particularly that produced by emotional factors. **metabolic b.,** the blocking of a biosynthetic pathway due to a genetic enzyme defect or to inhibition of an enzyme by a drug or other substance. **nerve b.,** regional anesthesia secured by injection of anesthetics in close proximity to the appropriate nerve. **parasacral b.,** regional anesthesia produced by injection of a local anesthetic around the sacral nerves as they emerge from the sacral foramina. **paravertebral b.,** infiltration of the cervicothoracic ganglion with procaine hydrochloride. **presacral b.,** anesthesia produced by injection of the local anesthetic into the sacral nerves on the anterior aspect of the sacrum. **pudendal b.,** anesthesia produced by blocking the pudendal nerves, accomplished by injection of the local anesthetic into the tuberosity of the ischium. **sacral b.,** anesthesia produced by injection of the local anesthetic into the extradural space of the spinal canal. **saddle b.,** the production of anesthesia in a region corresponding roughly with the areas of the buttocks, perineum, and inner aspects of the thighs, by introducing the anesthetic agent low in the dural sac. **subarachnoid b.,** anesthesia produced by the injection of a local anesthetic into the subarachnoid space around the spinal cord. **vagal b., vagus nerve b.,** blocking of vagal impulses by injection of a solution of local anesthetic into the vagus nerve at its exit from the skull.

blockade (blok-ād′) 1. in pharmacology, the blocking of the effect of a neurotransmitter or hormone by a drug. 2. in histochemistry, a chemical reaction that modifies certain chemical groups and blocks a specific staining method. **adrenergic b.,** selective inhibition of the response to sympathetic impulses transmitted by epinephrine or norepinephrine at alpha or beta receptor sites of an effector organ or postganglionic adrenergic neuron. **cholinergic b.,** selective inhibition of cholinergic nerve impulses at autonomic ganglionic synapses, postganglionic parasympathetic effectors, or neuromuscular junction. **narcotic b.,** inhibition of the euphoric effects of narcotic drugs by the use of other drugs, such as methadone, in the treatment of addiction. **neuromuscular b.,** a failure in neuromuscular transmission that can be induced by a wide variety of disturbances at the myoneural junction.

blocker (blok′er) something that blocks or obstructs passage, activity, etc. α-**b.,** a drug that induces adrenergic blockade at α-adrenergic receptors. β-**b.,** a drug that induces adrenergic blockade at either β_1- or β_2-adrenergic receptors or at both. **calcium channel b.,** one of a group of drugs that inhibit the entry of calcium into cells or inhibit the mobilization of calcium from intracellular stores, resulting in slowing of atrioventricular and sinoatrial conduction and relaxation of arterial smooth and cardiac muscle; used in the treatment of angina, cardiac arrhythmias, and hypertension.

blocking (-ing) 1. interruption of an afferent nerve pathway; see *block.* 2. difficulty in recollection, or interruption of a train of thought or speech, due to emotional factors, usually unconscious.

blood (blud) the fluid circulating through the heart, arteries, capillaries, and veins, carrying nutriment and oxygen to body cells, and removing waste products and carbon dioxide. It consists of the liquid portion (the plasma) and the formed elements (erythrocytes, leukocytes, and platelets). **aerated b., arterial b.,** that which carries oxygen to the tissues through the systemic arteries. **citrated b.,** blood treated with sodium citrate to prevent its coagulation. **cord b.,** that contained in umbilical vessels at time of delivery of the infant. **occult b.,** that present in such small quantities that it is detectible only by chemical tests or by spectroscopic or microscopic examination. **splanchnic b.,** that circulating in thoracic, abdominal, and pelvic viscera, further distinguished on the basis of specific organ, e.g., pulmonary, hepatic, splenic. **venous b.,** blood that has given up its oxygen to the tissues and is carrying carbon dioxide back through the systemic veins for gas-exchange in the lungs. **whole b.,** that from which none of the elements has been removed, especially that drawn from a selected donor under aseptic conditions, containing citrate ion or heparin.

blood group (blud′grōōp) 1. an erythrocytic allotype (or phenotype) defined by one or more cellular antigenic groupings controlled by allelic genes. A considerable number of blood group systems are now known, the most widely used in matching blood for transfusion being the ABO and the Rh blood groups. 2. any characteristic, function, or trait of a cellular or fluid component of blood, considered as the expression (phenotype or allotype) of the actions and interactions of dominant genes, and useful in medicolegal and other studies of human inheritance; such characteristics include the antigenic groups of erythrocytes, leukocytes, platelets, and plasma proteins.

blood plasma (blud plaz′mah) the fluid portion of the blood, in which the microscopically visible formed elements (erythrocytes, leukocytes, blood platelets) are suspended.

blood pressure (blud presh′er) see under *pressure.*

blood serum (blud sēr′um) the clear liquid that separates from blood when it is allowed to clot completely, and is therefore blood plasma from which fibrogen has been removed during clotting.

blood type (blud′ tīp) see *blood group.*

blowpipe (blo′pīp) a tube through which a current of air is forced upon a flame to concentrate and intensify the heat.

blue (bloo) 1. one of the principal colors of the visible spectrum, lying between green and violet; the color of the clear sky. 2. a dye of blue color. **aniline b.,** a mixture of the trisulfonates of triphenyl rosaniline and of diphenyl rosaniline. **brilliant cresyl b.,** an oxazin dye, usually $C_{15}H_{16}N_3OCl$, used in staining blood. **methylene b.,** dark green crystals or crystalline powder with a bronze-like luster, $C_{16}H_{18}ClN_3\cdot S\cdot 3H_2O$, used as an antidote in cyanide poisoning, in the treatment of methemoglobinemia, and as a stain and an indicator. **Prussian b.,** an amorphous blue powder, $Fe_4[Fe(CN)_6]_3$. **toluidine b.,** the chloride salt or zinc chloride double salt of aminodimethylaminotoluphenazthionium chloride; useful as a stain for demonstrating basophilic and metachromatic substances.

B.M.A. British Medical Association.

B.M.R. basal metabolic rate.

BNA Basle Nomina Anatomica, a system of anatomic nomenclature adopted at the annual meeting of the German Anatomic Society in 1895; superseded by *Nomina Anatomica.*

B.O.A. British Orthopaedic Association.

body (bod′e) 1. the trunk, or animal frame, with its organs. 2. the largest and most important part of any organ. 3. any mass or collection of material. **acetone b's,** ketone b's. **alkapton b's,** a class of substances with an affinity for alkali, found in urine and causing alkaptonuria; the compound most commonly found, and most commonly referred to by the term, is homogentisic acid. **aortic b's,** small neurovascular structures on either side of the aorta in the region of the aortic arch, containing chemoreceptors that play a role in reflex regulation of respiration. **b's of Arantius,** small tubercles, one at the center of the free margin of each of the three cusps of the aortic and pulmonary valves. **Aschoff b's,** submiliary collections of cells and leukocytes in the interstitial tissues of the heart in rheumatic myocarditis. **asteroid b.,** an irregularly star-shaped inclusion body found in the giant cells in sarcoidosis and other diseases. **Auer b's,** finely granular, lamellar bodies having acid-phosphatase activity, found in the cytoplasm of myeloblasts, myelocytes, monoblasts, and granular histiocytes, rarely in plasma cells, and virtually pathognomonic of leukemia. **Barr b.,** sex chromatin. **basal b.,** a modified centriole that occurs at the base of a flagellum or cilium. **Cabot's ring b's,** lines in the form of loops or figures-of-8, seen in stained erythrocytes in severe anemias. **carotid b.,** a small neurovascular structure lying in the bifurcation of the right and left carotid arteries, containing chemoreceptors that monitor oxygen content in blood and help to regulate respiration. **chromatoid b.,** 1. a dense, deeply staining rodlike accumulation of RNA in the cysts of some amebas. 2. a dense mass near the distal centriole of a spermatozoon. **ciliary b.,** the thickened part of the vascular tunic of the eye, connecting the choroid and iris. **Döhle's inclusion b's,** small bodies seen in the cytoplasm of neutrophils in many infectious diseases, burns, aplastic anemia, and other disorders, and after administration of toxic agents. **Donovan's b's,** encapsulated bacteria (*Calymmatobacterium granulomatis*) found in lesions of granuloma inguinale. **fruiting b.,** a specialized structure, as an apothecium, which produces spores. **geniculate b., lateral,** an eminence of the metathalamus, just lateral to the medial geniculate body, marking the end of the optic tract. **geniculate b., medial,** an eminence of metathalamus just lateral to the superior colliculi, concerned with hearing. **Hassall's b's,** see under *corpuscle.* **Golgi b.,** see under *complex.* **Heinz b's, Heinz-Ehrlich b's,** inclusion bodies resulting from oxidative injury to and precipitation of hemoglobin; seen in the presence of certain abnormal hemoglobins and erythrocytes with enzyme deficiencies. **hyaloid b.,** vitreous b. **immune b.,** antibody. **inclusion b's,** round, oval, or irregular shaped bodies in the cytoplasm and nuclei of cells, in disease due to viral infection, such as rabies, smallpox, etc. **ketone b's,** the substances acetone, acetoacetic acid, and β-hydroxybutyric acid; except for acetone (which may arise spontaneously from acetoacetic acid), they are normal metabolic products of lipid within the liver, and are oxidized by muscles; excessive production leads to urinary secretion of these bodies, as in diabetes mellitus. **Leishman-Donovan b's,** round or oval bodies found in the reticuloendothelial cells, especially those of the spleen and liver, in kala-azar; they are nonflagellate intracellular forms of *Leishmania donovani.* Also used to designate similar forms of *L. tropica* found in macrophages in lesions of cutaneous leishmaniasis. **mamillary b.,** either of the pair of small spherical masses in the interpeduncular fossa of the midbrain, forming part of the hypothalamus. **Masson b's,** cellular tissue that fills the pulmonary alveoli and alveolar ducts in rheumatic pneumonia; they may be modified Aschoff bodies. **metachromatic b's,** see under *granule.* **Negri b's,** round or oval inclusion bodies seen in the cytoplasm and sometimes in the processes of neurons of rabid animals after death. **Nissl b's,** large granular basophilic bodies found in the cytoplasm of neurons, composed of rough endo-

plasmic reticulum and free polyribosomes. **olivary b.,** olive (2). **pacchionian b's,** arachnoid granulations. **para-aortic b's,** enclaves of chromaffin cells near the sympathetic ganglia along the abdominal aorta, serving as chemoreceptors responsive to oxygen, carbon dioxide, and hydrogen in concentration and which help control respiration. **pineal b.,** a small conical structure attached by a stalk to the posterior wall of the third ventricle. It secretes melatonin. **pituitary b.,** see under *gland.* **polar b's,** small cells consisting of a tiny bit of cytoplasm and a nucleus, resulting from unequal division of the primary oocyte (*first polar b.*) and, if fertilization occurs, of the secondary oocyte (*second polar b.*). 2. metachromatic granules located at the ends of bacteria. **quadrigeminal b's,** corpora quadrigemina. **Russell b's,** globular plasma cell inclusions, representing aggregates of immunoglobulins synthesized by the cell. **trachoma b's,** inclusion bodies found in clusters in the cytoplasm of the epithelial cells of the conjunctiva in trachoma. **vermiform b's,** peculiar sinuous invaginations of the plasma membrane of Kupffer cells of the liver. **vitreous b.,** the transparent gel filling the inner portion of the eyeball between the lens and retina.

boil (boil) furuncle. **Aleppo b., Delhi b., Natal b., Oriental b.,** cutaneous leishmaniasis.

bolometer (bo-lom′it-er) 1. an instrument for measuring the force of the heart beat. 2. an instrument for measuring minute degrees of radiant heat.

bolus (bo′lus) 1. a rounded mass of food or pharmaceutical preparation ready to swallow, or such a mass passing through the gastrointestinal tract. 2. a concentrated mass of pharmaceutical preparation, e.g., an opaque contrast medium, given intravenously. 3. a mass of scattering material, such as wax or paraffin, placed between the radiation source and the skin to achieve a precalculated isodose pattern in the tissue irradiated.

bombesin (bom′bah-sin) a tetradecapeptide neurotransmitter and hormone found in the brain and gut.

bond (bond) the linkage between atoms or radicals of a chemical compound, or the mark indicating the number and attachment of the valencies of an atom in constitutional formulas, represented by a pair of dots or a line between atoms, e.g., H—O—H, H—C≡C—H or H:O:H, H:C:::C:H. **coordinate covalent b.,** a covalent bond in which one of the bonded atoms furnishes both of the shared electrons. **covalent b.,** a chemical bond between two atoms or radicals formed by the sharing of a pair (single bond), 2 pairs (double bond), or 3 pairs of electrons (triple bond). **disulfide b.,** a strong covalent bond, —S—S—, important in linking polypeptide chains in proteins, the linkage arising as a result of the oxidation of the sulfhydryl (SH) groups of two molecules of cysteine. **peptide b.,** a ·CO·NH· linkage formed between the carboxyl group of one amino acid and the amino group of another; it is an amide linkage joining amino acids to form peptides.

bone (bōn) 1. the hard, rigid form of connective

tissue constituting most of the skeleton of vertebrates, composed chiefly of calcium salts. 2. any distinct piece of the skeleton of the body. See *Table of Bones* for regional listing and alphabetical listing of common names of bones of the body, and see Plates II and III. **ankle b.,** talus. **basiotic b.,** a small bone in the fetus between the basilar process and the basisphenoid. **brittle b's,** osteogenesis imperfecta. **cartilage b.,** bone developing within cartilage, ossification taking place within a cartilage model. **cheek b.,** zygomatic b. **coffin b.,** the third phalanx of the horse's foot. **collar b.,** clavicle. **cortical b.,** the compact bone of the shaft of a bone that surrounds the marrow cavity. **flat b.,** one whose thickness is slight, sometimes consisting of only a thin layer of compact bone, or of two layers with intervening cancellous bone and marrow; usually curved rather than flat. **funny b.,** the region of the median condyle of the humerus where it is crossed by the ulnar nerve. **heel b.,** calcaneus. **hip b.,** os coxae. **incisive b.,** the portion of the maxilla bearing the incisors; developmentally, it is the premaxilla, which in humans later fuses with the maxilla, but in most other vertebrates persists as a separate bone. **jaw b.,** the mandible or maxilla, especially the mandible. **jugal b.,** zygomatic b. **lingual b.,** hyoid b. **malar b.,** zygomatic b. **marble b's,** osteopetrosis. **mastoid b.,** see under *process*. **pelvic b.,** os coxae. **petrous b.,** the petrous portion of the temporal bone. **pneumatic b.,** bone that contains air-filled spaces. **premaxillary b.,** premaxilla. **pterygoid b.,** see under *process*. **rider's b.,** localized ossification of the inner aspect of the lower end of the tendon of the adductor muscle of the thigh; sometimes seen in horseback riders. **semilunar b.,** lunate b. **shin b.,** tibia. **squamous b.,** the upper forepart of the temporal bone, forming an upright plate. **sutural b's,** variable and irregularly shaped bones in the sutures between the bones of the skull. **thigh b.,** femur. **turbinated b.,** nasal conchae. **tympanic b.,** the part of the temporal bone surrounding the middle ear. **unciform b.,** hamate b. **wormian b's,** sutural b's.

Boophilus (bo-of′ĭ-lus) a genus of hard-bodied ticks primarily parasitic on cattle. *B. annula′tus* (*B. bo′vis*) and *B. mi′croplus* are vectors of *Babesia bigemina*, the cause of a fever in cattle; *B. decolora′tus* is a vector of *Anaplasma marginale*, the cause of gallsickness in cattle.

booster (boost′er) see under *dose*.

boot (boot) an encasement for the foot; a protective casing or sheath. **Gibney b.,** an adhesive tape support used in treatment of sprains and other painful conditions of the ankle, the tape being applied in a basket-weave fashion with strips placed alternately under the sole of the foot and around the back of the leg. **Unna's paste b.,** a dressing for varicose ulcers, consisting of a paste made from gelatin, zinc oxide, glycerin; the entire leg is covered with paste and covered with spiral bandages, applied in alternate layers until a rigid boot is made.

borate (bor′āt) a salt of boric acid.

borax (bor′aks) sodium borate.

borborygmus (bor″bah-rig′mus) a rumbling noise caused by propulsion of gas through the intestines.

border (bor′der) a bounding line, edge, or surface. **brush b.,** a specialization of the free surface of a cell, consisting of minute cylindrical processes (microvilli) that greatly increase the surface area. **vermilion b.,** the exposed red portion of the upper or lower lip.

Bordetella (bor″dah-tel′ah) a genus of bacteria (family Brucellaceae), including *B. bronchisep′tica,* a common cause of bronchopneumonia in guinea pigs and other rodents, in swine, and in lower primates; *B. parapertus′sis,* found occasionally in whooping cough; and *B. pertus′sis,* the cause of whooping cough in man.

boric acid (bor′ik) a crystalline powder, H_3BO_3, used as a buffer. Its sodium salt (*sodium borate,* or *borax*) is used as an alkalizing agent in pharmaceuticals.

boron (bor′on) chemical element (*see table*), at. no. 5, symbol B.

Borrelia (bor-el′e-ah) a genus of bacteria (family Treponemataceae), parasitic in many animals, some species causing relapsing fever in man and animals; it includes *B. anseri′na,* the etiologic agent of fowl spirochetosis; *B. recurren′tis,* an etiologic agent of relapsing fever; and *B. vincen′tii,* parasitic in the human mouth, occurring in large numbers with a fusiform bacillus in necrotizing ulcerative gingivitis and in necrotizing ulcerative gingivostomatitis.

borreliosis (bor-el″e-o′sis) infection with *Borrelia;* see *relapsing fever*.

boss (bos) a rounded eminence.

bot (bot) the larva of botflies, which may be parasitic in the stomach of animals and sometimes man.

Bothriocephalus (both″re-o-sef′ah-lus) *Diphyllobothrium*.

botryoid (bah′tre-oid) shaped like a bunch of grapes.

bottle (bot′l) a hollow narrow-necked vessel of glass or other material. **wash b.,** 1. a flexible squeeze-bottle with delivery tube, or one with two tubes through the cork, so arranged that blowing into one forces a stream of liquid from the other; used in washing chemical materials. 2. one containing some washing fluid, through which gases are passed for the purpose of freeing them from impurities.

botuliform (bah-choo′lĭ-form) sausage-shaped.

botulin (bah′choo-lin) a neurotoxin produced by *Clostridium botulinum,* sometimes found in imperfectly canned or preserved foods.

botulism (bah′choo-lizm) an extremely severe type of food poisoning due to a neurotoxin (botulin) produced by *Clostridium botulinum* in improperly canned or preserved foods. **infant b.,** that affecting infants, thought to result from toxin produced in the gut by ingested organisms, rather than from preformed toxins. **wound b.,** a form resulting from infection of a wound with *Clostridium botulinum*.

bougie (boo-zhe′) a slender, flexible, hollow or solid, cylindrical instrument for introduction into the urethra or other tubular organ, usually for calibrating or dilating constricted areas.

TABLE OF BONES, LISTED BY REGIONS OF THE BODY

REGION	NAME	TOTAL NUMBER	REGION	NAME	TOTAL NUMBER
Axial skeleton			Upper limb (×2)		64
	Skull	21	Shoulder	scapula	
	(eight paired–16)			clavicle	
	inferior nasal concha		Upper arm	humerus	
	lacrimal		Lower arm	radius	
	maxilla			ulna	
	nasal			carpal (8)	
	palatine			(capitate)	
	parietal			(hamate)	
	temporal			(lunate)	
	zygomatic			(pisiform)	
	(five unpaired–5)		Wrist	(scaphoid)	
	ethmoid			(trapezium)	
	frontal			(trapezoid)	
	occipital			(triquetral)	
	sphenoid		Hand	metacarpal (5)	
	vomer		Fingers	phalanges (14)	
	Ossicles of each ear	6	Lower limb (×2)		62
	incus		Pelvis	hip bone (1)	
	malleus			(ilium)	
	stapes			(ischium)	
	Lower jaw			(pubis)	
	mandible	1	Thigh	femur	
	Neck		Knee	patella	
	hyoid	1	Leg	tibia	
	Vertebral column	26		fibula	
	cervical vertebrae (7)			tarsal (7)	
	(atlas)			(calcaneus)	
	(axis)			(cuboid)	
	thoracic vertebrae (12)		Ankle	(cuneiform, medial)	
	lumbar vertebrae (5)			(cuneiform, intermediate)	
	sacrum (5 fused)			(cuneiform, lateral)	
	coccyx (4–5 fused)			(navicular)	
	Chest			(talus)	
	sternum	1	Foot	metatarsal (5)	
	ribs (12 pairs)	24	Toes	phalanges (14)	

COMMON NAME*	NA EQUIVALENT†	REGION	DESCRIPTION	ARTICULATIONS
astragalus. *See* talus				
atlas	atlas	neck	first cervical vertebra, ring of bone supporting the skull	with occipital b. and axis
axis	axis	neck	second cervical vertebra, with thick process (odontoid process) around which first cervical vertebra pivots	with atlas above and third cervical vertebra below
calcaneus	calcaneus	foot	the "heel bone," or irregular cuboidal shape, largest of the tarsal bones	with talus and cuboid b.
capitate b.	o. capitatum	wrist	with second, third, and fourth metacarpal b's, and hamate, lunate, trapezoid, and scaphoid b's	
carpal b's	oss. carpi	wrist	see *capitate, hamate, lunate, pisiform b's, scaphoid, trapezium, trapezoid, and triquetral b's*	
clavicle	clavicula	shoulder	elongated, slender, curved bone (collar bone) lying horizontally at root of neck, in upper part of thorax	with sternum and ipsilateral scapula and cartilage of first rib
coccyx	o. coccygis	lower back	triangular bone formed usually by fusion of last 4 (sometimes 3 or 5) (coccygeal) vertebrae	with sacrum
concha, inferior nasal	concha nasalis inferior	skull	thin, rough plate of bone attached by one edge to side of each nasal cavity, the free edge curling downward	with ethmoid and ipsilateral lacrimal and palatine b's and maxilla
cuboid b.	o. cuboideum	foot	pyramidal bone, on lateral side of foot, in front of calcaneus	with calcaneus, lateral cuneiform b., fourth and fifth metatarsal b's, occasionally with navicular b.
cuneiform b., intermediate	o. cuneiforme intermedium	foot	smallest of 3 cuneiform b's, located between medial and lateral cuneiform b's	with navicular, medial and lateral cuneiform b's, and second metatarsal b.
cuneiform b., lateral	o. cuneiforme laterale	foot	wedge-shaped bone at lateral side of foot, intermediate in size between medial and intermediate cuneiform b's	with cuboid, navicular, intermediate cuneiform b's and second, third, and fourth metatarsal b's
cuneiform b., medial	o. cuneiforme mediale	foot	largest of 3 cuneiform b's, at medial side of foot	with navicular, intermediate cuneiform, and first and second metatarsal b's
epistropheus. *See* axis				
ethmoid b.	o. ethmoidale	skull	unpaired bone in front of sphenoid b. and below frontal b., forming part of nasal septum and superior and medial conchae of nose	with sphenoid and frontal b's, vomer, and both lacrimal, nasal, and palatine b's maxillae, and inferior nasal conchae

*b. = bone; b's = (pl.) bones.
†o. = os; oss. = (L.pl.) ossa.

87

TABLE OF BONES—*Continued*

COMMON NAME*	NA EQUIVALENT†	REGION	DESCRIPTION	ARTICULATIONS
fabella		knee	sesamoid b. in lateral head of gastrocnemius muscle	with femur
femur	femur	thigh	longest, strongest, heaviest bone of the body (thigh b.)	proximally with hip b., distally with patella and tibia
fibula	fibula	leg	lateral and smaller of 2 bones of leg	proximally with tibia, distally with tibia and talus
frontal b.	o. frontale	skull	unpaired bone constituting anterior part of skull	with ethmoid and sphenoid b's, and both parietal, nasal, lacrimal, and zygomatic b's, and maxillae
hamate b.	o. hamatum	wrist	most medial of 4 bones of distal row of carpal b's	with fourth and fifth metacarpal b's and lunate, capitate, and triquetral b's
hip b.	o. coxae	pelvis and hip	broadest bone of skeleton, composed originally of 3 bones which become fused together in acetabulum: *ilium*, broad, flaring, uppermost portion; *ischium*, thick, three-sided part behind and below acetabulum and behind obturator foramen; *pubis*, consisting of body (expanded anterior portion), inferior ramus (extending backward and fusing with ramus of ischium) and superior ramus (extending from body to acetabulum)	with femur, anteriorly with its fellow (at symphysis pubis), posteriorly with sacrum
humerus	humerus	arm	long bone of upper arm	proximally with scapula, distally with radius and ulna
hyoid b.	o. hyoideum	neck	U-shaped bone at root of tongue, between mandible and larynx	none; attached by ligaments and muscles to skull and larynx
ilium	o. ilii	pelvis	see *hip b.*	
incus	incus	ear	middle ossicle of chain in the middle ear, so named because of its resemblance to an anvil	with malleus and stapes
innominate b. See hip b.				
ischium	o. ischii	pelvis	see *hip b.*	
lacrimal b.	o. lacrimale	skull	thin, uneven scale of bone near rim of medial wall of each orbit	with ethmoid and frontal b's, and ipsilateral inferior nasal concha and maxilla
lunate b.	o. lunatum	wrist	second from thumb side of 4 bones of proximal row of carpus	with radius, and capitate, hamate, scaphoid, and triquetral b's
malleus	malleus	ear	most lateral ossicle of chain in middle ear, so named because of its resemblance to a hammer	with incus; fibrous attachment to tympanic membrane
mandible	mandibula	lower jaw	horseshoe-shaped bone carrying lower teeth	with temporal b's
maxilla	maxilla	skull (upper jaw)	paired bone, below orbit and at either side of nasal cavity, carrying upper teeth	with ethmoid and frontal b's, vomer, fellow maxilla, and ipsilateral inferior nasal concha and lacrimal, nasal, palatine, and zygomatic b's

maxilla, inferior. *See* mandible				
maxilla, superior. *See* maxilla				
metacarpal b's	oss. metacarpi	hand	five miniature long bones of hand proper, slightly concave on palmar surface	first—trapezium and proximal phalanx of thumb; second—third metacarpal b, trapezium, trapezoid, capitate, and proximal phalanx of index finger (second digit); third—second and fourth metacarpal b's, capitate and proximal phalanx of middle finger (third digit); fourth—third and fifth metacarpal b's, capitate, hamate, and proximal phalanx of ring finger (fourth digit); fifth—fourth metacarpal b., hamate b. and proximal phalanx of little finger (fifth digit)
metatarsal b's	oss. metatarsi	foot	five miniature long bones of foot, concave on plantar and slightly convex on dorsal surface	first—medial cuneiform b., proximal phalanx of great toe, and occasionally with second metatarsal b.; second—medial, intermediate, and lateral cuneiform b's, third and occasionally with first metatarsal b., and proximal phalanx of second toe; third—lateral cuneiform b., second and fourth metatarsal b's and proximal phalanx of third toe; fourth—lateral cuneiform b., cuboid b., third and fifth metatarsal b's and proximal phalanx of fourth toe; fifth—cuboid b., fourth metatarsal b., and proximal phalanx of fifth toe
multangulum majus. *See* trapezium; trapezoid b.				
nasal b.	o. nasale	skull	paired bone, the two uniting in median plane to form bridge of nose	with frontal and ethmoid b's, fellow of opposite side, and ipsilateral maxilla
navicular b.	o. naviculare	foot	bone at medial side of tarsus, between talus and cuneiform b's	with talus and 3 cuneiform b's occasionally with cuboid b.
occipital b.	o. occipitale	skull	unpaired bone constituting back and part of base of skull	with sphenoid b. and atlas and both parietal and temporal b's
os magnum. *See* capitate b.				

TABLE OF BONES—*Continued*

COMMON NAME*	NA EQUIVALENT†	REGION	DESCRIPTION	ARTICULATIONS
palatine b.	o. palatinum	skull	paired bone, the two forming posterior portions of bony palate	with ethmoid and sphenoid b's, vomer, fellow of opposite side, and ipsilateral inferior nasal concha and maxilla
parietal b.	o. parietale	skull	paired bone between frontal and occipital b's, forming superior and lateral parts of skull	with frontal, occipital, sphenoid, fellow parietal, and ipsilateral temporal b's
patella	patella	knee	small, irregularly rectangular compressed (sesamoid) bone over anterior aspect of knee (kneecap)	with femur
phalanges (proximal, middle, and distal phalanges)	oss. digitorum (phalanx proximalis, phalanx media, and phalanx distalis)	fingers and toes	miniature long bones, two only in thumb and great toe, three in each of other fingers and toes	proximal phalanx of each digit with corresponding metacarpal or metatarsal b., and phalanx distal to it; other phalanges with phalanges proximal and distal (if any) to them
pisiform b.	o. pisiforme	wrist	medial and palmar of 4 bones of proximal row of capal b's	with triquetral b
pubic b.	o. pubis	pelvis	see *hip b.*	
radius	radius	forearm	lateral and shorter of 2 bones of forearm	proximally with humerus and ulna; distally with ulna and lunate and scaphoid b's
ribs	oss. costalia	chest	12 pairs of thin, narrow, curved long bones, forming posterior and lateral walls of chest	all posteriorly with thoracic vertebrae; upper 7 pairs (true ribs) with sternum; lower 5 pairs (false ribs) by costal cartilages, with rib above or (lowest 2—floating ribs) unattached anteriorly
sacrum	o. sacrum	lower back	wedge-shaped bone formed usually by fusion of 5 vertebrae below lumbar vertebrae, constituting posterior wall of pelvis	with fifth lumbar vertebra above, coccyx below, and with ilium at each side
scaphoid	o. scaphoideum	wrist	most lateral of 4 bones of proximal row of carpal b's	with radius, trapezium, and trapezoid capitate and lunate b's
scapula	scapula	shoulder	wide, thin, triangular bone (shoulder blade) opposite second to seventh ribs in upper part of back	with ipsilateral clavicle and humerus
sesamoid b's	oss. sesamoidea	chiefly hands and feet	small, flat, round bones related to joints between phalanges or between digits and metacarpal or metatarsal b's; include also 2 at knee (fabella and patella)	
sphenoid b.	o. sphenoidale	base of skull	unpaired, irregularly shaped bone, constituting part of sides and base of skull and part of lateral wall or orbit	with frontal, occipital, and ethmoid b's, vomer and both parietal, temporal, palatine, and zygomatic b's
stapes	stapes	ear	most medial ossicle of chain in middle ear, so named because of its resemblance to a stirrup	with incus; ligamentous attachment to fenestra vestibuli

Term	Latin	Region	Definition	Articulation
sternum	sternum	chest	elongated flat bone, forming anterior wall of chest, consisting of 3 segments: *manubrium* (topmost segment), *body* (in youth composed of 4 separate segments joined by cartilage), and *xiphoid process* (lowermost segment)	with both clavicles and upper 7 pairs of ribs
talus	talus	ankle	the "ankle bone," second largest of tarsal b's	with tibia, fibula, calcaneus, and navicular b.
tarsal b's	oss. tarsi	ankle and foot	see *calcaneus, cuboid, intermediate, lateral,* and *medial cuneiform b's, naviular b.,* and *talus*	
temporal b.	o. temporale	skull	irregularly shaped bone, one on either side, forming part of side and base of skull, and containing middle and inner ear	with occipital, sphenoid, mandible, and ipsilateral parietal and zygomatic b's
tibia	tibia	leg	medial and larger of 2 bones of lower leg (shin b.)	proximally with femur and fibula, distally with talus and fibula
trapezium	o. trapezium	wrist	most lateral of 4 bones of distal row of carpal b's	with first and second metacarpal b's and trapezoid and scaphoid b's
trapezoid b.	o. trapezoideum	wrist	second from thumb side of 4 bones of distal row of carpal b's	with second metacarpal b. and capitate, trapezium, and scaphoid b's
triquetral b.	o. triquetrum	wrist	third from thumb side of 4 bones of proximal row of carpal b's	with hamate, lunate, and pisiform b's and articular disk
turbinate b., inferior. See concha, inferior nasal				
ulna	ulna	forearm	medial and longer of 2 bones of forearm	proximally with humerus and radius, distally with radius and articular disk
vertebrae (cervical, thoracic [dorsal], lumbar, sacral and coccygeal)	vertebrae (vertebrae cervicales, vertebrae thoracicae, vertebrae lumbales, vertebrae sacrales, vertebrae coccygeae)	back	separate segments of vertebral column: about 33 in the child; uppermost 24 remain separate as true, movable vertebrae; the next 5 fuse to form the sacrum; the lowermost 3–5 fuse to form the coccyx	except first cervical (atlas) and fifth lumbar, each vertebra articulates with adjoining vertebrae above and below; the first cervical articulates with the occipital b. and second cervical vertebra (axis); the fifth lumbar with the fourth lumbar vertebra and sacrum; the thoracic vertebrae articulate also with the heads of the ribs
vomer	vomer	skull	thin bone forming posterior and posteroinferior part of nasal septum	with ethmoid and sphenoid b's and both maxillae and palatine b's
zygomatic b.	o. zygomaticum	skull	bone forming hard part of cheek and lower, lateral portion of rim of each orbit	with frontal and sphenoid b's and ipsilateral maxilla and temporal b.

bulbous b., one with a bulb-shaped tip. **filiform b.,** one of very slender caliber. **soluble b.,** one that will melt or dissolve *in situ*.

bouton (boo-taw′) [Fr.] button. **b's terminaux,** synaptic end-feet.

bovine (bo′vin) pertaining to, characteristic of, or derived from the ox (cattle).

bowel (bow′il) the intestine.

bowleg (bo′leg) genu varum; an outward curvature of one or both legs near the knee.

B.P. 1. blood pressure. 2. British Pharmacopoeia, a publication of the General Medical Council, describing and establishing standards for medicines, preparations, materials, and articles used in the practice of medicine, surgery, or midwifery.

b.p. boiling point.

bp base pair.

B.P.A. British Paediatric Association.

Bq becquerel.

Br chemical symbol, *bromine.*

brace (brās) an orthopedic appliance or apparatus (an orthosis) used to support, align, or hold parts of the body in correct position; also, usually in the plural, an orthodontic appliance for correction of malaligned teeth.

brachi(o)- word element [L., Gr.], *arm.*

brachialgia (bra″ke-al′je-ah) pain in the arm.

brachiocephalic (-o-sah-fal′ik) pertaining to the arm and head.

brachiocubital (-ku′bit'l) pertaining to the arm and elbow or forearm.

brachium (bra′ke-um), pl. *bra′chia* [L.] 1. the arm; specifically, the arm from shoulder to elbow. 2. an armlike process or structure. **b. colli′culi inferio′ris,** fibers of the auditory pathway connecting the inferior quadrigeminal body to the medial geniculate body. **b. colli′culi superio′ris,** fibers connecting the optic tract and lateral geniculate body with the superior quadrigeminal body. **b. conjuncti′vum [cerebel′li],** superior cerebellar peduncle. **b. op′ticum,** one of the processes extending from the corpora quadrigemina to the optic thalamus. **b. pon′tis,** middle cerebellar peduncle.

brachy- word element [Gr.], *short.*

brachybasia (brak″e-ba′ze-ah) a slow, shuffling, short-stepped gait.

brachycardia (-kar′de-ah) bradycardia.

brachydactyly (-dak′tĭ-le) abnormal shortness of fingers and toes.

brachygnathia (brak″ig-na′the-ah) abnormal shortness of the lower jaw.

brachymetropia (-mě-trop′pe-ah) myopia. **brachymetrop′ic,** adj.

brachyphalangia (-fah-lan′je-ah) abnormal shortness of one or more of the phalanges.

brachytherapy (-thě′rah-pe) treatment with ionizing radiation whose source is applied to the surface of the body or located a short distance from the area being treated.

brady- word element [Gr.], *slow.*

bradyarrhythmia (brad″e-ah-rith′me-ah) bradycardia associated with an irregularity in the heart rhythm.

bradycardia (-kar′de-ah) slowness of the heart beat, as evidenced by slowing of the pulse rate to less than 60. **bradycar′diac,** adj.

bradydiastole (-di-as′tah-le) abnormal prolongation of the diastole.

bradyesthesia (-es-the′ze-ah) slowness or dullness of perception.

bradykinesia (-ki-ne′ze-ah) abnormal slowness of movement; sluggishness of physical and mental responses. **bradykinet′ic,** adj.

bradykinin (-ki′nin) a nonapeptide kinin formed from kallindin II by the action of kallikrein; it is a very powerful vasodilator and increases capillary permeability; in addition, it constricts smooth muscle and stimulates pain receptors.

bradypnea (-ne′ah) abnormal slowness of breathing.

bradysphygmia (-sfig′me-ah) bradycardia.

bradystalsis (-stal′sis) abnormal slowness of peristalsis.

bradytachycardia (-tak″e-kar′de-ah) alternating attacks of bradycardia and tachycardia.

bradytocia (-to′she-ah) slow parturition.

brain (brān) encephalon; that part of the central nervous system contained within the cranium, comprising the forebrain, midbrain, and hindbrain, and developed from the anterior part of the embryonic neural tube; see also *cerebrum.*

brain stem (brān′stem) the stemlike portion of the brain connecting the cerebral hemispheres with the spinal cord, and comprising the pons, medulla oblongata, and midbrain; considered by some to include the diencephalon.

brainwashing (brān′wash″ing) systematic emotional and mental conditioning of an individual or of a group, designed to secure attitudes and beliefs conformable to the wishes of those administering the conditioning, accomplished by means of propaganda, torture, drugs, distorted psychiatric procedures, or by other means.

branch (branch) ramus; a division or offshoot from a main stem, especially of blood vessels, nerves, or lymphatics.

branchial (brang′ke-al) pertaining to or resembling gills of a fish or derivatives of homologous parts in higher forms.

Branhamella (bran″hah-mel′ah) a genus of aerobic, nonmotile, non–spore-forming cocci. The type species, *B. catarrhalis,* is a normal inhabitant of the nasopharynx, which occasionally causes disease.

brash (brash) heartburn. **water b.,** heartburn with regurgitation of sour fluid or almost tasteless saliva into the mouth. **weaning b.,** diarrhea in infants occurring as a result of weaning.

breast (brest) the front of the chest, especially its modified glandular structure, the mamma. See *mammary gland.* **chicken b.,** pigeon b. **funnel b.,** see under *chest.* **pigeon b.,** prominence of the sternum due to obstruction to infantile respiration or to rickets.

breast-feeding (brest′fēd′ing) the nursing of an infant at the mother's breast.

breath (breth) the air taken in and expelled by

the expansion and contraction of the thorax. **liver b.,** hepatic fetor.

breathing (brēth′ing) the alternate inspiration and expiration of air into and out of the lungs. **frog b., glossopharyngeal b.,** respiration unaided by the primary or ordinary accessory muscles of respiration, the air being "swallowed" into the lungs by the tongue and muscles of the pharynx; used by patients with chronic muscle paralysis to augment their breathing. **intermittent positive pressure b.,** the active inflation of the lungs during inspiration under positive pressure from a cycling valve.

breech (brēch) the buttocks.

bregma (breg′mah) the point on the surface of the skull at the junction of the coronal and sagittal sutures. **bregmat′ic,** adj.

Brethine (breth′ēn) trademark for preparations of terbutaline sulfate.

bretylium tosylate (brah-til′e-um) an adrenergic blocking agent, $C_{18}H_{24}BrNO_3S$, used as an antiarrhythmic in certain cases of ventricular tachycardia or fibrillation.

brevicollis (brev″ĭ-kol′is) shortness of the neck.

bridge (brij) 1. a dental prosthesis bearing one or more artificial teeth, attached to adjacent natural teeth. 2. pons. 3. a protoplasmic structure uniting adjacent elements of a cell, similar in plants and animals. **cytoplasmic b.,** 1. protoplasmic b. 2. intercellular b. **disulfide b.,** see under *bond*. **extension b.,** a bridge having an artificial tooth attached beyond the point of anchorage of the bridge. **intercellular b.,** 1. protoplasmic b. 2. a misnomer for the junction of epithelial cells at a desmosome, which was formerly thought to constitute a cytoplasmic bridge. **protoplasmic b.,** a strand of protoplasm connecting two secondary spermatocytes, occurring as a result of incomplete cytokinesis. **b. of Varolius,** pons (2).

bridgework (brij′werk) a partial denture retained by attachments other than clasps. **fixed b.,** one retained with crowns or inlays cemented to the natural teeth. **removable b.,** one retained by attachments allowing removal.

brim (brim) the edge of the superior strait of the pelvis.

brisement (brēz-maw′) [Fr.] the breaking up or tearing of anything. **b. forcé,** the breaking up or tearing of a bony ankylosis.

broach (brōch) a fine barbed instrument for dressing a tooth canal or extracting the pulp.

bromelain (bro′mah-lān) a proteolytic and milk-clotting enzyme derived from the pineapple plant, *Ananas sativus*. In the plural, a concentrate of these enzymes, used as an anti-inflammatory agent. Also used in tenderizing meat, preparing protein hydrolysates, and chill-proofing beer.

bromide (bro′mīd) any binary compound of bromine. Bromides produce depression of the central nervous system, and were once widely used for their sedative effect. Because overdosage causes serious mental disturbances they are now seldom used, except occasionally in grand mal seizures. See also *brominism*.

bromine (bro′mēn) chemical element (*see table*), at. no. 35, symbol Br.

brominism (bro′min-izm) poisoning by excessive use of bromine or its compounds; symptoms include acne, headache, coldness of arms and legs, fetid breath, sleeplessness, weakness, and impotence.

bromocriptine (bro‴mo-krip′tēn) a dopamine agonist, an ergot alkaloid used to suppress prolactin secretion and thereby to inhibit lactation and stimulate ovulation.

bromodiphenhydramine (-di″fen-hi′drah-min) an antihistaminic, $C_{17}H_{20}BrNO$, used as the hydrochloride salt.

bromomenorrhea (-men″or-e′ah) menstruation characterized by an offensive odor.

brompheniramine (brōm″fen-ir′ah-mēn) an antihistaminic, $C_8H_9BrN_2$, used as the maleate salt.

Bromsulphalein (brōm-sul′fah-lin) trademark for a preparation of sulfobromophthalein.

bronchadenitis (brongk″ad-in-īt′is) inflammation of the bronchial glands.

bronchi (bron′ki) plural of *bronchus*.

bronchial (brong′ke-il) pertaining to or affecting one or more bronchi.

bronchiectasis (-ek′tah-sis) chronic dilatation of one or more bronchi.

bronchiocele (brong′ke-o-sēl″) dilatation or swelling of a bronchiole.

bronchiocrisis (brong″ke-o-kri′sis) bronchial crisis.

bronchiole (brong′ke-ōl) one of the finer subdivisions of the branched bronchial tree. **respiratory b.,** the final branch of a bronchiole.

bronchiolectasis (brong″ke-ōl-ek′tah-sis) dilatation of the bronchioles.

bronchiolus (brong-ki′ah-lus), pl. *bronchi′oli* [L.] bronchiole.

bronchiospasm (brong′ke-o-spazm″) bronchospasm.

bronchitis (brong-kīt′is) inflammation of one or more bronchi. **bronchit′ic,** adj. **acute b.,** a bronchitic attack with a short, severe course, due to exposure to cold, breathing of irritants, or acute infection, and marked by fever, pain in the chest (especially on coughing), dyspnea, and coughing. **catarrhal b.,** acute bronchitis with profuse mucopurulent discharge. **chronic b.,** a long-continued, recurrent inflammation due to repeated attacks of acute bronchitis or to chronic general disease, and marked by coughing, expectoration, and secondary changes in lung tissue. **croupous b.,** a form marked by violent cough and paroxysms of dyspnea, in which casts of the bronchial tubes are expectorated with Charcot-Leyden crystals and eosinophil cells. **fibrinous b.,** croupous b. **infectious avian b.,** an acute, highly contagious, respiratory viral disease of chickens. **b. obli′terans,** that in which the smaller bronchi become filled with nodules composed of fibrinous exudate.

bronchocandidiasis (brong″ko-kan″dĭ-di′ah-sis) candidiasis of the respiratory tree, occurring in a mild afebrile form manifested as chronic bronchitis, and in a usually fatal form resembling tuberculosis.

bronchocele (brong′kah-sēl) localized dilatation of a bronchus.

bronchoconstrictor (-kun-strik′ter) 1. narrowing the lumina of the air passages of the lungs. 2. an agent that causes such constriction.

bronchodilator (-di-lāt′er) 1. expanding the lumina of the air passages of the lungs. 2. an agent which causes dilatation of the bronchi.

bronchoesophageal (-ah-sof″ah-je′al) pertaining to or communicating with a bronchus and the esophagus.

bronchoesophagoscopy (-ah-sof″ah-gos′kah-pe) instrumental examination of the bronchi and esophagus.

bronchofiberscope (-fi′ber-skōp) a flexible bronchoscope utilizing fiberoptics.

bronchogenic (-jen′ik) originating in bronchi.

bronchography (brong-kog′rah-fe) radiography of the lungs after instillation of an opaque medium in the bronchi. **bronchograph′ic,** adj.

broncholithiasis (brong″ko-lĭ-thi′ah-sis) a condition in which calculi are present within the lumen of the tracheobronchial tree.

bronchology (brong-kol′ah-je) the study and treatment of diseases of the tracheobronchial tree. **broncholog′ic,** adj.

bronchomalacia (brong″ko-mah-la′she-ah) a deficiency in the cartilaginous wall of the trachea or a bronchus that may lead to atelectasis or obstructive emphysema.

bronchomotor (-mōt′er) affecting the caliber of the bronchi.

bronchomucotropic (-mu″ko-trop′ik) augmenting secretion by the respiratory mucosa.

bronchopancreatic (-pan″kre-at′ik) communicating with a bronchus and the pancreas, as a bronchopancreatic fistula.

bronchophony (brong-kof′ah-ne) the sound of the voice as heard through the stethoscope applied over a healthy large bronchus.

bronchoplasty (brong′ko-plas″te) plastic surgery of a bronchus; surgical closure of a bronchial fistula.

bronchoplegia (brong″ko-ple′je-ah) paralysis of the muscles of the walls of the bronchial tubes.

bronchopleural (-plōōr′il) pertaining to a bronchus and the pleura, or communicating with a bronchus and the pleural cavity.

bronchopneumonia (-noo-mo′ne-ah) inflammation of the lungs, usually beginning in the terminal bronchioles.

bronchopulmonary (-pul′mun-ĕ-re) pertaining to the bronchi and the lungs.

bronchorrhaphy (brong-kor′ah-fe) suture of a bronchus.

bronchoscope (brong′kah-skōp) an instrument for inspecting the interior of the tracheobronchial tree and carrying out endobronchial diagnostic and therapeutic maneuvers, such as taking specimens for culture and biopsy and removing foreign bodies. **bronchoscop′ic,** adj. **fiberoptic b.,** bronchofiberscope. **fiberoptic b.,** bronchofibroscopy.

bronchospasm (brong′kah-spazm) spasmodic contraction of the smooth muscle of the bronchi, as occurs in asthma.

bronchospirometry (-spi-rom′ĕ-tre) determination of vital capacity, oxygen intake, and carbon dioxide excretion of a single lung, or simultaneous measurements of the function of each lung separately. **differential b.,** measurement of the function of each lung separately.

bronchostenosis (-stah-no′sis) stricture or cicatricial diminution of the caliber of a bronchial tube.

bronchostomy (brong-kos′tah-me) the surgical creation of an opening through the chest wall into the bronchus.

bronchotracheal (brong″ko-tra′ke-il) pertaining to the bronchi and trachea.

bronchovesicular (-vah-sik′u-ler) pertaining to the bronchi and alveoli.

bronchus (brong′kus), pl. *bron′chi* [L.] one of the larger passages conveying air to (right or left principal bronchus) and within the lungs (lobar and segmental bronchi).

brow (brow) the forehead, or either lateral half of it.

B.R.S. British Roentgen Society.

Brucella (broo-sel′ah) a genus of schizomycetes (family Brucellaceae). **B. abor′tus,** the causative agent of infectious abortion in cattle and the commonest cause of brucellosis in man. **B. bronchisep′tica,** *Bordetella bronchiseptica.* **B. meliten′sis,** a causative agent of brucellosis, occurring primarily in goats. **B. o′vis,** the causative agent of an infectious disease in sheep. **B. su′is,** a species found in swine, which is capable of producing severe disease in man.

brucella (broo-sel′ah), pl. *brucel′lae.* Any member of *Brucella.* **brucel′lar,** adj.

Brucellaceae (broo″sel-a′se-e) a family of schizomycetes (order Eubacteriales), some genera of which are parasites of and pathogenic for warm-blooded animals, including man and birds.

brucellosis (broo″sel-o′sis) a generalized infection of man involving primarily the reticuloendothelial system, caused by species of *Brucella.*

Brugia (broo′je-ah) a genus of filarial worms, including *B. malayi,* a species similar to, and often found in association with, *Wuchereria bancrofti,* which causes human filariasis and elephantiasis throughout Southeast Asia, the China Sea, and eastern India.

bruit (brwe, brōōt) a sound or murmur heard in auscultation, especially an abnormal one. **aneurysmal b.,** blowing sound heard over an aneurysm. **placental b.,** see under *souffle.*

bruxism (bruk′sizm) grinding of the teeth, especially during sleep.

B.S. Bachelor of Surgery; Bachelor of Science; breath sounds; blood sugar.

BSA body surface area.

BSP Bromsulphalein.

B.T.U. British thermal unit.

bubo (bu′bo) an enlarged and inflamed lymph node, particularly in the axilla or groin, due to such infections as plague, syphilis, gonorrhea, lymphogranuloma venereum, and tuberculosis. **bubon′ic,** adj. **climatic b.,** lymphogranuloma venereum. **indolent b.,** a hard, nearly painless bubo that shows no tendency to break. **pestilential b.,** that associated with plague. **sympathetic b.,** bubo due to friction and injury.

bubonalgia (bu″bo-nal′je-ah) pain in the groin.

bubonocele (bu-bon′ah-sēl) inguinal or femoral hernia forming a swelling in the groin.

bucardia (bu-kar′de-ah) cor bovinum.

bucca (buk′ah) [L.] the cheek.

bucco- word element [L.], *cheek.*

buccoclusion (-kloo″zhin) malocclusion in which the dental arch or a quadrant or group of teeth is buccal to the normal.

buccoversion (-ver′zhin) position of a tooth lying buccally to the line of occlusion.

buckling (buk′ling) the process or an instance of becoming crumpled or warped. **scleral b.,** a technique for repair of a detached retina, in which indentations or infoldings of the sclera are made over the tears in the retina to promote adherence of the retina to the choroid.

buclizine (bu′klĭ-zēn) an antihistamine, $C_{28}H_{33}$-ClN_2, used mainly as an antinauseant in the management of motion sickness.

bud (bud) any small part of the embryo or adult metazoon more or less resembling the bud of a plant and presumed to have potential for growth and differentiation. **end b.,** the remnant of the primitive knot, from which arises the caudal part of the trunk. **limb b.,** a swelling on the trunk of an embryo that becomes a limb. **periosteal b.,** vascular connective tissue from the periosteum growing through apertures in the periosteal bone collar into the cartilage matrix of the primary center of ossification. **tail b.,** 1. the primordium of the caudal appendage. 2. end b. **taste b.,** one of the end organs of the gustatory nerve containing the receptor surfaces for the sense of taste. **ureteric b.,** an outgrowth of the mesonephric duct giving rise to all but the nephrons of the permanent kidney. **b. of urethra,** bulb of penis.

buffer (buf′er) 1. a chemical system that prevents changes in hydrogen ion concentration. 2. a physical or physiological system that tends to maintain constancy.

buiatrics (bu″e-at′riks) the treatment of diseases of cattle.

bulb (bulb) a rounded mass or enlargement. **bul′bar,** adj. **b. of aorta,** the enlargement of the aorta at its point of origin from the heart. **auditory b.,** the membranous labyrinth and cochlea. **b. of corpus cavernosum,** bulb of penis. **b. of hair,** the bulbous expansion at the proximal end of a hair in which the hair shaft is generated. **olfactory b.,** the bulblike expansion of the olfactory tract on the under surface of the frontal lobe of each cerebral hemisphere; the olfactory nerves enter it. **b. of penis,** the enlarged proximal part of the corpus spongiosum. **b. of urethra,** b. of penis. **b. of vestibule of vagina, vestibulovaginal b.,** a body consisting of paired masses of erectile tissue, one on either side of the vaginal opening.

bulbar (bul′ber) pertaining to a bulb; pertaining to or involving the medulla oblongata, as bulbar paralysis.

bulbitis (bul-bīt′is) inflammation of the bulb of the penis.

bulbourethral (bul″bo-ūr-e′thril) pertaining to the bulb of the urethra (bulb of penis).

bulbus (bul′bus), pl. *bul′bi* [L.] bulb.

bulimia (bu-lim′e-ah) a mental disorder affecting adolescent girls and young women, characterized by binge eating alternating with normal eating or fasting, but without the extreme loss of weight as in anorexia nervosa. *bulimic,* adj.

bulla (bul′ah), pl. *bul′lae* [L.] a blister; a circumscribed, fluid-containing, elevated lesion of the skin, usually more than 5 mm. in diameter. **bul′late, bul′lous,** adj.

bullosis (bul-o′sis) the production of, or a condition characterized by, bullous lesions.

BUN blood urea nitrogen; see *urea nitrogen.*

bundle (bun′d′l) a collection of fibers or strands, as of muscle fibers, or a fasciculus or band of nerve fibers. **fundamental b., ground b.,** that part of the white matter of the spinal cord bordering the gray matter and containing fibers that travel for a distance of only a few segments of the cord. **b. of His,** a band of cardiac muscle fibers connecting the atria with the ventricles of the heart. **Keith's b.,** a bundle of fibers in the wall of the right atrium between the openings of the venae cavae. **medial forebrain b.,** a group of nerve fibers containing the midbrain tegmentum and elements of the limbic system. **sinoatrial b.,** Keith's b. **Thorel's b.,** a bundle of muscle fibers in the human heart connecting the sinoatrial and atrioventricular nodes. **b. of Vicq d'Azyr,** a band of fibers from the mamillary body to the anterior nucleus of the thalamus.

bundle branch (bun′d′l branch) a branch of the bundle of His.

bunion (bun′yin) an abnormal prominence on the inner aspect of the first metatarsal head, with bursal formation, and resulting in displacement of the great toe. **tailor's b.,** bunionette.

bunionette (-et′) enlargement of the lateral aspect of the fifth metatarsal head.

Bunostomum (bu″no-sto′mum) a genus of hookworms parasitic in ruminants.

buphthalmos (būf-thal′mos) abnormal enlargement of the eyes; see *infantile glaucoma.*

bupivacaine (bu-piv′ah-kān) a local anesthetic, $C_{18}H_{28}N_2O$, used for peripheral nerve block, and sympathetic, caudal, or epidural block.

bur, burr (ber) a form of drill used for creating openings in bone or similar hard material.

buret, burette (bu-ret′) a graduated glass tube used to deliver a measured amount of liquid.

burn (bern) injury to tissues caused by the contact with heat, flame, chemicals, electricity, or radiation. First degree burns show redness; second degree burns show vesication; third degree burns show necrosis through the entire skin. Burns of the first and second degree are partial-thickness burns, those of the third are full-thickness burns.

burner (bern′er) the part of a lamp, stove, or furnace from which the flame issues. **Bunsen b.,** a gas burner in which the gas is mixed with air before ignition, in order to give complete oxidation.

burnishing (ber'nish-ing) a dental procedure somewhat related to polishing and abrading.

bursa (ber'sah), pl. *bur'sae, bursas* [L.] a fluid-filled sac or saclike cavity situated in places in tissues where friction would otherwise occur. **bur'sal**, adj. **b. of Achilles (tendon)**, one between the calcaneal tendon and the back of the calcaneus. **b. anseri'na**, one between the tendons of the sartorius, gracilis, and semitendinosus muscles, and the tibial collateral ligments. **Calori's b.**, one between the trachea and the arch of the aorta. **Fleischmann's b.**, one beneath the tongue. **His' b.**, the dilatation at the end of the archenteron. **iliac b.**, one at the point of insertion of the iliopsoas muscle into the lesser trochanter. **Luschka's b.**, b. pharyngea (1). **b. muco'sa**, synovial b. **omental b.**, **b. omenta'lis**, the lesser sac of the peritoneum. **b. pharyn'gea, pharyngeal b.**, an inconstant blind sac located above the pharyngeal tonsil in the midline of the posterior wall of the nasopharynx; it represents persistence of an embryonic communication between the anterior tip of the notochord and the roof of the pharynx. **popliteal b.**, one in the popliteal space beneath the tendon of the semimembranosus and the tendon of the inner head of the gastrocnemius. **prepatellar b.**, one of the bursae in front of the patella; it may be subcutaneous, subfascial, or subtendinous in location. **subcromial b., b. subacromia'lis**, one between the acromion and the insertion of the supraspinatus muscle, extending between the deltoid and greater tubercle of the humerus. **subdeltoid b., b. subdeltoi'dea**, one between the deltoid and the shoulder joint capsule, usually connected to the subacromial bursa. **synovial b., b. synovia'lis**, a closed synovial sac interposed between surfaces that glide upon each other; it may be subcutaneous, submuscular, subfascial, or subtendinous in location.

bursitis (ber-sīt'is) inflammation of a bursa; specific types of bursitis are named according to the bursa affected, e.g., prepatellar bursitis, subacromial bursitis, etc. **calcific b.**, see under *tendinitis.* **ischiogluteal b.**, inflammation of the bursa over the ischial tuberosity, characterized by sudden onset of excruciating pain over the center of the buttock and down the back of the leg. **subacromial b., subdeltoid b.**, inflammation and calcification of the subacromial or subdeltoid bursa. **Thornwaldt's b.**, chronic inflammation of the pharyngeal bursa.

bursotomy (ber-sot'ah-me) incision of a bursa.

busulfan (bu-sul'fan) an antineoplastic, C_6H_{14}-O_6S_2, used in treating myelocytic leukemia.

butabarbital (būt''ah-bar'bit-al) a short- to intermediate-acting barbiturate, $C_{10}H_{15}N_2O_3$; its sodium salt is used as a sedative and hypnotic.

butacaine (-kān) a local anesthetic, $C_{18}H_{30}N_2O_2$; the sulfate salt is used as a topical anesthetic in the eye and on mucous membranes, in solution or as ointment.

butalbital (bu-tal'bit-al) a sedative, $C_{11}H_{16}N_2$-O_3.

butamben (bu-tam'ben) a local anesthetic, C_{11}-$H_{15}NO_2$, applied topically in the treatment of painful skin conditions.

butane (bu'tān) an aliphatic hydrocarbon from petroleum, C_4H_{10}, occurring as a colorless flammable gas.

butaperazine (būt''ah-per'ah-zēn) a phenothiazine derivative, $C_{24}H_{31}N_3OS$, used as an antipsychotic drug.

Butazolidin (būt''ah-zol'ĭ-din) trademark for a preparation of phenylbutazone.

Butisol (būt'ĭ-sol) trademark for preparations of butabarbital.

butorphanol (bu-tor'fah-nōl) a synthetic opioid, $C_{21}H_{29}NO_2$, having analgesic and antitussive properties.

buttock (but'ok) either of the two fleshy prominences formed by the gluteal muscles on the lower part of the back.

button (but'′n) 1. a knoblike elevation or structure. 2. a spool- or disk-shaped device used in surgery for construction of intestinal anastomosis. **Jaboulay's b.**, a device used for lateral intestinal anastomosis. **mescal b's**, transverse slices of the flowering heads of a Mexian cactus, *Lophophora williamsii*, whose major active principle is mescaline. **Murphy's b.**, a metallic device used for connecting the ends of a dividing intestine.

butyl (būt'′l) a hydrocarbon radical, C_4H_9. **b. chloride**, a clear colorless volatile liquid, C_4-H_9Cl, used as a veterinary anthelmintic.

butylparaben (būt'''il-par'ah-ben) an antifungal agent, $C_{11}H_{14}O_3$, used as a pharmaceutic preservative.

butyrate (būt'ĭ-rāt) a salt of butyric acid.

butyric acid (bu-tir'ik) a saturated fatty acid, C_3H_7 COOH, found in butter, sweat, feces, and urine, and in traces in the spleen and blood.

butyroid (būt'ĭ-roid) resembling or having the consistency of butter.

butyrophenone (būt''ĭ-ro-fe'nōn) a chemical class of major tranquilizers especially useful in the treatment of manic and moderate to severe agitated states and in the control of the vocal utterances and tics of Gilles de la Tourette's syndrome.

bypass (bi'pas) an auxiliary flow; a shunt; a surgically created pathway circumventing the normal anatomical pathway, as an aortoiliac or a jejunal bypass.

byssinosis (bis''ĭ-no'sis) pneumoconiosis due to inhalation of cotton dust. **byssinot'ic**, adj.

C

C chemical symbol, *carbon;* cervical vertebrae; complement; coulomb; cytosine or cytidine.

C. cathode (cathodal); Celsius or centigrade (scale); cervical; clearance; clonus; closure; contraction; cylinder.

c. contact; *centi.*

CA cardiac arrest; coronary artery.

Ca chemical symbol, *calcium.*

cac(o)- word element [Gr.], *bad; ill.*

cacesthesia (kak″is-the′ze-ah) any morbid sensation or disorder of sensibility.

cachectin (kah-kek′tin) a hormonelike protein, produced by macrophages, that releases fat and reduces the concentration of enzymes required for the storage and production of fat. When bacterial endotoxins cause its release, it can induce shock.

cachet (kah-sha′) a disk-shaped wafer or capsule enclosing a dose of medicine.

cachexia (kah-kek′se-ah) a profound and marked state of constitutional disorder; general ill health and malnutrition. **cachec′tic,** adj. **c. hypophysiopri′va,** the train of symptoms resulting from total deprivation of pituitary function, including loss of sexual function, bradycardia, hypothermia, and coma. **malarial c.,** the physical signs resulting from antecedent attacks of severe malaria, including anemia, sallow skin, yellow sclera, splenomegaly, hepatomegaly, and, in children, retardation of growth and puberty. **pachydermic c.,** myxedema. **pituitary c.,** see *panhypopituitarism.*

cachinnation (kak″ĭ-na′shin) excessive, hysterical laughter.

cacodylic acid (kak″o-dil′ik) a crystalline compound, $(CH_3)_2ASO \cdot OH$, used as an herbicide.

cacogeusia (kak″o-gu′se-ah) a bad taste; a complaint of some patients with idiopathic epilepsy or those receiving antipsychotic agents or lithium, and a somatic delusion in psychoses.

cacomelia (-me′le-ah) congenital deformity of a limb.

cacumen (kah-ku′min), pl. *cacu′mina* [L.] 1. the top or apex of an organ. 2. the top of a plant. 3. culmen.

cadaver (kah-dav′er) a dead body; generally applied to a human body preserved for anatomical study. **cadav′eric, cadav′erous,** adj.

cadaverine (-in) a relatively nontoxic ptomaine, $C_5H_{14}N_2$, formed by decarboxylation of lysine; it is sometimes one of the products of *Vibrio proteus* and of *V. cholerae,* and occasionally found in the urine in cystinuria.

cadmium (kad′me-um) chemical element (*see table*), at. no. 48, symbol Cd; its salts are poisonous. Inhalation of cadmium fumes causes pulmonary edema, followed by proliferative interstitial pneumonia, and is associated with various degrees of lung damage; poisoning may also be due to ingestion of foods contaminated by cadmium-plated containers, causing violent gastrointestinal symptoms.

caduceus (kah-doo′se-us) the wand of Hermes or Mercury; used as a symbol of the medical profession and as the emblem of the Medical Corps of the U.S. Army. See also *staff of Aesculapius.*

cae- for words beginning thus, see also those beginning *ce-.*

caffeine (kah-fēn′) a central nervous system stimulant, $C_8H_{10}N_4O_2$, from coffee, tea, guarana, and maté.

cage (kāj) a box or enclosure. **thoracic c.,** the bony structure enclosing the thorax, consisting of the ribs, vertebral column, and sternum.

cal calorie.

calamine (kal′ah-mīn) a preparation of zinc and ferric oxides, used topically as a protectant.

calamus (kal′ah-mus) 1. a reed or reedlike structure. 2. the peeled, dried rhizome of *Acorus calamus;* mild aromatic. **c. scripto′rius,** the lowest portion of the floor of the fourth ventricle, situated between the restiform bodies.

calcaneoapophysitis (kal-ka″ne-o-ah-pof″ĭ-sĭt′is) inflammation of the posterior part of the calcaneus, marked by pain and swelling.

calcaneoastragaloid (-ah-strag′ah-loid) pertaining to the calcaneus and astragalus.

calcaneodynia (-din′e-ah) pain in the heel.

calcaneus (kal-ka′ne-us) [L.] see *Table of Bones.* **calca′neal, calca′nean,** adj.

calcar (kal′kar) a spur or spur-shaped structure. **c. a′vis,** the lower of two medial elevations in the posterior horn of the lateral cerebral ventricle, produced by the lateral extension of the calcarine sulcus.

calcareous (kal-kār′e-us) pertaining to or containing lime; chalky.

calcarine (kal′kar-in) 1. spur-shaped. 2. pertaining to the calcar.

calcemia (kal-se′me-ah) hypercalcemia.

calcibilia (kal″sĭ-bil′e-ah) presence of calcium in the bile.

calcic (kal′sik) of or pertaining to lime or calcium.

calciferol (kal-sif′er-ol) 1. see *vitamin D.* 2. ergocalciferol.

calcific (kal-sif′ik) forming lime.

calcification (kal″sĭ-fĭ-ka′shin) the deposit of calcium salts in a tissue. **dystrophic c.,** the deposition of calcium in abnormal tissue, such as scar tissue or atherosclerotic plaques, without abnormalities of blood calcium. **Mönckeberg's c.,** see under *arteriosclerosis.*

calcinosis (kal″sĭ-no′sis) a condition characterized by abnormal deposition of calcium salts in the tissues. **c. circumscrip′ta,** localized deposition of calcium in small nodules in subcutaneous tissues or muscle. **c. universa′lis,** widespread deposition of calcium in nodules or plaques in the dermis, panniculus, and muscles.

calcipexis, calcipexy (kal″sĭ-pek′sis; kal′sĭ-pek″se) fixation of calcium in the tissues. **calcipec′tic, calcipex′ic,** adj.

calciphylaxis (-fi-lak′sis) the formation of calcified tissue in response to administration of a challenging agent after induction of a hypersensitive state. **calciphylac′tic,** adj.

calciprivia (-priv′e-ah) deprivation or loss of calcium. **calcipri′vic,** adj.

calcitonin (-to′nin) a polypeptide hormone secreted by C cells of the thyroid gland, and sometimes of the thymus and parathyroids, which lowers calcium and phosphate concentration in plasma and inhibits bone resorption.

calcium (kal′se-um) chemical element (see table), at. no. 20, symbol Ca. Calcium phosphate salts form the dense hard material of teeth and bones. The calcium(II) ion is involved in many physiologic processes. A normal blood calcium level is essential for normal function of the heart, nerves, and muscles. It is involved in blood coagulation (in which connection it is called coagulation Factor IV). **c. carbonate,** an insoluble salt, $CaCO_3$, occurring naturally in shells, limestone, and chalk; used as an antacid. **c. chloride,** a salt, $CaCl_2 2H_2O$, used as a calcium replenisher and as an antidote for magnesium poisoning. **c. gluconate,** $C_{12}H_{22}CaO_{14}$, a calcium replenisher and oral antidote for fluoride or oxalic acid poisoning. **c. glycerophosphate,** a calcium and phosphorus dietary supplement. **c. hydroxide,** a base, $Ca(OH)_2$, used in solution as a topical astringent. **c. levulinate,** a salt used infrequently as a calcium supplement. **c. mandelate,** $C_{16}H_{14}CaO_6$, a urinary antiseptic. **c. oxalate,** a compound occurring in urine as crystals and in certain calculi. **c. oxide,** lime (1). **c. pantothenate,** calcium salt of the dextrorotatory isomer of pantothenic acid; used as a growth-promoting vitamin. **c. phosphate,** one of three salts containing calcium and the phosphate radical: dibasic and tribasic c. phosphate are used as sources of calcium; monobasic c. phosphate is used in fertilizers and as a calcium and phosphorus supplement. **c. propionate,** a salt used as an antifungal preservative in foods and as a topical antifungal agent.

calcospherite (kal″ko-sfēr′it) one of the minute globular bodies formed during calcification by chemical union of calcium particles and albuminous matter of cells.

calculosis (-lo′sis) lithiasis.

calculus (kal′ku-lus), pl. cal′culi [L.] an abnormal concretion, usually composed of mineral salts, occurring within the animal body. **cal′culous,** adj. **biliary calculi,** stones of the gallbladder (cholelithiasis) composed almost entirely of the excessive blood pigment liberated by hemolysis, with calcium deposits in some. **dental c.,** calcium phosphate and carbonate, with organic matter, deposited on tooth surfaces. **fusible c.,** a urinary calculus composed of phosphates of ammonium, calcium, and magnesium, which fuses to a black mass when tested under the blowpipe. **lung c.,** a concretion formed in the bronchi by accretion about an inorganic nucleus, or from calcified portions of lung tissue or adjacent lymph nodes. **renal c.,** one in the kidney. **salivary c.,** one in a salivary gland or duct. **urinary c.,** one in any part of the

urinary tract. **vesical c.,** one in the urinary bladder.

calefacient (kal″i-fa′shint) causing a sensation of warmth; an agent that so acts.

calf (kaf) sura; the fleshy back part of the leg below the knee.

caliber (kal′i-ber) the diameter of the opening of a canal or tube.

calibration (kal″i-bra′shin) determination of the accuracy of an instrument, usually by measurement of its variation from a standard, to ascertain necessary correction factors.

calicectasis (kal″i-sek′tah-sis) dilatation of a calix of the kidney.

calicivirus (kal″i-si-vi′rus) any of a subgroup of picornaviruses, including the virus of vesicular exanthem.

caliculus (kah-lik′u-lus), pl. cali′culi [L.] a small cup or cup-shaped structure.

californium (kal″i-for′ne-um) chemical element (see table), at. no. 98, symbol Cf.

calipers (kal′i-perz) an instrument with two bent or curved legs used for measuring thickness or diameter of a solid.

calisthenics (kal″is-then′iks) systematic exercise for attaining strength and gracefulness.

calix (ka′liks), pl. ca′lices [L.] a cup-shaped organ or cavity, e.g., one of the recesses of the pelvis of the kidney which enclose the pyramids. **calice′al,** adj.

Calliphora (kal-if′or-ah) a genus of flies, the blowflies or bluebottle flies, which deposit their eggs in decaying matter, on wounds, or in body openings; the maggots are a cause of myiasis.

callosity (kah-los′it-e) a callus (1).

callosum (kah-lo′sum) corpus callosum. **callo′sal,** adj.

callus (kal′us) 1. localized hyperplasia of the horny layer of the epidermis due to pressure or friction. 2. an unorganized network of woven bone formed about the ends of a broken bone, which is absorbed as repair is completed (provisional c.), and ultimately replaced by true bone (definitive c.).

calmative (kah′mah-tiv, kal′) 1. sedative; allaying excitement. 2. an agent having such effects.

calmodulin (kal-mod′u-lin) a calcium-binding protein present in all nucleated cells, thought to be an essential mediator of most calcium-sensitive cellular processes.

calomel (kal′ah-mel) a heavy, white, impalpable powder, Hg_2Cl, used as a cathartic.

calor (kal′er) [L.] heat; one of the cardinal signs of inflammation.

caloric (kah-lo′rik) pertaining to heat or to calories.

calorie (kal′ah-re) any of a variety of units of heat defined as the amount of heat required to raise 1 gm. of water 1° C. at a specified temperature; the calorie used in chemistry and biochemistry is equal to 4.184 joules. Abbreviated cal. **large c.,** kilocalorie; the calorie used in metabolic studies. **small c.,** calorie.

calorigenic (kah-lor″i-jen′ik) producing or increasing production of heat or energy; increasing oxygen consumption.

calorimeter (kal″ah-rim′it-er) an instrument for measuring the amount of heat produced in any system or organism.

calsequestrin (kal″sĭ-kwes′trin) a calcium-binding protein rich in carboxylate side chains, occurring on the inner membrane surface of the sarcoplasmic reticulum.

calvaria (kal-va′re-ah) the domelike superior portion of the cranium, comprising the superior portions of the frontal, parietal, and occipital bones.

calvarium (kal-va′re-um) calvaria.

calx (kalks) 1. lime or chalk. 2. the heel.

calyculus (kah-lik′u-lus), pl. *calyc′uli* [L.] caliculus.

Calymmatobacterium (kah-lim″ah-to-bak-te′re-um) a genus of bacteria (family Brucellaceae), composed of pleomorphic nonmotile, gram-negative rods. **C. granulo′matis**, the species causing granuloma inguinale in man. Called also *Donovania granulomatis*. See also *Donovan's bodies*.

camera (kam′er-ah), pl. *cam′erae* [L.] a cavity or chamber. **c. ante′rior bul′bi**, anterior chamber of the eye. **c. o′culi**, either the anterior or the posterior chamber of the eye. **c. poste′rior bul′bi**, posterior chamber of the eye. **c. vi′trea bul′bi**, vitreous chamber.

cAMP cyclic adenosine monophosphate.

camphor (kam′fer) 1. a ketone derived from the Asian tree *Cinnamomum camphora* or produced synthetically; used topically as an antipruritic. 2. any compound with characteristics similar to those of camphor.

campimeter (kam-pim′it-er) an apparatus for mapping the central portion of the visual field on a flat surface.

campotomy (kam-pot′ah-me) the stereotaxic surgical technique of producing a lesion in Forel's fields, beneath the thalamus, for correction of tremor in Parkinson's disease.

camptocormia (kamp″tah-kor′me-ah) a static deformity consisting of forward flexion of the trunk.

camptodactyly (-dak′tĭ-le) permanent flexion of one or more fingers.

camptomelia (-me′le-ah) bending of the limbs, producing permanent bowing or curving of the affected part. **camptome′lic**, adj.

Campylobacter (kam′pĭ-lo-bak″ter) a genus of bacteria, family Spirillaceae, made up of gram-negative, non–spore-forming, motile, spirally curved rods, which are microaerophilic to anaerobic. **C. fe′tus**, a species, certain subspecies of which cause acute gastroenteritis in man and abortion in sheep and cattle.

camsylate (kam′sĭ-lāt) USAN contraction for camphorsulfonate.

canal (kah-nal′) a relatively narrow tubular passage or channel. **adductor c.**, a fascial tunnel in the middle third of the medial part of the thigh, containing the femoral vessels and saphenous nerve. **Alcock's c.**, a tunnel formed by a splitting of the obturator fascia, which encloses the pudendal vessels and nerve. **alimentary c.**, the musculomembranous digestive tube extending from the mouth to the anus; see Plate IV.

anal c., the terminal portion of the alimentary canal, from the rectum to the anus. **Arnold's c.**, a channel in the petrous portion of the temporal bone for passage of the vagus nerve. **atrioventricular c.**, the common canal connecting the primitive atrium and ventricle; it sometimes persists as a congenital anomaly. **birth c.**, the canal through which the fetus passes in birth. **caroticotympanic c's**, tiny passages in the temporal bone connecting the carotid canal and the tympanic cavity, carrying communicating twigs between the internal carotid and tympanic plexuses. **carotid c.**, a tunnel in the petrous portion of the temporal bone that transmits the internal carotid artery to the cranial cavity. **cochlear c.**, see under *duct*. **condylar c.**, an occasional opening in the condylar fossa for transmission of the transverse sinus. **c. of Cuvier**, ductus venosus. **Dorello's c.**, an occasional opening in the temporal bone through which the abducens nerve and inferior petrosal sinus enter the cavernous sinus. **facial c.**, a canal for the facial nerve in the petrous portion of the temporal bone. **femoral c.**, the medial part of the femoral sheath lateral to the base of the lacunar ligament. **Gartner's c.**, see under *duct*. **genital c.**, any canal for the passage of ova or for copulatory use. **haversian c.**, any of the anastomosing channels of the haversian system in compact bone, containing blood and lymph vessels and nerves. **c. of Huguier**, a small canal opening into the facial canal just before its termination, transmitting the chorda tympani nerve. **Huschke's c.**, a canal formed by the tubercles of the tympanic ring, usually disappearing during childhood. **hyaloid c.**, a passage running from in front of the optic disk to the lens of the eye; in the fetus, it transmits the hyaloid artery. **hypoglossal c.**, an opening in the occipital bone, transmitting the hypoglossal nerve and a branch of the posterior meningeal artery. **incisive c.**, one of the small canals opening into the incisive fossa of the hard palate, transmitting the nasopalatine nerves. **infraorbital c.**, a small canal running obliquely through the floor of the orbit, transmitting the infraorbital vessels and nerve. **inguinal c.**, the oblique passage in the lower anterior abdominal wall, through which passes the round ligament of the uterus in the female, and the spermatic cord in the male. **interdental c's**, channels in the alveolar process of the mandible between the roots of the central and lateral incisors, for passage of anastomosing blood vessels between the sublingual and inferior dental arteries. **interfacial c's**, a labyrinthine system of expanded intercellular spaces between desmosomes. **Löwenberg's c.**, the part of the cochlear duct above the membrane of Corti. **medullary c.**, 1. vertebral c. 2. see under *cavity*. **nasolacrimal c.**, a canal formed by the maxilla laterally and the lacrimal bone and inferior nasal concha medially, transmitting the nasolacrimal duct. **neurenteric c.**, a temporary communication in the embryo between the cavities of the yolk sac and the amnion. **c. of Nuck**, a pouch of peritoneum extending into the inguinal canal, accompanying the round ligament in the female, or the testis in its descent into the scrotum in the male; usually obliterated in the female. **nutrient c. of bone,** haversian c. **perivascular c.,** a lymph space about a blood vessel. **c. of Petit,** zonular spaces. **portal c.,** a space within the capsule of Glisson and liver substance, containing branches of the portal vein, of the hepatic artery, and of the hepatic duct. **pterygoid c.,** a canal in the sphenoid bone transmitting the pterygoid vessels and nerves. **pterygopalatine c.,** a passage in the sphenoid and palatine bones for the greater palatine vessels and nerve. **pyloric c.,** the short narrow part of the stomach extending from the gastroduodenal junction to the pyloric antrum. **root c.,** that part of the pulp cavity extending from the pulp chamber to the apical foramen. **sacculocochlear c.,** the canal connecting the saccule and cochlea. **sacral c.,** the continuation of the vertebral canal through the sacrum. **semicircular c's,** three long canals (anterior, lateral, and posterior) of the bony labyrinth. **spiral c. of cochlea,** cochlear duct. **spiral c. of modiolus,** a canal following the course of the bony spiral lamina of the cochlea and containing the spiral ganglion. **tarsal c.,** see under *sinus.* **tympanic c.,** see under *canaliculus.* **uterine c.,** the cavity of the uterus. **vertebral c.,** the canal formed by the series of vertebral foramina together, enclosing the spinal cord and meninges. **Volkmann's c's,** canals communicating with the haversian canals, for passage of blood vessels through bone. **c. of Wirsung,** pancreatic duct. **zygomaticotemporal c.,** see under *foramen.*

canaliculus (kan″ah-lik′u-lus), pl. *canali′culi* [L.] an extremely narrow tubular passage or channel. **canalic′ular,** adj. **apical c.,** one of the numerous tubular invaginations arising from the clefts between the microvilli of the proximal convoluted tubule of the kidney and extending downward into the apical cytoplasm. **bone canaliculi,** branching tubular passages radiating like wheel spokes from each bone lacuna to connect with the canaliculi of adjacent lacunae, and with the haversian canal. **cochlear c.,** see under *aqueduct.* **dental canaliculi,** minute channels in dentin, extending from the pulp cavity to the overlying cement and enamel. **intercellular c.,** one located between adjacent cells, such as one of the secretory capillaries, or canaliculi, of the gastric parietal cells. **intracellular canaliculi of parietal cells,** a system of canaliculi that seem to be intracellular but are formed by deep invaginations of the surface of the gastric parietal cells rather than extending into the cytoplasm of the cell. **lacrimal c.,** the short passage in an eyelid, beginning at the lacrimal point and draining tears from the lacrimal lake to the lacrimal sac. **mastoid c.,** a small channel in the temporal bone transmitting the tympanic branch of the vagus nerve. **tympanic c.,** a small opening on the inferior surface of the petrous portion of the temporal bone, transmitting the tympanic branch of the glossopharyngeal nerve and a small artery.

canalis (kah-nal′is), pl. *cana′les* [L.] a canal or channel.

canalization (kan″il-i-za′shin) 1. the formation of canals, natural or morbid. 2. the surgical establishment of canals for drainage.

cancellus (kan-sel′us), pl. *cancel′li* [L.] the lattice-like structure in bone; any structure arranged like a lattice.

cancer (kan′ser) any malignant, cellular tumor; cancers are divided into two broad categories of carcinoma and sarcoma. **can′cerous,** adj. **epithelial c.,** carcinoma.

canceremia (kan″ser-e′me-ah) the presence of cancer cells in the blood.

cancerigenic (kan″ser-i-jen′ik) giving rise to a malignant tumor.

cancriform (kang′kri-form) resembling cancer.

cancroid (kang′kroid) 1. cancer-like. 2. a skin cancer of a low grade of malignancy.

cancrum (kang′krum) [L.] canker. **c. o′ris,** see *noma.* **c. puden′di,** see *noma.*

candela (kan-del′ah) the SI unit of luminous intensity. Abbreviated cd.

candicidin (kan″di-sīd′′n) an antifungal antibiotic produced by a strain of *Streptomyces griseus;* used for the treatment of vaginal candidiasis.

Candida (kan′did-ah) a genus of yeastlike fungi that are commonly part of the normal flora of the mouth, skin, intestinal tract, and vagina, but can cause a variety of infections (see *candidiasis*). *C. al′bicans* is the usual pathogen.

candidiasis (-di′ah-sis) infection by fungi of the genus *Candida,* generally *C. albicans,* most commonly involving the skin, oral mucosa (thrush), respiratory tract, and vagina; rarely there is a systemic infection or endocarditis.

candidid (kan′did-id) a secondary skin eruption that is the expression of hypersensitivity to infection with *Candida* elsewhere on the body.

candidin (-in) a skin test antigen derived from *Candida albicans,* used in testing for the development of delayed-type hypersensitivity to the microorganism.

canine (ka′nīn) 1. of pertaining to, or characteristic of a dog. 2. a canine tooth.

canities (kah-nish′e-ēz) grayness or whiteness of the scalp hair.

canker (kang′ker) an ulceration, especially of the lip or oral mucosa.

cannabinoid (kan-ab′ĭ-noid) any of the principles of *Cannabis,* including tetrahydrocannabinol, cannabinol, and cannabidiol.

Cannabis (kan′ah-bis) a genus of plants, hemp, including *C. in′dica,* an Asiatic variety of common hemp and *C. sati′va,* the common hemp. See *cannabis.*

cannabis (kan′ah-bis) the dried flowering tops of hemp plants (*Cannabis sativa*), which have euphoric principles (tetrahydrocannabinols); classified as a hallucinogen and prepared as bhang, ganja, hashish, and marihuana.

cannula (kan′u-lah) a tube for insertion into a duct or cavity; during insertion its lumen is usually occupied by a trocar.

canthitis (kan-thīt'is) inflammation of the canthus.

canthoplasty (kan'thah-plas"te) plastic surgery of a canthus.

canthotomy (kan-thot'ah-me) incision of a canthus.

canthus (kan'this), pl. *can'thi* [L.] the angle at either end of the fissure between the eyelids.

C.A.P. College of American Pathologists.

cap (kap) a protective covering for the head or for a similar structure; a structure resembling such a covering. **acrosomal c.**, acrosome. **cradle c.**, crusta lactea. **duodenal c.**, the part of the duodenum adjacent to the pylorus, forming the superior flexure. **enamel c.**, the enamel organ after it covers the top of the growing tooth papilla. **head c.**, the doubled-layered caplike structure over the upper two-thirds of the acrosome of a spermatozoon, consisting of the collapsed acrosomal vesicle. **knee c.**, patella; see *Table of Bones*. **skull c.**, calvaria.

capacitance (kah-pas'it-ins) 1. the property of being able to store an electric charge. 2. the ratio of charge to potential in a conductor.

capacitation (kah-pas"ĭ-ta'shin) the process by which spermatozoa become capable of fertilizing an ovum after it reaches the ampullar portion of the uterine tube.

capacity (kah-pas'it-e) the power to hold, retain, or contain, or the ability to absorb; usually expressed numerically as the measure of such ability. **functional residual c.**, the amount of air remaining at the end of normal quiet respiration. **heat c.**, thermal c. **inspiratory c.**, the volume of gas that can be taken into the lungs in a full inspiration, starting from the resting inspiratory position; equal to the tidal volume plus the inspiratory reserve volume. **maximal breathing c.**, the greatest volume of gas that can be breathed per minute by voluntary effort. **thermal c.**, the amount of heat absorbed by a body in being raised 1° C. **total lung c.**, the amount of gas contained in the lung at the end of a maximal inspiration. **virus neutralizing c.**, the ability of a serum to inhibit the infectivity of a virus. **vital c.**, the volume of gas that can be expelled from the lungs from a position of full inspiration, with no limit to duration of inspiration; equal to inspiratory capacity plus expiratory reserve volume.

capillarectasia (kap"ĭ-lar"ek-ta'ze-ah) dilatation of capillaries.

Capillaria (kap"il-la're-ah) a genus of parasitic nematodes, including *C. contor'ta*, found in domestic fowl; *C. hepat'ica*, found in the liver of rats and other mammals, including man; and *C. philippinen'sis*, found in the human intestine in Luzon, causing severe diarrhea, malabsorption, and high mortality.

capillariasis (kap"ĭ-lah-ri'ah-sis) infection with nematodes of the genus *Capillaria*, especially *C. philippinensis*.

capillariomotor (kap"ĭ-lar"e-o-mōt'er) pertaining to the functional activity of the capillaries.

capillarity (kap"ĭ-lar'it-e) the action by which the surface of a liquid in contact with a solid, as in a capillary tube, is elevated or depressed.

capillary (kap'ĭ-ler"e) 1. pertaining to or resembling a hair. 2. one of the minute vessels connecting the arterioles and venules, the walls of which act as a semipermeable membrane for interchange of various substances between the blood and tissue fluid; see Plate IX. **arterial c's**, minute vessels lacking a continuous muscular coat, intermediate in structure and location between arterioles and capillaries. **continuous c's**, one of the two major types of capillaries, found in muscle, skin, lung, central nervous system, and other tissues, characterized by the presence of an uninterrupted endothelium and a continuous basal lamina, and by fine filaments and numerous pinocytotic vesicles. **fenestrated c's**, one of the two major types of capillaries, found in the intestinal mucosa, renal glomeruli, pancreas, endocrine glands, and other tissues, and characterized by the presence of circular fenestrae or pores that penetrate the endothelium; these pores may be closed by a very thin diaphragm. **lymph c., lymphatic c.**, one of the minute vessels of the lymphatic system; see Plate IX. **secretory c.**, one of the extremely fine intercellular canaliculi situated between adjacent gland cells, such as the gastric parietal cells, being formed by the apposition of grooves in the surfaces of the cells and opening into the gland's lumen. **venous c's**, minute vessels lacking a muscular coat, intermediate in structure and location between venules and capillaries.

capillus (kah-pil'us), pl. *capil'li* [L.] a hair; used in the plural to designate the aggregate of hair on the scalp.

capitate (kap'ĭ-tāt) head-shaped.

capitation (kap"ĭ-ta'shin) the annual fee paid to a physician or group of physicians by each participant in a health plan.

capitatum (kap"ĭ-tāt-um) the capitate bone; see *Table of Bones*.

capitellum (kap"ĭ-tel'um) capitulum.

capitonnage (kap"ĭ-to-nahzh') [Fr.] closure of a cyst by applying sutures to approximate the opposing surfaces of the cavity.

capitulum (kah-pit'u-lum), pl. *capit'ula* [L.] a small eminence on a bone, as on the distal end of the humerus, by which it articulates with another bone. **capit'ular**, adj.

Capnocytophaga (kap"no-si-tof'ah-gah) a genus of anaerobic, gram-negative, rod-shaped bacteria that have been implicated in the pathogenesis of periodontal disease; they closely resemble *Bacteroides ochraceus*.

capotement (kah-pōt-maw') [Fr.] a splashing sound heard in dilatation of the stomach.

cappie (kap'e) a disease of young sheep characterized by thinning of the bones of the scalp, possibly due to phosphorus-deficient diet.

capping (cap'ing) 1. the provision of a protective or obstructive covering. 2. the formation of a polar cap on the surface of a cell concerned with immunologic responses, occurring as a result of movement of components on the cell surface into clusters or patches that coalesce to form the cap. The process is produced by reaction of antibody with the cell membrane and appears to involve cross-linking of antigenic determinants. **pulp c.,** the covering of an exposed or nearly exposed dental pulp with some material to provide protection against external influences and to encourage healing.

capreomycin (kap″re-o-mi′sin) a polypeptide antibiotic produced by *Streptomyces capreolus*, which is active against human strains of *Mycobacterium tuberculosis* and has four microbiologically active components.

capric acid (kap′rik) a rancid-smelling saturated fatty acid, $C_9H_{19}COOH$, in butter and coconut oil.

caproate (kap′ro-āt) 1. any salt or ester of caproic acid (hexanoic acid). 2. USAN contraction for hexanoate.

caproic acid (kah-pro′ik) a saturated fatty acid, $C_5H_{11}COOH$, in milk fat and some plant oils, used in manufacture of artificial flavors.

caprylate (kap′rĭ-lāt) any salt of caprylic acid.

caprylic acid (kah-pril′ik) a saturated fatty acid, C_7H_5COOH, found in goat- and cow-milk fat and in some seed oils; used in manufacture of perfumes.

capsid (kap′sid) the shell of protein that protects the nucleic acid of a virus; it is composed of structural units, or capsomers.

capsitis (kap-sīt′is) inflammation of the capsule of the crystalline lens.

capsomer, capsomere (kap′so-mer; -mēr) a morphological unit of the capsid of a virus.

capsula (kap′su-lah), pl. *cap′sulae* [L.] capsule.

capsule (kap′sūl) 1. an enclosing structure, as a soluble container enclosing a dose of medicine. 2. a cartilaginous, fatty, fibrous, membranous structure enveloping another structure, organ, or part. **cap′sular,** adj. **articular c.,** the saclike envelope enclosing the cavity of a synovial joint. **auditory c.,** the cartilaginous capsule of the embryo that becomes the bony labyrinth of the inner ear. **bacterial c.,** an envelope of gel surrounding a bacterial cell, usually polysaccharide but sometimes polypeptide in nature; it is associated with the virulence of pathogenic bacteria. **c's of brain,** see *external c.* and *internal c.* **cartilage c.,** a basophilic zone of cartilage matrix bordering on a lacuna and its enclosed cartilage cells. **external c.,** the layer of white fibers between the putamen and claustrum. **Glisson's c.,** the connective tissue sheath accompanying the hepatic ducts and vessels through the hepatic portal. **glomerular c., c. of glomerulus,** the globular dilatation forming the beginning of a uriniferous tubule within the kidney and surrounding the glomerulus. **internal c.,** a fanlike mass of white fibers separating the lentiform nucleus laterally from the head of the caudate nucleus, the dorsal thalamus, and the tail of the caudate nucleus medially. **joint c.,** articular c. **c. of lens,** the elastic envelope covering the lens of the eye. **optic c.,** the embryonic structure from which the sclera develops. **otic c.,** the skeletal element enclosing the inner ear mechanism. In the human embryo, it develops as cartilage at various ossification centers and becomes completely bony and unified at about the 33rd week of fetal life. **renal c., adi-**

pose, the investment of fat surrounding the fibrous capsule of the kidney, continuous at the hilus with the fat in the renal sinus. **renal c., fibrous,** the connective tissue investment of the kidney, continuous through the hilus to line the renal sinus. **Tenon's c.,** the connective tissue enveloping the posterior eyeball.

capsulectomy (kap″sūl-ek′tah-me) excision of a capsule, especially a joint capsule or lens capsule.

capsulitis (kap″sūl-īt′is) inflammation of a capsule, as that of the lens. **adhesive c.,** adhesive inflammation between the joint capsule and the peripheral articular cartilage of the shoulder, with obliteration of the subdeltoid bursa, characterized by increasing pain, stiffness, and limitation of motion.

capsuloma (kap″su-lo′mah) a capsular or subcapsular tumor of the kidney.

capsuloplasty (kap′sul-o-plas″te) plastic repair of a joint capsule.

capsulotomy (kap″su-lot′ah-me) incision of a capsule, as that of the lens or of a joint.

caput (kap′ut), pl. *cap′ita* [L.] the head; a general term applied to the expanded or chief extremity of an organ or part. **c. co′li,** the cecum. **c. gallina′ginis,** the verumontanum. **c. medu′sae,** dilated cutaneous veins around the umbilicus, seen mainly in the newborn and in patients suffering from cirrhosis of the liver. **c. succeda′neum,** edema occurring in and under the fetal scalp during labor.

C.A.R. Canadian Association of Radiologists.

caramiphen (kah-ram′ĭ-fen) an anticholinergic, $C_{18}H_{28}ClNO_2$, used as the hydrochloride salt in parkinsonism.

carbamate (kar′bah-māt) any ester of carbamic acid.

carbamazepine (kar″bah-maz′ĭ-pēn) an anticonvulsant and analgesic, $C_{15}H_{12}N_2O$, used in the treatment of pain associated with trigeminal neuralgia and in epilepsy manifested by certain types of seizures.

carbamic acid (kar-bam′ik) NH_2COOH, the parent acid of urethan.

carbamide (kar-bam′īd) urea in anhydrous, lyophilized, sterile powder form; injected intravenously in dextrose or invert sugar solution to induce diuresis.

carbaminohemoglobin (kar-bam″ĭ-no-he″mo-glo′bin) a combination of carbon dioxide and hemoglobin, CO_2HHb, being one of the forms in which carbon dioxide exists in the blood.

carbamoyl (kar-bam′ah-wil) the radical NH_2—CO—; see *carbamoyltransferase.*

carbamoyltransferase (-trans′fer-ās) an enzyme that catalyzes the transfer of carbamoyl, as from carbamoylphosphate to *L*-ornithine to form orthophosphate and citrulline in the synthesis of urea.

carbaspirin calcium (karb-as′pĭ-rin) an analgesic, $C_{19}H_{18}CaN_2O_9$, which also has antipyretic properties.

carbarsone (kar-bar′sōn) an arsenical compound, $C_7H_9AsN_2O_4$, used as an antiamebic.

carbenicillin (kar″ben-ĭ-sil′in) a semisynthetic antibiotic of the penicillin group, prepared as both the disodium and the potassium salt and used in urinary tract infections.

carbidopa (kar″bĭ-do′pah) an inhibitor of decarboxylation of levodopa in extracerebral tissues, $C_{10}H_{14}N_2O_4$.

carbinol (kar′bĭ-nol) methanol.

carbinoxamine (kar″bin-ok′sah-mēn) a potent antihistaminic, $C_{16}H_{19}ClN_2O$; used in the treatment of allergic disorders.

carbo (kar′bo) [L.] charcoal.

carbohydrase (kar″bo-hi′drās) any of a group of enzymes that catalyze the hydrolysis of higher carbohydrates to lower forms.

carbohydrate (-hi′drāt) a compound of carbon, hydrogen, and oxygen, the latter two usually in the proportion of water $(CH_2O)_n$; the most important carbohydrates are the starches, sugars, celluloses, and gums. They are classified into mono-, di-, tri-, poly-, and heterosaccharides.

carbol-fuchsin (kar″bol-fōōk′sin) a stain for microorganisms, containing basic fuchsin and dilute phenol; see also under *solution*.

carbolic acid (kar-bol′ik) phenol.

carbolism (kar′bah-lizm) phenol poisoning; see *phenol* (1).

carbomer (kar′bah-mer) a polymer of acrylic acid, cross-linked with a polyfunctional agent; a suspending agent.

carbon (kar′bin) chemical element (*see table*), at. no. 6, symbol C. **c. dioxide,** an odorless, colorless gas, CO_2, resulting from oxidation of carbon, and formed in the tissues and eliminated by the lungs; used with oxygen to stimulate respiration, and in solid form (*carbon dioxide snow*) as an escharotic. **c. monoxide,** an odorless gas, CO, formed by burning carbon or organic fuels with a scanty supply of oxygen; inhalation causes central nervous system damage and asphyxiation by combining irreversibly with blood hemoglobin. **c. tetrachloride,** a clear, colorless, mobile liquid; the inhalation of its vapors can depress central nervous system activity and cause degeneration of the liver and kidneys.

carbonate (-āt) a salt of carbonic acid.

carbonic acid (kar-bon′ik) an aqueous solution of carbon dioxide, H_2CO_3.

carbonic anhydrase (kar-bon′ik an′hi-drās) an enzyme that catalyzes the decomposition of carbonic acid into carbon dioxide and water, facilitating the transfer of carbon dioxide from tissues to blood and from blood to alveolar air.

carbonyl (kar′bah-nil) the bivalent organic radical, C:O, characteristic of aldehydes, ketones, carboxylic acid, and esters.

γ**-carboxyglutamic acid** (kar-bok″se-gloo-tam′ik) an amino acid occurring in biologically active prothrombin, and formed in the liver in the presence of vitamin K by carboxylation of glutamic acid residues in prothrombin precursor molecules.

carboxyhemoglobin (kar-bok″se-he″mo-glo′bin) hemoglobin combined with carbon monoxide, which occupies the sites on the hemoglobin molecule that normally bind with oxygen and which is not readily displaced from the mole-

cule; exposure to carbon monoxide thus results in cellular anoxia.

carboxyl (kar-bok′sil) the monovalent radical —COOH, occurring in those organic acids termed carboxylic acids.

carboxylase (kar-bok′sĭ-lās) an enzyme that catalyzes the removal of carbon dioxide from the carboxyl group of alpha amino keto acids.

carboxylation (kar-bok″sil-a′shin) the addition of a carboxyl group, as to pyruvate to form oxaloacetate.

carboxylesterase (-es″ter-ās) an enzyme that catalyzes the hydrolysis of the esters of carboxylic acids.

carboxylic acid (kar-bok-sil′ik) an organic compound containing the carboxy group (RCOOH), which is weakly ionized in solution forming a carboxylate ion (RCOO⁻).

carboxyltransferase (-trans′fer-ās) an enzyme that catalyzes carboxylation.

carboxy-lyase (kar-bok′se-li′ās) any of a group of lyases that catalyze the removal of a carboxyl group; it includes the carboxylases and decarboxylases.

carboxymyoglobin (-mi″ah-glo′bin) a compound formed from myoglobin on exposure to carbon monoxide.

carboxypeptidase (-pep′tĭ-dās) an exopeptidase that acts only on the peptide linkage of a terminal amino acid containing a free carboxyl group.

carbromal (kar-bro′mal) a sedative and hypnotic, $C_7H_{13}BrN_2O_2$.

carbuncle (kar′bunk'l) a necrotizing infection of skin and subcutaneous tissues composed of a cluster of furuncles, usually due to *Staphylococcus aureus*, with multiple drainage sinuses. **carbunc′ular,** adj. **malignant c.,** anthrax.

carcinectomy (kar″sĭ-nek′tah-me) excision of carcinoma.

carcinoembryonic (kar″sin-o-em″bre-on′ik) relating to carcinoma and to the embryonic state; see under *antigen*.

carcinogen (kar-sin′ah-jen) any substance which causes cancer. **carcinogen′ic,** adj.

carcinogenicity (-jĕ-nis′it-e) the ability or tendency to produce cancer.

carcinoid (kar′sĭ-noid) argentaffinoma.

carcinolysis (kar″sĭ-nol′ĭ-sis) destruction of cancer cells. **carcinolyt′ic,** adj.

carcinoma (kar″sĭ-no′mah) a malignant new growth made up of epithelial cells tending to infiltrate surrounding tissues and to give rise to metastases. **adenocystic c., adenoid cystic c.,** cylindroma; carcinoma marked by cylinders or bands of hyaline or mucinous stroma separated or surrounded by nests or cords of small epithelial cells, occurring in the mammary and salivary glands, and mucous glands of the respiratory tract. **alveolar c.,** see under *adenocarcinoma*. **basal cell c.,** an epithelial tumor of the skin that seldom metastasizes but has potentialities for local invasion and destruction. **bronchogenic c.,** carcinoma of the lung, so called because it arises from the epithelium of the bronchial tree. **cholangiocellular c.,** primary carcinoma of the liver originating in bile duct cells. **chorionic c.,** choriocarcinoma. **colloid c.,** mucinous c. **embryonal c.,** a highly malignant, primitive form of carcinoma, probably of germinal cell or teratomatous derivation, usually arising in a gonad. **epidermoid c.,** that in which the cells tend to differentiate in the same way as those of the epidermis; i.e., they tend to form prickle cells and undergo cornification. **hair matrix c.,** basal cell c. **hepatocellular c.,** primary carcinoma of the liver cells. **Hürthle cell c.,** see under *tumor.* **c. in si′tu,** a neoplastic entity wherein the tumor cells have not invaded the basement membrane but are still confined to the epithelium of origin; popularly applied to such cells in the uterine cervix. **large-cell c.,** a bronchogenic tumor of undifferentiated (anaplastic) cells of large size. **medullary c.,** that composed mainly of epithelial elements with little or no stroma. **mucinous c.,** adenocarcinoma producing significant amounts of mucin. **nasopharyngeal c.,** a malignant tumor arising in the epithelial lining of the space behind the nose (nasopharynx) and occurring at high frequency in southern China. The Epstein-Barr virus has been implicated as a causative agent. **oat cell c.,** small-cell c. **papillary c.,** carcinoma in which there are papillary excrescences. **renal cell c.,** carcinoma of the renal parenchyma, composed of tubular cells in varying arrangements. **scirrhous c.,** carcinoma with a hard structure owing to the formation of dense connective tissue in the stroma. **c. sim′plex,** an undifferentiated carcinoma. **small-cell c.,** a radiosensitive tumor composed of small, oval, undifferentiated cells that are intensely hematoxyphilic and typically bronchogenic. **spindle cell c.,** squamous cell carcinoma marked by fusiform development of rapidly proliferating cells. **squamous cell c.,** that arising from squamous epithelium and having cuboid cells.

carcinomatosis (kar″sĭ-no″mah-to′sis) the condition of widespread dissemination of cancer throughout the body.

carcinosarcoma (-sar-ko′mah) a malignant tumor composed of carcinomatous and sarcomatous tissues. **embryonal c.,** Wilms' tumor.

carcinosis (kar″sĭ-no′sis) carcinomatosis. **miliary c.,** that marked by development of numerous nodules resembling miliary tuberculosis.

cardi(o)- word element [Gr.], *heart.*

cardia (kar′de-ah) 1. the cardiac opening. 2. the cardiac part of the stomach, surrounding the esophagogastric junction and distinguished by the presence of cardiac glands.

cardiac (kar′de-ak) 1. pertaining to the heart. 2. pertaining to the cardia.

cardialgia (kar″de-al′je-ah) cardiodynia.

cardiectasis (kar″de-ek′tah-sis) dilatation of the heart.

cardioaccelerator (kar″de-o-ak-sel′er-āt-er) quickening the heart action; an agent that so acts.

cardioangiology (-an″je-ol′ah-je) the medical specialty dealing with the heart and blood vessels.

Cardiobacterium (kar″de-o-bak-tē′re-um) a genus of gram-negative, facultatively anaerobic, fermentative, rod-shaped bacteria, part of the normal flora of the nose and throat, and also isolated from the blood. **C. ho′minis,** a species that is an etiologic agent of endocarditis.

cardiocele (kar′de-o-sēl″) hernial protrusion of the heart through a fissure of the diaphragm or through a wound.

cardiocentesis (kar″de-o-sen-te′sis) surgical puncture of the heart.

cardiochalasia (-kah-la′ze-ah) relaxation or incompetence of the sphincter action of the cardiac opening of the stomach.

cardiocirrhosis (-sir-ro′sis) cirrhosis of the liver complicating heart disease, with recurrent intractable congestive heart failure.

cardiodiosis (-di-o′sis) dilatation of the cardiac opening of the stomach.

cardiodynamics (-di-nam′iks) study of the forces involved in the heart's action.

cardiodynia (-din′e-ah) pain in the heart.

cardioesophageal (-ĕ-sof″ah-je′al) pertaining to the cardia of the stomach and the esophagus, as the cardioesophageal junction or sphincter.

cardiogram (kar′de-o-gram″) a tracing of a cardiac event produced by cardiography. **apex c.,** the record produced by apex cardiography. **precordial c.,** kinetocardiogram.

cardiography (kar″de-ah′grah-fe) the graphic recording of a physical or functional aspect of the heart, e.g., electrocardiography, kinetocardiography, phonocardiography, vibrocardiography. **apex c.,** the graphic recording of low-frequency pulsations at the anterior chest wall over the apex of the heart. **ultrasonic c.,** echocardiography. **vector c.,** vectorcardiography.

cardioinhibitor (-in-hib′it-er) an agent that restrains the heart's action.

cardiokinetic (-ki-net′ik) 1. exciting or stimulating the heart. 2. an agent that so acts.

cardiokymography (-ki-mah′grah-fe) the recording of the motion of the heart by means of the electrokymograph. **cardiokymograph′ic,** adj.

cardiology (-ol′ah-je) the study of the heart and its functions.

cardiolysis (-ol′ĭ-sis) the operation of freeing the heart from its adhesions to the sternal periosteum in adhesive mediastinopericarditis.

cardiomalacia (kar″de-o-mah-la′she-ah) morbid softening of the muscular substance of the heart.

cardiomegaly (-meg′ah-le) hypertrophy of the heart.

cardiomelanosis (-mel″ah-no′sis) melanosis of the heart.

cardiomotility (-mo-til′it-e) the movements of the heart; motility of the heart.

cardiomyoliposis (-mi″o-lĭ-po′sis) fatty degeneration of the heart muscle.

cardiomyopathy (-mi-op′ah-the) a general diagnostic term designating primary myocardial disease. **alcoholic c.,** a congestive cardiomyopathy resulting in cardiac enlargement and low cardiac output occurring in chronic alcoholics;

the heart disease in beriberi (thiamine deficiency) is also associated with alcoholism. **congestive c.,** a syndrome characterized by cardiac enlargement, especially of the left ventricle, myocardial dysfunction, and congestive heart failure. **infiltrative c.,** myocardial disease resulting from deposition in the heart tissue of abnormal substances, as may occur in amyloidosis, hemochromatosis, etc.

cardiomyopexy (-mi′o-pek″se) surgical removal of the epicardium and application of a pedicled flap of adjacent muscle to the denuded myocardium and pericardium, as a means of supplying collateral circulation to the heart.

cardioneurosis (-nōōr-o′sis) neurocirculatory asthenia.

cardio-omentopexy (-o-men′tah-pek″se) suture of a portion of the omentum to the heart.

cardiopaludism (-pal′u-dizm) heart disease due to malaria.

cardiopathy (kar″de-op′ah-the) any disorder or disease of the heart.

cardiopericardiopexy (kar″de-o-pĕ″re-kar′de-o-pek″se) surgical establishment of adhesive pericarditis, for relief of coronary disease.

cardioplasty (kar′de-o-plas″te) esophagogastroplasty.

cardioplegia (kar″de-o-ple′je-ah) arrest of myocardial contractions, as by use of chemical compounds or cold in cardiac surgery. **cardiople′gic,** adj.

cardiopneumatic (-noo-mat′ik) of or pertaining to the heart and respiration.

cardioptosis (kar″de-op′tah-sis) downward displacement of the heart.

cardiopuncture (-punk′cher) cardiocentesis.

cardiorrhaphy (kar″de-or′ah-fe) suture of the heart muscle.

cardiorrhexis (kar″de-o-rek′sis) rupture of the heart.

cardiosclerosis (-skler-o′sis) fibrous induration of the heart.

cardioselective (-sah-lek′tiv) having greater activity on heart tissue than on other tissue.

cardiospasm (kar′de-o-spazm″) achalasia of the esophagus.

cardiosphygmograph (kar″de-o-sfig′mah-graf) a combination of the cardiograph and sphygmograph for recording the movements of the heart and an arterial pulse.

cardiosplenopexy (-splen′ah-pek″se) suture of the splenic parenchyma to the denuded surface of the heart for revascularization of the myocardium.

cardiotachometer (-tah-kom′it-er) an instrument for continuously portraying or recording the heart rate.

cardiotherapy (-thĕ′rah-pe) the treatment of diseases of the heart.

cardiotocography (-tah-kog′rah-fe) the monitoring of the fetal heart rate and uterine contractions, as during delivery.

cardiotomy (kar″de-ot′ah-me) 1. surgical incision of the heart. 2. surgical incision into the cardia.

cardiotonic (kar″de-o-ton′ik) having a tonic effect on the heart; an agent that so acts.

cardiotopometry (-tah-pom′ĭ-tre) measurement of the area of cardiac dullness.

cardiotoxic (-tok′sik) having a poisonous or deleterious effect upon the heart.

cardiovalvulotome (-val′vu-lah-tōm″) an instrument for incising a heart valve.

cardioversion (kar″de-o-ver′zhin) the restoration of normal rhythm of the heart by electrical shock.

cardioverter (-vert′er) an energy-storage capacitor-discharge type of condenser which is discharged with an inductance; it delivers a direct-current shock which restores normal rhythm of the heart.

carditis (kar-dīt′is) inflammation of the heart; myocarditis.

cardivalvulitis (kar″dĭ-val″vu-līt′is) inflammation of the heart valves.

caries (ka′re-ēz, kār′ez) decay, as of bone or teeth. **ca′rious,** adj. **dental c.,** a destructive process causing decalcification of the tooth enamel and leading to continued destruction of enamel and dentin, and cavitation of the tooth.

carina (kah-ri′nah), pl. **cari′nae** [L.] a ridgelike structure. **c. tra′cheae,** a downward and backward projection of the lowest tracheal cartilage, forming a ridge between the openings of the right and left principal bronchi. **c. urethra′lis vagi′nae,** the column of rugae in the lower anterior wall of the vagina, immediately below the urethra.

cariogenesis (kar″e-o-jen′i-sis) development of caries.

carisoprodol (kar″i-so′pro-dol) an analgesic and skeletal muscle relaxant, $C_{12}H_{24}N_2O_4$.

carminative (kar-min′it-iv) 1. relieving flatulence. 2. an agent that relieves flatulence.

carmine (kar′min) a red coloring matter used as a histologic stain. **indigo c.,** indigotinsulfonate sodium.

carminic acid (kar-min′ik) the active principle of carmine and cochineal, $C_{22}H_{20}O_{13}$.

carminophil (kar″min′ah-fil) 1. easily stainable with carmine. 2. a cell or element readily taking a stain from carmine.

carmustine (kar-mus′tēn) BCNU; a nitrosourea, $C_5H_9Cl_2N_3O_2$, used as an antineoplastic agent.

carnitine (kar′nĭ-tēn) a betaine derivative involved in the transport of fatty acids into mitochondria, where they are metabolized.

carnivore (kar′nĭ-vor) any animal that eats primarily flesh, particularly mammals of the order Carnivora, which includes cats, dogs, bears, etc. **carniv′orous,** adj.

carnosinase (kar′no-sĭ-nās) an enzyme that hydrolyzes carnosine (amino-acyl-L-histidine) and other dipeptides containing L-histidine into their constituent amino acids.

carnosine (kar′no-sin) a dipeptide, $C_9H_{14}N_4O_2$, composed of beta-alanine and histidine, found in skeletal muscle of vertebrates.

carnosinemia (kar″no-sĭ-ne′me-ah) excessive amounts of carnosine in the blood; it has been associated with a progressive neurologic disease characterized by severe mental defect and myoclonic seizures, and is probably due to a genetic deficiency of carnosinase in the serum.

carnosinuria (-sin-ūr′e-ah) an aminoaciduria characterized by excess of carnosine in the urine; it occurs in carnosinemia or may be dietary in origin, especially in young children.

caro (ka′ro), pl. *car′nes* [L.] flesh, or muscular tissue.

carotenase (kar-ot′in-ās) an enzyme that converts carotene into vitamin A.

carotene (kar′ah-tēn) a yellow or red pigment from carrots, sweet potatoes, milk and body fat, egg yolk, etc.; it is a chromolipoid hydrocarbon existing in several forms (α-, β-, and γ-carotene), which can be converted into vitamin A in the body.

carotenemia (kar″ah-tin-e′me-ah) presence of excessive carotene in the blood; sometimes occurring in sufficient amounts to cause yellowing of the skin.

carotenodermia (kah-rot″in-o-der′me-ah) yellowness of the skin due to carotenemia.

carotenoid (kah-rot′in-oid) 1. any member of a group of red, orange, or yellow pigmented polyisoprenoid lipids found in carrots, sweet potatoes, green leaves, and some animal tissues; examples are the carotenes, lycopene, and xanthophyll. 2. marked by yellow color. 3. lipochrome.

carotenosis (kar″ah-tin-o′sis) deposition of carotene in tissues, especially the skin.

caroticotympanic (kah-rot″ĭ-ko-tim-pan′ik) pertaining to carotid canal and tympanum.

carotid (kah-rot′id) pertaining to the carotid artery, the principal artery of the neck; see *Table of Arteries.*

carotodynia (kah-rot″ah-din′e-ah) tenderness along the course of the carotid artery.

carp (karp) a fruiting body of a fungus.

carpal (kar′p'l) pertaining to the carpus.

carpectomy (kar-pek′tah-me) excision of a carpal bone.

carphenazine (kar-fen′ah-zēn) a major tranquilizer, $C_{24}H_{31}N_3O_2$, used as the maleate salt.

carphology (kar-fol′ah-je) involuntary picking at the bedclothes, seen in grave fevers and in conditions of great exhaustion.

carpitis (kar-pīt′is) inflammation of the synovial membranes of the bones of the carpal joint in domestic animals, producing swelling, pain, and lameness.

carpoptosis (-to′sis) wristdrop.

carpus (kar′pus) the joint between the arm and hand, made up of eight bones; the wrist. Also, the corresponding forelimb joint in quadrupeds.

carrier (kar′e-er) 1. one who harbors disease organisms in his body without manifest symptoms, thus acting as a carrier or distributor of infection; also, a heterozygote, i.e., one who carries a recessive gene, autosomal or sex-linked, and its normal allele. 2. a substance in a cell which can accept electrons and so be reduced and be reoxidized.

carrier-free (kar′e-er-fre″) a term denoting a radioisotope of an element in pure form, i.e., undiluted with a stable isotope carrier.

cart (kart) a vehicle for conveying patients or equipment and supplies in a hospital. **crash c.**, resuscitation c. **dressing c.**, one containing all supplies necessary for changing dressings of surgical or injured patients. **resuscitation c.**, one containing all equipment for initiating emergency resuscitation.

cartilage (kart′ĭ-lij) a specialized, fibrous connective tissue present in adults, and forming the temporary skeleton in the embryo, providing a model in which the bones develop, and constituting a part of the organism's growth mechanism; the three most important types are hyaline cartilage, elastic cartilage, and fibrocartilage. Also, a general term for a mass of such tissue in a particular site in the body. **alar c's,** the cartilages of the wings of the nose. **aortic c.**, the second costal cartilage on the right side. **arthrodial c., articular c.,** that lining the articular surface of synovial joints. **arytenoid c's,** the two pyramid-shaped cartilages of the larynx. **connecting c.**, that connecting the surfaces of an immovable joint. **corniculate c.**, a nodule of cartilage at the apex of each arytenoid cartilage. **costal c.**, a bar of hyaline cartilage that attaches a rib to the sternum in the case of true ribs, or to the immediately above rib in the case of the upper false ribs. **cricoid c.**, a ringlike cartilage forming the lower and back part of the larynx. **cuneiform c.**, either of the paired cartilages, one on either side in the aryepiglottic fold. **dentinal c.**, the substance remaining after the lime salts of dentin have been dissolved in an acid. **diarthrodial c.**, articular c. **elastic c.**, cartilage whose matrix contains yellow elastic fibers. **ensiform c.**, xiphoid process. **epactal c's,** one or more small cartilages in the lateral wall of the nose. **floating c.**, a detached portion of semilunar cartilage in the knee joint. **hyaline c.**, a flexible semitransparent substance with an opalescent tint, composed of a basophilic, fibril-containing substance with cavities in which the chondrocytes occur. **interosseous c.**, connecting c. **Jacobson's c.**, vomeronasal c. **mandibular c.**, **Meckel's c.**, the ventral cartilage of the first branchial arch. **parachordal c.**, one of the two embryonic cartilages beside the occipital part of the notochord. **permanent c.**, cartilage which does not normally become ossified. **precursory c.**, temporary c. **Reichert's c.**, the dorsal cartilage of the second branchial arch. **Santorini's c.**, corniculate c. **semilunar c.**, one of the two interarticular cartilages of the knee joint. **sesamoid c's,** small cartilages found in the thyrohyoid ligament (*sesamoid c. of larynx*), on either side of the nose (*sesamoid c. of nose*), and occasionally in the vocal ligaments (*sesamoid c. of vocal ligament*). **slipping rib c.**, a loosened or deformed cartilage whose slipping over an adjacent rib cartilage may produce discomfort or pain. **tarsal c.**, see under *plate.* **temporary c.**, cartilage that is being replaced by bone or that is destined to be replaced by bone. **thyroid c.**, the shield-shaped cartilage of the larynx. **triticeous c.**, a small cartilage in the thyrohyoid ligament. **tympanomandibular c.,** Meckel's c. **vomeronasal c.,** either of the two strips of cartilage of the nasal septum supporting the vomeronasal organ. **Weitbrecht's c.,** a pad of fibrocartilage sometimes present within the articular cavity of the acromioclavicular joint. **Wrisberg's c.,** cuneiform c. **xiphoid c.,** see under *process.* **Y c.,** Y-shaped cartilage within the acetabulum, joining the ilium, ischium, and pubes. **yellow c.,** elastic c.

cartilago (kart″ĭ-lah′go), pl. *cartila′gines* [L.] cartilage.

caruncle (kar′unk'l) a small fleshy eminence, often abnormal. **hymenal c's,** small elevations of the mucous membrane around the vaginal opening, being relics of the torn hymen. **lacrimal c.,** the red eminence at the medial angle of the eye. **myrtiform c's,** hymenal c's. **sublingual c.,** an eminence on either side of the frenulum of the tongue, on which the major sublingual duct and the submandibular duct open. **urethral c.,** a polypoid, deep red growth on the mucous membrane of the urinary meatus in women.

caruncula (kah-runk′u-lah), pl. *carun′culae* [L.] caruncle.

carver (kar′ver) a tool for producing anatomic form in artificial teeth and dental restorations.

caryo- for words beginning thus, see those beginning *karyo-*.

casanthranol (kah-san′thrah-nōl) a purified mixture of the anthranol glycosides derived from *Cascara sagrada;* a cathartic.

cascade (kas-kād′) a series (as in a physiological process) which, once initiated, continues to the end, each step being triggered by the preceding one, sometimes with cumulative effect.

cascara (kas-kar′ah) bark. **c. sagra′da,** dried bark of the shrub *Rhamnus purshiana,* used as a cathartic.

case (kās) an instance of a disease. **index c.,** the case of the original patient (propositus or proband) that stimulates investigation of other members of the family to discover a possible genetic factor. In epidemiology, the first case of a contagious disease. **trial c.,** a box containing lenses, arranged in pairs, a trial spectacle frame, and other devices used in testing vision.

caseation (ka″se-a′shin) 1. the precipitation of casein. 2. necrosis in which tissue is changed into a dry mass resembling cheese.

case history (kās his′ter-e) the data concerning an individual, his family, and environment, including his medical history that may be useful in analyzing and diagnosing his case or for instructional purposes.

casein (ka′se-in, ka′sēn) a phosphoprotein, the principal protein of milk, the basis of curd and of cheese. NOTE: In British nomenclature casein is called *caseinogen,* and paracasein is called *casein.*

caseinogen (ka″se-in′ah-jen) the British term for casein.

caseworm (kās′werm) echinococcus.

cassette (kās-set′) [Fr.] a light-proof housing for x-ray film, containing front and back intensify-

ing screens, between which the film is placed; a magazine for film or magnetic tape.

cast (kast) 1. a positive copy of an object, e.g., a mold of a hollow organ (a renal tubule, bronchiole, etc.), formed of effused plastic matter and extruded from the body, as a urinary cast; named according to constituents, as epithelial, fatty, waxy, etc. 2. a positive copy of the tissues of the jaws, made in an impression, and over which denture bases or other restorations may be fabricated. 3. to form an object in a mold. 4. a stiff dressing or casing, usually made of plaster of Paris, used to immobilize body parts. 5. strabismus. **dental c.,** see *cast* (2). **hanging c.,** one applied to the arm in fracture of the shaft of the humerus, suspended by a sling looped around the neck. **quarter c.,** a cut in the quarter of a horse's hoof. **urinary c.,** one formed from gelled protein in the renal tubules, which becomes molded to the tubular lumen.

castrate (kas′trāt) 1. to deprive of the gonads, rendering the individual incapable of reproduction. 2. a castrated individual.

castration (kas-tra′shin) excision of the gonads, or their destruction as by radiation or parasites. **female c.,** bilateral oophorectomy, or spaying. **male c.,** bilateral orchiectomy. **parasitic c.,** defective sexual development due to parasitic infestation in early life.

casualty (kazh′oo-il-te, kazh′il-te) 1. an accident; an accidental wound; death or disablement from an accident; also the person so injured. 2. in the armed forces, one missing from his unit as a result of death, injury, illness, capture, because his whereabouts are unknown, or other reasons.

casuistics (kazh-oo-is′tiks) the recording and study of cases of disease.

CAT computerized axial tomography.

cat(a)- word element [Gr.], *down; lower; under; against; along with; very.*

catabasis (kah-tab′ah-sis) the stage of decline of a disease. **catabat′ic,** adj.

catabiosis (kat″ah-bi-o′sis) the normal senescence of cells. **catabiot′ic,** adj.

catabolism (kah-tab′ah-lizm) any destructive process by which complex substances are converted by living cells into more simple compounds, with release of energy. **catabol′ic,** adj.

catabolize (-līz) to subject to catabolism; to undergo catabolism.

catacrotism (kah-tak′rah-tizm) a pulse anomaly in which a small additional wave or notch appears in the descending limb of the pulse tracing. **catacrot′ic,** adj.

catadicrotism (kat″ah-di′krah-tizm) a pulse anomaly in which two small additional waves or notches appear in the descending limb of the pulse tracing. **catadicrot′ic,** adj.

catagen (kat′ah-jen) the brief portion in the hair growth cycle in which growth (anagen) stops and resting (telogen) starts.

catagenesis (kat″ah-jen′ĭ-sis) involution or retrogression. **catagenet′ic,** adj.

catalase (kat′ah-lās) a crystalline enzyme which catalyzes the decomposition of hydrogen perox-

catalepsy

ide; found in almost all cells except certain anaerobic bacteria. **catalat′ic,** adj.

catalepsy (-lep″se) a condition of diminished responsiveness usually characterized by trancelike states and by a waxy rigidity of the muscles (flexibilitas cerea) so that the patient tends to remain in any position in which he is placed; it occurs in organic and psychological disorders and under hypnosis. **catalep′tic,** adj.

catalysis (kah-tal′ĭ-sis) increase in the velocity of a chemical reaction or process produced by the presence of a substance that is not consumed in the net chemical reaction or process; *negative catalysis* denotes the slowing down or inhibition of a reaction or process by the presence of such a substance. **catalyt′ic,** adj.

catamnesis (kat″am-ne′sis) the follow-up history of a patient after he is discharged from treatment or a hospital.

cataphasia (kat″ah-fa′ze-ah) speech disorder with constant repetition of a word or phrase.

cataphora (kah-taf′or-ah) lethargy with intervals of imperfect waking.

cataphoria (kat″ah-for′e-ah) a permanent downward turning of the visual axis of both eyes after visual functional stimuli have been removed. **cataphor′ic,** adj.

cataphylaxis (-fĭ-lak′sis) movement of leukocytes and antibodies to the site of an infection. **cataphylac′tic,** adj.

cataplasia (-pla′ze-ah) atrophy in which tissues revert to earlier, more embryonic conditions.

cataplexy (kat′ah-plek″se) a condition marked by abrupt attacks of muscular weakness and hypotonia triggered by such emotional stimuli as mirth, anger, fear, etc., often associated with narcolepsy. **cataplec′tic,** adj.

Catapres (kat′ah-pres) trademark for a preparation of clonidine hydrochloride.

cataract (kat′ah-rakt) an opacity of the crystalline lens of the eye or its capsule. **catarac′tous,** adj. **after-c.,** a recurrent capsular cataract. **atopic c.,** cataract occurring, most often in the second to third decade, in those with longstanding atopic dermatitis. **black c.,** see *senile nuclear sclerotic c.* **blue c., blue dot c.,** a condition in which small blue punctate opacities are scattered throughout the nucleus and cortex of the lens. **brown c., brunescent c.,** see *senile nuclear sclerotic c.* **capsular c.,** one consisting of an opacity in the capsule of the lens. **complicated c.,** secondary c. **congenital c.,** 1. a general term for common, usually bilateral opacities present at birth; they may be mild or severe and may or may not impair vision depending upon their size, density, and location. 2. developmental c. **coronary c.,** one in which white punctate or flakelike opacities form a ring or crown around the lens, the center of the lens and the extreme periphery remaining clear. **cortical c.,** an opacity in the cortex of the lens. **cuneiform c.,** the most common senile cataract, consisting of white, wedgelike opacities distributed like spokes around the periphery of the cortex. **cupuliform c.,** a senile cataract in the posterior cortex of the lens just under the capsule. **developmental c.,** small, common

opacities occurring in youth as a result of heredity, malnutrition, toxicity, or inflammation; they seldom affect vision. **electric c.,** anterior subcapsular opacities that may occur within days after a severe shock to the head. **glassblowers' c.,** heat c. **heat c.,** posterior subcapsular opacities caused by chronic exposure to infrared (heat) radiation. **hypermature c.,** one with a swollen, milky cortex, the result of autolysis of the lens fibers of a mature cataract. **lamellar c.,** an opacity affecting only certain layers between the cortex and nucleus of the lens. **lenticular c.,** opacity of the lens not affecting the capsule. **mature c.,** one producing swelling and opacity of the entire lens. **membranous c.,** a condition in which the lens substance has shrunk, leaving remnants of the capsule and fibrous tissue formation. **morgagnian c.,** a mature cataract in which the cortex has become completely liquefied and the nucleus moves freely within the lens. **nuclear c.,** one in which the opacity is in the central nucleus of the eye. **overripe c.,** hypermature c. **polar c.,** one seated at the center of the anterior (*anterior polar c.*) or posterior (*posterior polar c.*) pole of the lens. **pyramidal c.,** a conoid anterior cataract with its apex projecting forward into the aqueous humor. **radiation c.,** subcapsular opacities caused by ionizing radiation, e.g., x-rays, or by nonionizing radiation, e.g., infrared (heat) rays, ultraviolet rays, microwaves. **ripe c.,** mature c. **secondary c.,** one resulting from disease, e.g., iridocyclitis; degeneration, e.g., chronic glaucoma, retinal detachment; or from surgery, e.g., glaucoma filtering, retinal reattachment. **senile c.,** the cataract of old persons. **senile nuclear sclerotic c.,** a slowly increasing hardening of the nucleus, beginning between ages 50 and 60, the opacity, usually bilateral, appearing brown or black, and the lens becoming inelastic and unable to accommodate. **snowflake c.,** one marked by numerous grayish or bluish white flaky opacities, often seen in young diabetics. **total c.,** an opacity of all the fibers of a lens. **toxic c.,** that due to exposure to a toxic drug, e.g., naphthalene. **traumatic c.,** opacification of the lens due to injury to the eye. **zonular c.,** lamellar c.

cataracta (kat″ah-rak′tah) cataract. **c. brune′scens,** brown cataract. **c. ceru′lea,** blue dot cataract.

catarrh (kah-tahr′) inflammation of a mucous membrane (particularly of the head and throat), with free discharge. **catar′rhal,** adj.

catatonia (kat″ah-to′ne-ah) catatonic schizophrenia. **cataton′ic,** adj.

catatricrotism (-tri′krot-izm) a pulse anomaly in which three small additional waves or notches appear in the descending limb of the pulse tracing. **catatricrot′ic,** adj.

catechol (kat′ah-kol) a compound, *o*-dihydroxybenzene, $C_6H_4(OH)_2$, used as a reagent and comprising the aromatic portion in the synthesis of catecholamines.

catecholamine (kat″ah-kol-ah-mēn″) any of a group of sympathomimetic amines (including dopamine, epinephrine, and norepinephrine), the aromatic portion of whose molecule is catechol.

catecholaminergic (kath″ah-kol-am″in-er′jik) activated by or secreting catecholamines.

catelectrotonus (kat″ah-lek-trot′ah-nus) increase of nerve or muscle irritability near the cathode during passage of an electric current.

Catenabacterium (kah-te″nah-bak-tēr′e-um) formerly, a genus of anaerobic, gram-positive schizomycetes (tribe Lactobacilleae) found in the intestinal tract and occasionally associated with purulent infections.

catgut (kat′gut) an absorbable sterile strand obtained from collagen derived from healthy mammals, used as a surgical ligature.

catharsis (kah-thar′sis) 1. a cleansing or purgation. 2. in psychiatry, the expression and discharge of repressed emotions and ideas.

cathartic (kah-thart′ik) 1. causing bowel evacuation; an agent that so acts. 2. producing catharsis. **bulk c.,** one stimulating bowel evacuation by increasing fecal volume. **lubricant c.,** one that acts by softening the feces and reducing friction between them and the intestinal wall. **saline c.,** one that increases fluidity of intestinal contents by retention of water by osmotic forces and indirectly increases motor activity. **stimulant c.,** one that directly increases motor activity of the intestinal tract.

catheter (kath′it-er) a tubular, flexible instrument passed through body channels for withdrawal of fluids from (or introduction of fluids into) a body cavity. **angiographic c.,** one through which a contrast medium is injected for visualization of the vascular system of an organ. **cardiac c.,** a long, fine catheter designed for passage, usually through a peripheral blood vessel, into the chambers of the heart under roentgenologic control. **central venous c.,** a long, fine catheter introduced into a large vein for the purposes of administering parenteral fluids or for measurement of central venous pressure. **double-current c.,** a catheter having two channels; one for injection and one for removal of fluid. **faucial c.,** a eustachian catheter for passage through the fauces. **female c.,** a short catheter for passage through the female urethra. **Foley c.,** an indwelling catheter retained in the bladder by a balloon which may be inflated with air or liquid. **Gouley's c.,** a solid, curved steel catheter grooved on its inferior surface so that it can be passed over a guide through a urethral stricture. **indwelling c.,** one held in position in the urethra. **prostatic c.,** one with a short angular tip for passing an enlarged prostate **self-retaining c.,** one so constructed as to be retained at will and to effect bladder drainage. **Swan-Ganz c.,** a soft, flow-directed catheter with a balloon at the tip for measuring pulmonary arterial pressures. **toposcopic c.,** a miniature catheter that can pass through narrow tortuous vessels to convey chemotherapy directly to brain tumors. **two-way c.,** a double-channel catheter used in irrigation. **vertebrated c.,** one made in small sections fitted together so as to be flexible. **winged c.,** one with two projections on the end to retain it in the bladder.

catheterization (kath″it-er-i-za′shin) passage of a catheter into a body channel or cavity. **cardiac c.,** passage of a small catheter through a vein in an arm or leg or the neck and into the heart, permitting the securing of blood samples, determination of intracardiac pressure, and detection of cardiac anomalies.

cathexis (kah-thek′sis) the charge or attachment of mental or emotional energy upon an idea or object. **cathec′tic,** adj.

cathode (kath′ōd) 1. the negative electrode, from which electrons are emitted and to which positive ions are attracted. 2. the electrode through which current leaves a nerve or other substance. **cathod′ic,** adj.

cation (kat′i-on) a positively charged ion. **cation′ic,** adj.

cauda (kaw′dah), pl. *cau′dae* [L.] a tail or taillike appendage. **c. cerebel′li,** vermis cerebelli. **c. equi′na,** the collection of spinal roots descending from the lower spinal cord and occupying the vertebral canal below the cord.

caudad (kaw′dad) directed toward the tail or distal end; opposite to cephalad.

caudal (kaw′d'l) 1. pertaining to a cauda. 2. situated more toward the cauda, or tail, than some specified reference point; toward the inferior (in humans) or posterior (in animals) end of the body.

caudatum (kaw-dat′-um) the caudate nucleus.

caul (kawl) a piece of amnion sometimes enveloping a child's head at birth.

causalgia (kaw-zal′je-ah) a burning pain, often with trophic skin changes, due to peripheral nerve injury.

caustic (kaws′tik) 1. burning or corrosive; destructive to living tissues. 2. having a burning taste. 3. an escharotic or corrosive agent.

cauterant (kawt′er-int) 1. any caustic material or application. 2. caustic.

cautery (kawt′er-e) 1. the application of a caustic agent or other agent to destroy tissue. 2. an agent used for such purpose. **actual c.,** 1. a red-hot iron used as a cauterizing agent. 2. the application of an agent that actually burns tissue. **cold c.,** cauterization by carbon dioxide. **galvanic c.,** galvanocautery. **potential c.,** **virtual c.,** cauterization by an escharotic.

cava (ka′vah) 1. plural of *cavum.* 2. a vena cava. **ca′val,** adj.

caveola (ka″ve-o′lah), pl. *caveo′lae* [L.] one of the minute pits or incuppings of the cell membrane formed during pinocytosis.

caverna (ka-ver′nah), pl. *caver′nae* [L.] a cavity.

caverniloquy (kav″er-nil′o-kwe) low-pitched pectoriloquy indicative of a pulmonary cavity.

cavernitis (-nīt′is) inflammation of the corpora cavernosum or corpus spongiosum of the penis.

cavernoma (-no′mah) cavernous hemangioma.

cavernous (kav′er-nus) pertaining to a hollow, or containing hollow spaces.

cavitary (kav′ĭ-tĕ-re) characterized by the presence of a cavity or cavities.

cavitas (kav′ĭ-tas), pl. *cavita′tes* [L.] cavity.

cavitis (ka-vīt′is) inflammation of a vena cava.

cavity (kav′it-e) a hollow place or space, or a

potential space, within the body or one of its organs; in dentistry, the lesion produced by caries. **abdominal c.,** the cavity of the body between the diaphragm and pelvis, containing the abdominal organs. **absorption c's,** cavities in developing compact bone due to osteoclastic erosion, usually occurring in the areas laid down first. **amniotic c.,** the closed sac between the embryo and the amnion, containing the amniotic fluid. **cleavage c.,** blastocoele. **complex c.,** a carious lesion involving three or more surfaces of a tooth in its prepared state. **compound c.,** a carious lesion involving two surfaces of a tooth in its prepared state. **cotyloid c.,** acetabulum. **cranial c.,** the space enclosed by the bones of the cranium. **dental c.,** the carious defect (lesion) produced by destruction of enamel and dentin in a tooth. **glenoid c.,** a depression in the lateral angle of the scapula for articulation with the humerus. **marrow c., medullary c.,** the cavity in the diaphysis of a long bone containing the marrow. **nasal c.,** the proximal part of the respiratory tract, separated by the nasal septum and extending from the nares to the pharynx. **oral c.,** the cavity of the mouth, bounded by the jaw bones and associated structures (muscles and mucosa). **pelvic c.,** the space within the walls of the pelvis. **pericardial c.,** the potential space between the epicardium and the parietal layer of the serous pericardium. **peritoneal c.,** the potential space between the parietal and the visceral peritoneum. **pleural c.,** the potential space between the parietal and the visceral pleura. **pleuroperitoneal c.,** the temporarily continuous coelomic cavity in the embryo that is later partitioned by the developing diaphragm. **prepared c.,** a lesion from which all carious tissue has been removed, preparatory to filling of the tooth. **pulp c.,** the pulp-filled central chamber in the crown of a tooth. **Rosenmüller's c.,** a wide, slitlike lateral extension of the nasopharynx, cranial and dorsal to the pharyngeal orifice of the auditory tube. **serous c.,** a coelomic cavity, like that enclosed by the pericardium, peritoneum, or pleura, not communicating with the outside body, whose lining membrane secretes a serous fluid. **sigmoid c.,** either of two depressions in head of the ulna for articulation with the humerus and radius. **simple c.,** a carious lesion whose preparation involves only one tooth surface. **somatic c.,** the intraembryonic portion of the coelom. **tension c's,** cavities of the lung in which the air pressure is greater than that of the atmosphere. **thoracic c.,** the part of the ventral body cavity between the neck and the diaphragm. **tympanic c.,** middle ear. **uterine c.,** the flattened space within the uterus communicating proximally on either side with the uterine tubes and below with the vagina. **yolk c.,** the space between the embryonic disk and the yolk of the developing ovum of some animals.

cavum (ka′vum), pl. **ca′va** [L.] cavity.

cavus (ka′vus) [L.] hollow.

c.b.c. complete blood (cell) count.

cc. cubic centimeter.

CCNU lomustine.

C.D. curative dose.

C.D.₅₀ median curative dose.

Cd 1. chemical symbol, *cadmium.* 2. caudal or coccygeal.

cd candela.

CDC Centers for Disease Control.

Ce chemical symbol, *cerium.*

ceasmic (se-az′mik) characterized by persistence of embryonic fissures after birth.

cecectomy (se-sek′tah-me) excision of the cecum.

cecitis (se-sīt′is) inflammation of the cecum.

ceco- word element [L.], *cecum.*

cecocele (se′ko-sēl) a hernia containing part of the cecum.

cecocolostomy (-kol-os′tah-me) surgical anastomosis of the cecum and colon.

cecoileostomy (-il″e-os′tah-me) ileocecostomy.

cecoplication (se″ko-pli-ka′shin) plication of the cecal wall to correct ptosis or dilatation.

cecorrhaphy (se-kor′ah-fe) suture or repair of the cecum.

cecosigmoidostomy (se″ko-sig″moid-os′tah-me) formation, usually by surgery, of an opening between the cecum and sigmoid.

cecostomy (se-kos′tah-me) surgical creation of an artificial opening or fistula into the cecum.

cecum (se′kum) 1. the first part of the large intestine, forming a dilated pouch distal to the ileum and proximal to the colon, and giving off the vermiform appendix. 2. any blind pouch.

cefadroxil (sef″ah-droks′il) a semisynthetic cephalosporin antibiotic, $C_{16}H_{17}N_3O_5S$.

cefazolin (sah-faz′ah-lin) a semisynthetic cephalosporin antibiotic, $C_{14}H_{14}N_8O_4S_3$, effective against a wide range of gram-negative and gram-positive bacteria.

cefotaxime (sef″o-tak′sem) a semisynthetic broad-spectrum cephalosporin antibiotic active against many organisms that have become resistant to penicillin, cephalosporin, and aminoglycoside antibiotics.

cefoxitin (sah-foks′it-in) a semisynthetic cephalosporin antibiotic, especially effective against gram-negative organisms, with strong resistance to degradation by β-lactamase.

ceftazidime (sef′ta-zĭ-dēm) a cephalosporin derivative with high activity against *Pseudomonas* spp.

-cele word element [Gr.], *tumor; hernia; cavity.*

celi(o)- word element [Gr.], *abdomen; through the abdominal wall.*

celiectomy (sēl″e-ek′tah-me) 1. excision of the celiac branches of the vagus nerve. 2. excision of an abdominal organ.

celiocolpotomy (-kol-pot′ah-me) incision into the abdomen through the vagina.

celiogastrotomy (-gas-trot′ah-me) incision through the abdominal wall into the stomach.

celioma (sēl″e-o′mah) a tumor of the abdomen.

celiomyositis (sēl″e-o-mi″ah-sīt′is) inflammation of the abdominal muscles.

celiopathy (sēl″e-op′ah-the) any abdominal disease.

celioscopy (sēl″e-os′kah-pe) examination of an abdominal cavity through an endoscope.

celiotomy (sēl″e-ot′ah-me) incision into the abdominal cavity. **vaginal c.,** incision into the abdominal cavity through the vagina.

celitis (se-lit′is) any abdominal inflammation.

cell (sel) 1. any of the protoplasmic masses making up organized tissue, consisting of a nucleus surrounded by cytoplasm enclosed in a cell or plasma membrane. It is the fundamental, structural, and functional unit of living organisms. In some of the lower forms of life, such as bacteria, a morphological nucleus is absent, although nucleoproteins (and genes) are present. 2. a small, more or less closed space. **accessory c's,** macrophages involved in the processing and presentation of antigens making them more immunogenic. **acid c's,** parietal c's. **acinar c.** or **acinous c.,** any of the cells lining an acinus, especially the zymogen-secreting cells of the pancreatic acini. **adventitial c's,** macrophages that occur along the walls of blood vessels. **air c.,** one containing air, as in the lungs or auditory tube. **alpha c's,** 1. cells situated in the periphery of the islets of Langerhans, which secrete glucagon. 2. the acidophils of the adenohypophysis. **alveolar c.,** any cell of the walls of the pulmonary alveoli; often restricted to the cells of the alveolar epithelium (squamous alveolar cells and great alveolar cells) and alveolar phagocytes. **Alzheimer's c's,** 1. giant astrocytes with large prominent nuclei found in the brain in hepatolenticular degeneration and hepatic coma. 2. degenerated astrocytes. **amacrine c.,** see *amacrine* (2). **Anichkov's (Anitschkow's) c.,** see under *myocyte*. **APUD c's** (*a*mine *p*recursor *u*ptake and *d*ecarboxylation), a group of cells that manufacture polypeptides and biogenic amines serving as hormones or neurotransmitters. The polypeptide production is linked to the uptake of a precursor amino acid and its decarboxylation to an amine. **argentaffin c's,** enterochromaffin cells that reduce ammoniacal silver solutions without additional treatment with a reducing agent; the reducing substance is serotonin. **Arias-Stella c's,** columnar cells in the endometrial epithelium which have a hyperchromatic enlarged nucleus and which appear to be associated with chorionic tissue in an intrauterine or extrauterine site. **band c.,** a late metamyelocyte in which the nucleus is in the form of a curved or coiled band. **basal c.,** an early keratinocyte, present in the basal layer of the epidermis. **basal granular c's,** APUD cells located at the base of the epithelium at many places in the gastrointestinal tract. **basket c.,** a neuron of the cerebral cortex whose fibers form a basket-like nest in which a Purkinje cell rests. **beaker c.,** goblet c. **beta c's,** 1. basophilic cells of the pancreas that secrete insulin and make up most of the bulk of the islands of Langerhans; they contain granules that are soluble in alcohol. 2. basophilic cells of the anterior pituitary. **Betz c's,** large pyramidal ganglion cells forming a layer of the gray matter of the brain. **bipolar c.,** a neuron with two processes. **blood c's,** see under *corpuscle.* **bone c.,** osteocyte.

bristle c's, the hair cells associated with the auditory and cochlear nerves. **burr c.,** a form of spiculed mature erythrocyte, the echinocyte, having multiple, small projections evenly spaced over the cell circumference; observed in azotemia, gastric carcinoma, and bleeding peptic ulcer. **cartilage c's,** chondrocytes. **chief c's,** 1. columnar or cuboidal epithelial cells that line the lower portions of the gastric glands; they secrete pepsin. 2. pinealocytes. 3. the most abundant parenchymal cells of the parathyroid; their cytoplasm does not stain. Cf. *oxyphil c's.* **chromaffin c's,** cells staining readily with chromium salts, especially those of the adrenal medulla and similar cells occurring in widespread accumulations throughout the body in various organs, whose cytoplasm shows fine brown granules when stained with potassium bichromate. **chromophobe c's,** faintly staining cells in the adenohypophysis, which may be transitionally degranulated cells that have just released their secretory granules. **Claudius' c's,** cuboidal cells, which along with Böttcher's cells form the floor of the external spiral sulcus, external to the organ of Corti. **columnar c.,** an elongate epithelial cell. **committed c.,** a lymphocyte which, after contact with antigen, is obligated to follow an individual course of development leading to antibody synthesis or immunological memory. **Corti's c's,** the cells of the organ of Corti. **daughter c.,** one formed by division of a mother cell. **decidual c.,** a connective-tissue cell of the uterine mucous membrane, enlarged and specialized during pregnancy. **Deiters' c's,** 1. the outer phalangeal cells of the organ of Corti. 2. neuroglia c's. **delta c's,** 1. cells in the islets of Langerhans filled with small blue-staining secretory granules. 2. gonadotropes. **dendritic c.,** cells with long cytoplasmic processes in the lymph nodes and germinal centers of the spleen; such processes, which extend along lymphoid cells, retain antigen molecules for extended periods of time. **dust c's,** alveolar macrophages. **effector c.,** any cell, such as an activated lymphocyte or plasma cell, which is instrumental in causing antigen disposal accomplished by either a cell-mediated or a humoral immunological response. **enamel c.,** ameloblast. **enterochromaffin c's,** chromaffin cells of the intestinal mucosa that stain with chromium salts and are impregnable with silver; they are sites of synthesis and storage of serotonin. **epithelioid c's,** 1. large polyhedral cells of connective tissue origin. 2. highly phagocytic, modified macrophages, resembling epithelial cells, which are characteristic of granulomatous inflammation. 3. pinealocytes. **eukaryotic c.,** a cell with a true nucleus; see *eukaryote.* **fat c.,** a connective tissue cell specialized for the synthesis and storage of fat; such cells are bloated with globules of triglycerides, the nucleus being displaced to one side and the cytoplasm seen as a thin line around the fat droplet. **foam c's,** cells with a vacuolated appearance due to the presence of complex lipoids; seen notably in xanthoma. **follicle c's, follicular c's,** epithelial cells located in thyroid or ovarian follicles. **G c's,** granular enterochromaffin cells in the mucosa of the pyloric part of the stomach, a source of gastrin. **ganglion c.,** a large nerve cell, especially one of those of the spinal ganglia. **Gaucher's c.,** a large cell characteristic of Gaucher's disease, with eccentrically placed nuclei and fine wavy fibrils parallel to the long axis of the cell. **germ c.,** the cells of an organism whose function it is to reproduce the kind, i.e., an ovum or spermatozoon, or an immature stage of either. **ghost c.,** 1. a keratinized denucleated cell with an unstained, shadowy center where the nucleus has been. 2. erythroclast. **giant c.,** 1. any very large cell, such as the megakaryocyte of bone marrow. 2. any of the very large, multinucleate, modified macrophages, which may be formed by coalescence of epithelioid cells or by nuclear division without cytoplasmic division of monocytes, e.g., those characteristic of granulomatous inflammation and those that form around large foreign bodies. **glial c's,** neuroglia c's. **glomus c's,** the specific cells of the carotid body, which contain many dense-cored vesicles, occurring in clusters surrounded by other cells with no cytoplasmic granules. **goblet c., goblet mucous c.,** a unicellular mucous gland found in the epithelium of various mucous membranes, especially those of the respiratory passages and intestines. **Golgi's c's,** see under *neuron*. **granular c.,** one containing granules, such as a keratinocyte in the stratum granulosum of the epidermis, when it contains a dense collection of darkly staining granules. **granule c's,** a diminutive cell found in the granular layers of the cerebral and cerebellar cortices. **granulosa c's,** ovarian follicular cells in the stratum granulosum. **gustatory c's,** taste c's. **hair c's,** sensory epithelial cells with long hairlike processes (kinocilia or stereocilia) found in the organ of Corti and the vestibular labyrinth. **hairy c.,** one of the abnormal large cells found in the blood in leukemic reticuloendotheliosis, having numerous irregular cytoplasmic villi that give the cell a flagellated or hairy appearance. **heart failure c's, heart lesion c's,** macrophages containing granules of iron, found in the pulmonary alveoli and sputum in congestive heart failure. **HeLa c's,** cells of the first continuously cultured carcinoma strain, descended from a human cervical carcinoma. **helmet c.,** an abnormal red cell form resembling a helmet, seen in hemolytic anemia. **helper c.,** a subtype of T lymphocytes which cooperate with B lymphocytes in the synthesis of antibody to many antigens; they play an integral role in immunoregulation. **Hensen's c's,** tall supporting cells constituting the outer border of the organ of Corti. **hepatic c's, hepatic parenchymal c's,** the polyhedral epithelial cells that constitute the parenchyma of a hepatic lobule. **Hürthle c's,** large eosinophilic cells sometimes found in the thyroid gland; see also under *tumor.* **interdental c's,** cells found in the spiral limbus between the dens acustici, which secrete the tectorial membrane of the cochlear duct. **interstitial c's,** 1. Leydig's c's. 2. large epithelioid cells in the ovarian stroma, believed to have a secretory function, derived from the theca interna of atretic ovarian follicles. 3. cells found in the perivascular areas and

between the cords of pinealocytes in the pineal body. 4. nerve cells with short, branching processes that interlace with other processes to form an irregular feltwork in the enteric plexuses, submucosa, and interior of the villi of the intestinal tract. 5. fat-storing c's of liver. **intestinal absorptive c.,** one of the cells of the intestinal epithelium, having a brush border made up of many closely packed parallel microvilli, and believed to be associated with absorption, particularly of macromolecules. **islet c's,** the cells composing the islets of Langerhans. **juxtaglomerular c's,** specialized cells containing secretory granules, located in the tunica media of the afferent glomerular arterioles, thought to stimulate aldosterone secretion and to play a role in renal autoregulation. These cells secrete the enzyme renin. **K c's, killer c's,** cells that are morphologically indistinguishable from small lymphocytes, but which have cytotoxic activity against target cells coated with specific IgG antibody. **Kupffer's c's,** large, stellate or pyramidal, intensely phagocytic cells lining the walls of the hepatic sinusoids and forming part of the reticuloendothelial system. **lacunar c.,** a variant of the Reed-Sternberg cell, primarily associated with nodular sclerosing Hodgkin's disease. **Langerhans' c's,** 1. dendritic clear cells of the granular layer of the epidermis that resemble melanocytes but lack tyrosinase. 2. spindle-shaped cells in the acini of the pancreas. **LE c.,** a mature neutrophilic polymorphonuclear leukocyte, which has phagocytized a spherical, homogeneous-appearing inclusion, itself derived from another neutrophil; a characteristic of lupus erythematosus, but also found in analogous connective tissue disorders. **Leydig's c's,** 1. interstitial cells of the testis, which secrete testosterone. 2. mucous cells that do not pour their secretion out over the epithelial surface. **luteal c's, lutein c's,** the plump, pale-staining, polyhedral cells of the corpus luteum. **lymph c.,** lymphocyte. **lymphoid c's,** lymphocytes and plasma cells. **mast c.,** a connective tissue cell capable of elaborating basophilic, metachromatic cytoplasmic granules that contain histamine, heparin, hyaluronic acid, slow-reacting substance of anaphylaxis, and, in some species, serotonin. **mastoid c's,** air spaces of various size and shape in the mastoid process of the temporal bone. **mother c.,** one that divides to form new, or daughter, cells. **mucous c's,** cells which secrete mucus or mucin. **muscle c.,** see under *fiber.* **myoid c's,** cells in the seminiferous tubules which are presumed to be contractile and to be responsible for the rhythmic shallow contractions of the tubules. **nerve c.,** neuron. **neuroglia c's, neuroglial c's,** the branching, non-neural cells of the neuroglia; they are of three types: astroglia (macroglia), oligodendroglia, and microglia. **nevus c.,** a small oval or cuboidal cell with a deeply staining nucleus and scanty pale cytoplasm, sometimes containing melanin granules, possibly derived from Schwann cells or from embryonal nevoblasts; they are clustered in rounded masses (called *theques*) in the epidermis, and reach the dermis by a kind of centripetal extrusion *(abtropfung).* **Niemann-**

Pick c's, Pick's c's. **NK c's,** natural killer cells; cells capable of mediating cytotoxic reactions without themselves being specifically sensitized against the target. **null c's,** lymphocytes that lack the surface antigens characteristic of B and T lymphocytes; such cells are seen in active systemic lupus erythematosus and other disease states. **nurse c's, nursing c's,** Sertoli's c's. **olfactory c's,** a set of specialized cells of the mucous membranes of the nose, which are receptors of smell. **osteoprogenitor c's,** relatively undifferentiated cells found on or near all of the free surfaces of bone, which, under certain circumstances, undergo division and transform into osteoblasts or coalesce to give rise to osteoclasts. **oxyntic c's,** parietal c's. **oxyphil c's, oxyphilic c's,** acidophilic cells found, along with the more numerous chief cells, in the parathyroid glands. **packed human blood c's, packed red blood c's (human),** whole blood from which plasma has been removed; used therapeutically in blood transfusions. **Paget c's,** degenerating cells, swollen, rounded, and pigmented, found in the epidermis in Paget's disease of the nipple and in extramammary Paget's disease. **Paneth's c's,** narrow, pyramidal, or columnar epithelial cells with a round or oval nucleus close to the base of the cell, occurring in the fundus of the crypts of Lieberkühn; they contain large secretory granules that may contain peptidase. **parafollicular c's,** ovoid epithelial cells located in the thyroid follicles; they secrete the hormone calcitonin. **parietal c's,** large spheroidal or pyramidal cells that are the source of gastric hydrochloric acid and are the site of intrinsic factor production. **peptic c's,** chief c's (1). **peritubular contractile c's,** myoid c's. **pheochrome c's,** chromaffin c's. **Pick's c's,** round, oval, or polyhedral cells with foamy, lipid-containing cytoplasm, found in the bone marrow and spleen in Niemann-Pick disease. **plasma c.,** a spherical or ellipsoidal cell with a single nucleus containing chromatin, an area of perinuclear clearing, and generally abundant, sometimes vacuolated cytoplasm; they are involved in the synthesis, storage, and release of antibody. **polychromatic c's, polychromatophil c's,** immature erythrocytes staining with both acid and basic stains in a diffuse mixture of blue-gray and pink. **pre-B c's,** lymphoid cells that are immature and contain cytoplasmic IgM; they develop into B lymphocytes. **pre-T c.,** a T-lymphocyte precursor before undergoing induction of the maturation process in the thymus; it lacks the characteristics of a mature T lymphocyte. **prickle c.,** a cell with delicate radiating processes connecting with similar cells, being a dividing keratinocyte of the prickle-cell layer of the epidermis. **prokaryotic c.,** a cell without a true nucleus; see *prokaryote.* **pulmonary epithelial c's,** extremely thin nonphagocytic squamous cells with flattened nuclei, constituting the outer layer of the alveolar wall in the lungs. **Purkinje's c's,** large branching neurons in the middle layer of the cerebellar cortex. **red c., red blood c.,** erythrocyte. **Reed-Sternberg c's,** giant histiocytic cells, typically multinucleate, which are the common histologic characteristic of Hodgkin's disease. **reticular c's,** the cells forming the reticular fibers of connective tissue; those forming the framework of lymph nodes, bone marrow, and spleen form part of the reticuloendothelial system and may differentiate into macrophages. **reticuloendothelial c.,** see under *system.* **Rieder's c.,** a myeloblast seen in acute leukemia, having a nucleus with several wide and deep indentations suggesting lobulation. **Schwann c.,** any of the large nucleated cells whose cell membrane spirally enwraps the axons of myelinated peripheral neurons supplying the myelin sheath between two nodes of Ranvier. **segmented c.,** a mature granulocyte in which the nucleus is divided into definite lobes joined by a filamentous connection. **seminoma c.,** a large, round-to-polygonal cell occurring in fairly well-differentiated sheets or cords in classical seminoma of the testis. **Sertoli's c's,** cells in the testicular tubules to which the spermatids become attached and which support, protect, and apparently nourish the spermatids until they develop into mature spermatozoa. **sickle c.,** a crescentic or sickle-shaped erythrocyte; see also under *anemia.* **somatic c's,** the cells of the somatoplasm; undifferentiated body cells. **sperm c.,** a spermatozoon. **squamous c.,** a flat, scalelike epithelial cell. **stab c., staff c.,** band c. **stellate c.,** any star-shaped cell, as a Kupffer cell or astrocyte, having many filaments extending in all directions. **stem c.,** a generalized mother cell whose descendants specialize, often in different directions, as an undifferentiated mesenchymal cell that may be considered to be a progenitor of the blood and fixed-tissue cells of the bone marrow. **Sternberg-Reed c's,** Reed-Sternberg c's. **suppressor c's,** lymphoid cells, especially T lymphocytes, that inhibit humoral and cell-mediated immune responses. They play an integral role in immunoregulation, and are believed to be operative in various autoimmune and other immunological disease states. **synovial c's,** fibroblasts lying between the cartilaginous fibers in the synovial membrane of a joint. **target c.,** 1. an abnormally thin erythrocyte which, when stained, shows a dark center and a peripheral ring of hemoglobin, separated by a pale unstained ring containing less hemoglobin, as seen in certain anemias, thalassemias, hemoglobinopathies, obstructive jaundice, and the postsplenectomy state. 2. any cell selectively affected by a particular agent, such as a hormone or drug. **taste c's,** cells in taste buds associated with the nerves of taste. **tendon c's,** flattened cells of connective tissue occurring in rows between the primary bundles of the tendons. **visual c's,** the neuroepithelial elements of the retina. **white c., white blood c.,** leukocyte.

cella (sel′ah), pl. *cel′lae* [L.] cell.

celloidin (sĕ-loi′din) a concentrated preparation of pyroxylin, used in microscopy for embedding specimens for section cutting.

cellula (sel′u-lah), pl. *cel′lulae* [L.] cell.

cellularity (sel″u-lăr′it-e) the state of a tissue or other mass as regards the number of constituent cells.

cellule (-ūl) a small cell.

cellulifugal (-lif′u-gil) directed away from a cell body.

cellulipetal (-lip′it-il) directed toward a cell body.

cellulitis (-līt′is) inflammation of the soft or connective tissue, in which a thin, watery exudate spreads through the cleavage planes of interstitial and tissue spaces; it may lead to ulceration and abscess. **anaerobic c.,** inflammation of the subcutaneous tissue in which the infecting bacteria, most commonly *Clostridium perfringens,* proliferate and produce gas in the tissue (but not in muscle); the onset is gradual, pain is absent, and systemic symptoms are not severe. **clostridial c.,** anaerobic c. **dissecting c.,** inflammation with suppuration spreading between layers of the involved tissue. **gangrenous c.,** that leading to death of the tissue followed by bacterial invasion and putrefaction. **gaseous c.,** inflammation due to a gas-producing organism and presence of gas in the tissues. **pelvic c.,** parametritis.

celluloid (sel′u-loid) a plastic compound of pyroxylin and camphor.

celluloneuritis (sel″u-lo-noo-rīt′is) inflammation of neurons.

cellulose (sel′u-lōs) a carbohydrate, $(C_6H_{10}O_5)_n$, forming the skeleton of most plant structures and plant cells. **absorbable c., oxidized c.,** an absorbable oxidation product of cellulose, used as a local hemostatic.

celom (sel′lom) coelom.

celoschisis (se-los′kĭ-sis) congenital fissure of the abdominal wall.

celosomia (se″lo-so′me-ah) congenital fissure or absence of the sternum, with hernial protrusion of the viscera.

celothelioma (-the″le-o′mah) mesothelioma.

celotomy (se-lot′ah-me) herniotomy.

celovirus (sel″o-vi′rus) CELO virus.

celozoic (-zo′ik) inhabiting the intestinal canal of the body; said of parasites.

cement (se-ment′) 1. a substance that produces a solid union between two surfaces. 2. in dentistry, a filling material used to aid the retention of gold castings and to insulate the tooth pulp. 3. cementum. **dental c.,** cementum.

cementicle (se-men′tĭ-k′l) a small, discrete globular mass of cementum in the region of a tooth root.

cementoblast (se-men′tah-blast) a large cuboidal cell, found between the fibers on the surface of the cementum, which is active in cementum formation.

cementoblastoma (se-men″to-blas-to′mah) an odontogenic fibroma whose cells are developing into cementoblasts and in which there is only a small proportion of calcified tissue.

cementocyte (se-men′to-sīt) a cell in the lacunae of cellular cementum, frequently having long processes radiating from the cell body toward the periodontal surface of the cementum.

cementogenesis (se-men″to-jen′ĭ-sis) development of cementum on the root dentin of a tooth.

cementoma (se″men-to′mah) a mass of cementum lying free at the apex of a tooth, probably a reaction to injury.

cementum (se-men′tum) the bonelike connective tissue covering the root of a tooth and assisting in tooth support.

cenesthesia (sen″es-the′ze-ah) the general feeling or sense of conscious existence; the sense of normal functioning of body organs. **cenesthe′sic, cenesthet′ic,** adj.

ceno- word element [Gr.], *new; empty; common.*

cenosis (se-no′sis) a morbid discharge. **cenot′ic,** adj.

cenosite (se′no-sīt) coinsite.

censor (sen′ser) 1. a member of a committee on ethics or for critical examination of a medical or other society. 2. the psychic influence which prevents unconscious thoughts and wishes coming into consciousness.

center (sen′ter) 1. the middle point of a body. 2. a collection of neurons concerned with performance of a particular function. **accelerating c.,** one in the brain stem involved in acceleration of the heart. **apneustic c.,** a nerve center in the brain stem controlling normal respiration. **auditory c.,** the center for hearing, in the more anterior of the transverse temporal gyri. **Broca's c.,** speech c. **cardioinhibitory c.,** one in the medulla oblongata that exerts an inhibitory influence on the heart. **c's of chondrification,** dense aggregations of embryonic mesenchymal cells at sites of future cartilage formation. **ciliospinal c.,** one in the lower cervical and upper dorsal portions of the spinal cord involved in dilatation of the pupil. **community mental health c.,** a mental health facility or group of affiliated agencies that provide various psychotherapeutic services to a designated geographic area. **coughing c.,** one in the medulla oblongata above the respiratory center, which controls the act of coughing. **deglutition c.,** a nerve center in the medulla oblongata that controls the function of swallowing. **C's for Disease Control (CDC),** an agency of the U.S. Department of Health and Human Services, which serves as a center for the control, prevention, and investigation of diseases. **epiotic c.,** the center of ossification forming the mastoid process. **epiphyseal c.,** secondary c. of ossification. **facial c.,** one in the lower part of the ascending frontal convolution, controlling facial movements. **germinal c.,** the area in the center of a lymph nodule containing aggregations of actively proliferating lymphocytes. **health c.,** 1. a community health organization for creating health work and coordinating the efforts of all health agencies. 2. an educational complex consisting of a medical school and various allied health professional schools. **medullary respiratory c.,** one in the medulla oblongata that coordinates respiratory movements. **motor c.,** any center that originates, controls, inhibits, or maintains motor impulses. **nerve c.,** an aggregation, in brain or spinal cord, of cell bodies of neurons. **ossification c.,** any point at which the process of ossification begins in a bone; in a long bone there is a *primary center* for the diaphysis and one *secondary center* for each epiphysis.

pneumotaxic c., one in the upper pons that rhythmically inhibits inspiration. **reflex c.,** any center in the brain or spinal cord in which a sensory impression is changed into a motor impulse. **respiratory c's,** a series of the centers (the apneustic, pneumotaxic, and medullary respiratory c's) in the medulla and pons that coordinate respiratory movements. **Setschenow's c's,** reflex inhibitory centers in the medulla oblongata and spinal cord. **speech c.,** one in the left (or right) inferior frontal gyrus concerned with aspects of speech. **swallowing c.,** deglutition c. **thermoregulatory c's,** hypothalamic centers regulating the conservation and dissipation of heat. **vasomotor c's,** centers in the tuber cinereum, medulla oblongata, and spinal cord, believed to regulate the contraction and dilatation of blood vessels. **Wernicke's c.,** the speech center in the cortex of the left temporo-occipital convolution. **word c.,** one concerned with the recognition of words, different areas being involved for recognition of written and of spoken words.

centesimal (sen-tes′ĭ-mal) divided into hundredths.

-centesis word element [Gr.], *puncture and aspiration of.*

centi- word element [L.], *hundred;* used in naming units of measurement to indicate one hundredth (10^{-2}) of the unit designated by the root with which it is combined; symbol c.

centigrade (sen′tĭ-grād) having 100 gradations (steps or degrees), as the Celsius (centigrade) scale; abbreviated C.

centigram (-gram) one hundredth of a gram; abbreviated cg.

centigray (sen′ti-grā″) a unit of absorbed radiation dose equal to one hundredth of a gray, or 1 rad; abbreviated cGy.

centiliter (-lēt″er) one hundredth of a liter; abbreviated cl.

centimeter (-mēt″er) one hundredth of a meter, or approximately 0.3937 inch; abbreviated cm. **cubic c.,** a unit of capacity, being that of a cube each side of which measures 1 cm.; abbreviated cc., cm.³, or cu. cm.

centipoise (sen″tĭ-poiz) one hundredth of a poise.

centistoke (sen′tĭ-stōk) one hundreth of a stoke.

centrad (sen′trad) toward a center.

centrencephalic (sen″tren-sah-fal′ik) pertaining to the center of the encephalon.

centriciput (sen-tris′ĭ-put) the central part of the upper surface of the head, located between the occiput and sinciput.

centrifugate (sen-trif′u-gāt) material subjected to centrifugation.

centrifugation (sen-trif″u-ga′shin) the process of separating lighter portions of a solution, mixture, or suspension from the heavier portions by centrifugal force.

centrifuge (sen′trĭ-fūj) 1. a machine by which centrifugation is effected. 2. to subject to centrifugation.

centrilobular (sen″trĭ-lob′u-ler) pertaining to the central portion of a lobule.

centriole (sen′tre-ōl) either of the two cylindrical organelles located in the centrosome and containing nine triplets of microtubules arrayed around their edges; centrioles migrate to opposite poles of the cell during cell division and serve to organize the spindles. They are capable of independent replication and of migrating to form basal bodies.

centripetal (sen-trip′it′l) moving toward a center.

centro- word element [L., Gr.], *center; a central location.*

centrokinesia (sen″tro-ki-ne′se-ah) movement originating from central stimulation. **centrokinet′ic,** adj.

centromere (sen′tro-mēr) the clear constricted portion of the chromosome at which the chromatids are joined and by which the chromosome is attached to the spindle during cell division. **centromer′ic,** adj.

centrosclerosis (sen″tro-skler-o′sis) osteosclerosis of the marrow cavity of a bone.

centrosome (sen′tro-sōm) a specialized area of condensed cytoplasm containing the centrioles and playing an important part in mitosis.

centrostaltic (sen″tro-stal′tik) pertaining to a center of motion.

centrum (sen′trum), pl. *cen′tra* [L.] 1. a center. 2. the body of a vertebra.

cephal(o)- word element [Gr.], *head.*

cephalad (sef′ah-lad) toward the head.

cephalalgia (sef″al-al′je-ah) headache.

cephaledema (-ĭ-de′mah) edema of the head.

cephalexin (sef″ah-lek′sin) a semisynthetic analogue, $C_{16}H_{17}N_3O_4S$, of the natural cephalosporin C, used in the treatment of infections of the urinary and respiratory tracts and of skin and soft tissues due to sensitive pathogens.

cephalhematocele (sef″al-he-mat′ah-sēl) a hematocele under the pericranium, communicating with one or more dural sinuses.

cephalhematoma (-he″mah-to′mah) a subperiosteal hemorrhage limited to the surface of one cranial bone; a usually benign condition seen in the newborn as a result of bone trauma.

cephalhydrocele (-hi′dro-sēl) a serous or watery accumulation under the pericranium.

cephalic (sĕ-fal′ik) pertaining to the head, or to the head end of the body.

cephalin (sef′ah-lin) a group of phosphoglycerides in which phosphatidic acid is linked to ethanolamine (phosphatidyl ethanolamine) or to serine (phosphatidyl serine); the cephalins are found particularly in brain and nervous tissue and have blood-coagulating properties.

cephalitis (sef″ah-lit′is) encephalitis.

cephalocele (sĕ-fal′ah-sēl) protrusion of a part of the cranial contents.

cephalocentesis (sef″ah-lo-sen-te′sis) surgical puncture of the head.

cephalodactyly (-dak′tĭ-le) malformation of the head and digits.

cephaloglycin (-gli′sin) a semisynthetic analogue, $C_{18}H_{19}N_3O_6S$, of cephalosporin C, used in the treatment of acute and chronic urinary infections due to sensitive pathogens.

cephalogram (-gram) an x-ray image of the structures of the head; cephalometric radiograph.

cephalogyric (-ji′rik) pertaining to turning motions of the head.

cephalometer (sef″ah-lom′it-er) an instrument for measuring the head; an orienting device for positioning the head for radiographic examination and measurement.

cephalometry (sef″ah-lom′ĭ-tre) scientific measurement of the dimensions of the head.

cephalomotor (sef″ah-lo-mōt′er) moving the head; pertaining to motions of the head.

Cephalomyia (-mi′yah) *Oestrus.*

cephalonia (sef″ah-lo′ne-ah) a condition in which the head is abnormally enlarged, with sclerotic hyperplasia of the brain.

cephalopathy (sef″ah-lop′ah-the) any disease of the head.

cephalopelvic (sef″ah-lo-pel′vik) pertaining to the relationship of the fetal head to the maternal pelvis.

cephaloridine (sef″ah-lor′ĭ-dēn) a semisynthetic antibiotic, $C_{19}H_{17}N_3O_4S_2$, of the natural antibiotic cephalosporin C, used in the treatment of infections of the bones, joints, skin, soft tissues, and major organ and tissue systems due to sensitive pathogens.

cephalosporin (sef″ah-lo-spor′in) any of a group of broad-spectrum, penicillinase-resistant antibiotics from *Cephalosporium,* including cephalexin, cephaloridine, cephaloglycin, and cephalothin, which share the nucleus 7-aminocephalosporanic acid.

cephalosporinase (-spor′in-ās) an enzyme that hydrolyzes the CO—NH bond in the lactam ring of cephalosporin, converting it to an inactive product.

Cephalosporium (-spor′e-um) a genus of soil-inhabiting fungi (family Moniliaceae); some species are the source of the cephalosporins.

cephalostat (sef′ah-lo-stat″) a head-positioning device which assures reproducibility of the relations between an x-ray beam, a patient's head, and an x-ray film.

cephalothin (-thin″) a semisynthetic analogue, $C_{16}H_{16}N_2O_6S_2$, of the natural antibiotic cephalosporin C, effective against a wide range of gram-positive and gram-negative bacteria.

cephalotomy (sef″ah-lot′ah-me) 1. the cutting up of the fetal head to facilitate delivery. 2. dissection of the fetal head.

cephapirin (sef″ah-pi′rin) a semisynthetic analogue, $C_{17}H_{16}N_3O_6S_2$, of the natural antibiotic cephalosporin C, effective against a wide range of gram-negative and gram-positive bacteria.

cephradine (sef′rah-dēn) a semisynthetic analogue, $C_{16}H_{19}N_3O_4S$, of the natural antibiotic cephalosporin C; used in the treatment of infections of the urinary tract, skin, and soft tissues due to sensitive pathogens.

ceramics (sah-ram′iks) the modeling and processing of objects made of clay or similar materials. **dental c.,** the use of porcelain and similar materials in restorative dentistry.

ceramidase (sah-ram′ĭ-dās) an enzyme occurring in most mammalian tissue that catalyzes the reversible acylation-deacylation of ceramides.

ceramide (ser′ah-mīd) any of a group of naturally occurring sphingolipids in which the NH_2 group of sphingosine is acylated with a fatty acyl CoA derivative to form an *N*-acylsphingosine. **galactosyl c.,** cerebroside. **c. glucoside,** the major sphingolipid accumulated in Gaucher's disease. **c. trihexoside,** the major sphingolipid accumulated in Fabry's disease.

cerato- for words beginning thus, see also those beginning *kerato-.*

Ceratophyllus (ser″ah-tof′ĭ-lus) a genus of fleas.

cercaria (ser-ka′re-ah), pl. *cerca′riae* [Gr.] the final, free-swimming larval stage of a trematode parasite.

cerclage (ser-klahzh′) [Fr.] encircling of a part with a ring or loop, as for correction of an incompetent cervix uteri or fixation of adjacent ends of a fractured bone.

cercus (ser′kus) a bristle-like structure.

cerea flexibilitas (sēr′e-ah flek″sĭ-bil′ĭ-tas) waxy flexibility; see under *flexibility.*

cerebellifugal (ser″ah-bel-lif′u-g′l) conducting away from the cerebellum.

cerebellipetal (-lip′it′l) conducting toward the cerebellum.

cerebellospinal (ser″ah-bel″o-spi′nil) proceeding from the cerebellum to the spinal cord.

cerebellum (ser″ah-bel′um) the part of the metencephalon situated on the back of the brain stem, to which it is attached by three cerebellar peduncles on each side; it consists of a median lobe (vermis) and two lateral lobes (the hemispheres).

cerebral (ser′ah-bril, sah-re′bril) pertaining to the cerebrum.

cerebration (ser″ah-bra′shin) functional activity of the brain.

cerebrifugal (-brif′u-g′l) conducting or proceeding away from the cerebrum.

cerebripetal (-brip′it′l) conducting or proceeding toward the cerebrum.

cerebritis (-brīt′is) inflammation of the cerebrum.

cerebroma (ser″ah-bro′mah) any abnormal mass of brain substance.

cerebromacular (ser″ah-bro-mak′u-ler) pertaining to or affecting the brain and the macula retinae.

cerebromalacia (-mah-la′she-ah) abnormal softening of the substance of the cerebrum.

cerebromeningitis (-men″in-jīt′is) meningoencephalitis.

cerebronic acid (ser″ah-bron′ik) the principal hydroxy acid from the brain, $C_{24}H_{48}O_3$, a constituent of sphingomyelin.

cerebropathia (-path′e-ah) [L.] cerebropathy. **c. psy′chica toxe′mica,** Korsakoff's psychosis.

cerebrophysiology (ser″ah-bro-fiz″e-ol′ah-je) the physiology of the cerebrum.

cerebropontile (-pon′tīl) pertaining to cerebrum and pons.

cerebrosclerosis (-skler-o′sis) morbid hardening of the substance of the cerebrum.

cerebroside (sah-re'bro-sīd) a general designation for sphingolipids in which sphingosine is combined with galactose or glucose; found chiefly in nervous tissue.

cerebrosis (ser''ah-bro'sis) any disease of the cerebrum.

cerebrospinant (-spi'nant) an agent which affects the brain and spinal cord.

cerebrotomy (ser''ah-brot'ah-me) anatomy or dissection of the brain.

cerebrum (ser'ah-brum, sah-re'brum) the main portion of the brain, occupying the upper part of the cranial cavity; its two hemispheres, united by the corpus callosum, form the largest part of the central nervous system in man. The term is sometimes applied to the postembryonic forebrain and midbrain together or to the entire brain.

cerium (sēr'e-um) chemical element (*see table*), at. no. 58, symbol Ce.

ceroplasty (sēr'o-plas''te) the making of anatomical models in wax.

ceruloplasmin (sah-roo''lo-plaz'min) an alpha₂-globulin of plasma, being a glycoprotein in which most of the plasma copper is transported.

cerumen (sah-roo'men) earwax; the waxlike substance found within the external meatus of the ear. **ceru'minal, ceru'minous,** adj.

ceruminolysis (sah-roo''mĭ-nol'ĭ-sis) dissolution or disintegration of cerumen in the external auditory meatus. **ceruminolyt'ic,** adj.

cervic(o)- word element [L.], *neck; cervix.*

cervicectomy (ser''vĭ-sek'tah-me) excision of the cervix uteri.

cervicitis (-sīt'is) inflammation of the cervix uteri.

cervicobrachialgia (ser''vĭ-ko-brak''e-al'je-ah) pain in the neck radiating to the arm, due to compression of nerve roots of the cervical spinal cord.

cervicocolpitis (-kol-pīt'is) inflammation of the cervix uteri and vagina.

cervicovesical (ser''vĭ-ko-ves'ĭ-k'l) relating to the cervix uteri and urinary bladder.

cervix (ser'viks), pl. *cer'vices* [L.] neck; the front portion of the neck (collum), or a constricted part of an organ (e.g., cervix uteri). **incompetent c.,** one that is abnormally prone to dilate in the second trimester of pregnancy, resulting in premature expulsion of the fetus. **c. u'teri,** the narrow lower end of the uterus, between the isthmus and the opening of the uterus into the vagina. **c. vesi'cae,** the lower, constricted part of the urinary bladder, proximal to the opening of the urethra.

cesium (se'ze-um) chemical element (*see table*), at. no. 55, symbol Cs.

cesticidal (ses''tĭ-sīd'l) destructive to cestodes.

Cestoda (ses-tōd'ah) a subclass of Cestoidea comprising the true tapeworms, which have a head (scolex) and segments (proglottides). The adults are endoparasitic in the alimentary tract and associated ducts of various vertebrate hosts; their larvae may be found in various organs and tissues.

Cestodaria (ses''to-da're-ah) a subclass of tapeworms, the unsegmented tapeworms of the class Cestoidea, which are endoparasitic in the intestines and coelom of various primitive fishes and rarely in reptiles.

cestode (ses'tōd) 1. any individual of the class Cestoidea, especially any member of the subclass Cestoda. 2. cestoid.

Cestoidea (ses-toid'e-ah) a class of tapeworms (phylum Platyhelminthes), characterized by the absence of a mouth or digestive tract, and by a noncuticular layer covering their bodies.

cetalkonium chloride (set''al-ko'ne-um) a cationic quaternary ammonium surfactant, $C_{25}H_{46}ClN$, used as a topical anti-infective and disinfectant.

cetrimonium bromide (sĕ''trĭ-mo'ne-um) a quaternary ammonium antiseptic and detergent, $C_{19}H_{42}BrN$, applied topically to the skin to cleanse wounds, as a preoperative disinfectant, and to treat seborrhea of the scalp; also used to cleanse and to store surgical instruments.

cetylpyridinium chloride (se''til-pi''rĭ-din'e-um) a cationic disinfectant, $C_{21}H_{38}ClN \cdot H_2O$, used as a local anti-infective administered sublingually or applied topically to intact skin and mucous membranes, and as a preservative in pharmaceutical preparations.

CF cardiac failure; Christmas factor.

Cf chemical symbol, *californium.*

C.F.T. complement fixation test.

cg. centigram.

C.G.S., c.g.s. centimeter-gram-second (system), a system of measurements based on the centimeter as the unit of length, the gram as the unit of mass, and the second as the unit of time.

cGy centigray.

chafe (chāf) irritation of the skin, as by rubbing together of opposing skin folds.

chagasic (chah-gas'ik) pertaining to or due to Chagas' disease.

chagoma (chah-go'mah) a skin tumor occurring in Chagas' disease.

chain (chān) A collection of objects linked end to end. **branched c.,** an open chain of atoms, usually carbon, with one or more side chains attached to it. **H c., heavy c.,** any of the large polypeptide chains of five classes that, paired with the light chains, make up the antibody molecule. Heavy chains bear the antigenic determinants that differentiate the immunoglobulin classes. **J c.,** a polypeptide occurring in polymeric IgM and IgA molecules. **light c.,** either of the two small polypeptide chains (molecular weight 22,000) that, when linked to heavy chains by disulfide bonds, make up the antibody molecule; they are of two types, kappa and lambda, which are unrelated to immunoglobulin class differences. **side c.,** a chain of atoms attached to a larger chain or to a ring.

chalasia (kah-la'ze-ah) relaxation of a bodily opening, such as the cardiac sphincter (a cause of vomiting in infants).

chalazion (kah-la'ze-on) a small eyelid mass due to inflammation of a meibomian gland.

chalcosis (kal-ko'sis) copper deposits in tissue.

chalicosis (kal″ĭ-ko′sis) pneumoconiosis due to inhalation of fine particles of stone.

chalone (kal′ōn) 1. a group of tissue-specific water-soluble substances that are produced within a tissue and that inhibit mitosis of cells of that tissue and whose action is reversible. 2. (*obs.*) a substance which neutralizes the action of a hormone; inhibitory hormone.

chamaecephaly (kam″ah-sef′ah-le) the condition of having a low flat head, i.e., a cephalic index of 70 or less. **chamaecephal′ic,** adj.

chamber (chām′ber) an enclosed space. **anterior c.,** the part of the aqueous-containing space of the eyeball between the cornea and iris. **aqueous c.,** the part of the eyeball filled with aqueous humor; see *anterior c.* and *posterior c.* **counting c.,** a shallow glass chamber specially ruled to facilitate the counting of discrete particles in the sample under study. **diffusion c.,** an apparatus for separating a substance by means of a semipermeable membrane. **Haldane c.,** an air-tight chamber in which animals are confined for metabolic studies. **hyperbaric c.,** an enclosed space in which gas (oxygen) can be raised to greater than atmospheric pressure. **ionization c.,** an enclosure containing two or more electrodes between which an electric current may be passed when the enclosed gas is ionized by radiation; used for determining the intensity of roentgen and other rays. **posterior c.,** that part of the aqueous-containing space of the eyeball between the iris and the lens. **pulp c.,** the natural cavity in the central portion of the tooth crown that is occupied by the dental pulp. **relief c.,** the recess in a denture surface that rests on the oral structures, to reduce or eliminate pressure. **Thoma-Zeiss counting c.,** a device for counting blood or other cells. **vitreous c.,** the vitreous-containing space in the eyeball, bounded anteriorly by the lens and ciliary body and posteriorly by the posterior wall of the eyeball.

chancre (shang′ker) 1. the primary sore of syphilis, also known as *hard, hunterian,* or *true chancre,* at the site of entry of the infection. 2. the primary cutaneous lesion of such diseases as sporotrichosis and tuberculosis. **hard c., hunterian c.,** chancre (1). **c. re′dux,** chancre developing on the scar of a healed primary chancre. **soft c.,** chancroid. **sporotrichotic c.,** the primary lesion at the site of inoculation in the cutaneous lymphatic form of sporotrichosis. **true c.,** chancre (1). **tuberculous c.,** a brownish red papule which develops into an indurated nodule or plaque, representing the initial cutaneous infection of the tubercle bacillus into the skin or mucosa.

chancroid (shang′kroid) a nonsyphilitic venereal disease transmitted by direct contact, and caused by *Hemophilus ducreyi.* It begins as a painless macule on the genitalia, which enlarges and becomes pustular; an ulcer forms with a shaggy base and adjacent bubo formation. **phagedenic c.,** chancroid with a tendency to slough. **serpiginous c.,** a variety tending to spread in curved lines.

character (kar′ik-ter) a quality indicative of the nature of an object or an organism; in genetics, the expression of a gene or group of genes in a phenotype. **acquired c.,** a noninheritable modification produced in an animal as a result of its own activities or of environmental influences. **dominant c.,** a mendelian character that is expressed when it is transmitted by a single gene. **mendelian c's,** in genetics, the separate and distinct traits exhibited by an organism and dependent on its genetic constitution. **primary sex c's,** those characters of the male and female concerned directly in reproduction. **recessive c.,** a mendelian character that is expressed only when transmitted by both genes (one from each parent) determining the trait. **secondary sex c's,** those characters specific to the male and female but not directly concerned in reproduction. **sex-conditioned c., sex-influenced c.,** an autosomal trait whose full expression is conditioned by the sex of the individual, e.g., human baldness. **sex-linked c.,** one transmitted consistently to individuals of one sex only, being carried in the sex chromosome.

characteristic (kar″ik-ter-is′tik) 1. character. 2. typical of an individual or other entity. **demand c's,** behavior exhibited by the subject of an experiment in an attempt to accomplish certain goals as a result of cues communicated by the experimenter (expectations or hypothesis).

charcoal (char′kōl) carbon prepared by charring other organic material. **activated c.,** residue of destructive distillation of various organic materials, treated to increase its adsorptive power; used as a general purpose antidote. **animal c.,** charcoal prepared from bone, which is purified (*purified animal c.*) by removal of materials dissolved in hot hydrochloric acid and water; adsorbent and decolorizer.

charleyhorse (char′le-hors) soreness and stiffness in a muscle, especially the quadriceps, due to overstrain or contusion.

chart (chart) a record of data in graphic or tabular form. **reading c.,** a chart printed in gradually increasing type sizes, used in testing acuity of near vision. **Reuss' color c's,** charts with colored letters printed on colored backgrounds, used in testing color vision. **Snellen's c.,** a chart with block letters in gradually decreasing sizes, used in testing visual acuity.

Ch.B. [L.] *Chirur′giae Baccalau′reus* (Bachelor of Surgery).

ChE cholinesterase.

check-bite (chek′bīt) a sheet of hard wax or modeling compound placed between the teeth, used to check occlusion of the teeth.

cheek (chēk) bucca; a fleshy protuberance, especially the fleshy portion of either side of the face. Also, the inner surface of the cheeks. **cleft c.,** facial cleft caused by developmental failure of union between the maxillary and primitive frontonasal processes.

cheil(o)- word element [Gr.], *lip.*

cheilectropion (ki″lek-tro′pe-on) eversion of the lip.

cheilitis (ki-līt′is) inflammation of the lips. **actinic c.,** pain and swelling of the lips and development of a scaly crust on the vermilion border after exposure to actinic rays. **solar c.,**

involvement of the lips after exposure to actinic rays; it may be acute (*actinic c.*), or chronic, with alteration of the epithelium and sometimes fissuring or ulceration.

cheilognathoprosoposchisis (ki″lo - na″tho-pros″o-pos′kĭ-sis) congenital oblique facial cleft continuing into the lip and upper jaw.

cheiloplasty (ki′lo-plas″te) surgical repair of a defect of the lip.

cheilorrhaphy (ki-lor′ah-fe) suture of the lip; surgical repair of harelip.

cheiloscopy (ki-los′kah-pe) study of the configuration of the vermilion border of the lips to identify individual patterns (lip-print patterns).

cheiloschisis (ki-los′kĭ-sis) harelip.

cheilosis (ki-lo′sis) fissuring and dry scaling of the vermilion surface of the lips and angles of the mouth, a characteristic of riboflavin deficiency. **angular c.,** perlèche.

cheilostomatoplasty (ki″lo-sto-mat′ah-plas″te) surgical restoration of the lips and mouth.

cheir(o)- word element [Gr.], *hand.* See also words beginning *chir*(o)-.

cheirarthritis (ki″rar-thrīt′is) inflammation of the joints of the hands and fingers.

cheirognostic (ki″rog-nos′tik) pertaining to the ability to distinguish stimuli as originating on the right or left side of the body.

cheirokinesthesia (ki″ro-kin″es-the′ze-ah) the subjective perception of movements of the hand, especially in writing.

cheiromegaly (-meg′ah-le) abnormal enlargement of the hands and fingers.

cheiroplasty (ki′ro-plas″te) plastic surgery on the hand.

cheiropompholyx (-pom′fah-liks) pompholyx.

cheirospasm (ki′ro-spazm) spasm of the muscles of the hand.

chelate (ke′lāt) to combine with a metal in complexes in which the metal is part of a ring. By extension, a chemical compound in which a metallic ion is sequestered and firmly bound into a ring within the chelating molecules. Chelates are used in chemotherapy of metal poisoning.

chem(o)- word element [Gr.], *chemical; chemistry.*

chemabrasion (kēm-ah-bra′zhin) superficial destruction of the epidermis and the dermis by application of a cauterant to the skin; done to remove scars, tattoos, etc.

chemexfoliation (kēm′eks-fo″le-a″shin) chemabrasion.

chemical (kem′ĭ-k′l) 1. pertaining to chemistry. 2. a substance composed of chemical elements, or obtained by chemical processes.

chemist (kem′ist) 1. an expert in chemistry. 2. (British) pharmacist.

chemistry (kem′is-tre) the science dealing with the elements and atomic relations of matter, and of various compounds of the elements. **colloid c.,** chemistry dealing with the nature and composition of colloids. **inorganic c.,** that branch of chemistry dealing with compounds not occurring in the plant or animal worlds. **organic c.,** that branch of chemistry dealing with carbon-containing compounds.

chemoattractant (ke″mo-ah-trak′tint) a chemotactic agent that induces an organism or a cell (e.g., a leukocyte) to migrate toward it.

chemoautotroph (-awt′o-trōf) a chemoautotrophic microorganism.

chemoautotrophic (-awt″o-trof′ik) capable of synthesizing cell constituents from carbon dioxide with energy from inorganic reactions.

chemocautery (-kawt′er-e) cauterization by application of a caustic substance.

chemodectoma (-dek-to′mah) a tumor of the chemoreceptor system, e.g., a carotid body tumor.

chemohormonal (-hor-mo′nil) pertaining to drugs having hormonal activity.

chemokinesis (-ki-ne′sis) increased activity of an organism caused by a chemical substance.

chemolithotrophic (-lith″o-trof′ik) deriving energy from the oxidation of inorganic compounds of iron, nitrogen, sulfur, or hydrogen; said of bacteria.

chemoluminescence (-loo″mĭ-nes′ins) luminescence produced by direct transformation of chemical energy into light energy.

chemonucleolysis (-noo″kle-ol′ĭ-sis) dissolution of a portion of the nucleus pulposus of an intervertebral disk by injection of a chemolytic agent (e.g., chymopapain) for treatment of a herniated intervertebral disk.

chemo-organotroph (-or′gah-no-trōf″) an organism that derives its energy and carbon from organic compounds.

chemopallidectomy (-pal″ĭ-dek′tah-me) chemical destruction of tissue of the globus pallidus.

chemoprophylaxis (-pro″fĭ-lak′sis) prevention of disease by chemical means.

chemopsychiatry (-si-ki′ah-tre) the treatment of mental and emotional disorders by drugs.

chemoreceptor (-re-sep′ter) a receptor sensitive to stimulation by chemical substances.

chemosensitive (-sen′sĭ-tiv) sensitive to changes in chemical composition.

chemosensory (-sen′sah-re) relating to the perception of chemicals, as in odor detection.

chemoserotherapy (-sēr″o-thĕ′rah-pe) treatment of infection by drugs and serum.

chemosis (ke-mo′sis) edema of the conjunctiva of the eye.

chemosterilant (ke″mo-stĕ′rĭ-lant) a chemical compound which upon ingestion causes sterility of an organism.

chemosurgery (-ser′jer-e) destruction of tissue by chemical means for therapeutic purposes.

chemosynthesis (-sin′thĭ-sis) the building up of chemical compounds under the influence of chemical stimulation, specifically the formation of carbohydrates from carbon dioxide and water as a result of energy derived from chemical reactions. **chemosynthet′ic,** adj.

chemotaxin (-tak′sin) a substance, e.g., a complement component, that induces chemotaxis.

chemotaxis (-tak′sis) taxis in response to the influence of chemical stimulation. **chemotac′-tic,** adj. **leukocyte c.,** the response of leukocytes to products formed in immunologic reactions, wherein leukocytes are attracted to and accumulate at the site of the reaction; a part of the inflammatory response.

chemotherapy (-thĕ′rah-pe) treatment of disease by chemical agents.

chemotic (ke-mot′ik) 1. pertaining to or affected with chemosis. 2. an agent that increases lymph production in the ocular conjunctiva.

chemotrophic (-trof′ik) deriving energy from the oxidation of organic (chemo-organotrophic) or inorganic (chemolithotrophic) compounds; said of bacteria.

chemotropism (ke-mah′trah-pizm) tropism due to chemical stimulation. **chemotrop′ic,** adj.

chenodeoxycholic acid (ke″no-de-ok″se-kol′ik) a primary bile acid, $C_{24}H_{40}O_4$, administered as an anticholelithogenic agent.

chenodiol (ke″no-di′ol) chenodeoxycholic acid.

chenotherapy (-thĕ′rah-pe) treatment with chenodeoxycholic acid, to dissolve gallstones.

cherubism (cher′ĭ-bizm) hereditary and progressive bilateral swelling at the angle of the mandible, sometimes involving the entire jaw, imparting a cherubic look to the face, in some cases enhanced by upturning of the eyes.

chest (chest) the thorax, especially its anterior aspect. **flail c.,** one whose wall moves paradoxically with respiration, owing to multiple fractures of the ribs. **funnel c.,** a congenital abnormality in which the sternum is depressed. **pigeon c.,** see under *breast.*

chiasm (ki′azm) a decussation or X-shaped crossing. **optic c.,** the structure in the forebrain formed by the decussation of the fibers of the optic nerve from each half of each retina.

chiasma (ki-az′mah), pl. *chias′mata* [L.; Gr.] chiasm; in genetics, the points at which members of a chromosome pair are in contact during the prophase of meiosis and because of which recombination, or crossing over, occurs on separation.

chickenpox (chik′en-poks) varicella; a highly contagious disease caused by the herpes zoster virus, characterized by vesicular eruptions appearing over a period of a few days to a week after an incubation period of 17–21 days; usually benign in children, but in infants and adults may be accompanied by severe symptoms.

chigger (chig′er) the six-legged red larva of mites of the family Trombiculidae (e.g., *Eutrombicula alfreddugèsi, E. splendens, Trombicula autumnalis*), which attach to their host's skin, and whose bite produces a wheal with intense itching and severe dermatitis. Some species are vectors of the rickettsiae of scrub typhus.

chigoe (chig′o) the flea, *Tunga penetrans*, of subtropical and tropical America and Africa; the pregnant female burrows into the skin of the feet, legs, or other part of the body, causing intense irritation and ulceration, sometimes leading to spontaneous amputation of a digit.

chilblain (chil′blān) a recurrent localized itching, swelling, and painful erythema of the fingers, toes, or ears, caused by mild frostbite.

chill (chil) a sensation of cold, with convulsive shaking of the body.

Chilomastix (ki″lo-mas′tiks) a genus of parasitic

protozoa found in the intestines of vertebrates, including *C. mesni′li,* a very common species found as a commensal in the human cecum and colon.

Chilopoda (ki-lop′ah-dah) a class of the phylum Arthropoda, including the centipedes.

chimera (ki-me′rah) an organism with different cell populations derived from different zygotes of the same or different species, occurring spontaneously or produced artificially.

chin (chin) the anterior prominence of the lower jaw; the mentum.

chionablepsia (ki″ah-nah-blep′se-ah) snow blindness.

chir(o)- word element [Gr.], *hand.* See also words beginning *cheir(o)-.*

chiropodist (ki-rop′ah-dist) podiatrist.

chiropody (ki-rop′ah-de) podiatry.

chiropractic (ki″rah-prak′tik) a system of therapeutics that attributes disease to irritation of the nervous system, and attempts to restore normal function by manipulation of the body structures, especially those of the vertebral column.

chirurgenic (ki″rur-jen′ik) arising as a result of a surgical procedure.

chi-square (ki′skwār) see under *test.*

chitin (kīt′in) a horny polysaccharide, the principal constituent of the shells of arthropods and shards of beetles, and found in certain fungi.

Chlamydia (klah-mid′e-ah) a genus of the family Chlamydiaceae. **C. psitta′ci,** a species, strains of which cause psittacosis, ornithosis, and a variety of diseases in animals. **C. tracho′matis,** a species, various strains of which cause trachoma, inclusion conjunctivitis, urethritis, bronchopneumonia of laboratory mice, proctitis, and lymphogranuloma venereum.

Chlamydiaceae (klah-mid″e-a′se-e) a family of bacteria (order Chlamydiales) consisting of small coccoid microorganisms that have a unique, obligately intracellular developmental cycle and are incapable of synthesizing ATP. They induce their own phagocytosis by host cells, in which they then form intracytoplasmic colonies. They are parasites of birds and mammals (including man). The family contains a single genus, *Chlamydia.*

Chlamydiales (klah-mid′e-al-ēz) an order of coccoid, gram-negative, parasitic microorganisms that multiply within the cytoplasm of vertebrate host cells by a unique development cycle.

chlamydiosis (klah-mid″e-o′sis) any infection or disease caused by *Chlamydia.*

Chlamydobacteriaceae (klah-mi″do-bak-tēr″e-a′se-e) in former systems of classification, a family of bacteria made up of the genera *Leptothrix, Sphaerotilus,* and *Toxothrix.*

Chlamydobacteriales (-bak-tēr″e-a′lēz) in former systems of classification, an order of bacteria made up of nonpigmented filamentous bacteria.

chlamydospore (klam′ĭ-do-spor″) a thickwalled intercalary or terminal asexual spore formed by the rounding-up of a cell; it is not shed.

chloasma (klo-az′mah) melasma. **c. gravida′-rum,** see under *melasma.* **c. uteri′num,** melasma gravidarum.

chloracne (klor-ak′ne) an acneiform eruption due to exposure to chlorine compounds.

chloral (klo′ril) 1. an oily liquid, $Cl_3C\cdot CHO$, with a pungent, irritating odor, prepared by the mutual action of alcohol and chlorine; used in manufacture of chloral hydrate and DDT. 2. c. hydrate. **c. betaine,** an adduct formed by the reaction of chloral hydrate with betaine; used as a sedative. **c. hydrate,** a crystalline substance used as a hypnotic.

chlorambucil (klor-am′bu-sil) an antineoplastic, $C_{14}H_{19}Cl_2NO_2$, from nitrogen mustard.

chloramphenicol (klor″am-fen′ĭ-kol) an antibacterial and antirickettsial, $C_{11}H_{12}Cl_2N_2O_5$.

chlorcyclizine (klor-si′klĭ-zēn) an antihistaminic, $C_{18}H_{21}ClN_2$, used as the hydrochloride salt.

chlordane (klor′dān) a poisonous substance of the chlorinated hydrocarbon group, used as an insecticide.

chlordiazepoxide (klor″di-az″ah-pok′sīd) a minor tranquilizer, $C_{16}H_{14}ClN_3O$.

chloremia (klo-re′me-ah) 1. chlorosis. 2. hyperchloremia.

chloretic (klo-ret′ik) an agent which accelerates the flow of bile.

chlorhexidine (-hek′sĭ-dēn) an antibacterial, $C_{22}H_{30}Cl_2N_{10}$, effective against a wide variety of gram-negative and gram-positive organisms.

chlorhydria (-hi′dre-ah) an excess of hydrochloric acid in the stomach.

chloride (klo′rīd) a salt of hydrochloric acid; any binary compound of chlorine in which the latter is the negative element. **ferric c.,** $FeCl_3\cdot 6H_2O$; used as a reagent and topically as an astringent and styptic.

chloridorrhea (klor″īd-ah-re′ah) diarrhea with an excess of chlorides in the stool.

chlorinated (klo′rĭ-nat″id) charged with chlorine.

chlorine (klo′rēn) chemical element (*see table*), at. no. 17, symbol Cl.

chlorite (klo′rīt) a salt of chlorous acid; disinfectant and bleaching agent.

chlormerodrin (klor-mĕ′rah-drin) a mercurial diuretic, $C_5H_{11}ClHgN_2O_2$. **c. Hg 197,** chlormerodrin tagged with radioactive mercury (^{197}Hg); used as a diagnostic aid in renal function determination. **c. Hg 203,** chlormerodrin tagged with radioactive mercury (^{203}Hg); used as a diagnostic aid in renal function determination.

chlormezanone (-mez′ah-nōn) a muscle relaxant and tranquilizer, $C_{11}H_{12}ClNO_3S$.

chloroform (klo′rah-form) a colorless, mobile liquid, $CHCl_3$, with ethereal odor and sweet taste, used as a solvent; once widely used as an inhalation anesthetic and analgesic, and as an antitussive, carminative, and counterirritant.

chlorolabe (klor′ah-lāb) the pigment in retinal cones that is more sensitive to the green portion of the spectrum than are the other pigments (cyanolabe and erythrolabe).

chloroleukemia (klo″ro-loo-ke′me-ah) myelogenous leukemia in which no specific tumor masses are observed at autopsy, but the body organs and fluids show a definite green color.

chloroma (klo-ro′mah) a malignant, green-colored tumor arising from myeloid tissue.

Chloromycetin (klo″ro-mi-sēt′in) trademark for preparations of chloramphenicol.

chloromyeloma (-mi″ah-lo′mah) chloroma with multiple growths in bone marrow.

chlorophenol (klo″ro-fe′nol) a topical antiseptic, $C_6H_4Cl\cdot OH$, prepared by the action of chlorine on phenol.

chlorophyll (klo′rah-fil) any of a group of green pigments containing a magnesium-porphyrin complex that are involved in oxygen-producing photosynthesis. Preparations of water-soluble chlorophyll derivatives are applied topically for deodorization of skin lesions and administered orally to deodorize ulcerative lesions and the urine and feces in colostomy, ileostomy, or incontinence.

chloroplast (-plast) any of the chlorophyll-bearing bodies of plant cells.

chloroprivic (klo″ro-pri′vik) deprived of chlorides; due to loss of chlorides.

chloroprocaine (-pro′kān) a local anesthetic, $C_{13}H_{19}ClN_2O_2$, used as the hydrochloride salt.

chloropsia (klo-rop′se-ah) defect of vision in which objects appear to have a greenish tinge.

chloroquine (klo′rah-kwin) an antimalarial and lupus erythematosus suppressant, $C_{18}H_{26}ClN_3$.

chlorosis (klo-ro′sis) a once common disorder that usually affected adolescent females, and was believed to be associated with iron deficiency anemia, and characterized by greenish yellow discoloration of the skin and by hypochromic erythrocytes. **chlorot′ic,** adj.

chlorothiazide (klo″ro-thi′ah-zīd) a diuretic and antihypertensive, $C_7H_6ClN_3O_4S_2$.

chlorotrianisene (-tri-an′ĭ-sēn) a long-acting synthetic estrogen, $C_{23}H_{21}ClO_3$, used for treatment of vasomotor symptoms or urogenital atrophy associated with menopause and for palliative treatment of prostatic carcinoma.

chloroxine (klo-rok′sēn) an antibacterial, $C_9H_5-Cl_2NO$, used in the topical treatment of dandruff and seborrheic dermatitis of the scalp.

chlorpheniramine (klor″fen-ir′ah-mēn) an antihistaminic, $C_{16}H_{19}ClN_2$, used as the maleate salt.

chlorphenesin carbamate (klor-fen′ah-sin) a centrally acting skeletal muscle relaxant, $C_{10}-H_{12}ClNO_4$, used in skeletal muscle spasms and trauma to tendons and ligaments.

chlorphenoxamine (klor″fen-ok′sah-mēn) a compound, $C_{18}H_{22}ClNO$, used as the hydrochloride salt to reduce muscular rigidity in parkinsonism.

chlorphentermine (klor-fen″ter-mēn) a sympathomimetic amine, $C_{10}H_{14}ClN$, used as an anorexic agent.

chlorpromazine (-pro′mah-zēn) a phenothiazine derivative, $C_{17}H_{19}ClN_2S$, used as an antiemetic and tranquilizer.

chlorpropamide (-pro′pah-mīd) an oral hypoglycemic, $C_{10}H_{13}ClN_2O_3S$.

chlorprothixene (klor″-pro-thik′sēn) a major tranquilizer, $C_{18}H_{18}ClNS$.

chlortetracycline (-tĕ-trah-si′klēn) an antibiotic obtained from *Streptomyces aureofaciens;* the hydrochloride salt is used as an antibacterial and antiprotozoal.

chlorthalidone (klor-thal′ĭ-dōn) a diuretic, C_{14}-$H_{11}ClN_2O_4S$.

Chlor-Trimeton (-tri′mĕ-ton) trademark for preparations of chlorpheniramine.

chloruresis (klor″ūr-e′sis) excretion of chlorides in the urine. **chloruret′ic,** adj.

chloruria (klo-rūr-e-ah) excess chlorides in the urine.

chlorzoxazone (klor-zok′sah-zōn) a skeletal muscle relaxant, $C_7H_4ClNO_2$.

Ch.M. [L.] *Chirur′giae Magis′ter* (Master of Surgery).

choana (ko-a′nah), pl. *choa′nae* [L.] 1. any funnel-shaped cavity or infundibulum. 2. [pl.] the paired openings between the nasal cavity and the nasopharynx.

Choanotaenia (ko-a″no-te′ne-ah) a genus of tapeworms, including *C. infundi′bulum,* an important parasite of chickens and turkeys.

choke (chōk) 1. to interrupt respiration by obstruction or compression, or the resulting condition. 2. [pl.] a burning sensation in the substernal region, with uncontrollable coughing, occurring during decompression.

chol(o)- word element [Gr.], *bile.*

cholagogue (ko′lah-gog) an agent that stimulates gallbladder contraction to promote bile flow. **cholagog′ic,** adj.

cholangeitis (ko-lan″je-īt′is) cholangitis.

cholangiectasis (-ek′tah-sis) dilatation of a bile duct.

cholangiocarcinoma (ko-lan″je-o-kar″sĭ-no′mah) cholangiocellular carcinoma.

cholangioenterostomy (-en″ter-os′tah-me) surgical anastomosis of a bile duct to the intestine.

cholangiogastrostomy (-gas-tros′tah-me) anastomosis of a bile duct to the stomach.

cholangiography (kol-an″je-og′rah-fe) radiography of the bile ducts.

cholangiohepatoma (kol-an″je-o-hep″ah-to′-mah) primary carcinoma of the liver of mixed liver cell and bile duct cell origin.

cholangiole (kol-an′je-ōl) one of the fine terminal elements of the bile duct system. **cholangi′olar,** adj.

cholangiolitis (kol-an″je-o-līt′is) inflammation of the cholangioles. **cholangiolit′ic,** adj.

cholangioma (-o′mah) cholangiocellular carcinoma.

cholangiostomy (kol″an-je-os′tah-me) fistulization of a bile duct.

cholangiotomy (-ot′ah-me) incision into a bile duct.

cholangitis (kol″an-jīt′is) inflammation of a bile duct. **cholangit′ic,** adj.

cholanopoiesis (kol″ah-no-poi-e′sis) the synthesis of bile acids or of their conjugates and salts by the liver.

cholanopoietic (-poi-et′ik) 1. promoting chola-

nopoiesis. 2. an agent that promotes cholanopoiesis.

cholate (ko′lāt) a salt or ester of cholic acid.

chole- word element [Gr.], *bile.*

cholecalciferol (ko″le-kal-sif′er-ol) vitamin D_3, an oil-soluble antirachitic vitamin.

cholecyst (ko′lah-sist) the gallbladder.

cholecystagogue (ko″lah-sis′tah-gog) an agent that promotes evacuation of the gallbladder.

cholecystalgia (-sis-tal′je-ah) biliary colic.

cholecystectasia (-sis″tek-ta′ze-ah) distention of the gallbladder.

cholecystectomy (-sis-tek′tah-me) excision of the gallbladder.

cholecystenterostomy (-sis″ten-ter-os′tah-me) formation of a new communication between the gallbladder and the intestine.

cholecystis (-sis′tis) the gallbladder. **cholecys′tic,** adj.

cholecystitis (-sis-tīt′is) inflammation of the gallbladder. **emphysematous c.,** that due to gas-producing organisms, marked by gas in the gallbladder lumen, often infiltrating into the gallbladder wall and surrounding tissues.

cholecystocolostomy (-sis″to-ko-los′tah-me) anastomosis of the gallbladder and colon.

cholecystoduodenostomy (-doo″o-dah-nos′tah-me) anastomosis of the gallbladder and duodenum.

cholecystogastrostomy (-gas-tros′tah-me) anastomosis between the gallbladder and stomach.

cholecystogram (-sis′tah-gram) a roentgenogram of the gallbladder.

cholecystography (-sis-tog′rah-fe) roentgenography of the gallbladder. **cholecystograph′ic,** adj.

cholecystojejunostomy (-sis″to-je-joo-nos′tah-me) anastomosis of the gallbladder and jejunum.

cholecystokinetic (-ki-net′ik) stimulating contraction of the gallbladder.

cholecystokinin (-kin′in) a polypeptide hormone secreted in the small intestine that stimulates gallbladder contraction and secretion of pancreatic enzymes.

cholecystolithiasis (-lĭ-thi′ah-sis) cholelithiasis.

cholecystopexy (-sis′tah-pek″se) surgical suspension or fixation of the gallbladder.

cholecystorrhaphy (-sis-tor′ah-fe) suture or repair of the gallbladder.

cholecystostomy (-sis-tos′tah-me) the creation of an opening into the gallbladder for drainage.

cholecystotomy (-sis-tot′ah-me) incision of the gallbladder.

choledochal (kol′ah-dok'l) pertaining to the common bile duct.

choledochectomy (kol″ah-do-kek′tah-me) excision of part of the common bile duct.

choledochitis (-kīt′is) inflammation of the common bile duct.

choledocho- word element [Gr.], *common bile duct.*

choledochoduodenostomy (kol-ed″o-kah-doo″

od-in-os′tah-me) surgical anastomosis of the common bile duct to the duodenum.

choledochoenterostomy (-en″ter-os′tah-me) anastomosis of the bile duct to the intestine.

choledochogastrostomy (-gas-tros′tah-me) anastomosis of the bile duct to the stomach.

choledochojejunostomy (-je-joo-nos′tah-me) anastomosis of the bile duct to the jejunum.

choledocholithiasis (-lĭ-thi′ah-sis) calculi in the common bile duct.

choledocholithotomy (-lĭ-thot′ah-me) incision into common bile duct for removal of stone.

choledochoplasty (kol-ed′ah-kah-plas″te) plastic repair of the common bile duct.

choledochorrhaphy (kol-ed″o-kor′ah-fe) suture or repair of the common bile duct.

choledochostomy (-kos′tah-me) creation of an opening into the common bile duct for drainage.

choledochotomy (-kot′ah-me) incision into the common bile duct.

choledochus (kol-ed′ah-kus) the common bile duct.

Choledyl (kōl′ah-dil) trademark for a preparation of oxtriphylline.

choleic (ko-le′ik) pertaining to the bile.

cholelith (ko′lah-lith) gallstone.

cholelithiasis (ko″le-lĭ-thi′ah-sis) the presence or formation of gallstones.

cholelithotomy (-lĭ-thot′ah-me) incision of the biliary tract for removal of gallstones.

cholelithotripsy (-lith′ah-trip″se) crushing of a gallstone.

cholemesis (ko-lem′ĕ-sis) vomiting of bile.

cholemia (ko-le′me-ah) bile or bile pigment in the blood. **chole′mic,** adj.

choleperitoneum (ko″le-per″ĭ-tah-ne′um) the presence of bile in the peritoneum.

cholepoiesis (-poi-e′sis) the formation of bile in the liver. **cholepoiet′ic,** adj.

cholera (kol′er-ah) Asiatic cholera; an acute infectious disease endemic and epidemic in Asia, caused by *Vibrio cholerae,* marked by severe diarrhea with extreme fluid and electrolyte depletion, and by vomiting, muscle cramps, and prostration. **Asiatic c.,** see *cholera.* **chicken c.,** see *fowl c.* **fowl c.,** hemorrhagic septicemia due to *Pasteurella multocida,* affecting all domestic fowl and other fowl worldwide. **hog c.,** an acute, highly infectious, fatal viral disease of swine. **pancreatic c.,** a condition marked by profuse watery diarrhea, hypokalemia, and usually achlorhydria, and due to an islet-cell tumor (other than beta cell) of the pancreas.

choleragen (kol′er-ah-jen) the exotoxin produced by the cholera vibrio, thought to stimulate electrolyte and water secretion into the small intestine.

choleraic (kol″ah-ra′ik) of, pertaining to, or of the nature of cholera.

choleresis (ko-ler′ĕ-sis) the secretion of bile by the liver.

choleretic (ko″ler-et′ik) stimulating bile production by the liver; an agent that so acts.

choleria (ko-ler′e-ah) an irritable or hostile temperament.

cholerine (kol′er-ēn) 1. the earliest stage of cholera. 2. a relatively mild form of cholera.

choleroid (-oid) resembling cholera.

cholestasis (ko″lah-sta′sis) stoppage or suppression of bile flow, having intrahepatic or extrahepatic causes. **cholestat′ic,** adj.

cholesteatoma (-ste″ah-to′mah) a cystlike mass with a lining of stratified squamous epithelium filled with desquamating debris frequently including cholesterol, which occurs in the meninges, central nervous system, and bones of the skull, but most commonly in the middle ear and mastoid region.

cholesteatosis (-ste-ah-to′sis) fatty degeneration due to cholesterol esters.

cholesterol (ko-les′ter-ol) a fatlike steroid alcohol, $C_{27}H_{45}OH$, found in animal fats, bile, blood, brain tissue, milk, egg yolk, myelin sheaths of nerve fibers, liver, kidneys, and adrenal glands. It constitutes a large part of most gallstones and occurs in atheroma of the arteries, in various cysts, and in carcinomatous tissue. Most of the body's cholesterol is synthesized in the liver, but some is absorbed from the diet. It is a precursor of bile acids and is important in the synthesis of steroid hormones.

cholesterolemia (ko-les″ter-ol-e′me-ah) hypercholesterolemia.

cholesterolosis (-o′sis) cholesterosis.

cholesteroluria (-ūr′e-ah) the presence of cholesterol in the urine.

cholesterosis (ko-les″ter-o′sis) abnormal deposition of cholesterol in tissues.

choletherapy (ko″le-ther′ah-pe) treatment by administration of bile salts.

choleuria (-ūr′e-ah) choluria.

cholic acid (ko′lik) an acid, $C_{24}H_{40}O_5$, formed in the liver from cholesterol; it plays, with other bile acids, an important role in digestion.

choline (ko′lēn) a quaternary amine, $HOCH_2$-$CH_2N(CH_3)_3{}^+$, which occurs in the phospholipid phosphatidylcholine and the neurotransmitter acetylcholine, and is an important methyl donor in intermediary metabolism. Choline is a lipotropic agent, a substance that decreases liver fat content by increasing phospholipid turnover. **c. acetylase, c. acetyltransferase,** an enzyme that brings about the synthesis of acetylcholine. **c. magnesium trisalicylate,** a combination of choline salicylate and magnesium salicylate, used as an antiarthritic. **c. salicylate,** the choline salt of salicylic acid, $C_{12}H_{19}$-NO_4, having analgesic, antipyretic, and anti-inflammatory properties.

cholinergic (ko″lin-er′jik) parasympathomimetic: activated or transmitted by choline (acetylcholine); said of nerve fibers that liberate acetylcholine at a synapse when a nerve impulse passes, i.e., the parasympathetic fibers. Also, an agent that produces such an effect.

cholinesterase (-es′ter-ās) 1. an enzyme that catalyzes the hydrolysis of acylcholine to choline and an anion. 2. acetylcholinesterase.

cholinoceptive (ko″lin-o-sep′tiv) pertaining to the sites on effector organs that are acted upon by cholinergic transmitters.

cholinoceptor (-sep′ter) cholinergic receptor.

cholinolytic (-lit′ik) 1. blocking the action of acetylcholine, or of cholinergic agents. 2. an agent that blocks the action of acetylcholine in cholinergic areas, i.e., organs supplied by parasympathetic nerves, and voluntary muscles.

cholinomimetic (-mi-met′ik) having an action similar to acetylcholine; parasympathomimetic.

choluria (ko-lu′re-ah) the presence of bile in the urine; discoloration of the urine with bile pigments. **cholu′ric**, adj.

cholylglycine (ko″lil-gli′sēn) a conjugated form of one of the bile acids that yields glycine and cholic acid on hydrolysis.

chondr(o)- word element [Gr.], *cartilage.*

chondral (kon′dril) pertaining to cartilage.

chondralgia (kon-dral′je-ah) pain in a cartilage.

chondrectomy (kon-drek′tah-me) surgical removal of a cartilage.

chondrio- word element [Gr.], *cartilage; granule.*

chondritis (kon-drīt′is) inflammation of a cartilage.

chondroadenoma (kon″dro-ad″in-o′mah) adenochondroma.

chondroangioma (-an″je-o′mah) a benign mesenchymoma containing chondromatous and angiomatous elements.

chondroblast (kon′dro-blast) an immature cartilage-producing cell.

chondroblastoma (kon″dro-blas-to′mah) a benign tumor arising from young chondroblasts in the epiphysis of a bone.

chondrocalcinosis (-kal″sĭ-no′sis) the presence of calcium salts, especially calcium pyrophosphate, in the cartilaginous structures of one or more joints; when accompanied by attacks of goutlike symptoms, it is known as *pseudogout.*

chondrocostal (kon″dro-kos′til) pertaining to the ribs and costal cartilages.

chondrocranium (-kra′ne-um) the cartilaginous cranial structure of the embryo.

chondrocyte (kon′dro-sīt) a mature cartilage cell embedded in a lacuna within the cartilage matrix.

chondrodermatitis (kon″dro-der″mah-tīt′is) an inflammatory process affecting cartilage and skin; used to mean *c. nodula′ris chron′ica hel′i-cis,* a condition marked by a painful nodule on the helix of the ear.

chondrodynia (-din′e-ah) pain in a cartilage.

chondrodysplasia (-dis-pla′ze-ah) enchondromatosis. **c. puncta′ta,** a heterogeneous group of hereditary bone dysplasias, the common characteristic of which is stippling of the epiphyses in infancy.

chondrodystrophia (-dis-tro′fe-ah) chondrodystrophy. **c. feta′lis,** achondroplasia.

chondrodystrophy (-dis′trah-fe) a disorder of cartilage formation.

chondroepiphysitis (-ep″ĭ-fiz-īt′is) inflammation involving the epiphyseal cartilages.

chondrofibroma (-fi-bro′mah) a fibroma with cartilaginous elements.

chondrogenesis (-jen′ĭ-sis) formation of cartilage.

chondroid (kon′droid) resembling cartilage.

chondroitin (kon-dro′ĭ-tin) a mucopolysaccharide, $C_{18}H_{27}NO_{14}$; its sulfate ester is widespread in connective tissue, particularly cartilage, and in the cornea.

chondrolipoma (kon″dro-lĭ-po′mah) a benign tumor with cartilaginous and fatty tissue.

chondroma (kon-dro′mah) a tumor or tumor-like growth of cartilage cells. **joint c.,** a mass of cartilage in the synovial membrane of a joint. **c. sarcomato′sum,** chondrosarcoma. **synovial c.,** a cartilaginous body formed in a synovial membrane.

chondromalacia (kon″dro-mah-la′she-ah) abnormal softening of cartilage.

chondromatosis (-mah-to′sis) formation of multiple chondromas. **synovial c.,** a rare condition in which cartilage is formed in the synovial membrane of joints, tendon sheaths, or bursae, sometimes becoming detached and producing a number of loose bodies.

chondromere (kon′dro-mēr) a cartilaginous vertebra of the fetal vertebral column.

chondrometaplasia (kon″dro-met″ah-pla′ze-ah) a condition characterized by metaplastic activity of the chondroblasts.

chondromyoma (-mi-o′mah) a benign tumor of myomatous and cartilaginous elements.

chondromyxoma (-mik-so′mah) myxoma with cartilaginous elements.

chondromyxosarcoma (-mik″so-sar-ko′mah) a sarcoma containing cartilaginous and mucous tissue.

chondro-osseous (-os′e-us) composed of cartilage and bone.

chondro-osteodystrophy (-os″te-o-dis′trah-fe) Morquio's syndrome.

chondropathy (kon-drop′ah-the) disease of cartilage.

chondrophyte (kon′dro-fīt) a cartilaginous growth at the articular extremity of a bone.

chondroplasia (kon″dro-pla′ze-ah) the formation of cartilage by specialized cells (chondrocytes).

chondroplast (kon′dro-plast) chondroblast.

chondroplasty (-plas″te) plastic repair of cartilage.

chondroporosis (kon″dro-por-o′sis) the formation of sinuses or spaces in cartilage.

chondrosarcoma (-sar-ko′ma) a malignant tumor derived from cartilage cells or their precursors. **central c.,** one within a bone.

chondrosis (kon-dro′sis) cartilage formation.

chondrosteoma (kon″dros-te-o′mah) osteochondroma.

chondrosternoplasty (-stern′o-plas″te) surgical correction of funnel chest.

chondrotomy (kon-drot′ah-me) the dissection or surgical division of cartilage.

chondroxiphoid (kon″dro-zi′foid) pertaining to the xiphoid process.

chonechondrosternon (ko″ne-kon″dro-stern′on) funnel chest.

chord (kord) cord.

chorda (kor′dah), pl. *chor′dae* [L.] a cord or

sinew. **chor′dal,** adj. **c. dorsa′lis,** notochord. **c. guberna′culum,** gubernacular cord; a portion of the gubernaculum testis or of the round ligament of the uterus that develops in the inguinal crest and adjoining body wall. **c. mag′na,** Achilles tendon. **chor′dae tendi′neae,** tendinous cords connecting the two atrioventricular valves to the appropriate papillary muscles in the heart ventricles. **c. tym′pani,** a nerve originating from the intermediate nerve, distributed to the submandibular, sublingual, and lingual glands and anterior two-thirds of the tongue; it is a parasympathetic and special senory nerve. **c. umbilica′lis,** umbilical cord. **c. voca′lis,** see *vocal cords.* **chor′dae willis′ii,** Willis' cords.

Chordata (kor-dāt′ah) a phylum of the animal kingdom comprising all animals having a notochord during some developmental stage.

chordate (kor′dāt) 1. an animal of the Chordata. 2. having a notochord.

chordee (kor′de) downward deflection of the penis, due to a congenital anomaly or to urethral infection.

chorditis (kor-dīt′is) inflammation of the vocal or the spermatic cords.

chordoma (kor-do′mah) a malignant tumor arising from the embryonic remains of the notochord.

chordoskeleton (kor′′do-skel′it-in) the part of the skeleton formed about the notochord.

chordotomy (kor-dot′ah-me) cordotomy (2).

chorea (kor-e′ah) the ceaseless occurrence of rapid, jerky involuntary movements. **chore′ic,** adj. **acute c.,** Sydenham's c. **chronic c.,** Huntington's c. **hereditary c., Huntington's c.,** a hereditary disease marked by chronic progressive chorea and mental deterioration. **Sydenham's c.,** a self-limited disorder, occurring between the ages of 5 and 15, or during pregnancy, linked with rheumatic fever, and marked by involuntary movements that gradually become severe, affecting all motor activities.

choreiform (kor-e′ĭ-form) resembling chorea.

choreoathetosis (kor′′e-o-ath′′ah-to′sis) a condition characterized by choreic and athetoid movements. **choreoath′etoid,** adj.

choreophrasia (-fra′ze-ah) meaningless repetition of words or phrases.

chorioadenoma (-ad′′in-o′mah) adenoma of the chorion. **c. destru′ens,** a hydatidiform mole in which molar chorionic villi enter the myometrium or parametrium or, rarely, are transported to distant sites, most often the lungs.

chorioallantois (-ah-lan′to-is) an extraembryonic structure formed by union of the chorion and allantois, which by means of vessels in the associated mesoderm serves in gas exchange. In reptiles and birds, it is a membrane apposed to the shell; in many mammals, it forms the placenta. **chorioallanto′ic,** adj.

chorioamnionitis (-am′′ne-o-nīt′is) inflammation of fetal membranes.

chorioangioma (-an′′je-o′mah) an angioma of the chorion.

choriocapillaris (-kap′′ĭ-la′ris) lamina choriocapillaris.

choriocarcinoma (-kar′′sĭ-no′mah) a malignant neoplasm of trophoblastic cells, formed by abnormal proliferation of the placental epithelium, without production of chorionic villi.

choriocele (kor′e-o-sēl′′) protrusion of the chorion through an aperture.

chorioepithelioma (kor′′e-o-ep′′ĭ-the′′le-o′mah) choriocarcinoma.

choriogenesis (-jen′ĭ-sis) the development of the chorion.

chorioid (kor′e-oid) choroid.

chorioma (kor′′e-o′mah) any trophoblastic proliferation, benign or malignant.

choriomeningitis (kor′′e-o-men′′in-jīt′is) cerebral meningitis with lymphocytic infiltration of the choroid plexus. **lymphocytic c.,** viral meningitis, occurring in adults between the ages of 20 and 40, during the fall and winter.

chorion (ko′re-on) the outermost of the fetal membranes, composed of trophoblast lined with mesoderm; it develops villi, becomes vascularized by allantoic vessels, and forms the fetal part of the placenta. **chorion′ic,** adj. **c. frondo′sum,** the part of chorion covered by villi. **c. lae′ve,** the nonvillous, membranous part of the chorion. **shaggy c.,** c. frondosum.

Chorioptes (ko′′re-op′tēz) a genus of parasitic mites infesting domestic animals and causing a kind of mange.

chorioretinal (kor′′e-o-ret′in-il) pertaining to the choroid and retina.

chorioretinitis (-ret′′ĭ-nīt′is) inflammation of the choroid and retina.

chorioretinopathy (-ret′′in-op′ah-the) a noninflammatory process involving both the choroid and retina.

chorista (ko-ris′tah) defective development due to, or marked by, a displaced primordium.

choristoma (ko′′ris-to′mah) a mass of histologically normal tissue in an abnormal location.

choroid (ko′roid) the middle, vascular coat of the eye, between the sclera and the retina. **choroid′al,** adj.

choroidea (ko-roi′de-ah) choroid.

choroideremia (ko-roi′′der-e′me-ah) an X-linked primary choroidal degeneration which, in males, eventually leads to blindness as degeneration of the retinal pigment epithelium progresses to complete atrophy; in females, it is nonprogressive and vision is usually normal.

choroiditis (ko′′roi-dīt′is) inflammation of the choroid.

choroidocyclitis (ko-roi′′do-sik-līt′is) inflammation of the choroid and ciliary processes.

chrom(o)- word element [Gr.], *color.*

chromaffin (kro-maf′in) staining strongly with chromium salts, as certain cells of the adrenal glands, along sympathetic nerves, etc.

chromaffinoma (kro-maf′′ĭ-no′mah) 1. any tumor containing chromaffin cells. 2. pheochromocytoma.

chromaffinopathy (-nop′ah-the) disease of the chromaffin system.

chromat(o)- word element [Gr.], *color; chromatin.*

chromate (kro′māt) any salt of chromic acid.

chromatic (kro-mat′ik) 1. pertaining to color; stainable with dyes. 2. pertaining to chromatin.

chromatid (kro′mah-tid) either of two parallel, spiral filaments joined at the centromere which make up a chromosome.

chromatin (kro′mah-tin) the substance of chromosomes, the portion of the cell nucleus that stains with basic dyes. See *euchromatin* and *heterochromatin.* **sex c.,** Barr body; the persistent mass of the inactivated X chromosome in cells of normal females.

chromatin-negative (kro″mah-tin-neg′ah-tiv) lacking sex chromatin, a characteristic of the nuclei of cells in a normal male.

chromatin-positive (-poz′it-iv) containing sex chromatin, a characteristic of the nuclei of cells in a normal female.

chromatism (kro′mah-tizm) abnormal pigment deposits.

chromatogenous (kro″mah-toj′i-nus) producing color or coloring matter.

chromatography (kro″mah-tog′rah-fe) a method of separating and identifying the components of a complex mixture by differential movement through a two-phase system, in which the movement is effected by a flow of a liquid or a gas (mobile phase) which percolates through an adsorbent (stationary phase) or a second liquid phase. **chromatograph′ic** adj. **adsorption c.,** that in which the stationary phase is an adsorbent. **column c.,** that in which the various solutes of a solution are allowed to travel down an absorptive column, the individual components being absorbed by the stationary phase. **gas c. (GC),** that in which an inert gas moves the vapors of the materials to be separated through a column of inert material. **gas-liquid c. (GLC),** gas chromatography in which the sorbent is a nonvolatile liquid coated on a solid support. **gas-solid c. (GSC),** gas chromatography in which the sorbent is an inert porous solid. **gel-filtration c., gel-permeation c.,** exclusion c. **ion-exchange c.,** that using resins to which are coupled either cations or anions that will exchange with other cations or anions in the material passed through their meshwork. **molecular sieve c.,** exclusion c. **paper c.,** that using a sheet of blotting paper, usually filter paper, for the adsorption column. **partition c.,** a method using the partition of the solutes between two liquid phases (the original solvent and the film of solvent on the adsorption column). **thin-layer c.,** chromatography through a thin layer of inert material, such as cellulose.

chromatolysis (kro″mah-tol′i-sis) disintegration of Nissl bodies of a neuron as a result of injury, fatigue, or exhaustion.

chromatophil (kro-mat′ah-fil) a cell or structure which stains easily. **chromatophil′ic,** adj.

chromatophore (-for) any pigmentary cell or color-producing plastid.

chromatopsia (kro″mah-top′se-ah) a visual defect in which (*a*) colorless objects appear to be tinged with color, or (*b*) colors are imperfectly perceived.

chromatoptometry (kro″mah-top-tom′i-tre) measurement of color perception.

chromaturia (kro″mah-tūr′e-ah) abnormal coloration of the urine.

chromesthesia (kro″mes-the′ze-ah) association of imaginary color sensations with actual sensations of taste, hearing, or smell.

chromhidrosis (kro″mĭ-dro′sis) secretion of colored sweat.

chromic acid (kro-mik) a dibasic acid, H_2CrO_4.

chromidrosis (kro″mĭ-dro′sis) chromhidrosis.

chromium (kro′me-um) chemical element (*see table*), at. no. 24, symbol Cr. **c.-51,** a radioisotope of chromium having a half-life of 27.8 days; used to label red blood cells to determine red cell volume and red cell survival time. Symbol ^{51}Cr. **c. oxide,** a substance used in dentistry as a polishing agent, especially for stainless steel. **c. trioxide,** chromic acid.

Chromobacterium (kro″mo-bak-tēr′e-um) a genus of schizomycetes (family Rhizobiaceae) that characteristically produce a violet pigment.

chromoblast (kro′mo-blast) an embryonic cell which develops into a pigment cell.

chromoblastomycosis (kro″mo-blas″to-mi-ko′-sis) chromomycosis.

chromoclastogenic (-klas″tah-jen′ik) inducing chromosomal disruption or damage.

chromocyte (kro′mah-sīt) any colored cell or pigmented corpuscle.

chromocystoscopy (kro″mo-sis-tos′kah-pe) cystoscopy of the ureteral orifices after oral administration of a dye which is excreted in the urine.

chromodacryorrhea (-dak″re-or-e′ah) the shedding of bloody tears.

chromogen (kro′mah-jen) any substance giving origin to a coloring matter.

chromogenesis (kro″mo-jen′ĭ-sis) the formation of color or pigment.

chromomere (kro′mo-mēr) 1. any of the bead-like granules occurring in series along a chromonema. 2. granulomere.

chromomycosis (kro″mo-mi-ko′sis) a chronic fungal infection of the skin, producing wartlike nodules or papillomas that may ulcerate.

chromonema (-ne′mah), pl. *chromone′mata.* The central thread of a chromatid, along which lie the chromomeres. **chromone′mal,** adj.

chromophil (kro′mo-fil) any easily stainable cell or tissue. **chromophil′ic,** adj.

chromophobe (-fōb) any cell or tissue not readily stainable, applied especially to the chromophobe cells of the anterior pituitary gland.

chromophobia (kro″mo-fo′be-ah) the quality of staining poorly with dyes. **chromopho′bic,** adj.

chromophore (kro′mo-for) any chemical group whose presence gives a decided color to a compound and which unites with certain other groups (auxochromes) to form dyes.

chromophoric (kro″mo-for′ik) 1. bearing color. 2. pertaining to a chromophore.

chromophose (kro′mo-fōs) sensation of color.

chromoscopy (kro-mos′kah-pe) diagnosis of renal function by color of the urine after administration of dyes. **gastric c.,** diagnosis of gastric function by the color of the gastric contents; a test for achylia gastrica.

chromosome (kro′mah-sōm) in animal cells, a structure in the nucleus containing a linear thread of DNA which transmits genetic information and is associated with RNA and histones; during cell division the material composing the chromosome is compactly coiled, making it visible with appropriate staining and permitting its movement in the cell with minimal entanglement; each organism of a species is normally characterized by the same number of chromosomes in its somatic cells, 46 being the number normally present in man, including the two (XX or XY) which determine the sex of the organism. In bacterial genetics, a closed circle of double-stranded DNA which contains the genetic material of the cell and is attached to the cell membrane; the bulk of this material forms a compact bacterial nucleus. **chromoso′mal,** adj. **bivalent c.,** see *bivalent* (2). **homologous c′s,** a matching pair of chromosomes, one from each parent, with the same gene loci in the same order. **Ph¹ c., Philadelphia c.,** an abnormality of chromosome 22, characterized by shortening of its long arms (the missing portion probably translocated to chromosome 9) and present in marrow cells of patients with chronic myelocytic leukemia. **ring c.,** a chromosome in which both ends have been lost (deletion) and the two broken ends have reunited to form a ring-shaped figure. **sex c′s,** those associated with sex determination, in mammals constituting an unequal pair, the X and the Y chromosome. **somatic c.,** autosome. **X c.,** a sex chromosome, carried by half the male gametes and all female gametes; female diploid cells have two X chromosomes. **Y c.,** a sex chromosome, carried by half the male gametes and none of the female gametes; male diploid cells have an X and a Y chromosome.

chron(o)- word element [Gr.], *time.*

chronaxie, chronaxy (kro′nak-se) the minimum time an electric current must flow at a voltage twice the rheobase to cause a muscle to contract.

chronic (kron′ik) persisting for a long time.

chronobiology (kron″o-bi-ol′ah-je) the scientific study of the effect of time on living systems and of biological rhythms. **chronobiolog′ic, chronobiolog′ical,** adj.

chronognosis (kron″og-no′sis) perception of the lapse of time.

chronograph (kron′ah-graf) an instrument for recording small intervals of time.

chronotaraxis (kron″o-tar-ak′sis) disorientation in relation to time.

chronotropism (kro-nah′trah-pizm) interference with regularity of a periodical movement, such as the heart's action. **chronotro′pic,** adj.

chrys(o)- word element [Gr.], *gold.*

chrysiasis (krĭ-si′ah-sis) deposition of gold in living tissue.

chrysoderma (kris″o-der′mah) permanent pigmentation of the skin due to gold deposit.

Chrysomyia (-mi′yah) a genus of flies whose lar-

vae may be secondary invaders of wounds or internal parasites of man.

Chrysops (kris′ops) a genus of bloodsucking tropical flies, the grove flies, including *C. disca′- lis,* a vector of tularemia in the western United States, and *C. sila′cea,* an intermediate host of *Loa loa.*

chylangioma (ki-lan″je-o′mah) a tumor of intestinal lymph vessels filled with chyle.

chyle (kīl) the milky fluid taken up by the lacteals from food in the intestine, consisting of lymph and triglyceride fat (chylomicrons) in a stable emulsion, and passed into the veins by the thoracic duct, becoming mixed with blood.

chylectasia (ki″lek-ta′ze-ah) dilatation of a chylous vessel, e.g., a lacteal.

chylemia (ki-le′me-ah) the presence of chyle in the blood.

chylifacient (ki″lĭ-fa′shint) forming chyle.

chyliferous (ki-lif′er-us) 1. forming chyle. 2. conveying chyle.

chylocele (ki′lo-sēl) elephantiasis scroti.

chylocyst (-sist) cisterna chyli.

chyloderma (ki″lo-der′mah) elephantiasis filariensis.

chylomediastinum (ki″lo-me″de-as-ti′num) the presence of chyle in the mediastinum.

chylomicron (-mi′kron) a stable droplet containing triglyceride fat, cholesterol, phospholipids, and protein, found in intestinal lymphatics (lacteals) and blood during and after meals.

chylomicronemia (-mi″kron-e′me-ah) an excess of chylomicrons in the blood.

chylopericardium (-per″ĭ-kar′de-um) the presence of effused chyle in the pericardium.

chyloperitoneum (-per″ĭ-ton-e′um) the presence of effused chyle in the peritoneal cavity.

chylophoric (-for′ik) conveying chyle.

chylopneumothorax (-noo″mo-thor′aks) the presence of chyle and air in the pleural cavity.

chylothorax (-thor′aks) the presence of effused chyle in the pleural cavity.

chylous (ki′lus) pertaining, mingled with, or of the nature of chyle.

chyluria (kīl-ūr′e-ah) the presence of chyle in the urine, giving it a milky appearance, due to obstruction between the intestinal lymphatics and the thoracic duct, which causes rupture of renal lymphatics into the renal tubules.

chyme (kim) the semifluid, creamy material produced by digestion of food.

chymification (ki″mĭ-fĭ-ka′shin) conversion of food into chyme; gastric digestion.

chymodenin (ki″mo-de′nin) a polypeptide secreted by the duodenum that specifically stimulates pancreatic secretion of chymotrypsinogen.

chymopapain (-pah-pa′in) a proteolytic enzyme (a sulfhydryl proteinase) from the tropical tree *Carica papaya,* used in chemonucleolysis.

chymotrypsin (-trip′sin) an endopeptidase with action similar to that of trypsin, produced in the intestine by activation of chymotrypsinogen by trypsin; a product crystallized from an extract of the pancreas of the ox is used clinically for enzymatic zonulolysis and debridement.

chymotrypsinogen (-trip-sin′ah-jen) the inactive precursor of chymotrypsin, the form in which it is secreted by the pancreas.

C.I. Colour Index.

Ci abbreviation for *curie* recommended by the International Commission on Radiological Units and Measurements.

cib. [L.] *ci'bus* (food).

cicatrectomy (sik″ah-trek′tah-me) excision of a cicatrix.

cicatricial (sik″ah-trish′il) pertaining to or of the nature of a cicatrix.

cicatrix (sĭ-ka′triks, sik′ah-triks), pl. *cica'trices* [L.] a scar; the fibrous tissue left after the healing of a wound. **vicious c.,** one causing deformity or impairing the function of an extremity.

cicatrization (sik″ah-tri-za′shin) the formation of a cicatrix or scar.

-cide word element [L.], *destruction or killing* (homicide); *an agent which kills or destroys* (germicide). **-ci′dal,** adj.

CIF clone-inhibiting factor.

cili(o)- word element [L.], *cilia; ciliary* (*body*).

cilia (sil′e-ah), sing. *cil'ium* [L.] 1. the eyelids or their outer edges. 2. the eyelashes. 3. minute hairlike processes that extend from a cell surface, composed of nine pairs of microtubules around a core of two microtubules. They beat rhythmically to move the cell or to move fluid or mucus over the surface.

ciliarotomy (sil″e-er-ot′ah-me) surgical division of the ciliary zone.

ciliary (sil′e-ĕ″re) pertaining to or resembling cilia; used particularly in reference to certain eye structures, as the ciliary body or muscle.

Ciliata (sil″e-a′tah) a class of protozoa (subphylum Ciliophora) whose members possess cilia throughout the life cycle; a few species are parasitic.

ciliate (sil′e-āt) 1. having cilia. 2. any individual of the Ciliophora.

ciliectomy (sil″e-ek′tah-me) 1. excision of a portion of the ciliary body. 2. excision of the portion of the eyelid containing the roots of the lashes.

Ciliophora (sil″e-of′ah-rah) a phylum of protozoa whose members possess cilia during some developmental stage and usually have two kinds of nuclei (a micro- and a macronucleus); it includes the Kinetofragminophorea, Oligohymenophorea, and Polyhymenophorea.

cilium (sil′e-um) singular of *cilia*.

Cillobacterium (sil″o-bak-tēr′e-um) in former systems of classification, a genus of bacteria of the family Lactobacillaceae, now assigned to the genus *Eubacterium*.

cillosis (sil-o′sis) spasms of the eyelid.

cimbia (sim′be-ah) a white band running across the ventral surface of the crus cerebri.

cimetidine (si-met′ĭ-dēn) an antagonist to histamine H_2 receptors, $C_{10}H_{16}N_6S$, which inhibits gastric acid secretion in response to all stimuli; used in the treatment of peptic ulcer.

Cimex (si′meks) a genus of blood-sucking insects (order Hemiptera), the bedbugs; it includes *C. boue'ti* of West Africa and South America, *C. lectula'rius*, the common bedbug of temperate regions, and *C. rotunda'tus* of the tropics.

cinchona (sin-ko′nah) the dried bark of the stem or root of various South American trees of the genus *Cinchona;* it is the source of quinine, cinchonine, and other alkaloids.

cinchonism (-nizm) toxicity due to cinchona alkaloid overdosage; symptoms are tinnitus and slight deafness, photophobia and other visual disturbances, mental dullness, depression, confusion, headache, and nausea.

cine- word element [Gr.], *movement;* see also words beginning *kine-*.

cineangiocardiography (sin″e-an″je-o-kar″-de-og′rah-fe) the photographic recording of fluoroscopic images of the heart and great vessels by motion picture techniques.

cineangiography (-an″je-og′rah-fe) the photographic recording of fluoroscopic images of the blood vessels by motion picture techniques. **radionuclide c.,** that in which a sample of human serum albumin labeled with a radioisotope (technetium-99m) is injected into the peripheral blood and then a scintillation camera records emitted radiation over the chest area, the heart movements being shown on a video tube.

cineradiography (-ra″de-og′rah-fe) the making of a motion picture record of successive images appearing on a fluoroscopic screen.

cinerea (sĭ-ne′re-ah) the gray matter of the nervous system. **cine′real,** adj.

cinesi- for words beginning thus, see those beginning *kinesi-*.

cingulectomy (sing″gu-lek′tah-me) bilateral extirpation of the anterior half of the gyrus cinguli.

cingulumotomy (sing″gu-lum-ot′ah-me) the creation of precisely placed lesions in the cingulum of the frontal lobe, for relief of intractable pain.

cingulum (sing′gu-lum), pl. *cin'gula* [L.] 1. an encircling structure or part; a girdle. 2. a bundle of association fibers encircling the corpus callosum close to the median plane, interrelating the cingulate and hippocampal gyri. 3. the lingual lobe of an anterior tooth. **cing′ulate,** adj.

circadian (ser″kah-de′an, ser-ka′de-an) denoting a 24-hour period; see under *rhythm*.

circinate (ser′sĭ-nāt) resembling a ring, or circle.

circle (ser′k'l) a round structure or part. **Berry's c's,** charts with circles on them for testing stereoscopic vision. **defensive c.,** the coexistence of two conditions which tend to have an antagonistic or inhibiting effect on each other. **c. of Haller,** a circle of arteries in the sclera at the site of the entrance of the optic nerve. **Minsky's c.,** a device for the graphic recording of eye lesions. **sensory c.,** a body area within which it is impossible to distinguish separately the impressions arising from two sites of stimulation. **Weber's c's,** circles on the skin delineating the distance at which two simultaneously applied points can be separately distinguished. **c. of Willis,** the anastomotic loop of vessels near the base of the brain.

circling (serk′ling) movement in a circle; a name applied to listeriosis in sheep, because of the tendency of affected animals to move in a circle.

circulation (serk″u-la′shin) movement in a regular course, as the movement of blood through the heart and blood vessels. **allantoic c.,** fetal circulation through the umbilical vessels. **collateral c.,** that carried on through secondary channels after obstruction of the principal channel supplying the part. **enterohepatic c.,** the cycle in which bile salts and other substances excreted by the liver are absorbed by the intestinal mucosa and returned to the liver via the portal circulation. **extracorporeal c.,** circulation of blood outside the body, as through an artificial kidney or a heart-lung apparatus. **fetal c.,** that propelled by the fetal heart through the fetus, umbilical cord, and placental villi. **first c.,** primitive c. **hypophyseoportal c.,** that passing from the capillaries of the median eminence of the hypothalamus into the portal vessels to the sinusoids of the adenohypophysis. **intervillous c.,** the flow of maternal blood through the intervillous space of the placenta. **lesser c.,** pulmonary c. **omphalomesenteric c.,** vitelline c. **persistent fetal c.,** pulmonary hypertension in the postnatal period secondary to right-to-left shunting of the blood through the foramen ovale and ductus arteriosus. **placental c.,** the fetal circulation; also, the maternal circulation through the intervillous space. **portal c.,** a general term denoting the circulation of blood through larger vessels from the capillaries of one organ to those of another; applied to the passage of blood from the gastrointestinal tract and spleen through the portal vein to the liver. **primitive c.,** the earliest circulation by which nutriment and oxygen are conveyed to the embryo. **pulmonary c.,** the flow of blood from the right ventricle through the pulmonary artery to the lungs, where carbon dioxide is exchanged for oxygen, and back through the pulmonary vein to the left atrium. **systemic c.,** the general circulation, carrying oxygenated blood from the left ventricle to the body tissues, and returning venous blood to the right atrium. **umbilical c.,** allantoic c. **vitelline c.,** the circulation through the blood vessels of the yolk sac.

circulus (serk′u-lus), pl. *cir′culi* [L.] a circle.

circum- word element [L.], *around.*

circumcision (serk″um-sizh′in) removal of the foreskin, or prepuce. **female c.,** incision of the fold of skin over the glans clitoridis; clitoridotomy.

circumduction (-duk′shin) circular movement of a limb or of the eye.

circumflex (serk′um-fleks) curved like a bow.

circuminsular (serk″um-in′su-ler) surrounding, situated, or occurring about the insula.

circumlental (-len′til) situated or occurring around the lens.

circumrenal (-re′nil) around the kidney.

circumscribed (serk′um-skrībd) bounded or limited; confined to a limited space.

circumstantiality (serk″um-stan″she-al′it-e) a disturbance in the flow of thought in which the patient's conversation is characterized by unnecessary elaboration of many trivial details.

circumvallate (-val′āt) surrounded by a ridge or trench, as the vallate papillae.

cirrhosis (sĭ-ro′sis) interstitial inflammation of an organ, particularly the liver; see *c. of liver.* **cirrhot′ic,** adj. **alcoholic c.,** cirrhosis in alcoholics, due to associated nutritional deficiency or chronic excessive exposure to alcohol as a hepatotoxin. **atrophic c.,** that in which the liver is decreased in size, seen in posthepatic or postnecrotic cirrhosis and in some alcoholics. **biliary c.,** cirrhosis of the liver from chronic bile retention, due to obstruction or infection of the major extra- or intrahepatic bile ducts (*secondary biliary c.*), or of unknown etiology (*primary biliary c.*), and sometimes occurring after administration of certain drugs. **fatty c.,** a form in which liver cells become infiltrated with fat. **Laënnec's c.,** cirrhosis of the liver associated with alcohol abuse. **c. of liver,** a group of liver diseases marked by loss of normal hepatic architecture, with fibrosis and nodular regeneration. **metabolic c.,** cirrhosis of the liver associated with metabolic diseases, such as hemochromatosis, Wilson's disease, glycogen storage disease, galactosemia, and disorders of amino acid metabolism. **portal c.,** Laënnec's c. **posthepatic c.,** that (usually macronodular) resulting as a sequel to acute hepatitis. **postnecrotic c.,** that which follows submassive necrosis of the liver (subacute yellow atrophy) due to toxic or viral hepatitis; the reticulin framework of normal lobules collapses and may be replaced by broad bands of fibrous tissue separating regeneration nodules (multilobular liver) of varying size.

cirrus (sir′us), pl. *cir′ri* [L.] a slender, usually flexible, appendage, as the muscular retractile copulatory organ of certain trematodes, or one of the organs of locomotion of ciliate protozoa, which are composed of fused cilia.

cirsectomy (ser-sek′tah-me) excision of a portion of a varicose vein.

cirsoid (ser′soid) resembling a varix.

cirsomphalos (ser-som′fah-los) caput medusae.

cis (sis) in organic chemistry, denoting an isomer with similar atoms or radicals on the same side; in genetics, having two mutant genes of a pseudoallele on the same chromosome. Cf. *trans.*

cisplatin (sis′plah-tin) an antineoplastic, Cl_2H_6-N_2Pt, used in the treatment of metastatic testicular and ovarian cancer.

cistern (sis′tern) a closed space serving as a reservoir for fluid, e.g., one of the enlarged spaces of the body containing lymph or other fluid. **cister′nal,** adj. **terminal c's,** pairs of transversely oriented channels that are confluent with the sarcotubules, which together with an intermediate T tubule constitute a triad of skeletal muscle.

cisterna (sis-ter′nah), pl. *cister′nae* [L.] cistern. **c. cerebellomedulla′ris,** the enlarged subarachnoid space between the undersurface of the cerebellum and the posterior surface of the medulla oblongata. **c. chy′li,** the dilated part of the thoracic duct at its origin in the lumbar region. **perinuclear c.,** the space separating the inner from the outer nuclear membrane.

cisternography (sis″ter-nog′rah-fe) radiography of the basal cistern of the brain after subarachnoid injection of a contrast medium.

cistron (sis′tron) the smallest unit of genetic material that must be intact to transmit genetic information; traditionally synonymous with gene.

citrate (sĭ′trāt, sĭ′trāt) a salt of citric acid.

citric acid (sĭ′trik) a tricarboxylic acid, $CH_2(COOH)C(OH)(COOH)CH_2COOH$, occurring in citrus fruits and acting as an antiscorbutic and diuretic. It functions as an anticoagulant in the blood preservatives, acid citrate dextrose and citrate phosphate dextrose, and is a metabolic intermediate in the tricarboxylic acid cycle.

citronella (sĭ″tron-el′ah) a fragrant grass, the source of a volatile oil (citronella oil) used in perfumes and insect repellents.

citrulline (sĭ-trul′ēn) an alpha-amino acid involved in urea production; formed from ornithine and itself converted into arginine in the urea cycle.

citrullinuria (sĭ-trul″in-ūr′e-ah) presence in the urine of large amounts of citrulline, with increased levels also in both plasma and cerebrospinal fluid.

cittosis (sĭ-to′sis) pica.

Cl chemical symbol, *chlorine.*

cladosporiosis (klad″o-spo″re-o′sis) any infection with *Cladosporium,* e.g., black degeneration of the brain, chromomycosis, and tinea nigra.

Cladosporium (-spo′re-um) a genus of imperfect fungi (order Moniliales). *C. herbarum* produces "black spot" on meat in cold storage, growing at a temperature of 18° F. (−8° C.); *C. carrioni* is an agent of chromomycosis; *C. wernecki* and *C. mansoni* are agents of tinea nigra; *C. trichoides* causes black degeneration of the brain.

clairvoyance (klār-voi′ins) [Fr.] extrasensory perception in which knowledge of objective events is acquired without the use of the senses.

clamp (klamp) a surgical device for compressing a part or structure. **rubber dam c's,** metallic devices used to retain the dam on a tooth.

clap (klap) gonorrhea.

clapotement (klah-pōt-maw′) [Fr.] a splashing sound, as in succussion.

clarificant (klah-rif′ĭ-kint) a substance which clears a liquid of turbidity.

clasp (klasp) a device to hold something.

class (klas) 1. a taxonomic category subordinate to a phylum and superior to an order. 2. a group of variables all of which show a value falling between certain limits.

classification (klas″sĭ-fĭ-ka′shin) the systematic arrangement of similar entities on the basis of certain differing characteristics. **adansonian c.,** numerical taxonomy. **Angle's c.,** a classification of dental malocclusion based on the mesiodistal position of the mandibular dental arch and teeth relative to the maxillary dental arch and teeth; see under *malocclusion.* **Bergey's c.,** a system of classifying bacteria by Gram reaction, metabolism, and morphology. **Caldwell-Moloy c.,** classification of female pelves as gynecoid, android, anthropoid, and platypelloid; see under *pelvis.* **Gell and Coombs c.,** a classification of immune mechanisms of tissue injury. **Lancefield c.,** the classification of hemolytic streptococci into groups on the basis of serologic action. **New York Heart Association (NYHA) c.,** a functional and therapeutic classification of physical activity for cardiac patients. **Wagener-Barker c.,** a classification of hypertension and arteriolosclerosis based on retinal changes.

clastic (klas′tik) 1. undergoing or causing division. 2. separable into parts.

clastogenic (klas″tah-jen′ik) causing disruption or breakages, as of chromosomes.

clastothrix (klas′tah-thriks) trichorrhexis nodosa.

clathrate (klath′rāt) 1. having the shape of a lattice; pertaining to clathrate compounds. 2. [pl.] inclusion complexes in which molecules of one type are trapped within cavities of the crystalline lattice of another substance.

claudication (klaw″dĭ-ka′shin) limping; lameness. **intermittent c.,** pain, tension, and weakness in the legs on walking, which intensifies to produce lameness and is relieved by rest; it is seen in occlusive arterial disease. **venous c.,** intermittent claudication due to venous stasis.

claustrophilia (klaws″trah-fil′e-ah) an abnormal desire to be in a closed room or space.

claustrophobia (-fo′be-ah) morbid fear of closed places.

claustrum (klaws′trum), pl. *claus′tra* [L.] the thin layer of gray matter lateral to the external capsule, separating it from the white matter of the insula.

clava (kla′vah) gracile tubercle.

Claviceps (klav′ĭ-seps) a genus of parasitic fungi that infest various plant seeds. *C. purpu′rea* is the source of ergot.

clavicle (klav′ĭ-k'l) see *Table of Bones.* **clavic′ular,** adj.

clavicotomy (klav″ĭ-kot′ah-me) surgical division of the clavicle.

clavicula (klah-vik′u-lah) [L.] clavicle.

clavus (kla′vus), pl. *cla′vi* [L.] a corn.

clawfoot (klaw′foot) a high-arched foot with the toes hyperextended at the metatarsophalangeal joint and flexed at the distal joints.

clawhand (-hand) flexion and atrophy of the hand and fingers.

clearance (klēr′ins) the act of clearing; specifically, complete removal by the kidneys of a solute or solution from a specific volume of blood per unit of time. **creatinine c.,** the volume of plasma cleared of creatinine after parenteral administration of a specified amount of the substance. **inulin c.,** an expression of the renal efficiency in eliminating inulin from the blood. **urea c.,** blood-urea c.

cleavage (klēv′ij) division into distinct parts; the early successive splitting of a fertilized ovum into smaller cells (blastomeres) by mitosis.

cleft (kleft) a fissure, especially one occurring during the embryonic development. **branchial c's,** the slitlike openings in the gills of fish between the branchial arches; also, the homologous branchial grooves between the branchial arches of mammalian embryos. **synaptic c.,** a narrow extracellular cleft between the pre- and postsynaptic cell membranes at the synapse. **visceral c's,** branchial c's.

cleid(o)- word element [Gr.], *clavicle.*

cleidocranial (klī″do-kra′ne-il) pertaining to the clavicle and the head.

cleidotomy (kli-dot′ah-me) surgical division of the clavicle of the fetus in difficult labor to facilitate delivery.

clemastine (klem′as-tēn) an antihistaminic, $C_{21}H_{26}ClNO$, used in the treatment of allergic rhinitis and allergic skin disorders.

click (klik) a brief, sharp sound, especially any of the short, dry clicking heart sounds during systole, indicative of various heart conditions.

clidinium bromide (klĭ-din′e-um) an anticholinergic, $C_{22}H_{26}BrNO_3$.

climacteric (kli-mak′ter-ik, kli″mak-tĕ′rik) the syndrome of endocrine, somatic, and psychic changes occurring at menopause; it may also accompany normal diminution of sexual activity in the male.

climatology (kli″mah-tol′ah-je) the study of natural environmental conditions (e.g., rainfall, temperature) in specific regions of the earth.

climatotherapy (kli″mah-to-ther′ah-pe) treatment of disease by means of a favorable climate.

climax (kli′maks) the period of greatest intensity, as in the course of a disease.

clindamycin (klin″dah-mi′sin) a semisynthetic derivative of lincomycin, $C_{18}H_{33}ClN_2O_5S$; used as an antibacterial and antiparasitic agent.

clinic (klin′ik) 1. a clinical lecture; examination of patients before a class of students; instruction at the bedside. 2. an establishment where patients are admitted for study and treatment by a group of physicians practicing medicine together. **ambulant c.,** one for patients not confined to the bed. **dry c.,** a clinical lecture with case histories, but without patients present.

clinical (klin′ĭ-k'l) pertaining to a clinic or to the bedside; pertaining to or founded on actual observation and treatment of patients, as distinguished from theoretical or basic sciences.

clinician (klĭ-nish′in) an expert clinical physician and teacher. **nurse c.,** see under *nurse.*

clinicopathologic (klin″ĭ-ko-path″ah-loj′ik) pertaining to symptoms and pathology of disease.

Clinistix (klin′ĭ-stiks) trademark for glucose oxidase reagent strips used to test for glucose in urine.

Clinitest (-test) trademark for alkaline copper sulfate reagent tablets used to test for reducing substances, e.g., sugars, in urine.

clinocephaly (kli″no-sef′ah-le) congenital flatness or concavity of the vertex of the head.

clinodactyly (-dak′til-e) permanent deviation or deflection of one or more fingers.

clinoid (kli′noid) bed-shaped.

clip (klip) a metallic device for approximating the edges of a wound or for the prevention of bleeding from small individual blood vessels.

cliseometer (klis″e-om′it-er) an instrument for

measuring the angles between the axis of the body and that of the pelvis.

clition (klit′e-on) the midpoint of the anterior border of the clivus.

clitoridectomy (klit″ah-rĭ-dek′tah-me) excision of the clitoris.

clitoridotomy (-dot′ah-me) incision of the clitoris; female circumcision.

clitorimegaly (-meg′ah-le) enlargement of the clitoris.

clitoris (klit′ah-ris) the small, elongated, erectile body in the female, situated at the anterior angle of the rima pudendi and homologous with the penis in the male.

clitorism (klit′ah-rizm) 1. hypertrophy of the clitoris. 2. persistent erection of the clitoris.

clitoritis (klit″ah-rīt′is) inflammation of the clitoris.

clitoroplasty (klit′er-o-plas″te) plastic surgery of the clitoris.

clivography (kli-vog′rah-fe) radiographic visualization of the clivus, or posterior cranial fossa.

clivus (kli′vus), pl. *cli′vi* [L.] a bony surface in the posterior cranial fossa sloping upward from the foramen magnum to the dorsum sellae.

cloaca (klo-a′kah), pl. *cloa′cae* [L.] 1. a common passage for fecal, urinary, and reproductive discharge in most lower vertebrates. 2. the terminal end of the hindgut before division into rectum, bladder, and genital primordia in mammalian embryos. 3. an opening in the involucrum of a necrosed bone. **cloa′cal,** adj.

cloacogenic (klo″ah-ko-jen′ik) originating from the cloaca or from persisting cloacal remnants; said of a group of rare transitional-cell nonkeratinizing epidermoid anal cancers.

clock (klok) a device for measuring time. **biological c.,** the physiologic mechanism which governs the rhythmic occurrence of certain biochemical, physiologic, and behavioral phenomena in living organisms.

clofibrate (klo-fi′brāt) an anticholesterolemic, $C_{12}H_{15}ClO_3$.

clomiphene (klo′mĭ-fēn) a nonsteroid estrogen analogue, $C_{26}H_{28}ClNO$, used as the citrate salt to stimulate ovulation.

clonality (klo-nal′ĭ-te) the ability to form clones.

clonazepam (klo-naz′ĕ-pam) a benzodiazepine derivative, $C_{15}H_{10}ClN_3O_3$, used as an oral anticonvulsant.

clone (klōn) 1. the genetically identical progeny produced by the natural or artificial asexual reproduction of a single organism, cell, or gene, e.g., plant cuttings, a cell culture descended from a single cell, or genes reproduced by recombinant DNA technology. 2. to establish or produce such a line of progeny. **clo′nal,** adj.

clonidine (klo′nĭ-dēn) a centrally acting antihypertensive agent, $C_9H_9Cl_2N_3$.

clonism (klon′izm) a succession of clonic spasms.

clonogenic (klo″nah-jen′ik) giving rise to a clone of cells.

clonograph (klon′ah-graf) an instrument for recording spasmodic movements of parts and tendon reflexes.

Clonopin (-pin) trademark for a preparation of clonazepam.

clonorchiasis (klo″nor-ki′ah-sis) infection of the biliary passages with the liver fluke *Clonorchis sinensis,* causing inflammation of the biliary tree, proliferation of the biliary epithelium, and progressive portal fibrosis; extension into the liver parenchyma causes fatty changes and cirrhosis.

Clonorchis (klo-nor′kis) a genus of Asiatic liver flukes.

clonospasm (klon′ah-spazm) clonic spasm.

clonus (klo′nus) alternate involuntary muscular contraction and relaxation in rapid succession. **clon′ic,** adj. **ankle c., foot c.,** a series of abnormal reflex movements of the foot, induced by sudden dorsiflexion, causing alternate contraction and relaxation of the triceps surae muscle. **toe c.,** abnormal rhythmic movement of the big toe, induced by suddenly extending the first phalanx. **wrist c.,** spasmodic movement of the hand, induced by forcibly extending the hand at the wrist.

clorazepate (klo-raz′ah-pāt) one of the benzodiazepine tranquilizers, $C_{16}H_{13}ClN_2O_4$.

clortermine hydrochloride (klor-ter′mēn) an adrenergic, $C_{10}H_{14}ClN \cdot HCl$, used as an anorexic.

Clostridium (klo-strid′e-um) a genus of anaerobic spore-forming bacteria (family Bacillaceae). **C. bifermen′tans,** a species common in feces, sewage, and soil and associated with gas gangrene. **C. botuli′num,** the causative agent of botulism, divided into six types (A through F) which elaborate immunologically distinct toxins. **C. diffi′cile,** a species often occurring transiently in the gut of infants, but whose toxin causes pseudomembranous enterocolitis in those receiving prolonged antibiotic therapy. **C. histoly′ticum,** a species found in feces and soil. **C. kluy′veri,** a species used in the study of both microbial synthesis and microbial oxidation of fatty acids. **C. no′vyi,** an important cause of gas gangrene. **C. oedema′tiens,** *C. novyi.* **C. perfrin′gens,** the most common etiologic agent of gas gangrene, differentiable into several different types: type A (classic gangrene in man), B (lamb dysentery), C (struck in sheep), D (enterotoxemia in sheep), E (enterotoxemia in lambs and calves), F (enteritis necroticans in man). **C. ramo′sum,** a species found in human and animal infections and in feces, one of the most commonly isolated clostridia in clinical specimens. **C. sporo′genes,** a species widespread in nature, reportedly associated with pathogenic anaerobes in gangrenous infections. **C. ter′tium,** a species found in feces, sewage, and soil and present in some gangrenous infections. **C. te′tani,** a common inhabitant of soil and human and horse intestines, and the cause of tetanus in man and domestic animals. **C. welch′ii,** British name for *C. perfringens.*

clostridium (klo-strid′ĭ-um), pl. *clostrid′ia* [Gr.] an individual of the genus *Clostridium.*

closylate (klo′sĭ-lāt) USAN contraction for *p*-chlorobenzesulfonate.

clot (klot) 1. a semisolidified mass of coagulum,

as of blood or lymph. 2. to form such a mass. **agonal c., agony c.,** one formed in the heart during the death agony. **antemortem c.,** one formed in the heart or in a large vessel before death. **blood c.,** one formed of blood, either in or out of the body. **chicken fat c.,** a yellow-appearing blood clot, due to settling out of erythrocytes before clotting. **currant jelly c.,** a reddish clot, due to the presence of erythrocytes enmeshed in it. **laminated c.,** a blood clot formed by successive deposits, giving it a layered appearance. **passive c.,** one formed in the sac of an aneurysm through which the blood has stopped circulating. **plastic c.,** one formed from the intima of an artery at the point of ligation, forming a permanent obstruction of the artery. **postmortem c.,** one formed in the heart or in a large blood vessel after death.

clotrimazole (klo-trim′ah-zōl) a topical antifungal agent, $C_{22}H_{17}ClN_2$.

cloxacillin (kloks″ah-sil′in) a semisynthetic penicillin; used to treat staphylococcal infections due to penicillinase-positive organisms.

clubbing (klub′ing) proliferation of soft tissue about the terminal phalanges of fingers or toes, without osseous change.

clubfoot (-foot) a congenitally deformed foot; see *talipes.*

clubhand (-hand) a hand deformity analogous to clubfoot; talipomanus.

clumping (klump′ing) the aggregation of particles, such as bacteria, into irregular masses.

clunis (kloo′nis), pl. *clu′nes* [L.] buttock.

clysis (kli′sis) the administration other than orally of any of several solutions to replace lost body fluid, supply nutriment, or raise blood pressure; also, the solution so administered.

clyster (klis′ter) an enema.

C.M. [L.] *Chirur′giae Magis′ter* (Master in Surgery).

Cm chemical symbol, *curium.*

cm. centimeter.

cm.² square centimeter.

cm.³ cubic centimeter.

CMA Certified Medical Assistant.

C.M.A. Canadian Medical Association.

CMI cell-mediated immunity.

C.N.A. Canadian Nurses' Association.

cnemial (ne′me-il) pertaining to the shin.

C.N.M. Certified Nurse-Midwife; see *nurse-midwife.*

CNS central nervous system.

Co chemical symbol, *cobalt.*

C.O.A. Canadian Orthopaedic Association.

CoA coenzyme A.

coacervation (ko-as-er-va′shin) the separation of a mixture of two liquids, one or both of which are colloids, into two phases, one of which, the coacervate, contains the colloidal particles, the other being an aqueous solution, as when gum arabic is added to gelatin.

coadaptation (ko″ad-ap-ta′shin) the correlated changes in two interdependent organs.

coagglutination (ko″ah-gl $\overline{oo}$ t″in-a′shin) the aggregation of particulate antigens combined with agglutinins of more than one specificity.

coagglutinin (ko″ah-glōōt′in-in) partial agglutinin.

coagulability (ko-ag″u-lah-bil′it-e) the capability of forming or of being formed into clots.

coagulant (ko-ag′u-lint) promoting or accelerating coagulation of blood; an agent that so acts.

coagulase (-lās) an antigenic substance of bacterial origin, produced by staphylococci, which may be causally related to thrombus formation.

coagulate (-lāt) 1. to cause to clot. 2. to become clotted.

coagulation (ko-ag″u-la′shin) 1. formation of a clot. 2. in surgery, the disruption of tissue by physical means to form an amorphous residuum, as in electrocoagulation and photocoagulation. **blood c.,** the sequential process by which the multiple coagulation factors of blood interact, resulting in formation of an insoluble clot, divisible into three stages: (1) formation of intrinsic and extrinsic prothrombin converting principle; (2) formation of thrombin; (3) formation of stable fibrin polymers. **diffuse intravascular c., disseminated intravascular c. (DIC),** a disorder characterized by reduction in the elements involved in blood coagulation due to their use in widespread blood clotting within the vessels. In the late stages, it is marked by profuse hemorrhaging. **electric c.,** destruction of tissue by application of a bipolar current delivered by a needle point.

coagulopathy (ko-ag″u-lop′ah-the) any disorder of blood coagulation. **consumption c.,** disseminated intravascular coagulation.

coagulum (ko-ag′u-lum), pl. *coa′gula* [L.] a clot. **closing c.,** the clot that closes the gap made in the uterine lining by the implanting blastocyst.

coalescence (ko″ah-les′ins) the fusion or blending of parts.

coapt (ko′apt) to approximate, as the edges of a wound.

coarctate (ko-ark′tāt) 1. to press close together; contract. 2. pressed together; restrained.

coarctation (ko″ark-ta′shin) narrowing. **c. of aorta,** a local malformation marked by deformed aortic media, causing narrowing of the lumen of the vessel. **reversed c.,** pulseless disease.

coat (kōt) tunica; a membrane or other tissue covering or lining an organ. **buffy c.,** the thin yellowish layer of leukocytes overlying the packed erythrocytes in centrifuged blood. **corneoscleral c.,** the corneosclera.

cobalamin (ko-bal′ah-min) a cobalt-containing complex common to the vitamin B_{12} group.

cobalt (ko′bawlt) chemical element (*see table*), at. no. 27, symbol Co. **c.-57,** a radioisotope of cobalt with a half-life of 270 days; used as a label for cyanocobalamin. Symbol ⁵⁷Co. **c.-60,** a radioisotope of cobalt with a half-life of 5.27 years and a principal gamma ray energy of 1.33 MeV; used in radiation therapy. Symbol ⁶⁰Co.

cocaine (ko-kān′, ko′kān) an alkaloid, $C_{17}H_{21}$-NO_4, obtained from leaves of various species of *Erythroxylon* (coca plants) or produced synthetically; used as a local anesthetic.

cocarcinogen (ko″kar-sin′o-jen) an agent that increases the effect of a carcinogen by direct concurrent local effect on the tissue.

cocarcinogenesis (ko-kar″sĭ-no-jen′ĭ-sis) the development, according to one theory, of cancer only in preconditioned cells as a result of conditions favorable to its growth.

cocci (kok′si) plural of *coccus.*

Coccidia (kok-sid′e-ah) a subclass of parasitic protozoa comprising the orders Agamococcidiida, Protoccidiida, and Eucoccidiida.

coccidia (kok-sid′e-ah) plural of *coccidium.*

Coccidioides (kok-sid″e-oi′dēz) a genus of pathogenic fungi, including *C. im′mitis,* the cause of coccidioidomycosis.

coccidioidin (-din) a sterile preparation containing by-products of growth products of *Coccidioides immitis,* injected intracutaneously as a test for coccidioidomycosis.

coccidioidoma (-do′mah) residual pulmonary granulomatous nodules seen roentgenographically as solid round foci in coccidioidomycosis.

coccidioidomycosis (-oi″do-mi-ko′sis) infection with *Coccidioides immitis,* occurring as a respiratory infection, due to spore inhalation, varying in severity from that of a common cold to symptoms resembling those of influenza (*primary c.*), or as a virulent and severe, chronic, progressive, granulomatous disease resulting in involvement of cutaneous and subcutaneous tissues, viscera, central nervous system, and lungs (*secondary c.*).

coccidiosis (-o′sis) infection by coccidia. In man, applied to the presence of *Isospora hominis* or *I. belli* in stools; it is often asymptomatic, rarely causing a severe watery mucous diarrhea.

coccidium (kok-sid′e-um), pl. *coccid′ia* [L.] any member of the order Coccidia.

coccigenic (kok″sĭ-jen′ik) produced by cocci.

coccobacillus (kok″o-bah-sil′us) an oval bacterial cell intermediate between the coccus and bacillus forms. **coccobac′illary,** adj.

coccobacteria (-bak-tēr′e-ah) a common name for spheroid bacteria, or for bacterial cocci.

coccus (kok′us), pl. *coc′ci* [L.] a spherical bacterium, less than 1 μ in diameter. **coc′cal,** adj.

coccyalgia (kok″se-al′je-ah) coccygodynia.

coccygeal (kok-sij′e-il) pertaining to or located in the region of the coccyx.

coccygectomy (kok″sĭ-jek′tah-me) excision of the coccyx.

coccygodynia (-go-din′e-ah) pain in the coccyx and neighboring region.

coccygotomy (-got′ah-me) incision of the coccyx.

coccyx (kok′siks) see *Table of Bones.*

cochineal (koch′ĭ-nēl) dried female insects of *Coccus cacti,* enclosing young larvae; used as a coloring agent for pharmaceuticals and as a biological stain.

cochlea (kok′le-ah) a spiral tube forming part of the inner ear, which is the essential organ of hearing. See Plate XII. **coch′lear,** adj.

cochleariform (kok″le-ar′ĭ-form) spoon-shaped.

cochleotopic (kok″le-ah-top′ik) relating to the

organization of the auditory pathways and auditory area of the brain.

Cochliomyia (-mi′ah) a genus of flies, including *C. hominivo′rax,* the screw-worm fly, which deposits its eggs on animal wounds; after hatching, the larvae burrow into the wound and feed on living tissue.

coctolabile (kok″tah-la′bil) capable of being altered or destroyed by heating.

coctostabile (-sta′bil) not altered by heating to the boiling point of water.

code (kōd) 1. a set of rules for regulating conduct. 2. a system by which information can be communicated. **genetic c.,** the arrangement of nucleotides in the polynucleotide chain of a chromosome governing transmission of genetic information to proteins, i.e., determining the sequence of amino acids in the polypeptide chain making up each protein synthesized by the cell. **triplet c.,** the three-base sequence in the DNA molecule that codes for one amino acid.

codeine (ko′dēn) an alkaloid, $C_{18}H_{21}NO_3 \cdot H_2O$, obtained from opium or prepared from morphine by methylation; used as a narcotic analgesic and as an antitussive. The phosphate and sulfate salts are soluble in water.

codominance (ko-dom′ĭ-nins) the full expression in a heterozygote of both alleles of a pair with neither influenced by the other, as in a person with blood group AB. **codom′inant,** adj.

codon (ko′don) a series of three adjacent bases in one polynucleotide chain of a DNA or RNA molecule, which codes for a specific amino acid.

coe- for words beginning thus, see also those beginning *ce-*.

coefficient (ko″ah-fish′int) 1. an expression of the change or effect produced by variation in certain factors, or of the ratio between two different quantities. 2. a number or figure put before a chemical formula to indicate how many times the formula is to be multiplied. **c. of absorption,** the volume of a gas absorbed by a unit volume of a liquid at 0° C. and a pressure of 760 mm. Hg. **biological c.,** the amount of potential energy consumed by the body at rest. **correlation c.,** a measure of the relationship between two statistical variables, most commonly expressed as their covariance divided by the standard deviation of each. **phenol c.,** a measure of the bactericidal activity of a chemical compound in relation to phenol; expressed as a ratio of the activity of a dilution of the unknown to that of phenol when both dilutions kill in 10 mins. but not in 5 mins. under the specified conditions. **sedimentation c.,** the rate in centimeters per second per unit centrifugal field at which a particle (e.g., protein) in solution travels in the analytical ultracentrifuge. A rate of 1×10^{-13} cm./second/unit centrifugal field is defined as one Svedberg unit (S). **c. of thermal conductivity,** a number indicating the quantity of heat passing in a unit of time through a unit thickness of a substance when the difference in temperature is 1° C. **c. of thermal expansion,** the change in volume per unit volume of a substance produced by a 1° C. temperature increase.

-coele word element [Gr.], *cavity; space.*

Coelenterata (se-len″ter-āt′ah) a phylum of invertebrates which includes the hydras, jellyfish, sea anemones, and corals.

coelenterate (se-len′ter-āt) 1. pertaining or belonging to the Coelenterata. 2. any member of the Coelenterata.

coeloblastula (se″lo-blas′tu-lah) the common type of blastula, consisting of a hollow sphere composed of blastomeres.

coelom (se′lom) body cavity, especially the cavity in the mammalian embryo between the somatopleure and splanchnopleure, which is both intra- and extraembryonic; the principal cavities of the trunk arise from the intraembryonic portion. **coelom′ic,** adj.

coelomate (sēl′ah-māt) 1. having a coelom. 2. an individual of the Eucoelomata; eucoelomate.

coelosomy (sēl″ah-so′me) a developmental anomaly marked by protrusion of the viscera from and their presence outside the body cavity.

coenurosis (sēn″ūr-o′sis) gid.

Coenurus (se-nu′rus) a genus of certain tapeworm larva, including *C. cerebra′lis,* the larva of *Multiceps multiceps,* which causes gid.

coenurus (se-nu′rus) the larval stage of tapeworms of the genus *Multiceps,* a semitransparent, fluid-filled, bladder-like organism that contains multiple scoleces attached to the inner surface of its wall and that does not form brood capsules. It develops in various parts of the host body, especially in the central nervous system.

coenzyme (ko-en′zīm) an organic molecule, containing phosphorus and vitamins, sometimes separable from the enzyme protein; a coenzyme and an apoenzyme must unite in order to function (as a holoenzyme). **c. A,** a coenzyme essential for carbohydrate and fat metabolism; among its constituents are pantothenic acid and a terminal SH group forming thioester linkages with various acids, e.g., acetic acid (acetyl CoA) and fatty acids (acyl CoA); abbreviated CoA. **c. Q,** any of a group of quinones with isoprenoid units in the side chains (the ubiquinones), occurring in the lipid fraction of mitochondria and serving, along with the cytochromes, as an intermediate in electron transport, and similar in structure and function to vitamin K_1.

coeur (ker) [Fr.] heart. **c. en sabot** (on sǎ-bo′) a heart whose shape on a radiograph resembles that of a wooden shoe; seen in tetralogy of Fallot.

cofactor (ko′fak-ter) an element or principle, e.g., a coenzyme, with which another must unite in order to function.

Cogentin (ko-jen′tin) trademark for preparations of benztropine mesylate.

cognition (kog-nish′in) that operation of the mind process by which we become aware of objects of thought and perception, including all aspects of perceiving, thinking, and remembering. **cog′nitive,** adj.

cohesion (ko-he′zhin) the force causing various particles to unite. **cohe′sive,** adj.

cohort (ko′hort) in statistics, a group of individuals of the same age who are followed for a long time to determine the incidence of disease (or other statistical variable) at different ages.

coil (koil) a winding structure or spiral.

coinosite (koi′nah-sīt) a free commensal organism.

coitophobia (ko″it-ah-fo′be-ah) morbid fear of coitus.

coitus (ko′it-us) sexual connection per vaginam between male and female. **co′ital,** adj. **c. incomple′tus, c. interrup′tus,** that in which the penis is withdrawn from the vagina before ejaculation. **c. reserva′tus,** that in which ejaculation of semen is purposely suppressed.

col (kol) a depression in the interdental tissues just below the interproximal contact area, connecting the buccal and lingual papillae.

colchicine (kol′chĭ-sēn) an alkaloid, $C_{22}H_{25}NO_6$, from the tree *Colchicum autumnale* (meadow saffron), used as a suppressant for gout.

cold (kōld) 1. privation, or relatively low degree, of heat. 2. common cold; a catarrhal disorder of the upper respiratory tract, which may be viral, a mixed infection, or an allergic reaction, and marked by acute coryza, slight temperature rise, chilly sensations, and general indisposition. **common c.,** see *cold* (2). **rose c.,** a form of seasonal hay fever caused by the pollen of roses.

coldsore (kōld′sor) see *herpes simplex.*

colectomy (ko-lek′tah-me) excision of the colon or of a portion of it.

Colesiota (ko-le″se-ōt′ah) a genus of microorganisms of uncertain classification, including *C. conjuncti′vae,* the agent causing infectious ophthalmia of sheep.

Colettsia (ko-let′se-ah) a genus of microorganisms of uncertain classification, including *C. pe′coris,* a parasitic species found in the conjunctiva of domestic animals.

colibacillosis (-lo′sis) infection with *Escherichia coli.*

colibacillus (ko″lĭ-bah-sil′us) *Escherichia coli.*

colic (kol′ik) 1. acute paroxysmal abdominal pain. 2. pertaining to the colon. **appendicular c.,** vermicular c. **biliary c.,** colic due to passage of gallstones along the bile duct. **Devonshire c.,** lead c. **gallstone c.,** biliary c. **gastric c.,** pain in the stomach. **hepatic c.,** biliary c. **infantile c.,** benign paroxysmal abdominal pain during the first 3 months of life. **lead c.,** colic due to lead poisoning. **menstrual c.,** dysmenorrhea. **ovarian c.,** ovarian pain. **painter's c.,** lead c. **renal c.,** pain due to thrombosis of the renal vein or artery, dissection of the renal artery, renal infarction, intrarenal mass lesions, or passage of a stone within the collecting system. **salivary c.,** pain in the region of the salivary gland in cases of salivary calculus. **sand c.,** chronic indigestion. **uterine c.,** severe colic arising in the uterus at the menstrual period. **vermicular c.,** pain in the vermiform appendix caused by catarrhal inflammation due to blockage of the outlet of the appendix.

colica (kol′ĭ-kah) [L.] colic.

colicin (kol′ĭ-sin) a protein secreted by colicinogenic strains of *Escherichia coli* and other enteric bacteria; lethal to related, sensitive bacteria.

colicky (kol′ik-e) pertaining to colic.

colicoplegia (ko″lĭ-ko-ple′je-ah) combined lead colic and lead paralysis.

colicystitis (-sis-tīt′is) cystitis due to *Escherichia coli.*

colicystopyelitis (-sis″to-pi″ah-līt′is) inflammation of the bladder and renal pelvis due to *Escherichia coli.*

coliform (kol′ĭ-form) pertaining to fermentative gram-negative enteric bacilli, sometimes restricted to those fermenting lactose, i.e., *Escherichia, Klebsiella, Enterobacter,* and *Citrobacter.*

colinephritis (ko″lĭ-ne-frĭt′is) nephritis due to *Escherichia coli.*

coliphage (kol′ĭ-fāj) any bacteriophage that infects *Escherichia coli.*

colipuncture (-punk″cher) colocentesis.

colipyelitis (-pi″ah-līt′is) pyelitis caused by *Escherichia coli.*

colisepsis (-sep′sis) infection with *Escherichia coli.*

colistimethate (ko-lis″tĭ-meth′āt) a colistin derivative; the sodium salt, $C_{49}H_{89}N_{13}NaO_{22}S_4$, is used as an antibacterial.

colistin (ko-lis′tin) an antibiotic produced by *Bacillus polymyxa* var. *colistinus,* related to polymyxin, and used to treat urinary tract infections; the water-soluble sulfate salt, effective against several gram-negative bacilli but not against *Proteus,* is used as an intestinal antibacterial.

colitides (ko-lit′ĭ-dēz) plural of *colitis;* inflammatory disorders of the colon, collectively.

colitis (ko-līt′is) inflammation of the colon. **amebic c.,** colitis due to *Entamoeba histolytica;* amebic dysentery. **antibiotic-associated c.,** see under *enterocolitis.* **granulomatous c.,** transmural colitis with the formation of noncaseating granulomas. **ischemic c.,** acute vascular insufficiency of the colon, affecting the portion supplied by the inferior mesenteric artery; symptoms include pain at the left iliac fossa, bloody diarrhea, low-grade fever, and abdominal distention and tenderness. **mucous c.,** a chronic noninflammatory disease marked by excessive secretion of mucus and disordered colonic motility, with colic, constipation, and/or diarrhea with mucus. **regional c., segmental c.,** transmural or granulomatous inflammatory disease of the colon; regional enteritis involving the colon. It may be associated with ulceration, strictures, or fistulas. **transmural c.,** inflammation of the full thickness of the bowel, rather than mucosal and submucosal disease, usually with the formation of noncaseating granulomas. It may be confined to the colon, segmentally or diffusely, or may be associated with small bowel disease (regional enteritis). Clinically, it may resemble ulcerative colitis, but the ulceration is often longitudinal or deep, the disease is often segmental, stricture formation is common, and fistulas, particularly in the perineum, are a frequent complication. **ulcerative c.,** chronic ulceration in the colon, chiefly of the mucosa and submucosa, manifested by cramp-

colitoxemia

136

ing abdominal pain, rectal bleeding, and loose discharges of blood, pus, and mucus with scanty fecal particles.

colitoxemia (ko″lĭ-tok-se′me-ah) toxemia due to infection with *Escherichia coli.*

colitoxin (-tok′sin) a toxin from *Escherichia coli.*

collagen (kol′ah-jen) the protein substance of the white fibers (collagenous fibers) of skin, tendon, bone, cartilage, and all other connective tissue; composed of molecules of tropocollagen. **collag′enous**, adj.

collagenase (kol-laj′ĭ-nās) an enzyme that catalyzes the degradation of collagen.

collagenation (kol-laj″ĭ-na′shin) the appearance of collagen in developing cartilage.

collagenitis (ko-laj′in-īt′is) inflammatory involvement of collagen fibers in the fibrous component of connective tissue, characterized by pain, swelling, low-grade fever, and by increased erythrocyte sedimentation rate.

collagenoblast (kol-laj′in-o-blast″) a cell arising from a fibroblast and which, as it matures, is associated with collagen production; it may also form cartilage and bone by metaplasia.

collagenocyte (-sīt″) a mature collagen-producing cell.

collagenogenic (kol-laj″ĭ-no-jen′ik) pertaining to or characterized by collagen production; forming collagen or collagen fibers.

collagenolysis (kol″ah-jen-ol′ĭ-sis) dissolution or digestion of collagen. **collagenolyt′ic**, adj.

collagenosis (kol″ah-jĭ-no′sis) collagen disease.

collapse (kah-laps′) 1. a state of extreme prostration and depression, with failure of circulation. 2. abnormal falling in of the walls of a part or organ. **circulatory c.**, shock; circulatory insufficiency without congestive heart failure.

collateral (kol-lat′er-il) 1. secondary or accessory; not direct or immediate. 2. a small side branch, as of a blood vessel or nerve.

colliculectomy (kah-lik″u-lek′tah-me) excision of the colliculus seminalis.

colliculitis (-lit′is) inflammation about the colliculus seminalis.

colliculus (kah-lik′u-lus), pl. *collic′uli* [L.] a small elevation. **c. semina′lis**, a prominent portion of the male urethral crest on which are the opening of the prostatic utricle and, on either side, the orifices of the ejaculatory ducts.

collimation (kol″ĭ-ma′shin) in microscopy, the process of making light rays parallel; the adjustment of optical axes with respect to each other. In radiology, the elimination of the more divergent portion of an x-ray beam.

colliquative (kah-lik′wah-tiv) characterized by excessive liquid discharge, or by liquefaction of tissue.

collodiaphyseal (kol″o-di″ah-fiz′e-il) pertaining to the neck and shaft of a long bone, especially the femur.

collodion (kah-lo′de-on) a syrupy liquid compounded of pyroxylin, ether, and alcohol, which dries to a transparent, tenacious film; used as a topical protectant, applied to the skin to close small wounds, abrasions, and cuts, to hold surgical dressings in place, and to keep medica-

tions in contact with the skin. **flexible c.**, a preparation of collodion, camphor, and castor oil; used as a topical protectant. **salicylic acid c.**, flexible collodion containing salicylic acid; used topically as a keratolytic.

colloid (kol′oid) a chemical system composed of a continuous medium (continuous phase) throughout which are distributed small particles, 1 to 1000 nm in size (disperse phase), that do not settle out under the influence of gravity. **stannous sulfur c.**, a sulfur colloid containing stannous ions formed by reacting sodium thiosulfate with hydrochloric acid, then adding stannous ions; a diagnostic aid (bone, liver, and spleen imaging).

collum (kol′um), pl. *col′la* [L.] the neck, or a necklike part. **c. distor′tum**, torticollis. **c. val′gum**, coxa valga.

collutory (kol′u-tor-e) mouthwash or gargle.

collyrium (kah-lir′e-um), pl. *colly′ria* [L.] a lotion for the eyes; an eye wash.

colo- word element [Gr.], *colon.*

coloboma (kol″ah-bo′mah) an absence or defect of some ocular tissue, due to failure of a part of the fetal fissure to close; it may affect the choroid, ciliary body, eyelid, iris, lens, optic nerve, or retina. **bridge c.**, coloboma of the iris in which a strip of iris tissue bridges over the fissure. **Fuchs′ c.**, a small, crescent-shaped defect of the choroid at the lower edge of the optic disk. **c. lo′buli**, fissure of the ear lobe.

colocentesis (-sen-te′sis) surgical puncture of the colon.

colocholecystostomy (-ko″le-sis-tos′tah-me) cholecystocolostomy.

coloclyster (ko″lo-klis′ter) an enema injected into the colon through the rectum.

colocolostomy (-kah-los′tah-me) surgical anastomosis between two portions of the colon.

colocutaneous (-ku-ta′ne-us) pertaining to the colon and skin, or communicating with the colon and the cutaneous surface of the body.

colofixation (-fik-sa′shin) the fixation or suspension of the colon in cases of ptosis.

colon (ko′lin) the part of the large intestine extending from the cecum to the rectum. See Plate IV. **colon′ic**, adj. **ascending c.**, the portion of the colon passing cephalad from the cecum to the right colic flexure. **descending c.**, the portion of the colon passing caudad from the left colic flexure to the sigmoid colon. **iliac c.**, the part of the descending colon lying in the left iliac fossa and continuous with the sigmoid colon. **irritable c.**, mucous colitis. **left c.**, the distal portion of the large intestine, developed embryonically from the hindgut and functioning in the storage and elimination from the body of nonabsorbed residue of ingested material. **pelvic c.**, sigmoid c. **right c.**, the proximal portion of the large intestine, developed embryonically from the terminal portion of the midgut and functioning in absorption of ingested material. **sigmoid c.**, that portion of the left colon situated in the pelvis and extending from the descending colon to the rectum. **spastic c.**, mucous colitis. **transverse c.**, that portion of the large intestine passing transversely across the upper part of the abdomen, between the right and left colic flexures.

colonitis (-īt′is) colitis.

colonopathy (-op′ah-the) any disease or disorder of the colon.

colonorrhea (-re′ah) mucous colitis.

colonoscopy (ko″lin-os′kah-pe) endoscopic examination of the colon, either transabdominally during laparotomy, or transanally by means of a fiberoptic endoscope.

colony (kol′ah-ne) a discrete group of organisms, as a collection of bacteria in a culture.

colopexy (ko′lah-pek″se) surgical fixation or suspension of the colon.

coloplication (ko″lah-pli-ka′shin) the operation of taking a reef in the colon.

coloproctectomy (-prok-tek′tah-me) surgical removal of the colon and rectum.

coloproctostomy (-prok-tos′tah-me) colorectostomy.

coloptosis (ko″lop-to′sis) downward displacement of the colon.

colopuncture (ko′lo-punk″cher) colocentesis.

color (kul′er) 1. a property of a surface or substance due to absorption of certain light rays and reflection of others within the range of wavelengths (roughly 370–760 mμ) adequate to excite the retinal receptors. 2. radiant energy within the range of adequate chromatic stimuli of the retina, i.e., between the infrared and ultraviolet. 3. a sensory impression of one of the rainbow hues. **complementary c′s,** a pair of colors the sensory mechanisms for which are so linked that when they are mixed on the color wheel they cancel each other out, leaving neutral gray. **confusion c′s,** different colors liable to be mistakenly matched by persons with defective color vision, and hence used for detecting different types of color vision defects. **primary c′s,** (a) according to the Newton theory, the seven rainbow hues: violet, indigo, blue, green, yellow, orange, red; (b) in painting and printing, blue, yellow, red; (c) according to the Helmholz theory, red, green, blue. **pure c.,** one whose stimulus consists of homogeneous wavelengths, with little or no admixture of wavelengths of other hues.

colorectostomy (-rek-tos′tah-me) formation of an opening between the colon and rectum.

colorectum (-rek′tum) the distal 10 inches (25 cm.) of the bowel, including the distal portion of the colon and the rectum, regarded as a unit. **colorec′tal,** adj.

colorimeter (kul″er-im′it-er) an instrument for measuring color differences, especially one for measuring the color of blood in order to determine the proportion of hemoglobin.

colorrhaphy (kol-or′ah-fe) suture of the colon.

colosigmoidostomy (ko″lo-sig″moid-os′tah-me) surgical anastomosis of a formerly remote portion of the colon to the sigmoid.

colostomy (kol-os′tah-me) the surgical creation of an opening between the colon and the body surface; also, the opening (stoma) so created. **dry c.,** that performed in the left colon, the discharge from the stoma consisting of soft or formed fecal matter. **ileotransverse c.,** surgi-

cal anastomosis between the ileum and the transverse colon. **wet c.,** colostomy in (a) the right colon, the drainage from which is liquid, or (b) the left colon following anastomosis of the ureters to the sigmoid or descending colon so that urine is also expelled through the same stoma.

colostrum (kol-os′trum) the thin, yellow, milky fluid secreted by the mammary gland a few days before or after parturition.

colotomy (kol-ot′ah-me) incision of the colon.

colovesical (-ves′ĭ-kil) pertaining to or communicating with the colon and bladder.

colp(o)- word element [Gr.], *vagina.*

colpalgia (kol-pal′je-ah) pain in the vagina.

colpectasia (kol″pek-ta′ze-ah) distention or dilatation of the vagina.

colpectomy (kol-pek′tah-me) excision of the vagina.

colpeurysis (kol-pūr′ĭ-sis) dilatation of the vagina.

colpitis (kol-pīt′is) inflammation of the vagina; vaginitis.

colpocele (kol′pah-sēl) vaginal hernia.

colpocleisis (kol″pah-kli′sis) surgical closure of the vaginal canal.

colpocystitis (-sis-tīt′is) inflammation of the vagina and bladder.

colpocystocele (-sis′to-sēl) hernia of the bladder into the vagina.

colpocytogram (-sīt′ah-gram) differential listing of cells observed in vaginal smears.

colpocytology (-si-tol′ah-je) the study of cells exfoliated from the epithelium of the vagina.

colpohyperplasia (-hi″per-pla′ze-ah) excessive growth of the mucous membrane and wall of the vagina.

colpomicroscope (-mi′krah-skōp) an instrument for microscopic examination of the tissues of the cervix *in situ.*

colpoperineoplasty (-per″ĭ-ne′o-plas″te) plastic repair of the vagina and perineum.

colpoperineorrhaphy (-per″ĭ-ne-or′ah-fe) suture of the ruptured vagina and perineum.

colpopexy (kol′pah-pek″se) suture of a relaxed vagina to the abdominal wall.

colpoptosis (kol″pop-to′sis) prolapse of the vagina.

colporrhagia (kol″pah-ra′je-ah) hemorrhage from the vagina.

colporrhaphy (kol-por′ah-fe) 1. suture of the vagina. 2. the operation of denuding and suturing the vaginal wall to narrow the vagina.

colporrhexis (kol″por-ek′sis) laceration of the vagina.

colposcope (kol′pah-skōp) a speculum for examining the vagina and cervix by means of a magnifying lens.

colpospasm (kol′pah-spazm) vaginal spasm.

colpostenosis (kol″po-stĕ-no′sis) contraction or narrowing of the vagina.

colpostenotomy (-stĕ-not′ah-me) a cutting operation for stricture of the vagina.

colpotomy (kol-pot′ah-me) incision of the vagina with entry into the cul-de-sac.

colpoxerosis (kol″po-zēr-o′sis) abnormal dryness of the vulva and vagina.

colt-ill (kōlt′il) see under *ill.*

columella (kol″u-mel′ah), pl. *columel′lae* [L.] a little column. **c. co′chleae,** modiolus. **c. na′si,** the fleshy external end of the nasal septum.

column (kol′um) an anatomical part in the form of a pillar-like structure. **anal c's,** vertical folds of mucous membrane at the upper half of the anal canal. **anterior c.,** the anterior portion of the gray substance of the spinal cord, in transverse section seen as a horn. **c's of Bertin,** renal c's. **c. of Burdach,** fasciculus cuneatus of the spinal cord. **Clarke's c.,** nucleus thoracicus. **enamel c's,** adamantine prisms. **c. of Goll,** fasciculus gracilis of spinal cord. **gray c's,** the longitudinally oriented parts of the spinal cord in which the nerve cell bodies are found, comprising the gray substance of the spinal cord. **lateral c.,** the lateral portion of the spinal cord, in transverse section seen as a horn; present only in the thoracic and upper lumbar regions. **c's of Morgagni,** anal c's. **posterior c.,** the posterior portion of gray substance of the spinal cord, in transverse section seen as a horn. **posteroexternal c.,** the outer wider portion of the posterior column of the cord. **rectal c's,** anal c's. **renal c's,** inward extensions of the cortical substance of the kidney between contiguous renal pyramids. **c. of Sertoli,** an elongated Sertoli cell in the parietal layer of the seminiferous tubules. **spinal c.,** vertebral c. **vertebral c.,** the rigid structure in the midline of the back, composed of the vertebrae.

columna (ko-lum′nah), pl. *colum′nae* [L.] column.

columnization (kol″um-nĭ-za′shin) support of the prolapsed uterus by tampons.

colypeptic (ko″lĭ-pep′tik) kolypeptic.

coma (ko′mah) 1. a state of profound unconsciousness from which the patient cannot be aroused, even by powerful stimuli. 2. a comet-shaped image caused by light passing obliquely through a lens. **co′matose,** adj. **alcoholic c.,** stupor accompanying severe alcoholic intoxication. **alpha c.,** coma in which there are electroencephalographic findings of dominant alpha-wave activity. **apoplectic c.,** the stupor accompanying stroke. **diabetic c.,** the coma of severe diabetic acidosis. **hepatic c.,** coma accompanying hepatic encephalopathy. **irreversible c.,** brain death. **Kussmaul's c.,** the coma and air hunger of diabetic acidosis. **metabolic c.,** the coma accompanying metabolic encephalopathy. **trance c.,** lethargy produced by hypnosis. **uremic c.,** lethargic state due to uremia. **c. vigil,** apparent wakefulness with absent or grossly diminished response to external stimuli.

combustion (kom-bus′chin) rapid oxidation with emission of heat.

comedo (kom′ĭ-do), pl. *comedo′nes.* A plug of keratin and sebum within the dilated orifice of a hair follicle frequently containing the bacteria *Corynebacterium acnes, Staphylococcus albus,* and *Pityrosporon ovale.*

comedogenic (kom″ĭ-do-jen′ik) producing comedones.

comedomastitis (mas-tīt′is) mammary duct ectasia.

comes (ko′mēz), pl. *co′mites* [L.] an artery or vein accompanying a nerve trunk.

commensal (kom-men′sil) 1. living on or within another organism, and deriving benefit without harming or benefiting the host. 2. a parasite that causes no harm to the host.

commensalism (-izm) symbiosis in which one population (or individual) is benefited and the other is neither benefited nor harmed.

comminuted (kom′in-ōot″id) broken or crushed into small pieces, as a comminuted fracture.

commissura (kom″ĭ-su′rah), pl. *commissu′rae* [L.] commissure. **c. cerebel′li,** pons (2). **c. mag′na,** corpus callosum.

commissure (kom″ĭ-shoor) a site of union of corresponding parts; specifically, the sites of junction between adjacent cusps of the heart valves. **anterior c. of cerebrum,** the band of fibers connecting the parts of the two cerebral hemispheres. **Gudden's c.,** see *supraoptic c's.* **Meynert's c.,** see *supraoptic c's.* **middle c. of cerebrum,** band of gray matter joining the optic thalami; it develops as a secondary adhesion and may be absent. **posterior c. of cerebrum,** a large fiber bundle crossing from one side of the cerebrum to the other dorsal where the aqueduct opens into the third ventricle. **supraoptic c's,** commissural fibers crossing the midline of the human brain dorsal to the caudal border of the optic chiasm, representing the combined commissures of Gudden and Meynert.

commissurorrhaphy (kom″ĭ-shoor-or′ah-fe) suture of the components of a commissure, to lessen the size of the orifice.

commissurotomy (-ot′ah-me) surgical incision or digital disruption of the components of a commissure to increase the size of the orifice; commonly done to separate adherent, thickened leaflets of a stenotic mitral valve.

communicable (kom-u′nĭ-kah-b'l) capable of being transmitted from one person to another.

communicans (kom-u′nĭ-kans) [L.] communicating.

community (kom-u′nit-e) a body of individuals living in a defined area or having a common interest or organization. **biotic c.,** an assemblage of populations living in a defined area. **therapeutic c.,** a structured mental hospital employing group therapy and encouraging the patient to function within social norms.

compaction (kom-pak′shin) a complication of labor in twin births in which there is simultaneous full engagement of the leading fetal poles of both twins, so that the true pelvic cavity is filled and further descent is prevented.

Compazine (kom′pah-zēn) trademark for preparations of prochlorperazine.

compensation (kom″pin-sa′shin) the counterbalancing of any defect. In psychoanalysis, the mechanism by which an approved character trait is put forward to hide from the ego the existence of an opposite trait. In cardiology, the maintenance of an adequate blood flow without distressing symptoms. **compen′satory,** adj.

dosage c., in genetics, the mechanism by which the effect of the two X chromosomes of the normal female is rendered identical to that of the one X chromosome of the normal male.

complaint (kom-plānt′) a disease, symptom, or disorder. **chief c.,** the symptom or group of symptoms about which the patient first consults the doctor; the presenting symptom.

complement (kom′plĕ-ment) a series of enzymatic proteins in normal serum that combine with antigen-antibody complex; complement comprises nine functioning components symbolized as C1 through C9, which cause lysis of cells and destruction of bacteria, and are involved in immunological and biological activities.

complementation (kom″plĭ-men-ta′shin) in genetics, the restoration of wild-type function as a result of two distinct mutations on the same chromosome. In virology, the interaction of two defective bacteriophages resulting in replication of both.

complex (kom′pleks) 1. the sum or combination of various things, like or unlike, as a complex of symptoms; see *syndrome.* 2. a group of associated, partially or wholly repressed ideas, usually outside of awareness, which can evoke emotional forces that influence an individual's behavior. 3. that portion of an electrocardiogram representing the systole of an atrium or ventricle. **AIDS-related c. (ARC),** a complex of signs and symptoms representing a less severe form of human immunodeficiency virus infection than acquired immune deficiency syndrome, characterized by chronic generalized lymphadenopathy, fever, weight loss, prolonged diarrhea, minor opportunistic infections, cytopenia, and T-cell abnormalities of the kind associated with AIDS. **anomalous c.,** a complex varying from the normal type, as an electrocardiographic complex. **antigen-antibody c.,** a complex formed by the binding of antigen to antibody. **atrial c.,** the portion (P wave) of the electrocardiogram produced by excitation of the atrium. **avian leukosis c.,** see *avian leukosis.* **calcarine c.,** calcar avis. **castration c.,** the fear (usually fantasied) of damage to or loss of sexual organs as punishment for forbidden sexual desires. **Eisenmenger c.,** a defect of the interventricular septum with severe pulmonary hypertension, hypertrophy of the right ventricle, and latent or overt cyanosis. **factor IX c.,** a sterile, freeze-dried powder containing coagulation Factors II, VII, IX, and X, extracted from plasma of healthy human donors. **Ghon c.,** primary c. (1). **Golgi c.,** Golgi apparatus; a complex cellular organelle consisting mainly of a number of flattened sacs (cisternae) and associated vesicles, involved in the synthesis of glycoproteins, lipoproteins, membrane-bound proteins, and lysosomal enzymes. The sacs form primary lysosomes and secretory vacuoles. **immune c.,** antigen-antibody c. **inferiority c.,** unconscious feelings of inferiority, producing timidity or, as a compensation, exaggerated aggressiveness and expression of superiority (*superiority c.*). **Lutembacher's c.,** see under *syndrome.* **major histocompatibility c. (MHC),**

the chromosomal region containing genes that control the histocompatibility antigens. In man, it controls the HLA antigens. **pore c.,** a nuclear pore and its annulus considered together. **primary c.,** the combination of a parenchymal pulmonary lesion (*Ghon focus*) and a corresponding lymph node focus, occurring in primary tuberculosis, usually in children. Similar lesions may also be associated with other mycobacterial infections and with fungal infections. 2. the primary cutaneous lesion at the site of infection in the skin, e.g., chancre in syphilis and tuberculous chancre. **primary inoculation c., primary tuberculous c.,** tuberculous chancre. **symptom c.,** syndrome. **synaptonemal c.,** the structure formed by the synapsis of homologous chromosomes during the zygotene stage of meiosis I. **ventricular c.,** the portion (Q, R, S, and T waves) of the electrocardiogram produced by excitation of the ventricles.

complexion (kom-plek′shin) the color and appearance of the skin of the face.

compliance (kom-pli′ins) the quality of yielding to pressure without disruption, or an expression of the ability to do so, as an expression of the distensibility of an air- or fluid-filled organ, e.g., lung or urinary bladder, in terms of unit of volume change per unit of pressure change.

complication (kom″plĭ-ka′shin) 1. disease(s) concurrent with another disease. 2. occurrence of several diseases in the same patient.

compos mentis (kom′pos men′tis) [L.] sound of mind; sane.

compound (kom′pownd) 1. made up of two or more parts or ingredients. 2. a substance made up of two or more materials. 3. in chemistry, a substance consisting of two or more elements in union. **inorganic c.,** a compound of chemical elements containing no carbon atoms. **organic c.,** a compound of chemical elements containing carbon atoms. **organometallic c.,** one in which carbon is linked to a metal. **quaternary ammonium c.,** an organic compound containing a quaternary ammonium group, a nitrogen atom carrying a single positive charge bonded to four carbon atoms, e.g., choline.

compress (kom′pres) a pad or bolster of folded linen or other material, applied with pressure; sometimes medicated, it may be wet or dry, or hot or cold.

compression (kom-presh′in) 1. act of pressing upon or together; the state of being pressed together. 2. in embryology, the shortening or omission of certain developmental stages.

compromised (kom′prah-mīzd) lacking adequate resistance to infection, or lacking the ability to mount an adequate immune response, owing to a course of treatment (irradiation, etc.) or to an underlying disorder (leukemia, etc.).

compulsion (kom-pul′shin) an overwhelming urge to perform an irrational act or ritual. **compulsive,** adj. **repetition c.,** in psychoanalytic theory, the impulse to reenact earlier emotional experiences.

conarium (ko-na′re-um) the pineal body.

conation (ko-na′shin) in psychology, the power

that impels effort of any kind; the conscious tendency to act. **con′ative,** adj.

concanavalin (kon″kah-nav′ah-lin) either of two phytohemagglutinins isolated along with canavalin from the meal of the Jack bean (*Canavalia ensiformis* and other species of *Canavalia*), which agglutinate the blood of mammals as a result of reaction with polyglucosans. *Concanavalin A* has been shown to inhibit the growth of ascites tumors.

concave (kon′kāv) rounded and somewhat depressed or hollowed out.

concavoconcave (kon-ka″vo-kon′kāv) concave on each of two opposite surfaces.

concavoconvex (-kon′veks) having one concave and one convex surface.

conceive (kon-sēv′) 1. to become pregnant. 2. take in, grasp, or form in the mind.

concentrate (kon′sin-trāt) 1. to bring to a common center; to gather at one point. 2. to increase the strength by diminishing the bulk of, as of a liquid; to condense. 3. a drug or other preparation that has been strengthened by evaporation of its nonactive parts.

concentration (kon″sin-tra′shin) 1. increase in strength by evaporation. 2. the ratio of the mass or volume of a solute to the mass or volume of the solution or solvent. **hydrogen ion c.,** the degree of concentration of hydrogen ions in a solution; related approximately to the pH of the solution by the equation $(H^+) = 10^{-pH}$. **mass c.,** the mass of a constituent substance divided by the volume of the mixture, as milligrams per liter (mg/l), etc. **molar c., substance c.,** the amount of a constituent substance in moles (millimoles or micromoles) divided by the volume of the mixture, as millimoles per liter (mmol/l), etc.

concept (kon′sept) the image of a thing held in the mind.

conception (kon-sep′shin) 1. the onset of pregnancy, the implantation of the blastocyst; the formation of a viable zygote. 2. concept.

conceptus (kon-sep′tus) all the derivatives of a fertilized ovum at any developmental stage from fertilization until birth, including extraembryonic membranes and the embryo or fetus.

concha (kong′kah), pl. *con′chae* [L.] a shell-shaped structure. **c. of auricle,** the hollow of the auricle of the external ear, bounded anteriorly by the tragus and posteriorly by the anthelix. **c. bullo′sa,** a cystic distention of the middle nasal concha. **ethmoidal c., inferior,** nasal c., middle. **ethmoidal c., superior,** nasal c., superior. **ethmoidal c., supreme,** nasal c., supreme. **nasal c., inferior,** a bone forming the lower part of the lateral wall of the nasal cavity. **nasal c., middle,** the lower of two bony plates projecting from the inner wall of the ethmoid labyrinth and separating the superior from the middle meatus of the nose. **nasal c., superior,** the upper of two bony plates projecting from the inner wall of the ethmoid labyrinth and forming the upper boundary of the superior meatus of the nose. **nasal c., supreme,** a third bony plate occasionally found projecting from the inner wall of the ethmoid labyrinth, above

the two usually found. **c. santori′ni,** nasal c., supreme. **sphenoidal c.,** a thin curved plate of bone at the anterior and lower part of the body of the sphenoid bone, on either side, forming part of the roof of the nasal cavity.

conclination (kon″klĭ-na′shin) inward rotation of the upper pole of the vertical meridian of each eye.

concordance (kon-kord′ins) in genetics, the occurrence of a given trait in both members of a twin pair. **concor′dant,** adj.

concrescence (kon-kres′ins) a growing together of parts originally separate.

concretio (kon-kre′she-o) concretion. **c. cor′dis,** adhesive pericarditis in which the pericardial cavity is obliterated.

concretion (kon-kre′shin) 1. a calculus or inorganic mass in a natural cavity or in tissue. 2. abnormal union of adjacent parts. 3. a process of becoming harder or more solid.

concussion (kon-kush′in) a violent shock or jar, or the condition resulting from such an injury. **c. of the brain,** loss of consciousness, transient or prolonged, due to a blow to the head; there may be transient amnesia, vertigo, nausea, weak pulse, and slow respiration. **c. of the labyrinth,** deafness with tinnitus due to a blow on or explosion near the ear. **pulmonary c.,** mechanical damage to the lungs caused by an explosion. **c. of the spinal cord,** transient spinal cord dysfunction caused by mechanical injury.

condensation (kon″din-sa′shin) 1. the act of rendering, or the process of becoming, more compact; in dentistry, the packing of filling materials into a tooth cavity. 2. the fusion of events, thoughts, or concepts to produce a new and simpler concept. 3. the process of passing from a gaseous to a liquid or solid phase.

condenser (kon-den′ser) 1. a vessel or apparatus for condensing gases or vapors. 2. a device for illuminating microscopic objects. 3. an apparatus for concentrating energy or matter. 4. a dental instrument used to pack plastic filling material into the prepared cavity of a tooth.

conditioning (-ing) learning in which a response is elicited by a neutral stimulus which previously has been repeatedly presented in conjunction with the stimulus that originally elicited the response.

condom (kon′dum) a sheath or cover to be worn over the penis in coitus to prevent impregnation or infection.

conductance (kon-duk′tins) ability to conduct energy or material; in studies of respiration, an expression of the amount of air reaching the alveoli per unit of time per unit of pressure, the reciprocal of resistance.

conduction (kon-duk′shin) conveyance of energy, as of heat, sound, or electricity. **aerial c.,** conduction of sound waves to the organ of hearing through the air. **aerotympanal c.,** conduction of sound waves to the ear through the air and the tympanum. **air c.,** aerial c. **bone c.,** conduction of sound waves to the inner ear through the bones of the skull. **saltatory c.,** the passage of a potential from node to node of a nerve fiber, rather than along the membrane.

conduit (kon′dit) a channel for the passage of fluids. **ileal c.,** the surgical anastomosis of the ureters to one end of a detached segment of ileum, the other end being used to form a stoma on the abdominal wall.

condylarthrosis (kon″dil-ar-thro′sis) a modification of the spheroidal form of synovial joint in which the articular surfaces are ellipsoidal rather than spheroid.

condyle (kon′dīl) a rounded projection on a bone, usually for articulation with another bone. **con′dylar,** adj.

condylion (kon-dil′e-on) the most lateral point on the surface of the head of the mandible.

condyloma (kon″dil-o′mah) an elevated lesion of the skin. **condylo′matous,** adj. **c.** acumina′-**tum,** a small, pointed papilloma of viral origin, usually occurring on the mucous membrane or skin of the external genitals or in the perianal region. **flat c.,** c. latum. **giant c.** acumina′tum, Buschke-Löwenstein tumor. **c. la′tum,** a broad, flat syphilitic condyloma on the folds of moist skin, especially about the genitals and anus.

condylotomy (-lot′ah-me) transection of a condyle.

condylus (kon′dil-us), pl. *con′dyli* [L.] condyle.

cone (kōn) 1. a solid figure or body having a circular base and tapering to a point, especially one of the conelike bodies of the retina. 2. in radiology, a conical or open-ended cylindrical structure used as an aid in centering the radiation beam and as a guide to source-to-film distance. 3. surgical c. **ether c.,** a cone-shaped device used over the face in administration of inhalation anesthesia. **c. of light,** the triangular light reflex on the membrana tympani. **retinal c's,** highly specialized conical or flask-shaped outer segments of the visual cells, which, with the retinal rods, form the light-sensitive elements of the retina. **surgical c.,** a cone of tissue removed surgically, as in partial excision of the cervix uteri. **twin c's,** retinal cone cells in which two cells are blended.

conexus (kon-ek′sus) a connecting structure.

confabulation (kon-fab″u-la′shin) telling imaginary experiences to fill gaps in memory.

confection (kon-fek′shin) a medicated sweetmeat or electuary.

confinement (kon-fīn′mint) restraint within a specific area, especially at childbirth.

conflict (kon′flikt) a painful state of consciousness due to clash between opposing emotional forces, found to a certain extent in every person. **extrapsychic c.,** that between the self and the external environment. **intrapsychic c.,** that between forces within the personality.

confluence (kon′floo-ins) a running together; a meeting of streams. **con′fluent,** adj. **c. of sinuses,** the dilated point of confluence of the superior sagittal, straight, occipital, and two transverse sinuses of the dura mater.

confusion (kon-fu′zhin) disturbed orientation in regard to time, place, or person, sometimes accompanied by disordered consciousness.

congener (kon′jĕ-ner) something closely related to another thing, as a member of the same genus, a muscle having the same function as another, or a chemical compound closely related to another in composition and exerting similar or antagonistic effects, or something derived from the same source or stock. **congener′ic, congen′erous,** adj.

congenic (kon-jen′ik) of or relating to a strain of animals developed from an inbred (isogenic) strain by repeated matings with animals from another stock that have a foreign gene, the final congenic strain then presumably differing from the original inbred strain by the presence of this gene.

congenital (kon-jen′ĭ-til) present at and existing from the time of birth.

congestion (kon-jes′chin) abnormal accumulation of blood in a part. **conges′tive,** adj. **hypostatic c.,** congestion of a dependent part of the body or an organ due to gravitational forces, as in venous insufficiency. **passive c.,** that due to lack of vital power or to obstruction of escape of blood from the part. **pulmonary c.,** engorgement of the pulmonary vessels, with transudation of fluid into the alveolar and interstitial spaces; it occurs in cardiac disease, infections, and certain injuries. **venous c.,** passive c.

conglobation (kon″glo-ba′shin) the act of forming, or the state of being formed, into a rounded mass. **conglo′bate,** adj.

conglutination (kon-gloot″in-a′shin) 1. the adherence of tissues to each other. 2. agglutination of erythrocytes that is dependent upon both complement and antibodies.

coniofibrosis (ko″ne-o-fi-bro′sis) pneumoconiosis with exuberant growth of connective tissue in the lungs.

coniosis (ko″ne-o′sis) a diseased state due to inhalation of dust.

coniosporosis (ko″ne-o-spor-o′sis) a condition characterized by asthmatic symptoms and acute pneumonitis, caused by inhalation of spores of *Coniosporium corticale,* a fungus growing under the bark of certain trees; observed in workers engaged in peeling logs.

coniotoxicosis (-tok″sĭ-ko′sis) pneumoconiosis in which the irritant affects the tissues directly.

conization (ko″ni-za′shin) the removal of a cone of tissue, as in partial excision of the cervix uteri. **cold c.,** that done with a cold knife, as opposed to electrocautery, to better preserve the histologic elements.

conjugata (kon″ju-gāt′ah) the conjugate diameter of the pelvis. **c. ve′ra,** the true conjugate diameter of the pelvis.

conjugate (kon′jug-āt) 1. paired, or equally coupled; working in unison. 2. a conjugate diameter of the pelvic inlet; used alone usually to denote the true conjugate diameter; see under *diameter.*

conjugation (kon″jug-a′shin) a joining. In unicellular organisms, a form of sexual reproduction in which two individuals join in temporary union to transfer genetic material. In biochemistry, the joining of a toxic substance with some natural substance of the body to form a detoxified product for elimination.

conjunctiva (kon″junk-ti′vah), pl. *conjuncti′vae* [L.] the delicate membrane lining the eyelids and covering the eyeball. **conjuncti′val,** adj.

conjunctivitis (kon-junk″tĭ-vīt′is) inflammation of the conjunctiva. **acute contagious c.,** pinkeye; a highly contagious form of conjunctivitis caused by *Hemophilus aegyptius.* **acute hemorrhagic c.,** a contagious form due to infection with enteroviruses. **allergic c., anaphylactic c.,** hay fever. **atopic c.,** allergic conjunctivitis of the immediate type, due to airborne allergens such as pollens, dusts, spores, and animal hair. **gonococcal c., gonorrheal c.,** a severe form due to infection with gonococci. **granular c.,** trachoma. **inclusion c.,** conjunctivitis affecting newborn infants, caused by a strain of *Chlamydia trachomatis,* beginning as acute purulent conjunctivitis and leading to papillary hypertrophy of the palpebral conjunctiva. **phlyctenular c.,** that marked by small vesicles surrounded by a reddened zone. **spring c., vernal c.,** that usually occurring in the spring.

conjunctivoma (kon-junk″tĭ-vo′mah) a tumor of the eyelid composed of conjunctival tissue.

conjunctivoplasty (kon″junk-ti′vo-plas″te) plastic repair of the conjunctiva.

connection (kon-ek′shin) 1. the act of connecting or state of being connected. 2. anything that connects; a connector.

connector (kon-nek′ter) a device which joins together two separate parts or units, e.g., the bilateral parts of a removable partial denture.

conoid (ko′noid) cone-shaped.

consanguinity (kon″sang-gwin′it-e) blood relationship; kinship. **consanguin′eous,** adj.

conscience (kon′shins) one's set of moral values, the conscious part of the superego.

conscious (kon′shus) capable of responding to sensory stimuli and having subjective experiences; awake; aware.

consciousness (-nes) the state of being conscious; responsiveness of the mind to impressions made by the senses. **double c.,** see *multiple personality.*

conservative (kon-serv′ah-tiv) designed to preserve health, restore function, and repair structures by nonradical methods.

consolidation (kon-sol″ĭ-da′shin) solidification; the process of becoming or the condition of being solid; said especially of the lung as it fills with exudate in pneumonia.

constant (kon′stint) 1. not failing; remaining unaltered. 2. a quantity that is not subject to change. **association c.,** a measure of the extent of a reversible association between two molecular species. **Avogadro's c.,** see under *number.* **binding c.,** association c. **Michaelis c.,** a constant representing the substrate concentration at which the velocity of an enzyme reaction is half the maximal velocity; symbol K_m. **sedimentation c.,** a measure, commonly expressed in Svedberg units, of the relative sedimentation rate of molecules under an induced gravitational field, as in a centrifuge; symbol S.

constipation (kon″stĭ-pa′shin) infrequent or difficult evacuation of feces. **constipa′ted,** adj.

constitution (kon″stĭ-too′shin) 1. the make-up or functional habit of the body. 2. the arrangement of atoms in a molecule.

constriction (kon-strik′shin) 1. a narrowing or compression of a part; a stricture. 2. a diminution in range of thinking or feeling, associated with diminished spontaneity.

consultation (kon″sul-ta′shin) a deliberation by two or more physicians about diagnosis or treatment in a particular case.

consumption (kon-sump′shin) 1. the act of consuming, or the process of being consumed. 2. wasting of the body; formerly, tuberculosis of the lungs. **luxus c.,** ingestion of excess protein which does not form part of the tissues but remains in the body as a reserve supply.

contact (kon′takt) 1. a mutual touching of two bodies or persons. 2. an individual known to have been sufficiently near an infected person to have been exposed to the transfer of infectious material. **balancing c.,** the contact between the upper and lower occlusal surfaces of the teeth on the side opposite the working contact. **complete c.,** contact of the entire adjoining surfaces of two teeth. **direct c., immediate c.,** the contact of a healthy person with a person having a communicable disease, the disease being transmitted as a result. **indirect c., mediate c.,** that achieved through some intervening medium, as propagation of a communicable disease through the air or by means of fomites. **occlusal c.,** contact between the upper and lower teeth when the jaws are closed. **proximal c., proximate c.,** touching of the proximal surfaces of two adjoining teeth. **working c.,** that between the upper and lower teeth on the side toward which the mandible has been moved in mastication.

contactant (kon-tak′tint) an allergen capable of inducing delayed contact-type hypersensitivity of the epidermis after contact.

contagion (kon-ta′jin) 1. the spread of disease from person-to-person. 2. a contagious disease. **direct c., immediate c.,** communication of disease by direct contact with a sick person. **mediate c.,** communication of disease through an intervening object or person. **psychic c.,** communication of psychological symptoms through mental influence.

contaminant (kon-tam′in-int) something that causes contamination.

contamination (kon-tam″in-a-shin) 1. the soiling or making inferior by contact or mixture. 2. the deposition of radioactive material in any place where it is not desired.

content (kon′tent) that which is contained within a thing. **latent c.,** the part of a dream hidden in the unconsciousness. **manifest c.,** the part of a dream remembered after awakening.

continence (kon′tin-ens) ability to control natural impulses. **con′tinent,** adj.

contra- word element [L.], *against; opposed.*

contra-angle (kon″trah-ang′g′l) an angulation by which the working point of a surgical instrument is brought close to the long axis of its shaft.

contra-aperture (-ap′er-cher) a second opening

made in an abscess to facilitate the discharge of its contents.

contraceptive (-sep′tiv) 1. diminishing the likelihood of or preventing conception. 2. an agent that so acts. **intrauterine c.,** see *contraceptive device.* **oral c.,** a hormonal compound taken orally in order to block ovulation and prevent the occurrence of pregnancy.

contractile (kon-trak′til) able to contract in response to a suitable stimulus.

contractility (kon″trak-til′ĭ-te) capacity for becoming short in response to a suitable stimulus.

contraction (kon-trak′shin) a drawing together; a shortening or shrinkage. **Braxton Hicks c's,** light, usually painless, irregular uterine contractions during pregnancy, gradually increasing in intensity and frequency and becoming more rhythmic during the third trimester. **carpopedal c.,** the condition due to chronic shortening of the muscles of the fingers, toes, arms, and legs in tetany. **cicatricial c.,** the shrinkage and spontaneous closing of open skin wounds. **clonic c.,** muscular contraction alternating with relaxation. **closing c.,** contraction occurring at the point of application of the stimulus when the electrical circuit is closed. **Dupuytren's c.,** see under *contracture.* **hourglass c.,** contraction of an organ, as the stomach or uterus, at or near the middle. **idiomuscular c.,** contraction due to direct electrical stimulation of a wasted muscle. **isometric c.,** muscle contraction without appreciable shortening or change in distance between its origin and insertion. **isotonic c.,** muscle contraction without appreciable change in the force of contraction; the distance between the muscle's origin and insertion becomes lessened. **opening c.,** contraction occurring at the point of application of the stimulus when the electrical circuit is opened. **paradoxical c.,** contraction of a muscle caused by the passive approximation of its extremities. **postural c.,** the state of muscular tension and contraction which just suffices to maintain the posture of the body. **tetanic c.,** sustained muscular contraction without intervals of relaxation. **tonic c.,** tetanic c. **twitch c.,** the all-or-none response of muscle cells to a single stimulus. **uterine c.,** contraction of the uterus during labor. **Volkmann's c.,** see under *contracture.* **wound c.,** the shrinkage and spontaneous closure of open skin wounds.

contracture (kon-trak′cher) abnormal shortening of muscle tissue, rendering the muscle highly resistant to passive stretching. **Dupuytren's c.,** flexion deformity of the fingers or toes, due to shortening, thickening, and fibrosis of the palmar or plantar fascia. **ischemic c.,** muscular contracture and degeneration due to interference with the circulation from pressure, or from injury or cold. **organic c.,** permanent and continuous contracture. **Volkmann's c.,** contraction of the fingers and sometimes of the wrist, or of analogous parts of the foot, with loss of power, after severe injury or improper use of a tourniquet.

contrafissure (kon″trah-fish′er) a fracture in a part opposite the site of the blow.

contraincision (-in-sizh′in) counterincision to promote drainage.

contraindication (-in″dĭ-ka′shin) any condition which renders a particular line of treatment improper or undesirable.

contralateral (-lat′er-il) pertaining to, situated on, or affecting the opposite side.

contrecoup (kon″truh-koo′) [Fr.] denoting an injury, as to the brain, occurring at a site opposite to the point of impact.

control (kon-trōl′) 1. the governing or limitation of certain objects or events. 2. a standard against which experimental observations may be evaluated, as a procedure identical to the experimental procedure except for absence of the one factor being studied; also any individual of the group exhibiting the standard characteristics. **aversive c.,** in behavior therapy, the use of unpleasant stimuli to change undesirable behavior. **birth c.,** deliberate limitation of childbearing by measures to control fertility and to prevent conception. **stimulus c.,** any influence of the environment on behavior.

Controlled Substances Act a federal law that regulates the prescribing and dispensing of psychoactive drugs, including narcotics, hallucinogens, depressants, and stimulants.

contuse (kon-tōōz′) to bruise; to wound by beating.

conus (ko′nus), pl. *co′ni* [L.] 1. a cone or cone-shaped structure. 2. posterior staphyloma of the myopic eye. **c. arterio′sus,** the anterosuperior portion of the right ventricle of the heart, at the entrance to the pulmonary trunk. **c. medulla′ris,** the cone-shaped lower end of the spinal cord, at the level of the upper lumbar vertebrae. **c. termina′lis,** c. medullaris. **co′ni vasculo′si,** lobules of epididymis.

convalescence (kon″vah-les′ins) the stage of recovery from an illness, operation, or injury.

convection (kon-vek′shin) the act of conveying or transmission, specifically transmission of heat in a liquid or gas by circulation of heated particles.

convergence (kon-ver′jins) the coordinated inclination of the two lines of sight towards their common point of fixation, or that point itself. **conver′gent,** adj. **negative c.,** outward deviation of the visual axes. **positive c.,** inward deviation of the visual axes.

conversion (kon-ver′zhin) 1. the transformation of emotions into physical manifestations. 2. manipulative correction of malposition of a fetal part during labor.

convertase (kon-ver′tās) an enzyme that converts a substance to its active state.

convertin (kon-ver′tin) coagulation Factor VII.

convex (kon′veks) having a rounded, somewhat elevated surface.

convexoconcave (kon-vek″so-kon′kāv) having one convex and one concave surface.

convexoconvex (-kon′veks) convex on two surfaces.

convolution (kon″vol-oo′shin) a tortuous irregularity or elevation caused by the infolding of a structure upon itself. **Broca's c.,** inferior frontal gyrus. **Heschl's c.,** anterior transverse temporal gyrus.

convulsion (kon-vul′shin) an involuntary contraction or series of contractions of the voluntary muscles. **central c.,** one not excited by any external cause, but due to a lesion of the central nervous system. **clonic c.,** one marked by alternating contraction and relaxation of the muscles. **coordinate c.,** one marked by clonic movements resembling healthy, purposeful movements. **epileptiform c.,** convulsion marked by loss of consciousness. **essential c.,** central c. **febrile c's,** those associated with high fever, occurring in infants and children. **hysterical c., hysteroid c.,** conversion hysteria with symptoms resembling convulsions. **mimetic c., mimic c.,** facial spasm or tic. **puerperal c.,** involuntary spasms in women just before, during, or just after childbirth. **salaam c.,** nodding spasm. **tetanic c.,** tonic spasm with loss of consciousness. **uremic c.,** convulsion due to uremia, or retention in the blood of material that should have been eliminated by the kidneys.

Cooperia (koo-pe′re-ah) a genus of parasitic nematodes.

coordination (ko-or″din-a′shin) the harmonious functioning of interrelated organs and parts.

COPD chronic obstructive pulmonary disease.

cope (kōp) in dentistry, the upper or cavity side of a denture flask.

coping (kōp′ing) a thin, metal covering or cap, such as the plate of metal applied over the prepared crown or root of a tooth prior to attaching an artificial crown.

copiopia (kop″e-o′pe-ah) eyestrain.

copolymer (ko-pol′ĭ-mer) a polymer containing monomers of more than one kind.

copper (kop′er) chemical element (*see table*), at. no. 29, symbol Cu. **c. sulfate,** cupric sulfate.

copperhead (-hed) 1. a venomous snake (a pit viper), *Agkistrodon contortrix,* of the United States, having a brown to copper-colored body with dark bands. 2. a very venomous elapid snake, *Denisonia superba,* of Australia, Tasmania, and the Solomon Islands.

coproantibody (kop″ro-an′tĭ-bod-e) an antibody (chiefly IgA) present in the intestinal tract, associated with immunity to enteric infection.

coprolalia (-la′le-ah) the utterance of obscene words, especially words relating to feces.

coprolith (kop′rah-lith) hard fecal concretion in the intestine.

coprophobia (-fo′be-ah) abnormal repugnance to defecation and to feces.

coproporphyria (-por-fir′e-ah) hereditary porphyria marked by excessive excretion of coproporphyrin, chiefly in the feces.

coproporphyrin (-por′fĭ-rin) a porphyrin formed in the blood-forming organs and intestine and found in the urine and feces in coproporphyrinuria.

coproporphyrinuria (-por″fĭ-rin-ūr′e-ah) the presence of coproporphyrin in the urine.

coprostasis (kop-ros′tah-sis) fecal impaction.

coprozoa (kop″rah-zo′ah) protozoa found in feces outside the body, but not in the intestines.

copula (kop′u-lah) any connecting part or structure.

copulation (kop″u-la′shin) sexual congress or coitus; usually applied to the mating process in animals lower than man.

cor (kor) [L.] heart. **c. adipo′sum,** a heart that has undergone fatty degeneration or that has an accumulation of fat around it. **c. bilocula′re,** a two-chambered heart with one atrium and one ventricle, and a common atrioventricular valve. **c. bovi′num,** a greatly enlarged heart due to a hypertrophied left ventricle. **c. hirsu′tum,** c. villosum. **c. pseudotrilocula′re biatria′tum,** a congenital anomaly in which the heart functions as a three-chambered heart, the blood passing from the right to the left atrium and thence to the left ventricle and aorta. **c. pulmona′le,** heart disease due to pulmonary hypertension secondary to disease of the lung or its blood vessels, with hypertrophy of the right ventricle. **c. triatria′tum,** a heart with three atrial chambers, the pulmonary veins emptying into an accessory chamber above the true left atrium and communicating with it by a small opening. **c. trilocula′re,** three-chambered heart. **c. trilocula′re biatria′tum,** a three-chambered heart with two atria communicating, by the tricuspid and mitral valves, with a single ventricle. **c. trilocula′re biventricula′re,** a three-chambered heart with one atrium and two ventricles. **c. villo′sum,** a roughened state of the pericardium, due to an exudate on its surface, occurring in pericarditis.

coracidium (kor″ah-sid′e-um), pl. *coracid′ia* [L.] the individual free-swimming or free-crawling, spherical, ciliated embryo of certain tapeworms, e.g., *Diphyllobothrium latum.*

coracoid (kor′ah-koid) 1. like a crow's beak. 2. the coracoid process.

corasthma (kor-az′mah) hay fever.

cord (kord) any long, cylindrical, flexible structure. **Braun's c's,** strings of cells which have been observed in the kidney of the early embryo. **Ferrein's c's,** the lower, or true, vocal cords. **genital c.,** in the embryo, the midline fused caudal part of the two urogenital ridges, each containing a mesonephric and paramesonephric duct. **gubernacular c.,** chorda gubernaculum. **sexual c's,** the seminiferous tubules during the early fetal stage. **spermatic c.,** the structure extending from the abdominal inguinal ring to the testis, comprising the pampiniform plexus, nerves, ductus deferens, testicular artery, and other vessels. **spinal c.,** that part of the central nervous system lodged in the vertebral canal, extending from the foramen magnum to the upper part of the lumbar region; see Plates XI and XIV. **umbilical c.,** the structure connecting the fetus and placenta, and containing the vessels through which fetal blood passes to and from the placenta. **vocal c's,** folds of mucous membrane in the larynx; the superior pair being called the *false,* and the inferior pair the *true,* vocal cords. **Willis' c's,** fibrous bands traversing the inferior angle of the superior sagittal sinus.

cordectomy (kor-dek′tah-me) excision of a cord, as of a vocal cord.

corditis (kor-dīt′is) inflammation of the spermatic cord.

cordotomy (kor-dot′ah-me) 1. section of a vocal cord. 2. surgical division of the anterolateral tracts of the spinal cord.

Cordran (kor′dran) trademark for a preparation of flurandrenolide.

core(o)- word element [Gr.], *pupil of eye.*

coreclisis (kor″ah-kli′sis) iridencleisis.

corectasis (kor-ek′tah-sis) dilation of the pupil.

corectome (ko-rek′tōm) cutting instrument for iridectomy.

corectomedialysis (ko-rek″to-me″de-al′ĭ-sis) surgical creation of an artificial pupil by detaching the iris from the ciliary ligament.

corectopia (kor″ek-to′pe-ah) abnormal location of the pupil of the eye.

coredialysis (ko″re-di-al′ĭ-sis) surgical separation of the external margin of the iris from the ciliary body.

corelysis (ko-rel′ĭ-sis) operative destruction of the pupil; especially detachment of adhesions of the pupillary margin of the iris from the lens.

coremorphosis (ko″re-mor-fo′sis) surgical formation of an artificial pupil.

coreoplasty (ko′re-o-plas″te) any plastic operation on the pupil.

corepressor (ko″re-pres′er) in genetic theory, a small molecule that combines with an aporepressor to form the complete repressor.

corium (ko′re-um) the dermis; the layer of the skin deep to the epidermis, consisting of a bed of vascular connective tissue, and containing the nerves and organs of sensation, the hair roots, and sebaceous and sweat glands.

corn (korn) a horny induration and thickening of the stratum corneum, caused by friction and pressure and forming a conical mass pointing down into the corium, producing pain and irritation. **hard c.,** one usually located on the outside of the little toe or the upper surfaces of the other toes. **soft c.,** one between the toes, kept softened by moisture, often leading to painful inflammation under the corn.

cornea (kor′ne-ah) the transparent anterior part of the eye. See Plate XIII. **cor′neal,** adj. **conical c.,** keratoconus.

corneosclera (-skle′rah) the cornea and sclera regarded as one organ.

corneous (kor′ne-us) hornlike or horny; consisting of keratin.

corniculum (kor-nik′u-lum) [L.] corniculate cartilage.

cornification (kor″nĭ-fi-ka′shin) 1. conversion into keratin, or horn. 2. conversion of epithelium to the stratified squamous type.

cornu (kor′nu), pl. *cor′nua* [L.] horn; a hornlike excrescence or projection; in anatomical nomenclature, a structure that appears hornshaped, especially in section. **c. ammo′nis,** hippocampus. **c. cuta′neum,** a horny excrescence on human skin. **c. sacra′le,** either of two hook-shaped processes extending down from the arch of the last sacral vertebra.

cornual, cornuate (kor′nu-il; kor′nu-āt) pertaining to a horn, especially to the horns of the spinal cord.

corona (kor-o′nah), pl. *coro′nae* [L.] a crown; in anatomical nomenclature, a crownlike eminence or encircling structure. **coro′nal,** adj. **dental c., c. den′tis,** the crown of a tooth; anatomical crown. **c. glan′dis pe′nis,** rim around proximal part of glans penis. **c. radia′ta,** 1. the radiating crown of projection fibers passing from the internal capsule to every part of the cerebral cortex. 2. an investing layer of radially elongated follicle cells surrounding the zona pellucida. **c. ve′neris,** a ring of syphilitic sores around the forehead.

coronad (kor′ah-nad) toward the crown of the head or any corona.

coronary (kor′ah-ner″e) encircling like a crown; applied to vessels, ligaments, etc., especially to the arteries of the heart, and to pathologic involvement of them.

coronavirus (kor″on-ah-vi′rus) any of a group of morphologically similar, ether-sensitive viruses, probably RNA, causing infectious bronchitis of birds, hepatitis in mice, gastroenteritis in swine, and respiratory infections in humans.

coroner (kor′on-er) an officer who holds inquests in regard to violent, sudden, or unexplained deaths.

coronoidectomy (kor″ah-noi-dek′tah-me) surgical removal of the coronoid process of the mandible.

coroscopy (ko-ros′kah-pe) retinoscopy.

corotomy (ko-rot′ah-me) iridotomy.

corpulency (kor′pu-lin-se) undue fatness.

corpus (kor′pus), pl. *cor′pora* [L.] body. **c. adipo′sum buc′cae,** sucking pad. **c. al′bicans,** white fibrous tissue that replaces the regressing corpus luteum in the human ovary in the latter half of pregnancy, or soon after ovulation when pregnancy does not supervene. **c. amyg-daloi′deum,** a small mass of subcortical gray matter within the tip of the temporal lobe, anterior to the inferior horn of the lateral ventricle of the brain; it is part of the limbic system. **c. callo′sum,** an arched mass of white matter in the depths of the longitudinal fissure, composed of transverse fibers connecting the cerebral hemispheres. **c. caverno′sum,** either of the columns of erectile tissue forming the body of the clitoris (*c. cavernosum clitoridis*) or penis (*c. cavernosum penis*). **c. fimbria′tum,** band of white matter bordering the lateral edge of the lower cornu of the lateral ventricle of the cerebrum. **c. hemorrha′gicum,** 1. an ovarian follicle containing blood. 2. a corpus luteum containing a blood clot. **c. lu′teum,** a yellow glandular mass in the ovary formed by an ovarian follicle that has matured and discharged its ovum. **c. spongio′sum pe′nis,** a column of erectile tissue forming the urethral surface of the penis, in which the urethra is found. **c. stria′tum,** a subcortical mass of gray and white substance in front of and lateral to the thalamus in each cerebral hemisphere. **c. vi′treum,** the vitreous body of the eye.

corpuscle (kor′pus′l) any small mass or body.

corpus′cular, adj. **Alzheimer's c's,** compound granular corpuscles in the oligodendroglia of the brain. **blood c's,** formed elements of the blood, i.e., erythrocytes and leukocytes. **corneal c's,** star-shaped corpuscles within the corneal spaces. **genital c's,** small encapsulated nerve endings in the mucous membranes in the genital region. **Golgi's c's,** encapsulated end-organs found in a tendon at its junction with muscular fibers. **Hassall's c's,** spherical or ovoid bodies found in the medulla of the thymus, composed of concentric arrays of epithelial cells which contain keratohyalin and bundles of cytoplasmic filaments. **lamellated c's,** large encapsulated nerve endings found throughout the body, concerned with perception of different sensations. **malpighian c's,** renal c's. **Meissner's c's,** tactile c's. **Merkel's c's,** tactile corpuscles in the submucosa of the tongue and mouth. **Pacini's c's, pacinian c's,** lamellated corpuscles concerned in perception of pressure. **Purkinje's c's,** large, branched nerve cells composing the middle layer of the cortex of the cerebellum. **red c., red blood c.,** erythrocyte. **renal c's,** bodies forming the beginning of nephrons, each consisting of the glomerulus and glomerular capsule. **tactile c's,** medium-sized nerve endings in the skin, chiefly in the palms and soles. **thymus c's,** Hassall's c's. **white blood c.,** leukocyte.

corpusculum (kor-pus′ku-lum), pl. *corpus′cula* [L.] corpuscle.

correction (kor-ek′shin) a setting right, e.g., the provision of lenses for improvement of vision, or an arbitrary adjustment made in values or devices in performance of experiments.

correlation (kor″il-a′shin) in neurology, the union of afferent impulses within a nerve center to bring about an appropriate response. In statistics, the degree of association of variable phenomena, as intelligence and birth order.

correspondence (kor″is-pon′dins) the condition of being in agreement or conformity. **anomalous retinal c.,** a condition in which disparate points on the retinas of the two eyes come to be associated sensorially. **harmonious retinal c.,** the condition in which the corresponding points on the retinas of the two eyes are associated sensorially. **retinal c.,** the state concerned with the impingement of image-producing stimuli on the retinas of the two eyes.

corrin (kor′in) a tetrapyrrole ring system resembling the porphyrin ring system. The cobalamins contain a corrin ring system.

corrosive (kor-o′siv) destructive to the texture or substance of the tissues; an agent that so acts.

cortex (kor′teks), pl. *cor′tices* [L.] an outer layer, as the bark of the trunk or the rind of a fruit, or the outer layer of an organ or other structure, as distinguished from its inner substance. **cor′tical,** adj. **adrenal c.,** the outer, firm layer comprising the larger part of the adrenal gland; it secretes various hormones; it secretes many steroid hormones including mineralocorticoids, glucocorticoids, androgens, 17-ketosteroids, and progestins. **cerebellar c.,** the superficial gray matter of the cerebellum. **cerebral c., c.**

cer′ebri, the convoluted layer of gray substance covering each cerebral hemisphere; see *archipallium, paleopallium,* and *neopallium.* **c. len′tis,** the softer, external part of the lens of the eye. **motor c.,** the area of the frontal lobe of the cerebral cortex concerned with primary motor control of the body. **provisional c.,** the cortex of the fetal adrenal gland that undergoes involution in early fetal life. **renal c.,** the outer part of the substance of the kidney, composed mainly of glomeruli and convoluted tubules. **striate c.,** the primary visual cortex; the part of the occipital lobe of the cerebral cortex that is the primary receptive area for vision. **c. of thymus,** the outer part of each lobule of the thymus; it consists chiefly of closely packed lymphocytes (thymocytes) and surrounds the medulla. **visual c.,** the area of the occipital lobe of the cerebral cortex concerned with vision.

corticate (kor′tǐ-kāt) having a cortex or bark.

corticectomy (kor″tǐ-sek′tah-me) excision of an area of cerebral cortex (scar or microgyrus) in treatment of focal epilepsy.

corticifugal (-sif′u-g'l) proceeding, conducting, or moving away from the cortex.

corticipetal (-sip′it′l) proceeding, conducting, or moving toward the cortex.

corticobulbar (-bul′ber) pertaining to or connecting the cerebral cortex and the medulla oblongata or brainstem.

corticoid (kor′tǐ-koid) corticosteroid; a steroid hormone of the adrenal cortex.

corticosteroid (-ster′oid) any of the steroids elaborated by the adrenal cortex (excluding the sex hormones) or any synthetic equivalents; divided, according to their predominant biological activity, into two major groups: *glucocorticoids,* chiefly involved in carbohydrate, fat, and protein metabolism, and *mineralocorticoids,* involved in the regulation of electrolyte and water balance; used clinically for hormonal replacement therapy, for suppression of ACTH secretion, as anti-inflammatory agents, and to suppress the immune response.

corticosterone (kor″tǐ-kos′ter-ōn) a mineralocorticoid with some glucocorticoid activity, $C_{21}H_{30}O_4$.

corticotensin (-ten′sin) a polypeptide purified from kidney extract that exhibits a vasopressor effect when given intravenously.

corticotrope (kor′tǐ-ko-trōp) a cell of the anterior pituitary gland that secretes ACTH.

corticotrophin (-tro′fin) corticotropin.

corticotropin (-tro′pin) a hormone secreted by the anterior pituitary gland, having a stimulating effect on the adrenal cortex; a preparation from the anterior pituitary gland of mammals is used for diagnostic testing of adrenocortical function and to stimulate adrenocortical hormone release to treat some diseases.

cortilymph (kor′tǐ-limf″) the fluid filling the intercellular spaces of the organ of Corti.

cortisol (-sol) the major natural glucocorticoid elaborated by the adrenal cortex. See *hydrocortisone* for therapeutic uses.

cortisone (-sōn) a glucocorticoid with significant mineralocorticoid activity, isolated from the adrenal cortex, largely inactive in man until converted to hydrocortisone (cortisol); the acetate is used as an anti-inflammatory agent and for adrenal replacement therapy.

corundum (kor-un′dum) native aluminum oxide, Al_2O_3, used in dentistry as an abrasive and polishing agent.

coruscation (kor″us-ka′shin) the sensation as of a flash of light before the eyes.

corymbiform (ko-rim′bĭ-form) clustered; said of lesions grouped around a single, usually larger, lesion.

Corynebacteriaceae (ko-ri″ne-bak-tēr″e-a′se-e) in former systems of classification, a family of coryneform bacteria, related to the actinomycetes, and consisting of the genera *Arthrobacter, Cellulomonas, Corynebacterium, Erysipelothrix, Listeria,* and *Microbacterium.*

Corynebacterium (-bak-tēr′e-um) a genus of bacteria including *C. ac′nes,* a species present in acne lesions, *C. diphthe′riae,* the etiologic agent of diphtheria, *C. minutis′simum,* the etiologic agent of erythrasma, *C. pseudodiphtheri′ticum,* a nonpathogenic species present in the respiratory tract, and *C. pseudotuberculo′sis,* which sometimes causes pseudotuberculosis in domestic animals.

coryneform (-form) denoting or resembling organisms of the family Corynebacteriaceae.

coryza (ko-ri′zah) profuse discharge from the mucous membrane of the nose. **infectious avian c.,** an acute respiratory disease of chickens characterized chiefly by nasal discharge, sneezing, and edema of the face, and caused by *Hemophilus gallinarum.*

coryzavirus (ko-ri″zah-vi′rus) rhinovirus.

C.O.S. Canadian Ophthalmological Society.

cosmetic (koz-met′ik) 1. beautifying; tending to preserve, restore, or confer comeliness. 2. a beautifying substance or preparation.

cost(o)- word element [L.], *rib.*

costa (kos′tah), pl. *cos′tae* [L.] 1. a rib. 2. a thin, firm, rodlike structure running along the base of the undulating membrane of certain flagellates. **cos′tal,** adj.

costalis (kos-ta′lis) [L.] costal.

costive (kos′tiv) 1. pertaining to, characterized by, or producing constipation. 2. an agent that depresses intestinal motility.

costocervical (kos″to-serv′ĭ-k'l) pertaining to ribs and neck.

costochondral (-kon′dril) pertaining to a rib and its cartilage.

costogenic (-jen′ik) arising from a rib, especially from a defect of the marrow of the ribs.

costoscapularis (-skap″u-la′ris) the serratus anterior muscle.

costosternoplasty (-stern′o-plas″te) surgical repair of funnel chest, a segment of rib being used to support the sternum.

costotransversectomy (-trans″ver-sek′to-me) excision of a part of a rib along with the transverse process of a vertebra.

cosyntropin (ko-sin-tro′pin) a synthetic corticotropin used in the screening of adrenal insuffi-

ciency on the basis of plasma cortisol response after intramuscular or intravenous injection.

cothromboplastin (ko-throm″bo-plas′tin) coagulation Factor VII.

co-trimoxazole (ko″tri-moks′ah-zōl) a mixture of trimethoprim and sulfamethoxazole.

cotton (kot′n) a textile material derived from the seeds of cultivated varieties of *Gossypium.* **absorbable c., absorbent c.,** purified c. **collodion c.,** pyroxylin. **purified c.,** purified cotton, bleached and sterilized; used as a surgical dressing.

cotyledon (kot″ĭ-le′d′n) any subdivision of the uterine surface of the placenta.

cotyloid (kot′ĭ-loid) cup-shaped.

cough (kof) 1. sudden noisy expulsion of air from lungs. 2. to produce such an expulsion of air. **dry c.,** cough without expectoration. **ear c.,** reflex cough produced by disease of the ear. **hacking c.,** a short, frequent, shallow and feeble cough. **productive c.,** cough attended with expectoration of material from the bronchi. **reflex c.,** cough due to irritation of some remote organ. **stomach c.,** cough caused by reflex irritation from stomach disorder. **wet c.,** productive cough. **whooping c.,** see under W.

coulomb (koo′lom) the unit of electrical charge, defined as the quantity of electrical charge transferred by 1 ampere in 1 second.

Coumadin (koo′mah-din) trademark for a preparation of warfarin.

coumarin (koo′mah-rin) 1. a principle extracted from the tonka bean from which several anticoagulants are derived that inhibit hepatic synthesis of vitamin K–dependent coagulation factors. 2. any of these derivatives.

count (kownt) a numerical computation or indication. **Addis c.,** determining the number of erythrocytes, leukocytes, epithelial cells, casts, and protein content in an aliquot of a 12-hour urine specimen. **blood c.,** determining the number of formed elements in a measured volume of blood, usually a cubic millimeter (as of red blood cells, white blood cells, or platelet count). **differential c.,** a count on a stained blood smear, of the proportion of different types of leukocytes (or other cells), expressed in percentages. **platelet c.,** the total number of platelets per cubic millimeter of blood by counting the platelets on a stained blood film.

counter (kown′ter) an instrument to compute numerical value; in radiology, a device for enumerating ionizing events. **Coulter c.,** an automatic instrument used in enumeration of formed elements in the peripheral blood. **Geiger c., Geiger-Müller c.,** an amplifying device that indicates the presence of ionizing particles. **scintillation c.,** a device for indicating the emission of ionizing particles, permitting determination of the concentration of radioactive isotopes in the body or other substance.

countercurrent (kown′ter-kur″int) flowing in an opposite direction.

counterextension (-eks-ten′shun) traction in a proximal direction coincident with traction in opposition to it.

counterimmunoelectrophoresis (-im″u-no-e-

counterincision

---

lek″tro-for-e′sis) immunoelectrophoresis in which the antigen and antibody migrate in opposite directions.

counterincision (-in-sizh′in) a second incision made to promote drainage or to relieve tension on the edges of a wound.

counterirritation (-ir″ĭ-ta′shin) superficial irritation intended to relieve some other irritation.

counteropening (-o″pin-ing) a second incision made across an earlier one to promote drainage.

counterpulsation (-pul-sa′shin) a technique for assisting the circulation and decreasing the work of the heart, by synchronizing the force of an external pumping device with cardiac systole and diastole. **intraaortic balloon c.,** circulatory support provided by a balloon inserted into the thoracic aorta, which is inflated during diastole and deflated during systole.

counterstain (-stān) a stain applied to render the effects of another stain more discernible.

countertraction (-trak″shin) traction opposed to another traction; used in reduction of fractures.

countertransference (kown″ter-trans-fer′ens) in psychoanalysis, the emotional reaction aroused in the physician by the patient.

coup (koo) [Fr.] stroke. **c. de fouet** (koo duh fwa) ["stroke of the whip"] rupture of the plantaris muscle accompanied by a sharp disabling pain. **c. de sabre** (koo duh sahbr) ["saber stroke"] resembling the scar of a saber wound; used to designate such a lesion of linear scleroderma on the forehead and scalp.

coupling (kup′ling) in genetics, occurrence in a double heterozygote on the same chromosome of the two mutant alleles of interest; in cardiology, serial occurrence of a normal heart beat followed closely by a premature beat.

covalence (ko-va′lins) a chemical bond between two atoms in which electrons are shared between the two nuclei. **cova′lent,** adj.

covariance (ko-vār′e-ins) the expected value of the product of the deviations of corresponding values of two random variables from their respective means.

coverglass (kuv′er-glas) a thin glass plate that covers a mounted microscopical object or a culture.

coverslip (-slip) coverglass.

cowperitis (kow″per-īt′is) inflammation of Cowper's (bulbourethral) glands.

cowpox (kow′poks) a mild eruptive disease of milk cows, confined to the udder and teats, due to vaccinia virus, and transmissible to man.

coxa (kok′sah), pl. *cox′ae* [L.] the hip; loosely, the hip joint. **c. mag′na,** broadening of the head and neck of the femur. **c. pla′na,** osteochondrosis of the capitular epiphysis of the femur. **c. val′ga,** deformity of the hip with increase in the angle of inclination between the neck and shaft of the femur. **c. va′ra,** deformity of the hip with decrease in the angle of inclination between the neck and shaft of the femur.

coxalgia (kok-sal′je-ah) 1. hip-joint disease. 2. pain in the hip.

coxarthropathy (koks″ar-throp′ah-the) hip-joint disease.

Coxiella (kok″se-el′ah) a genus of rickettsiae, including *C. burnet′ii,* the etiologic agent of Q fever.

coxofemoral (-fem′ah-ril) pertaining to the hip and thigh.

coxotuberculosis (kok″so-too-berk″u-lo′sis) hip-joint disease.

coxsackievirus (kok-sak′e-vi″rus) one of a group of viruses producing, in man, a disease resembling poliomyelitis, but without paralysis.

C. Ped. Certified Pedorthist.

CPK creatine phosphokinase.

c.p.m. counts per minute.

CPR cardiopulmonary resuscitation.

c.p.s. cycles per second.

CR conditioned reflex (response).

Cr chemical symbol, *chromium.*

cradle (kra′d′l) a frame placed over the body of a bed patient for application of heat or cold or for protecting injured parts from contact with bed covers.

Craigia (kra′ge-ah) a genus of flagellate protozoa; its flagellate stages are thought by some to be *Chilomastix mesnili,* and its ameboid stages *Entamoeba coli.*

cramp (kramp) a painful spasmodic muscular contraction. **heat c.,** spasm with pain, weak pulse, and dilated pupils; seen in workers in intense heat. **intermittent c.,** intermittent abnormal muscular contractions. **recumbency c's,** cramping in legs and feet occurring while resting or during light sleep. **writers' c.,** an occupational neurosis marked by spasmodic contraction of the muscles of the fingers, hand, and forearm, with neuralgic pain.

crani(o)- word element [L.], *skull.*

craniad (kra′ne-ad) in a cranial direction; toward the anterior (in animals) or superior (in humans) end of the body.

craniocele (kra′ne-o-sēl″) protrusion of part of the brain through the skull.

cranioclasis (kra″ne-ok′lah-sis) craniotomy (2).

cranioclasty (-klas″te) craniotomy (2).

craniocleidodysostosis (kra″ne-o-kli″do-dis″os-to′sis) cleidocranial dysostosis.

craniofenestria (-fen-es′tre-ah) defective development of the fetal skull, with areas in which no bone is formed.

craniolacunia (kra″ne-o-lah-ku′ne-ah) defective development of the fetal skull, with depressed areas on the inner surface.

craniomalacia (-mah-la′she-ah) abnormal softness of the bones of the skull.

craniopathy (-op′ah-the) any disease of the skull. **metabolic c.,** a condition characterized by lesions of the calvaria with multiple metabolic changes, and by headache, obesity, and visual disorders.

craniopharyngioma (-fah-rin″je-o′mah) a tumor arising from cell rests derived from the infundibulum of the hypophysis or Rathke's pouch.

cranioplasty (kra′ne-o-plas″te) any plastic operation on the skull.

craniorachischisis (kra″ne-o-rah-kis′kĭ-sis) congenital fissure of skull and spinal column.

cranioschisis (kra″ne-os′kĭ-sis) congenital fissure of the skull.

craniosclerosis (kra″ne-o-sklĕ-ro′sis) thickening of the bones of the skull.

craniostenosis (-ste-no′sis) deformity of the skull due to premature closure of the cranial sutures.

craniostosis (kra″ne-os-to′sis) congenital ossification of the cranial sutures.

craniosynostosis (kra″ne-o-sin″os-to′sis) premature closure of the sutures of the skull.

craniotabes (-ta″bēz) reduction in mineralization of the skull, with abnormal softness of the bone, usually affecting the occipital and parietal bones along the lambdoidal sutures.

craniotomy (kra″ne-ot′ah-me) 1. any operation on the cranium. 2. puncture of the skull and removal of its contents to decrease the size of the head of a dead fetus and aid delivery.

cranium (kra′ne-um), pl. *cra′nia* [L.] the skeleton of the head, variously construed as including all of the bones of the head, all except the mandible, or the eight bones forming the vault lodging the brain.

crater (krāt′er) an excavated area surrounded by an elevated margin.

cravat (krah-vat′) a triangular bandage.

cream (krēm) the fatty part of milk from which butter is prepared, or a fluid mixture of similar consistency; in pharmaceutical preparations, a semisolid emulsion of oil and water. **cold c.,** a preparation of spermaceti, white wax, mineral oil, sodium borate, and purified water, applied topically to skin; also used as a vehicle for medications.

crease (krēs) a line or slight linear depression. **flexion c., palmar c.,** any of the normal grooves across the palm which accommodate flexion of the hand by separating folds of tissue. **simian c.,** a single transverse palmar crease formed by fusion of the proximal and distal palmar creases; seen in congenital disorders such as Down's syndrome.

creatine (kre′ah-tin) a crystallizable nitrogenous compound synthesized in the body; phosphorylated creatine is an important storage form of high-energy phosphate. **c. kinase,** an enzyme of skeletal muscle, the myocardium, and brain tissue that catalyzes the transfer of a phosphate group from phosphocreatine to ADP, producing creatine and ATP. **c. phosphate,** phosphocreatine.

creatinine (kre-at′in-in) an anhydride of creatine, the end product of creatine metabolism, found in muscle and blood and excreted in urine.

cremasteric (kre″mas-tĕ′rik) pertaining to the cremaster muscle.

crena (kre′nah), pl. *cre′nae* [L.] a notch or cleft.

crenate, crenated (kre′nāt; kre′nāt-id) scalloped or notched.

crenation (kren-a′shin) the formation of abnormal notching around the edge of an erythrocyte; the notched appearance of an erythrocyte due to its shrinkage after suspension in a hypertonic solution.

crenocyte (kre′nah-sīt) a crenated erythrocyte.

crepitation (krep″ĭ-ta′shin) a dry, crackling sound or sensation, such as that produced by the grating of the ends of a fractured bone.

crepitus (krep′ĭ-tus) 1. the discharge of flatus from the bowels. 2. crepitation. 3. a crepitant rale. **c. re′dux,** crepitus heard in the resolving stage of pneumonia.

crescent (kres′int) 1. shaped like a new moon. 2. a crescent-shaped structure. **crescen′tic,** adj. **c's of Giannuzzi,** crescent-shaped patches of serous cells surrounding the mucous tubercles in mixed glands. **myopic c.,** a crescentic staphyloma in the fundus of the eye in myopia. **sublingual c.,** the crescent-shaped area on the floor of the mouth, bounded by the lingual wall of the mandible and the base of the tongue.

cresol (kre′sol) a mixture of isomeric cresols from coal tar, containing not more than 5% phenol; used as a disinfectant.

crest (krest) a projection, or projecting structure or ridge, especially one surmounting a bone or its border. **ampullar c.,** the most prominent part of a localized thickening of the membrane lining the ampullae of the semicircular ducts. **cross c.,** a ridge of enamel extending across the face of a tooth. **frontal c.,** a median ridge on the internal surface of the frontal bone. **iliac c.,** the thickened, expanded upper border of the ilium. **intertrochanteric c.,** a ridge on the posterior femur connecting the greater with the lesser trochanter. **lacrimal c., anterior,** the lateral margin of the groove on the posterior border of the frontal process of the maxilla. **lacrimal c., posterior,** a vertical ridge dividing the lateral or orbital surface of the lacrimal bone into two parts. **nasal c.,** a ridge on the internal border of the nasal bone. **neural c.,** a cellular band dorsolateral to the embryonic neural tube that gives origin to the cerebrospinal ganglia. **occipital c., external,** a ridge sometimes extending on the external surface of the occipital bone from the external protuberance toward the foramen magnum. **occipital c., internal,** a median ridge on the internal surface of the occipital bone, extending from the midpoint of the cruciform eminence toward the foramen magnum. **palatine c.,** a transverse ridge sometimes seen on the inferior surface of the horizontal plate of the palatine bone. **pubic c.,** the thick, rough anterior border of the body of the pubic bone. **sacral c., intermediate,** either of two indefinite ridges just medial to the dorsal sacral foramina. **sacral c., lateral,** either of two series of tubercles lateral to the dorsal sacral foramina. **sacral c., median,** a median ridge on the dorsal surface of the sacrum. **supramastoid c.,** the superior border of the posterior root of the zygomatic process of the temporal bone. **supraventricular c.,** a ridge on the inner wall of the right ventricle, marking off the conus arteriosus. **temporal c.,** a ridge extending upward and backward from the zygomatic process of the frontal bone. **turbinated c.,** a horizontal ridge on the internal surface of the palate bone.

urethral c., a prominent longitudinal mucosal fold along the posterior wall of the female urethra, or a median elevation along the posterior wall of the male urethra, lying between the prostatic sinuses. **c. of vestibule,** a ridge between the spherical and elliptical recesses of the vestibule, dividing posteriorly to bound the cochlear recess.

cretinism (krĕt′n-izm) arrested physical and mental development with dystrophy of bones and soft tissues, due to congenital lack of thyroid secretion. **athyreotic c.,** cretinism due to thyroid aplasia or destruction of the thyroid of the fetus in utero. **sporadic goitrous c.,** a genetic disorder in which enlargement of the thyroid gland is associated with deficient circulating thyroid hormone.

crevice (krev′is) a fissure. **gingival c.,** the space between the cervical enamel of a tooth and the overlying unattached gingiva.

crevicular (krĕ-vik′u-ler) pertaining to a crevice, especially the gingival crevice.

cribration (krĭ-bra′shin) 1. the quality of being cribriform. 2. the process or act of sifting or passing through a sieve.

cribriform (krib′rĭ-form) perforated like a sieve.

cribrum (kri′brum), pl. *cri′bra* [L.] lamina cribrosa of the ethmoid bone.

cricoid (kri′koid) 1. ring-shaped. 2. the cricoid cartilage.

cricothyreotomy (-thi″re-ot′ah-me) incision through the cricoid and thyroid cartilages.

cricothyrotomy (-thi-rot′ah-me) incision through the skin and cricothyroid membrane to secure a patent airway for emergency relief of upper airway obstruction.

cricotracheotomy (kri″ko-tra″ke-ot′ah-me) incision of the trachea through the cricoid cartilage.

cri du chat (kre-dŏŏ-shah) [Fr.] see under *syndrome.*

crinogenic (kri″no-jen′ik, krin″o-jen′ik) causing secretion in a gland.

crinophagy (krin-of′ah-je) the intracytoplasmic digestion of the contents (peptides, proteins) of secretory vacuoles, after the vacuoles fuse with lysosomes.

crisis (kri′sis), pl. *cri′ses* [L.] 1. the turning point of a disease for better or worse; especially a sudden change, usually for the better, in the course of an acute disease. 2. a sudden paroxysmal intensification of symptoms in the course of a disease. **addisonian c., adrenal c.,** fatigue, nausea, vomiting, and weight loss accompanying an acute attack of Addison's disease. **blast c.,** a sudden, severe change in the course of chronic myelocytic leukemia with an increase in the proportion of myeloblasts. **genital c. of newborn,** estrinization of the vaginal mucosa and hyperplasia of the breast, influenced by transplacentally acquired estrogens. **identity c.,** a period in the psychosocial development of an individual, usually occurring during adolescence, manifested by a loss of the sense of the sameness and historical continuity of one's self, and inability to accept the role the individual perceives as being expected of him by society. **thyroid c., thyrotoxic c.,** sudden and dangerous increase of symptoms of thyrotoxicosis.

crista (kris′tah), pl. *cris′tae* [L.] crest. **cris′tae cu′tis,** dermal ridges; ridges of the skin produced by the projecting papillae of the corium on the palm of the hand or sole of the foot, producing a fingerprint or footprint characteristic of the individual. **c. gal′li,** a thick, triangular process projecting upward from the cribriform plate of the ethmoid bone. **mitochondrial cristae,** numerous narrow, transverse infoldings of the inner membrane of a mitochondrion.

Crithidia (kri-thid′e-ah) a genus of parasitic protozoa found in the digestive tract of arthropods and other invertebrates.

C.R.N.A. Certified Registered Nurse Anesthetist.

cromolyn (kro′mol-in) a drug, $C_{23}H_{14}O_{11}$, used as the sodium salt in the prophylaxis of bronchial asthma and rhinitis associated with allergy.

cross (kros) 1. a cross-shaped figure or structure. 2. any organism produced by crossbreeding; a method of crossbreeding.

crossbite (kros′bīt) malocclusion in which the mandibular teeth are in buccal version (or complete lingual version in posterior segments) to the maxillary teeth.

crossbreeding (-brēd-ing) hybridization; the mating of organisms of different strains or species.

cross-eye (-i) esotropia.

crossing over (kros′ing o′ver) the exchanging of material between homologous chromosomes during the first meiotic division, resulting in new combinations of genes.

crossmatching (kros-mach′ing) see under *matching.*

cross-reactivity (kros″re-ak-tiv′it-e) the degree to which an antibody participates in cross-reactions.

crotalid (krot′ah-lid) 1. any snake of the family Crotalidae; a pit viper. 2. of or pertaining to the family Crotalidae.

Crotalidae (kro-tal′ĭ-de) a family of venomous snakes, the pit vipers.

Crotalus (krot′ah-lus) a genus of rattlesnakes.

crotamiton (krōt″ah-mi′ton) an acaricide, $C_{13}H_{17}NO$, used in the treatment of scabies and as an antipruritic.

crotaphion (kro-taf′e-on) the cranial point at the tip of great wing of sphenoid bone.

croup (krōōp) a condition of infants and children, due to obstruction of the larynx by allergy, foreign body, infection, or new growth, marked by a resonant barking cough, hoarseness, and persistent stridor. **croup′ous,** adj.

crown (krown) 1. the topmost part of an organ or structure, e.g., the top of the head. 2. artificial c. **anatomical c.,** the upper, enamel-covered part of a tooth. **artificial c.,** a reproduction of a crown affixed to the remaining natural structure of a tooth. **clinical c.,** the portion of a tooth exposed beyond the gingiva. **physiological c.,** the portion of a tooth distal to the gingival crevice or to the gum margin.

crowning (krown′ing) the appearance of a large segment of the fetal scalp at the vaginal orifice in childbirth.

cruciate (kroo′she-āt) shaped like a cross.

crucible (kroo′sĭ-b'l) a vessel for melting refractory substances.

cruciform (kroo′sĭ-form) cross-shaped.

crura (kroo′rah) plural of *crus*.

crus (krus), pl. *cru′ra* [L.] 1. the leg, from knee to foot. 2. a leglike part. **cru′ral**, adj. **c. ce′rebri**, a structure comprising fiber tracts descending from the cerebral cortex to form the longitudinal fascicles of the pons. **c. of clitoris**, the continuation of the corpus cavernosum of the clitoris, diverging posteriorly to be attached to the pubic arch. **crura of diaphragm**, two fibromuscular bands that arise from the lumbar vertebrae and insert into the central tendon of the diaphragm. **crura of fornix**, two flattened bands of white substance that unite to form the body of the fornix. **c. of penis**, the continuation of each corpus cavernosum of the penis, diverging posteriorly to be attached to the pubic arch.

crust (krust) a formed outer layer, especially of solid matter formed by drying of a bodily exudate or secretion. **milk c.**, crusta lactea.

crusta (krus′tah), pl. *crus′tae* [L.] 1. a crust. 2. crus cerebri. **c. lac′tea**, seborrhea of the scalp of nursing infants. **c. petro′sa**, cementum.

Crustacea (krus-ta′she-ah) a class of arthropods including the lobsters, crabs, shrimps, wood lice, water fleas, and barnacles.

crutch (kruch) a staff extending from the armpit to the ground, with a crosspiece at the top fitting under the arm and a crossbar for the hand, used to support the body in walking.

crux (kruks), pl. *cru′ces* [L.] cross. **c. of heart**, the intersection of the walls separating the right and left sides and the atrial and ventricular heart chambers. **cru′ces pilo′rum**, crosslike figures formed by the pattern of hair growth, the hairs lying in opposite directions.

cry(o)- word element [Gr.], *cold*.

cryalgesia (kri″al-je′ze-ah) pain on application of cold.

cryanesthesia (-an-es-the′ze-ah) loss of power of perceiving cold.

cryesthesia (-es-the′ze-ah) abnormal sensitiveness to cold.

crymoanesthesia (kri″mo-an″es-the′ze-ah) anesthesia produced by refrigeration.

crymodynia (-din′e-ah) rheumatic pain occurring in cold or damp weather.

cryoanalgesia (kri″o-an″al-je′ze-ah) the relief of pain by application of cold by cryoprobe to peripheral nerves.

cryobank (kri′o-bank″) a facility for freezing and preserving semen at low temperatures (usually –196.5° C.) for future use.

cryobiology (kri″o-bi-ol′ah-je) the science dealing with the effect of low temperatures on biological systems.

cryocrit (kri′o-krit) the percentage of the total volume of blood serum or plasma occupied by cryoprecipitates after centrifugation.

cryoextraction (kri″o-eks-trak′shin) applica-

tion of extremely low temperature for the removal of a cataractous lens.

cryoextractor (-eks-trak′ter) a cryoprobe used in cryoextraction.

cryofibrinogen (-fi-brin′ah-jen) an abnormal fibrinogen that precipitates at low temperatures and redissolves at 37° C.

cryofibrinogenemia (-fi-brin″ah-jen-e′me-ah) the presence of cryofibrinogen in the blood.

cryogenic (-jen′ik) producing low temperatures.

cryoglobulin (-glob′u-lin) an abnormal globulin that precipitates at low temperatures and redissolves at 37° C.

cryoglobulinemia (-glob″u-lin-e′me-ah) the presence in the blood of cryoglobulin, which is precipitated in the microvasculature on exposure to cold.

cryohypophysectomy (-hi″po-fiz-ek′tah-me) destruction of the pituitary gland by the application of cold.

cryopathy (kri-op′ah-the) a morbid condition caused by cold.

cryophilic (kri″o-fil′ik) psychrophilic.

cryoprecipitate (-pre-sip′ĭ-tāt) any precipitate that results from cooling.

cryopreservation (-prez″er-va′shin) maintenance of the viability of excised tissue or organs by storing at very low temperatures.

cryoprobe (kri′ah-prōb) an instrument for applying extreme cold to tissue.

cryoprotective (kri″o-pro-tek′tiv) capable of protecting against injury due to freezing, as glycerol protects frozen red blood cells.

cryoprotein (-pro′te-in, tēn) a blood protein that precipitates on cooling.

cryoscopy (kri-os′kah-pe) examination of fluids based on the principle that the freezing point of a solution varies according to the amount and nature of the solute. **cryoscop′ic**, adj.

cryospray (kri′ah-spra) the use of a liquid nitrogen spray in cryosurgery.

cryostat (-stat) 1. a device by which temperature can be maintained at a very low level. 2. in pathology and histology, a chamber containing a microtome for sectioning frozen tissue.

cryosurgery (kri″o-ser′jer-e) the destruction of tissue by application of extreme cold.

cryothalamectomy (-thal″ah-mek′tah-me) destruction of a portion of the thalamus by application of extreme cold.

cryotherapy (-ther′ah-pe) the therapeutic use of cold.

crypt (kript) a blind pit or tube on a free surface. **alveolar c.**, the bony compartment surrounding a developing tooth. **anal c's**, see under *sinus*. **enamel c.**, a space bounded by dental ledges on either side and usually by the enamel organ, and filled with mesenchyma. **c's of Fuchs**, **c's of iris**, pitlike depressions in the iris. **c's of Lieberkühn**, intestinal glands. **Luschka's c's**, deep indentations of the gallbladder mucosa which penetrate into the muscular layer of the organ. **c's of Morgagni**, anal sinuses. **synovial c.**, a pouch in the synovial membrane of a joint. **c's of tongue**, deep, irregular invaginations from the surface of the lingual tonsil. **tonsillar c's,** epithelium-lined clefts in the palatine tonsils.

crypt(o)- word element [Gr.], *concealed; crypt.*

crypta (krip′tah), pl. *cryp′tae* [L.] crypt.

cryptesthesia (krip″tes-the′ze-ah) subconscious perception of occurrences not ordinarily perceptible to the senses.

cryptitis (krip-tīt′is) inflammation of a crypt, especially the anal crypts.

cryptodeterminant (krip″to-de-ter′min-int) hidden determinant.

cryptococcosis (-kok-o′sis) infection by *Cryptococcus neoformans,* having a predilection for the brain and meninges but also invading the skin, lungs, and other parts.

Cryptococcus (-kok′us) a genus of yeastlike fungi, including *C. neofor′mans,* the cause of cryptococcosis in man.

cryptogenic (krip″tah-jen′ik) of obscure or doubtful origin.

cryptoglioma (-gli-o′mah) a stage of retinal glioma in which the eyeball shrinks, masking the presence of the growth.

cryptolith (krip′tah-lith) a concretion in a crypt.

cryptomenorrhea (krip″to-men″o-re′ah) the occurrence of menstrual symptoms without external bleeding, as in imperforate hymen.

cryptophthalmia, cryptophthalmos, cryptophthalmus (krip″tof-thal′me-ah; -thal′mos; -thal′mus) congenital absence of the palpebral fissure, the skin extending from the forehead to the cheek, and the eye malformed or rudimentary.

cryptopyic (-pi′ik) attended by concealed suppuration.

cryptorchid (krip-tor′kid) a person with undescended testes.

cryptorchidectomy (krip″tor-kid-ek′-tah-me) excision of an undescended testis.

cryptorchidopexy (krip-tor′kid-ah-pek″se) orchiopexy.

cryptorchism (krip-tor′kizm) failure of one or both testes to descend into the scrotum.

cryptosporidiosis (krip″to-spo-rid″e-o′sis) infection with protozoa of the genus *Cryptosporidium.* In humans, it is manifested as a rarely occurring self-limited diarrhea syndrome in immunocompetent patients and as a severe syndrome of prolonged, debilitating diarrhea, weight loss, fever, and abdominal pain, with occasional spread to the trachea and bronchial tree, in immunocompromised patients.

Cryptosporidium (krip″to-spo-rid′e-um) a genus of parasitic protozoa found in the intestinal tracts of many different vertebrates and the etiologic agent of cryptosporidiosis in humans.

crystal (kris′t'l) a naturally produced angular solid of definite form. **blood c's,** hematoidin crystals in the blood. **Charcot-Leyden c's,** crystalline structures, protein in nature, found wherever eosinophilic leukocytes are undergoing fragmentation, e.g., in bronchial secretions in bronchial asthma and in stools in some cases of intestinal parasitism.

crystalline (kris′til-in) 1. resembling a crystal in nature or clearness. 2. pertaining to crystals.

crystalluria (kris″til-ūr′e-ah) the excretion of crystals in the urine, causing renal irritation.

Crystodigin (kris″to-dij′in) trademark for preparations of digitoxin.

CS cesarean section; conditioned stimulus.

Cs chemical symbol, *cesium.*

C.S.A.A. Child Study Association of America.

CSF cerebrospinal fluid.

C.S.G.B.I. Cardiac Society of Great Britain and Ireland.

C.S.M. cerebrospinal meningitis.

CT computed tomography.

C.T.A. Canadian Tuberculosis Association.

Ctenocephalides (te″no-se-fal′ĭ-dēz) a genus of fleas, including *C. ca′nis,* frequently found on dogs, which may transmit the dog tapeworm to man, and *C. fe′lis,* commonly parasitic on cats.

C-terminal (ter′min-al) the end of the peptide chain carrying the free alpha carboxyl group of the last amino acid, conventionally written to the right.

CTL cytotoxic lymphocytes; cytotoxic T lymphocytes.

CTP cytidine triphosphate.

Cu chemical symbol, *copper* (L. *cuprum*).

cu. cubic.

cubitus (ku′bit-us) 1. elbow. 2. the upper limb distal to the humerus: the elbow, forearm, and hand. 3. ulna. **cu′bital,** adj. **c. val′gus,** deformity of the elbow in which it deviates away from the midline of the body when extended. **c. va′rus,** deformity of the elbow in which it deviates toward the midline of the body when extended.

cuboid (kūb′oid) resembling a cube.

cuff (kuf) a small, bandlike structure encircling a part or object. **musculotendinous c.,** one formed by intermingled muscle and tendon fibers. **rotator c.,** a musculotendinous structure encircling and giving strength to the shoulder joint.

cuffing (kuf′ing) formation of a cufflike surrounding border, as of leukocytes about a blood vessel, observed in certain infections.

cul-de-sac (kul-dĕ-sak′) [Fr.] a blind pouch. **Douglas′ c.,** rectouterine excavation.

culdocentesis (kul″do-sen-te′sis) transvaginal puncture of Douglas′ cul-de-sac for aspiration of fluid.

culdoscopy (kul-dos′kah-pe) visual examination of the female viscera through an endoscope introduced into the pelvic cavity through the posterior vaginal fornix.

Culex (ku′leks) a genus of mosquitoes found throughout the world, many species of which are vectors of disease-producing organisms.

culicide (ku′lĭ-sīd) an agent which destroys mosquitoes.

culicifuge (ku-lis′ĭ-fūj) an agent which repels mosquitoes.

culicine (ku-lĭ-sin, ku′lĭ-sīn) 1. a member of the genus *Culex* or related genera. 2. pertaining to, involving, or affecting mosquitoes of the genus *Culex* or related species.

culmen (kul'men), pl. *cul'mina* [L.] the anterior and upper part of the monticulus cerebelli.

cultivation (kul"tĭ-va'shin) the propagation of living organisms, especially the growing of cells in artificial media.

culture (kul'cher) 1. the propagation of microorganisms or of living tissue cells in media conducive to their growth. 2. to induce such propagation. 3. the product of such propagation. **cul'tural**, adj. **cell c.**, a growth of cells *in vitro;* although the cells proliferate they do not organize into tissue. **continuous flow c.**, the cultivation of bacteria in a continuous flow of fresh medium to maintain bacterial growth in logarithmic phase. **hanging-drop c.**, a culture in which the material to be cultivated is inoculated into a drop of fluid attached to a coverglass inverted over a hollow slide. **plate c.**, one grown on a medium, usually agar or gelatin, on a Petri dish. **primary c.**, a cell or tissue culture started from material taken directly from an organism, as opposed to that from an explant from an organism. **pure c.**, a culture of a single cell species, without presence of any contaminants. **slant c.**, one made on the surface of solidified medium in a tube which has been tilted to provide a greater surface area for growth. **stab c.**, one in which the medium is inoculated by thrusting a needle deep into its substance. **streak c.**, one in which the medium is inoculated by drawing an infected wire across it. **suspension c.**, a culture in which cells multiply while suspended in a suitable medium. **tissue c.**, maintenance or growth of tissue, organ primordia, or the whole or part of an organ *in vitro* so as to preserve its architecture and function. **type c.**, a culture of a species of microorganism usually maintained in a central collection of type or standard cultures.

culture medium (kul'cher mēd'e-um) any substance used to cultivate living cells.

cumulus (ku'mu-lus), pl. *cu'muli* [L.] a small elevation. **c. oo'phorus**, a mass of follicular cells surrounding the ovum in the vesicular ovarian follicle.

cuneate, cuneiform (ku'ne-āt; ku-ne'ĭ-form) wedge-shaped.

cuneus (ku'ne-us), pl. *cu'nei* [L.] a wedge-shaped lobule on the medial aspect of the occipital lobe of the cerebrum.

cuniculus (ku-nik'ūl-us), pl. *cunic'uli* [L.] a burrow in the skin made by the itch mite.

cunnilingus (kun"ĭ-ling'gus) [L.] oral stimulation of the female genitals.

cup (kup) a depression or hollow. **glaucomatous c.**, a form of optic disk depression peculiar to glaucoma. **optic c.**, physiologic c. **physiologic c.**, a slight depression sometimes observed in the optic disk.

cupola (ku'pah-lah) cupula.

cupping (kup'ing) the formation of a cup-shaped depression.

cuprous (ku'prus) pertaining to or containing monovalent copper.

cupruresis (ku"proo-re'sis) the urinary excretion of copper.

cupruretic (ku"proo-ret'ik) pertaining to or promoting the urinary excretion of copper.

cupula (ku'pu-lah), pl. *cu'pulae* [L.] a small, inverted cup or dome-shaped cap over a structure.

cupulolithiasis (ku"pu-lo-lĭ-thi'ah-sis) the presence of calculi in the cupula of the posterior semicircular duct.

cupulometry (ku"pu-lom'-ĭ-tre) a method of testing vestibular function in which subjects are accelerated in a rotational chair and the duration of postrotational vertigo and nystagmus are plotted against rates of angular momentum.

curare (koo-rah're) any of a wide variety of highly toxic extracts from various botanical sources, used originally as arrow poisons in South America. An extract of the shrub *Chondodendron tomentosum* has been used as a skeletal muscle relaxant.

curarization (ku"rar-i-za'shin) administration of curare (usually tubocurarine) to induce muscle relaxation by its blocking activity at the myoneural junction.

curarimimetic (koo-rah"re-mi-met'ik) producing effects similar to those of curare.

cure (kūr) 1. the treatment of any disease, or of a special case. 2. the successful treatment of a disease or wound. 3. a system of treating diseases. 4. a medicine effective in treating a disease.

curet (ku-ret') 1. a spoon-shaped instrument for cleansing a diseased surface. 2. to use a curet.

curettage (ku"rĕ-tahzh') [Fr.] the cleansing of a diseased surface, as with a curet. **medical c.**, induction of bleeding from the endometrium by administration and withdrawal of a progestational agent. **periapical c.**, removal with a curet of diseased periapical tissue without excision of the root tip. **suction c., vacuum c.**, removal of the uterine contents, after dilatation, by means of a hollow curet introduced into the uterus, through which suction is applied.

curettement (-ment) curettage. **physiologic c.**, enzymatic débridement.

curie (ku're) a unit of radioactivity, defined as the quantity of any radioactive nuclide in which the number of disintegrations per second is 3.700×10^{10}. Abbreviated Ci.

curie-hour (-owr") a unit of dose equivalent to that obtained by exposure for one hour to radioactive material disintegrating at the rate of 3.7×10^{10} atoms per second.

curium (ku're-um) a chemical element (*see table*), at. no. 96, symbol Cm.

current (kur'int) electric transmission in a circuit. **action c.**, the current generated in the cell membrane of a nerve or muscle by the action potential. **alternating c.**, a current which periodically flows in opposite directions. **direct c.**, a current flowing in one direction only.

curvatura (ker"vah-tu'rah), pl. *curvatu'rae* [L.] curvature.

curvature (ker'vah-cher) a nonangular deviation from a normally straight course. **greater c. of stomach,** the left or lateral and inferior border of the stomach, marking the inferior junction of the anterior and posterior surfaces.

lesser c. of stomach, the right or medial border of the stomach, marking the superior junction of the anterior and posterior surfaces. **Pott's c.,** abnormal posterior curvature of the spine due to tuberculous caries. **spinal c.,** abnormal deviation of the vertebral column.

curve (kerv) a line which is not straight, or which describes part of a circle, especially a line that represents varying values in a graph. **Barnes' c.,** the segment of a circle the center of which is the sacral promontory, its concavity being directed dorsally. **c. of Carus,** the normal axis of the pelvic outlet. **dental c.,** c. of occlusion. **dissociation c. of oxyhemoglobin,** a graphic curve representing the normal variation in the amount of oxygen which combines with hemoglobin as a function of the pressure of oxygen and carbon dioxide. **dye-dilution c.,** a graph representing the concentration of a fixed dose of a dye (as in the systemic circulation) at specific time intervals; used in studies of cardiac output. **growth c.,** the curve obtained by plotting increase in size or numbers against the elapsed time. **isodose c's,** lines delimiting body areas receiving the same quantity of radiation in radiotherapy. **muscle c.,** myogram. **Price-Jones c.,** a graphic curve representing the variation in the size of the red blood corpuscles. **temperature c.,** a graphic tracing showing the variations in body temperature. **tension c's,** lines observed in cancellous tissue of bones, determined by the exertion of stress during development.

cushion (koosh′in) a soft or padlike part. **endocardial c's,** elevations on the atrioventricular canal of the embryonic heart which later help form the interatrial septum. **intimal c's,** longitudinal thickenings of the intima of certain arteries, e.g., the penile arteries; they serve functionally as valves, controlling blood flow by occluding the lumen of the artery.

cusp (kusp) a pointed or rounded projection, such as on the crown of a tooth, or a segment of a cardiac valve. **semilunar c.,** any of the semilunar segments of the aortic valve (having posterior, right, and left cusps) or the pulmonary valve (having anterior, right, and left cusps).

cuspid (kus′pid) 1. having one cusp or point. 2. a canine tooth.

cuspis (kus′pis), pl. *cus′pides* [L.] a cusp.

cutaneous (ku-ta′ne-us) pertaining to the skin.

cutdown (kut′down) creation of a small incised opening, especially over a vein (*venous c.*), to facilitate venipuncture and permit passage of a needle or cannula for withdrawal of blood or administration of fluids.

cuticle (kūt′ĭ-k'l) 1. a layer of more or less solid substance covering the free surface of an epithelial cell. 2. eponychium (1). **dental c., enamel c.,** the calcified epithelial remnants on the tooth enamel after complete formation of the enamel.

cuticula (ku-tik′u-lah), pl. *cuti′culae* [L.] cuticle.

cutireaction (kūt″ĭ-re-ak′shin) an inflammatory or irritative reaction on the skin, occurring in certain infectious diseases, or on application

or injection of a preparation of the organism causing the disease.

cutis (kūt′is) the skin. **c. anseri′na,** transitory elevation of the hair follicles due to contraction of the arrectores pilorum muscles; a reflection of sympathetic nerve discharge. **c. elas′tica, c. hyperelas′tica,** Ehlers-Danlos syndrome. **c. lax′a,** a hereditary disorder in which the skin and subcutaneous tissues hypertrophy, so that the skin hangs in folds. **c. pen′dula,** c. laxa. **c. rhomboida′lis nu′chae,** thickening of the skin of the neck with striking accentuation of its markings, giving an appearance of diamond-shaped plaques. **c. ve′ra,** corium. **c. ver′ticis gyra′ta,** enlargement and thickening of the skin of the scalp, which lies in folds resembling gyri and sulci of the brain.

cuvette (ku-vet′) [Fr.] a glass container generally having well defined characteristics (dimensions, optical properties), to contain solutions or suspensions for study.

CV cardiovascular.

CVA cardiovascular accident; cerebrovascular accident.

CVP central venous pressure.

CVS cardiovascular system.

cyan(o)- word element [Gr.], *blue.*

cyanemia (si″an-e′me-ah) blueness of the blood.

cyanhemoglobin (si″an-he″mo-glo′bin) a compound formed by action of hydrocyanic acid on hemoglobin, giving the bright red color to blood.

cyanic acid (si-an′ik) a highly vesicant acid, HCNO.

cyanide (si′ah-nīd) 1. a compound containing the cyanide group (—CN) or ion (CN⁻). 2. hydrogen cyanide. **hydrogen c.,** see under *hydrogen.*

cyanmethemoglobin (si″an-met-he″mo-glo′bin) a crystalline substance formed by the action of hydrocyanic acid on methemoglobin in the cold, or on oxyhemoglobin at body temperature; the pigment most widely used in hemoglobinometry.

cyanmetmyoglobin (-mi″o-glo′bin) a compound formed from myoglobin by addition of the cyanide ion to yield reduction to the ferrous state.

Cyanobacteria (si″ah-no-bak-tēr′e-ah) Cyanophyceae.

cyanocobalamin (-ko-bal′ah-min) vitamin B₁₂; a hematopoietic vitamin found in liver, fish meal, eggs, and other natural sources, which combines with intrinsic factor for absorption and is needed for erythrocyte maturation. **radioactive c.,** a radiopharmaceutical used in the Schilling test for the diagnosis of pernicious anemia.

cyanolabe (si′ah-no-lāb″) the name proposed for the pigment in retinal cones that is more sensitive to the blue range of the spectrum than are chlorolabe and erythrolabe.

cyanophil (si-an′ah-fil) 1. cyanophilous. 2. a cell or other histologic element readily stainable with blue dyes.

Cyanophyceae (si″ah-no-fi′se-e) in some systems of classification, a division of the kingdom Procaryotae that includes the blue-green algae (blue-green bacteria), which are photosynthetic and fix nitrogen.

cyanopsia (si″ah-nop′se-ah) defect of vision in which objects appear tinged with blue.

cyanosed (si′ah-nōz, -nōst) cyanotic.

cyanosis (si″ah-no′sis) a bluish discoloration of skin and mucous membranes due to excessive concentration of reduced hemoglobin in the blood. **cyanot′ic,** adj. **autotoxic c.,** enterogenous c. **central c.,** that due to arterial unsaturation, the aortic blood carrying reduced hemoglobin. **enterogenous c.,** a syndrome due to absorption of nitrites and sulfides from the intestine, principally marked by methemoglobinemia and/or sulfhemoglobinemia associated with cyanosis, and accompanied by severe enteritis, abdominal pain, constipation or diarrhea, headache, dyspnea, dizziness, syncope, anemia, and, occasionally, digital clubbing and indicanuria. **peripheral c.,** that due to an excessive amount of reduced hemoglobin in the venous blood as a result of extensive oxygen extraction at the capillary level. **pulmonary c.,** central cyanosis due to poor oxygenation of the blood in the lungs. **c. re′tinae,** cyanosis of the retina, observable in certain congenital cardiac defects. **shunt c.,** central cyanosis due to the mixing of unoxygenated blood with arterial blood in the heart or great vessels.

cybernetics (si″ber-net′iks) the science of the processes of communication and control in the animal and in the machine.

cycl(o)- word element [Gr.], *round; recurring; ciliary body of the eye.*

cyclamate (si′klah-māt) any salt of cyclamic acid; the sodium and calcium salts have been widely used as non-nutritive sugar substitutes.

cyclandelate (si-klan′dil-āt) a vasodilator, C_{17}-$H_{24}O$, for peripheral vascular disease.

cyclarthrosis (si″klar-thro′sis) a pivot joint.

cyclase (si′klās) an enzyme that catalyzes the formation of a cyclic phosphodiester.

cycle (si′k′l) a succession or recurring series of events. **carbon c.,** the steps by which carbon (in the form of carbon dioxide) is extracted from the atmosphere by living organisms and ultimately returned to the atmosphere. It comprises a series of interconversions of carbon compounds beginning with the production of carbohydrates by plants during photosynthesis, proceeding through animal consumption, and ending and beginning again in the decomposition of the animal or plant or in the exhalation of carbon dioxide by animals. **cardiac c.,** a complete cardiac movement, or heart beat, including systole, diastole, and intervening pause. **cell c.,** the cycle of biochemical and morphological events occurring in a reproducing cell population; it consists of: the *S phase,* occurring toward the end of interphase, in which DNA is synthesized; the G_2 *phase,* a relatively quiescent period; the *M* phase, consisting of the four phases of mitosis; and the G_1 *phase* of interphase, which lasts until the S *phase* of the next cycle. **citric acid c.,** tricarboxylic acid c. **Cori c.,** the cycle in carbohydrate metabolism in which muscle glycogen is converted to lactate (glycolysis) during muscle activity and is carried by the blood to the liver, where it is converted to glucose (gluconeogenesis); the glucose

is then carried by the blood to muscle, where it is converted to muscle glycogen. **estrous c.,** the recurring periods of heat (estrus) in adult females of most mammals and the correlated changes in the reproductive tract from one period to another. **Krebs c.,** tricarboxylic acid c. **Krebs-Henseleit c.,** urea c. **menstrual c.,** the period of the regularly recurring physiologic changes in the endometrium, occurring during the reproductive period of female humans, culminating in partial shedding of the endometrium and some bleeding per vagina (menstruating). **mosquito c.,** that period in the life of a malarial parasite that is spent in the body of the mosquito host. **nitrogen c.,** the steps by which nitrogen is extracted from the nitrates of soil and water, incorporated as amino acids and proteins in living organisms, and ultimately reconverted to nitrates: (1) conversion of nitrogen to nitrates by bacteria; (2) the extraction of the nitrates by plants and the building of amino acids and proteins by adding an amino group to the carbon compounds produced in photosynthesis; (3) the ingestion of plants by animals, and (4) the return of nitrogen to the soil in animal excretions or on the death and decomposition of plants and animals. **ornithine c.,** urea c. **ovarian c.,** the sequence of physiologic changes in the ovary involved in ovulation. **reproductive c.,** the cycle of physiologic changes in the reproductive organs, from the time of fertilization of the ovum through gestation and parturition. **sex c., sexual c.,** 1. the physiologic changes recurring regularly in the genital organs of female mammals when pregnancy does not supervene. 2. the period of sexual reproduction in an organism which also reproduces asexually. **tricarboxylic acid c.,** the cyclic metabolic mechanism by which the complete oxidation of the acetyl moiety of acetyl-coenzyme A is effected; the process is the chief source of mammalian energy, during which carbon chains of sugars, fatty acids, and amino acid are metabolized to yield carbon dioxide, water, and high-energy phosphate bonds. **urea c.,** a cyclic series of reactions that produce urea, a major route for removal of the ammonia produced in the metabolism of amino acids in the liver and kidney. **uterine c.,** the phenomena occurring in the endometrium during the estrous or menstrual cycle, preparing it for implantation of the blastocyst. **vaginal c.,** the rhythmic alteration in the epithelial lining of the vagina in conjunction with the ovarian cycle.

cyclectomy (sĭ-klek′tah-me) 1. excision of a piece of the ciliary body. 2. excision of a portion of the ciliary border of the eyelid.

cyclic (sik′lik) pertaining to or occurring in a cycle or cycles; applied to chemical compounds containing a ring of atoms in the nucleus.

cyclitis (si-klīt′is) inflammation of the ciliary body.

cyclizine (si′klĭ-zēn) an antihistamine, $C_{18}H_{22}$-N_2; the hydrochloride salt is used as an antinauseant to prevent motion sickness.

cyclobenzaprine (si″klo-ben′zah-prēn) a muscle relaxant, $C_{20}H_{21}N$.

cyclochoroiditis (-ko″roi-dīt′is) inflammation of ciliary body and choroid.

cyclocryotherapy (-kri″o-thē′rah-pe) freezing of the ciliary body; done in the treatment of glaucoma.

cyclodialysis (-di-al′ĭ-sis) creation of a communication between the anterior chamber of the eye and the suprachoroidal space, in glaucoma.

cyclodiathermy (-di″ah-ther′me) destruction of a portion of the ciliary body by diathermy.

cycloid (si′kloid) 1. containing a ring of atoms; said of organic chemical compounds. 2. cyclothymic (2). 3. cyclothyme.

cyclokeratitis (si″klo-kĕ″rah-tīt′is) inflammation of cornea and ciliary body.

cyclomethycaine (-meth′ĭ-kān) a local anesthetic, $C_{22}H_{33}NO_3$.

cyclopentamine (-pen′tah-mēn) a sympathomimetic amine, $C_9H_{19}N$; used as a nasal decongestant in the form of the hydrochloride salt.

cyclophoria (-for′e-ah) heterophoria in which there is deviation of the eye from the anteroposterior axis in the absence of visual fusional stimuli. **minus c.,** incyclophoria. **plus c.,** excyclophoria.

cyclophosphamide (-fos′fah-mīd) a neoplastic suppressant, $C_7H_{15}Cl_2NO_2P \cdot H_2O$, used in the treatment of lymphomas and leukemias.

cyclopia (si-klo′pe-ah) a developmental anomaly marked by a single orbital fossa, with the globe absent, rudimentary, apparently normal, or duplicated, or the nose absent or present as a tubular appendix above the orbit.

cycloplegia (si″klo-ple′je-ah) paralysis of the ciliary muscle; paralysis of accommodation.

cyclopropane (-pro′pān) a colorless, highly inflammable and explosive gas, C_3H_6, used as an inhalation anesthetic.

Cyclops (si′klops) a genus of minute crustaceans, species of which are hosts of *Diphyllobothrium* and *Dracunculus.*

cyclops (si′klops) a monster exhibiting cyclopia.

cycloserine (si″klo-sĕ′rēn) an antibiotic, C_3H_6-N_2O_2, produced by *Streptomyces orchidaceus* or obtained synthetically; used as a tuberculostatic and in treatment of urinary tract infections.

cyclosis (si-klo′sis) movement of the cytoplasm within a cell, without deformation of the cell wall.

cyclosporin A (si″klo-spor′in) cyclosporine.

cyclosporine (si″klo-spor′in) a cyclic peptide from an extract of soil fungi with immunosuppressant (inhibition of T cell function) and antifungal effects; used to prevent rejection in organ transplant recipients.

cyclotate (si′klo-tāt) USAN contraction for 4-methylbicyclo[2.2.2]oct-2-ene-1-carboxylate.

cyclothiazide (si″klo-thi′ah-zīd) a diuretic and antihypertensive, $C_{14}H_{16}ClN_3O_4S_2$.

cyclothymia (si″klo-thi′me-ah) a mood disorder characterized by numerous hypomanic and depressive periods with symptoms like those of manic and major depressive episodes but of lesser severity.

cyclotomy (si-klot′ah-me) incision of the ciliary muscle.

cyclotron (si′klah-tron) an apparatus for accelerating protons or deutrons to high energies by means of a constant magnet and an oscillating electric field.

cyclotropia (si″klo-tro′pe-ah) permanent deviation of an eye around the anteroposterior axis in the presence of visional fusional stimuli, resulting in diplopia. **negative c.,** incyclotropia. **positive c.,** excyclotropia.

cycrimine (si′krī-mēn) an anticholinergic, C_{19}-$H_{29}NO$, used as the hydrochloride salt in the treatment of parkinsonism.

cyesis (si-e′sis) pregnancy. **cyet′ic,** adj.

cylindroid (sil′in-droid) 1. shaped like a cylinder. 2. a urinary cast of various origins, which tapers to a slender tail that is often twisted or curled upon itself.

cylindroma (sil″in-dro′mah) 1. adenoid cystic carcinoma. 2. a benign skin tumor on the face and scalp, consisting of cylindrical masses of epithelial cells surrounded by a thick band of hyaline material. **cylindrom′atous,** adj.

cymbocephaly (sim″bo-sef′ah-le) scaphocephaly.

cynanche (sĭ-nan′ke) severe sore throat with threatened suffocation.

cynophobia (sin″o-fo′be-ah) morbid fear of dogs.

cyotrophy (si-ah′trah-fe) nutrition of the fetus.

cypionate (sip′e-o-nāt) USAN contraction for cyclopentanepropionate.

cyproheptadine (si″pro-hep′tah-dēn) a histamine and serotonin antagonist, $C_{21}H_{21}N$; its hydrochloride salt is used as an antipruritic and antihistaminic.

cyrtometer (sir-tom′it-er) a device for measuring curved surfaces of the body.

cyrtosis (sir-to′sis) 1. kyphosis. 2. distortion of the bones.

Cys cysteine.

cyst (sist) 1. any closed epithelium-lined cavity or sac, normal or abnormal, usually containing liquid or semisolid material. 2. a stage in the life cycle of certain parasites, during which they are enveloped in a protective wall. **adventitious c.,** one formed about a foreign body or exudate. **alveolar c's,** dilatations of pulmonary alveoli, which may fuse by breakdown of their septa to form large air cysts (pneumatoceles). **aneurysmal bone c.,** a solitary lesion of bone which causes a bulging of the overlying cortex, resembling somewhat the saccular protrusion of the aortic wall in aortic aneurysm. **arachnoid c.,** a fluid-filled cyst between the layers of the leptomeninges, lined with arachnoid membrane, most commonly occurring in the sylvian fissure. **Baker's c.,** a swelling behind the knee due to escape of synovial fluid that has become enclosed in a sac or membrane. **Blessig's c's,** cystic spaces formed at the periphery of the retina. **blue dome c.,** a benign retention cyst of the breast which shows a blue color. **Boyer's c.,** an enlargement of the subhyoid bursa. **bronchogenic c.,** a spherical cyst of bronchial origin lined with bronchial epithelium which may contain secretory elements, generally found in the mediastinum or the lung. **choledochal c.,** a congenital cystic dilatation of the common bile duct, which may cause pain in the right upper quadrant, jaundice, fever, or vomiting, or be asymptomatic. **dentigerous c.,** an odontogenic cyst surrounding the crown of a tooth, originating after the crown is completely formed. **dermoid c.,** a teratoma, usually benign, representing a disorder of embryologic development, characterized by the presence of mature ectodermal elements, consisting of a fibrous wall lined with stratified epithelium, and containing a keratinous material and hair and sometimes other elements, such as bone, tooth, and nerve tissue. Dermoid cysts are found most often in the ovary. **echinococcus c.,** hydatid c. **epidermal c., epidermal inclusion c., epidermoid c.,** an epithelial cyst of the skin due to proliferation of surface epidermal cells within the corium, arising from occluded pilosebaceous follicles. **exudation c.,** one formed by an exudate in a closed cavity. **follicular c.,** one due to occlusion of the duct of a follicle or small gland, especially one formed by enlargement of a graafian follicle as a result of accumulated transudate. **globulomaxillary c.,** one within the maxilla at the junction of the globular portion of the medial nasal process and the maxillary process. **hydatid c.,** the larval cyst stage of the tapeworms *Echinococcus granulosus* and *E. multilocularis*, containing daughter cysts with many scoleces. **median anterior maxillary c.,** one in or near the incisive canal, arising from proliferation of epithelial remnants of the nasopalatine duct. **median palatal c.,** one in the midline of the hard palate, between the lateral palatal processes. **meibomian c.,** a cyst of the meibomian gland, sometimes applied to a chalazion. **myxoid c.,** a nodular lesion usually overlying a distal interphalangeal finger joint in the dorsolateral or dorsomesial position, consisting of focal mucinous degeneration of the collagen of the dermis; not a true cyst, lacking an epithelial wall, it does not communicate with the underlying synovial space. **Naboth's c's, nabothian c's,** see under *follicle*. **nasoalveolar c., nasolabial c.,** a fissural cyst arising outside the bones at the junction of the globular portion of the medial nasal process, the lateral nasal process, and the maxillary process, sometimes secondarily involving the maxilla. **osseous hydatid c's,** hydatid cysts formed by the larvae of *Echinococcus granulosus* in bone, which may become weakened and eroded by the exuberant growth. **pilar c.,** an epithelial cyst clinically indistinguishable from an epidermal cyst, almost always found on the scalp, and arising from the outer root sheath of the hair follicle. **piliferous c., pilonidal c.,** a hair-containing sacrococcygeal dermoid cyst or sinus, often opening at a postanal dimple. **preauricular c., congenital,** one due to imperfect fusion of the first and second branchial arches in formation of the auricle, communicating with a pitlike depression in front of the helix and above the tragus (ear pit). **radicular c.,** an epithelium-lined sac, which may contain cholesterol, at the apex of a tooth. **sarcosporidian c's,** cylindrical cysts containing parasitic spores, found in muscles of those infected with *Sarcocystis*. **sebaceous c.,** a retention cyst of a sebaceous gland, containing cheesy, yellow, fatty material, usually occurring on the face, neck, scalp, or trunk. **solitary bone c.,** a pathologic bone space in the metaphyses of long bones of growing children; of disputed origin, it may be either empty or filled with fluid and have a delicate connective tissue lining. **sterile c.,** a true hydatid cyst that fails to produce brood capsules. **subchondral c.,** a bone cyst within the fused epiphysis beneath the articular plate. **sublingual c.,** ranula. **tarry c.,** 1. one resulting from hemorrhage into a corpus luteum. 2. a bloody cyst resulting from endometriosis. **tarsal c.,** chalazion. **theca-lutein c.,** a cyst of the ovary in which the cystic cavity is lined with theca interna cells. **unicameral bone c.,** solitary bone c. **wolffian c.,** a cyst of the broad ligament developed from vestiges of the wolffian body, or mesonephros.

cyst(o)- word element [Gr.], *cyst; bladder.*

cystadenocarcinoma (sis-tad″in-o-kar″sĭ-no′mah) adenocarcinoma with cyst formation.

cystadenoma (sis-tad″in-o′mah) cystoma blended with adenoma. **mucinous c.,** a multilocular, usually benign, tumor produced by ovarian epithelial cells and having mucin-filled cavities. **papillary c.,** any tumor producing patterns that are both papillary and cystic. **serous c.,** a cystic tumor of the ovary with thin, clear yellow serum and some solid tissue.

cystalgia (sis-tal′je-ah) pain in the bladder.

γ-**cystathionase** (sis″tah-thi′ah-nās) a pyridoxal phosphate–containing enzyme that catalyzes the hydrolysis of cystathionine to cysteine, ammonia, and 2-oxobutyrate.

cystathionine (-nēn) a thio-ester of homocysteine and serine, occurring as an intermediate in cystine synthesis.

cystathioninuria (-thi″o-nin-ūr′e-ah) a genetic disorder of cystathionine metabolism marked by increased concentrations in the urine, due to deficiency of γ-cystathionase; mental retardation is seen in some instances.

cystectasia (sis″tek-ta′ze-ah) dilatation of the bladder.

cystectomy (sis-tek′tah-me) 1. excision of a cyst. 2. excision or resection of the bladder.

cysteic acid (sis-te′ik) an intermediate product in the oxidation of cysteine to taurine.

cysteine (sis′te-in) a sulfur-containing amino acid produced by enzymatic or acid hydrolysis of proteins, readily oxidized to cystine; sometimes found in urine.

cystic (sis′tik) 1. pertaining to or containing cysts. 2. pertaining to the urinary bladder or to the gallbladder.

cysticercosis (sis″tĭ-ser-ko′sis) infection with cysticerci. In man, infection with the larval forms (*Cysticercus cellulosae*) of *Taenia solium*.

cysticercus (-ser′kus), pl. *cysticer′ci* [Gr.] a larval form of tapeworm.

cystigerous (sis-tij′er-us) containing cysts.

cystine (sis′tēn, sis′tin) a sulfur-containing amino acid produced by digestion or acid hydrolysis of proteins, sometimes found in the urine and kidneys, and readily reduced to two molecules of cysteine.

cystinosis (-o′sis) a hereditary disorder of childhood marked by osteomalacia, aminoaciduria, phosphaturia, and deposition of cystine throughout the tissues of the body.

cystinuria (-ūr′e-ah) a hereditary condition of persistent excessive urinary excretion of cystine and the other amino acids lysine, ornithine, and arginine, due to impairment of renal tubular reabsorption.

cystistaxis (-stak′sis) oozing of blood from the mucous membrane into the bladder.

cystitis (sis-tit′is) inflammation of the urinary bladder. **catarrhal c., acute,** that resulting from injury, irritation of foreign bodies, gonorrhea, etc., and marked by burning in the bladder, pain in the urethra, and painful micturition. **c. follicula′ris,** that in which the bladder mucosa is studded with nodules containing lymph follicles. **c. glandula′ris,** that in which the mucosa contains mucin-secreting glands. **interstitial c., chronic,** a bladder condition with an inflammatory lesion, usually in the vertex, and involving the entire thickness of the wall. **c. papillomato′sa,** that with papillomatous growths on the inflamed mucous membrane.

cystitomy (sis-tit′ah-me) surgical division of the lens capsule.

cystocarcinoma (-kar″sin-o′mah) carcinoma associated with cysts.

cystocele (sis′to-sēl) herniation of the urinary bladder into the vagina.

cystoelytroplasty (-el′ĭ-tro-plas″te) surgical repair of a vesicovaginal injuries.

cystogastrostomy (-gas-tros′tah-me) surgical anastomosis of a cyst to the stomach for drainage.

cystography (sis-tog′rah-fe) radiography of the urinary bladder. **voiding c.,** radiography of the bladder while the patient is urinating.

cystoid (sis′toid) 1. resembling a cyst. 2. a cystlike, circumscribed collection of softened material, having no enclosing capsule.

cystojejunostomy (sis″to-je-joo-nos′tah-me) surgical anastomosis of a cyst to the jejunum.

cystolithectomy (sis″to-lĭ-thek′tah-me) surgical removal of a vesical calculus.

cystolithiasis (-lĭ-thi′ah-sis) formation of vesical calculi.

cystolithotomy (-lĭ-thot′ah-me) cystolithectomy.

cystometer (sis-tom′it-er) an instrument for studying the neuromuscular mechanism of the bladder by means of measurements of pressure and capacity.

cystometrography (-mĕ-trog′rah-fe) the graphic recording of intravesical volumes and pressures.

cystomorphous (-mor′fis) resembling a cyst or bladder.

cystopexy (sis′to-pek″se) fixation of the bladder to the abdominal wall.

cystoplasty (-plas″te) plastic repair of the bladder. **augmentation c.,** enlargement of the bladder by grafting to it a detached segment of intestine.

cystoplegia (sis″to-ple′je-ah) paralysis of the bladder.

cystoproctostomy (-prok-tos′tah-me) surgical creation of a communication between the urinary bladder and the rectum.

cystoptosis (sis″top-to′sis) prolapse of part of the inner bladder into the urethra.

cystopyelitis (sis″to-pi″il-īt′is) inflammation of the bladder and renal pelvis.

cystorrhaphy (sis-tor′ah-fe) suture of the bladder.

cystorrhea (sis″tor-e′ah) mucous discharge from the bladder.

cystosarcoma (-sar-ko′mah) an unusually large fibroadenoma of the mammary gland, with a cellular, sarcoma-like stoma; it is locally aggressive and sometimes metastasizes.

cystoscopy (sis-tos′kah-pe) visual examination of the urinary tract with an endoscope.

cystostomy (sis-tos′tah-me) surgical formation of an opening into the bladder.

cystoureteritis (sis″to-ūr-ēt″er-īt′is) inflammation of the urinary bladder and ureters.

cystourethrography (-ūr″ēth-rog′rah-fe) roentgenography of the urinary bladder and urethra. **chain c.,** that in which a sterile beaded metal chain is introduced via a modified catheter into the bladder and urethra; used in evaluating anatomical relationships of the bladder and urethra.

cystourethroscope (-ūr-ēth′rah-skōp″) an instrument for examining the posterior urethra and bladder.

cyt(o)- word element [Gr.], *a cell.*

cytapheresis (sīt″ah-fer-e′sis) a procedure in which cells of one or more kinds (leukocytes, platelets, etc.) are separated from whole blood and retained, the plasma and other formed elements being retransfused into the donor; it includes leukapheresis and thrombocytapheresis.

cytarabine (si-tār′ah-bēn) an antimetabolite, $C_9H_{13}N_3O_5$, which inhibits DNA synthesis, and hence has antineoplastic and antiviral properties.

-cyte word element [Gr.], *a cell.*

cytidylic acid (sīt″ĭ-dil′ik) cytidine monophosphate.

cytidine (sīt′ĭ-dēn) a nucleoside consisting of cytosine and ribose, a constituent of RNA. **c. triphosphate (CTP),** an energy-rich nucleotide that provides energy in the biosynthesis of certain cellular constituents.

cytoarchitectonic (-ar″kĭ-tek-ton′ik) pertaining to cellular structure or the arrangement of cells in tissue.

cytochalasin (-kal′ah-sin) any of a group of fungal metabolites that affect the motility of polymorphonuclear leukocytes.

cytochemistry (-kem′is-tre) the identification and localization of the different chemical compounds and their activities within the cell.

cytochrome (si′tah-krōm) any of a class of hemoproteins, widely distributed in animal and plant tissues, whose main function is electron transport; distinguished according to their prosthetic group as *a, b, c,* and *d.*

cytocide (sīt′ah-sīd) an agent which destroys cells. **cytoci′dal,** adj.

cytoclasis (si-tok′lah-sis) the destruction of cells. **cytoclas′tic,** adj.

cytodiagnosis (sīt″o-di″ag-no′sis) diagnosis based on examination of cells. **cytodiagnos′tic,** adj.

cytodifferentiation (-dif″er-en″she-a′shin) the development of specialized structures and functions in embryonic cells.

cytodistal (-dis′t′l) denoting that part of an axon remote from the cell body.

cytogenetics (-jĕ-net′iks) that branch of genetics devoted to the cellular constituents concerned in heredity, i.e., the chromosomes. **cytogenet′ical,** adj. **clinical c.,** the branch of cytogenetics concerned with relations between chromosomal abnormalities and pathologic conditions.

cytogenous (si-toj′in-is) producing cells.

cytoglycopenia (sīt″o-gli″ko-pe′ne-ah) deficient glucose content of body or blood cells.

cytohistogenesis (-his″to-jen′is-is) the development of the structure of cells.

cytohistology (-his-tol′ah-je) the combination of cytologic and histologic methods. **cytohistolog′ic,** adj.

cytoid (si′toid) resembling a cell.

cytokinesis (-ki-ne′sis) the division of the cytoplasm during the division of eukaryotic cells.

cytology (si-tol′ah-je) the study of cells, their origin, structure, function, and pathology. **cytolog′ic,** adj. **aspiration biopsy c. (ABC),** the microscopic study of cells obtained from superficial or internal lesions by suction through a fine needle. **exfoliative c.,** microscopic examination of cells desquamated from a body surface or lesion as a means of detecting malignancy and microbiologic changes, to measure hormonal levels, etc. Such cells are obtained by aspiration, washing, smear, or scraping.

cytolysin (si-tol′ĭ-sin) a substance or antibody that produces cytolysis.

cytolysis (si-tol′ĭ-sis) the dissolution of cells. **cytolyt′ic,** adj. **immune c.,** cell lysis produced by antibody with the participation of complement.

cytolysosome (sīt″o-li′so-sōm) autophagosome.

cytomegalovirus (-meg″ah-lo-vi′rus) any of a group of highly host-specific herpesviruses, infecting man, monkeys, or rodents, producing unique large cells with intranuclear inclusions; the virus specific for man causes cytomegalic inclusion disease, and it has been associated with a syndrome resembling infectious mononucleosis.

cytometaplasia (sīt″o-met″ah-pla′ze-ah) alteration in the function or form of cells.

cytometry (si-tom′ĭ-tre) the counting of blood cells.

cytomorphology (sīt″o-mor-fol′ah-je) the morphology of body cells.

cytomorphosis (-mor-fo′sis) the changes through which cells pass in development.

cytopathic (sīt″o-path′ik) pertaining to or characterized by pathologic changes in cells.

cytopathogenesis (-path″o-jen′is-is) production of pathologic changes in cells. **cytopathogenet′ic,** adj.

cytopathogenic (-jen′ik) capable of producing pathologic changes in cells.

cytopathologist (-pah-thol′ah-jist) an expert in the study of cells in disease; a cellular pathologist.

cytopenia (-pe′ne-ah) deficiency in the cells of the blood.

cytophagocytosis (sīt″o-fag″o-si-to′sis) cytophagy.

cytophagy (si-tof′ah-je) the ingestion of cells by phagocytes.

cytophilic (sīt″ah-fil′ik) having an affinity for cells.

cytophylaxis (-fi-lak′sis) 1. the protection of cells against cytolysis. 2. increase in cellular activity.

cytopipette (-pi-pet′) a pipette for taking cytological smears.

cytoplasm (sīt′ah-plazm) the protoplasm of a cell exclusive of that of the nucleus (nucleoplasm). **cytoplas′mic,** adj.

cytoproximal (sīt″o-prok′sĭ-mil) denoting that part of an axon nearer to the cell body.

cytosine (sīt′o-sēn) the base oxyaminopyrimidine, $C_4H_5N_3O$, a component of nucleic acid. **c. arabinoside,** cytarabine.

cytoskeleton (sīt″o-skel′it-on) a conspicuous internal reinforcement in the cytoplasm of a cell, consisting of tonofibrils, filaments of the terminal web, and other microfilaments. **cytoskel′etal,** adj.

cytosol (sīt′ah-sol) the liquid medium of the cytoplasm, i.e., cytoplasm minus organelles and nonmembranous insoluble components. **cytosol′ic,** adj.

cytosome (-sōm) the body of a cell apart from its nucleus.

cytostatic (sīt″ah-stat′ik) 1. suppressing the growth and multiplication of cells. 2. an agent that so acts.

cytostome (sīt′ah-stōm) the cell mouth; the aperture through which food enters certain protozoa.

cytotaxis (sīt″ah-tak′sis) the movement and arrangement of cells with respect to a specific source of stimulation. **cytotac′tic,** adj.

cytothesis (si-toth′is-is) restitution of cells to their normal condition.

cytotoxin (-tok′sin) a toxin or antibody having a specific toxic action upon cells of special organs.

cytotrophoblast (-trof′ah-blast) the cellular (inner) layer of the trophoblast.

cytotropism (si-tah′trah-pizm) 1. cell movement in response to external stimulation. 2. the tendency of viruses, bacteria, drugs, etc., to exert their effect upon certain cells of the body. **cytotrop′ic,** adj.

cytozoic (sīt″ah-zo′ik) living within or attached to cells; said of parasites.

cytula (sī′tūl-lah) the impregnated ovum.

cyturia (sī-tūr′e-ah) the presence of cells of any sort in the urine.

D

D chemical symbol, *deuterium;* symbol, *diopter.*

D. density; [L.] *dex'ter* (right); dose; duration.

D- chemical prefix (small capital) specifying that the substance corresponds in chemical configuration to the standard substance D-glyceraldehyde. Opposed to L-. For carbohydrates, the configuration of the highest numbered asymmetric carbon atoms determines whether the substance is D- or L-; for amino acids, the lowest numbered asymmetric carbon atom is the key.

d- chemical abbreviation, *dextrorotatory.*

2,4-D a toxic chlorphenoxy herbicide (2,4-dichlorophenoxyacetic acid), a component of Agent Orange.

dacarbazine (dah-kar'bah-zēn) a cytotoxic alkylating agent used as an antineoplastic primarily for treatment of malignant melanoma and in combination chemotherapy for Hodgkin's disease and sarcomas.

dacry(o)- word element [Gr.], *tears* or *the lacrimal apparatus of the eye.*

dacryagogic (dak"re-ah-goj'ik) 1. inducing a flow of tears. 2. serving as a channel for discharge of secretion of the lacrimal glands.

dacryoadenalgia (dak"re-o-ad"in-al'je-ah) pain in a lacrimal gland.

dacryoadenectomy (-ad"in-ek'tah-me) excision of a lacrimal gland.

dacryoblennorrhea (-blen"or-e'ah) mucous flow from the lacrimal apparatus.

dacryocyst (-sist") the lacrimal sac.

dacryocystectomy (-sis-tek'tah-me) excision of the wall of the lacrimal sac.

dacryocystoblennorrhea (-sis"to-blen"or-e'ah) chronic catarrhal inflammation of the lacrimal sac, with constriction of the lacrimal gland.

dacryocystocele (-sis'tah-sēl) hernial protrusion of the lacrimal sac.

dacryocystorhinostenosis (-sis"to-ri"no-stĕ-no'sis) narrowing of the duct leading from the lacrimal sac to the nasal cavity.

dacryocystorhinostomy (-ri-nos'tah-me) surgical creation of an opening between the lacrimal sac and nasal cavity.

dacryocystostenosis (-stĕ-no'sis) narrowing of the lacrimal sac.

dacryocystostomy (-sis-tos'tah-me) creation of a new opening into the lacrimal sac.

dacryohemorrhea (-he"mor-e'ah) the discharge of tears mixed with blood.

dacryolith (dak're-o-lith") a lacrimal calculus.

dacryoma (dak"re-o'mah) a tumor-like swelling due to obstruction of the lacrimal duct.

dacryops (dak're-ops) 1. a watery state of the eye. 2. distention of a lacrimal duct by contained fluid.

dacryopyosis (-pi-o'sis) suppuration of the lacrimal apparatus.

dacryoscintigraphy (-sin-tig'rah-fe) scintigraphy of the lacrimal ducts.

dacryostenosis (-stin-o'sis) stricture or narrowing of a lacrimal duct.

dacryosyrinx (-sir'inks) 1. a lacrimal duct. 2. a lacrimal fistula. 3. a syringe for irrigating the lacrimal ducts.

dactinomycin (dak"tĭ-no-mi'sin) actinomycin D, an antibiotic derived from several species of *Streptomyces,* $C_{62}H_{86}N_{12}O_{16}$; used as an antineoplastic.

dactyl (dak'til) a digit.

dactyl(o)- word element [Gr.], *a digit; a finger or toe.*

dactylography (dak"til-og'rah-fe) the study of fingerprints.

dactylogryposis (dak"til-o-grĭ-po'sis) permanent flexion of the fingers.

dactylolysis (dak"til-ol'ĭ-sis) 1. surgical correction of syndactyly. 2. loss or amputation of a digit. **d. sponta'nea,** spontaneous loss of digits, as in ainhum or in leprosy.

dactyloscopy (dak"til-os'kah-pe) examination of fingerprints for identification.

dactylus (dak'til-us), pl. *dac'tyli* [L.] a digit.

Dalmane (dal'mān) trademark for a preparation of flurazepam hydrochloride.

dalton (dawl'tin) an arbitrary unit of mass, being $\frac{1}{12}$ the mass of the nuclide of carbon-12, equivalent to 1.657×10^{-24} gm.

daltonism (-izm) red-green blindness.

dam (dam) rubber dam; a thin sheet of latex rubber used to isolate teeth from mouth fluids during dental therapy.

damping (damp'ing) steady diminution of the amplitude of successive vibrations of a specific form of energy, as of electricity.

danazol (dah'nah-zōl) an anterior pituitary suppressant, $C_{22}H_{27}NO_2$.

D and C dilatation (of cervix) and curettage (of uterus).

dander (dan'der) small scales from the hair or feathers of animals, which may be a cause of allergy in sensitive persons.

dandruff (dan'druf) 1. dry scaly material shed from the scalp; applied to that normally shed from the scalp epidermis as well as to the excessive scaly material associated with disease. 2. seborrheic dermatitis of the scalp.

DANS 1-dimethylaminonaphthalene-5-sulfonyl chloride; a fluorochrome employed in immunofluorescence studies of tissues and cells.

dantrolene (dan'trol-ēn) a skeletal muscle relaxant, $C_{14}H_{10}N_4O_5$.

dapsone (dap'sōn) an antibacterial, $C_{12}H_{12}N_2$-O_2S, used as a leprostatic and a dermatitis herpetiformis suppressant.

dartos (dart′os) the contractile tissue under the skin of the scrotum.

Darvocet (dar′vo-set) trademark for fixed combination preparations of propoxyphene napsylate and acetaminophen.

Darvon (dar′von) trademark for a preparation of propoxyphene.

darwinism (dar′win-izm) the theory of evolution according to which higher organisms have been developed from lower ones through the influence of natural selection.

daughter (dawt′er) 1. decay product. 2. arising from cell division, as a daughter cell.

db decibel.

D.C. direct current; Doctor of Chiropractic.

D & C dilatation (of cervix) and curettage (of uterus).

D.D.S. Doctor of Dental Surgery.

DDT dichloro-diphenyl-trichloroethane, a powerful insect poison; used in dilution as a powder or in an oily solution as a spray.

de- word element [L.], *down; from;* sometimes negative or privative, and often intensive.

deacylase (de-as′il-ās) any hydrolase that catalyzes the removal of an acyl group.

deaf (def) lacking the sense of hearing or not having the full power of hearing.

deafferentation (de-af″er-en-ta′shun) the elimination or interruption of sensory nerve fibers.

deaf-mute (def′mūt) a person unable to hear or speak.

deafness (def′nis) lack or loss, complete or partial, of the sense of hearing. See also *hearing loss.* **acoustic trauma d.,** that due to blast injury. **apoplectiform d.,** Meniere's disease in which the hearing impairment is sudden in onset and fluctuates. **cerebral d.,** that due to a brain lesion. **conduction d.,** that due to defect of the sound-conducting apparatus. **functional d.,** apparent deafness due to defective functioning of the auditory apparatus without organic lesions. **hysterical d.,** that which may appear or disappear in a hysterical patient without discoverable cause. **labyrinthine d.,** that due to disease of the labyrinth. **Michel's d.,** congenital deafness due to total lack of development of the inner ear. **Mondini's d.,** congenital deafness due to dysgenesis of the organ of Corti, with partial aplasia of the bony and membranous labyrinth and a resultant flattened cochlea. **nerve d., neural d.,** that due to a lesion of the auditory nerve on the central neural pathways. **pagetoid d.,** that occurring in osteitis deformans (Paget's disease) of the bones of the skull. **perceptive d.,** that due to a lesion in the sensory mechanism (cochlea) of the ear or to a lesion of the acoustic nerve or central neural pathways or to a combination of such lesions. **transmission d.,** conduction d. **word d.,** auditory aphasia; receptive aphasia in which sounds are heard but convey no meaning to the mind.

deamidase (de-am′ĭ-dās) an enzyme that splits amides to form a carboxylic acid and ammonia.

deamidization (de-am″ĭ-diz-a′shin) liberation of the ammonia from an amide.

deaminase (de-am′ĭ-nās) an enzyme causing deamination, or removal of the amino group from

organic compounds, named according to its substrate as *adenosine d., cytidine d., guanine d.,* etc.

deamination (de-am″ĭ-na′shin) removal of the amino group, —NH_2, from a compound.

deanol acetamidobenzoate (de′ah-nol as″etam″ĭ-do-ben′zo-āt) a cerebral stimulant with parasympathomimetic activity, $C_{13}H_{20}N_2O_4$; used as an antidepressant in the treatment of certain behavior and learning disorders in children.

death (deth) the cessation of life; permanent cessation of all vital bodily functions. **black d.,** bubonic plague. **brain d.,** irreversible coma; irreversible brain damage as manifested by absolute unresponsiveness to all stimuli, absence of all spontaneous muscle activity, and an isoelectric electroencephogram for 30 minutes, all in the absence of hypothermia or intoxication by central nervous system depressants. **cot d., crib d.,** sudden infant death syndrome. **somatic d.,** cessation of all vital cellular activity.

debility (de-bil′it-e) lack or loss of strength; weakness.

débridement (da-brēd-maw′) [Fr.] the removal of foreign material or devitalized tissue from or adjacent to a traumatic or infected lesion until surrounding healthy tissue is exposed.

debris (dĭ-bre′) [Fr.] devitalized tissue or foreign matter. In dentistry, soft foreign material loosely attached to a tooth surface.

debt (det) something owed. **oxygen d.,** the oxygen that must be used in the oxidative energy processes after strenuous exercise to reconvert lactic acid to glucose and decomposed ATP and creatine phosphate to their original states.

deca- word element [Gr.], *ten;* used in naming units of measurement to indicate a quantity 10 times the unit designated by the root with which it is combined.

decalcification (de-kal″sĭ-fĭ-ka′shin) 1. loss of calcium salts from a bone or tooth. 2. the process of removing calcareous matter.

decamethonium (dek″ah-mĕ-tho′ne-um) a muscle relaxant, $C_{16}H_{38}N_2$, used in surgical anesthesia and in electroshock treatment, in the form of its bromide or iodide salt.

decannulation (de-kan″u-la′shin) the removal of a cannula.

decantation (de″kan-ta′shin) the pouring of a clear supernatant liquid from a sediment.

decapitation (de-kap″ĭ-ta′shin) the removal of the head, as of an animal, fetus, or bone.

decarboxylase (de″kar-bok′sĭ-lās) any of the lyase class of enzymes that catalyze the removal of a carbon dioxide molecule from a compound.

decavitamin (dek″ah-vīt′ah-min) a combination of vitamins in capsular or tablet form, each of which contains vitamins A and D, ascorbic acid, calcium pantothenate, cyanocobalamin, folic acid, niacinamide, pyridoxine hydrochloride, riboflavin, thiamine hydrochloride, and a suitable form of alpha tocopherol.

decay (de-ka′) 1. the decomposition of dead matter. 2. the process of decline, as in aging. **beta d.,** disintegration of the nucleus of an unstable radionuclide in which the mass number is unchanged, but atomic number is changed by 1, as a result of emission of a negatively or positively charged (beta) particle.

decerebrate (de-sĕ′rĕ-brāt) to eliminate cerebral function by transecting the brain stem or by ligating the common carotid arteries and basilar artery at the center of the pons; an animal so prepared, or a brain-damaged person with similar neurologic signs.

decholesterolization (de-ko-les″ter-ol-iz-a′-shin) reduction of blood cholesterol levels.

deci- word element [L.], *one-tenth;* used in naming units of measurement to indicate one-tenth of the unit designated by the root with which it is combined (10^{-1}); symbol d.

decibel (des′ĭ-bel) a unit used to express the ratio of two powers, usually electric or acoustic powers, equal to one-tenth of a bel; one decibel equals approximately the smallest difference in acoustic power the human ear can detect.

decidua (de-sij′oo-ah) the endometrium of the pregnant uterus, all of which, except the deepest layer, is shed at parturition. **decid′ual**, adj. **basal d., d. basa′lis,** that portion on which the implanted ovum rests. **capsular d., d. capsula′ris,** that portion directly overlying the implanted ovum and facing the uterine cavity. **menstrual d., d. menstrua′lis,** the hyperemic uterine mucosa shed during menstruation. **parietal d., d. parieta′lis,** the decidua exclusive of the area occupied by the implanted ovum. **d. reflex′a,** capsular decidua. **d. seroti′na,** basal d. **d. subchoria′lis,** the maternal component of the tissue comprising the closing ring of Winkler-Waldeyer. **true d., d. ve′ra,** parietal d.

deciduation (de-sij″oo-a′shin) the shedding of the decidua.

deciduitis (-īt′is) a bacterial disease leading to changes in the decidua.

deciduosis (-o′sis) the presence of decidual tissue or of tissue resembling the endometrium of pregnancy in an ectopic site.

deciliter (des′ĭ-lēt″er) one tenth of a liter, one hundred milliliters.

declination (dek″lĭ-na′shin) cyclophoria.

declive (de-kliv′) a slope or a slanting surface. In anatomy, the part of the vermis of the cerebellum just caudal to the primary fissure. **declivis** (de-kli′vis) [L.] decline.

decoloration (de-kul″er-a′shin) 1. removal of color; bleaching. 2. lack or loss of color.

decompensation (de″kom-pen-sa′shin) 1. inability of the heart to maintain adequate circulation, marked by dyspnea, venous engorgement, and edema. 2. in psychiatry, failure of defense mechanisms resulting in progressive personality disintegration.

decomposition (de-kom″poz-ish′in) the separation of compound bodies into their constituent principles.

decompression (de″kom-presh′in) removal of pressure, especially from deep-sea divers and caisson workers to prevent bends, and from persons ascending to great heights. **cardiac d., d.** of heart. **cerebral d.,** relief of intracranial pressure by removal of a skull flap and incision of the dura mater. **d. of heart,** pericardiotomy with evacuation of a hematoma. **nerve d.,** relief of pressure on a nerve by surgical removal of the constricting fibrous or bony tissue. **d. of pericardium,** d. of heart. **d. of spinal cord,** surgical relief of pressure on the spinal cord, which may be due to hematoma, bone fragments, etc.

decongestant (de″kon-jes′tint) 1. tending to reduce congestion or swelling. 2. an agent that reduces congestion or swelling.

decontamination (de″kon-tam-ĭ-na′shin) the freeing of a person or object of some contaminating substance, e.g., war gas, radioactive material, etc.

decortication (de-kor″tĭ-ka′shin) 1. removal of the outer covering from a plant, seed, or root. 2. removal of portions of the cortical substance of a structure or organ.

decrudescence (de″kroo-des′ins) diminution or abatement of the intensity of symptoms.

decubitus (de-ku′bit-is), pl. *decu′bitus.* 1. an act of lying down; the position assumed in lying down. 2. decubitus ulcer. **decu′bital,** adj. **dorsal d.,** lying on the back. **lateral d.,** lying on one side, designated *right lateral decubitus* when the subject lies on the right side and *left lateral decubitus* when he lies on the left side. **ventral d.,** lying on the stomach.

decussatio (de″kus-a′she-o), pl. *decussatio′nes* [L.] decussation.

decussation (de″kus-a′shin) a crossing over; the intercrossing of fellow parts or structures in the form of an X. **Forel's d.,** the ventral tegmental decussation of the rubrospinal and rubroreticular tracts in the mesencephalon. **fountain d. of Meynert,** the dorsal tegmental decussation of the tectospinal tract in the mesencephalon. **d. of the pyramids,** the anterior part of the lower medulla oblongata in which most of the fibers of the pyramids intersect.

dedifferentiation (de-dif″er-en″she-a′shin) regression from a more specialized or complex form to a simpler state.

de-epicardialization (de″ep-ĭ-kar″dĭ-il-iz-a′-shin) a surgical procedure for the relief of intractable angina pectoris, in which epicardial tissue is destroyed by application of a caustic agent to promote development of collateral circulation.

defecation (def″ĭ-ka′shin) 1. the evacuation of fecal matter from the rectum. 2. the removal of impurities, as chemical defecation.

defect (de′fekt, dĭ-fekt′) an imperfection, failure, or absence. **acquired d.,** a non-genetic imperfection arising secondarily, after birth. **aortic septal d.,** a congenital anomaly in which there is abnormal communication between the ascending aorta and pulmonary artery just above the semilunar valves. **atrial septal d., atrioseptal d.,** a congenital anomaly in which there is persistent patency of the atrial septum, owing to failure of closure of the ostium primum or ostium secundum. **birth d.,** one present at birth, whether a morphological defect (dysmorphism) or an inborn error of metabolism. **congenital d.,** birth d. **cortical d.,** a benign, symptomless, circumscribed rarefaction of cortical bone, detected radiographically. **endocardial cushion d's,** a spectrum of septal defects resulting from imperfect fusion of the endocardial cushions, and ranging from persistent ostium primum to persistent common atrioventricular canal; see *atrial septal d.* and *atrioventricularis communis.* **filling d.,** any localized defect in the contour of the stomach, duodenum, or intestine, as seen in the roentgenogram after barium enema. **genetic d.,** see under *disease.* **neural-tube d.,** a developmental anomaly resulting in anencephaly or spina bifida. **retention d.,** a defect in the power of recalling or remembering names, numbers, or events. **septal d.,** a defect in a cardiac septum resulting in an abnormal communication between the opposite chambers of the heart. **ventricular septal d.,** a congenital cardiac anomaly in which there is persistent patency of the ventricular septum in either the muscular or fibrous portions, most often due to failure of the bulbar septum to completely close the interventricular foramen.

defeminization (de-fem″ĭ-niz-a′shin) loss of female sexual characteristics.

defense (dĭ-fens′) behavior directed to protection of the individual from injury. **character d.,** any character trait, e.g., a mannerism, attitude, or affectation, which serves as a defense mechanism. **insanity d.,** a legal concept that a person cannot be convicted of a crime if he lacked criminal responsibility by reason of insanity at the time of commission of the crime.

deferens (def′er-ens) [L.] deferent.

deferentectomy (def″er-en-tek′tah-me) excision of a ductus deferens.

deferential (def″er-en′shil) pertaining to the ductus deferens.

deferoxamine (dĕ″fer-oks′ah-mēn) an iron-chelating agent, $C_{25}H_{48}N_2O_8$, isolated from *Streptomyces pilosus;* used as an antidote in iron poisoning.

defervescence (def″er-ves′ins) the period of abatement of fever.

defibrillation (de-fib″ril-a′shin) 1. termination of atrial or ventricular fibrillation, usually by electroshock. 2. separation of tissue fibers by blunt dissection.

defibrination (de-fi″brĭ-na′shin) removal of fibrin from the blood.

deficiency (de-fish′in-se) a lack or shortage; a condition characterized by presence of less than normal or necessary supply or competence.

deficit (def′ĭ-sit) a lack or deficiency. **oxygen d.,** see *anoxemia, anoxia,* and *hypoxia.*

defluvium (de-floo′ve-um) [L.] a falling out, as of the hair.

defluxion (de-fluk′shin) 1. a sudden disappearance. 2. a copious discharge, as of catarrh. 3. a falling out, as of hair.

deformability (de-form″ah-bil′it-e) the ability of cells, such as erythrocytes, to change shape as they pass through narrow spaces, such as the microvasculature.

deformity (de-form′it-e) distortion of any part or general disfigurement of the body; malforma-

tion. **Akerlund d.,** an indentation (in addition to the niche) in the duodenal cap in the radiograph in duodenal ulcer. **Arnold-Chiari d.,** protrusion of the cerebellum and medulla oblongata down into the spinal canal through the foramen magnum. **Madelung's d.,** radial deviation of the hand secondary to overgrowth of the distal ulna or shortening of the radius. **reduction d.,** congenital absence of a portion or all of a body part, especially of the limbs. **silver-fork d.,** see under *fracture.* **Sprengel's d.,** congenital elevation of the scapula, due to failure of descent of the scapula to its normal thoracic position during fetal life. **Volkmann's d.,** see under *disease.*

Deg. degeneration; degree.

degenerate 1. (de-jen′er-āt) to change from a higher to a lower form. 2. (de-jen′er-it) characterized by degeneration. 3. a person whose moral or physical state is below the normal.

degeneration (de-jen″er-a′shin) deterioration; change from a higher to a lower form, especially change of tissue to a lower or less functionally active form. **degen′erative,** adj. Abercrombie's d., amyloid d. **adipose d.,** fatty d. **amyloid d.,** that with deposit of lardacein in the tissues; indicates impaired nutritive function, and is seen in wasting diseases. **ascending d.,** wallerian degeneration affecting centripetal nerve fibers and progressing toward the brain or spinal cord. **calcareous d.,** degeneration of tissue with deposit of calcareous material. **caseous d.,** caseation (2). **cellulose d.,** amyloid d. **cerebromacular d., cerebroretinal d.,** degeneration of brain cells and of the macula retinae. **congenital macular d.,** hereditary macular degeneration, marked by the presence of a cystlike lesion that in the early stages resembles egg yolk. **Crooke's hyaline d.,** degeneration of basophils of the pituitary gland, in which they lose their specific granulations and the cytoplasm becomes progressively hyalinized; a constant finding in Cushing's syndrome, but also occurring in Addison's disease. **descending d.,** wallerian degeneration extending peripherally along nerve fibers. **disciform macular d.,** a form of macular degeneration occurring in persons over 40 years of age, in which sclerosis involving the macula and retina is produced by hemorrhages between Bruch's membrane and the pigment epithelium. **fibrinous d.,** necrosis with deposit of fibrin within the cells of the tissue. **gray d.,** degeneration of the white substance of the spinal cord, in which it loses myelin and assumes a gray color. **hepatolenticular d.,** a hereditary disorder of copper metabolism, marked by a pigmented ring at the outer margin of the cornea, degenerative changes in the brain, cirrhosis of the liver, splenomegaly, tremor, rigidity, contractures, psychic disturbances, dysphagia, and increasing weakness and emaciation. **hyaline d.,** a regressive change in cells in which the cytoplasm takes on a homogeneous, glassy appearance; also used loosely to describe the histologic appearance of tissues. **lattice d. of retina,** a frequently bilateral, usually benign asymptomatic condition, characterized by patches of fine gray or white lines that intersect at irregular intervals in the peripheral retina, usually associated with numerous, round, punched-out areas of retinal thinning or retinal holes. **mucoid d.,** that with deposit of myelin and lecithin in the cells. **parenchymatous d.,** cloudy swelling. **polypoid d.,** development of polypoid growths on a mucous membrane. **spongy d. of central nervous system, spongy d. of white matter,** a rare hereditary form of leukodystrophy marked by early onset, widespread demyelination and vacuolation of the cerebral white matter giving rise to a spongy appearance, and by severe mental retardation, megalocephaly, atony of the neck muscles, spasticity of the arms and legs, and blindness; death usually occurs at about 18 months of age. **subacute combined d. of spinal cord,** degeneration of both the posterior and lateral columns of the spinal cord, producing various motor and sensory disturbances; it is due to vitamin B_{12} deficiency and usually associated with pernicious anemia. **transneuronal d.,** atrophy of certain neurons after interruption of afferent axons or death of other neurons to which they send their efferent output. **waxy d.,** amyloid d. **Zenker's d.,** hyaline degeneration and necrosis of striated muscle.

degloving (de-gluv′ing) intra-oral surgical exposure of the bony mandibular chin; it can be performed in the posterior region if necessary.

deglutition (de″gloo-tish′in) swallowing.

degradation (dĕg″grah-da′shin) conversion of a chemical compound to one less complex as by splitting off one or more groups of atoms.

degustation (de″gus-ta′shin) tasting

dehiscence (de-his′ins) a splitting open. **wound d.,** separation of the layers of a surgical wound.

dehydratase (de-hi′drah-tās) any lyase (hydro-lyase) that catalyzes the removal of H_2O, leaving double bonds (or adding groups to double bonds).

dehydrocholesterol (de-hi″dro-kol-es′ter-ol) a sterol present in skin which, on ultraviolet irradiation, produces vitamin D. **7-d., activated,** cholecalciferol.

dehydrocholic acid (-ko′lik) an acid, $C_{24}H_{34}O_5$, formed by oxidation of cholic acid and derived from natural bile acids; used as a choleretic.

11-dehydrocorticosterone (-kor″tĭ-kos′ter-ōn) one of the least active of the glucocorticoids produced by the adrenal cortex, $C_{21}H_{28}O_4$.

dehydroepiandrosterone (-ep″ĭ-an-dros′ter-ōn) an androgen, $C_{19}H_{28}O_2$, occurring in normal human urine and synthesized from cholesterol; abbreviated DHA.

dehydrogenase (de-hi′dro-jin-ās″) an enzyme that mobilizes the hydrogen of a substrate so that it can pass to a hydrogen acceptor. **glucose-6-phosphate d. (G6PD),** an enzyme of the pentose phosphate pathway which, with $NADP^+$ as coenzyme, catalyzes the dehydrogenation of glucose-6-phosphate to 6-phosphogluconolactone. **lactate d. (LDH),** an enzyme that catalyzes the interconversion of lactate and pyruvate. It is widespread in tissues and is abundant in kidney, skeletal muscle, liver, and

myocardium, appearing in elevated concentrations in the blood when these tissues are injured.

dehydroretinal (de-hi″dro-ret′in-il) the aldehyde of dehydroretinol, derived from the visual pigment porphyropsin, found in fresh-water fishes and certain vertebrates and amphibians; its metabolic role is analogous to that of rhodopsin in other animals.

dehydroretinol (-ret′ĭ-nol) vitamin A_2; the form, $C_{20}H_{28}O$, of vitamin A found in the retina and liver of fresh-water fishes and certain invertebrates and amphibians; it differs from retinol (vitamin A_1) in having one more conjugated double bond and has approximately one-third the biological activity of retinol.

deionization (de-i″on-i-za′shin) the production of a mineral-free state by the removal of ions.

déjà vu (da′zhah voo′) [Fr.] an illusion that a new situation is a repetition of a previous experience.

dejecta (de-jek′tah) excrement.

dejection (de-jek′shun) 1. a mental state marked by depression and melancholy. 2. discharge of feces; defecation. 3. excrement; feces.

delactation (de″lak-ta′shin) 1. weaning. 2. cessation of lactation.

delamination (de-lam″in-a′shin) separation into layers, as of the blastoderm.

de-lead (de-led′) to induce the removal of lead from tissues and its excretion in the urine by the administration of chelating agents.

deleterious (del″ĭ-tēr′e-is) injurious; harmful.

deletion (de-le′shin) in genetics, loss of genetic material from a chromosome.

delinquent (de-lin′kwint) characterized by antisocial, illegal, or criminal conduct; a person exhibiting such conduct, especially a minor (*juvenile d.*).

deliquescence (del″ĭ-kwes′ins) dampness or liquefaction from the absorption of water from air. **deliques′cent,** adj.

delirium (dĕ-lēr′e-um) a mental disturbance of relatively short duration usually reflecting a toxic state, marked by illusions, hallucinations, delusions, excitement, restlessness, and incoherence. **d. tre′mens,** an acute mental disturbance marked by delirium with trembling and excitement, attended by anxiety, mental distress, sweating, gastrointestinal symptoms, and precordial pain; a form of alcoholic psychosis seen after withdrawal from heavy alcohol intake.

delivery (de-liv′er-e) expulsion or extraction of the child and fetal membranes at birth. **abdominal d.,** delivery of an infant through an incision made into the intact uterus through the abdominal wall. **breech d.,** delivery in which the fetal buttocks present first. **forceps d.,** extraction of the child from the maternal passages by application of forceps to the fetal head; designated *low* or *midforceps delivery* according to the degree of engagement of the fetal head and *high* when engagement has not occurred. **postmortem d.,** delivery of a child after death of the mother. **spontaneous d.,** birth of an infant without any aid from an attendant.

delle (del'ah) the clear area in the center of a stained erythrocyte.

dellen (del'in) saucer-shaped excavations at the periphery of the cornea, usually on the temporal side.

delmadinone acetate (del-mad'ĭ-nōn) a progestin, antiandrogen, and antiestrogen, $C_{23}H_{27}ClO_4$; used in veterinary medicine.

delomorphous (del"o-mor'fus) having definitely formed and well-defined limits, as a cell or tissue.

delta (delt'ah) 1. the fourth letter of the Greek alphabet, Δ or δ; used in chemical names to denote the fourth of a series of isomeric compounds or the carbon atom fourth from the carboxyl group, or to denote the fourth of any series. 2. a triangular area.

deltoid (del'toid) 1. triangular. 2. the deltoid muscle.

delusion (de-loo'zhin) a false personal belief based on incorrect inference about external reality and firmly maintained in spite of incontrovertible and obvious proof or evidence to the contrary. **delu'sional,** adj. **depressive d.,** a delusion of unworthiness or futility. **expansive d.,** abnormal belief in one's own greatness, goodness, or power. **d. of grandeur,** delusional conviction of one's own importance, power, wealth, etc., as in megalomania, dementia paralytica, and paranoid schizophrenia. **d. of negation, nihilistic d.,** a depressive delusion that the self or part of the self, part of the body, other persons, or the whole world has ceased to exist. **d. of persecution,** a morbid belief on the part of a patient that he is being persecuted, slandered, and injured. **systematized d.,** a delusion formulated in a logical manner; a delusion having a logical structure.

deme (dēm) a population of very similar organisms interbreeding in nature and occupying a circumscribed area.

demecarium (dem"ĭ-kār'e-um) a cholinesterase inhibitor, $C_{32}H_{52}N_4O_4$, used as the bromide salt in the treatment of glaucoma and convergent strabismus.

demeclocycline (dem"ĭ-klo-si'klēn) a broad-spectrum antibiotic of the tetracycline group, $C_{21}H_{21}ClN_2O_8$, produced by a mutant strain of *Streptomyces aureofaciens* or semisynthetically; the base and the hydrochloride salt are used as antibacterials.

dementia (de-men'she-ah) organic loss of intellectual function. **Alzheimer's d.,** see under *disease*. **Binswanger's d.,** that due to demyelination of the subcortical white matter of the brain with sclerotic changes in the blood vessels supplying it. **dialysis d.,** a progressive encephalopathy marked by dysarthria with nominal aphasia, dementia, myoclonic jerking, grand mal seizures, and psychosis, occurring in persons undergoing chronic hemodialysis, and probably due to high levels of aluminum in the water used in the dialysis fluid. **paralytic d., d. paraly'tica,** a chronic meningoencephalitis marked by degeneration of the cortical neurons, progressive dementia, and generalized paralysis, which, if untreated, is ultimately fatal.

d. prae'cox, in the U.S., a former name for schizophrenia; commonly used in Europe to denote process schizophrenia. **presenile d.,** Alzheimer's disease. **senile d.,** see under *psychosis*.

Demerol (dem'er-ol) trademark for preparations of meperidine.

demineralization (de-min"er-il-iz-a'shin) excessive elimination of mineral or organic salts from tissues of the body.

Demodex (dem'ah-deks) a genus of mites parasitic within the hair follicles of the host, including the species *D. folliculo'rum* in man, and *D. ca'nis* and *D. e'qui,* which cause mange in dogs and horses, respectively.

demography (de-mog'rah-fe) the statistical science dealing with populations, including matters of health, disease, births, and mortality.

demulcent (de-mul'sint) 1. soothing; bland. 2. a soothing mucilaginous or oily medicine or application.

demyelination (de-mi"ĭ-lin-a'shin) destruction, removal, or loss of the myelin sheath of a nerve or nerves.

denasality (de"na-zal'it-e) hyponasality.

denaturation (de-na"cher-a'shin) a change in the usual nature of a substance, as by the addition of methanol or acetone to alcohol to render it unfit for drinking, or the change in molecular structure of proteins due to splitting of hydrogen bonds caused by heat or certain chemicals.

dendr(o)- word element [Gr.], *tree; treelike.*

dendraxon (den-drak'son) a nerve cell whose axon splits up into terminal filaments immediately after leaving the cell.

dendrite (den'drīt) one of the threadlike extensions of the cytoplasm of a neuron; dendrites branch into treelike processes and compose most of the receptive surface of a neuron.

dendritic (den-drit'ik) 1. branched like a tree. 2. pertaining to or possessing dendrites.

dendrodendritic (den"dro-den-drit'ik) referring to a synapse between dendrites of two neurons.

dendron (den'dron) dendrite.

dendrophagocytosis (den"dro-fag"o-si-to'sis) the absorption by microglial cells of broken portions of astrocytes.

denervation (de"ner-va'shin) interruption of the nerve connection to an organ or part.

dengue (den'ge) an infectious, eruptive, febrile, viral disease of tropical areas, transmitted by *Aedes* mosquitoes, and marked by severe pains in the head, eyes, muscles, and joints, sore throat, catarrhal symptoms, and sometimes a skin eruption and painful swellings of parts.

denial (dī-ni'il) a defense mechanism in which the existence of intolerable actions, ideas, etc., is unconsciously denied.

denidation (de"ni-da'shin) degeneration and expulsion of the endometrium during the menstrual cycle.

dens (dens), pl. *den'tes* [L.] a tooth or toothlike structure. **d. in den'te,** a malformed tooth caused by invagination of the crown before it is calcified, giving the appearance of a "tooth within a tooth."

densitometry (den″sĭ-tom′ĭ-tre) determination of variations in density by comparison with that of another material or with a certain standard.

density (den′sit-e) 1. the ratio of the mass of a substance to its volume. 2. the quality of being compact or dense. 3. the quantity of matter in a given space. 4. the quantity of electricity in a given area, volume, or time. 5. the degree of darkening of exposed and processed photographic or x-ray film, expressed as the logarithm of the opacity of a given area of the film.

dent(o)- word element [L.], *tooth; toothlike.*

dentalgia (den-tal′je-ah) toothache.

dentate (den′tāt) notched; tooth-shaped.

dentes (den′tēz) [L.] plural of *dens.*

dentia (den′she-ah) a condition relating to development or eruption of the teeth. **d. prae′cox,** premature eruption of the teeth; presence of teeth in the mouth at birth. **d. tar′da,** delayed eruption of the teeth, beyond the usual time for their appearance.

dentibuccal (den″tĭ-buk′′l) pertaining to the cheek and teeth.

denticle (den′tĭ-k'l) 1. a small toothlike process. 2. a distinct calcified mass within the pulp chamber of a tooth.

dentifrice (den′tĭ-fris) a preparation for cleansing and polishing the teeth; it may contain a therapeutic agent, such as fluoride, to inhibit dental caries.

dentilabial (den″tĭ-la′be-il) pertaining to the teeth and lips.

dentin (den′tin) the chief substance of the teeth, surrounding the tooth pulp and covered by enamel on the crown and by cementum on the roots. **den′tinal,** adj. **adventitious d.,** secondary d. **circumpulpar d.,** the inner portion of dentin, adjacent to the pulp, consisting of thinner fibrils. **cover d.,** the peripheral portion of dentin, adjacent to the enamel or cementum, consisting of coarser fibers than the circumpulpar dentin. **irregular d.,** secondary d. **mantle d.,** cover d. **opalescent d.,** dentin giving an unusual translucent or opalescent appearance to the teeth, as occurs in dentinogenesis imperfecta. **primary d.,** dentin formed before the eruption of a tooth. **secondary d.,** new dentin formed in response to stimuli associated with the normal aging process or with pathological conditions, such as caries or injury, or cavity preparation. **transparent d.,** dentin in which some dentinal tubules have become sclerotic or calcified, producing the appearance of translucency.

dentinogenesis (den″tin-o-jen′is-is) the formation of dentin. **d. imperfec′ta,** a hereditary condition marked by imperfect formation and calcification of dentin, giving the teeth a brown or blue opalescent appearance.

dentinogenic (-jen′ik) forming or producing dentin.

dentinoma (den″tĭ-no′mah) a tumor of odontogenic origin, consisting mainly of dentin.

dentinum (den-ti′num) dentin.

dentist (den′tist) a person with a degree in dentistry and authorized to practice dentistry.

dentistry (den′tis-tre) 1. that branch of the healing arts concerned with the teeth, oral cavity, and associated structures, including prevention, diagnosis, and treatment of disease and restoration of defective or missing tissue. 2. the work done by dentists, e.g., the creation of restorations, crowns and bridges, and surgical procedures performed in and about the oral cavity. **operative d.,** dentistry concerned with restoration of parts of the teeth that are defective as a result of disease, trauma, or abnormal development to a state of normal function, health, and esthetics. **pediatric d.,** pedodontics. **preventive d.,** dentistry concerned with maintenance of a normal masticating mechanism by fortifying the structures of the oral cavity against damage and disease. **prosthetic d.,** prosthodontics. **restorative d.,** dentistry concerned with the restoration of existing teeth that are defective because of disease, trauma, or abnormal development to normal function, health, and appearance; it includes crown and bridgework.

dentition (den-tish′in) the teeth in the dental arch; ordinarily used to designate the natural teeth in position in their alveoli. **deciduous d.,** the teeth that erupt first and are later replaced by the permanent dentition. **mixed d.,** the complement of teeth in the jaws after eruption of some of the permanent teeth, but before all the deciduous teeth are shed. **permanent d.,** the teeth that erupt and take their places after the deciduous teeth are lost. **precocious d.,** abnormally accelerated appearance of the deciduous or permanent teeth. **primary d.,** deciduous d. **retarded d.,** abnormally delayed appearance of the deciduous or permanent teeth.

dentoalveolar (den″to-al-ve′ah-ler) pertaining to a tooth and its alveolus.

dentofacial (-fa′shil) of or pertaining to the teeth and alveolar process and the face.

dentotropic (-trop′ik) turning toward or having an affinity for tissues composing the teeth.

dentulous (den′tu-lus) having natural teeth.

denture (den′cher) a complement of teeth, either natural or artificial; ordinarily used to designate an artificial replacement for the natural teeth and adjacent tissues. **complete d.,** an appliance replacing all the teeth of one jaw, as well as associated structures of the jaw. **implant d.,** one constructed with a metal substructure embedded within the underlying soft structures of the jaws. **interim d.,** a denture to be used for a short interval of time for reasons of esthetics, mastication, occlusal support, convenience, or to condition the patient to the acceptance of an artificial substitute for missing natural teeth until more definite prosthetic dental treatment can be provided. **overlay d.,** a complete denture supported both by soft tissue (mucosa) and by a few remaining natural teeth that have been altered, as by insertion of a long or short coping, to permit the denture to fit over them. **partial d.,** a removable (*removable partial d.*) or permanently attached (*fixed partial d.*) appliance replacing one or more missing teeth in one jaw and receiving support and retention from underlying tissues and some or all of the remaining teeth. **provisional d.,** an interim denture used for the purpose of conditioning the patient to the acceptance of an artificial substitute for missing natural teeth. **transitional d.,** a partial denture which is to serve as a temporary prosthesis and to which teeth will be added as more teeth are lost and which will be replaced after postextraction tissue changes have occurred.

denudation (de″noo-da′shin) the stripping or laying bare of any part.

deodorant (de-o′der-int) an agent that masks offensive odors.

deorsumduction (de-or″sum-duk′shin) infraduction.

deorsumvergence (-ver′jins) infravergence.

deorsumversion (-ver′zhin) infraversion.

deossification (de-os″ĭ-fĭ-ka′shin) loss or removal of the mineral elements of bone.

deoxy- chemical prefix designating a compound containing one less oxygen atom than the reference substance; see also words beginning *desoxy-*.

deoxycholic acid (de-ok″se-ko′lik) one of the bile acids, capable of forming soluble, diffusible complexes with fatty acids.

deoxyhemoglobin (-he″mo-glo′bin) hemoglobin not combined with oxygen, formed when oxyhemoglobin releases its oxygen to the tissues.

deoxyribonuclease (-ri″bo-noo′kle-ās) an enzyme that catalyzes the hydrolysis (depolymerization) of deoxyribonucleic acid (DNA).

deoxyribonucleic acid (DNA) (-noo-kle′ik) a nucleic acid that on hydrolysis yields adenine, guanine, cytosine, thymine, deoxyribose, and phosphoric acid; it is the carrier of genetic information for all organisms except RNA viruses. See *Watson-Crick helix.*

deoxyribonucleoprotein (-noo″kle-o-pro″te-in) a nucleoprotein in which the sugar is D-2-deoxyribose.

deoxyribonucleoside (-noo′kle-o-sīd) a nucleoside having a purine or pyrimidine base bonded to deoxyribose.

deoxyribonucleotide (-noo′kle-o-tīd) a nucleotide having a purine or pyrimidine base bonded to deoxyribose, which in turn is bonded to a phosphate group.

deoxyribose (-ri″bōs) an aldopentose, $CH_2 \cdot OH \cdot (CHOH)_2 \cdot CH_2 \cdot CHO$, found in deoxyribonucleic acids, deoxyribonucleotides, and deoxyribonucleosides.

dependence (de-pend′ins) the psychophysical state of a drug user in which the usual or increasing doses of the drug are required to prevent the onset of withdrawal symptoms. **substance d., psychoactive,** psychoactive substance abuse (q.v.) in which either tolerance or withdrawal is present.

dependency (de-pend′in-se) reliance on others for love, affection, mothering, comfort, security, food, warmth, shelter, protection, and the like—the so-called dependency needs.

dependent (de-pend′int) 1. pertaining to dependence or to dependency. 2. hanging down.

depersonalization (de-per″sun-il-iz-a′shin) alteration in the perception of self so that the usual sense of one's own reality is temporarily lost or changed; it may be a manifestation of a neurosis or another mental illness or can occur in mild form in normal persons.

depilatory (dĕ-pil′ah-tor″e) 1. having the power to remove hair. 2. an agent for removing or destroying hair.

depolarization (de-po″ler-iz-a′shin) the process or act of neutralizing polarity.

depolymerization (de-pol″ĭ-mer-iz-a′shin) the conversion of a compound into one of smaller molecular weight and different physical properties without changing the percentage relations of the elements composing it.

deposit (de-poz′it) 1. sediment or dregs. 2. extraneous inorganic matter collected in the tissues or in an organ of the body.

depot (de′po, dep′o) a body area in which a substance, e.g., a drug, can be accumulated, deposited, or stored and from which it can be distributed.

depressant (de-pres′int) diminishing any functional activity; an agent that so acts. **cardiac d.,** an agent that depresses the rate or force of contraction of the heart.

depression (de-presh′in) 1. a hollow or depressed area; downward or inward displacement. 2. a lowering or decrease of functional activity. 3. in psychiatry, a morbid sadness, dejection, or melancholy. **agitated d.,** psychotic depression accompanied by more or less constant activity. **anaclitic d.,** impairment of an infant's physical, social, and intellectual development which sometimes follows a sudden separation from his mother. **congenital chondrosternal d.,** congenital deformity with a deep, funnel-shaped depression in the anterior chest wall. **endogenous d.,** any depression that is not a reactive depression; the term implies that some intrinsic biological process rather than environmental influence is the cause. **involutional d.,** see under *melancholia.* **major d.,** a mental disorder characterized by the occurrence of one or more major depressive episodes and the absence of any history of manic or hypomanic episodes. **pacchionian d's,** small pits on the internal cranium on either side of the groove for the superior sagittal sinus, occupied by the arachnoid granulations. **reactive d.,** depression due to some external situation, and relieved when that situation is removed. **situational d.,** reactive d.

depressor (de-pres′er) anything that depresses, as a muscle, agent, or instrument, or an afferent nerve whose stimulation causes a fall in blood pressure.

deprivation (dep-rĭ-va′shin) loss or absence of parts, powers, or things that are needed. **emotional d.,** deprivation of adequate interpersonal and/or environmental experience, usually in the early developmental years. **sensory d.,** deprivation of usual external stimuli and the opportunity for perception.

depth (depth) distance measured perpendicularly downward from a surface. **focal d., d. of focus,** the measure of the power of a lens to yield clear images of objects at different distances.

derangement (de-rānj′mint) 1. mental disorder. 2. disarrangement of a part or organ.

dereism (de′re-izm) mental activity in which fantasy runs unhampered by logic and experience. **dereis′tic,** adj.

derepression (de″re-presh′in) 1. elevation of the level of an enzyme above the normal, either by lowering of the corepressor concentration or by a mutation that decreases the formation of aporepressor or the response to the complete repressor. 2. the inhibition of the repressor substance produced by the regulator genes with the result that the operator gene is free to initiate the process of polypeptide formation.

derivative (de-riv′ah-tiv) a chemical substance derived from another substance either directly or by modification or partial substitution.

derma (derm′ah) corium.

dermabrasion (derm″ah-bra′zhin) planing of the skin done by mechanical means, e.g., sandpaper, wire brushes, etc.; see *planing.*

Dermacentor (-sent′er) a genus of ticks that are important transmitters of disease. **D. albipic′tus,** a species found in Canada and the United States, parasitic on cattle, horses, moose, and elk. **D. anderso′ni,** a species parasitic on various wild mammals, responsible for transmitting Rocky Mountain spotted fever, Colorado tick fever, and tularemia to man and for causing tick paralysis. **D. varia′bilis,** the chief vector of Rocky Mountain spotted fever in the central and eastern United States, the dog being the principal host of the adults, but also parasitic on cattle, horses, rabbits, and man. **D. venus′tus,** *D. andersoni.*

Dermanyssus (derm″ah-nis′is) a genus of mites, including *D. galli′nae,* the bird mite, poultry (chicken or fowl) mite, or chicken louse, which sometimes infests man.

dermat(o)- word element [Gr.], *skin.*

dermatitis (derm″ah-tīt′is), pl. *dermati′tides.* Inflammation of the skin. **actinic d.,** that due to exposure to actinic radiation, such as that from the sun, ultraviolet waves, or x- or gamma radiation. **ammonia d.,** diaper dermatitis attributed to skin irritation due to the ammonia decomposition products of urine. **atopic d.,** a chronic pruritic eruption of unknown etiology; allergic, hereditary, and psychogenic factors appear to be involved. **berlock d.,** dermatitis, typically of the neck, face, and breast, with drop-shaped or quadrilateral patches or streaks, induced by sequential exposure to perfume or other toilet articles and then to sunlight. **contact d.,** 1. acute dermatitis due to contact with a substance to which the person is allergic or sensitive; when severe, called *d. venenata.* 2. primary-irritant (nonallergic) d. **exfoliative d.,** virtually universal erythema, desquamation, scaling, and itching of the skin, and loss of hair. **d. exfoliati′va neonato′rum,** exfoliative dermatitis supervening in bullous impetigo of the newborn. **d. herpetifor′mis,** chronic dermatitis marked by successive crops of grouped, symmetrical, erythematous, papular, vesicular, eczematous, or bullous lesions, accompanied by itching and burning; a granular deposition of IgA around the lesion almost always occurs. **infectious eczematoid d.,** a pustular eczematoid eruption frequently following or occurring coincidentally with some pyogenic process. **livedoid d.,** severe local pain, swelling, livedoid changes, and local increase in temperature due to temporary or prolonged local ischemia resulting from accidental arterial obliteration from intragluteal administration of medications. **meadow d., meadow-grass d.,** phototoxic dermatitis marked by an eruption of vesicles and bullae arranged in streaks and bizarre configurations, caused by exposure to sunlight after contact with meadow grass, usually *Agrimonia eupatoria.* **photoallergic contact d., photocontact d.,** allergic contact dermatitis caused by the action of sunlight on skin sensitized by contact with a substance capable of causing this reaction, such as a halogenated salicylanilide, sandalwood oil, or hexachlorophene. **phototoxic d.,** erythema followed by hyperpigmentation of sun-exposed areas of the skin, resulting from sequential exposure to agents containing photosensitizing substances, such as coal tar and certain perfumes, drugs, or plants containing psoralens, and then to sunlight. **poison ivy d., poison oak d., poison sumac d.,** allergic contact dermatitis due to exposure to plants of the genus *Rhus,* which contain urushiol, a skin-sensitizing agent. **primary-irritant d.,** that induced by a substance acting as an irritant rather than as a sensitizer or allergen. **radiation d.,** radiodermatitis. **rat-mite d.,** that due to a bite of the rat-mite, *Ornithonyssus bacoti.* **d. re′pens,** acrodermatitis continua. **rhus d.,** poison ivy, poison oak, or poison sumac dermatitis. **roentgen-ray d.,** radiodermatitis. **schistosome d.,** swimmer's itch. **seborrheic d., d. seborrhe′ica,** a chronic pruritic dermatitis with erythema, dry, moist, or greasy scaling, and yellow crusted patches on various areas, especially the scalp, with exfoliation of an excessive amount of dandruff. **stasis d.,** a chronic eczematous dermatitis, which initially involves the inner aspect of the lower leg just above the internal malleolus and which later may entirely or partially involve the lower leg, marked by edema, pigmentation, and commonly ulceration; it is due to venous insufficiency. **uncinarial d.,** ground itch. **d. venena′ta,** see *contact d.* (1). **x-ray d.,** radiodermatitis.

dermatoautoplasty (derm″ah-to-awt′o-plas″te) autotransplantation of skin.

Dermatobia (derm″ah-to′be-ah) a genus of botflies, including *D. hominis,* whose larvae are parasitic in the skin of man, mammals, and birds.

dermatofibrosarcoma (derm″mah-to-fi″brosar-ko′mah) a fibrosarcoma of the skin.

dermatoglyphics (derm″ah-to-glif′iks) the study of the patterns of ridges of the skin of the fingers, palms, toes, and soles; of interest in anthropology and law enforcement as a means of establishing identity and in medicine, both clinically and as a genetic indicator, particularly of chromosomal abnormalities.

dermatographism (derm″ah-tog′rah-fizm) urticaria due to physical allergy, in which moderately firm stroking or scratching of the skin with a dull instrument produces a pale, raised welt or wheal, with a red flare on each side. **dermatograph'ic,** adj. **black d.,** black or greenish streaking of the skin caused by deposit of fine metallic particles abraded from jewelry by various dusting powders. **white d.,** linear blanching of (usually erythematous) skin of persons with atopic dermatitis in response to firm stroking with a blunt instrument.

dermatoheteroplasty (derm″ah-to-het′er-o-plas″te) the grafting of skin derived from an individual of another species.

dermatology (-tol′ah-je) the medical specialty concerned with the diagnosis and treatment of skin diseases.

dermatolysis (-tol′ĭ-sis) cutis laxa.

dermatome (derm′ah-tōm) 1. an instrument for cutting thin skin slices for grafting. 2. the area of skin supplied with afferent nerve fibers by a single posterior spinal root. 3. the lateral part of an embryonic somite.

dermatomere (derm′ah-to-mēr″) any segment or metamere of the embryonic integument.

dermatomycosis (derm″ah-to-mi-ko′sis) a superficial fungal infection of the skin or its appendages.

dermatomyoma (-mi-o′mah) a dermal leiomyoma.

dermatomyositis (-mi″o-sīt′is) a collagen disease marked by nonsuppurative inflammation of the skin, subcutaneous tissue, and muscles, with necrosis of muscle fibers.

dermatopathic (-path′ik) pertaining or attributable to disease of the skin, as dermatopathic lymphadenopathy.

dermatopathy (derm″ah-top′ah-the) dermopathy.

Dermatophagoides (derm″ah-tof″ah-goi′dēs) a genus of sarcoptiform mites, usually found on the skin of chickens. *D. pteronyssimus* (house dust mite) acts as an antigen and produces allergic asthma in atopic persons.

dermatopharmacology (derm″ah-to-far″mah-kol′ah-je) pharmacology as applied to dermatologic disorders.

dermatophilosis (-fi-lo′sis) an actinomyotic disease caused by *Dermatophilus congolensis*, affecting cattle, sheep, horses, goats, deer, and sometimes man. In man, it is marked by painless pustules on the hands and arms; the lesions break down and form shallow red ulcers which regress spontaneously, leaving some scarring. In sheep, it is marked by exudative red scaling lesions that form pyramidal masses.

Dermatophilus (derm″ah-tof′ĭ-lus) 1. *Tunga.* 2. a genus of pathogenic actinomycetes. **D. con-golen'sis,** the etiologic agent of dermatophilosis. **D. pe'netrans,** *Tunga penetrans* (chigoe).

dermatophyte (derm′ah-to-fīt″) a fungus parasitic upon the skin, including *Microsporum, Epidermophyton,* and *Trichophyton.*

dermatophytid (derm″ah-tof′it-id) a secondary skin eruption which is an expression of hypersensitivity to a dermatophyte, especially *Epidermophyton,* infection, occurring on an area remote from the site of infection.

dermatophytosis (derm″ah-to-fi-to′sis) a fungous infection of the skin; often used to refer to tinea pedis (athlete's foot).

dermatoplasty (derm′ah-to-plas″te) a plastic operation on the skin; operative replacement of destroyed or lost skin. **dermatoplas'tic,** adj.

dermatosis (derm″ah-to′sis) any skin disease, especially one not characterized by inflammation. **d. papulo'sa ni'gra,** a form of seborrheic keratosis seen chiefly in blacks, with multiple miliary pigmented papules usually on the cheek bones, but sometimes occurring more widely on the face and neck. **progressive pigmentary d.,** a slowly progressive purpuric and pigmentary disease of the skin affecting chiefly the shins, ankles, and dorsum of the feet. **subcorneal pustular d.,** a bullous dermatosis resembling dermatitis herpetiformis, with single and grouped vesicles and pustules beneath the horny layer of the skin.

dermatosparaxis (derm″ah-to-spah-rak′sis) a disease of cattle and sheep related to the Ehlers-Danlos syndrome of humans, in which the skin is fragile and very easily torn; the defect may reside in an abnormally low activity of the enzyme procollagen peptidase.

dermatozoon (-zo′on) any animal parasite on the skin; an ectoparasite.

dermis (derm′is) the true skin, or corium. **der'-mal, der'mic,** adj.

dermoblast (derm′ah-blast) that part of the mesoblast developing into the true skin.

dermoid (derm′oid) 1. skinlike. 2. dermoid cyst.

dermoidectomy (derm″oi-dek′tah-me) excision of a dermoid cyst.

dermomyotome (der″mo-mi′ah-tōm) all but the sclerotome of a mesodermal somite; the primordium of skeletal muscle and, perhaps, of corium.

dermopathy (derm-op′ah-the) any skin disorder. **diabetic d.,** any of several cutaneous manifestations of diabetes.

dermosynovitis (derm″o-sin″o-vīt′is) inflammation of skin overlying an inflamed bursa or tendon sheath.

dermovascular (-vas′kūl-er) pertaining to the blood vessels of the skin.

desaturation (de-sach″er-a′shin) the process of introducing a double bond between carbon atoms of a fatty acid.

descemetocele (des″ĕ-met′o-sēl) hernia of Descemet's membrane.

descensus (de-sen′sus) pl. *descen'sus* [L.] downward displacement or prolapse. **d. tes'tis,** normal migration of the testis from its fetal position in the abdominal cavity to its location within the scrotum, usually during the last three months of gestation. **d. u'teri,** prolapse of the uterus.

desensitization (de-sen″sit-iz-a′shin) 1. the prevention or reduction of immediate hypersensitivity reactions by administration of graded doses of allergen. 2. in behavior therapy, the treatment of phobias and related disorders by intentionally exposing the patient, in imagination or in real life, to emotionally distressing stimuli.

deserpidine (de-serp′ĭ-dēn) an alkaloid of *Rauwolfia canescens*, $C_{32}H_{38}N_2O_8$; used as an antihypertensive and tranquilizer.

desexualize (de-sek′shoo-il-īz) to deprive of sexual characters; to castrate.

desferrioxamine (des-fer′e-ok′sah-mēn) deferoxamine.

desiccant (des′ĭ-kint) 1. promoting dryness. 2. an agent that promotes dryness.

desipramine (des-ip′rah-mēn) a metabolite of imipramine, $C_{18}H_{22}N_2$; the hydrochloride salt is used as an antidepressant.

deslanoside (des-lan′o-sīd) a cardiotonic glycoside, $C_{47}H_{74}O_{19}$, obtained from lanatoside C; used where digitalis is recommended.

desm(o)- word element [Gr.], *ligament.*

desmitis (dez-mīt′is) inflammation of a ligament.

desmocranium (dez″mo-kra′ne-um) the mass of mesoderm at the cranial end of the notochord in the early embryo, forming the earliest stage of the skull.

desmogenous (dez-moj′ah-nus) of ligamentous origin.

desmography (dez-mog′rah-fe) a description of ligaments.

desmoid (dez′moid) 1. an uncapsulated, locally invasive, and rarely metastasizing fibromatous tumor arising in the muscle sheath, usually of the abdominal wall, which closely resembles fibrosarcoma. 2. fibrous or fibroid.

desmolase (dez′mo-lās) any enzyme that catalyzes the addition or removal of some chemical group to or from a substrate without hydrolysis.

desmopathy (dez-mop′ah-the) any disease of the ligaments.

desmoplasia (dez″mo-pla′ze-ah) the formation and development of fibrous tissue. **desmoplas′tic,** adj.

desmosome (dez′mo-sōm) a circular, dense body that forms the site of attachment between certain epithelial cells, especially those of stratified epithelium of the epidermis, which consists of local differentiations at the apposing cell membranes.

desmotomy (dez-mot′ah-me) incision or division of a ligament.

desonide (des′o-nīd) a synthetic corticosteroid, $C_{24}H_{36}O_6$, used as a topical anti-inflammatory in the treatment of steroid-responsive dermatoses.

desorb (de-sorb′) to remove a substance from the state of absorption or adsorption.

desoximetasone (des-ok″se-met′ah-sōn) an anti-inflammatory, antipruritic, and vasoconstrictive corticosteroid; used topically to relieve inflammation in corticosteroid-responsive dermatoses.

desoxy- for words beginning thus, see also those beginning *deoxy-.*

desoxycorticosterone (des-ok″se-kor″tĭ-kos′-ter-ōn) a mineralocorticoid secreted in small amounts by the human adrenal cortex, $C_{21}H_{30}O_3$, which has no glucocorticoid activity; used in the form of the acetate and pivalate esters as replacement therapy in adrenocortical insufficiency and for treatment of salt-losing adrenogenital syndrome.

despeciate (de-spe′se-āt) to undergo despeciation; to subject to (as by chemical treatment) or to undergo loss of species antigenic characteristics.

desquamation (des″kwah-ma′shin) the shedding of epithelial elements, chiefly of the skin, in scales or sheets. **desquam′ative,** adj.

dest. [L.] *destilla′ta* (distilled).

desulfhydrase (de″sulf-hi′drās) an enzyme that removes hydrogen sulfide from a compound.

detachment (de-tach′mint) the condition of being separated or disconnected. **d. of retina, retinal d.,** separation of the inner layers of the retina from the pigment epithelium.

detector (de-tek′ter) an instrument or apparatus for revealing the presence of something. **lie d.,** polygraph.

detergent (de-terj′int) 1. purifying, cleansing. 2. an agent that purifies or cleanses.

determinant (de-term′ĭ-nint) a factor that establishes the nature of an entity or event. **antigenic d.,** the structural component of an antigen molecule responsible for its specific interaction with antibody molecules elicited by the same or related antigen. **hidden d.,** an antigenic determinant in an unexposed region of a molecule so that it is prevented from interacting with receptors on lymphocytes, or with antibody molecules, and is unable to induce an immune response; it may appear following stereochemical alterations of molecular structure.

determination (de-term″ĭ-na′shin) the establishment of the exact nature of an entity or event. **sex d.,** the process by which the sex of an organism is fixed; associated, in man, with the presence or absence of the Y chromosome. **embryonic d.,** the loss of pluripotentiality in any embryonic part and its start on the way to an unalterable fate.

determinism (de-term′ĭ-nizm) the theory that all phenomena are the result of antecedent conditions and that nothing occurs by chance.

detoxification (de-tok′sĭ-fĭ-ka′shin) 1. reduction of the toxic properties of a substance. 2. treatment designed to assist in recovery from the toxic effects of a drug. **metabolic d.,** reduction of the toxicity of a substance by chemical changes induced in the body, producing a compound less poisonous or more readily eliminated.

detrition (de-trish′in) the wearing away, as of teeth, by friction.

detritus (de-trīt′is) particulate matter produced by or remaining after the wearing away or disintegration of a substance or tissue.

detruncation (de″trung-ka′shin) decollation; decapitation, especially of a fetus.

detrusor (de-troo′zer) a general term for a body part, e.g., a muscle, that pushes down.

detumescence (de″tu-mes′ins) the subsidence of congestion and swelling.

deutan (doo′tan) a person exhibiting deuteranomalopia or deuteranopia.

deuteranomaly (doōt″er-ah-nom′ah-le) deuteranomalopia. **deuteranom′alous,** adj.

deuteranopia, deuteranopsia (dōōt″er-ah-no′-pe-ah; -ah-nop′se-ah) defective color vision, with confusion of greens and reds, and retention of the sensory mechanism for two hues only—blue and yellow. **deuteranop′ic,** adj.

deuterium (doo-tēr′e-um) see *hydrogen.*

Deuteromycetes (-mi-sēt′ēz) an imperfect fungus.

deuteroplasm (dōōt′er-o-plazm″) the passive or inactive materials in protoplasm, especially reserve foodstuffs, such as yolk.

deuteropathy (dōōt″er-op′ah-the) a disease that is secondary to another disease.

devascularization (de-vas″ku-ler-ĭ-za′shin) interruption of circulation of blood to a part due to obstruction of blood vessels supplying it.

development (de-vel′up-mint) the process of growth and differentiation. **developmen′tal,** adj. **cognitive d.,** the development of intelligence, conscious thought, and problem-solving ability that begins in infancy. **psychosexual d.,** 1. development of the individual's sexuality as affected by biological, cultural, and emotional influences from prenatal life onward throughout life. 2. in psychoanalysis, libidinal maturation from infancy through adulthood (including the oral, anal, and genital stages). **psychosocial d.,** the development of the personality, and the acquisition of social attitudes and skills, from infancy through maturity.

deviant (de′ve-int) 1. varying from a determinable standard. 2. a person with characteristics varying from what is considered standard or normal.

deviation (de″ve-a′shin) variation from the regular standard or course. In ophthalmology, a tendency for the visual axes of the eyes to fall out of alignment due to muscular imbalance. **complement d.,** inhibition of complement-mediated immune hemolysis in the presence of excess antibody. **conjugate d.,** deflection of the eyes in the same direction at the same time. **immune d.,** modification of the immune response to an antigen by previous inoculation of the same antigen. **standard d.,** in standardized tests, a measure of deviations from a central value, determined as the square root of the average of the squares of all deviations from the mean; symbol σ.

device (dĭvīs′) something contrived for a specific purpose. **contraceptive d.,** one used to prevent conception, as a diaphragm or condom to prevent entrance of spermatozoa into the uterine cervix, or one inserted into the uterus (*intrauterine d.*) to prevent implantation of a fertilized ovum. **intrauterine d. (IUD),** a plastic or metallic device inserted in the uterus to prevent implantation of the fertilized ovum; available in various shapes, including loops, coils, bows, rings, shields, springs, M's, and T's.

deviometer (de″ve-om′it-er) an instrument for measuring the deviation in strabismus.

devitalize (de-vīt′il-īz) to deprive of life or vitality.

dexamethasone (dek″sah-meth′ah-sōn) a synthetic glucocorticoid, $C_{22}H_{29}FO_5$, used primarily as an anti-inflammatory in various condi-

tions, including collagen diseases and allergic states; it is the basis of a screening test in the diagnosis of Cushing's syndrome.

dexbrompheniramine (deks″brōm-fen-ir′ah-mēn) the bromine analogue of dexchlorpheniramine, $C_{16}H_{19}BrN_2$, used as an antihistaminic in the form of the maleate salt.

dexchlorpheniramine (-klōr-fen-ir′ah-mēn) the dextrorotatory isomer of chlorpheniramine, $C_{18}H_{19}ClN_2$, used as an antihistaminic in the form of the maleate salt.

Dexedrine (dek′sĭ-drēn) trademark for preparations of dextroamphetamine.

Dexon (dek′son) trademark for a synthetic suture material, polyglycolic acid, a polymer that is completely absorbable and nonirritating.

dexpanthenol (deks-pan′thĭ-nōl) the D(+) form of panthenol, $C_9H_{19}NO_4$, the alcoholic analogue of pantothenic acid, which is claimed to be a precursor of coenzyme A. Used to increase peristalsis in atony and paralysis of the lower intestine and to help relieve gas retention and abdominal distention in certain conditions; also used topically to stimulate healing of the lesions of various dermatologic lesions.

dexter (dek′ster) [L.] right; on the right side.

dextr(o)- word element [L.], *right.*

dextrad (dek′strad) to or toward the right side.

dextral (dek′stril) pertaining to the right side.

dextrality (dek-stral′it-e) the preferential use of the right member of the major paired organs of the body.

dextran (dek′stran) a water-soluble polysaccharide of glucose (dextrose) produced by the action of *Leuconostoc mesenteroides* on sucrose; used as a plasma volume extender.

dextranomer (deks-tran′ah-mer) small beads of highly hydrophilic dextran polymers, used in débridement of secreting wounds, such as venous stasis ulcers; the sterilized beads are poured over secreting wounds to absorb wound exudates and prevent crust formation.

dextrin (dek′strin) a carbohydrate formed during the hydrolysis of starch to sugar.

dextrin-1,6-glucosidase (deks″trin-gloo-ko′sĭ-dās) dextrin 6-glucanohydrolase: an enzyme that catalyzes the hydrolysis of α-1-6-glucan links in dextrins containing short 1,6-linked side chains.

dextrinosis (dek″strin-o′sis) accumulation in the tissues of an abnormal polysaccharide. **limit d.,** Forbes' disease.

dextrinuria (dek″strin-ūr′e-ah) presence of dextrin in the urine.

dextroamphetamine (dek″stro-am-fet′ah-mēn) the dextrorotatory isomer of amphetamine, having more central nervous system stimulating effect than the levorotatory (levamfetamine) or racemic forms of amphetamine; abuse of this drug may lead to dependence.

dextrocardia (-kar′de-ah) location of the heart in the right side of the thorax, the apex pointing to the right. **mirror-image d.,** location of the heart in the right side of the chest, the atria being transposed and the right ventricle lying anteriorly and left of the left ventricle.

dextroclination (-klĭ-na′shin) rotation of the upper poles of the vertical meridians of the eyes to the right.

dextroduction (dek″stro-duk′shin) movement of an eye to the right.

dextrogastria (-gas′tre-ah) displacement of the stomach to the right.

dextrogram (dek′stro-gram) an electrocardiographic tracing showing right axis deviation, indicative of right ventricular hypertrophy.

dextrogyration (dek″stro-ji-ra′shin) rotation to the right.

dextromanual (-man′u-il) right-handed.

dextromethorphan (-meth′or-fan) a synthetic morphine derivative, $C_{18}H_{25}NO$, used as an antitussive in the form of the hydrobromide salt.

dextroposition (dek″stro-po-zish′in) displacement to the right.

dextrorotatory (-rōt′ah-tor″e) turning the plane of polarization to the right.

dextrose (dek′strōs) a monosaccharide, C_6H_{12}-$O_6 \cdot H_2O$, usually obtained by hydrolysis of starch; used chiefly as a fluid and nutrient replenisher, and also as a diuretic and alone or in combination with other agents for various other clinical purposes. Known as D-*glucose* in biochemistry and physiology.

dextrosinistral (dek″stro-sin′is-tril) extending from right to left; also applied to a left-handed person trained to use the right hand in certain performances.

dextrothyroxine (-thi-rok′sin) the dextrorotatory isomer of thyroxine, used as an oral anticholesteremic, mainly to treat hypercholesteremia in euthyroid patients.

dextroversion (-ver′zhin) 1. version to the right, especially movement of the eyes to the right. 2. location of the heart in the right chest, the left ventricle remaining in the normal position on the left, but lying anterior to the right ventricle.

DFP diisopropyl fluorophosphate; see *isofluro-phate.*

di- word element [Gr., L.], *two.*

dia- word element [Gr.], *through; between; apart; across; completely.*

diabetes (di″ah-bēt′ēz) any disorder characterized by excessive urine excretion. **adult-onset d.,** maturity-onset d. When used alone, the term refers to *diabetes mellitus.* **bronze d., bronzed d.,** hemochromatosis. **chemical d.,** a mild abnormality of carbohydrate tolerance manifested by hyperinsulinemia or hyperglycemia only when the patient is subjected to stress loads of glucose. **gestational d.,** that in which onset or recognition of impaired glucose tolerance occurs during pregnancy. **growth-onset d.,** juvenile d. **d. insi′pidus,** a metabolic disorder due to deficiency of antidiuretic hormone, resulting in failure of tubular reabsorption of water in the kidney and the consequent passage of a large amount of urine and great thirst. **d. insi′pidus, nephrogenic,** a congenital and familial form of diabetes insipidus due to failure of the renal tubules to reabsorb water; there is excessive production of antidiuretic hormone but the tubules fail to respond to it. **insu-**lin-dependent d. (IDD), juvenile d., juvenile-onset d., ketosis-prone d., severe diabetes mellitus, usually having an abrupt onset before the age of 25 and tending to be difficult to control and unstable (''brittle''); plasma insulin is often deficient, ketoacidosis occurs frequently, and oral hypoglycemics and diet are almost never effective, daily injections of insulin being almost always required. **latent d.,** chemical d. **maturity-onset d.,** non-insulin-dependent d. **d. melli′tus (DM),** a metabolic disorder in which there is inability to oxidize carbohydrates, due to disturbance of the normal insulin mechanism, producing hyperglycemia, glycosuria, polyuria, thirst, hunger, emaciation, weakness, acidosis, sometimes leading to dyspnea, lipemia, ketonuria, and finally coma. **non-insulin-dependent d. (NIDD),** a mild, often asymptomatic form of diabetes mellitus with onset after 40; pancreatic insulin reserve is diminished but is nearly always sufficient to prevent ketoacidosis, and dietary control is usually effective. **phosphate d.,** vitamin D–resistant rickets. **puncture d.,** a form produced by puncturing the floor of the fourth ventricle in the medulla oblongata. **renal d.,** see under *glycosuria.* **subclinical d.,** a state characterized by an abnormal glucose tolerance test result, but without clinical signs of diabetes.

diabetid (-bēt′id) a cutaneous manifestation of diabetes; diabetic dermopathy.

diabetogenic (-bet″ah-jen′ik) producing diabetes.

diabetogenous (-be-toj′ĭ-nus) caused by diabetes.

Diabinese (di-ab′ĭ-nēs) trademark for preparations of chlorpropamide.

diabrotic (di″ah-brot′ik) 1. ulcerative; caustic. 2. a corrosive or escharotic substance.

diaclasis (di″ak′lah-sis) osteoclasis.

diacrisis (di-ak′rĭ-sis) 1. diagnosis. 2. a disease marked by a morbid state of the secretions. 3. a critical discharge or excretion.

diadochokinesia (di″ah-do″ko-ki-ne′ze-ah) the function of arresting one motor impulse and substituting one that is diametrically opposite.

diagnose (di′ag-nōs) to identify or recognize a disease.

diagnosis (di″ag-no′sis) determination of the nature of a cause of a disease. **diagnos′tic,** adj. **clinical d.,** diagnosis based on signs, symptoms, and laboratory findings during life. **differential d.,** the determination of which one of several diseases may be producing the symptoms. **physical d.,** diagnosis based on information obtained by inspection, palpation, percussion, and auscultation. **serum d.,** serodiagnosis.

diagnostics (di″ag-nos′tiks) the science and practice of diagnosis of disease.

diagram (di′ah-gram) a graphic representation, in simplest form, of an object or concept, made up of lines and lacking pictorial elements. **vector d.,** a diagram representing the direction and magnitude of electromotive forces of the heart for one entire cycle, based on analysis of the scalar electrocardiogram.

diakinesis (di″ah-ki-ne′sis) the stage of first

meiotic prophase in which the nucleolus and nuclear envelope disappear and the spindle fibers form.

dialysance (-li'sins) the minute rate of net exchange of solute molecules passing through a membrane in dialysis.

dialysis (di-al'ĭ-sis) the process of separating crystalloids and colloids in solution by the difference in their rates of diffusion through a semipermeable membrane: crystalloids pass through readily, colloids very slowly or not at all. See also *hemodialysis.* **equilibrium d.,** a technique of determination of the association constant of hapten-antibody reactions. **lymph d.,** removal of urea and other elements from lymph collected from the thoracic duct, treated outside the body, and later reinfused. **peritoneal d.,** dialysis through the peritoneum, the dialyzing solution being introduced into and removed from the peritoneal cavity, as either a continuous or an intermittent procedure.

dialyzer (di'ah-līz''er) a hemodialyzer.

diameter (di-am'ĭt-er) the length of a straight line passing through the center of a circle and connecting opposite points on its circumference. **anteroposterior d.,** the distance between two points located on the anterior and posterior aspects, respectively, of the structure being measured, such as the true conjugate diameter of the pelvis or occipitofrontal diameter of the skull. **Baudelocque's d.,** external conjugate d. **conjugate d.,** see *pelvic d.* **cranial d's,** distances measured between certain landmarks of the skull, such as *biparietal,* that between the two parietal eminences; *bitemporal,* that between the two extremities of the coronal suture; *cervicobregmatic,* that between the center of the anterior fontanel and the junction of the neck with the floor of the mouth; *frontomental,* that between the forehead and chin; *occipitofrontal,* that between the external occipital protuberance and most prominent midpoint of the frontal bone; *occipitomental,* that between the external occipital protuberance and the most prominent midpoint of the chin; *suboccipitobregmatic,* that between the lowest posterior point of the occiput and the center of the anterior fontanel. **extracanthic d.,** the distance between the lateral points of junction of the upper and lower eyelids. **intercanthic d.,** the distance between the medial points of junction of the upper and lower eyelids. **pelvic d.,** any diameter of the pelvis, such as *diagonal conjugate,* joining the posterior surface of the pubis to the tip of the sacral promontory; *external conjugate* joining the depression under the last lumbar spine to the upper margin of the pubis; *true (internal) conjugate,* the anteroposterior diameter of the pelvic inlet, measured from the upper margin of the pubic symphysis to the sacrovertebral angle; *oblique,* joining the one sacroiliac articulation to the iliopubic eminence of the other side; *transverse* (of inlet), joining the two most widely separated points of the pelvic inlet; *transverse* (of outlet) joining the medial surfaces of the ischial tuberosities.

diamniotic (di''am-ne-ot'ik) having or developing within separate amniotic cavities, as diamniotic twins.

Diamox (di'ah-moks) trademark for preparations of acetazolamide.

diapause (di'ah-pawz) a state of inactivity and arrested development accompanied by greatly decreased metabolism, as in many eggs, insect pupae, and plant seeds; it is a mechanism for surviving adverse winter conditions.

diapedesis (di''ah-pĭ-de'sis) the outward passage of blood cells through intact vessel walls.

diaphemetric (-fĕ-mĕ'trik) pertaining to measurement of tactile sensibility.

diaphoresis (di''ah-for-e'sis) perspiration, especially profuse perspiration.

diaphoretic (-for-et'ik) 1. pertaining to, characterized by, or promoting diaphoresis. 2. an agent that promotes diaphoresis.

diaphragm (di'ah-fram) 1. the musculomembranous partition separating the abdominal and thoracic cavities and serving as a major inspiratory muscle. 2. any separating membrane or structure. 3. a disk with one or more openings or with an adjustable opening, mounted in relation to a lens or source of radiation, by which part of the light or radiation may be excluded from the area. 4. contraceptive d. **diaphragmat'ic,** adj. **Bucky d., Bucky-Potter d.,** a device used in radiography to prevent scattered radiation from reaching the film, thereby securing better contrast and definition. **contraceptive d.,** a device of molded rubber or other soft plastic material, fitted over the cervix uteri to prevent entrance of spermatozoa. **pelvic d.,** the portion of the floor of the pelvis formed by the coccygeus muscles and the levator muscles of the anus, and their fascia. **polyarcuate d.,** one showing abnormal scalloping of the margins on radiographic visualization. **urogenital d.,** the musculomembranous layer superficial to the pelvic diaphragm, extending between the ischiopubic rami and surrounding the urogenital ducts. **vaginal d.,** contraceptive d.

diaphragma (di''ah-frag'mah), pl. *diaphragmata* [Gr.] diaphragm (1).

diaphragmitis (-frag-mīt'is) inflammation of the diaphragm.

diaphysectomy (-fĭ-zek'tah-me) excision of part of a diaphysis.

diaphysis (di-af'ĭ-sis), pl. *diaph'yses* [Gr.] 1. the shaft of a long bone, between the epiphyses. 2. the portion of a long bone formed from a primary center of ossification.

diaphysitis (di''ah-fĭ-zīt'is) inflammation of a diaphysis.

diapophysis (di''ah-pof'ĭ-sis) an upper transverse process of a vertebra.

diapyesis (-pi-e'sis) suppuration. **diapyet'ic,** adj.

diarrhea (-re'ah) abnormally frequent evacuation of watery stools. **diarrhe'al, diarrhe'ic,** adj. **choleraic d.,** that with serous stools, accompanied by circulatory collapse, thus resembling cholera. **familial chloride d.,** severe watery diarrhea with an excess of chloride in the stool, beginning in early infancy, marked by distended abdomen, lethargy, and retarded growth and mental development, and accompanied by alkalosis and hypokalemia; maternal hydramnios is often associated. It is due to impairment of chloride-bicarbonate exchange in the lower bowel. **lienteric d.,** diarrhea marked by stools containing undigested food. **osmotic d.,** that due to the presence of osmotically active nonabsorbable solutes, e.g., magnesium sulfate, in the intestine. **parenteral d.,** diarrhea due to infections outside the gastrointestinal tract. **summer d.,** acute diarrhea in children during the intense heat of summer. **traveler's d.,** diarrhea among travelers, particularly in those visiting tropical or subtropical areas where sanitation is poor; it is currently considered to be due to infection with *Escherichia coli.* **tropical d.,** see under *sprue.*

diarthric (di-ar'thrik) pertaining to or affecting two different joints; biarticular.

diarthrosis (-thro'sis), pl. *diarthro'ses* [Gr.] a synovial joint.

diarticular (-tik'u-ler) diarthric.

diaschisis (di-as'ki-sis) loss of function and electrical activity due to cerebral lesions in areas remote from the lesion but neuronally connected to it.

diascope (di'ah-skōp) a glass or clear plastic plate pressed against the skin for observing changes produced in the underlying skin after the blood vessels are emptied and the skin is blanched.

diastase (di'ah-stās) a combination of enzymes produced during germination of seeds, and contained in malt; it converts starch into maltose and then into dextrose.

diastasis (di-as'tah-sis) 1. dislocation or separation of two normally attached bones between which there is no true joint. Also, separation beyond the normal between associated bones, as between the ribs. 2. diastasis cordis, the rest period of the cardiac cycle, occurring just before systole.

diastema (di"ah-ste'mah) a space or cleft.

diastematocrania (-stem"ah-to-kra'ne-ah) longitudinal congenital fissure of the cranium.

diastematomyelia (-mi-e'le-ah) abnormal congenital division of the spinal cord by a bony spicule or fibrous band protruding from a vertebra or two, each of the halves surrounded by a dural sac.

diastematopyelia (-pi-e'le-ah) congenital median fissure of the pelvis.

diastole (di-as'tah-le) the dilatation, or the period of dilatation, of the heart, especially of the ventricles. **diastol'ic,** adj.

diastrophic (di"ah-strah'fik) bent or curved; said of structures, such as bones, deformed in such manner.

diataxia (-tak'se-ah) ataxia affecting both sides of the body. **cerebral d., d. cerebra'lis infanti'lis,** infantile cerebral ataxic paralysis.

diathermy (-therm'e) the heating of body tissues due to their resistance to the passage of high-frequency electromagnetic radiation, electric current, or ultrasonic waves. In *medical d.* the tissues are warmed, in *surgical d.* tissue is destroyed. **short-wave d.,** diathermy with high-frequency current of wavelength less than 30 meters.

diathesis (di-ath'ĭ-sis) an unusual constitutional susceptibility or predisposition to a particular disease. **diathet'ic,** adj.

diatom (di'ah-tom) a unicellular microscopic form of alga having a cell wall of silica.

diatomaceous (di"ah-to-ma'shis) composed of diatoms; said of earth composed of the silicious skeletons of diatoms.

diatrizoate (-tri-zo'āt) any salt of diatrizoic acid; used in the form of its meglumine and sodium salts as a radiopaque contrast medium.

diazepam (di-az'ah-pam) a benzodiazepine tranquilizer, $C_{16}H_{13}ClN_2O$, used as a sedative, skeletal muscle relaxant, and anticonvulsant, to produce anesthesia, and in the management of alcohol withdrawal symptoms and delirium tremens.

diazo- (di-az'o) the group —N=N—.

diazotize (-tīz) to introduce the diazo group into a compound.

diazoxide (di"az-ok'sīd) an antihypertensive, C_8-$H_7ClN_2O_2S$, structurally related to chlorothiazide but having no diuretic properties; because it inhibits release of insulin, it is also used orally in hypoglycemia due to hyperinsulinism.

dibasic (di-ba'sik) containing two replaceable hydrogen atoms, or furnishing two hydrogen ions.

dibothriocephaliasis (di-both"re-o-sef"ah-li'-ah-sis) diphyllobothriasis.

Dibothriocephalus (-sef'ah-lus) *Diphyllobothrium.*

dibucaine (di'bu-kān) a local anesthetic, $C_{20}H_{29}$-N_3O_2, used topically and intraspinally in the form of the base and as the hydrochloride salt; the latter is also used intramuscularly for infiltration anesthesia.

dicentric (di-sen'trik) 1. pertaining to, developing from, or having two centers. 2. having two centromeres.

dichorial (di-ko're-il) dichorionic.

dichorionic (di-ko"re-on'ik) having two distinct chorions; said of dizygotic twins.

dichroism (di'kro-izm) the quality or condition of showing one color in reflected and another in transmitted light. **dichro'ic,** adj.

dichromasy (di-kro'mah-se) defective color vision in which one of the three cone pigments is missing. See *protanopia* and *deuteranopia.*

dichromate (di-kro'māt) a salt containing the bivalent Cr_2O_7 radical.

dichromatic (di"kro-mat'ik) pertaining to or characterized by dichromasy.

dichromatism (di-kro'mah-tizm) 1. the quality of existing in or exhibiting two different colors. 2. dichromasy.

dichromatopsia (di"kro-mah-top'se-ah) dichromasy.

dicloxacillin (di-kloks"ah-sil'in) a semisynthetic penicillinase-resistant penicillin, $C_{19}H_{16}$-Cl_2N_3S; used primarily in the treatment of infections due to penicillinase-producing staphylococci.

dicoelous (di-se′lus) 1. hollowed on each of two sides. 2. having two cavities.

Dicrocoelium (dik″ro-sēl′e-um) a genus of flukes, including *D. dentri′ticum*, which has been found in human biliary passages.

dicrotism (di′krot-izm) the occurrence of two sphygmographic waves or elevations to one beat of the pulse. **dicrot′ic,** adj.

Dictyocaulus (dik″te-o-kaw′lus) a genus of nematode parasites of the bronchial tree of horses, sheep, goats, cattle, and deer.

dictyotene (-o-tēn″) the protracted stage resembling suspended prophase in which the primary oocyte persists from late fetal life until discharged from the ovary at or after puberty.

dicumarol (di-koo′mah-rol) a coumarin anticoagulant, $C_{19}H_{12}O_6$, which acts by inhibiting the hepatic synthesis of vitamin K–dependent coagulation factors. It is the etiologic agent of the hemorrhagic disease in animals known as *sweet clover disease.*

dicyclomine (di-si′klo-mēn) an anticholinergic, $C_{19}H_{35}NO_2$, used as a gastrointestinal antispasmodic.

didelphia (di-del′fe-ah) the condition of having a double uterus.

didymalgia (did″ĭ-mal′je-ah) pain in a testis.

didymitis (-mīt′is) inflammation of a testis.

didymous (did′ĭ-mus) occurring in pairs.

didymus (did′ĭ-mus) a testis; also used as a word termination designating a fetus with duplication of parts or one consisting of conjoined symmetrical twins.

die (di) a form used in the construction of something, as a positive reproduction of the form of a prepared tooth in a suitable hard substance.

diecious (di-e′shus) sexually distinct; denoting species in which male and female genitals do not occur in the same individual. In botany, having staminate and pistillate flowers on separate plants.

dieldrin (di-el′drin) an insecticide, $C_{12}H_8Cl_6O$.

diencephalon (di″en-sef′ah-lon) 1. the posterior part of the forebrain, consisting of the hypothalamus, thalamus, metathalamus, and epithalamus; the subthalamus is often recognized as a distinct division. 2. the posterior of the two brain vesicles formed by specialization in embryonic development. See also *brain stem.*

dienestrol (di″en-es′trol) a synthetic estrogen, $C_{18}N_{18}O_2$, used mainly in the treatment of atrophic vaginitis and kraurosis vulvae.

Dientamoeba (di-ent″ah-me′bah) a genus of amebas commonly found in the colon and appendix of man, including *D. fra′gilis,* a species that has been associated with diarrhea.

dieresis (di-er′ah-sis) 1. the division or separation of parts normally united. 2. the surgical separation of parts.

diet (di′it) the customary amount and kind of food and drink taken by a person from day to day; more narrowly, a diet planned to meet specific requirements of the individual, including or excluding certain foods. **acid-ash d.,** one of meat, fish, eggs, and cereals with little fruit or vegetables and no cheese or milk. **alkali-ash d.,** one of fruit, vegetables, and milk with as little as possible of meat, fish, eggs and cereals. **balanced d.,** one containing foods which furnish all the nutritive factors in proper proportion for adequate nutrition. **bland d.,** one that is free of irritating or stimulating foods. **diabetic d.,** one prescribed in diabetes mellitus, usually limited in the amount of sugar or readily available carbohydrate. **elimination d.,** one for diagnosis of food allergy, based on sequential omission of foods that might cause the symptoms. **Feingold d.,** one that avoids all foods containing artificial color and flavoring and limits the intake of fruits and vegetables in which salicylates occur naturally (e.g., apples, apricots, blackberries, cucumbers, grapes, oranges, peaches, plums, raspberries, tea, and tomatoes). It is used in the control of hyperactivity in children. **gouty d.,** one for mitigation of gout, restricting nitrogenous, especially high-purine foods, and substituting dairy products, with prohibition of wines and liquors. **high caloric d.,** one furnishing more calories than needed to maintain weight, often more than 3500–4000 calories per day. **high fat d.,** ketogenic d. **high fiber d.,** one relatively high in dietary fibers, which decreases bowel transit time and relieves constipation. **high protein d.,** one containing large amounts of protein, consisting largely of meat, fish, milk, legumes, and nuts. **ketogenic d.,** one containing large amounts of fat, with minimal amounts of protein and carbohydrate. **low calorie d.,** one containing fewer calories than needed to maintain weight, e.g., less than 1200 calories per day for an adult. **low fat d.,** one containing limited amounts of fat. **low fiber d.,** low residue d. **low purine d.,** one for mitigation of gout, omitting meat, fowl, and fish and substituting milk, eggs, cheese, and vegetable protein. **low residue d.,** one giving the least possible fecal residue. **low salt d., low sodium d.,** one containing very little sodium chloride; often prescribed for hypertension and edematous states. **protein-sparing d.,** one consisting only of liquid proteins or liquid mixtures of proteins, vitamins, and minerals, and containing no more than 600 calories; designed to maintain a favorable nitrogen balance. **purine-free d.,** see *low purine d.* **salt-free d.,** low salt d. **Sippy d.,** one for peptic ulcer and conditions requiring a smooth diet, at first consisting of only milk and cream, with gradual addition of other foods, the amounts increasing until on day 28 the patient is placed on the regular ward diet.

dietetic (di″ah-tet′ik) pertaining to diet or proper food.

dietetics (-iks) the science of diet and nutrition.

diethylcarbamazine (di-eth″il-kar-bam′ah-zēn) an antifilarial agent, $C_{10}H_{21}N_3O$, used as the citrate salt.

diethylenetriaminepentaacetic acid (DTPA) (di-eth″il-ēn-tri-am″in-pen″tah-ah-sēt′ik) a chelating agent used in nuclear medicine in preparing radiopharmaceuticals, e.g., ^{99m}Tc-DTPA.

diethylpropion (-pro′pe-on) an adrenergic, C_{13}-

$H_{19}NO$, structurally related to amphetamine: used as an anorexic.

diethylstilbestrol (-stil-bes′trol) a synthetic nonsteroidal estrogen, $C_{18}H_{20}O_2$, used to relieve vasomotor symptoms associated with menopause in female hypogonadism, atrophic vaginitis, kraurosis vulvae, female castration, primary ovarian failure, palliative treatment of female breast carcinoma, and to relieve the symptoms of prostatic carcinoma.

diethyltoluamide (-tol-u′ah-mīd) an arthropod repellent, $C_{12}H_{17}NO$.

diethyltryptamine (DET) (-trip′tah-mēn) a synthetic hallucinogenic substance closely related to dimethyltryptamine.

dietitian (di″ah-tish′in) one skilled in the use of diet in health and disease.

dietotherapy (di″ah-to-ther′ah-pe) the regulation of diet in treating disease.

differentiation (dif″er-en″she-a′shin) 1. the distinguishing of one thing from another. 2. the act or process of acquiring completely individual characters, as occurs in progressive diversification of embryonic cells and tissues. 3. increase in morphological or chemical heterogeneity.

diffraction (dĭ-frak′shin) the bending or breaking up of a ray of light into its component parts.

diffusate (dĭ-fu′zāt) material that has diffused through a membrane.

diffuse 1. (dĭ-fūs′) not definitely limited or localized. 2. (dĭ-fūz′) to pass through or to spread widely through a tissue or substance.

diffusion (dĭ-fu′zhin) 1. the process of becoming diffused, or widely spread; the spontaneous movement of molecules or other particles in solution, owing to their random thermal motion, to reach a uniform concentration throughout the solvent, a process requiring no addition of energy to the system. 2. dialysis. **double d.,** an immunodiffusion test in which both antigen and antibody diffuse into a common area so that, if the antigen and antibody are interacting, they combine to form bands of precipitate. **gel d.,** a test in which antigen and antibody diffuse toward one another through a gel medium to form a precipitate.

diflorasone diacetate (di-flor′ah-sōn) a corticosteroid, $C_{26}H_{32}F_2O_7$, used topically in treatment of certain dermatoses.

digastric (di-gas′trik) 1. having two bellies. 2. digastric muscle.

digenetic (di″jah-net′ik) having two stages of multiplication, one sexual in the mature forms, the other asexual in the larval stages.

digestion (di-jes′chin) 1. the act or process of converting food into chemical substances that can be absorbed and assimilated. 2. the subjection of a substance to prolonged heat and moisture, so as to disintegrate and soften it. **diges′tive,** adj. **artificial d.,** digestion carried on outside the body. **gastric d.,** digestion by the action of gastric juice. **gastrointestinal d.,** the gastric and intestinal digestions together. **intestinal d.,** digestion by the action of intestinal juices. **pancreatic d.,** digestion by the action of pancreatic juice. **peptic d.,** gastric d. **primary d.,**

gastrointestinal d. **salivary d.,** the change of starch into maltose by the saliva.

digit (dij′it) a finger or toe. **dig′ital,** adj.

Digitalis (dij″ĭ-tal′is) a genus of herbs; *D. lana′ta,* a Balkan species, yields digoxin and lanatoside, and the leaves of *D. purpu′rea,* the purple foxglove, furnish digitalis.

digitalis (dij″ĭ-tal′is) the dried leaf of *Digitalis purpurea;* used as a cardiotonic agent.

digitalization (dij″it-al-i-za′shun) the administration of digitalis to produce and then maintain optimal therapeutic concentrations of its cardiotonic glycosides.

digitate (dij′ĭ-tāt) having digit-like branches.

digitation (dij″ĭ-ta′shin) 1. a finger-like process. 2. surgical creation of a functioning digit by making a cleft between two adjacent metacarpal bones, after amputation of some or all of the fingers.

digitigrade (-grād″) characterized by walking or running on the toes; applied to animals whose digits only touch the ground, the back part of the foot being raised, as horses and cattle.

digitonin (dij″ĭ-to′nin) a saponin, $C_{55}H_{90}O_{29}$, from *Digitalis purpurea;* used as a reagent to precipitate cholesterol.

digitoxin (dij″ĭ-tok′sin) a cardiotonic glycoside, $C_{41}H_{64}O_{13}$, from *Digitalis purpurea* and other *Digitalis* species; used in the treatment of congestive heart failure.

digitus (dij′it-us), pl. *di′giti* [L.] a digit.

diglyceride (di-glis′er-īd) a glyceride containing two fatty acid molecules in ester linkage.

digoxin (dĭ-gok′sin) a cardiotonic glycoside, C_{41}-$H_{64}O_{14}$, from the leaves of *Digitalis lanata;* used in the treatment of congestive heart failure.

dihydric (di-hi′drik) having two hydrogen atoms in each molecule.

dihydrocodeine (di-hi″dro-ko′dēn) a narcotic analgesic and antitussive, $C_{18}H_{23}NO_3$.

dihydroergotamine (-er-got′ah-mēn) an antiadrenergic, $C_{33}H_{37}N_5O_5$, produced by the catalytic hydrogenation of ergotamine; used as a vasoconstrictor in the treatment of migraine.

dihydrotachysterol (-tah-kis′ter-ol) a synthetic reduction product of tachysterol, $C_{28}H_{46}O$; used as an antihypocalcemic agent in the treatment of hypocalcemic tetany.

dihydrotestosterone (-tes-tos′ter-ōn) an androgen formed in peripheral tissue by the action of 5α-reductase on testosterone; thought to be the androgen responsible for external virilization during embryogenesis, for development of male secondary characteristics at puberty, and for adult male sexual function.

dihydroxyaluminum (di″hi-drok″se-ah-loo′-min-um) an aluminum compound having two hydroxyl groups in a molecule; available as d. *aminoacetate* and d. *sodium carbonate,* which are used as antacids.

dihydroxycholecalciferol (-ko″le-kal-sif′er-ol) a group of active metabolites of cholecalciferol (vitamin D_3). 1,25-Dihydroxycholecalciferol increases intestinal absorption of calcium and phosphate, enhances bone resorption, and prevents rickets, and, because of these activities at sites distant from the site of its synthesis, is considered to be a hormone.

diiodotyrosine (-ti′rah-sēn) an organic iodine-containing precursor of thyroxine, liberated from thyroglobulin by hydrolysis.

diktyoma (dik″te-o′mah) a tumor of the ciliary epithelium resembling embryonic retinal tissue in structure.

dilaceration (di-las″er-a′shin) a tearing apart, as of a cataract. In dentistry, an abnormal angulation or curve in the root or crown of a formed tooth.

Dilantin (di-lan′tin) trademark for phenytoin.

dilatation (dil″ah-ta′shun) 1. the condition, as of an orifice or tubular structure, of being dilated or stretched beyond normal dimensions. 2. the act of dilating or stretching. **d. of heart,** compensatory enlargement of the cavities of the heart, with thinning of its walls.

dilation (di-la′shun) 1. the act of dilating or stretching. 2. dilatation.

dilator (di-lāt′er) a structure (muscle) that dilates, or an instrument used to dilate.

diluent (dil′oo-int) 1. diluting. 2. an agent that dilutes or renders less potent or irritant.

dilution (di-loo′shin) 1. reduction of concentration of an active substance by admixture of a neutral agent. 2. a substance that has undergone dilution. **serial d.,** 1. the progressive dilution of a substance in a series of tubes in predetermined ratios. 2. a method of obtaining a pure bacterial culture by rapid transfer of an exceedingly small amount of material from one nutrient medium to a succeeding one of the same volume.

dimenhydrinate (di″men-hi′drĭ-nāt) an antihistaminic, $C_{17}H_{21}NO \cdot C_7H_7ClN_4O_2$, used as an antiemetic.

dimer (di′mer) 1. a compound formed by combination of two identical molecules. 2. a capsomer having two structural subunits.

dimercaprol (di″mer-kap′rol) a metal complexing agent, $C_3H_8OS_2$; used as an antidote to poisoning by arsenic, gold, mercury, and sometimes other metals.

Dimetane (di′mah-tān) trademark for preparations of brompheniramine.

Dimetapp (di′mah-tap) trademark for a fixed combination preparation of brompheniramine maleate, phenylephrine hydrochloride, and phenylpropanolamine hydrochloride.

dimethicone (di-meth′ĭ-kōn) 1. a silicone oil used as a skin protective; available as ointment, spray, and cream. 2. simethicone.

dimethindene (di″meth-in′dēn) an antihistaminic, $C_{20}H_{24}N_2$, used as the maleate salt.

dimethisoquin (di″mĕ-thi′so-kwin) a local anesthetic, $C_{17}H_{24}N_2O$; the hydrochloride salt is used topically to relieve pain, itching, and burning of the skin.

dimethyl- having two methyl groups in the molecule.

dimethyl sulfoxide (DMSO) (di-meth′il sulfok′sīd) DMSO; a powerful solvent, C_2H_6OS, which has the ability to penetrate plant and animal tissues and to preserve living cells during freezing; it has been proposed as a topical analgesic and anti-inflammatory agent and to increase penetrability of other substances.

dimethyltryptamine (DMT) (di-meth″il-trip′tah-mēn) a hallucinogenic substance, $C_{12}H_{16}$-N_2, derived from the plant *Prestonia amazonica.*

dimetria (di-me′tre-ah) a condition characterized by double uterus.

dimorphism (di-mor′fizm) the quality of existing in two distinct forms. **dimor′phic, dimor′phous,** adj. **sexual d.,** 1. physical or behavioral differences associated with sex. 2. having some properties of both sexes, as in the early embryo and in some hermaphrodites.

dinoflagellate (-flaj′il-āt) 1. of or pertaining to the order Dinoflagellida. 2. any individual of the order Dinoflagellida.

Dinoflagellida (di″no-flah-jel′ĭ-dah) an order of minute plantlike, chiefly marine protozoa, which are an important component of plankton. They may be present in sea water in such vast numbers that they cause a discoloration (red tide), which may result in the death of marine animals, including fish, by exhaustion of their oxygen supply. Some species secrete a powerful neurotoxin that can cause a severe toxic reaction in humans who ingest shellfish that feed on the toxin-producing organisms.

dinucleotide (di-nook′le-o-tīd″) one of the cleavage products into which a polynucleotide may be split, itself composed of two mononucleotides.

Dioctophyma (di-ok″to-fi′mah) a genus of nematodes, including *D. rena′le,* the kidney worm, found in dogs, cattle, horses, and other animals, and rarely in man; it is highly destructive to kidney tissue.

dioctyl calcium sulfosuccinate (di-ok′til kal′-se-um sul″fo-suk′sin-āt) docusate calcium.

dioctyl sodium sulfosuccinate (di-ok′til so′de-um sul″fo-suk′sin-āt) docusate sodium.

diolamine (di-ol′ah-mēn) USAN contraction for diethanolamine.

diopter (di-op′ter) a unit for refractive power of lenses, being the reciprocal of the focal length expressed in meters; symbol D. **prism d.,** a unit of prismatic deviation, being the deflection of 1 cm. at a distance of one meter; symbol Δ.

dioptometry (di-op-tom′ĭ-tre) the measurement of ocular accommodation and refraction.

dioptric (di-op′trik) pertaining to refraction or to transmitted and refracted light; refracting.

diovulatory (di-ov′u-lah-to″re) ordinarily discharging two ova in one ovarian cycle.

dioxide (di-ok′sīd) an oxide with two oxygen atoms.

dioxin (di-ok′sin) any of the heterocyclic hydrocarbons present as a trace contaminant in herbicides; thought to have oncogenic and teratogenic properties.

dioxybenzone (di-ok″sĭ-ben′zōn) a topical sunscreening agent, $C_{14}H_{12}O_4$.

dioxyline (di-ok′sĭ-lēn) a coronary and peripheral vasodilator, $C_{22}H_{25}NO_4$, used as the phosphate salt.

dipeptidase 178

dipeptidase (di-pep'tĭ-dās) an enzyme that catalyzes the hydrolysis of the peptide linkage in a dipeptide.

diperodon (di-per'ah-don) a surface anesthetic and analgesic, $C_{22}H_{27}N_3O_4$, used as the hydrochloride salt.

Dipetalonema (di-pet''ah-lo-ne'mah) a genus of nematode parasites (superfamily Filarioidea), including *D. per'stans* and *D. strepto'ca*, species primarily parasitic in man, other primates serving as reservoir hosts.

diphasic (di-fa'zik) having two phases.

diphemanil (di-fe'mah-nil) an anticholinergic, $C_{21}H_{27}NO_4S$, used to inhibit gastric secretion and motility, relieve pylorospasm, control sweating, and relieve pruritus.

diphenhydramine (di''fen-hi'drah-min) an antihistaminic, $C_{17}H_{21}NO$, used as the hydrochloride salt in the treatment of allergic symptoms and for its sedative, antiemetic, antitussive, local anesthetic, and anticholinergic effects.

diphenidol (di-fen'ĭ-dōl) an antiemetic, $C_{21}H_{27}$-NO.

diphenoxylate (-ok'sĭ-lāt) an antiperistaltic derived from meperidine, $C_{30}H_3N_2O_2$; the hydrochloride salt is used as an antidiarrheal.

diphenylpyraline (-pi'rah-lēn) an antihistaminic, $C_{18}H_{23}NO$, used as the hydrochloride salt.

diphtheria (dif-thēr'e-ah) an acute infectious disease caused by *Corynebacterium diphtheriae* and its toxin, affecting the membranes of the nose, throat, or larynx, and marked by formation of a gray-white pseudomembrane, with fever, pain, and, in the laryngeal form, aphonia and respiratory obstruction. The toxin may also cause myocarditis and neuritis. **diphthe'rial, diphther'ic, diphtherit'ic,** adj.

diphtheroid (dif'ther-oid) 1. resembling diphtheria or the diphtheria bacillus. 2. any member of *Corynebacterium* other than *C. diphtheriae*. 3. pseudodiphtheria.

diphyllobothriasis (di-fil''o-both-ri'ah-sis) infection with *Diphyllobothrium*.

Diphyllobothrium (-both're-um) a genus of large tapeworms, including *D. la'tum* (broad or fish tapeworm), found in the intestine of man, cats, dogs, and other fish-eating mammals; its first intermediate host is a crustacean and the second a fish, the infection in man being acquired by eating inadequately cooked fish.

diphyodont (dif'e-o-dont'') having two dentitions, a deciduous and a permanent.

diplacusis (dip''lah-koo'sis) the perception of a single auditory stimulus as two separate sounds. **binaural d.,** different perception by the two ears of a single auditory stimulus. **disharmonic d.,** binaural diplacusis in which a pure tone is heard differently in the two ears. **echo d.,** binaural diplacusis in which a sound of brief duration is heard at different times in the two ears. **monaural d.,** diplacusis in which a pure tone is heard in the same ear as a split tone of two frequencies.

diplegia (di-ple'je-ah) paralysis of like parts on either side of the body. **diple'gic,** adj.

diplobacillus (dip''lo-bah-sil'us) a short, rod-shaped organism occurring in pairs.

diploblastic (-blas'tik) having two germ layers.

diplocardia (-kar'de-ah) separation of the two halves of the heart.

Diplococcus (-kok'us) former name for a genus of bacteria (tribe Streptococceae), the species of which have been assigned to other genera. **D. pneumo'niae,** *Streptococcus pneumoniae.*

diplococcus (-kok'us), pl. *diplococ'ci*. 1. any of the spherical, lanceolate, or coffee-bean-shaped bacteria occurring usually in pairs as a result of incomplete separation after cell division in a single plane. 2. any organism of the genus *Diplococcus.*

diploë (dip'lo-e) the spongy layer between the inner and outer compact layers of the flat bones of the skull. **diploet'ic, diplo'ic,** adj.

diploid (dip'loid) 1. having two sets of chromosomes, as normally found in the somatic cells; in man, the diploid number is 46. 2. an individual or cell having two full sets of homologous chromosomes.

diplomyelia (dip''lo-mi-e'le-ah) lengthwise fissure and seeming doubleness of the spinal cord.

diplonema (-ne'mah) the double chromosomes in the diplotene stage.

diplopia (dĭ-plo'pe-ah) the perception of two images of a single object. **binocular d.,** double vision in which the images of an object are formed on noncorresponding points of the retinas. **crossed d.,** diplopia in which the image belonging to the right eye is displaced to the left of the image belonging to the left eye. **direct d.,** that in which the image belonging to the right eye appears to the right of the image belonging to the left eye. **heteronymous d.,** crossed d. **homonymous d.,** direct d. **horizontal d.,** that in which the images lie in the same horizontal plane, being either direct or crossed. **monocular d.,** perception by one eye of two images of a single object. **paradoxical d.,** crossed d. **torsional d.,** that in which the upper pole of the vertical axis of one image is inclined toward or away from that of the other. **vertical d.,** that in which one image appears above the other in the same vertical plane.

diplosome (dip'lo-sōm) the two centrioles of a mammalian cell.

diplotene (dip'lo-tēn) the stage of the first meiotic prophase, following the pachytene, in which the two chromosomes in each bivalent begin to repel one another and a split occurs between the chromosomes.

dipole (di'pōl) 1. a molecule having charges of equal and opposite sign. 2. a pair of electric charges or magnetic poles separated by a short distance.

dipsesis (dip-se'sis) excessive thirst. **dipset'ic,** adj.

dipsia (dip'se-ah) thirst; often used as a suffix to denote thirst or the physiological state leading to ingestion of fluids.

dipsogen (dip'sah-jen) an agent or measure that induces thirst and promotes ingestion of fluids. **dipsogen'ic,** adj.

dipsomania (-ma'ne-ah) alcoholism.

dipsosis (dip-so′sis) excessive thirst.

Diptera (dip′ter-ah) an order of insects, including flies, gnats, and mosquitoes.

dipterous (-us) 1. having two wings. 2. pertaining to insects of the order Diptera.

Dipylidium (dip″ĭ-lid′e-um) a genus of tapeworms. *D. cani′num,* the dog tapeworm, is parasitic in dogs and cats and is occasionally found in man.

dipyridamole (di″pi-rid′ah-mōl) a coronary vasodilator, $C_{24}H_{40}N_8O_4$.

director (dĭ-rek′ter) a grooved instrument for guiding a surgical instrument.

Dirofilaria (di″ro-fĭ-la′re-ah) a genus of filarial nematodes (superfamily Filarioidea), including *D. immit′is,* the heartworm, found in the right heart and veins of the dog, wolf, and fox.

dirofilariasis (-fil″ah-ri′ah-sis) infection with organisms of the genus *Dirofilaria.*

dis- word element [L.], *reversal* or *separation;* [Gr.], *duplication.*

disability (dis″ah-bil′it-e) 1. inability to function normally, physically or mentally; incapacity. 2. anything that causes disability. 3. as defined by the federal government: "inability to engage in any substantial gainful activity by reason of any medically determinable physical or mental impairment which can be expected to last or has lasted for a continuous period of not less than 12 months." **developmental d.,** a substantial handicap of indefinite duration, with onset before the age of 18 years, and attributable to mental retardation, autism, cerebral palsy, epilepsy, or other neuropathy.

disaccharidase (di-sak′ah-rĭ-dās″) an enzyme that catalyzes the hydrolysis of disaccharides.

disaccharide (di-sak′ah-rīd) any of a class of sugars yielding two monosaccharides on hydrolysis.

disarticulation (dis″ar-tik″ūl-a′shin) amputation or separation at a joint.

disc (disk) disk.

discharge (dis-charj′) 1. a setting free, or liberation. 2. matter or force set free. 3. an excretion or substance evacuated.

discission (dĭ-sish′in) incision, or cutting into, as of a soft cataract.

disclination (dis″klin-a′shin) extorsion.

discoblastula (dis″ko-blas′tūl-ah) the specialized blastula formed by cleavage of a fertilized telolecithal ovum, consisting of a cellular cap (blastoderm) separated by the blastocele from a floor of uncleaved yolk.

discogenic (-jen′ik) caused by derangement of an intervertebral disk.

discoid (dis′koid) 1. disk-shaped. 2. a disklike medicated tablet. 3. a dental instrument with a disklike or circular blade.

discopathy (dis-kop′ah-the) any disease of an intervertebral disk.

discoplacenta (dis″ko-plah-sen′tah) a discoid placenta.

discordance (dis-kord′ans) the occurrence of a given trait in only one member of a twin pair. **discor′dant,** adj.

discrete (dis-krēt′) made up of separated parts or

characterized by lesions which do not become blended.

discus (dis′kus), pl. *dis′ci* [L.] disk. **d. oo′phorus, d. ovi′gerus, d. proli′gerus,** cumulus oophorus.

discutient (dis-ku′shint) scattering, or causing a disappearance; a remedy that so acts.

disease (dĭ-zēz′) any deviation from or interruption of the normal structure or function of any body part, organ, or system that is manifested by a characteristic set of symptoms and signs and whose etiology, pathology, and prognosis may be known or unknown. **Adams' d., Adams-Stokes d.,** sudden attacks of unconsciousness, with or without convulsions, due to heart block. **Addison's d.,** bronzelike pigmentation of the skin, severe prostration, progressive anemia, low blood pressure, diarrhea, and digestive disturbance, due to adrenal hypofunction. **Albers-Schönberg d.,** osteopetrosis. **allogeneic d.,** graft-versus-host reaction occurring in immunosuppressed animals receiving injections of allogeneic lymphocytes. **Alper's d.,** poliodystrophy cerebri. **alpha-chain d.,** heavy chain disease characterized by a serum paraprotein composed of incomplete heavy chains without light chains of IgA. Free incomplete alpha chains appear in the serum and patients exhibit severe malabsorption syndrome with chronic diarrhea, steatorrhea, weight loss, hypocalcemia, and lymphadenopathy. **Alzheimer's d.,** progressive degenerative disease of the brain, of unknown cause, and characterized by diffuse atrophy throughout the cerebral cortex. **Andersen's d.,** amylopectinosis. **Apert-Crouzon d.,** acrocephalosyndactyly type I. **Aran-Duchenne d.,** spinal muscular atrophy. **Australian X d.,** an acute epidemic encephalitis of viral origin observed in Australia during the summer months between 1917 and 1926, resembling Japanese B encephalitis symptomatically and pathologically. **autoimmune d.,** any of a group of disorders in which tissue injury is associated with humoral or cell-mediated responses to the body's own constituents; they may be systemic or organ-specific. **Ayerza's d.,** a form of polycythemia vera marked by chronic cyanosis, chronic dyspnea, chronic bronchitis, bronchiectasis, hepatosplenomegaly, hyperplasia of bone marrow, and associated with sclerosis of the pulmonary artery. **Bang's d.,** infectious abortion in cattle. **Banti's d.,** congestive splenomegaly; originally, a primary disease of the spleen with splenomegaly and pancytopenia, now considered secondary to portal hypertension. **Barlow's d.,** scurvy in infants. **Barraquer's d.,** partial lipodystrophy. **Basedow's d.,** Graves' d. **Bayle's d.,** general paresis. **Bazin's d.,** erythema induratum. **Bechterew's d.,** rheumatoid spondylitis. **Behçet's d.,** see under *syndrome.* **Benson's d.,** asteroid hyalosis. **Berger's d.,** IgA glomerulonephritis. **Bernhardt's d.,** meralgia paresthetica. **Besnier-Boeck d.,** sarcoidosis. **Best's d.,** congenital macular degeneration. **Bielschowsky-Jansky d.,** late infantile form of amaurotic idiocy. **Biermer's d.,** pernicious anemia. **black d.,** a fatal disease of sheep, and sometimes of man, in the United States and Australia, due to *Clostridium novyi*, marked by necrotic areas in the liver. **Blocq's d.**, astasia-abasia. **Bloodgood's d.**, cystic d. of breast. **Blount's d.**, tibia vara. **Boeck's d.**, sarcoidosis. **Borna d.**, a fatal enzootic encephalitis of viral origin, affecting horses, cattle, and sheep. **Bornholm d.**, epidemic pleurodynia. **Bowen's d.**, intraepidermal squamous cell carcinoma, often occurring in multiple primary sites. **Breda's d.**, yaws. **Brill's d.**, a recrudescence of typhus occurring as long as 70 years after the initial acute episode of epidemic typhus; it is milder than the primary infection. **Brill-Symmers d.**, giant follicular lymphoma. **broad-beta d.**, hyperlipoproteinemia (type III); so called because on electrophoresis the lipoproteins show a broad band of beta lipoproteins. **Busse-Buschke d.**, cryptococcosis. **Caffey's d.**, infantile cortical hyperostosis. **caisson d.**, decompression sickness. **Calvé-Perthes d.**, osteochondrosis of capitular epiphysis of femur. **Camurati-Engelmann d.**, diaphyseal dysplasia. **Canavan's d.**, spongy degeneration of the central nervous system. **canine parvovirus d.**, an acute, often fatal gastroenteritis of dogs due to a parvovirus. **Carrión's d.**, an infectious disease in South America due to *Bartonella bacilliformis*, usually transmitted by the sandfly *Phlebotomus verrucarum*, appearing in an acute febrile anemic stage (*Oroya fever*) followed by a nodular skin eruption (*verruga peruana*). **cat-scratch d.**, see under *fever*. **Chagas' d.**, **Chagas-Cruz d.**, trypanosomiasis due to *Trypanosoma cruzi*; it runs an acute course in children and a chronic course in adults. **Charcot-Marie-Tooth d.**, progressive neuropathic (peroneal) muscular atrophy. **Christmas d.**, Factor IX deficiency; see *coagulation factors*, under *factor*. **chronic granulomatous d.**, chronic suppurative lymphadenitis, eczematoid dermatitis, hepatosplenomegaly, and chronic pulmonary disease associated with a genetically determined defect in the intracellular bactericidal function of leukocytes. **chronic obstructive pulmonary d. (COPD),** any disorder marked by persistent obstruction of bronchial air flow. **circling d.**, see *circling*. **Coats' d.**, chronic progressive retinopathy usually affecting boys; there is an exudative retinal detachment associated with telangiectatic blood vessels and multiple hemorrhages; it may lead to total retinal detachment, iritis, glaucoma, and cataract. **collagen d.**, any of a group of diseases characterized by widespread pathologic changes in connective tissue; they include lupus erythematosus, dermatomyositis, scleroderma, polyarteritis nodosa, thrombotic purpura, rheumatic fever, and rheumatoid arthritis. Cf. *collagen disorder*. **communicable d.**, a disease the causative agents of which may pass or be carried from one person to another directly or indirectly. **Concato's d.**, progressive malignant polyserositis with large effusions into the pericardium, pleura, and peritoneum. **constitutional d.**, one involving a system of organs or one with widespread symptoms. **Cori's d.**, Forbes' d. **Cowden's d.**, a heriditary disease marked by multiple ectodermal,

mesodermal, and endodermal nevoid and neoplastic anomalies. **Creutzfeldt-Jakob d.**, a usually fatal, transmissible spongiform viral encephalopathy, occurring in middle life. **Crigler-Najjar d.**, see under *syndrome*. **Crohn's d.**, a chronic granulomatous inflammatory disease commonly involving the terminal ileum with scarring and thickening of the bowel wall, often leading to intestinal obstruction and fistula and abscess formation. Called also *regional enteritis* or *regional ileitis*. **Crouzon's d.**, craniofacial dysostosis. **Cruveilhier's d.**, 1. simple ulcer of the stomach. 2. spinal muscular atrophy. **Cushing's d.**, Cushing's syndrome in which the hyperadrenocorticism is secondary to excessive pituitary secretion of adrenocorticotropic hormone. **cystic d. of breast**, a form of mammary dysplasia with formation of cysts of various sizes containing a semitransparent, turbid fluid that imparts a brown to blue color (blue dome cyst) to the unopened cysts. **cytomegalic inclusion d.**, an infection due to cytomegalovirus and marked by nuclear inclusion bodies in enlarged infected cells. In the congenital form, there is hepatosplenomegaly with cirrhosis, and microcephaly with mental or motor retardation. Acquired disease may cause a clinical state similar to infectious mononucleosis. When acquired by blood transfusion, postperfusion syndrome results. **deficiency d.**, a condition caused by dietary or metabolic deficiency, including all diseases due to an insufficient supply of essential nutrients. **degenerative joint d.**, osteoarthritis. **Dejerine's d.**, **Dejerine-Sottas d.**, progressive hypertrophic interstitial neuropathy. **demyelinating d.**, any condition characterized by destruction of myelin. **diverticular d.**, a general term including the prediverticular state, diverticulosis, and diverticulitis. **Duchenne's d.**, 1. spinal muscular atrophy. 2. progressive bulbar paralysis. 3. tabes dorsalis. **Duchenne-Aran d.**, spinal muscular atrophy. **Duhring's d.**, dermatitis herpetiformis. **Duke's d.**, a febrile disease of childhood marked by an exanthematous eruption, probably a mild form of scarlet fever. **Duplay's d.**, see under *bursitis*. **Durand-Nicolas-Favre d.**, lymphogranuloma venereum. **Duroziez's d.**, congenital mitral stenosis. **Ebstein's d.**, see under *anomaly*. **Economo's d.**, lethargic encephalitis. **epizootic d.**, one affecting a large number of animals in some particular region within a short period of time. **Erb's d.**, progressive muscular atrophy. **Erb-Goldflam d.**, myasthenia gravis. **Eulenburg's d.**, paramyotonia congenita. **extrapyramidal d.**, any of a group of clinical disorders marked by abnormal involuntary movements, alterations in muscle tone, and postural disturbances; they include parkinsonism, chorea, athetosis, etc. **Fabry's d.**, a sphingolipidosis transmitted as an X-linked recessive trait, in which trihexosyl ceramide is deposited in various tissues, especially the kidneys; the deficient enzyme is α-galactosidase A. **Fanconi's d.**, see under *syndrome*. **Farber's d.**, a hereditary sphingolipidosis, transmitted as an autosomal dominant trait, due to deficiency of the enzyme ceramidase. **Feer's d.**, acrodynia. **fibrocystic d. of pancreas,** cystic fibrosis.

fifth venereal d., lymphogranuloma venereum. flint d., chalicosis. focal d., a localized disease. foot-and-mouth d., an acute, contagious viral disease of wild and domestic cloven-footed animals, very rarely of man, marked by a vesicular eruption on the lips, buccal cavity, pharynx, legs, and feet, sometimes involving the udder or teats. Forbes' d., glycogenosis (type III) in which a deficiency of the debrancher enzyme dextrin-1,6-glucosidase affects the heart and liver, with hepatomegaly, hypoglycemia, acidosis, stunted growth, and doll facies. Fothergill's d., 1. scarlatina anginosa. 2. trigeminal neuralgia. fourth d., Duke's d. fourth venereal d., 1. gangrenous balanitis. 2. granuloma inguinale. Fox-Fordyce d., a persistent and recalcitrant, itchy, papular eruption, chiefly of the axillae and pubes, due to inflammation of apocrine sweat glands. Freiberg's d., osteochondrosis of the head of the second metatarsal bone. Friedländer's d., endarteritis obliterans. Friedreich's d., paramyoclonus multiplex. functional d., one involving functions without detectable tissue damage. Garré's d., sclerosing nonsuppurative osteomyelitis. Gaucher's d., a hereditary disorder of glucocerebroside metabolism, marked by the presence of Gaucher's cells in the marrow, and by hepatosplenomegaly and erosion of the cortices of long bones and pelvis. The adult form is associated with moderate anemia and thrombocytopenia, and yellowish pigmentation of the skin; in the infantile form there is, in addition, marked central nervous system impairment; in the juvenile form there are rapidly progressive systemic manifestations but moderate central nervous system involvement. genetic d., a general term for any disorder caused by a genetic mechanism, comprising chromosome aberrations (or anomalies), mendelian (or monogenic or single-gene) disorders, and multifactorial disorders. Gierke's d., glycogenosis (type I) in which deficiency of the hepatic enzyme glucose-6-phosphatase results in liver and kidney involvement, with hepatomegaly, hypoglycemia, hyperuricemia, and gout. Gilbert's d., a familial, benign elevation of bilirubin levels without evidence of liver damage or hematologic abnormalities. Gilles de la Tourette's d., see under syndrome. Glanzmann's d., see thrombasthenia. glycogen storage d., a group of genetically determined disorders of glycogen metabolism, marked by abnormal storage of glycogen in the body tissues. See Gierke's d. (type I), Pompe's disease (type II), Forbes' d. (type III), amylopectinosis (type IV), McArdle's d. (type V), Hers' d. (type VI), Tarui's d. (type VII). In type VIII, defective hepatic phosphorylase kinase causes hepatomegaly, but no other symptoms. graft-versus-host d., graft-versus-host reaction. Graves' d., an association of hyperthyroidism, goiter, and exophthalmos, with accelerated pulse rate, profuse sweating, nervous symptoms, psychic disturbances, emaciation, and elevated basal metabolism. Greenfield's d., infantile metachromatic leukodystrophy. Gull's d., atrophy of the thyroid gland with myxedema. Günther's d., congenital erythro-

poietic porphyria. H d., Hartnup d. Hailey-Hailey d., benign familial pemphigus. Hand's d., Hand-Schüller-Christian d. hand-foot-and-mouth d., a mild, highly infectious viral disease of children, with vesicular lesions in the mouth and on the hands and feet. Hand-Schüller-Christian d., chronic idiopathic histiocytosis, with multifocal histiocytic lipogranulomas of bone and of the skin and viscera; the histiocytes contain abundant cholesterol. Hansen's d., leprosy. Hartnup's d., a genetically determined disorder of intestinal and renal transport of neutral alpha-amino acids, marked by a pellagra-like skin rash, with transient cerebellar ataxia, constant renal aminoaciduria, and other biochemical abnormalities. Hashimoto's d., struma lymphomatosa. heavy-chain d., a condition marked by the presence of heavy-chain fragments of immunoglobulins in the serum. It occurs in three forms: IgG (γ-chain), IgA (α-chain), and IgM (μ-chain). Heine-Medin d., the major form of poliomyelitis. hemoglobin d., any of a group of hereditary molecular diseases, characterized by the presence of various abnormal hemoglobins in the red blood cells; the homozygous form is manifested by hemolytic anemia. hemolytic d. of newborn, erythroblastosis fetalis. hemorrhagic d. of newborn, a self-limited hemorrhagic disorder of the first few days of life, due to deficiency of vitamin K–dependent coagulation Factors II, VII, IX, and X. Hers' d., glycogenosis (type VI), in which a deficiency of liver phosphorylase affects the liver and leukocytes, with hepatomegaly, moderate hypoglycemia, mild acidosis, and growth retardation. Heubner-Herter d., nontropical sprue of children. hip-joint d., tuberculosis of the hip joint. Hippel's d., von Hippel's d. Hirschsprung's d., congenital megacolon. His' d., His-Werner d., trench fever. Hodgkin's d., a malignant condition marked clinically by painless, progressive enlargement of lymph nodes, spleen, and general lymphoid tissue; other symptoms may include anorexia, lassitude, weight loss, fever, pruritus, night sweats, and anemia. Reed-Sternberg cells are characteristically present. hoof-and-mouth d., foot-and-mouth d. hookworm d., infection with the hookworm Ancylostoma duodenale or Necator americanus, the larvae of which enter the body through the skin or are ingested with contaminated food or water, and migrate to the small intestine where, as adults, they attach to the intestinal mucosa and ingest blood; symptoms may include abdominal pain, diarrhea, colic or nausea, and anemia. In dogs, it is caused by Uncinaria stenocephala. Hutchinson-Gilford d., progeria. hyaline membrane d., a disorder of newborn infants, usually premature, characterized by the formation of a hyaline-like membrane lining the terminal respiratory passages. Extensive atelectasis is attributed to lack of surfactant. See respiratory distress syndrome of newborn. hydatid d., an infection, usually of the liver, due to larval forms of tapeworms of the genus Echinococcus, marked by development of expanding cysts. immune-complex d's, those caused by the formation of immune complexes in tissues or by the deposition of circulating immune complexes in tissues, resulting in acute or chronic inflammation. **immunodeficiency d.,** one caused by functional impairment of components of the immune system, including deficiency or malfunctioning of a cell population, lack of antibody response, or complement abnormality. **infectious d.,** one due to organisms ranging in size from viruses to parasitic worms; it may be contagious in origin, result from nosocomial organisms, or be due to endogenous microflora from the nose and throat, skin, or bowel. **inflammatory bowel d.,** any idiopathic inflammatory disease of the bowel. **intercurrent d.,** one occurring during the course of another disease with which it has no connection. **iron-storage d.,** hemochromatosis. **Johne's d.,** a usually fatal, chronic enteritis of cattle, but also affecting sheep, goats, and deer, caused by *Mycobacterium paratuberculosis.* **juvenile Paget's d.,** hyperphosphatasia. **Kahler's d.,** multiple myeloma. **Kashin-Beck d.,** a disabling degenerative disease of the peripheral joints and spine, endemic in eastern Siberia, northern China, and Korea; believed to be caused by ingestion of cereal grains infected with the fungus *Fusarium sporotrichiella.* **Katayama d.,** schistosomiasis japonica. **Kienböck's d.,** 1. slowly progressive osteochondrosis of the lunate bone; it may affect other wrist bones. 2. traumatic cavitation of the spinal cord. **kinky hair d.,** Menkes' syndrome. **Klippel's d.,** arthritic general pseudoparalysis. **Köhler's bone d.,** 1. osteochondrosis of the tarsal navicular bone in children. 2. thickening of the shaft of the second metatarsal bone and changes about its articular head, with pain in the second metatarsophalangeal joint on walking or standing. **Krabbe's d.,** a familial form of leukoencephalopathy beginning in infancy, in which ceramide galactoside accumulates in the tissues owing to deficiency of β-galactosidase. Pathologically, there is rapidly progressive cerebral demyelination and large globoid bodies (swollen with accumulated cerebroside) in the white substance. **Kufs' d.,** the late juvenile form of amaurotic idiocy. **Kugelberg-Welander d.,** a hereditary juvenile form of muscular atrophy, due to lesions of the anterior horns of the spinal cord, with onset principally between 2 and 17 years of age; it is marked by atrophy and weakness of the proximal muscles of the lower extremities and pelvic girdle, followed by involvement of the distal muscles and muscular twitchings. **Kümmell's d.,** compression fracture of vertebra, with symptoms occurring a few weeks after injury, including spinal pain, intercostal neuralgia, motor disturbances of the legs, and kyphosis which is painful on pressure and easily reduced by extension. **Kyasanur Forest d.,** a highly fatal viral disease of monkeys in the Kyasanur Forest of India, communicable to man, in whom it produces hemorrhagic symptoms. **Leber's d.,** see under *amaurosis* and *atrophy.* **legionnaires' d.,** an often fatal disease caused by a gram-negative bacillus (*Legionella pneumophila*), not spread by person-to-person contact, and characterized by high fever, gastrointestinal pain, headache, and

pneumonia; there may also be involvement of the kidneys, liver, and nervous system. **Leiner's d.,** erythroderma desquamativum. **Leriche's d.,** Sudeck's atrophy. **Letterer-Siwe d.,** a nonlipid reticuloendotheliosis of early childhood, marked by a hemorrhagic tendency, eczematoid skin eruption, hepatosplenomegaly with lymph node involvement, and progressive anemia. **Libman-Sacks d.,** atypical verrucous endocarditis. **Lignac-Fanconi d.,** Fanconi's syndrome (2). **Lindau's d., Lindau-von Hippel d.,** von Hippel-Lindau d. **Little's d.,** congenital spastic stiffness of the limbs, a form of cerebral spastic paralysis due to lack of development of the pyramidal tracts. **Lobstein's d.,** see *osteogenesis imperfecta.* **Lowe's d.,** oculocerebrorenal syndrome. **lumpy skin d.,** a highly infectious viral disease of cattle in Africa, which may result in permanent sterility or death, marked by the formation of nodules on the skin and sometimes on the mucous membranes. **Lutz-Splendore-Almeida d.,** paracoccidioidomycosis. **Lyme d.,** a recurrent multisystemic disorder caused by the spirochete *Borrelia burgdorferi,* the vector being the tick *Ixodes dammini,* and characterized by lesions of erythema chronicum migrans followed by arthritis of the large joints, myalgia, and neurologic and cardiac manifestations. **lysosomal storage d.,** any inborn error of metabolism characterized by (1) a defect in a lysosomal hydrolase, (2) intracellular accumulation of the unmetabolized substrate, (3) clinical progression affecting multiple tissues and organs, (4) considerable phenotypic variation within a disease. **McArdle's d.,** glycogenosis (type V) in which a deficiency of muscle phosphorylase affects the skeletal muscles, with muscle cramps and a depressed blood lactate level during exercise. **Madelung's d.,** 1. see under *deformity.* 2. see under *neck.* **maple syrup urine d. (MSUD),** a hereditary disease involving an enzyme defect in the metabolism of the branched chain amino acids, marked clinically by mental and physical retardation, feeding difficulties, and a characteristic odor of maple syrup or curry in the urine. **Marburg virus d.,** a severe, often fatal, viral hemorrhagic fever first reported in Marburg, Germany, among laboratory workers exposed to African green monkeys. **Marchiafava- Micheli d.,** paroxysmal nocturnal hemoglobinuria; see *intermittent hemoglobinuria.* **Marie's d.,** acromegaly. **Marie-Bamberger d.,** hypertrophic pulmonary osteoarthropathy. **Marie-Strümpell d.,** rheumatoid spondylitis. **Marie-Tooth d.,** progressive neuropathic (peroneal) muscular atrophy. **Mediterranean d.,** see β-*thalassemia.* **medullary cystic d.,** familial juvenile nephronophthisis. **Meniere's d.,** deafness, tinnitus, and dizziness, in association with nonsuppurative disease of the labyrinth. **mental d.,** see under *disorder.* **Merzbacher-Pelizaeus d.,** familial centrolobar sclerosis. **metabolic d.,** one caused by a disruption of a normal metabolic pathway because of a genetically determined enzyme defect. **Meyer's d.,** adenoid vegetations of the pharynx. **Mikulicz's d.,** benign, self-limited lymphocytic infiltration and enlargement of the lacrimal and salivary glands of uncertain etiology. **Milroy's d.,** hereditary permanent lymphedema of the legs due to lymphatic obstruction. **Minamata d.,** a severe neurologic disorder due to alkyl mercury poisoning, leading to severe permanent neurologic and mental disabilities or death; once prevalent among those who ate contaminated seafood from Minamata Bay, Japan. **mixed connective tissue d.,** a combination of scleroderma, myositis, systemic lupus erythematosus, and rheumatoid arthritis, and marked serologically by the presence of antibody against extractable nuclear antigen. **Möbius' d.,** periodic migraine with paralysis of the oculomotor muscles. **molecular d.,** any disease in which the pathogenesis can be traced to a single molecule, usually a protein, which is either abnormal in structure or present in reduced amounts. **Mondor's d.,** phlebitis affecting the large subcutaneous veins normally crossing the lateral chest wall and breast from the epigastric or hypochondriac region to the axilla. **Monge's d.,** chronic mountain sickness. **Morquio's d.,** see under *syndrome.* **Morquio-Ullrich d.,** Morquio's syndrome. **Morton's d.,** see under *toe.* **mosaic d's,** infectious viral diseases of plants, marked by mottling of the foliage. **motor neuron d.,** any disease of a motor neuron, including spinal muscular atrophy, progressive bulbar paralysis, amyotrophic lateral sclerosis, and lateral sclerosis. **Newcastle d.,** a viral disease of birds, including domestic fowl, characterized by respiratory and gastrointestinal or pneumonic and encephalitic symptoms; also transmissible to man. **Nicolas-Favre d.,** lymphogranuloma venereum. **Niemann's d., Niemann-Pick d.,** a hereditary disease with massive hepatosplenomegaly, brownish yellow discoloration of skin, nervous system involvement, and the presence in the liver, spleen, lungs, lymph nodes, and bone marrow of foamy reticular cells containing phospholipids. **Norrie's d.,** an X-linked disorder consisting of bilateral blindness from retinal malformation, mental retardation, and deafness. **notifiable d.,** one required to be reported to federal, state or local health officials when diagnosed, because of infectiousness, severity, or frequency of occurrence. **oasthouse urine d.,** methionine malabsorption syndrome. **occupational d.,** disease due to various factors involved in one's employment. **Oguchi's d.,** a form of hereditary night blindness occurring in Japan. **Oppenheim's d.,** amyotonia congenita. **organic d.,** one associated with demonstrable change in a bodily organ or tissue. **Osgood-Schlatter d.,** osteochondrosis of the tuberosity of the tibia. **Osler's d.,** 1. polycythemia vera. 2. hereditary hemorrhagic telangiectasia. **Owren's d.,** coagulation Factor V deficiency. **Paget's d.,** 1. (of bone) osteitis deformans. 2. (of breast) an inflammatory cancerous affection of the areola and nipple. 3. an extramammary counterpart of Paget's disease (2), usually involving the vulva, and sometimes other sites, as the perianal and axillary regions. **Parkinson's d.,** paralysis agitans. **parrot d.,** psittacosis. **Parrot's d.,** see under *pseudoparalysis.* **Parry's d.,** Graves' d. **pearl d.,** tuberculosis of the peri-

toneum and mesentery of cattle. **Pelizaeus-Merzbacher d.,** familial centrolobar sclerosis. **Pellegrini's d., Pellegrini- Stieda d.,** calcification of medial collateral ligament of knee due to trauma. **periodontal d.,** any disease or disorder of the periodontium. **Perthes' d.,** osteochondrosis of capitular femoral epiphysis. **Pfeiffer's d.,** infectious mononucleosis. **Pick's d.,** 1. lobar atrophy. 2. ascites and fibrotic liver disease associated with constrictive pericarditis. **polycystic d. of kidneys, polycystic renal d.,** a heritable disorder marked by cysts scattered throughout both kidneys, occurring in two forms: an *infantile* form, transmitted as an autosomal recessive trait, which may be congenital or appear at any time during childhood; and an *adult* form, transmitted as an autosomal dominant trait, marked by progressive deterioration of renal function. **polycystic ovary d.,** Stein-Leventhal syndrome. **Pompe's d.,** glycogenosis (type II) in which deficiency of the enzyme α-1,4-glucosidase results in generalized glycogen accumulation, with cardiomegaly, cardiorespiratory failure, and death; affected children appear imbecilic and are hypotonic. **Pott's d.,** tuberculosis of the spine, with osteitis or caries of the vertebrae, marked by stiffness of the spine, pain on motion, tenderness on pressure, and prominence of certain vertebral spines. **pulseless d.,** progressive obliteration of the brachiocephalic trunk and left subclavian and left common carotid arteries above their origin in the aortic arch, leading to loss of the pulse in both arms and carotids and to symptoms associated with ischemia of the brain, eyes, face, and arms. **Raynaud's d.,** a primary or idiopathic vascular disorder, most often affecting women, marked by bilateral attacks of Raynaud's phenomenon. **Recklinghausen's d.,** 1. neurofibromatosis. 2. (of bone) osteitis fibrosa cystica generalisata. **rheumatic heart d.,** the most important manifestation and sequel to rheumatic fever, consisting chiefly of valvular deformities. **rheumatoid d.,** a systemic condition best known by its articular involvement (rheumatoid arthritis) but emphasizing nonarticular changes, e.g., pulmonary interstitial fibrosis, pleural effusion, and lung nodules. **Ritter's d.,** dermatitis exfoliativa neonatorum. **Roger's d.,** a ventricular septal defect; the term is usually restricted to small, asymptomatic defects. **Rokitansky's d.,** acute yellow atrophy of the liver. **runt d.,** a graft-versus-host disease produced by immunologically competent cells in a foreign host that is unable to reject them, resulting in gross retardation of host development and in death. **Sandhoff's d.,** a type of GM_2 gangliosidosis resembling Tay-Sachs disease, seen in non-Jews, marked by a progressively more rapid course, and due to a defect in the enzymes hexosaminidase A and B. **Schamberg's d.,** progressive pigmentary dermatosis. **Schilder's d.,** a subacute or chronic leukoencephalopathy of children and adolescents, with massive destruction of the white substance of the cerebral hemispheres; clinical symptoms include blindness, deafness, bilateral spasticity, and mental deterioration. **Schönlein's d.,** see under *purpura.*

Schönlein-Henoch d., see under *purpura.*
secondary d., 1. a morbid condition occurring subsequent to or as a consequence of another disease. 2. one due to introduction of incompatible, immunologically competent cells into a host rendered incapable of rejecting them by heavy exposure to ionizing radiation. **self-limited d.,** one which by its very nature runs a limited and definite course. **serum d.,** see under *sickness.* **severe combined immunodeficiency d. (SCID),** a group of rare congenital disorders in which the functional capacities of both the humoral (B-lymphocyte) and cell-mediated (T-lymphocyte) components of the immune system are absent or severely depressed. **sexually transmitted d.,** any of a diverse group of infections caused by biologically dissimilar pathogens and transmitted by sexual contact; for some of these diseases, sexual contact is the only important mode of transmission, while for others transmission by nonsexual means is also possible. **sickle-cell d.,** any disease associated with the presence of hemogloblin S. **Simmonds' d.,** see *panhypopituitarism.* **sixth d.,** exanthema subitum. **sixth venereal d.,** lymphogranuloma venereum. **Smith-Strang d.,** methionine malabsorption syndrome. **Spielmeyer-Vogt d.,** the juvenile form of amaurotic idiocy. **Steinert's d.,** myotonic dystrophy. **stiff lamb d.,** stiffness and lameness of lambs, due to infection with *Erysipelothrix insidiosa.* **Still's d.,** juvenile rheumatoid arthritis. **Stokes-Adams d.,** Adams-Stokes d. **storage d.,** a metabolic disorder in which a specific substance (a lipid, a protein, etc.) accumulates in certain cells in unusually large amounts. **storage pool d.,** a blood coagulation disorder due to failure of the platelets to release ADP in response to aggregating agents (collagen, epinephrine, exogenous ADP, thrombin, etc.); characterized by mild bleeding episodes, prolonged bleeding time, and reduced aggregation response to collagen or thrombin. **Strümpell's d.,** 1. hereditary lateral sclerosis with the spasticity mainly limited to the legs. 2. polioencephalomyelitis. **Strümpell-Leichtenstern d.,** hemorrhagic encephalitis. **Strümpell-Marie d.,** rheumatoid spondylitis. **Sturge-Weber d.,** see under *syndrome.* **Stuttgart d.,** leptospirosis affecting dogs. **Sutton's d.,** 1. (*a*) halo nevus; (*b*) periadenitis mucosa necrotica recurrens. 2. granuloma fissuratum. **sweet clover d.,** a hemorrhagic disease of animals, especially cattle, caused by ingestion of spoiled sweet clover, which contains the anticoagulant dicumarol. **Swift's d.,** acrodynia. **Takayasu's d.,** pulseless d. **Tangier d.,** a familial disorder characterized by a deficiency of high-density lipoproteins in the blood serum, with storage of cholesterol esters in the tonsils and other tissues. **Tarui's d.,** glycogenosis (type VII) in which defective phosphofructokinase affects muscle and erythrocytes, with temporary weakness and cramping of skeletal muscle after exercise. **Tay-Sachs d. (TSD),** the most common GM_2 gangliosidosis, occurring almost exclusively among northeast European Jews, and specifically characterized by infantile onset (3–6 months), doll-like facies, cherry-red macular spot (90+ per cent of the infants), early blindness, hyperacusis, macrocephaly, seizures, and hypotonia; the children die between 2 and 5 years of age. **Teschen d.,** infectious porcine encephalomyelitis. **Thomsen's d.,** myotonia congenita. **thyrotoxic heart d.,** heart disease associated with hyperthyroidism, marked by atrial fibrillation, cardiac enlargement, and congestive heart failure. **trophoblastic d.,** any of a group of disorders that have their origin in the placenta, including hydatidiform mole, chorioadenoma destruens, and gestational choriocarcinoma. **tsutsugamushi d.,** scrub typhus. **tunnel d.,** decompression sickness. **vagabonds' d.,** discoloration of the skin in persons subjected to louse bites over long periods. **venereal d.,** a contagious disease usually acquired in sexual intercourse or other genital contact, including syphilis, gonorrhea, chancroid, granuloma inguinale, lymphogranuloma venereum, and balanitis gangrenosa. **veno-occlusive d. of liver,** acute or chronic, partial or complete occlusion of the branches of the hepatic veins by endophlebitis and thrombosis, leading to centrolobular necrosis, fibrosis, and ascites; most often seen in children. **Vogt-Spielmeyer d.,** the juvenile form of amaurotic idiocy. **Volkmann's d.,** congenital deformity of the foot due to tibiotarsal dislocation. **von Hippel-Lindau d.,** a hereditary condition marked by angiomatosis of the retina and cerebellum, which may be associated with similar lesions of the spinal cord and cysts of the viscera; neurologic symptoms, including seizures and mental retardation, may be present. **von Willebrand's d.,** a congenital hemorrhagic diathesis, inherited as an autosomal dominant trait, characterized by a prolonged bleeding time, deficiency of coagulation Factor VIII, and often impairment of adhesion of platelets on glass beads, associated with epistaxis and increased bleeding after trauma or surgery, menorrhagia, and postpartum bleeding. **Waldenström's d.,** osteochondrosis of the capitular femoral epiphysis. **Weber-Christian d.,** nodular nonsuppurative panniculitis. **Weil's d.,** leptospiral jaundice. **Werlhof's d.,** idiopathic thrombocytopenia purpura. **Wernicke's d.,** see under *encephalopathy.* **Westphal-Strümpell d.,** hepatolenticular degeneration. **Whipple's d.,** intestinal lipodystrophy, a malabsorption syndrome marked by diarrhea, steatorrhea, skin pigmentation, arthralgia and arthritis, lymphadenopathy, central nervous system lesions, and infiltration of the intestinal mucosa with macrophages containing PAS-positive material. **white muscle d.,** 1. muscular dystrophy in calves, due to vitamin E deficiency. 2. stiff lamb d. **Whitmore's d.,** melioidosis. **Wilson's d.,** hepatolenticular degeneration. **Wolman's d.,** a lysosomal storage disease due to acid lipase deficiency, occurring in infants, and associated with involvement and calcification of the adrenal glands, failure to thrive, vomiting, diarrhea, hepatomegaly, splenomegaly, foam cells in the bone marrow and other tissues, and early death. **woolsorter's d.,** inhalation anthrax. **x d.,** 1. hyperkeratosis (3). 2. aflatoxicosis.

disengagement (dis″in-gāj′mint) emergence of the fetus from the vaginal canal.

disequilibrium (-e-kwĭ-lib′re-um) unstable equilibrium. **linkage d.**, a genetic phenomenon in which certain phenotypic combinations are much more common than expected on the basis of gene frequencies of individual genes.

disgerminoma (dis-jerm″in-o′mah) dysgerminoma.

dish (dish) a shallow vessel of glass or other material for laboratory work. **evaporating d.**, a laboratory vessel, usually wide and shallow, in which material is evaporated by exposure to heat. **Petri d.**, a shallow glass dish for growing bacterial cultures.

disinfectant (-in-fek′tint) 1. freeing from infection. 2. an agent that disinfects, particularly one used on inanimate objects.

disinfestation (-in-fes-ta′shin) destruction of insects, rodents, or other animal forms present on the person or his clothes or in his surroundings, and which may transmit disease.

disintegrant (dis-in′tĭ-grint) an agent used in pharmaceutical preparation of tablets, which causes them to disintegrate and release their medicinal substances on contact with moisture.

Disipal (dis′ĭ-pal) trademark for a preparation of orphenadrine.

disjunction (dis-junk′shin) the act or state of being disjoined. In genetics, the moving apart of bivalent chromosomes at the first anaphase of meiosis. **craniofacial d.**, Le Fort III fracture.

disk (disk) a circular or rounded flat plate. **articular d.**, a pad of fibrocartilage or dense fibrous tissue present in some synovial joints. **Bowman's d's**, flat, disklike plates making up striated muscle fibers. **choked d.**, papilledema. **cupped d.**, a pathologically depressed optic disk. **embryonic d.**, a flattish area in a cleaved ovum in which the first traces of the embryo are seen. **gelatin d.**, a disk or lamina of gelatin variously medicated, used chiefly in eye diseases. **germ d., germinal d.**, embryonic d. **Hensen's d.**, H band. **intervertebral d's**, layers of fibrocartilage between the bodies of adjacent vertebrae. **intra-articular d's**, fibrous structures within the capsules of diarthrodial joints. **optic d.**, the intraocular part of the optic nerve formed by fibers converging from the retina and appearing as a pink to white disk. **Placido's d.**, a disk marked with concentric circles, used in examining the cornea. **slipped d.**, popular term for herniation of an intervertebral disk.

diskectomy (dis-kek′tah-me) excision of an intervertebral disk.

diskitis (dis-kīt′is) inflammation of a disk, especially of an intervertebral disk.

diskography (dis-kog′rah-fe) radiography of the vertebral column after injection of radiopaque material into an intervertebral disk.

dislocation (dis″lo-ka′shin) displacement of a part. **complete d.**, one completely separating the surfaces of a joint. **compound d.**, one in which the joint communicates with the air through a wound. **pathologic d.**, one due to paralysis, synovitis, infection, or other disease. **simple d.**, one in which there is no communication with the air through a wound. **subspinous d.**, dislocation of the head of the humerus into the space below the spine of the scapula.

dismemberment (dis-mem′ber-mint) amputation of a limb or a portion of it.

disocclude (dis″ah-klōōd′) to grind a tooth so that it does not touch its antagonist in the other jaw in any masticatory movements.

disorder (dis-or′der) a derangement or abnormality of function; a morbid physical or mental state. **adjustment d.**, maladaptive reaction to identifiable stress (divorce illness), which will, supposedly, remit when the stress ceases or when the patient adapts. **affective d's**, mood d's. **anxiety d's**, mental disorders in which anxiety and avoidance behavior predominate, i.e., panic disorder, agoraphobia, social phobia, simple phobia, obsessive compulsive disorder, post-traumatic stress disorder, and generalized anxiety disorder. **attention-deficit hyperactivity d.**, a controversial childhood mental disorder with onset before age seven, and characterized by restlessness, distractibility, inability to follow instructions, excessive talking, and other disruptive behavior. **autistic d.**, a pervasive developmental disorder with onset in infancy, differing from childhood schizophrenia in its early onset, lack of delusions or hallucinations or incoherence or loosening of associations or mental retardation in the presence of intelligent, responsive facies. **behavior d.**, conduct d. **bipolar d.**, 1. a mood disorder characterized by manic episodes and major depressive disorders. 2. bipolar disorder and cyclothymia. **body dysmorphic d.**, a somatoform disorder characterized by a normal-looking person's preoccupation with an imagined defect in appearance. **character d.**, a personality d. **collagen d.**, an inborn error of metabolism involving abnormal structure or metabolism of collagen, e.g., the Marfan syndrome, cutis laxa. Cf. *collagen disease*. **conduct d.**, mental disorders of childhood and adolescence marked by persistent violation of the rights of others and of age-appropriate societal norms or rules. **conversion d.**, a somatoform disorder characterized by conversion symptoms (loss or alteration of physical function suggesting physical illness) with no physiological basis; the psychological basis is suggested by exacerbation of symptoms during psychological stress, relief from tension (primary gain), or outside support or attention (secondary gains). **depersonalization d.**, a dissociative disorder not secondary to another mental disorder, e.g., agoraphobia, and characterized by feelings of detachment from one's body or thoughts. **depressive d's**, mental illnesses characterized by major depression without a manic episode or an unequivocal hypomanic episode. **dissociative d's**, hysterical neuroses characterized by sudden, temporary alterations in identity, memory, or consciousness, segregating normally integrated parts of one's personality from one's dominant identity, as in *multiple personality disorder, psychogenic fugue, psychogenic amnesia*, and *depersonalization disorder*. **factitious d.**, a mental disorder marked by repeated, knowing simulation of physical symptoms (Munchausen syndrome) or psychological ones (Ganser syndrome) solely to obtain treatment. **functional d.,** a disorder not associated with any clearly defined physical or structural change, i.e., having no organic basis. **generalized anxiety d.,** an anxiety disorder (q.v.) characterized by unrealistic or excessive worry about one's circumstances, e.g., one's finances or the safety of one's children. **identity d.,** severe subjective distress in late adolescence over inability to reconcile aspects of the self into a coherent whole, uncertainty over the future, one's career, ethics, and the like. **induced psychotic d.,** a delusional system developing in a second person with a close relationship with another person who has a psychotic disorder with prominent delusions. **intermittent explosive d.,** a functional mental disorder characterized by multiple discrete episodes of loss of control of aggressive impulses resulting in serious assault or destruction of property that are out of keeping with the individual's normal personality. **major mood d's,** bipolar disorder and major depression. **manic-depressive d.,** bipolar d. **mental d.,** a psychiatric illness with behavioral or psychologic manifestations, measured in terms of deviation from a norm. **mood d's,** those mental illnesses characterized by disturbances of mood as seen in full or partial manic or depressive syndromes, i.e., the *bipolar disorders, depressive disorders,* and the *organic mood syndrome.* **mendelian d.,** a genetic disease showing a mendelian pattern of inheritance, caused by a single mutation in the structure of DNA, which causes a single basic defect with pathologic consequences. **monogenic d.,** mendelian d. **multifactorial d.,** one caused by genetic and nongenetic environmental factors, e.g., diabetes mellitus. **multiple personality d.,** see *multiple personality,* under *personality.* **organic mental d's,** a particular organic brain syndrome of known or presumed etiology, such as Alzheimer's disease. **overanxious d.,** one of childhood or adolescence, marked by excessive worry or fear unrelated to a specific situation. **panic d.,** an anxiety disorder characterized by attacks of panic (anxiety), fear or terror, by feelings of unreality, or by fears of dying, or losing control together with somatic signs such as dyspnea, choking, palpitations, dizziness, vertigo, flushing or pallor, and sweating. **paranoid d's,** see *paranoia.* **personality d.,** see *personality* and specific personality disorders, under *personality,* and see *organic personality syndrome,* under *syndrome.* **pervasive developmental d's,** disorders in which there is impaired development of reciprocal social interaction, of verbal and nonverbal communication, and of imaginative activity, as in autistic disorder. **post-traumatic stress d.,** an anxiety disorder caused by an event beyond normal human experience, such as rape, combat, death camps, or natural disasters, and characterized by reexperiencing the trauma in recurrent intrusive flashbacks and nightmares, by "emotional anesthesia," hyperalertness and difficulty in sleeping, remembering, or concentrating, and by guilt about survival when others died or about things one had to do to survive. **psychoactive substance use d's,** mental disorders with maladaptive behavior from regular use of mood- or behavior-altering substances. See *psychoactive substance abuse,* under *abuse,* and *psychoactive substance dependence,* under *dependence.* **psychoactive substance–induced organic mental d's,** ten syndromes associated with psychoactive substances—*intoxication, withdrawal, delirium, dementia, amnestic disorder, delusional disorder, hallucinosis, mood disorder, perception disorder,* and *personality disorder.* **psychosomatic d.,** one in which the physical symptoms are caused or exacerbated by psychological factors, as in migraine headaches, lower back pain, gastric ulcer, or irritable bowel syndrome. **schizoaffective d.,** a diagnostic category for mental disorders with features of schizophrenia and mood disorders. **schizophreniform d.,** a mental disorder with the signs and symptoms of schizophrenia but of less than six months' duration. **separation anxiety d.,** distress in a child on being removed from his parents, home, or familiar surroundings. **sleep terror d.,** episodes of awakening early in the night with a panicky scream, autonomic symptoms, unresponsiveness to attempts to comfort, and amnesia of the event in the morning; quite common in children 3 to 5. **somatization d.,** classic hysteria (Briquet's syndrome); a somatoform disorder characterized by multiple somatic complaints vaguely or dramatically presented and not caused by physical illness; most patients are anxious and depressed and have interpersonal difficulties; many have histrionic (hysterical) personality traits. **somatoform d's** mental disorders characterized by symptoms suggesting physical disorders of psychogenic origin but not under voluntary control, e.g., body dysmorphic disorder, conversion disorder, hypochondriasis, somatization disorder, and somatoform pain disorder. **somatoform pain d.,** a somatoform disorder meeting the criteria of conversion disorder and characterized by a complaint of severe chronic pain inconsistent with neuroanatomy and pathophysiological mechanisms. **unipolar d's,** major depression and dysthymic disorder (depressive neurosis).

disorganization (-or″gin-iz-a′shin) the process of destruction of any organic tissue; any profound change in the tissues of an organ or structure which causes the loss of most or all of its proper characters.

disorientation (-o′re-en-ta′shin) the loss of proper bearings, or a state of mental confusion as to time, place, or identity. **spatial d.,** the inability of a pilot or other air crew member to determine spatial attitude in relation to the surface of the earth; it occurs in conditions of restricted vision, and results from vestibular illusions.

dispensary (-pen′ser-e) 1. a place for dispensation of free or low cost medical treatment. 2. any place where drugs and medicines are actually dispensed.

dispensatory (-pen′sah-tor″e) a book which describes medicines and their preparation and uses. **D. of the United States of America,** a collection of monographs on unofficial drugs and drugs recognized by the United States Pharmacopeia, the British Pharmacopoeia, and the National Formulary, also on general tests, processes, reagents, and solutions of the U.S.P. and N.F., as well as drugs used in veterinary medicine.

dispense (dis-pens′) to prepare medicines for and distribute them to their users.

disperse (-pers′) to scatter the component parts, as of a tumor or the fine particles in a colloid system; also, the particles so dispersed.

dispersion (-per′zhin) 1. the act of scattering or separating; the condition of being scattered. 2. the incorporation of one substance into another. 3. a colloid solution.

displacement (-plās′mint) removal to an abnormal location or position; in psychology, unconscious transference of an emotion from its original object onto a more acceptable substitute.

disproportion (dis″prah-por′shin) a lack of the proper relationship between two elements or factors. **cephalopelvic d.,** a condition in which the fetal head is too large for the mother's pelvis.

disruption (dis-rup′shin) the act of separating forcibly, or the state of being abnormally separated.

dissect (dĭ-sekt′, di-sekt′) to cut apart, or separate; especially, the exposure of structures of a cadaver for anatomical study.

dissection (dĭ-sek′shin) 1. the act of dissecting. 2. a part or whole of an organism prepared by dissecting. **blunt d.,** dissection accomplished by separating tissues along natural cleavage lines, without cutting. **sharp d.,** dissection accomplished by incising tissues with a sharp edge.

disseminated (dis-sem′in-āt″id) scattered; distributed over a considerable area.

dissociation (dĭ-so″se-a′shin) 1. the act of separating or the state of being separated. 2. an unconscious defense mechanism in which one or more groups of mental processes become separated from normal consciousness.

dissolution (dis″ah-loo′shin) 1. the process in which one substance is passed in another. 2. separation of a compound into its components by chemical action. 3. liquefaction. 4. death.

dissolve (dĭ-zolv′) 1. to cause a substance to pass into solution. 2. to pass into solution.

distad (dis′tad) in a distal direction.

distal (dis′t′l) remote; farther from any point of reference.

distalis (dis-ta′lis) [L.] distal.

distance (dis′tins) the measure of space intervening between two objects or two points of reference. **focal d.,** that from the focal point to the optical center of a lens or the surface of a concave mirror. **hearing d.,** the maximum distance at which sound-producing stimuli can be perceived by the ear. **interarch d.,** the vertical distance between the maxillary and mandibular arches under certain specified conditions of vertical dimension. **interocclusal d.,** the distance between the occluding surfaces of the maxillary and mandibular teeth with the man-

dible in physiologic rest position. **interocular d.,** the distance between the eyes, usually used in reference to the interpupillary distance. **working d.,** the distance between the front lens of a microscope and the object when the instrument is correctly focused.

distemper (dis-tem′per) a name for several infectious diseases of animals, especially *canine distemper,* a highly fatal viral disease of dogs, marked by fever, loss of appetite, and a discharge from the nose and eyes.

distichiasis (dis″tĭ-ki′ah-sis) the presence of a double row of eyelashes, one or both of which are turned in against the eyeball.

distillation (dis″til-a′shin) vaporization; the process of vaporizing and condensing a substance to purify the substance or to separate a volatile substance from less volatile substances. **destructive d., dry d.,** decomposition of a solid by heating in the absence of air, resulting in volatile liquid products. **fractional d.,** that attended by the successive separation of volatilizable substances in order of their respective volatility.

distobucco-occlusal (dis″to-buk″o-ŏ-kloo′z′l) pertaining to or formed by the distal, buccal, and occlusal surfaces of a tooth.

distobuccopulpal (-pul′p′l) pertaining to or formed by the distal, buccal, and pulpal walls of a tooth cavity.

distocclusion (-kloo′zhin) malrelation of the dental arches with the lower jaw in a distal or posterior position in relation to the upper.

distomiasis (-mi′ah-sis) infection due to trematodes or flukes.

distomolar (-mo′ler) a supernumerary molar; any tooth distal to a third molar.

distortion (dis-tor′shin) the state of being twisted out of normal shape or position; in psychiatry, the conversion of material offensive to the superego into acceptable form. **parataxic d.,** distortions in judgment and perception, particularly in interpersonal relations, based upon the need to perceive objects and relationships in accord with a pattern from earlier experience.

distraction (dis-trak′shin) 1. diversion of attention. 2. separation of joint surfaces without rupture of their binding ligaments and without displacement. 3. surgical separation of the two parts of a bone after the bone is transected.

distress (dis-tres′) anguish or suffering. **idiopathic respiratory d. of newborn,** see *respiratory distress syndrome of newborn.*

disturbance (dis-turb′ins) a departure or divergence from that which is considered normal. **emotional d.,** mental disorder. **sexual orientation d.,** direction of sexual interests toward persons of the same sex, affected persons being either disturbed by, in conflict with, or wishing to change their sexual orientation; to be distinguished from homosexuality and lesbianism.

disulfiram (di-sul′fĭ-ram) an antioxidant, $C_{10}H_{20}N_2S_4$, which inhibits the oxidation of the acetaldehyde metabolized from alcohol, resulting in high concentrations of acetaldehyde in the body. Used in the treatment of alcoholism because extremely uncomfortable symptoms occur when alcohol is drunk after the administration of disulfiram.

diuretic (di″ūr-et′ik) 1. increasing urine excretion or the amount of urine. 2. an agent that promotes urine secretion. **high-ceiling d., loop d.,** any diuretic that appears to exert its action on the sodium reabsorption mechanism of the ascending limb of the loop of Henle, resulting in excretion of urine isotonic with plasma. **osmotic d.,** a low-molecular-weight substance capable of remaining in high concentrations in the renal tubules, thereby contributing to the osmolality of the glomerular filtrate. **potassium-sparing d.,** one blocking the exchange of sodium for potassium and hydrogen ions in the distal tubule, increasing sodium and chloride excretion without increasing potassium excretion. **thiazide d.,** any of a group of synthetic compounds that effect diuresis by enhancing the excretion of sodium and chloride.

Diuril (di′ūr-il) trademark for preparations of chlorothiazide.

diurnal (di-ern′al) pertaining to or occurring during the daytime, or period of light.

divalent (di-va′lent) bivalent; carrying a valence of two.

divergence (di-verj′ins) a moving apart, or inclination away from a common point. **diver′gent,** adj.

diverticulectomy (di″ver-tik″ūl-ek′tah-me) excision of a diverticulum.

diverticulitis (di″ver-tik″ūl-īt′is) inflammation of a diverticulum.

diverticulosis (di″ver-tik″ūl-o′sis) the presence of diverticula in the absence of inflammation.

diverticulum (di″ver-tik″ūl-um), pl. *divertic′ula* [L.] a circumscribed pouch or sac occurring normally or created by herniation of the lining mucous membrane through a defect in the muscular coat of a tubular organ.

division (dĭ-vizh′in) the act of separating into parts. **cell d.,** fission of a cell. **direct cell d.,** see *amitosis.* **indirect cell d.,** see *meiosis* and *mitosis.* **maturation d.,** meiosis.

divulse (dĭ-vuls′) to pull apart forcibly.

divulsion (dĭ-vul′shin) the act of separating or pulling apart.

divulsor (dĭ-vul′ser) an instrument for dilating the urethra.

dizygotic (di″zi-got′ik) pertaining to or derived from two separate zygotes (fertilized ova).

dizziness (diz′e-nis) 1. a disturbed sense of relationship to space; a sensation of unsteadiness and a feeling of movement within the head; lightheadedness; dysequilibrium. 2. erroneous synonym for *vertigo.*

DL chemical prefix (small capitals) used with the D and L convention to indicate a racemic mixture of enantiomers.

DLE discoid lupus erythematosus.

D.M.D. Doctor of Dental Medicine.

D.M.R.D. Diploma in Medical Radio-Diagnosis (Brit.).

D.M.R.T. Diploma in Medical Radio-Therapy (Brit.).

DNA deoxyribonucleic acid. **recombinant DNA,** deoxyribonucleic acid that has been artificially introduced into a cell so that it alters the genotype and phenotype of the cell and is replicated along with the natural DNA.

DNase deoxyribonuclease.

D.O. Doctor of Osteopathy.

D.O.A. dead on admission (arrival).

doctor (dok′ter) a practitioner of medicine, as one graduated from a college of medicine, osteopathy, dentistry, chiropractic, optometry, podiatry or veterinary medicine, and licensed to practice.

docusate calcium (dok′u-sāt) an ionic surfactant, $C_{40}H_{74}CaO_{14}S_2$; used as a fecal softener.

docusate sodium (dok′u-sāt) an anionic surfactant, $C_{20}H_{37}NaO_7S$; used as a fecal softener.

dol (dōl) a unit of pain intensity.

dolich(o)- word element [Gr.], *long.*

dolichocephalic (dol″ĭ-ko-sĕ-fal′ik) long headed; having a cephalic index of 75.9 or less.

dolichopellic (-pel′ik) having a pelvic index of 95 or above.

Dolophine (do′lah-fēn) trademark for a preparation of methadone.

dolor (do′lor) [L.] pain; one of the cardinal signs of inflammation. **d. ca′pitis,** headache.

dolorific (do″lor-if′ik) producing pain.

dolorimeter (-im′it-er) an instrument for measuring pain in dols.

dolorogenic (dol-or″o-jen′ik) dolorific.

domain (do-mān′) in immunology, any of the homology regions of heavy or light polypeptide chains of immunoglobulins.

dominance (dom′in-ins) in genetics, the full phenotypic expression of a gene in both heterozygotes and homozygotes. **incomplete d.,** failure of one gene to be completely dominant, heterozygotes showing a phenotype intermediate between the two parents.

dominant (dom′in-int) 1. in genetics, capable of expression when carried by only one of a pair of homologous chromosomes. 2. a dominant allele or trait.

Donnatal (don′ah-tal) trademark for fixed combination preparations of phenobarbital, hyoscyamine sulfate, atropine sulfate, and hyoscine hydrobromide.

donor (do′ner) 1. an organism that supplies living tissue to be used in another body, as a person who furnishes blood for transfusion, or an organ for transplantation. 2. a substance or compound that contributes part of itself to another substance (acceptor). **general d.,** universal d. **hydrogen d.,** a substance or compound that gives up hydrogen to another substance. **universal d.,** a person with group O blood; such blood (blood cells preferred, rather than whole blood) is sometimes used in emergency transfusion.

dopa (do′pah) 3,4-dihydroxyphenylalanine, produced by oxidation of tyrosine by tyrosinase; it is the precursor of dopamine and an intermediate product in the biosynthesis of norepinephrine, epinephrine, and melanin. L-dopa, the naturally occurring form, and levodopa, the synthetic form, are used in parkinsonism and manganese poisoning.

dopamine (-mēn) a monoamine, $C_8H_{11}NO_2$, formed in the body by the decarboxylation of dopa; it is an intermediate product in the synthesis of norepinephrine, and acts as a neurotransmitter in the central nervous system. The hydrochloride salt is used to correct hemodynamic balance in the treatment of shock syndrome.

dopaminergic (-mēn-er′jik) activated or transmitted by dopamine; pertaining to tissues or organs affected by dopamine.

dopa-oxidase (-ok′sĭ-dās) an enzyme that oxidizes dopa to melanin in the skin, producing pigmentation.

dors(o)- word element [L.], *the back; the dorsal aspect.*

dorsad (dor′sad) toward the back.

dorsalis (dor-sa′lis) [L.] dorsal.

dorsiflexion (dor″sĭ-flek′shin) backward flexion or bending, as of the hand or foot.

dorsocephalad (dor″so-sef′ah-lad) toward the back of the head.

dorsoventral (-ven′tril) 1. pertaining to the back and belly surfaces of a body. 2. passing from the back to the belly surface.

dorsum (dor′sum), pl. *dor′sa* [L.] 1. the back; the posterior or superior surface of a body or body part, as of the foot or hand. 2. the aspect of an anatomical structure or part corresponding in position to the back; posterior in the human.

dosage (do′sij) the determination and regulation of the size, frequency, and number of doses.

dose (dōs) the quantity to be administered at one time, as a specified amount of medication or a given quantity of radiation. **absorbed d.,** that amount of energy from ionizing radiations absorbed per unit mass of matter, expressed in rads. **air d.,** the intensity of a roentgen-ray or gamma-ray beam in air, expressed in roentgens. **booster d.,** an amount of immunogen usually smaller than the original amount, given to maintain immunity. **curative d., median,** a dose that abolishes symptoms in 50% of test subjects; abbrev. C.D.$_{50}$. **divided d.,** a fraction of the total quantity of a drug prescribed to be given at intervals, usually during a 24-hour period. **effective d.,** that quantity of a drug that will produce the effects for which it is given. **effective d., median,** a dose that produces the desired effect in 50% of a population. **fatal d.,** lethal d. **infective d.,** that amount of pathogenic organisms that will cause infection in susceptible subjects. **infective d., median,** the amount of pathogenic microorganisms that will cause infection in 50% of the test subjects. **lethal d.,** that quantity of an agent that will or may be sufficient to cause death. **lethal d., median,** the quantity of an agent that will kill 50% of the test subjects; in radiology, the amount of radiation that will kill, within a specified period, 50% of individuals in a large group or population. **lethal d., minimum,** 1. the smallest amount of toxin that will kill an experimental animal. 2. the smallest quantity of diphtheria toxin that will kill a guinea pig of

250-gm. weight in 4 to 5 days when injected subcutaneously. **maximum d.,** the largest dose consistent with safety. **maximum permissible d.,** the largest amount of ionizing radiation that one may safely receive according to recommended limits in radiation protection guides. **minimum d.,** the smallest dose that will produce an appreciable effect. **permissible d.,** that amount of ionizing radiation which is not expected to lead to appreciable bodily injury. **threshold erythema d.,** the single skin dose that will produce in 80% of those tested a faint but definite erythema within 30 days, and in the other 20%, no visible reaction. Abbreviated T.E.D. **tolerance d.,** the largest quantity of an agent that may be administered without harm.

dosimetry (do-sim′ĭ-tre) scientific determination of amount, rate, and distribution of radiation emitted from a source of ionizing radiation.

dot (dot) a small spot or speck. **Gunn's d's,** white dots seen about the macula lutea on oblique illumination. **Maurer's d's,** irregular dots, staining red with Leishman's stain, seen in erythrocytes infected with *Plasmodium falciparum.* **Mittendorf's d.,** a congenital anomaly manifested as a small gray or white opacity just inferior and nasal to the posterior pole of the lens, representing the remains of the lenticular attachment of the hyaloid artery; it does not affect vision. **Trantas' d's,** small, white calcareous-looking dots in the limbus of the conjunctiva in vernal conjunctivitis.

double-blind (dub″l-blīnd′) denoting a study of the effects of a specific agent in which neither the administrator nor the recipient, at the time of administration, knows whether the active or an inert substance is given.

douche (dōōsh) [Fr.] a stream of water directed against a part of the body or into a cavity. **air d.,** a current of air blown into a cavity, particularly into the tympanum to open the eustachian tube.

douglasitis (dug″lah-sīt′is) inflammation of the rectouterine excavation (Douglas' cul-de-sac).

dowel (dow′l) a peg or pin for fastening an artificial crown or core to a natural tooth root, or affixing a die to a working model for construction of a crown, inlay, or partial denture.

doxapram (dok′sah-pram) a respiratory stimulant, $C_{24}H_{30}N_2O_2$, used as the hydrochloride salt.

doxepin (dok′sah-pin) a tricyclic compound, $C_{19}H_{21}NO$, having marked antianxiety and significant antidepressant activity; also used as an antipruritic in veterinary medicine.

doxorubicin (dok″so-roo′bĭ-sin) an antineoplastic antibiotic which binds to DNA and inhibits nucleic acid synthesis; used as the hydrochloride salt in the treatment of various leukemias, sarcomas, lymphomas, and neuroblastomas and of Wilms' tumor.

doxycycline (dok″se-si′klēn) a broad-spectrum antibiotic, $C_{22}H_{24}N_2O$, synthetically derived from oxytetracycline, active against a wide range of gram-positive and gram-negative organisms.

doxylamine (dok″sil-am′ēn) an antihistaminic, $C_{17}H_{22}N_2O$, used as the bisuccinate salt.

D.P. Doctor of Pharmacy; Doctor of Podiatry.

D.P.H. Diploma in Public Health.

DPT diphtheria-pertussis-tetanus; see under *vaccine.*

DR reaction of degeneration.

dr. dram.

drachm (dram) dram.

dracunculiasis, dracunculosis (drah-kung″-kūl-i′ah-sis; -o′sis) infection by nematodes of the genus *Dracunculus.*

Dracunculus (drah-kung′kūl-us) a genus of nematode parasites, including *D. medinen′sis* (guinea worm), a threadlike worm, 30–120 cm. long, widely distributed in India, Africa, and Arabia, inhabiting subcutaneous and intermuscular tissues of man and other animals.

draft (draft) potion or dose.

drain (drān) any device by which a channel or open area may be established for exit of fluids or purulent material from a cavity, wound, or infected area. **controlled d.,** a square of gauze, filled with gauze strips, pressed into a wound, the corners of the square and ends of the strips left protruding. **Mikulicz's d.,** a single layer of gauze, packed with several thick wicks of gauze, pushed into a wound cavity. **Penrose d.,** cigarette d. **stab wound d.,** one brought out through a small puncture wound at some distance from the operative incision, to prevent infection of the operation wound.

drainage (drān′ij) systematic withdrawal of fluids and discharges from a wound, sore, or cavity. **capillary d.,** that effected by strands of hair, catgut, spun glass, or other material of small caliber which acts by capillary attraction. **closed d.,** drainage of an empyema cavity carried out with protection against the entrance of outside air into the pleural cavity. **open d.,** drainage of an empyema cavity through an opening in the chest wall into which one or more rubber drainage tubes are inserted, the opening not being sealed against the entrance of outside air. **postural d.,** therapeutic drainage in bronchiectasis and lung abscess by placing the patient head downward so that the trachea will be inclined below the affected area. **through d.,** that effected by passing a perforated tube through the cavity, so that irrigation may be effected by injecting fluid into one aperture and letting it escape out of another. **tidal d.,** drainage of the urinary bladder by an apparatus which alternately fills the bladder to a predetermined pressure and empties it by a combination of siphonage and gravity flow.

dram (dram) a unit of measure in the avoirdupois (27.34 grains, $\frac{1}{16}$ ounce) or apothecaries' (60 grains, $\frac{1}{8}$ ounce) system. **fluid d.,** a unit of liquid measure of the apothecaries' system, containing 60 minims; equivalent to 3.697 ml.

Dramamine (dram′ah-mēn) trademark for preparations of dimenhydrinate.

drepanocytosis (drep″ah-no-si-to′sis) the presence of sickle cells in the blood.

dressing (dres′ing) any material used for covering and protecting a wound. **antiseptic d.,** gauze impregnated with antiseptic material. **occlusive d.,** one that seals a wound from contact with air or bacteria. **pressure d.,** one by which pressure is exerted on the covered area to prevent collection of fluids in underlying tissues.

drift (drift) a chance variation, as in gene frequency from one generation to another; the smaller the population, the greater are the random variations.

drip (drip) the slow, drop-by-drop infusion of a liquid. **Murphy d.,** the continuous drop by drop administration per rectum of saline solution. **postnasal d.,** drainage of excessive mucous or mucopurulent discharge from the postnasal region into the pharynx.

drocarbil (dro-kar′bil) a veterinary anthelmintic, $C_{16}H_{23}AsN_2O_7$.

dromograph (drom′ah-graf) a recording flowmeter for measuring blood flow.

dromostanolone propionate (dro″mo-stan′o-lōn) an androgenic, anabolic steroid, $C_{23}H_{36}O_3$; used as an antineoplastic agent in the palliative treatment of advanced metastatic, inoperable breast cancer in certain postmenopausal women.

dromotropic (-trop′ik) affecting conductivity of a nerve fiber.

drop (drop) 1. a minute sphere of liquid as it hangs or falls. 2. a descent or falling below the usual position.

droperidol (dro-per′ĭ-dol) a tranquilizer of the butyrophenone series, $C_{22}H_{22}FN_3O_2$, used as a narcoleptic preanesthetic, and, in combination with fentanyl citrate (known as *Innovar*), as a neuroleptanalgesic.

dropsy (drop′se) the abnormal accumulation of serous fluid in cellular tissues or in a body cavity.

Drosophila (dro-sof′il-ah) a genus of flies; the fruit flies. **D. melanogas′ter,** a small fly often seen around decaying fruit; used extensively in experimental genetics.

drowning (drown′ing) suffocation and death resulting from filling of the lungs with water or other substance.

Dr.P.H. Doctor of Public Health.

drug (drug) 1. any medicinal substance. 2. a narcotic. 3. to administer a drug to.

druggist (drug′ist) pharmacist.

drum (drum) 1. the middle ear. 2. the tympanic membrane.

drumhead (drum′hed) the tympanic membrane.

drumstick (-stik) a nuclear lobule attached by a slender strand to the nucleus of some polymorphonuclear leukocytes of normal females but not of normal males.

drusen (droo′zin) 1. hyaline excrescences in Bruch's membrane of the eye, usually due to aging. 2. rosettes of granules occurring in the lesions of actinomycosis.

duct (dukt) a passage with well-defined walls, especially a tubular structure for the passage of excretions or secretions. **duc′tal,** adj. **aberrant d.,** any duct that is not usually present or that takes an unusual course or direction. **alveolar**

d's, small passages connecting the respiratory bronchioles and alveolar sacs. **Bartholin's d.,** the larger of the sublingual ducts, which opens into the submandibular duct. **Bellini's d's,** the excretory or collecting portions of the renal tubules. **bile d's, biliary d's,** the passages for the conveyance of bile in and from the liver. **branchial d's,** the drawn-out branchial grooves which open into the temporary cervical sinus of the embryo. **cochlear d.,** a spiral tube in the bony canal of the cochlea, divided into the scala tympani and scala vestibuli by the lamina spiralis. **common bile d.,** the duct formed by the union of the cystic and hepatic ducts. **d's of Cuvier,** two short venous trunks in the fetus opening into the atrium of the heart; the right one becomes the superior vena cava. **cystic d.,** the passage connecting the gallbladder neck and the common bile duct. **deferent d.,** ductus deferens. **efferent d.,** any duct which gives outlet to a glandular secretion. **ejaculatory d.,** the duct formed by union of the ductus deferens and the duct of the seminal vesicle, opening into the prostatic urethra on the colliculus seminalis. **endolymphatic d.,** a canal connecting the membranous labyrinth of the ear with the endolymphatic sac. **excretory d.,** one that is merely conductive and not secretory. **Gartner's d.,** a closed rudimentary duct lying parallel to the uterine tube, into which transverse ducts of the epoophoron open; it is the remains of the part of the mesonephros that participates in formation of the reproductive organs. **genital d.,** see under *canal.* **hepatic d.,** the excretory duct of the liver, or one of its branches in the lobes of the liver. **interlobular d's,** channels between different lobules of a gland. **lacrimal d.,** see under *canaliculus.* **lactiferous d's,** ducts conveying the milk secreted by the mammary lobes to and through the nipples. **Luschka's d's,** tubular structures in the wall of the gallbladder; some are connected with bile ducts, but none with the lumen of the gallbladder. **lymphatic d's,** channels for conducting lymph. **lymphatic d., left, thoracic d. lymphatic d., right,** a vessel draining lymph from the upper right side of the body, receiving lymph from the right subclavian, jugular, and mediastinal trunks when those vessels do not open independently into the right brachiocephalic vein. **mesonephric d.,** an embryonic duct of the mesonephros, which in the male develops into the epididymis, ductus deferens and its ampulla, seminal vesicles, and ejaculatory duct and in the female is largely obliterated. **d. of Müller, müllerian d.,** paramesonephric d. **nasolacrimal d.,** the canal conveying the tears from the lacrimal sac to the inferior meatus of the nose. **omphalomesenteric d.,** yolk stalk. **pancreatic d.,** the main excretory duct of the pancreas, which usually unites with the common bile duct before entering the duodenum. **papillary d's,** the straight excretory or collecting portions of the renal tubules, which descend through the renal medulla to a renal papilla. **paramesonephric d.,** either of the paired embryonic ducts developing into the uterine tubes, uterus, and vagina in the female and becoming largely obliterated in the male.

parotid d., the duct by which the parotid gland empties into the mouth. **perilymphatic d.,** a small canal connecting the scala tympani of the cochlea with the subarachnoid space. **pronephric d.,** the duct of the pronephros, which later serves as the mesonephric duct. **prostatic d's,** ducts from the prostate, opening into or near the prostatic sinuses on the posterior urethra. **d's of Rivinus,** the small sublingual ducts which open into the mouth on the sublingual fold. **Santorini's d.,** a small inconstant duct draining a part of the head of the pancreas into the minor duodenal papilla. **secretory d.,** a smaller duct that is tributary to an excretory duct of a gland and that also has a secretory function. **semicircular d's,** the long ducts of the membranous labyrinth of the ear. **seminal d's,** the passages for conveyance of spermatozoa and semen. **d. of Steno, d. of Stensen,** parotid d. **submandibular d., submaxillary d.,** the duct that drains the submandibular gland and opens at the sublingual caruncle. **tear d.,** lacrimal canaliculus. **thoracic d.,** the canal that ascends from the cisterna chyli to the junction of the left subclavian and left internal jugular vein. **thyroglossal d.,** an embryonic duct extending between the thyroid primordium and the posterior tongue. **urogenital d's,** the paramesonephric and mesonephric ducts. **Wharton's d.,** submandibular d. **d. of Wirsung,** pancreatic d. **wolffian d.,** mesonephric d.

ductile (duk'til) susceptible of being drawn out without breaking.

duction (duk'shin) in ophthalmology, the rotation of an eye by the extraocular muscles around its horizontal, vertical, or anteroposterior axis.

ductule (duk'tūl) a minute duct.

ductulus (duk'tu-lus), pl. *duc'tuli* [L.] ductule.

ductus (duk'tus), pl. *duc'tus* [L.] duct. **d. arterio'sus,** fetal blood vessel which joins the aorta and pulmonary artery. **d. arterio'sus, patent,** abnormal persistence of an open lumen in the ductus arteriosus after birth. **d. choledo'chus,** common bile duct. **d. de'ferens,** the excretory duct of the testis which joins the excretory duct of the seminal vesicle to form the ejaculatory duct. **d. veno'sus,** a major blood channel that develops through the embryonic liver from the left umbilical vein to the inferior vena cava.

dull (dul) not resonant on percussion.

dumb (dum) unable to speak; mute.

dumping (dump'ing) see under *syndrome.*

duodenal (doo″o-de'nil) of or pertaining to the duodenum.

duodenectomy (doo″o-dĕ-nek'tah-me) excision of the duodenum, total or partial.

duodenitis (doo″o-dĕ-nīt'is) inflammation of the duodenal mucosa.

duodenocholedochotomy (doo″o-de″no-ko-led″o-kot'ah-me) incision of the duodenum and common bile duct.

duodenoenterostomy (-en″ter-os'tah-me) anastomosis of the duodenum to some other part of the small intestine.

duodenogram (doo-od″in-ah-gram) a roentgenogram of the duodenum.

duodenohepatic (doo-od″in-o-hĕ-pat′ik) pertaining to the duodenum and liver.

duodenojejunostomy (-jĕ″joo-nos′tah-me) anastomosis of the duodenum to the jejunum.

duodenoscope (doo″o-de′no-skōp) an endoscope for examining the duodenum.

duodenostomy (-nos′tah-me) surgical formation of a permanent opening into the duodenum.

duodenum (doo″o-de′num) the first or proximal portion of the small intestine, extending from the pylorus to the jejunum.

duplication (doo-pli-ka′shin) in genetics, the presence in the genome of additional genetic material (a chromosome or segment thereof, a gene or part thereof).

dupp (dup) a syllable used to represent the second heart sound in auscultation.

dural (dūr′′l) pertaining to the dura mater.

dura mater (dūr′ah māt′er) the outermost, toughest of the three meninges (membranes) of the brain and spinal cord.

duroarachnitis (dūr″o-ar″ak-nīt′is) inflammation of the dura mater and arachnoid.

D.V.M. Doctor of Veterinary Medicine.

dwarf (dwarf) an abnormally undersized person. **achondroplastic d.,** a dwarf having a relatively large head with saddle nose and brachycephaly, short extremities, and usually lordosis. **Amsterdam d.,** a dwarf affected with de Lange's syndrome. **ateliotic d.,** a dwarf with infantile skeleton, with persistent nonunion between epiphyses and diaphyses. **pituitary d.,** a dwarf whose condition is due to hypofunction of the anterior pituitary. **rachitic d.,** a person dwarfed by rickets, having a high forehead with prominent bosses, bent long bones, and Harrison's groove. **renal d.,** a dwarf whose failure to achieve normal bone maturation is due to renal failure.

Dy chemical symbol, *dysprosium.*

dyad (di′ad) a double chromosome resulting from the halving of a tetrad.

Dyazide (di′ah-zīd) trademark for a fixed combination preparation of triamterene and hydrochlorothiazide.

dyclonine (di′klo-nēn) a bactericidal and fungicidal local anesthetic, $C_{18}H_{27}NO_2$; used topically as the hydrochloride salt.

dydrogesterone (di″dro-jes′ter-ōn) an orally effective, synthetic progestin, $C_{21}H_{28}O_2$; used mainly in the diagnosis and treatment of primary amenorrhea and severe dysmenorrhea, and in combination with estrogen in dysfunctional menorrhagia.

dye (di) any colored substance containing auxochromes and thus capable of coloring substances to which it is applied; used for staining and coloring, as a test reagent, and as a therapeutic agent. **acid d., acidic d.,** one which is acidic in reaction and usually unites with positively charged ions of the material acted upon. **amphoteric d.,** one containing both reactive basic and reactive acidic groups, and staining both acidic and basic elements. **anionic d.,** acid d. **basic d.,** one which is basic in reaction and unites with negatively charged ions of the material acted upon. **cationic d.,** basic d.

dynamics (di-nam′iks) the scientific study of forces in action; a phase of mechanics.

dynamometer (di″nah-mom′it-er) an instrument for measuring the force of muscular contraction.

dyne (dīn) the metric unit of force, being that amount which would, during each second, produce an acceleration of 1 cm. per second in a particle of 1 gram mass.

dynein (di′ne-in) an ATP-splitting enzyme essential to the motility of cilia and flagella.

dyphilline (di-fil′in) a theophylline derivative, $C_{10}H_{14}N_4O_4$; used chiefly in the treatment of acute bronchial asthma and reversible bronchospasm associated with chronic bronchitis and emphysema.

dys- prefix [Gr.], *bad; difficult; disordered.*

dysacusis (dis″ah-koo′sis) 1. a hearing impairment in which the loss is not measurable in decibels, but in disturbances in discrimination of speech or tone quality, pitch, or loudness, etc. 2. a condition in which sounds produce discomfort.

dysaphia (dis-a′fe-ah) impairment of the sense of touch.

dysarteriotony (dis″ar-tēr″e-ot′ah-ne) abnormality of blood pressure.

dysarthria (dis-ar′thre-ah) imperfect articulation of speech due to disturbances of muscular control resulting from central or peripheral nervous system damage.

dysarthrosis (dis″ar-thro′sis) 1. deformity or malformation of a joint. 2. dysarthria.

dysautonomia (-awt-o-no′me-ah) a hereditary condition marked by defective lacrimation, skin blotching, emotional instability, motor incoordination, total absence of pain sensation, and hyporeflexia.

dysbarism (dis′bar-izm) any clinical syndrome due to difference between the surrounding atmospheric pressure and the total gas pressure in the tissues, fluids, and cavities of the body.

dysbasia (dis-ba′ze-ah) difficulty in walking, especially that due to nervous lesion.

dysbetalipoproteinemia (dis-ba″tah-lip″o-pro″te-in-e′me-ah) the accumulation of abnormal β-lipoproteins in the blood. **familial d.,** familial hyperlipoproteinemia, type III.

dyscephaly (-sef′ah-le) malformation of the cranium and bones of the face. **dyscephal′ic,** adj.

dyschezia (-ke′ze-ah) difficult or painful defecation.

dyschiria (-ki′re-ah) loss of power to tell which side of the body has been touched.

dyschondroplasia (dis″kon-dro-pla′ze-ah) enchondromatosis.

dyschromatopsia (-kro-mah-top′se-ah) disorder of color vision.

dyschromia (dis-kro′me-ah) any disorder of pigmentation of skin or hair.

dyscoria (-kor′e-ah) abnormality in the form or shape of the pupil or in the reaction of the two pupils.

dysembryoma (dis″em-bre-o′mah) teratoma.

dysencephalia splanchnocystica (dis-en″se-fa′le-ah splank″no-sis′tĭ-kah) Meckel's syndrome.

dysentery (dis′in-tĕ″re) any of a number of disorders marked by inflammation of the intestine, especially of the colon, with abdominal pain, tenesmus, and frequent stools containing blood and mucus. **dysenter′ic,** adj. **amebic d.,** amebic colitis. **bacillary d.,** dysentery caused by *Shigella.* **viral d.,** dysentery caused by a virus, occurring in epidemics and marked by acute watery diarrhea.

dysergia (dis-er′je-ah) motor incoordination due to defect of efferent nerve impulse.

dysesthesia (dis″es-the′ze-ah) 1. impairment of any sense, especially of the sense of touch. 2. an unpleasant abnormal sensation produced by normal stimuli. **auditory d.,** dysacusis (2).

dysfunction (dis-funk′shun) disturbance, impairment, or abnormality of functioning of an organ. **minimal brain d.,** attention-deficit hyperactivity disorder.

dysgammaglobulinemia (-gam″ah-glob″ūl-in-e′me-ah) an immunological deficiency state marked by selective deficiencies of one or more, but not all, classes of immunoglobulins. **dysgammaglobuline′mic,** adj.

dysgenesis (-jen′ĭ-sis) defective development; malformation. **gonadal d.,** Turner syndrome and its variants.

dysgerminoma (-jerm″in-o′mah) a malignant ovarian neoplasm, thought to be derived from primordial germ cells of the sexually undifferentiated embryonic gonad; it is the counterpart of the classical testicular seminoma.

dysgeusia (-gu′ze-ah) impairment of the sense of taste.

dysgnathia (dis-na′the-ah) any oral abnormality extending beyond the teeth to involve the maxilla or mandible, or both. **dysgnath′ic,** adj.

dysgraphia (-gra′fe-ah) inability to write properly; it may be part of a language disorder due to disturbance of the parietal lobe or of the motor system.

dyshematopoiesis (-hem″ah-to-poi-e′sis) defective blood formation. **dyshematopoiet′ic,** adj.

dyshesion (-he′zhin) 1. disordered cell adherence. 2. loss of intercellular cohesion; a characteristic of malignancy.

dyshidrosis (dis″hĭ-dro′sis) 1. pompholyx. 2. any disorder of eccrine sweat glands.

dyskaryosis (-kă-re-o′sis) abnormality of the nucleus of a cell. **dyskaryot′ic,** adj.

dyskeratoma (-ker-ah-to′mah) a dyskeratotic tumor. **warty d.,** a solitary brownish red nodule with a soft, yellowish, central keratotic plug, occurring on the face, neck, scalp, or axilla, or in the mouth; histologically it resembles an individual lesion of keratosis follicularis.

dyskeratosis (-ker-ah-to′sis) abnormal, premature, or imperfect keratinization of the keratinocytes. **dyskeratot′ic,** adj.

dyskinesia (-ki-ne′ze-ah) impairment of the power of voluntary movement. **dyskinet′ic,** adj. **biliary d.,** derangement of the filling and emptying mechanism of the gallbladder. **d. intermit′tens,** intermittent disability of the limbs due to impaired circulation. **d. tar′da, tardive d.,** involuntary repetitive movements of the facial, buccal, oral, and cervical musculature, affecting chiefly the elderly; induced by long-term use of antipsychotic agents, and may persist after withdrawal of the agent.

dyslalia (dis-la′le-ah) impairment of ability to speak associated with abnormality of external speech organs.

dyslexia (-lek′se-ah) impairment of ability to comprehend written language, due to a central lesion. **dyslex′ic,** adj.

dyslipoproteinemia (-lip″o-pro″te-in-e′me-ah) the presence of abnormal lipoproteins in the blood.

dyslogia (-lo′je-ah) impairment of the reasoning power; also, impairment of speech, due to mental disorders.

dysmaturity (dis″mah-chōōr′it-e) the condition of being small or immature for gestational age; said of fetuses that are the product of a pregnancy involving placental dysfunction. **pulmonary d.,** Wilson-Mikity syndrome.

dysmelia (dis-mēl′e-ah) malformation of a limb or limbs due to disturbance in embryonic development.

dysmenorrhea (dis″men-or-e′ah) painful menstruation. **dysmenorrhe′al,** adj. **congestive d.,** that accompanied by great congestion of the uterus. **essential d.,** that for which there is no demonstrable cause. **membranous d.,** that marked by membranous exfoliations derived from the uterus. **obstructive d.,** that due to mechanical obstruction to the discharge of menstrual fluid. **primary d.,** essential d. **secondary d.,** that due to a pelvic lesion. **spasmodic d.,** that due to spasmodic uterine contraction.

dysmetabolism (-mah-tab′o-lizm) defective metabolism.

dysmimia (-mim′e-ah) impairment of the power to express thought by gestures.

dysmorphism (-mor′fizm) 1. appearing under different morphologic forms. 2. an abnormality in morphologic development. **dysmor′phic,** adj.

dysodontiasis (-o-don-ti′ah-sis) defective, delayed, or difficult eruption of the teeth.

dysontogenesis (-on-to-jen′ĭ-sis) defective embryonic development. **dysontogenet′ic,** adj.

dysorexia (dis″o-rek′se-ah) impaired or deranged appetite.

dysosteogenesis (-os″te-o-jen′ĭ-sis) defective bone formation; dysostosis.

dysostosis (dis″os-to′sis) defective ossification; defect in the normal ossification of fetal cartilages. **cleidocranial d.,** a hereditary condition marked by defective ossification of the cranial bones, absence of the clavicles, and dental and vertebral anomalies. **craniofacial d.,** a hereditary condition marked by acrocephaly, exophthalmos, hypertelorism, strabismus, parrot-beaked nose, and hypoplastic maxilla. **mandibulofacial d.,** a hereditary disorder occurring in a complete form (*Franceschetti's syndrome*) with antimongoloid slant of the palpebral fissures, coloboma of the lower lid, micrognathia and hypoplasia of the zygomatic arches, and microtia, and in an incomplete form (*Treacher Collins syndrome*) with the same anomalies in lesser degree. **metaphyseal d.**, a skeletal abnormality in which the epiphyses are normal and the metaphyseal tissues are replaced by masses of cartilage, producing interference with enchondral bone formation. **d. mul′tiplex,** Hurler's syndrome. **orodigitofacial d.,** orofaciodigital syndrome.

dyspareunia (pah-ru′ne-ah) difficult or painful coitus.

dyspepsia (dis-pep′se-ah) impairment of the power or function of digestion; usually applied to epigastric discomfort after meals. **dyspep′tic,** adj.

dysphagia (-fa′je-ah) difficulty in swallowing.

dysphasia (-fa′ze-ah) impairment of speech, consisting in lack of coordination and failure to arrange words in their proper order; due to a central lesion.

dysphonia (-fo′ne-ah) any voice impairment; difficulty in speaking. **dysphon′ic,** adj.

dysphoria (-for′e-ah) disquiet; restlessness; malaise.

dyspigmentation (dis″pig-men-ta′shin) a disorder of pigmentation of skin or hair.

dysplasia (dis-pla′ze-ah) abnormality of development; in pathology, alteration in size, shape, and organization of adult cells. **dysplas′tic,** adj. **anhidrotic ectodermal d.,** congenital ectodermal defect. **anteroposterior facial d.,** defective development resulting in abnormal anteroposterior relations of the maxilla and mandible to each other or to the cranial base. **bronchopulmonary d.,** a chronic lung disease of infants, possibly related to oxygen toxicity or barotrauma, characterized by bronchiolar metaplasia and interstitial fibrosis. **chondroectodermal d.,** achondroplasia with defective development of skin, hair, and teeth, polydactyly, and defect of cardiac septum. **cretinoid d.,** a developmental abnormality characteristic of cretinism, consisting of retarded ossification and smallness of the internal and sexual organs. **diaphyseal d.,** thickening of the cortex of the midshaft area of the long bones, progressing toward the epiphyses, and sometimes also in the flat bones. **epiphyseal d.,** faulty growth and ossification of the epiphyses with roentgenographically apparent stippling and decreased stature, not associated with thyroid disease. **fibrous d. (of bone),** thinning of the cortex of bone and replacement of bone marrow by gritty fibrous tissue containing bony spicules, causing pain, disability, and gradually increasing deformity; only one bone may be involved (*monostotic fibrous d.*), with the process later affecting several or many bones (*polyostotic fibrous d.*). **hereditary ectodermal d.,** congenital ectodermal defect. **metaphyseal d.,** a disturbance in enchondral bone growth, failure of modeling causing the ends of the shafts to remain larger than normal in circumference. **spondyloepiphyseal d.,** hereditary dysplasia of the vertebrae and extremities resulting in dwarfism of the short-trunk type, often with shortened limbs due to epiphyseal abnormalities.

dyspnea (disp-ne′ah) labored or difficult breathing. **dyspne′ic,** adj. **paroxysmal nocturnal d.,** respiratory distress related to posture (especially reclining at night), usually attributed to congestive heart failure with pulmonary edema.

dyspraxia (-prak′se-ah) partial loss of ability to perform coordinated acts.

dysprosium (-pro′ze-um) chemical element (see table), at. no. 66, symbol Dy.

dysraphia, dysraphism (dis-ra′fe-ah; dis′rah-fizm) incomplete closure of a raphe; defective fusion, e.g., of the neural tube.

dysrhythmia (dis-rith′me-ah) a disturbance of rhythm. **cerebral d., electroencephalographic d.,** a disturbance or irregularity in the rhythm of the brain waves as recorded by electroencephalography.

dyssebacea (dis″se-ba′she-ah) disorder of sebaceous follicles; specifically, a condition seen (but not exclusively) in riboflavin deficiency, marked by greasy, branny seborrhea on the midface, with erythema in the nasal folds, canthi, or other skin folds.

dysspermia (-sperm′e-ah) impairment of the spermatozoa, or of the semen.

dysstasia (-sta′ze-ah) difficulty in standing. **dysstat′ic,** adj.

dyssynergia (dis″sin-er′je-ah) muscular incoordination. **d. cerebella′ris myoclon′ica,** dyssynergia cerebellaris progressiva associated with myoclonus epilepsy. **d. cerebella′ris progressi′va,** a condition marked by generalized intention tremors associated with disturbance of muscle tone and of muscular coordination; due to disorder of cerebellar function.

dystaxia (dis-tak′se-ah) difficulty in controlling voluntary movements.

dysthymia (dis-thi′me-ah) a chronic nonpsychotic mood disorder characterized by depression or a loss of interest and pleasure in one's normal activities, but whose symptoms are not severe enough for major depression.

dysthyroid, dysthyroidal (dis-thi′roid; dis″-thi-roid′′l) denoting defective functioning of the thyroid gland.

dystocia (dis-to′se-ah) abnormal labor or childbirth.

dystonia (-to′ne-ah) impairment of muscular tonus. **dyston′ic,** adj. **d. musculo′rum defor′mans,** a hereditary disorder marked by involuntary, irregular, clonic contortions of the muscles of the trunk and extremities, which twist the body forward and sideways grotesquely.

dystopia (-to′pe-ah) malposition; displacement.

dystrophia (-tro′fe-ah) [Gr.] dystrophy. **d. adiposogenita′lis,** adiposogenital dystrophy. **d. epithelia′lis cor′neae,** dystrophy of the corneal epithelium, with erosions. **d. myoto′nica,** myotonic dystrophy. **d. un′guium,** changes in the texture, structure, and/or color of the nails due to no demonstrable cause, but presumed to be attributable to some disturbance of nutrition.

dystrophoneurosis (-trof″o-noōr-o′sis) 1. any nervous order due to poor nutrition. 2. impairment of nutrition due to nervous disorder.

dystrophy (dis′trof-e) any disorder due to defective or faulty nutrition. **dystroph′ic,** adj. **adiposogenital d.,** a condition marked by adiposity of the feminine type, genital hypoplasia, changes in secondary sex characters, and metabolic disturbances; seen with lesions of the hypothalamus. **Becker's d., Becker's muscular d.,** a form closely resembling pseudohypertrophic muscular dystrophy but having a late onset and slowly progressive course; transmitted as an X-linked recessive trait. **Duchenne type muscular d.,** pseudohypertrophic muscular d. **Landouzy-Dejerine d.,** a relatively benign form of muscular dystrophy, with marked atrophy of the muscles of the face, shoulder girdle, and arm. **Leyden-Möbius muscular d. limb-girdle muscular d.,** slowly progressive muscular dystrophy, usually beginning in childhood, marked by weakness and wasting in the shoulder or pelvic girdle. **mus-**cular d., a group of genetically determined, painless, degenerative myopathies marked by muscular weakness and atrophy without nervous system involvement; see *pseudohypertrophic muscular d., Landouzy-Dejerine d.,* and *limb-girdle muscular d.* **myotonic d.,** a rare, slowly progressive, hereditary disease, marked by myotonia followed by muscular atrophy (especially of the face and neck), cataracts, hypogonadism, frontal balding, and cardiac disorders. **pseudohypertrophic muscular d.,** muscular dystrophy affecting the shoulder and pelvic girdles, beginning in childhood and marked by increasing weakness and pseudohypertrophy of the muscles, followed by atrophy and a peculiar swaying gait with the legs kept wide apart.

dysuria (dis-ūr′e-ah) painful or difficult urination. **dysu′ric,** adj.

E

EAC an abbreviation used in studies of complement in which E represents erythrocyte, A antibody, and C complement.

ear (ēr) the organ of hearing and of equilibrium, consisting of the external ear, the middle ear, and the internal ear. See Plate XII. **Blainville's e.,** congenital difference in size or shape of the ears. **Cagot e.,** one without a lower lobe. **cauliflower e.,** a partially deformed auricle due to injury and subsequent perichondritis. **diabetic e.,** mastoiditis complicating diabetes. **external e.,** the auricle and external meatus together. **glue e.,** a chronic condition marked by a collection of fluid of high viscosity in the middle ear, due to obstruction of the eustachian tube. **inner e., internal e.,** the vestibule, cochlea, and semicircular canals together. **middle e.,** an air space in the temporal bone containing the auditory ossicles; see Plate XII. **outer e.,** external e.

earwax (ēr′waks) cerumen.

eburnation (e″ber-na′shin) conversion of bone into a hard, ivory-like mass.

EBV Epstein-Barr virus.

ecaudate (e-kaw′dāt) tail-less.

ecbolic (ek-bol′ik) oxytocic.

eccentric (ek-sen′trik) situated or occurring or proceeding away from a center.

eccentrochondroplasia (ek-sen″tro-kon″dropla′ze-ah) Morquio's syndrome.

ecchondroma (ek″on-dro′mah) a hyperplastic growth of cartilaginous tissue on the surface of a cartilage or projecting under the periosteum of a bone.

ecchymoma (ek″ĭ-mo′mah) swelling due to blood extravasation.

ecchymosis (ek″ĭ-mo′sis), pl. *ecchymo'ses* [Gr.] a small hemorrhagic spot, larger than a petechia, in the skin or mucous membrane, forming a nonelevated, rounded or irregular, blue or purplish patch. **ecchymot′ic,** adj.

eccrine (ek′rin) exocrine, with special reference to ordinary sweat glands.

eccrisis (ek′rĭ-sis) excretion of waste products.

eccritic (ek-krit′ik) 1. promoting excretion. 2. an agent which promotes excretion.

eccyesis (ek″si-e′sis) ectopic pregnancy.

ECF-A eosinophil chemotactic factor of anaphylaxis; a primary mediator of Type I anaphylactic hypersensitivity.

ECG electrocardiogram.

ecgonine (ek′go-nin) the final basic product, $C_9H_{15}NO_3$, obtained by hydrolysis of cocaine and several related alkaloids.

Echinococcus (-kok′us) a genus of small tapeworms, including *E. granulo'sus,* usually parasitic in dogs and wolves, whose larvae (hydatids) may develop in mammals, forming hydatid tumors or cysts chiefly in the liver; and *E. multilocula'ris,* whose larvae form alveolar or multilocular cysts and whose adult forms usually parasitize the fox and wild rodents, although man is sporadically infected.

echo (ek′o) a repeated sound, produced by reverberation of sound waves; also, the reflection of ultrasonic, radio, and radar waves. **amphoric e.,** a resonant repetition of a sound heard on auscultation of the chest, occurring at an appreciable interval after the vocal sound. **metallic e.,** a ringing repetition of the heart sounds sometimes heard in patients with pneumopericardium and pneumothorax.

echoacousia (ek″o-ah-koo′ze-ah) the subjective experience of hearing echoes after normally heard sounds.

echocardiography (-kar″de-og′rah-fe) recording of the position and motion of the heart walls or internal structures of the heart by the echo obtained from beams of ultrasonic waves directed through the chest wall.

echoencephalography (-en-sef″ah-log′rah-fe) a

diagnostic technique in which pulses of ultrasonic waves are beamed through the head from both sides, and echoes from the midline structures of the brain are recorded graphically; shifts from the midline may indicate a centrally placed mass.

echography (ĕ-kog′rah-fe) ultrasonography; the use of ultrasound as a diagnostic aid. Ultrasound waves are directed at the tissues, and a record is made of the waves reflected back through the tissues, which indicate interfaces of different acoustic densities and thus differentiate between solid and cystic structures.

echolalia (ek″o-la′le-ah) automatic repetition by a patient of what is said to him.

echolucent (-loo′sint) permitting the passage of ultrasonic waves without echoes, the representative areas appearing black on the sonogram.

echopathy (ek-op′ah-the) automatic repetition by a patient of words or movements of others.

echophonocardiography (ek″o-fo″no-kar″de-og′rah-fe) the combined use of echocardiography and phonocardiography.

echopraxia (-prak′se-ah) the involuntary imitation of the movements of others.

echo-ranging (-rān′jing) in ultrasonography, determination of the position or depth of a body structure on the basis of the time interval between the moment an ultrasonic pulse is transmitted and the moment its echo is received.

echothiophate iodide (-thi′o-fāt) a cholinesterase inhibitor, $C_9H_{23}INO_3PS$, used in the treatment of glaucoma.

echovirus (-vi′rus) an enterovirus isolated from man, separable into many serotypes, certain of which are associated with human disease, especially aseptic meningitis.

eclampsia (ĕ-klamp′se-ah) convulsions and coma, rarely coma alone, occurring in a pregnant or puerperal woman, and associated with hypertension, edema, and/or proteinuria. **eclamp′tic,** adj. **puerperal e.,** that occurring after childbirth. **uremic e.,** that due to uremia.

eclampsism (ĕ-klamp′sizm) preeclampsia.

eclamptogenic (ĕ-klamp″to-jen′ik) causing convulsions.

ecology (e-kol′ah-je) the science of organisms as affected by environmental factors; study of the environment and life history of organisms. **ecolog′ic, ecolog′ical,** adj.

ecomania (e″ko-ma′ne-ah) an attitude of mind that is dominating toward family members but humble toward those in authority.

economy (e-kon′ah-me) the management of domestic affairs. **token e.,** in behavior therapy, a program of treatment in which the patient earns tokens, exchangeable for rewards, for appropriate personal and social behavior and loses tokens for antisocial behavior.

ecosystem (ek′o-sis″tim) the unit in ecology, comprising the living organisms and the nonliving elements interacting in a certain defined area.

ecotaxis (-tak″sis) the movement or "homing" of a circulating cell, e.g., a lymphocyte, to a specific anatomical compartment.

ECT electroconvulsive therapy.

ect(o)- word element [Gr.], *external; outside.*

ectad (ek′tad) directed outward.

ectasia (ek-ta′ze-ah) dilatation, expansion, or distention. **ectat′ic,** adj. **annuloaortic e.,** dilatation of the proximal aorta and the fibrous ring of the heart at the aortic orifice, marked by aortic regurgitation, and when severe by dissecting aneurysm; often associated with Marfan's syndrome. **mammary duct e.,** dilatation of the collecting ducts of the mammary gland, with inspissation of gland secretion and inflammatory changes in the tissues; a benign process associated with atrophy of the duct epithelium, it generally occurs during or after menopause.

ectethmoid (ek-teth′moid) one of the paired lateral masses of the ethmoid bone.

ecthyma (ek-thi′mah) a shallowly ulcerative form of impetigo, chiefly on the shins or forearms.

ectoantigen (ek″to-ant′ĭ-jen) 1. an antigen that seems to be loosely attached to the outside of bacteria. 2. an antigen formed in the ectoplasm (cell membrane) of a bacterium.

ectoblast (ek′to-blast) the ectoderm.

ectocardia (ek″to-kar′de-ah) congenital displacement of the heart.

ectocervix (-serv′iks) portio vaginalis. **ectocer′vical,** adj.

ectoderm (ek′to-derm) the outermost of the three primitive germ layers of the embryo; from it are derived the epidermis and epidermic tissues, such as the nails, hair, and glands of the skin, the nervous system, external sense organs and mucous membrane of the mouth and anus. **ectoder′mal, ectoder′mic,** adj.

ectodermosis (ek″to-der-mo′sis) a disorder based on congenital maldevelopment of organs derived from the ectoderm. **e. erosi′va pluriorificia′lis,** Stevens-Johnson syndrome.

ectoenzyme (-en′zīm) an extracellular enzyme.

ectogenous (ek-toj′ĭ-nus) introduced from without; arising from causes outside the organism.

ectomere (ek′tah-mēr) one of the blastomeres taking part in formation of the ectoderm.

ectomorphy (-mor″fe) a type of body build in which tissues derived from the ectoderm predominate; a somatotype in which both visceral and body structures are relatively slightly developed, the body being linear and delicate. **ectomor′phic,** adj.

-ectomy word element [Gr.], *excision; surgical removal.*

ectopia (ek-to′pe-ah) [Gr.] displacement or malposition, especially if congenital. **e. cor′dis,** congenital displacement of the heart outside the thoracic cavity. **e. len′tis,** abnormal position of the lens of the eye. **e. pupil′lae conge′nita,** congenital displacement of the pupil.

ectopic (ek-top′ik) 1. pertaining to ectopia. 2. located away from normal position. 3. arising from an abnormal site or tissue.

ectosteal (ek-tos′te-il) pertaining to or situated outside of a bone.

ectostosis (ek″to-sto′sis) ossification beneath the

perichondrium of a cartilage or the periosteum of a bone.

ectothrix (ek′to-thriks) a fungus that grows inside the shaft of a hair, but produces a conspicuous external sheath of spores.

ectro- word element [Gr.], *miscarriage; congenital absence.*

ectrogeny (ek-troj′ĭ-ne) congenital absence or defect of a part. **ectrojen′ic,** adj.

ectromelia (-me′le-ah) gross hypoplasia or aplasia of one or more long bones of one or more limbs. **ectromel′ic,** adj.

ectropion (ek-tro′pe-on) eversion or turning outward, as of the margin of an eyelid.

ectrosyndactyly (ek″tro-sin-dak′tĭ-le) a condition in which some digits are absent and those that remain are webbed.

eczema (ek′zĭ-mah) 1. a superficial inflammatory process involving primarily the epidermis, marked early by redness, itching, minute papules and vesicles, weeping, oozing, and crusting, and later by scaling, lichenification, and often pigmentation. 2. atopic dermatitis. **facial e. of ruminants,** a photosensitive disease of ruminants, particularly in New Zealand, due to ingestion of the spores of the mold *Pithomyces chartarum,* which contain sporidesmin. **e. herpe′ticum,** disseminated herpes simplex; see *Kaposi's varicelliform eruption.* **nummular e., e. nummula′re,** that in which the patches are coin shaped; it may be a form of neurodermatitis. **e. vaccina′tum,** a severe generalized vesiculopustular eruption due to the vaccinia virus, superimposed upon a preexisting chronic dermatitis.

E.D. effective dose; erythema dose.

ED₅₀ median effective dose; a dose that produces its effects in 50% of a population.

edema (ĭ-de′mah) an abnormal accumulation of fluid in intercellular spaces of the body. **angioneurotic e.,** angioedema. **cardiac e.,** a manifestation of congestive heart failure, due to increased venous and capillary pressures and often associated with renal sodium retention. **dependent e.,** edema affecting most severely the lowermost or dependent parts of the body. **e. neonato′rum,** a disease of premature and feeble infants resembling sclerema, marked by spreading edema with cold, livid skin. **pitting e.,** that in which pressure leaves a persistent depression in the tissues. **pulmonary e.,** diffuse extravascular accumulation of fluid in the pulmonary tissues and air spaces due to changes in hydrostatic forces in the capillaries or to increased capillary permeability; it is marked by intense dyspnea. **vasogenic e.,** that characterized by increased permeability of capillary endothelial cells; the most common form of brain edema.

edemagen (ĭ-de′mah-jen) an irritant that elicits edema by causing capillary damage but not the cellular response of true inflammation.

edentia (e-den′she-ah) absence of the teeth.

edentulous (-tu-lus) without teeth.

edetate (ed′it-āt) any salt of ethylenediaminetetraacetic acid (EDTA), including *e. disodium calcium,* used in the diagnosis and treatment of

lead poisoning, and *e. disodium,* used in the treatment of poisoning with lead and other heavy metals and, because of its affinity for calcium, in the treatment of hypercalcemia.

edetic acid (ah-det′ik) ethylenediaminetetraacetic acid.

edisylate (ĕ-dis′ĭ-lāt) USAN contraction for 1,2-ethanedisulfonate.

edrophonium (ed″ro-fo′ne-um) a cholinergic, $C_{10}H_{16}NO$, used in the form of the chloride salt as a curare antagonist and as a diagnostic agent in myasthenia gravis.

EDTA ethylenediaminetetraacetic acid.

educable (ej′ŏŏ-kah-b'l) capable of being educated; used with special reference to persons with mild retardation (I.Q. approximately 50–70).

EEE eastern equine encephalomyelitis.

EEG electroencephalogram.

E.E.N.T. eye-ear-nose-throat.

E.E.S. trademark for a preparation of erythromycin ethylsuccinate.

effacement (ĭ-fās′mint) the obliteration of features; said of the cervix during labor when it is so changed that only the external os remains.

effect (ĭ-fekt′) the result produced by an action. **Doppler e.,** the relationship of the apparent frequency of waves, as of sound, light, and radio waves, to the relative motion of the source of the waves and the observer, the frequency increasing as the two approach each other and decreasing as they move apart. **experimenter e's,** demand characteristics. **position e.,** in genetics, the changed effect produced by alteration of the relative positions of various genes on the chromosomes. **pressure e.,** the sum of the changes that are due to obstruction of tissue drainage by pressure. **Somogyi e.,** a rebound phenomenon occurring in diabetes: overtreatment with insulin induces hypoglycemia, which initiates the release of epinephrine, ACTH, glucagon, and growth hormone, which stimulate lipolysis, gluconeogenesis, and glycogenolysis, which, in turn, result in a rebound hyperglycemia and ketosis. **side e.,** see under S.

effectiveness (ĭ-fek′tiv-nis) the ability to produce a specific result or to exert a specific measurable influence. **relative biological e.,** an expression of the effectiveness of other types of radiation in comparison with that of gamma or roentgen rays; abbreviated RBE.

effector (ĭ-fek′ter) 1. a muscle or gland that contracts or secretes, respectively, in direct response to nerve impulses. 2. a molecule that binds to an enzyme with an effect on its catalytic activity; see also *activator* and *inhibitor.* **alloster′ic e.,** one that binds to an enzyme at a site other than the active site.

effemination (ĭ-fem″ĭ-na′shin) feminization.

efferent (ef′er-ent) conveying away from a center, as an efferent nerve.

effleurage (ef″lu-rahzh′) [Fr.] a stroking movement in massage.

efflorescent (ef″lor-es′int) becoming powdery by losing the water of crystallization.

effluvium (ĭ-floo′ve-um), pl. *efflu′via* [L.] 1. an outflowing or shedding, as of the hair. 2. an exhalation or emanation, especially one of noxious nature.

effusion (ĭ-fu′zhun) 1. escape of a fluid into a part; exudation or transudation. 2. effused material; an exudate or transudate.

egestion (e-jes′chin) the casting out of undigestible material.

egg (eg) 1. an ovum; a female gamete. 2. an oocyte. 3. a female reproductive cell at any stage before fertilization and its derivatives after fertilization and even after some development.

ego (e′go) that segment of the personality dominated by the reality principle, comprising integrative and executive aspects functioning to adapt the forces and pressures of the id and superego and the requirements of external reality by conscious perception, thought, and learning.

ego-alien (e″go-āl′yen) ego-dystonic.

egobronchophony (-brong-kof′ah-ne) increased vocal resonance with high-pitched bleating quality of the voice, heard on auscultation of the lungs, especially in pleural effusion.

egocentric (-sen′trik) having all one's ideas centered on one's self.

ego-dystonic (-dis-ton′ik) denoting any impulse, idea, or the like, that is repugnant to and inconsistent with an individual's conception of himself.

egoism (e′go-izm) 1. a healthy awareness and advancement of one's own interests. 2. the philosophical doctrine that self-interest is the proper basis for all human conduct. 3. egotism.

egomania (e″go-ma′ne-ah) morbid self-esteem.

ego-syntonic (e″go-sin-ton′ik) denoting any impulse, idea, or the like, that is in harmony with an individual's conception of himself.

egotism (e′go-tizm) overevaluation of one's self; selfishness.

Ehrlichia (ār-li′ke-ah) a genus of the tribe Ehrlichieae causing disease in dogs, cattle, and sheep.

Ehrlichieae (ār″lĭ-ki′e-e) a tribe of rickettsiae made up of organisms adapted for existence in invertebrates, chiefly arthropods, and pathogenic for certain mammals, including man.

eiconometer (i″kon-om′it-er) eikonometer.

eidetic (i-det′ik) denoting exact visualization of events or objects previously seen; a person having such an ability.

eidoptometry (i″dop-tom′ĭ-tre) measurement of the acuteness of visual perception.

eikonometer (i″ko-nom′it-er) an instrument for measuring the degree of aniseikonia.

Eimeria (i-me′re-ah) a genus of protozoa (order Eucoccidiida) found in the epithelial cells of man and animals, including pathogens of many economically important diseases of domestic animals.

einsteinium (īn-sti′ne-um) chemical element (*see table*), at. no. 99, symbol Es.

ejaculatio (e-jak″u-la′she-o) [L.] ejaculation. **e. prae′cox,** premature ejaculation in coitus.

ejaculation (e-jak″ūl-a′shin) forcible, sudden expulsion; especially expulsion of semen from the male urethra. **ejac′ulatory,** adj.

EKG electrocardiogram.

EKY electrokymogram.

elaboration (ĭ-lab″ah-ra′shun) 1. the process of producing complex substances out of simpler materials. 2. in psychiatry, an unconscious mental process of expansion and embellishment of detail, especially of a symbol or representation in a dream.

Elapidae (e-lap′ĭ-de) a family of usually terrestrial, venomous snakes, which have cylindrical tails and front fangs that are short, stout, immovable, and grooved. It includes cobras, kraits, coral snakes, Australian copperheads, Australian blacksnakes, brown snakes, tiger snakes, death adders, and mambas.

elastance (ĭ-las′tins) the quality of recoiling on removal of pressure without disruption, or an expression of the measure of the ability to do so in terms of unit of volume change per unit of pressure change. It is the reciprocal of compliance.

elastase (e-las′tās) a pancreatic protease formed from the proenzyme proelastase.

elasticin (e-las′tĭ-sin) elastin.

elastin (e-las′tin) a yellow scleroprotein, the essential constituent of elastic connective tissue; it is brittle when dry, but when moist is flexible and elastic.

elastofibroma (e-las″to-fi-bro′mah) a tumor consisting of both elastin and fibrous elements. **e. dor′si,** a tumor-like nodule of subscapular tissue occurring in old age.

elastolysis (e″las-tol′ĭ-sis) the digestion of elastic substance or tissue. **perifollicular e.,** see under *anetoderma.*

elastoma (ī″las-to′mah) a tumor or focal excess of elastic tissue fibers or abnormal collagen fibers of the skin.

elastometry (ī″las-tom′ĭ-tre) the measurement of elasticity.

elastorrhexis (-rek′sis) rupture of fibers composing elastic tissue.

elastosis (e″las-to′sis) 1. degeneration of elastic tissue. 2. degenerative changes in the dermal connective tissue with increased amounts of elastotic material. 3. any disturbance of the dermal connective tissue. **actinic e.,** degeneration of the elastic tissue of the dermis due to constant exposure to sunlight. **nodular e. of Favre–Racouchot,** actinic elastosis occurring chiefly in elderly men, with giant comedones, pilosebaceous cysts, and large folds of furrowed, yellowish skin in the periorbital region. **e. per′forans serpigino′sa,** perforating an elastic tissue defect, occurring alone or in association with other disorders, including Down's syndrome and Ehlers-Danlos syndrome, in which elastomas are extruded through small keratotic papules in the epidermis; the lesions are usually arranged in arcuate serpiginous clusters on the sides of the nape, face, or arms.

elastotic (e″las-tot′ik) 1. pertaining to or characterized by elastosis. 2. resembling elastic tissue; having the staining properties of elastin.

elation (ĭ-la′shin) emotional excitement marked by acceleration of mental and bodily activity.

Elavil (el′ah-vil) trademark for a preparation of amitriptyline hydrochloride.

elbow (el′bo) 1. the bend of the arm; the joint connecting the arm and forearm. 2. any angular bend. **capped e.,** a hygroma on the point of the elbow in horses or cattle. **little leaguer's e.,** medial epicondylitis of the elbow due to repeated stress on the flexor muscles of the forearm, often seen in adolescent ballplayers. **miner's e.,** enlargement of the bursa over the point of the elbow, due to resting the body weight on the elbow, as in mining. **pulled e.,** subluxation of the head of the radius distally under the round ligament. **tennis e.,** a painful condition of the outer elbow, due to inflammation or irritation of the extensor tendon attachment of the lateral humeral epicondyle.

electroaffinity (-ah-fin′it-e) electronegativity.

electroanalgesia (-an″al-je′ze-ah) the reduction of pain by electrical stimulation of a peripheral nerve or the dorsal column of the spinal cord.

electrobiology (-bi-ol′ah-je) the study of electric phenomena in living tissue.

electrocardiogram (-kar′de-ah-gram″) the record produced by electrocardiography. Abbreviated ECG or EKG. **scalar e.,** the tracing showing only changes in magnitude of voltage and polarity (positive or negative) with time.

electrocardiography (-kar″de-og′rah-fe) the making of graphic records of the variations in electrical potential caused by electrical activity of the heart muscle and detected at the body surface, as a method for studying the action of the heart muscle. **electrocardiograph′ic,** adj.

electrocautery (-kawt′er-e) an apparatus for cauterizing tissue by means of a platinum wire heated by electric current.

electrocoagulation (-ko-ag″ūl-a′shin) coagulation of tissue by means of an electric current.

electrocochleography (-kok″le-og′rah-fe) measurement of electrical potentials of the eighth cranial nerve in response to acoustic stimuli applied by an electrode to the external acoustic canal, promontory, or tympanic membrane.

electrocontractility (-kon″trak-til′it-e) contractility in response to electrical stimulation.

electroconvulsive (-kun-vul′siv) inducing convulsions by means of electricity.

electrocorticography (-kort″i-kog′rah-fe) electroencephalography with the electrodes applied directly to the cerebral cortex.

electrode (ĭ-lek′trōd) either of the two terminals of an electrically conducting system or cell. **active e.,** one smaller than an indifferent electrode, producing electrical stimulation in a concentrated area. **calomel e.,** one capable of both collecting and giving up chloride ions in neutral or acidic aqueous media, consisting of mercury in contact with mercurous chloride; used as a reference electrode in pH measurements. **depolarizing e.,** one having a resistance greater than that of the portion of the body enclosed in the circuit. **exciting e.,** active e. **hydrogen e.,** one made by depositing platinum black on platinum and then allowing it to absorb hydrogen gas to saturation; used in determination of hydrogen ion concentration. **impregnated e.,** one

with an absorbent tip impregnated with prescribed medicament. **indifferent e.,** one larger than an active electrode, dispersing electrical stimulation over a larger area. **negative e.,** cathode. **point e.,** an electrode having on one end a metallic point; used in applying current. **positive e.,** anode. **silent e.,** indifferent e. **therapeutic e.,** active e.

electrodermal (e-lek″tro-derm′′l) pertaining to the electrical properties of the skin, especially to changes in its resistance.

electrodesiccation (-des″ĭ-ka′shin) destruction of tissue by dehydration, done by means of a high-frequency electric current.

electrodialyzer (-di″ah-li′zer) a blood dialyzer utilizing an applied electric field and semipermeable membranes for separating the colloids from the solution.

electroencephalography (-en-sef″ah-log′rah-fe) the recording of changes in electric potential in various areas of the brain by means of electrodes placed on the scalp or on or in the brain itself. **electroencephalograph′ic,** adj.

electrofocusing (-fo′kus-ing) isoelectric focusing.

electrogastrography (-gas-trog′rah-fe) the recording of the electrical activity of the stomach as measured between its lumen and the body surface. **electrogastrograph′ic,** adj.

electrogram (ĭ-lek′trah-gram) any record produced by changes in electric potential. **His bundle e.,** an intracardiac electrocardiogram of potentials in the bundle of His, done through a cardiac catheter.

electrogustometry (ĭ-lek″tro-gus-tom′ĭ-tre) the testing of the sense of taste by application of galvanic stimuli to the tongue.

electrohemostasis (-he″mo-sta′sis) arrest of hemorrhage by electrocautery.

electrohysterography (-his″ter-og′rah-fe) recording of changes in electric potential associated with uterine contractions.

electroimmunodiffusion (-im″ūn-o-dif-u′zhin) immunodiffusion accelerated by application of an electric current.

electrokymography (-ki-mog′rah-fe) the photography on x-ray film of the motion of the heart or of other moving structures which can be visualized radiographically.

electrolysis (ĭ″lek-trol′ĭ-sis) destruction by passage of a galvanic current, as in disintegration of a chemical compound in solution or removal of excessive hair from the body.

electrolyte (ĭ-lek′tro-līt) a substance that dissociates into ions fused in solution, thus becoming capable of conducting electricity.

electromagnet (-mag′nit) a temporary magnet made by passing electric current through a coil of wire surrounding a core of soft iron.

electromyography (-mi-og′rah-fe) the recording and study of the electrical properties of skeletal muscle. **electromyograph′ic,** adj.

electron (ĭ-lek′tron) any of the negatively charged particles arranged in orbits around the nucleus of an atom and determining all of the atom's physical and chemical properties except mass and radioactivity. **electron′ic,** adj.

electronarcosis (ĭ-lek″tro-nar-ko′sis) anesthesia produced by passage of an electric current through electrodes placed on the temples.

electron-dense (ĭ-lek′tron-dens″) in electron microscopy, having a density that prevents electrons from penetrating.

electronegative (ĭ-lek″tro-neg′it-iv) bearing a negative electric charge.

electroneurography (-nōōr-og′rah-fe) the measurement of the conduction velocity and latency of peripheral nerves.

electroneuromyography (-nōōr″o-mi-og′rah-fe) electromyography in which the nerve of the muscle under study is stimulated by application of an electric current.

electronystagmography (-nis″tag-mog′rah-fe) electroencephalographic recordings of eye movements that provide objective documentation of induced and spontaneous nystagmus.

electro-oculogram (-ok′ūl-ah-gram″) the electroencephalographic tracings made while moving the eyes a constant distance between two fixation points, inducing a deflection of fairly constant amplitude; abbreviated EOG.

electro-olfactogram (-ol-fak′tah-gram) a recording of electrical potential changes detected by an electrode placed on the surface of the olfactory mucosa as the mucosa is subjected to an odorous stimulus. Abbreviated EOG.

electrophile (ĭ-lek′tro-fīl) an electron acceptor. **electrophil′ic,** adj.

electrophoresis (ĭ-lek″tro-for-e′sis) the movement of charged particles suspended in a liquid on various media (e.g., paper, starch, agar), under the influence of an applied electric field. **electrophoret′ic,** adj. **counter e.,** counterimmunoelectrophoresis.

electrophoretogram (-for-et′o-gram) the record produced on or in a supporting medium by bands of material which have been separated by the process of electrophoresis.

electroretinograph (-ret′in-ah-graf) an instrument to measure the electrical response of the retina to light stimulation; abbreviated ERG.

electroscission (-sish′in) cutting of tissue by means of the electric cautery.

electroscope (ĭ-lek′trah-skōp) an instrument for measuring radiation intensity.

electroshock (-shok) shock produced by applying electric current to the brain.

electrosleep (-slēp) see *cerebral electrotherapy.*

electrostriatogram (ĭ-lek″tro-stri-āt′ah-gram) an electroencephalogram showing differences in electric potential recorded at various levels of the corpus striatum.

electrosurgery (-serj′er-e) surgery performed by electrical methods; the active electrode may be a needle, bulb, or disk. **electrosur′gical,** adj.

electrotaxis (-tak′sis) taxis in response to electric stimuli.

electrotherapy (-ther′ah-pe) treatment of disease by means of electricity. **cerebral e.,** the use of low-intensity electricity, usually employing positive pulses or direct current in the treatment of insomnia, anxiety, and neurotic depression. Misleadingly called *electrosleep*—the treatment does not induce sleep.

electrotonic (-ton′ik) 1. pertaining to electrotonus. 2. denoting the direct spread of current in tissues by electrical conduction, without the generation of new current by action potentials.

electrotonus (ĭ-lek-trot′ah-nus) the altered electrical state of a nerve or muscle cell when a constant electric current is passed through it.

electroureterography (-ūr-ēt″er-og′rah-fe) electromyography in which the action potentials produced by peristalsis of the ureter are recorded.

electrovalence (ĭ-lek″tro-va′lins) 1. the number of charges an atom acquires by the gain or loss of electrons in forming an ionic bond. 2. the bonding resulting from such a transfer of electrons. **electrova′lent,** adj.

electrovert (ĭ-lek′tro-vert) to apply electricity to the heart or precordium to depolarize the heart and terminate a cardiac dysrhythmia.

electuary (ĭ-lek′choo-er″e) a medicinal preparation consisting of a powdered drug made into a paste with honey or syrup.

eledoisin (el-ĭ-doi′sin) an endecapeptide, $C_{54}H_{85}$-$N_{13}O_{15}S$, from a species of octopus (*Eledone*), which is a precursor of a large group of biologically active peptides; it has vasodilator, hypotensive, and extravascular smooth muscle stimulant properties.

eleidin (el-e′ĭ-din) a substance, allied to keratin, found in the stratum lucidum of the skin.

element (el′ĭ-mint) 1. any of the primary parts or constituents of a thing. 2. in chemistry, a simple substance which cannot be decomposed by chemical means and which is made up of atoms which are alike in their peripheral electronic configurations and so in their chemical properties and also in the number of protons in their nuclei, but which may differ in the number of neutrons in their nuclei and so in their mass number and in their radioactive properties. See *Table of Elements.* **formed e's (of the blood),** erythrocytes, leukocytes, and platelets. **trace e's,** chemical elements distributed throughout the tissues in very small amounts and that are either essential in nutrition, as cobalt, copper, etc., or harmful, as selenium.

eleo- word element [Gr.], *oil.*

elephantiasis (el″ĭ-fan-ti′ah-sis) elephantiasis filariensis; a chronic filarial disease, usually seen in the tropics, due to infection with *Brugia malayi* or *Wuchereria bancrofti,* marked by inflammation and obstruction of the lymphatics and hypertrophy of the skin and subcutaneous tissues, chiefly affecting the legs and external genitals. The term is often applied to hypertrophy and thickening of the tissues from any cause. **e. neuromato′sa,** neurofibroma. **e. nos′tras,** that due to either chronic streptococcal erysipelas or chronic recurrent cellulitis. **e. scro′ti,** that in which the scrotum is the main seat of the disease.

elevator (el′ĭ-vāt-er) an instrument for elevating tissues for removing osseous fragments or roots of teeth.

elimination (ĭ-lim″ĭ-na′shin) 1. the act of expul-

ELEMENT (DATE OF DISCOVERY)	SYMBOL	ATOMIC NUMBER	ATOMIC WEIGHT*	VALENCE	SPECIFIC GRAVITY OR DENSITY (Grams/Liter)	DESCRIPTIVE COMMENT
Actinium (1899)	Ac	89	[227]	3	10.07	radioactive element associated with uranium
Aluminum (1827)	Al	13	26.9815	3	2.6989	silvery-white metal, abundant in earth's crust, but not in free form
Americium (1944)	Am	95	[243]	3,4,5,6	13.67	fourth transuranium element discovered
Antimony (prehistoric)	Sb	51	121.75	3,5	6.691	exists in 4 allotropic forms
Argon (1894)	Ar	18	39.948	0?	1.7837 g/l	colorless, odorless gas
Arsenic (1250)	As	33	74.9216	3,5	5.73; 4.73; 1.97	(gray) semimetallic solid; (black); (yellow)
Astatine (1940)	At	85	[210]	1,3,5,7		radioactive halogen
Barium (1808)	Ba	56	137.34	2	3.5	silvery-white, alkaline earth metal
Berkelium (1949)	Bk	97	[247]	3,4		fifth transuranium element discovered
Beryllium (1798)	Be	4	9.0122	2	1.848	light, steel-gray metal
Bismuth (1753)	Bi	83	208.980	3,5	9.747	pinkish-white, crystalline, brittle metal
Boron (1808)	B	5	10.811	3	2.34, 2.37	crystalline or amorphous element, not occurring free in nature
Bromine (1826)	Br	35	79.909	1,3,5,7	3.12; 7.59 g/l	mobile, reddish-brown liquid, volatilizing readily; red vapor with disagreeable odor
Cadmium (1817)	Cd	48	112.40	2	8.65	soft, bluish-white metal
Calcium (1808)	Ca	20	40.08	2	1.55	metallic element, forming more than 3 per cent of earth's crust
Californium (1950)	Cf	98	[251]	2,3,4		sixth transuranium element discovered
Carbon (prehistoric)	C	6	12.01115	2,3,4	1.8-2.1; 1.9-2.3; 3.15-3.53	(amorphous) element widely distributed in nature; (graphite); (diamond)
Cerium (1803)	Ce	58	140.12	3,4	6.67-8.23	most abundant rare earth metal
Cesium (1869)	Cs	55	132.905	1	1.873	silvery-white, soft, alkaline metal
Chlorine (1774)	Cl	17	35.453	1,3,5,7	3.214 g/l	greenish-yellow gas of the halogen group
Chromium (1797)	Cr	24	51.996	2,3,6	7.18-7.20	steel-gray, lustrous, hard metal
Cobalt (1735)	Co	27	58.9332	2,3	8.9	brittle, hard metal
Copper (prehistoric)	Cu	29	63.54	1,2	8.96	reddish, lustrous, malleable metal
Curium (1944)	Cm	96	[247]	3,4	13.51	third transuranium element discovered
Dysprosium (1886)	Dy	66	162.50	3	8.536	rare earth metal with metallic bright silver luster
Einsteinium (1952)	Es	99	[252]	2,3		seventh transuranium element discovered
Element 106 (1974)		106	[263]			thirteenth transuranium element discovered; no name yet proposed
Erbium (1843)	Er	68	167.26	3	9.051	soft, malleable rare earth metal
Europium (1896)	Eu	63	151.96	2,3	5.259	lustrous, silvery-white rare earth metal
Fermium (1953)	Fm	100	[257]	2,3		eighth transuranium element discovered
Fluorine (1771)	F	9	18.9984	1	1.696 g/l	pale yellow, corrosive gas of the halogen group
Francium (1939)	Fr	87	[223]	1		product of alpha disintegration of actinium
Gadolinium (1880)	Gd	64	157.25	3	7.8, 7.895	lustrous, silvery-white rare earth metal
Gallium (1875)	Ga	31	69.72	2,3	5.907	beautiful, silvery-appearing metal

*Figures in brackets represent mass number of most stable isotope.

Table of Chemical Elements—*Continued*

ELEMENT (DATE OF DISCOVERY)	SYMBOL	ATOMIC NUMBER	ATOMIC WEIGHT*	VALENCE	SPECIFIC GRAVITY OR DENSITY (Grams/Liter)	DESCRIPTIVE COMMENT
Germanium (1886)	Ge	32	72.59	2,4	5.323	grayish-white, brittle metal
Gold (prehistoric)	Au	79	196.967	1,3	19.32	malleable yellow metal
Hafnium (1923)	Hf	72	178.49	4	13.29	gray metal associated with zirconium
Hahnium (1970) (*Element 105*)	Ha	105	[260]			twelfth transuranium element discovered
Helium (1895)	He	2	4.0026	0	0.177 g/l	inert gas
Holmium (1879)	Ho	67	164.930	3	8.803	relatively soft and malleable rare earth metal
Hydrogen (1766)	H	1	1.00797	1	0.08988 g/l 0.070	(gas) most abundant element in the universe (liquid)
Indium (1863)	In	49	114.82	1,2?,3	7.31	soft, silvery-white metal
Iodine (1811)	I	53	126.9044	1,3,5,7	4.93, 11.27 g/l	grayish-black, lustrous solid or violet-blue gas
Iridium (1803)	Ir	77	192.2	3,4	22.42	white, brittle metal of platinum family
Iron (prehistoric)	Fe	26	55.847	2,3,4,6	7.874	fourth most abundant element in earth's crust
Krypton (1898)	Kr	36	83.80	0	3.733 g/l	inert gas
Lanthanum (1839)	La	57	138.91	3	5.98–6.186	silvery-white, ductile, rare earth metal
Lawrencium (1961)	Lr	103	[260]	3		tenth transuranium element discovered
Lead (prehistoric)	Pb	82	207.19	2,4	11.35	bluish-white, lustrous, malleable metal
Lithium (1817)	Li	3	6.939	1	0.534	lightest of all metals
Lutetium (1907)	Lu	761	174.97	3	9.872	rare earth metal
Magnesium (1808)	Mg	12	24.312	2	1.738	silvery-white metallic element, eighth in abundance in earth's crust
Manganese (1774)	Mn	25	54.9380	1,2,3,4,6,7	7.21–7.44	exists in 4 allotropic forms
Mendelevium (1955)	Md	101	[258]	2,3		ninth transuranium element discovered
Mercury (prehistoric)	Hg	80	200.59	1,2	13.546	heavy, silvery-white metal, liquid at ordinary temperatures
Molybdenum (1782)	Mo	42	95.94	2,3,4?,5,6	10.22	silvery-white, very hard metal
Neodymium (1885)	Nd	60	144.24	3	6.80, 7.004	exists in 2 allotrophic forms
Neon (1898)	Ne	10	20.183	0?	0.89990 g/l	inert gas
Neptunium (1940)	Np	93	237.0482	3,4,5,6	20.45	first transuranium element discovered
Nickel (1751)	Ni	28	58.71	0,1,2,3	8.902	silvery-white, malleable metal
Niobium (1801)	Nb	41	92.906	2,3,4?,5	8.57	shiny white, soft ductile metal
Nitrogen (1772)	N	7	14.0067	3,5	1.2506 g/l	colorless, odorless, inert element, making up 78 per cent of the air
Nobelium (1958)	No	102	[259]	2,3		acceptance of this element considered premature
Osmium (1803)	Os	76	190.2	2,3,4,8	22.57	bluish-white, hard metal of platinum family
Oxygen (1774)	O	8	15.9994	2	1.429 g/l	colorless, odorless gas, third most abundant element in the universe
Palladium (1803)	Pd	46	106.4	2,3,4	12.02	steel-white metal of the platinum family
Phosphorus (1669)	P	15	30.9738	3,5	1.82 2.20 2.25–2.69	(white) waxy solid, transparent when pure (red) (black)
Platinum (1735)	Pt	78	195.09	1?,2,3,4	21.45	silvery-white, malleable metal

Element (discovery year)	Symbol	Atomic No.	Atomic weight	Valence	Density	Description
Plutonium (1940)	Pu	94				second transuranium element discovered
Polonium (1898)	Po	84	[210]	2,4,6	9.32	very rare natural element
Potassium (1807)	K	19	39.102	1	0.862	soft, silvery, alkali metal, seventh in abundance in earth's crust
Praseodymium (1885)	Pr	59	140.907	3,4	6.782, 6.64	soft, silvery rare earth metal
Promethium (1941)	Pm	61	[145]	3	7.22 ± 0.02	produced by irradiation of neodymium and praseodymium; identity established in 1945
Protactinium (1917)	Pa	91	231.0359	4,5	15.37	bright lustrous metal
Radium (1898)	Ra	88	226.0254	2	5.5	brilliant white, radioactive metal
Radon (1900)	Rn	86	[222]	0	9.73 g/l	heaviest known gas
Rhenium (1925)	Re	75	186.2	–1,2,3,4,5,6,7	21.02	silvery-white lustrous metal
Rhodium (1803)	Rh	45	102.905	–2,3,4,5	12.41	silvery-white metal of platinum family
Rubidium (1861)	Rb	37	85.47	1,2,3,4	1.532	soft, silvery-white, alkali metal
Ruthenium (1844)	Ru	44	101.07	0,1,2,3,4,5,6,7,8	12.41	hard white metal of platinum family
Rutherfordium (1969) *(Element 104)*	Rf	104	[261]			eleventh transuranium element discovered
Samarium (1879)	Sm	62	150.35	2,3	7.536–7.40	bright silver lustrous metal
Scandium (1879)	Sc	21	44.956	3	2.992	soft, silvery-white metal
Selenium (1817)	Se	34	78.96	2,4,6	4.79, 4.28	exists in several allotropic forms
Silicon (1823)	Si	14	28.086	4	2.33	a relatively inert element, second in abundance in earth's crust
Silver (prehistoric)	Ag	47	107.870	1,2	10.50	malleable, ductile metal with brilliant white luster
Sodium (1807)	Na	11	22.9898	1	0.971	most abundant of alkali metals, sixth in abundance in earth's crust
Strontium (1808)	Sr	38	87.62	2	2.54	exists in 3 allotropic forms
Sulfur (prehistoric)	S	16	32.064	2,4,6	1.957, 2.07	exists in several isotopic and many allotropic forms
Tantalum (1802)	Ta	73	180.948	2?,3,4,5	16.6	gray, heavy, very hard metal
Technetium (1937)	Tc	43	98.9062	3?,4,6,7	11.50	first element produced artificially
Tellurium (1782)	Te	52	127.60	2,4,6	6.24	silvery-white, lustrous element
Terbium (1843)	Tb	65	158.924	3,4	8.272	silvery-gray, malleable, ductile rare earth metal
Thallium (1861)	Tl	81	204.37	1,3	11.85	very soft, malleable metal
Thorium (1828)	Th	90	232.038	4	11.66	silvery-white, lustrous metal
Thulium (1879)	Tm	69	168.934	2,3		least abundant rare earth metal
Tin (prehistoric)	Sn	50	118.69	2,4	5.75, 7.31	(gray) malleable metal existing in 2 or 3 allotropic forms, changing from white to gray on cooling and back to white on warming (white)
Titanium (1791)	Ti	22	47.90	2,3,4	4.54	lustrous white metal
Tungsten (1783)	W	74	183.85	2,3,4,5,6	19.3	steel-gray to tin-white metal
Uranium (1789)	U	92	238.03	3,4,5,6	18.95	heavy, silvery-white metal
Vanadium (1801)	V	23	50.942	2,3,4,5	6.11	bright, white metal
Xenon (1898)	Xe	54	131.30	0?	5.887 g/l	one of the so-called rare or inert gases
Ytterbium (1878)	Yb	70	173.04	2,3	6.977, 6.54	exists in 2 allotropic forms
Yttrium (1794)	Y	39	88.905	3	4.45	rare earth metal with silvery metallic luster
Zinc (1746)	Zn	30	65.37	2	7.133	bluish-white, lustrous metal, malleable at 100–150°C
Zirconium (1789)	Zr	40	91.22	4	6.4	grayish-white, lustrous metal

TABLE OF ELEMENTS BY ATOMIC NUMBERS

1 hydrogen	16 sulfur	31 gallium	46 palladium	61 promethium	76 osmium
2 helium	17 chlorine	32 germanium	47 silver	62 samarium	77 iridium
3 lithium	18 argon	33 arsenic	48 cadmium	63 europium	78 plantinum
4 beryllium	19 potassium	34 selenium	49 indium	64 gadolinium	79 gold
5 boron	20 calcium	35 bromine	50 tin	65 terbium	80 mercury
6 carbon	21 scandium	36 krypton	51 antimony	66 dysprosium	81 thallium
7 nitrogen	22 titanium	37 rubidium	52 tellurium	67 holmium	82 lead
8 oxygen	23 vanadium	38 strontium	53 iodine	68 erbium	83 bismuth
9 fluorine	24 chromium	39 yttrium	54 xenon	69 thulium	84 polonium
10 neon	25 manganese	40 zirconium	55 cesium	70 ytterbium	85 astatine
11 sodium	26 iron	41 niobium	56 barium	71 lutetium	86 radon
12 magnesium	27 cobalt	42 molybdenum	57 lanthanum	72 hafnium	87 francium
13 aluminum	28 nickel	43 technetium	58 cerium	73 tantalum	88 radium
14 silicon	29 copper	44 ruthenium	59 praseodymium	74 tungsten	89 actinium
15 phosphorus	30 zinc	45 rhodium	60 neodymium	75 rhenium	90 thorium
					91 protactinium
					92 uranium
					93 neptunium
					94 plutonium
					95 americium
					96 curium
					97 berkelium
					98 californium
					99 einsteinium
					100 fermium
					101 mendelevium
					102 nobelium
					103 lawrencium
					104 rutherfordium
					105 hahnium
					106 element 106

sion or extrusion, especially expulsion from the body. 2. omission or exclusion.

ELISA (e-li′sah) Enzyme-Linked Immuno-Sorbent Assay; any enzyme immunoassay using an enzyme-labeled immunoreactant and an immunosorbent.

elixir (ĭ-lik′ser) a clear, sweetened, usually hydroalcoholic liquid containing flavoring substances and sometimes active medicinal agents, for oral use.

Elixophyllin (e-lik″so-fil′in) trademark for preparations of theophylline.

elliptocytosis (ĭ-lip″to-si-to′sis) a hereditary disorder in which the erythrocytes are largely elliptical and in which there is increased red cell destruction and anemia.

eluate (el′u-āt) the substance separated out by, or the product of, elution or elutriation.

elution (e-loo′shin) in chemistry, separation of material by washing; the process of pulverizing substances and mixing them with water in order to separate the heavier constituents, which settle out in solution, from the lighter.

elutriation (e-loo″tre-a′shun) purification of a substance by dissolving it in a solvent and pouring off the solution, thus separating it from the undissolved foreign material.

Em. emmetropia.

emaciation (ĭ-ma″she-a′shin) excessive leanness; a wasted condition of the body.

emasculation (ĭ-mas″kūl-a′shin) removal of the penis or testes.

embalming (em-bahm′ing) treatment of a dead body to retard decomposition.

embarrass (em-bar′is) to impede the function of; to obstruct.

embedding (em-bed′ing) fixation of tissue in a firm medium, in order to keep it intact during cutting of thin sections.

embolectomy (em″bol-ek′tah-me) surgical removal of an embolus from a blood vessel.

emboli (em′bol-i) plural of *embolus.*

embolism (em′bol-izm) the sudden blocking of an artery by a clot or foreign material which has been brought to its site of lodgment by the blood current. **air e.,** that due to air bubbles entering the veins after trauma or surgical procedures. **cerebral e.,** embolism of a cerebral artery. **coronary e.,** embolism of a coronary artery. **fat e.,** obstruction by a fat embolus, occurring especially after fractures of large bones. **infective e.,** obstruction by an embolus containing bacteria or septic poison. **miliary e.,** embolism affecting many small blood vessels. **paradoxical e.,** blockage of a systemic artery by a thrombus originating in a systemic vein that has passed through a defect in the interatrial or interventricular septum. **pulmonary e.,** obstruction of the pulmonary artery or one of its branches by an embolus.

embolization (em″bol-ĭ-za′shin) 1. the process or condition of becoming an embolus. 2. therapeutic introduction of a substance into a vessel in order to occlude it. **poppet e.,** embolization of the ball of a poppet valve used as a heart valve prosthesis.

embolus (em′bol-us), pl. *em′boli* [L.] a clot or other plug brought by the blood from another vessel and forced into a smaller one, thus obstructing the circulation. **fat e.,** one composed of oil or fat. **saddle e.,** one at the bifurcation of an artery, blocking both branches.

emboly (em′bol-e) invagination of the blastula to form the gastrula.

embrasure (em-bra′zher) the interproximal space occlusal to the area of contact of adjacent teeth in the same dental arch.

embryectomy (em″bre-ek′tah-me) excision of an extrauterine embryo or fetus.

embryo (em′bre-o) 1. in animals, those derivatives of the fertilized ovum that eventually become the offspring, during their period of most rapid growth, i.e., after the long axis appears until all major structures are represented. In man, the developing organism from about two weeks after fertilization to the end of the seventh or eighth week. 2. in plants, the element of the seed that develops into a new individual. **em′bryonal, embryon′ic,** adj. **presomite e.,** the embryo at any stage before the appearance of the first somite. **previllous e.,** the embryo before the appearance of the chorionic villi. **somite e.,** the embryo between the appearance of the first and the last somites.

embryocardia (em″bre-o-kar′de-ah) a symptom in which the heart sounds resemble those of the fetus, there being very little difference in the quality of the first and second sounds.

embryogeny (em″bre-ah′jin-e) the origin or development of the embryo. **embryogenet′ic, embryogen′ic,** adj.

embryology (em″bre-ol′ah-je) the science of the development of the individual during the embryonic stage and, by extension, in several or even all preceding and subsequent stages of the life cycle. **embryolog′ic,** adj.

embryoma (em″bre-o′mah) a general term applied to neoplasms thought to be derived from embryonic cells or tissues, including dermoid cysts, teratomas, embryonal carcinomas, etc. **e. of kidney,** Wilms′ tumor.

embryopathy (em″bre-op′ah-the) a morbid condition of the embryo or a disorder resulting from abnormal embryonic development. **rubella e.,** rubella syndrome.

embryoplastic (em″bre-o-plas″tik) pertaining to or concerned in formation of an embryo.

embryotomy (em″bre-ot′o-me) dissection of the fetus in difficult labor.

embryotoxon (em″bre-o-tok′son) a ringlike opacity at the margin of the cornea. **anterior e.,** embryotoxon. **posterior e.,** a developmental anomaly in which there is a ringlike opacity at Schwalbe′s ring, with thickening and anterior displacement of the latter; it is seen in Axenfeld′s syndrome and Rieger′s syndrome.

embryotroph (em′bre-o-trōf″) the total nutriment (histotroph and hemotroph) made available to the embryo.

embryotrophy (em″bre-ah′truf-e) the nutrition of the early embryo.

emedullate (e-mĕ-dul′āt) to remove bone marrow.

emergent (e-mer′jint) 1. coming out from a cavity or other part. 2. coming on suddenly.

emery (em′er-e) an abrasive substance consisting of corundum and various impurities, such as iron oxide.

emesis (em′ĭ-sis) the act of vomiting. Also used as a word termination, as in *hematemesis*.

emetic (ĭ-met′ik) 1. causing vomiting. 2. an agent that causes vomiting.

emetine (em′ĭ-tēn) an alkaloid, $C_{29}H_{40}N_2O_4$, derived from ipecac or produced synthetically; its hydrochloride salt is used as an antiamebic.

emetocathartic (em″ĭ-to-kah-thart′ik) both emetic and cathartic; an emetocathartic agent.

E.M.F. electromotive force.

-emia word element [Gr.], *condition of the blood.*

emigration (em″ĭ-gra′shin) the escape of leukocytes through the walls of small blood vessels; diapedesis.

eminence (em′ĭ-nins) a projection or boss.

eminentia (em″ĭ-nen′she-ah), pl. *eminen′tiae* [L.] eminence.

emiocytosis (e″me-o-si-to′sis) the ejection of material, e.g., insulin granules, from a cell.

emissary (em′ĭ-sĕ-re) affording an outlet, referring especially to the venous outlets from the dural sinuses through the skull.

emission (e-mish′in) a discharge; specifically an involuntary discharge of semen. **nocturnal e.,** reflex emission of semen during sleep.

emmenagogue (ĕ-men′ah-gog) an agent or measure that promotes menstruation.

emmenia (ĕ-me′ne-ah) the menses. **emmen′ic,** adj.

emmenology (em″ĭ-nol′ah-je) the sum of knowledge about menstruation and its disorders.

emmetropia (em″ĭ-tro′pe-ah) the ideal optical condition, parallel rays coming to a focus on the retina. **emmetrop′ic,** adj.

Emmonsia (ĕ-mon′se-ah) a genus of imperfect, saprophytic, soil fungi; two species, *E. cres′cens* and *E. par′va,* cause adiospiromycosis in rodents and man.

emollient (e-mol′yent) 1. softening or soothing. 2. an agent that softens or soothes the skin, or soothes an irritated internal surface.

emotion (e-mo′shin) a state of mental excitement characterized by alteration of feeling tone and by physiological and behavorial changes.

empathy (em′pah-the) the recognition of and entering into another's feelings. **empath′ic,** adj.

emperipolesis (em-per″ĭ-pol-e′sis) lymphocytic penetration of and movement within another cell.

emphysema (em″fĭ-se′mah) 1. a pathologic accumulation of air in tissues or organs. 2. pulmonary e. **atrophic e.,** overdistention and stretching of lung tissues due to atrophic changes. **bullous e.,** single or multiple large cystic alveolar dilatations of lung tissue. **centriacinar e., centrilobular e.,** focal dilatations of the respiratory bronchioles rather than alveoli, distributed throughout the lung in the midst of grossly normal lung tissue. **hypoplastic e.,** pulmonary emphysema due to a developmental abnormality, resulting in reduced number of alveoli, which are abnormally large. **interlobular e.,** accumulation of air in the septa between lobules of the lungs. **interstitial e.,** presence of air in the peribronchial and interstitial tissues of the lungs. **intestinal e.,** a condition marked by accumulation of gas under the serous tunic of the intestine. **lobar e., congenital, lobar e., infantile,** a condition characterized by overinflation, commonly affecting one of the upper lobes and causing respiratory distress in early life. **mediastinal e.,** pneumomediastinum. **obstructive e.,** overinflation of the lungs associated with partial bronchial obstruction which interferes with exhalation. **panacinar e., panlobular e.,** generalized obstructive emphysema affecting all lung segments, with atrophy and dilatation of the alveoli and destruction of the vascular bed. **pulmonary e.,** increase beyond normal in the size of the air space in the lungs distal to the terminal bronchioles. **subcutaneous e.,** the presence of air or gas in subcutaneous tissues. **surgical e.,** subcutaneous emphysema following an operation. **vesicular e.,** panacinar e.

empiricism (em-pir′ĭ-sizm) skill or knowledge based entirely on experience. **empir′ic, empir′ical,** adj.

Empirin (em′pĭ-rin) trademark for tablets containing acetylsalicylic acid, phenacetin, and caffeine.

emprosthotonos (em″pros-thot′ah-nos) tetanic forward flexure of the body.

empyema (em″pi-e′mah) accumulation of pus in a body cavity. **empye′mic,** adj.

emulgent (ĭ-mul′jint) 1. effecting a straining or purifying process. 2. a renal artery or vein. 3. a medicine that stimulates bile or urine flow.

emulsion (ĭ-mul′shin) a mixture of two immiscible liquids, one being dispersed throughout the other in small droplets; a colloid system in which both the dispersed phase and the dispersion medium are liquids.

emulsoid (ĭ-mul′soid) a colloid system in which the dispersion medium is liquid, usually water, and the disperse phase consists of highly complex organic substances, such as starch or glue, which absorb much water, swell, and become distributed throughout the dispersion medium.

E-Mycin (e-mi′sin) trademark for a preparation of erthromycin.

enamel (ĭ-nam′l) the white, compact, and very hard substance covering and protecting the dentin of a tooth crown.

enameloma (ĭn-am″il-o′mah) a small spherical nodule of enamel attached to a tooth at the cervical line or on the root.

enamelum (e-nam′el-um) [L.] enamel.

enanthate (en-an-thāt) USAN contraction of heptanoate.

enanthema (en″an-the′ma) an eruption upon a mucous surface. **enanthem′atous,** adj.

enantiobiosis (en-an″te-o-bio′sis) commensalism in which the associated organisms are mutually antagonistic.

enantiomorph (en-an′te-o-morf″) one of a pair

of isomeric substances, the structures of which are mirror opposites of each other.

enarthrosis (en″ar-thro′sis) a joint in which the rounded head of one bone is received into a socket in another, as in the hip bone.

encephal(o)- word element [Gr.], *brain.*

encephalalgia (en″sef-il-al′je-ah) pain within the head.

encephalatrophy (en″sef-il-ă′trof-e) atrophy of the brain.

encephalic (en″sĭ-fal′ik) 1. pertaining to the encephalon. 2. within the skull.

encephalitis (en″sef-il-īt′is) inflammation of the brain. **encephalit′ic,** adj. **acute disseminated e.,** postinfection e. **Economo's e.,** lethargic e. **equine e.,** 1. see under *encephalomyelitis.* 2. Borna disease. **herpes e.,** that caused by herpesvirus, resembling equine encephalomyelitis. **Japanese B e.,** a form of epidemic encephalitis of varying severity occurring in Japan and other Pacific islands, China, U.S.S.R., and probably much of the Far East. **lead e.,** encephalitis with cerebral edema due to lead poisoning. **lethargic e.,** a form of epidemic encephalitis characterized by increasing languor, apathy, and drowsiness. **postinfectious e., postvaccinal e.,** acute disseminated encephalomyelitis. **St. Louis e.,** a viral disease first observed in Illinois in 1932, closely resembling western equine encephalomyelitis clinically; it is usually transmitted by certain mosquitoes.

encephalitogenic (en″sef-il-it-ah-jen′ik) causing encephalitis.

encephalocele (en-sef′il-o-sēl″) hernial protrusion of brain substance through a congenital or traumatic opening of the skull.

encephalocystocele (en-sef″il-o-sis′tah-sēl) hernial protrusion of the brain distended by fluid.

encephalography (en-sef″il-og′rah-fe) roentgenography demonstrating the intracranial fluid-containing spaces after the withdrawal of cerebrospinal fluid and introduction of air or other gas; it includes pneumoencephalography and ventriculography.

encephaloid (en-sef′il-oid) 1. resembling brain or brain substance. 2. medullary carcinoma.

encephalolith (en-sef′il-o-lith″) a brain calculus.

encephalology (en-sef″il-ol′ah-je) the sum of knowledge regarding the brain, its functions, and its diseases.

encephaloma (en-sef″il-o′mah) 1. any swelling or tumor of the brain. 2. medullary carcinoma.

encephalomalacia (en-sef″il-o-mul-a′she-ah) softening of the brain.

encephalomeningitis (-men″in-jīt′is) meningoencephalitis.

encephalomeningocele (-mĕ-ning′go-sēl) meningocephalocele.

encephalomere (en-sef′il-o-mēr″) one of the segments making up the embryonic brain.

encephalometer (en″sef-ilom′it-er) an instrument used in locating certain of the brain regions.

encephalomyelitis (en-sef″ilo-mi″il-īt′is) inflammation of the brain and spinal cord. **acute disseminated e.,** inflammation of the brain and spinal cord after infection (especially measles) or, formerly, rabies vaccination. **benign myalgic e.,** a disease, usually occurring in epidemics, characterized by headache, fever, myalgia, muscular weakness, and emotional lability. **equine e.,** see *equine e., eastern, Venezuelan,* and *western.* **equine e., eastern,** a viral disease similar to western equine encephalomyelitis, but occurring in a region extending from New Hampshire to Texas and as far west as Wisconsin, and in Canada, Mexico, the Carribean, and parts of Central and South America. **equine e., Venezuelan,** a viral disease of horses and mules; the infection in man resembles influenza, with little or no indication of nervous system involvement; the causative agent was first isolated in Venezuela. **equine e., western,** a viral disease of horses and mules, communicable to man, occurring chiefly as a meningoencephalitis, with little involvement of the medulla or spinal cord; observed in the United States chiefly west of the Mississippi River. **infectious porcine e.,** a highly fatal disease of swine, due to a picornavirus, marked by flaccid ascending paralysis. **postinfectious e., postvaccinal e.,** acute disseminated e.

encephalomyeloneuropathy (-mi″il-o-nōōr-op′ah-the) a disease involving the brain, spinal cord, and peripheral nerves.

encephalomyeloradiculitis (-mi″il-o-rah-dik″ūl-īt′is) inflammation of the brain, spinal cord, and spinal nerve roots.

encephalomyeloradiculopathy (-mi″il-o-rah-dik″ūl-op′ah-the) a disease involving the brain, spinal cord, and spinal nerve roots.

encephalomyocarditis (-mi″o-kard-īt′is) a viral disease marked by degenerative and inflammatory changes in skeletal and cardiac muscle and by central lesions resembling those of poliomyelitis.

encephalon (en-sef′ah-lon) the brain.

encephalopathy (en-sef″il-op′ah-the) any degenerative brain disease. **biliary e., bilirubin e.,** kernicterus. **dialysis e.,** a degenerative disease of the brain associated with long-term use of hemodialysis, marked by speech disorders and constant myoclonic jerks, progressing to global dementia. **hepatic e.,** a condition, usually occurring secondarily to advanced liver disease, marked by disturbances of consciousness that may progress to deep coma (hepatic coma), psychiatric changes of varying degree, flapping tremor, and fetor hepaticus. **lead e.,** brain disease caused by lead poisoning. **myoclonic e. of childhood,** a neurologic disorder of unknown etiology with onset between ages 1 and 3, characterized by myoclonus of trunk and limbs and by opsoclonus with ataxia of gait, and intention tremor; some cases have been associated with occult neuroblastoma. **Wernicke's e.,** an inflammatory hemorrhagic form due to thiamine deficiency associated with chronic alcoholism, but also occurring as a complication of certain other diseases, with paralysis of the eye muscles, diplopia, nystagmus, ataxia, and mental changes ranging from deterioration and forgetfulness to delirium tremens and Korsakoff's psychosis.

encephalopyosis (-pi-o′sis) suppuration or abscess of the brain.

encephalorrhagia (-ra′je-ah) hemorrhage within or from the brain.

encephalosis (en″sef-ilo′sis) any organic brain disease.

encephalotomy (-lot′ah-me) 1. craniotomy (2). 2. dissection or anatomy of the brain.

enchondroma (en″kon-dro′mah) a benign growth of cartilage arising in the metaphysis of a bone. **enchondro′matous,** adj.

enclave (en′klāv) tissue detached from its normal connection and enclosed within another organ.

enclitic (en-klit′ik) having the planes of the fetal head inclined to those of the maternal pelvis.

encopresis (en″ko-pre′sis) incontinence of feces not due to organic defect or illness.

encyesis (en-si-e′sis) normal uterine pregnancy.

encyopyelitis (en-si″o-pi-il-īt′is) dilatation and edema of the ureters and renal pelvis during normal pregnancy, but seldom with all the classic signs of inflammation.

encysted (en-sist′id) enclosed in a sac, bladder, or cyst.

end(o)- word element [Gr.], *within; inward.*

endangium (en-dan′je-um) tunica intima (inner coat) of a blood vessel.

endaortitis (en″da-or-tīt′is) inflammation of the membrane lining the aorta.

endarterectomy (en″dart-er-ek′tah-me) excision of thickened atheromatous areas of the innermost coat of an artery.

endarteritis (en″dart-er-īt′is) inflammation of the innermost coat (tunica intima) of an artery.

end-artery (end-art′er-e) an artery that does not anastomose with other arteries.

endaural (-aw′r′l) within the ear.

end-body (end′bod-e) end-piece.

endbrain (-brān) telencephalon.

end-bulb (-bulb) one of the small encapsulated bodies at the end of sensory nerve fibers in skin, mucous membranes, muscles, and other areas.

endemic (en-dem′ik) 1. present in a community at all times. 2. a disease of low morbidity that is constantly present in a human community, but clinically recognizable in only a few.

endemoepidemic (en″de-mo-ep″ĭ-dem′ik) endemic, but occasionally becoming epidemic.

endergonic (en″der-gon′ik) characterized or accompanied by the absorption of energy; requiring the input of free energy.

end-feet (end′fēt) button- or knoblike terminal enlargements of naked nerve fibers which end in relation to dendrites of another cell.

endoaneurysmorrhaphy (en″do-an″u-riz-mor′ah-fe) opening of an aneurysmal sac and suture of the orifices.

endoappendicitis (-ah-pen″dĭ-sīt′is) inflammation of the mucous membrane of the vermiform appendix.

endoblast (en′do-blast) entoderm.

endobronchitis (en″do-brong-kīt′is) inflammation of the epithelial lining of the bronchi.

endocardial (-kard′e-il) 1. situated or occurring within the heart. 2. pertaining to the endocardium.

endocarditis (-kard-īt′is) exudative and proliferative inflammatory alterations of the endocardium, characterized by the presence of vegetations on the surface of the endocardium or in the endocardium itself, and most commonly involving a heart valve, but also affecting the inner lining of the cardiac chambers or the endocardium elsewhere. **endocardit′ic,** adj. **atypical verrucous e.,** nonbacterial endocarditis found in association with systemic lupus erythematosus. **bacterial e.,** infectious, endocarditis, acute or subacute, caused by various bacteria, including streptococci, staphylococci, enterococci, gonococci, gram-negative bacilli, etc. **infectious e., infective e.,** that due to infection with microorganisms, especially bacteria and fungi: the *acute* form may be due to staphylococci, pneumococci, gonococci, streptococci, and other bacteria or to other microorganisms; the *subacute* form may be caused by viridans streptococci, fungi, or other microorganisms. **Löffler's e., Löffler's parietal fibroplastic e.,** endocarditis associated with eosinophilia, marked by fibroplastic thickening of the endocardium, resulting in congestive heart failure, persistent tachycardia, hepatomegaly, splenomegaly, serous effusions into the pleural cavity, and edema of the limbs. **mycotic e.,** infectious endocarditis, usually subacute, due to various fungi, most commonly *Candida, Aspergillus,* and *Histoplasma.* **nonbacterial thrombotic e.,** that in which the vegetations, single or multiple, consist of fibrin and other blood elements. **prosthetic valve e.,** infectious endocarditis as a complication of implantation of a prosthetic valve in the heart; the vegetations usually occur along the line of suture. **rheumatic e.,** that associated with rheumatic fever. **rickettsial e.,** endocarditis caused by invasion of the heart valves with *Coxiella burnetii;* it is a sequela of Q fever, usually occurring in persons who have had rheumatic fever. **vegetative e., verrucous e.,** endocarditis, infectious or noninfectious, the characteristic lesions of which are vegetations or verrucae on the endocardium.

endocardium (en″do-kard′e-um) the endothelial lining membrane of the cavities of the heart and the connective tissue bed on which it lies.

endocervix (-serv′iks) 1. the mucous membrane lining the canal of the cervix uteri. 2. the region of the opening of the cervix into the uterine cavity. **endocer′vical,** adj.

endochondral (-kon′dril) situated, formed, or occurring within cartilage.

endocolitis (-kol-īt′is) inflammation of the mucous membrane of the colon.

endocranium (-kra′ne-um) the endosteal layer of the dura mater of the brain.

endocrine (en′dah-krin) 1. secreting internally. 2. pertaining to internal secretions; hormonal. See also under *system.*

endocrinologist (en″dah-krĭ-nol′ah-jist) an individual skilled in endocrinology, and in the diagnosis and treatment of disorders of the glands of internal secretion, i.e., the endocrine glands.

endocrinopathy (en″dah-krĭ-nop′ah-the) any disease due to disorder of the endocrine system. **endocrinopath′ic,** adj.

endocystitis (-sis-tīt′is) inflammation of the bladder mucosa.

endocytosis (-si-to′sis) the uptake by a cell of material from the environment by invagination of its plasma membrane; it includes both phagocytosis and pinocytosis.

endoderm (en′do-derm) entoderm.

Endodermophyton (en″do-der-mof′ĭ-ton) *Trichophyton.*

endodontics (-don′tiks) the branch of dentistry concerned with the etiology, prevention, diagnosis, and treatment of conditions that affect the tooth pulp, root, and periapical tissues.

endodontium (-don′she-um) dental pulp.

endodontology (-don-tol′ah-je) endodontics.

endoenteritis (-ent″er-īt′is) inflammation of the intestinal mucosa.

endogamy (en-dog′ah-me) 1. fertilization by union of separate cells having the same chromatin ancestry. 2. restriction of marriage to persons within the same community. **endog′amous,** adj.

endogenous (en-dah′jin-is) produced within or caused by factors within the organism.

endolaryngeal (-lah-rin′je-il) situated or occurring within the larynx.

endolymph (en′do-limf) the fluid within the membranous labyrinth. **endolymphat′ic,** adj.

endolysin (en-dol′ĭ-sin) a bactericidal substance in cells, acting directly on bacteria.

endometrial (en″do-me′tre-il) pertaining to the endometrium.

endometrioma (-me″tre-o′mah) a solitary non-neoplastic mass containing endometrial tissue.

endometriosis (-me″tre-o′sis) the aberrant occurrence of tissue which more or less perfectly resembles the endometrium, in various locations in the pelvic cavity. **endometriot′ic,** adj. **e. exter′na,** endometriosis. **e. inter′na,** adenomyosis. **ovarian e.,** that involving the ovary, either in the form of small superficial islands or in the form of epithelial ("chocolate") cysts of various sizes.

endometritis (-me-trīt′is) inflammation of the endometrium. **puerperal e.,** that following childbirth. **syncytial e.,** a benign tumor-like lesion with infiltration of the uterine wall by large syncytial trophoblastic cells. **tuberculous e.,** inflammation of the endometrium, usually also involving the uterine tubes, due to infection by *Mycobacterium tuberculosis,* with the presence of tubercles.

endometrium (-me′tre-um) the mucous membrane lining the uterus.

endomitosis (-mi-to′sis) reproduction of nuclear elements not followed by chromosome movements and cytoplasmic division. **endomitot′ic,** adj.

endomorph (en′do-morf) an individual having the type of body build in which entodermal tissues predominate: there is relative preponderance of soft roundness throughout the body, with large digestive viscera and fat accumulations, and with large trunk and thighs and tapering extremities.

endomysium (-mis′e-um) the sheath of delicate reticular fibrils surrounding each muscle fiber.

endoneuritis (-noōr-īt′is) inflammation of the endoneurium.

endoneurium (-noōr′e-um) the interstitial connective tissue in a peripheral nerve, separating individual nerve fibers. **endoneu′rial,** adj.

endonuclease (-nu′kle - ās) a nuclease that cleaves internal bonds of polynucleotides. **restriction e's,** enzymes that cleave large DNA molecules at specific sequences of four to six nucleotides.

endopelvic (-pel′vik) within the pelvis.

endopeptidase (-pep′tĭ-dās) a peptidase capable of acting on any peptide linkage in a peptide chain.

endopericarditis (-per″ĭ-kar-dīt′is) inflammation of the endocardium and pericardium.

endoperitonitis (-per″ĭ-ton-īt′is) inflammation of the serous lining of peritoneal cavity.

endophthalmitis (en″dof-thal-mīt′is) inflammation of the ocular cavities and their adjacent structures.

endophyte (en′do-fit) a parasitic plant organism living within its host's body.

endophytic (en″do-fit′ik) 1. pertaining to an endophyte. 2. growing inward; proliferating on the interior of an organ or structure.

endopolyploid (en″do-pol′ĭ-ploid) having reduplicated chromatin within an intact nucleus, with or without an increase in the number of chromosomes (applied only to cells and tissues).

endoreduplication (-re-doōp″lĭ-ka′shin) replication of chromosomes without subsequent cell division.

end organ (end″or′gin) one of the larger, encapsulated endings of sensory nerves.

endorphin (en-dor′fin) any of a group of endogenous polypeptide brain substances that bind to opiate receptors in various areas of the brain and thereby raise the pain threshold.

endosalpingoma (-sal″ping-go′mah) adenomyoma of the uterine tube.

endosalpingosis (-sal″ping-go′sis) 1. endometriosis involving the uterine tube. 2. ovarian endometriosis in which the abnormal mucosa resembles tubal mucosa rather than endometrium.

endoscope (en′do-skōp) an instrument for examining the interior of a hollow viscus.

endoscopy (en-dos′kah-pe) visual examination by means of an endoscope. **endoscop′ic,** adj. **peroral e.,** examination of organs accessible to observation through an endoscope passed through the mouth.

endoskeleton (en″do-skel′it-in) the cartilaginous and bony skeleton of the body, exclusive of that part of the skeleton of dermal origin.

endosmosis (en″dos-mo′sis) inward osmosis; inward passage of liquid through a membrane of a cell or cavity. **endosmot′ic,** adj.

endosome (en'do-sōm) a body thought to consist of deoxyribonucleic acid, observed in the vesicular nucleus of certain protozoa.

endosteal (en-dos'te-il) 1. pertaining to the endosteum. 2. occurring or located within a bone.

endosteoma (en-dos"te-o'mah) a tumor in the medullary cavity of a bone.

endosteum (en-dos'te-um) the tissue lining the medullary cavity of a bone.

endotendineum (en"do-ten-din'e-um) the delicate connective tissue separating the secondry bundles (fascicles) of a tendon.

endothelia (-thēl'e-ah) [Gr.] plural of *endothelium.*

endothelial (-thēl'e-il) pertaining to or made up of endothelium.

endothelioblastoma (en"do-thēl"e-o-blas-to'mah) a tumor derived from primitive vasoformative tissue, it includes hemangioendothelioma, angiosarcoma, lymphangioendothelioma, and lymphangiosarcoma.

endotheliochorial (-thēl"e-o-kor'e-il) denoting a type of placenta in which syncytial trophoblast embeds maternal vessels bared to their endothelial lining.

endotheliocyte (-thēl'e-o-sīt") endothelial leukocyte.

endothelioma (-thēl"e-o'mah) a tumor arising from the endothelial lining of blood vessels.

endotheliomatosis (-thēl"e-o"mah-to'sis) formation of multiple, diffuse endotheliomas.

endothelium (-thēl'e-um), pl. *endothe'lia* [Gr.] the layer of epithelial cells that lines the cavities of the heart and of the blood and lymph vessels, and the serous cavities of the body.

endothermal, endothermic (-ther'mil; -ther'-mik) 1. characterized by the absorption of heat. 2. pertaining to diathermy.

endothrix (-thriks) a dermatophyte whose growth and spore production are confined chiefly within the hair shaft.

endotoxemia (en"do-toks-ēm'e-ah) the presence of endotoxins in the blood, which may result in shock.

endotoxin (-tok'sin) a heat-stable toxin present in the intact bacterial cell but not in cell-free filtrates of cultures of intact bacteria. Endotoxins are lipopolysaccharide complexes that occur in the cell wall; they are pyrogenic and increase capillary permeability.

endotrachelitis (-tra"kil-īt'is) endocervicitis.

endovasculitis (-vas"kūl-īt'is) endangiitis.

end plate (end-plāt) a flattened expansion at the myoneural junction, where a myelinated motor nerve fiber joins a skeletal muscle fiber.

endrin (en'drin) a highly toxic insecticide of the chlorinated hydrocarbon group.

Enduron (en'du-ron) trademark for a preparation of methyclothiazide.

enema (en'ĭ-mah) 1. introduction of fluid into the rectum. 2. a solution introduced into the rectum to promote evacuation of feces or as a means of introducing nutrient or medicinal substances, or opaque material in roentgen examination of the lower intestinal tract. **analep-**tic e., an enema consisting of a pint of tepid water containing ½ teaspoonful of salt. **barium e., contrast e.,** a suspension of barium injected into and retained in the intestines during roentgenographic examination; intestinal deformities are demonstrated by filling defects revealed by the column of radiopaque barium. **double contrast e.,** injection and evacuation of a barium suspension, followed by inflation of the intestines with air, to facilitate roentgen visualization of the intestinal mucosa. **Fleet e.,** trademark for an enema containing, in each 100 ml., 16 gm. sodium biphosphate and 6 gm. sodium phosphate, packaged in a plastic squeeze bottle fitted with a 2-inch, prelubricated rectal tube.

energy (en'er-je) power which may be translated into motion, overcoming resistance, or effecting physical change; the ability to do work. **free e.,** the energy equal to the maximum amount of work that can be obtained from a process occurring under conditions of fixed temperature and pressure. **kinetic e.,** the energy of motion. **nuclear e.,** energy that can be liberated by changes in the nucleus of an atom (as by fission of a heavy nucleus or fusion of light nuclei into heavier ones with accompanying loss of mass). **potential e.,** energy at rest or not manifested in actual work.

enervation (en"er-va'shin) 1. lack of nervous energy. 2. removal of a nerve or a section of a nerve.

ENG electronystagmography.

engagement (en-gāj'mint) the entrance of the fetal head or presenting part into the superior pelvic strait.

engorgement (en-gorj'mint) local congestion; distention with fluids; hyperemia.

enhancement (en-hans'mint) immunologic enhancement; prolonged survival of tumor cells in animals immunized with antigens of the tumor because of "enhancing" or "facilitating" antibodies preventing an immune response against these antigens.

enkatarrhaphy (en"kah-tar'ah-fe) the operation of burying a structure by suturing together the sides of tissues adjacent to it.

enkephalin (en-kef'ah-lin) either of two pentapeptides (methionine e. and leucine e.) isolated from the brain that have potent opiate-like effects and probably serve as neurotransmitters.

enol (e'nol) one of two tautomeric forms of a substance, the other being the keto form; the enol is formed from the keto by migration of hydrogen from the adjacent carbon atom to the carbonyl group.

enolase (e'no-lās) an enzyme in glycolytic systems that changes phosphoglyceric acid into phosphopyruvic acid.

enostosis (en"os-to'sis) a morbid bony growth within a bone cavity or on the internal surface of the bone cortex.

ensiform (en'sĭ-form) sword-shaped; xiphoid.

enstrophe (en'stro-fe) inversion, especially of the margin of the eyelids.

E.N.T. ear, nose, and throat.

entad (en'tad) toward a center; inwardly.

entamebiasis (en''tah-me-bi'ah-sis) infection by *Entamoeba*.

Entamoeba (en''tah-me'bah) a genus of amebas parasitic in the intestines of vertebrates, including three species commonly parasitic in man: *E. co'li,* found in the intestinal tract; *E. gingiva'lis* (*E. bucca'lis*), found in the mouth; and *E. histoly'tica,* the cause of amebic dysentery and tropical abscess of the liver.

entasia (en-ta'ze-ah) a constrictive spasm; tonic spasm.

enter(o)- word element [Gr.], *intestines.*

enteralgia (en''ter-al'je-ah) pain in the intestine.

enterepiplocele (-e-pip'lo-sēl) enteroepiplocele.

enteric (en-tĕ'rik) pertaining to the small intestine.

enteric-coated (en-tĕ''rik-kōt'id) designating a special coating applied to tablets or capsules that prevents release and absorption of active ingredients until they reach the intestine.

enteritis (en''ter-īt'is) inflammation of the intestine, especially of the small intestine.

Enterobacteriaceae (-bak-tēr''e-a'se-e) a family of gram-negative, rod-shaped bacteria (order Eubacteriales) occurring as plant or animal parasites or as saprophytes.

enterobiasis (-bi'ah-sis) infection with nematodes of the genus *Enterobius,* especially *E. vermicularis.*

Enterobius (en''ter-o'be-us) a genus of intestinal nematodes (superfamily Oxyuroidea), including *E. vermicula'ris,* the seatworm or pinworm, parasitic in the upper large intestine, and occasionally in the female genitals and bladder; infection is frequent in children, sometimes causing itching.

enterocele (en'ter-o-sēl'') intestinal hernia.

enterocentesis (en''ter-o-sen-te'sis) surgical puncture of the intestine.

enteroclysis (en''ter-ok'lĭ-sis) the injection of liquids into the intestine.

enterococcus (en''ter-o-kok'us), pl. *enterococ'ci* [Gr.] any streptococcus of the human intestine.

enterocolectomy (-kol-ek'tah-me) resection of the intestine, including the ileum, cecum, and colon.

enterocolitis (-kol-īt'is) inflammation of the small intestine and colon. **antibiotic-associated e.,** that in which treatment with antibiotics alters the bowel flora and results in diarrhea or pseudomembranous enterocolitis. **hemorrhagic e.,** enterocolitis characterized by hemorrhagic breakdown of the intestinal mucosa, with inflammatory cell infiltration. **necrotizing e., pseudomembranous e.,** an acute inflammation of the bowel mucosa with the formation of pseudomembranous plaques overlying an area of superficial ulceration, with passage of the pseudomembranous material in the feces; it may result from shock and ischemia or be associated with antibiotic therapy.

enterocutaneous (-ku-ta'ne-us) pertaining to or communicating with the intestine and the skin, or surface of the body.

enterocyst (en'ter-o-sist'') a cyst proceeding from subperitoneal tissue.

enterocystoma (-sis-to'mah) vitelline cyst.

enteroenterostomy (-en''ter-os''tah-me) surgical anastomosis between two segments of the intestine.

enteroepiplocele (en''ter-o-ĕ-pip'lah-sēl) hernia of the small intestine and omentum.

enterogastrone (-gas'trōn) anthelone E; a hormone of the duodenum which mediates the humoral inhibition of gastric secretion and motility produced by ingestion of fat.

enterogenous (en''ter-ah'jin-is) 1. arising from the primitive foregut. 2. originating within the small intestine.

enteroglucagon (en''ter-o-gloo'kah-gon) a glucagon-like hyperglycemic agent released by the mucosa of the upper intestine in response to the ingestion of glucose; immunologically distinct from pancreatic glucagon but with similar activities.

enterography (en''ter-og'rah-fe) a description of the intestine.

enterohepatitis (en''ter-o-hep''ah-tīt'is) 1. inflammation of the intestine and liver. 2. histomoniasis of turkeys.

enterohepatocele (-hep'it-i-sēl'') an umbilical hernia containing intestine and liver.

enterohydrocele (-hi'drah-sēl) hernia with hydrocele.

enterokinesia (-ki''ne'se-ah) peristalsis. **enterokinet'ic,** adj.

enterolith (en'ter-o-lith'') a calculus in the intestine.

enterology (en''ter-ol'ah-je) scientific study of the intestine.

enterolysis (en''ter-ol'ĭ-sis) surgical separation of intestinal adhesions.

enteromerocele (-me'rah-sēl) femoral hernia.

enteromycosis (-mi-ko'sis) fungal disease of the intestine.

enteron (en'ter-on) the gut or alimentary canal; usually used in medicine with specific reference to the small intestine.

enteroparesis (en''ter-o-pah-re'sis, -pă'rĭ-sis) relaxation of the intestine resulting in dilatation.

enteropathogenesis (-path''ah-jen'ĭ-sis) the production of disease or disorder of the intestine.

enteropathy (en''ter-op'ah-the) any disease of the intestine. **gluten e.,** nontropical sprue.

enteropeptidase (en''ter-o-pep'tĭ-dās) an enzyme of the intestinal juice which activates the proteolytic enzyme of the pancreatic juice by converting trypsinogen into trypsin.

enteropexy (en'ter-o-pek''se) surgical fixation of the intestine to the abdominal wall.

enteroplasty (-plas''te) plastic repair of the intestine.

enteroplegia (en''ter-o-ple'je-ah) adynamic ileus.

enteroptosis (en''ter-op-to'sis) abnormal downward displacement of the intestine. **enteroptot'ic,** adj.

enterorrhagia (en″ter-o-ra′je-ah) intestinal hemorrhage.

enterorrhexis (en″ter-o-rek′sis) rupture of the intestine.

enteroscope (en′ter-ah-skōp″) an instrument for inspecting the inside of the intestine.

enterosepsis (en″ter-o-sep′sis) sepsis developed from the intestinal contents.

enterostaxis (-stak′sis) slow hemorrhage through the intestinal mucosa.

enterostenosis (-stĕ-no′sis) narrowing or stricture of the intestine.

enterostomy (en″ter-os′tah-me) formation of a permanent opening into the intestine through the abdominal wall. **enterosto′mal,** adj.

enterotoxemia (en″ter-o-tok-se′me-ah) a condition characterized by the presence in the blood of toxins produced in the intestines.

enterotoxin (-tok′sin) 1. a toxin specific for the cells of the intestinal mucosa. 2. a toxin arising in the intestine. 3. an exotoxin that is protein in nature and relatively heat-stable, produced by staphylococci.

enterotoxism (-tok′sizm) autointoxication of enteric origin.

enterotropic (-trop′ik) affecting the intestine.

enterovaginal (-vaj′ĭ-nil) pertaining to or communicating with the intestine and the vagina.

enterovenous (-ve′nis) communicating between the intestinal lumen and the lumen of a vein.

enterovesical (-ves′ĭ-k'l) pertaining to or communicating with the intestine and urinary bladder.

enterovirus (-vi′ris) one of a subgroup of the picornaviruses infecting the gastrointestinal tract and discharged in the excreta, including coxsackieviruses, echoviruses, and polioviruses. **enterovi′ral,** adj.

enterozoon (-zo′on) an animal parasite in the intestine. **enterozo′ic,** adj.

enthalpy (en′thal-pe) the heat content or chemical energy of a physical system; a thermodynamic function equal to the internal energy plus the product of the pressure and volume.

enthesis (en′thĭ-sis) 1. the use of artificial material in the repair of a defect or deformity of the body. 2. the site of attachment of a muscle or ligament to bone.

enthesopathy (en-thĕ-sop′ah-the) disorder of the muscular or tendinous attachment to bone.

enthetobiosis (en-thet″o-bi-o′sis) dependency on a mechanical implant, as on an artificial cardiac pacemaker.

ento- word element [Gr.], *within; inner.*

entoblast (en′to-blast) the entoderm.

entochoroidea (en″to-kor-oi′de-ah) the inner layer of the choroid.

entocornea (en″to-kor′ne-ah) Descemet's membrane.

entoderm (en′to-derm) the innermost of the three primitive germ layers of the embryo; from it are derived the epithelium of the pharynx, respiratory tract (except the nose), digestive tract, bladder, and urethra. **entoder′mal, entoder′mic,** adj.

entomion (en-to′me-on) the tip of mastoid angle of parietal bone.

entomology (en″tah-mol′ah-je) that branch of biology concerned with the study of insects.

entomophilous (-mof′ĭ-lus) fertilized by insect-borne pollen; said of certain flowers.

entopic (en-top′ik) occurring in the proper place.

entoptic (en-top′tik) originating within the eye.

entoptoscopy (en″top-tos′kah-pe) inspection of the interior of the eye.

entoretina (en″to-ret′ĭ-nah) the nervous or inner layer of the retina.

entozoon (en″to-zo′on) an internal animal parasite. **entozo′ic,** adj.

entropion (en-tro′pe-on) inversion, or the turning inward, as of the margin of an eyelid.

entropy (en′tro-pe) the measure of that part of the heat or energy of a system not available to perform work; entropy increases in all natural (spontaneous and irreversible) processes.

entypy (en′tĭ-pe) a method of gastrulation in which the entoderm lies external to the amniotic ectoderm.

enucleation (e-noo″kle-a′shin) removal of an organ or other mass intact from its supporting tissues, as of the eyeball from the orbit.

enuresis (en″ūr-e′sis) involuntary discharge of urine; usually referring to involuntary discharge of urine during sleep at night. **enuret′ic,** adj.

envelope (en′vah-lōp) an encompassing structure or membrane. In virology, a coat surrounding the capsid and usually furnished at least partially by the host cell. In bacteriology, the cell wall and the plasma membrane considered together. **nuclear e.,** the condensed double layer of lipids and proteins enclosing the cell nucleus and separating it from the cytoplasm; its two concentric membranes, inner and outer, are separated by a perinuclear space.

envenomation (en-ven″im-a′shin) the poisonous effects caused by the bites, stings, or effluvia of insects and other arthropods, or the bites of snakes.

environment (en-vi′rin-mint) the sum total of all the conditions and elements that make up the surroundings and influence the development of an individual.

enzootic (en″zo-ot′ik) 1. present in an animal community at all times, but occurring in only small numbers of cases. 2. a disease of low morbidity which is constantly present in an animal community.

enzygotic (en″zi-got′ik) developed from one zygote.

enzyme (en′zīm) a protein produced in a cell and capable of greatly accelerating by its catalytic action the chemical reaction of a substance (the substrate) for which it is often specific. Enzymes perform this function without being destroyed or altered. They are divided into six main groups: oxidoreductases, transferases, hydrolases, lyases, isomerases, and ligases. **allosteric e.,** one containing an allosteric site; see under *site.* **brancher e., branching e.,** α-glucan-branching glycosyltransferase: an enzyme involved in conversion of amylose to amylopectin;

deficiency causes amylopectinosis (glycogenosis, type IV). **constitutive e.,** one produced by a microorganism regardless of the presence or absence of the specific substrate. **debrancher e., debranching e.,** amylo-1,6-glucosidase: one acting on glucose residues of the glycogen molecule, it is important in glycogenolysis. Deficiency cause Forbes disease (glycogenosis, type III). **induced e., inducible e.,** one whose production requires or is stimulated by a specific small molecule, the *inducer,* which is the substrate of the enzyme or a compound structurally related to it. **proteolytic e.,** one that catalyzes the hydrolysis of proteins and various split products of proteins, the final product being small peptides and amino acids. **repressible e.,** one whose rate of production is decreased as the concentration of certain metabolites is increased. **respiratory e's,** enzymes of the mitochondria, e.g., cytochrome oxidase, which serve as catalysts for cellular oxidations.

enzymopathy (en″zi-mop′ah-the) an inborn error of metabolism consisting of defective or absent enzymes, as in the glycogenoses or the mucopolysaccharidoses.

EOG electro-olfactogram.

eonism (e′ah-nizm) transvestism in the male.

eosin (e′ah-sin) any of a class of rose-colored stains or dyes, all being bromine derivatives of fluorescein; *eosin Y,* the sodium salt of tetrabromfluorescein, is much used in histologic and laboratory procedures.

eosinopenia (e″ah-sin″o-pe′ne-ah) abnormal deficiency of eosinophils in the blood.

eosinophil (e″ah-sin′ah-fil) a granular leukocyte having a nucleus with two lobes connected by a thread of chromatin, and cytoplasm containing coarse, round granules of uniform size.

eosinophilopoietin (-fil″ah-poi′it-in) a peptide of low molecular weight that induces production of eosinophils.

eosinophilotactic (e″ah-sin-ah-fil″o-tak′tik) having the power of attracting eosinophils; chemotactic for eosinophils.

epactal (e-pak′til) 1. supernumerary. 2. any wormian bone.

epallobiosis (ep-al″o-bi-o′sis) dependency on an external life-support system, as on a heart-lung machine or hemodialyzer.

epaxial (ep-ak′se-il) situated upon or above an axis.

ependyma (e-pen′dĭ-mah) the membrane lining the cerebral ventricles and the central canal of the spine. **epen′dymal,** adj.

ependymoblast (ep″en-di′mo-blast) an embryonic ependymal cell.

ependymocyte (e-pen′dim-o-sīt) an ependymal cell.

ependymoma (e-pen″dĭ-mo′mah) a neoplasm, usually slow growing and benign, composed of differentiated ependymal cells.

Eperythrozoon (ep″ah-rith″ro-zo′on) a genus of the family Bartonellaceae; its members are of limited pathogenicity, infecting rodents, cattle, sheep, and swine.

ephapse (e-faps′) a point of lateral contact (other than a synapse) between nerve fibers across which impulses are conducted directly through the nerve membranes. **ephap′tic,** adj.

ephebiatrics (ĕ-fe″be-ă′triks) the branch of medicine which deals especially with the diagnosis and treatment of diseases and problems peculiar to youth.

ephebogenesis (ef″ĭ-bo-jen′is-is) the bodily changes occurring at puberty. **ephebogenet′ic,** adj.

ephedrine (ĕ-fed′rin, ef′ĕ-drin) an adrenergic, $C_{10}H_{15}NO$, extracted from several species of *Ephedra* or produced synthetically; used as a bronchodilator, antiallergic, central nervous system stimulant, mydriatic, and antihypotensive.

ephelis (ĕ-fel′is), pl. *ephe′lides* [Gr.] a freckle.

epi- word element [Gr.], *upon; over.*

epiandrosterone (ep″ĭ-an-dros′ter-ōn) an androgenic steroid less active than androsterone and excreted in small amounts in normal human urine.

epiblast (ep′ĭ-blast) 1. ectoderm. 2. ectoderm, except for the neural plate. **epiblas′tic,** adj.

epiblepharon (ep″ĭ-blef′ah-ron) a developmental anomaly in which a horizontal fold of skin stretches across the border of the eyelid, pressing the eyelashes inward, against the eyelid.

epiboly (e-pib′o-le) gastrulation in which smaller blastomeres at the animal pole of the fertilized ovum grow over and enclose the cells of the vegetal hemisphere.

epibulbar (ep″ĭ-bul′ber) situated upon the eyeball.

epicanthus (-kan′this) a vertical fold of skin on either side of the nose, sometimes covering the inner canthus; a normal characteristic in persons of certain races, but anomalous in others. **epican′thal, epican′thic,** adj.

epicardia (-kar′de-ah) the portion of the esophagus below the diaphragm.

epicardium (-kar′de-um) the visceral pericardium.

epichorion (-ko′re-on) the portion of the uterine mucosa enclosing the implanted conceptus.

epicondylalgia (-kon″dil-al′je-ah) pain in the muscles or tendons attached to the epicondyle of the humerus.

epicondyle (-kon′dĭl) an eminence upon a bone, above its condyle.

epicondylus (-kon′dil-us), pl. *epicon′dyli* [L.] epicondyle.

epicranium (-kra′ne-um) structures collectively which cover the skull.

epicrisis (-kri′sis) a secondary crisis.

epicritic (-krit′ik) determining accurately; said of cutaneous nerve fibers sensitive to fine variations of touch or temperature.

epicystotomy (-sis-tot′ah-me) cystotomy by the suprapubic method.

epicyte (ep′ĭ-sīt) cell membrane.

epidemic (ep″ĭ-dem′ik) 1. attacking many people in a region at the same time; widely diffused and rapidly spreading. 2. a disease of high morbidity which is only occasionally present in the human community.

epidemiology (-de″me-ol′ah-je) 1. the study of

the relationships of various factors determining the frequency and distribution of diseases in the human community. 2. the field of medicine dealing with the determination of specific causes of localized outbreaks of infection, toxic poisoning, or other disease of recognized etiology.

epidermidalization (-derm″id-il-iz-a′shin) development of epidermal cells (stratified epithelium) from mucous cells (columnar epithelium).

epidermis (-derm′is) the outermost and nonvascular layer of the skin, derived from the embryonic ectoderm, varying in thickness from 0.07–1.4 mm. On the palmar and plantar surfaces it comprises, from within outward, five layers: (1) *basal layer* (stratum basale), composed of columnar cells arranged perpendicularly; (2) *prickle-cell* or *spinous layer* (stratum spinosum), composed of flattened polyhedral cells with short processes or spines; (3) *granular layer* (stratum granulosum) composed of flattened granular cells; (4) *clear layer* (stratum lucidum), composed of several layers of clear, transparent cells in which the nuclei are indistinct or absent; and (5) *horny layer* (stratum corneum), composed of flattened, cornified, non-nucleated cells. In the epidermis of the general body surface, the clear layer is usually absent. **epider′mal, epider′mic,** adj.

epidermitis (-derm-it′is) inflammation of the epidermis.

epidermodysplasia (-derm″o-dis-pla′ze-ah) faulty development of the epidermis. **e. verrucifor′mis,** a condition due to a virus identical with or closely related to the virus of common warts, in which the lesions are red or red-violet and widespread, and tend to become malignant.

epidermoid (-derm′oid) 1. resembling the epidermis. 2. any tumor occurring in a noncutaneous site and formed by inclusion of epidermal elements.

epidermoidoma (-derm″oi-do′mah) a cerebral or meningeal tumor formed by inclusion of ectodermal elements at the time of closure of the neural groove.

epidermolysis (-der-mol′ĭ-sis) a loosened state of the epidermis with formation of blebs and bullae, occurring either spontaneously or at the site of trauma. **e. bullo′sa,** a variety with development of bullae and vesicles, often at the site of trauma; in the hereditary forms, there may be severe scarring after healing, or extensive denuded areas after rupture of the lesions.

epidermomycosis (-derm″o-mi-ko′sis) dermatophytosis.

Epidermophyton (-derm-of′it-on) a genus of fungi, including *E. flocco′sum,* which attacks both skin and nails but not hair, and is one of the causative agents of tinea cruris, tinea pedis (athlete's foot), and onychomycosis.

epidermophytosis (-derm″o-fi-to′sis) a fungal skin infection, especially one due to *Epidermophyton;* dermatophytosis.

epididymis (-did′im-is) an elongated, cordlike structure along the posterior border of the testis, whose elongated coiled duct provides for storage, transit, and maturation of spermatozoa and is continuous with the ductus deferens. **epidid′ymal,** adj.

epididymitis (-did″im-īt′is) inflammation of the epididymis.

epididymo-orchitis (-did″im-o-or-kīt′is) inflammation of the epididymis and testis.

epididymovasostomy (-did″im-o-vas-os′tah-me) surgical anastomosis of the epididymis to the ductus deferens.

epidural (ep″ĭ-dūr′il) situated upon or outside the dura mater.

epidurography (-dūr-og′rah-fe) radiography of the spine after a radiopaque medium has been injected into the epidural space.

epiestriol (-es′tre-ol) an estrogenic steroid found in pregnant women.

epigastrium (-gas′tre-um) the upper and middle region of the abdomen, located within the sternal angle. **epigas′tric,** adj.

epigastrocele (-gas′tro-sēl) epigastric hernia.

epigenesis (-jen′is-is) the development of an organism from an undifferentiated cell, consisting in the successive formation and development of organs and parts that do not preexist in the fertilized egg. **epigenet′ic,** adj.

epiglottidectomy (-glot″ĭ-dek′tah-me) excision of the epiglottis.

epiglottiditis (-glot″id-īt′is) inflammation of the epiglottis.

epiglottis (-glot′is) the lidlike cartilaginous structure overhanging the entrance to the larynx, guarding it during swallowing; see Plate IV. **epiglot′tic,** adj.

epilation (-la′shin) the removal of hair by the roots.

epilemma (-lem′ah) endoneurium.

epilepsia (ep″ĭ-lep′se-ah) epilepsy. **e. partia′lis contin′ua,** continuous clonic movements of a limited part of the body, due to an abnormal neuronal discharge.

epilepsy (ep′ĭ-lep″se) paroxysmal transient disturbances of brain function that may be manifested as episodic impairment or loss of consciousness, abnormal motor phenomena, psychic or sensory disturbances, or perturbation of the autonomic nervous system; symptoms are due to disturbance of the electrical activity of the brain. **focal e.,** minor epileptic seizures in which the seizures are predominately one-sided or local, or present localized features. **generalized e.,** epilepsy in which the seizures are generalized; they may have a focal onset or be generalized from the beginning. **grand mal e.,** epilepsy, often preceded by an aura, in which a sudden loss of conciousness is immediately followed by generalized convulsions. **jacksonian e.,** epilepsy marked by unilateral clonic movements that start in one muscle group and spread systematically to adjacent groups, reflecting the march of epileptic activity through the motor cortex. **myoclonus e.,** slowly progressive hereditary epilepsy beginning in childhood, with intermittent or continuous clonus of muscle groups, resulting in difficulties in voluntary movements; there is mental deterioration and the presence of Lafora bodies in various cells. **petit mal e.**, epilepsy seen especially in children, in which there is sudden momentary unconsciousness with only minor myoclonic jerks. **photogenic e.**, epilepsy in which seizures are induced by a flickering light. **post-traumatic e.**, recurring convulsions due to head injury. **psychomotor e.**, that associated with disease of the temporal lobe, with impaired consciousness of variable degree, the patient carrying out a series of coordinated acts that are out of place, bizarre, and serve no useful purpose and for which he is amnesic. **reflex e.**, an epileptic seizure occurring in response to a sensory stimulus. **sensory e.**, seizures manifested by hallucinations of sight, smell, or taste. **temporal lobe e.**, psychomotor e. **tonic e.**, seizure characterized by generalized rigidity.

epileptogenic (-lep″tah-jen′ik) causing an epileptic seizure.

epileptoid (-lep′toid) epileptiform.

epimandibular (-man-dib′u-ler) situated on the lower jaw.

epimenorrhagia (-men″ah-ra′je-ah) too frequent and excessive menstruation.

epimenorrhea (-men″ah-re′ah) abnormally frequent menstruation.

epimer (ep′ĭ-mer) either of two optical isomers that differ in the configuration around one asymmetrical carbon atom.

epimerase (ĕ-pim′er-ās″) an isomerase that catalyzes the inversion of asymmetric groups in substrates (epimers) having more than one center of asymmetry.

epimere (ep′ĭ-mēr) the dorsal portion of a somite, from which is formed muscles innervated by the dorsal ramus of a spinal nerve.

epimerite (ep″ĭ-mer′īt) an organelle of certain protozoa by which they attach themselves to epithelial cells.

epimerization (ĕ-pim″er-iz-a′shin) the changing of one epimeric form of a compound into another, as by enzymatic action.

epimorphosis (ep″ĭ-mor-fo′sis) the regeneration of a part of an organism by proliferation at the cut surface. **epimor′phic,** adj.

epimysium (-mis′e-um) the fibrous sheath around an entire skeletal muscle. See Plate XIV.

epinephrine (-nef′rin) a hormone, $C_9H_{13}NO_3$, secreted by the adrenal medulla in response to splanchnic stimulation, and stored in the chromaffin granules; it is released also in response to hypoglycemia. Epinephrine is a potent stimulator of the sympathetic nervous system (adrenergic receptors), and a powerful vasopressor, increasing blood pressure, stimulating the heart muscle, accelerating the heart rate, and increasing cardiac output. It also increases such metabolic activities as glycogenolysis and glucose release. It is used chiefly as a topical vasoconstrictor, cardiac stimulant, and bronchodilator. Called also *adrenaline* (Great Britain).

epinephros (-nef′ros) adrenal gland.

epineurium (-nōōr′e-um) the sheath of a peripheral nerve. **epineu′rial,** adj.

epipharynx (-fă′rinks) nasopharynx. **epipharyn′geal,** adj.

epiphenomenon (-fī-nom′ĭ-non) an accessory, exceptional, or accidental occurrence in the course of any disease.

epiphora (e-pif′or-ah) overflow of tears due to obstruction of lacrimal duct.

epiphysis (e-pif′ĭ-sis), pl. *epi′physes* [Gr.] 1. the end of a long bone, usually wider than the shaft, and either entirely cartilaginous or separated from the shaft by a cartilaginous disk. 2. part of a bone formed from a secondary center of ossification, commonly found at the ends of long bones on the margins of flat bones, and at tubercles and processes; during the period of growth, epiphyses are separated from the main portion of the bone by cartilage. **epiphys′eal,** adj. **e. ce′rebri,** pineal body. **stippled epiphyses,** epiphyseal dysplasia.

epiphysitis (e-pif″ĭ-sīt′is) inflammation of an epiphysis or of the cartilage joining the epiphysis to a bone shaft.

epiphyte (ep′ĭ-fit) an external plant parasite.

epiphytic (ep″ĭ-fit′ik) 1. pertaining to or caused by epiphytes. 2. a widely diffused outbreak of an infectious disease in plants.

epiplocele (e-pip′lah-sēl) omental hernia.

epiploenterocele (-en′ter-o-sēl″) a hernia containing intestine and omentum.

epiplomerocele (-mēr′ah-sēl) a femoral hernia containing omentum.

epiplomphalocele (ep″ĭ-plom-fal′ah-sēl) an umbilical hernia containing omentum.

epiploon (e-pip′lo-on), pl. *epi′ploa* [Gr.] the omentum. **epiplo′ic,** adj.

epiploscheocele (e″pĭ-plos′ke-o-sēl″) a scrotal hernia containing omentum.

epipygus (ep″ĭ-pi′gus) pygomelus.

episclera (-sklē′rah) the loose connective tissue between the sclera and the conjunctiva.

episcleritis (-sklē-rīt′is) inflammation of the episcleral and adjacent tissues.

episioperineoplasty (e-piz″e-o-pĕ″re-ne′o-plas″te) plastic repair of the vulva and perineum.

episioperineorrhaphy (-pĕ″re-ne-or′ah-fe) suture of the vulva and perineum.

episiorrhaphy (e-piz″e-or′ah-fe) 1. suture of the labia majora. 2. suture of a lacerated perineum.

episiostenosis (e-piz″e-o-stĭ-no′sis) narrowing of the vulvar orifice.

episiotomy (e-piz″e-ot′ah-me) surgical incision into the perineum and vagina for obstetrical purposes.

episode (ep′ĭ-sōd) a noteworthy happening occurring in the course of a continuous series of events. **acute schizophrenic e.**, acute schizophrenia. **major depressive e.**, a period marked by loss of interest and pleasure in one's ordinary activities, associated with disturbances in sleep and appetite, changes in weight, psychomotor agitation or retardation, difficulty in thinking and concentration, fatigue, feelings of worthlessness and hopelessness, and thoughts of death and suicide. **manic e.**, a period of predominant elevation, expansiveness, or irritation together with inflated self-esteem or grandiosity, decreased need of sleep, talkativeness, flight of ideas, distractability, hyperactivity, hypersexuality, and recklessness.

episome (-sōm) in bacterial genetics, any accessory extrachromosomal replicating genetic element that can exist either autonomously or integrated with the chromosome.

epispadias (ep″ĭ-spa′de-as) congenital absence of the upper wall of the urethra, occurring in both sexes, but more commonly in the male, the urethral opening being located anywhere on the dorsum of the penis. **epispa′diac, epispa′dial,** adj.

epistaxis (-stak′sis) nosebleed; hemorrhage from the nose, usually due to rupture of small vessels overlying the anterior part of the cartilaginous nasal septum.

episternum (-stern′um) a bone present in reptiles and monotremes that may be represented as part of the manubrium, or first piece of the sternum.

epistropheus (-stro′fe-us) axis (see *Table of Bones).*

epitendineum (-ten-din′e-um) the fibrous sheath covering a tendon.

epithalamus (-thal′ah-mus) the part of the diencephalon just superior and posterior to the thalamus, comprising the pineal body and adjacent structures; considered by some to include the stria medullaris.

epithelial (-thēl′e-al) pertaining to or composed of epithelium.

epithelialization (-thēl″e-il-iz-a′shin) healing by the growth of epithelium over a denuded surface.

epithelialize (-thēl′e-il-īz″) to cover with epithelium.

epitheliitis (-thēl″e-īt′is) inflammation of epithelium.

epitheliochorial (ep″ĭ-thēl″e-o-kor′e-il) denoting a type of placenta in which the chorion is apposed to the uterine epithelium but does not erode it.

epitheliolysin (-thēl″e-ol′ĭ-sin) a cytolysin formed in the serum in response to injection of epithelial cells from a different species; it is capable of destroying epithelial cells of animals of the donor species.

epitheliolysis (-thēl″e-ol′ĭ-sis) destruction of epithelial tissue. **epitheliolyt′ic,** adj.

epithelioma (-thēl″e-o′mah) any tumor derived from epithelium. **epithelio′matous,** adj. **malignant e.,** carcinoma.

epithelium (-thēl′e-um), pl. *epithe′lia* [Gr.] the cellular covering of internal and external body surfaces, including the lining of vessels and small cavities. It consists of cells joined by small amounts of cementing substances and is classified according to the number of layers and the shape of the cells. **ciliated e.,** that bearing vibratile cilia on the free surface. **columnar e.,** epithelium whose cells are of much greater height than width. **cubical e., cuboidal e.,** that composed of cube-shaped cells. **germinal e.,** thickened peritoneal epithelium covering the gonad from earliest development; formerly thought to give rise to germ cells. **glandular e.,** that composed of secreting cells. **laminated e.,**

stratified e. **olfactory e.,** pseudostratified epithelium lining the olfactory region of the nasal cavity, and containing the receptors for the sense of smell. **pseudostratified e.,** that in which the cells are so arranged that the nuclei occur at different levels, giving the appearance of being stratified. **seminiferous e.,** stratified epithelium lining the seminiferous tubules of the testis. **simple e.,** that composed of a single layer of cells. **squamous e.,** that composed of flattened platelike cells. **stratified e.,** that composed of cells arranged in layers. **transitional e.,** that characteristically found lining hollow organs that are subject to great mechanical change due to contraction and distention, originally thought to represent a transition between stratified squamous and columnar epithelium.

epitope (ep′ĭ-tōp) an antigenic determinant (see under *determinant)* of known structure.

epitrichium (ep″ĭ-trik′e-um) periderm.

epitrochlea (-trok′le-ah) the inner condyle of the humerus.

epitympanum (-tim′pah-num) the upper part of the tympanum. **epitympan′ic,** adj.

epizootic (-zo-ot′ik) 1. attacking many animals in any region at the same time; widely diffused and rapidly spreading. 2. a disease of high morbidity which is only occasionally present in an animal community.

epizootiology (-zo-ot″e-ol′ah-je) the scientific study of factors in the frequency and distribution of infectious diseases among animals.

eponychium (ep″on-ik′e-um) 1. the narrow band of epidermis extending from the nail wall onto the nail surface. 2. the horny fetal epidermis at the site of the future nail.

eponym (ep′ah-nim) a name or phrase formed from or including a person's name, as Hodgkin's disease. **eponym′ic, epon′ymous,** adj.

epoophoron (-of′ah-ron) a vestigial structure associated with the ovary.

epoxy (ĕ-pok′se) 1. containing one atom of oxygen bound to two different carbon atoms. 2. a resin composed of epoxy polymers and characterized by adhesiveness, flexibility, and resistance to chemical actions.

epulis (ĕ-pūl′is), pl. *epu′lides* [Gr.] any tumor of the gingiva.

Equanil (ek′wah-nil) trademark for preparations of meprobamate.

equation (e-kwa′zhin) an expression of equality between two parts. **Henderson-Hasselbalch e.,** a formula for calculating the pH of a buffer solution such as blood plasma,

$$pH = pK' + \log \frac{(BA)}{(HA)}; (HA) \text{ is the concentration}$$

of a weak acid; (BA) the concentration of a salt of this acid; pK′ the dissociation constant of the acid.

equiaxial (e″kwe-ak′se-il) having axes of the same length.

equilibration (e″kwĭ-lĭ-bra′shin) the achievement of a balance between opposing elements or forces. **occlusal e.,** modification of the occlusal stress, to produce simultaneous occlusal contacts, or to achieve harmonious occlusion.

equilibrium (e″kwĭ-lib′re-um) a state of balance between opposing forces or influences. **dynamic e.**, the condition of balance between varying, shifting, and opposing forces that is characteristic of living processes.

equine (e′kwīn) pertaining to, characteristic of, or derived from the horse.

equinovalgus (e-kwi″no-val′gus) talipes equinovalgus.

equinovarus (e-kwi″no-va′rus) talipes equinovarus.

equipotential (e″kwĭ-pah-ten′shil) having similar and equal power or capability.

equivalent (ĭ-kwiv′ah-lint) 1. of equal force, power, value, etc. 2. something that has equivalent properties. 3. chemical e. **chemical e.**, that weight in grams of a substance that will produce or react with 1 mole of hydrogen ion or 1 mole of electrons. Symbol Eq. **epilepsy e.**, any disturbance, mental or physical, which may take the place of an epileptic seizure.

equulosis (ĕ″kwōōl-o′sis) a purulent arthritis, synovitis, and enteritis, often with formation of kidney abscesses, affecting primarily foals; caused by *Actinobacillus equuli.*

Er chemical symbol, *erbium.*

erasion (e-ra′zhin) removal by scraping, or curettage.

erbium (er′be-im) chemical element (*see table*), at. no. 68, symbol Er.

erection (ĭ-rek′shin) the condition of being rigid and elevated, as erectile tissue when filled with blood.

erector (ĭ-rek′ter) [L.] a structure that erects, as a muscle which raises or holds up a part.

erethism (ĕ′rĭ-thizm) excessive irritability or sensibility to stimulation. **erethis′mic, erethis′tic,** adj.

erg (erg) a unit of work or energy, equivalent to 2.4×10^{-8} gram calories, or to 0.624×10^{12} electron volts.

ergasia (er-ga′ze-ah) any mentally integrated function, activity, reaction, or attitude of the individual.

ergastoplasm (er-gas′tah-plazm) granular endoplasmic reticulum.

ergocalciferol (er″go-kal-sif′er-ol) calciferol; vitamin D_2: an activation product, $C_{28}H_{44}O$, of ergosterol, produced by ultraviolet radiation of ergosterol; used as an antirachitic vitamin.

ergometer (er-gom′it-er) a dynamometer. **bicycle e.**, an apparatus for measuring the muscular, metabolic, and respiratory effects of exercise.

ergonomics (er″gah-nom′iks) the science relating to man and his work, including the factors affecting the efficient use of human energy.

ergonovine (-no′vin) an alkaloid, $C_{19}H_{23}N_3O_2$, from ergot or produced synthetically, used as an oxytocic and to relieve migraine.

ergostat (er′go-stat) a machine to be worked for muscular exercise.

ergosterol (er-gos′ter-ol) a sterol, $C_{28}H_{43} \cdot OH$, occurring in animal and plant tissues which, on ultraviolet irradiation becomes a potent antirachitic substance, ergocalciferol.

ergot (er′got) the dried sclerotium of the fungus *Claviceps purpurea,* which is developed on rye plants; ergot alkaloids are used as oxytocics and in treatment of migraine. See also *ergotism.*

ergotamine (er-got′ah-min) an alkaloid of ergot, $C_{33}H_{35}N_5O_5$; the tartrate salt is used for relief of migraine.

ergotism (er′go-tizm) chronic poisoning produced by ingestion of ergot, marked by cerebrospinal symptoms, spasms, cramps, or by a kind of dry gangrene.

eriodictyon (er″e-o-dik′te-on) the dried leaf of *Eriodictyon californicum,* used in pharmaceutical preparations.

erogenous (ĭ-roj′ĭ-nis) arousing erotic feelings.

erosion (ĭ-ro′zhin) an eating or gnawing away; a shallow or superficial ulceration; in dentistry, the wasting away or loss of substance of a tooth by a chemical process that does not involve known bacterial action. **ero′sive,** adj. **cervical e.**, destruction of the squamous epithelium of the vaginal portion of the cervix, due to irritation; the eroded area is covered by columnar epithelium.

erotic (ĭ-rot′ik) pertaining to sexual love or to lust.

erotism (er′o-tizm) a sexual instinct or desire; expression of one's instinctual energy or drive, especially the sex drive. **anal e.**, fixation of libido at (or regression to) the anal phase of infantile development, producing egotistic, dogmatic, stubborn, miserly character. **genital e.**, achievement and maintenance of libido at genital phase of psychosexual development, permitting acceptance of normal adult relationships and responsibilities. **oral e.**, fixation of libido at the oral phase of infantile development, producing passive, insecure, sensitive character.

erotogenic (ĭ-rōt″o-jen′ik) producing erotic feelings.

erotomania (-ma′ne-ah) exaggerated sexual behavior or reaction; preoccupation with sexuality.

erotopathy (er″o-top′ah-the) any perversion of the sexual impulse.

erotophobia (ĕ-rōt″o-fo′be-ah) morbid dread of sexual love.

eructation (e″ruk-ta′shin) belching; casting up wind from the stomach through the mouth.

eruption (ĭ-rup′shin) 1. the act of breaking out, appearing, or becoming visible, as eruption of the teeth. 2. visible efflorescent lesions of the skin due to disease, with redness, prominence, or both; a rash. **creeping e.**, larva migrans. **drug e.**, an eruption or a solitary lesion caused by a drug taken internally. **fixed e.**, a circumscribed inflammatory skin lesion(s) recurring at the same site(s) over a period of months or years; each attack lasts only a few days but leaves residual pigmentation which is cumulative. **Kaposi's varicelliform e.**, a generalized and serious vesiculopustular eruption of viral origin, superimposed on preexisting atopic dermatitis; it may be due to the herpes simplex virus (*eczema herpeticum*) or vaccinia (*eczema vaccinatum*).

ERV expiratory reserve volume.

erysipelas (er″ĭ-sip′ĭ-lis) a contagious disease of the skin and subcutaneous tissues due to infection with *Streptococcus pyogenes*, with redness and swelling of affected areas, constitutional symptoms, and sometimes vesicular and bullous lesions. **swine e.**, a contagious and highly fatal disease of pigs, caused by *Erysipelothrix insidiosa.*

erysipeloid (er″ĭ-sip′ĭ-loid) a dermatitis or cellulitis of the hand chiefly affecting fish handlers and caused by *Erysipelothrix insidiosa.*

Erysipelothrix (er″ĭ-sip′ĭ-lah-thriks″) a genus of gram-positive bacteria (family Corynebacteriaceae), containing the single species *E. insidio′sa* (*E. rhusiopath′iae*), the causative agent of swine erysipelas and erysipeloid.

erythema (er″ĭ-the′mah) redness of the skin due to congestion of the capillaries. **e. annula′re**, a type of erythema multiforme with ring-shaped lesions. **e. annula′re centri′fugum**, a chronic variant of erythema multiforme usually affecting the thighs and lower legs, with single or multiple erythematous-edematous papules that enlarge peripherally and clear in the center to produce annular lesions, which may coalesce. **e. chro′nicum mi′grans**, an annular erythema due to the bite of a tick (*Ixodes*); it begins as an erythematous plaque several weeks after the bite and spreads peripherally with central clearing. **cold e.**, a congenital hypersensitivity to cold seen in children, characterized by localized pain, widespread erythema, occasional muscle spasms, and vascular collapse on exposure to cold, and vomiting after drinking cold liquids. **epidemic arthritic e.**, Haverhill fever. **e. indura′tum**, chronic necrotizing vasculitis, usually occurring on the calves of young women; its association with tuberculosis is in dispute. **e. infectio′sum**, a mildly contagious, sometimes epidemic, disease of children between the ages of four and twelve, marked by a rose-colored, coarsely lacelike macular rash. **e. i′ris**, a type of erythema multiforme in which the lesions form concentric rings, producing a target-like appearance. **e. margina′tum**, a type of erythema multiforme in which the reddened areas are disk-shaped with elevated edges. **e. mi′grans**, geographic tongue. **e. multifor′me**, a symptom complex with highly polymorphic skin lesions, including macular papules, vesicles, and bullae; attacks are usually self-limited but recurrences are the rule. **e. nodo′sum**, an acute inflammatory skin disease marked by tender red nodules, usually on the shins, due to exudation of blood and serum. **e. nodo′sum lepro′sum**, a form of lepra reaction occurring in lepromatous and sometimes borderline leprosy, marked by the occurrence of tender, inflamed subcutaneous nodules; the reactions resemble multifocal Arthus reactions. **toxic e., e. tox′icum**, a generalized erythematous or erythematomacular eruption due to administration of a drug or to bacterial toxins or other toxic substances. **e. tox′icum neonato′rum**, a self-limited urticarial condition affecting infants in the first few days of life.

erythr(o)- word element [Gr.], *red; erythrocyte.*

erythrasma (er″ĭ-thraz′mah) a chronic bacterial infection of the major skin folds due to *Corynebacterium minutissimum*, marked by red or brownish patches on the skin.

erythredema polyneuropathy (ĭ-rith″rĭ-de′mah pol″ĭ-nōōr-op′ah-the) acrodynia.

erythremia (ĕ″rith-re′me-ah) polycythemia vera.

erythritol (ĭ-rith′rit-ol) a polyhydric alcohol, $C_4H_{10}O_4$, which is about twice as sweet as sucrose, found in algae, lichens, grasses, and several fungi.

erythrityl (ĭ-rith′rit-il) the univalent radical, C_4H_9, from erythritol. **e. tetranitrate**, a vasodilator used in angina pectoris and coronary insufficiency; because of its explosiveness it must be diluted, as with lactose.

erythroblast (ĭ-rith′ro-blast) originally, any nucleated erythrocyte, but now more generally used to designate the nucleated precursor from which an erythrocyte develops.

erythroblastoma (-blas-to′mah) a tumor-like mass composed of nucleated red blood cells.

erythroblastopenia (-blas″to-pe′ne-ah) abnormal deficiency of erythroblasts.

erythroblastosis (-blas-to′sis) 1. the presence of erythroblasts in the circulating blood. 2. avian leukosis marked by increased numbers of immature erythrocytes in the circulating blood. **erythroblastot′ic**, adj. **e. feta′lis, e. neonato′rum**, hemolytic anemia of the fetus or newborn due to transplacental transmission of maternally formed antibody against the fetus' erythrocytes, usually secondary to an incompatibility between the mother's Rh blood group and that of her offspring.

erythrochromia (-kro′me-ah) hemorrhagic, red pigmentation of the spinal fluid.

Erythrocin (ĭ-rith′rah-sin) trademark for preparations of erythromycin.

erythroclasis (ĕ″rith-rok′lah-sis) fragmentation of the red blood cells. **erythroclas′tic**, adj.

erythrocyanosis (ĭ-rith″ro-si″ah-no′sis) coarsely mottled bluish red discoloration on the legs and thighs, especially of girls; thought to be a circulatory reaction to exposure to cold.

erythrocytapheresis (-sīt″ah-fer′ĭ-sis) the withdrawal of blood, separation and retention of red blood cells, and retransfusion of the remainder into the donor.

erythrocyte (ĭ-rith′rah-sīt) a red blood cell or corpuscle; one of the formed elements in peripheral blood. Normally, in the human, the mature form is a non-nucleated, yellowish, biconcave disk, containing hemoglobin and transporting oxygen. For immature forms, see *normoblast.* **achromic e.**, a colorless erythrocyte. **basophilic e.**, one that takes the basic stain. **hypochromic e.**, one that contains less than normal concentration of hemoglobin and as a result appears paler than normal; it is usually also microcytic. **"Mexican hat" e.**, target cell. **normochromic e.**, one of normal color with a normal concentration of hemoglobin. **orthochromatic e.**, one that takes only the acid stain. **polychromatic e., polychromatophilic e.**, one that, on staining, shows shades of blue combined with tinges of pink. **target e.**, see under *cell.*

erythrocythemia (ĭ-rith″ro-si-the′me-ah) an increase in the number of erythrocytes in the blood, as in erythrocytosis.

erythrocytolysis (-si-tol′ĭ-sis) dissolution of erythrocytes and escape of the hemoglobin.

erythrocytorrhexis (-sīt″ah-rek′sis) the escape from erythrocytes of round, shiny granules and the splitting off of particles.

erythrocytoschisis (-si-tos′kĭ-sis) degeneration of erythrocytes into platelet-like bodies.

erythrocytosis (-si-to′sis) increase in the total red cell mass secondary to any of a number of nonhematogenic systemic disorders in response to a known stimulus (*secondary polycythemia*), in contrast to primary polycythemia (*polycythemia vera*). **leukemic e., e. megalosplen′ica,** polycythemia vera. **stress e.,** see under *polycythemia.*

erythroderma (-derm′ah) abnormal redness of the skin over widespread areas of the body. **congenital ichthyosiform e.,** a generalized hereditary dermatitis with scaling, which occurs in bullous and nonbullous forms. **e. desquamati′vum,** a condition resembling and probably identical with severe seborrheic dermatitis, affecting newborn breast-fed infants, characterized by generalized exfoliative dermatitis and marked erythroderma. **psoriatic e.,** **e. psoria′ticum,** a generalized psoriasis vulgaris, showing the chemical characteristics of exfoliative dermatitis.

erythrodontia (-don′she-ah) reddish brown pigmentation of the teeth.

erythrogenesis (-jen′ĭ-sis) the production of erythrocytes. **e. imperfec′ta,** congenital hypoplastic anemia (1).

erythrogenic (-jen′ik) 1. producing erythrocytes. 2. producing a sensation of red. 3. producing or causing erythema.

erythroid (ĕ′rith-roid) 1. of a red color; reddish. 2. pertaining to the developmental series of cells ending in erythrocytes.

erythrokeratodermia (ĕ-rith″ro-ker″ah-to-derm′ e-ah) a reddening and hyperkeratosis of the skin. **e. figura′ta varia′bilis, e. varia′bilis,** a rare hereditary disorder marked by circumscribed erythematous and hyperkeratotic plaques on the skin which vary in size and shape within hours or days; they appear shortly after birth and persist into adolescence or adulthood.

erythrokinetics (-ki-net′iks) the quantitative, dynamic study of in vivo production and destruction of erythrocytes.

erythrolabe (ĕ-rith′rah-lāb) the pigment in retinal cones that is more sensitive to the red range of the spectrum than are the other pigments (chlorolabe and cyanolabe).

erythroleukemia (ĕ-rith″ro-loo-ke′me-ah) a malignant blood dyscrasia, one of the myeloproliferative disorders, with atypical erythroblasts and myeloblasts in the peripheral blood.

erythromelalgia (-mel-al′je-ah) paroxysmal, bilateral vasodilation, particularly of the extrem-

ities, with burning pain and increased skin temperature and redness.

erythromycin (-mi′sin) a broad-spectrum antibiotic, $C_{37}H_{67}NO_{13}$, produced by a strain of *Streptomyces erythreus;* used against gram-positive bacteria and certain gram-negative bacteria.

erythron (ĕ′rith-ron) the circulating erythrocytes in the blood, their precursors, and all the body elements concerned in their production.

erythroneocytosis (ĕ-rith″ro-ne″o-si-to′sis) presence of immature erythrocytes in the blood.

erythropenia (-pe′ne-ah) deficiency in the number of erythrocytes.

erythrophage (ĕ-rith′rah-fāj) a phagocyte that ingests erythrocytes.

erythrophagia, erythrophagocytosis (-fa′je-ah; -fag″o-si-to′sis) phagocytosis of erythrocytes.

erythrophil (ĕ-rith′rah-fil) 1. a cell or other element that stains easily with red. 2. erythrophilous.

erythrophobia (ĕ-rith″ro-fo′be-ah) 1. a neurotic manifestation marked by blushing at the slightest provocation. 2. morbid aversion to red.

erythrophose (ĕ-rith′ro-fōz) any red phose.

erythrophthisis (ĕ-rith″rah-thi′sis) a condition characterized by severe impairment of the restorative power of the erythrocyte-forming tissues.

erythroplasia (-pla′ze-ah) a condition of the mucous membranes characterized by erythematous papular lesions. **e. of Queyrat,** squamous cell carcinoma *in situ,* manifested as a circumscribed, velvety, erythematous papular lesion on the glans penis, coronal sulcus, or prepuce, leading to scaling and superficial ulceration.

erythropoiesis (-poi-e′sis) the formation of erythrocytes. **erythropoiet′ic,** adj.

erythropoietin (-poi′it-in) a glycoprotein hormone secreted by the kidney in the adult and by the liver in the fetus, which acts on stem cells of the bone marrow to stimulate red blood cell production (erythropoiesis).

erythroprosopalgia (-pros″ah-pal′je-ah) a nervous disorder marked by redness and pain in the face.

erythrorrhexis (ĕ-rith″rah-rek′sis) erythrocytorrhexis.

erythrosine sodium (ĕ-rith′rah-sēn) a coloring agent, $C_{20}H_6I_4Na_2O_5$, used to disclose plaque on teeth.

erythrosis (ĕ″rith-ro′sis) 1. reddish or purplish discoloration of the skin and mucous membranes, as in polycythemia vera. 2. hyperplasia of the hematopoietic tissue.

erythrostasis (ĕ-rith″rah-sta′sis) the stoppage of erythrocytes in the capillaries, as in sickle cell anemia.

Es chemical symbol, *einsteinium.*

escape (es-kāp′) the act of becoming free. **nodal e.,** extrasystole in which the atrioventricular node is the pacemaker. **vagal e.,** the exhaustion of or adaptation to neural chemical mediators in the regulation of systemic arterial pressure. **ventricular e.,** extrasystole in which a ventricular pacemaker becomes effective before the sinoatrial pacemaker; it usually occurs with slow sinus rates and often, but not necessarily, with increased vagal tone.

eschar (es'kar) 1. a slough produced by a thermal burn, by a corrosive application, or by gangrene. 2. tache noire. **escharot'ic,** adj.

Escherichia (esh''ĭ-rik'e-ah) a genus of widely distributed, gram-negative bacteria (family Enterobacteriaceae, occasionally pathogenic for man. **E. co'li,** a species constituting the greater part of the normal intestinal flora of man and other animals; it is a frequent cause of urinary tract infections and epidemic diarrheal disease, especially in children.

Escherichieae (esh''er-ĭ-ki'e-e) in some taxonomic systems, a tribe of bacteria (family Enterobacteriaceae), comprising the genera *Escherichia* and *Shigella.*

escorcin (es-kor'sin) a brown powder, $C_9H_8O_4$, prepared from a substance extracted from the horse chestnut; used in detecting corneal and conjunctival lesions.

escutcheon (es-kuch'in) the pattern of distribution of the pubic hair.

Esidrix (es'ĭ-driks) trademark for a preparation of hydrochlorothiazide.

-esis word element, *state; condition.*

esmarch (es'mark) an Esmarch bandage.

eso- word element [Gr.], *within.*

esogastritis (-gas-trīt'is) inflammation of the gastric mucosa.

esophagectasia (ĭ-sof''ah-jek-ta'se-ah) dilatation of the esophagus.

esophagism (ĭ-sof'ah-jizm) spasm of the esophagus.

esophagitis (ĭ-sof''ah-jīt'is) inflammation of the esophagus. **peptic e.,** that due to a reflux of acid and pepsin from the stomach.

esophagocele (ĭ-sof'ah-go-sēl'') abnormal distention of the esophagus; protrusion of the esophageal mucosa through a rupture in the muscular coat.

esophagocoloplasty (ĭ-sof''ah-go-ko'lah-plas''te) excision of a portion of the esophagus and its replacement by a segment of the colon.

esophagodynia (-din'e-ah) pain in the esophagus.

esophagoesophagostomy (-ĭ-sof''ah-gos'tah-me) anastomosis between two formerly remote parts of the esophagus.

esophagogastric (-gas'trik) pertaining to the esophagus and the stomach.

esophagogastroplasty (-gas'trah-plas''te) plastic repair of the esophagus and stomach.

esophagogastrostomy (-gas-tros'tah-me) anastomosis of the esophagus to the stomach.

esophagojejunostomy (ĭ-sof''ah-go-je''jōōn-os'-tah-me) anastomosis of the esophagus to the jejunum.

esophagomyotomy (-mi-ot'ah-me) incision through the muscular coat of the esophagus.

esophagoplication (ĭ-sof''ah-go-pli-ka'shin) infolding of the wall of an esophageal pouch.

esophagorespiratory (ĭ-sof''ah-go-res-pir'ah-to''re) pertaining to or communicating with the esophagus and respiratory tract (trachea or a bronchus).

esophagoscopy (ĕ-sof''ah-gos'ko-pe) endoscopic examination of the esophagus.

esophagostenosis (-stī-no'sis) stricture of the esophagus.

esophagotomy (ĭ-sof''ah-got'ah-me) incision of the esophagus.

esophagus (ĭ-sof'ah-gis) the musculomembranous passage extending from the pharynx to the stomach. See Plate IV.

esophoria (es''o-for'e-ah) deviation of the visual axis toward that of the other eye in the absence of visual fusional stimuli.

esosphenoiditis (-sfe''noid-īt'is) osteomyelitis of the sphenoid bone.

esotropia (-tro'pe-ah) cross-eye; deviation of the visual axis of one eye toward that of the other eye. **esotrop'ic,** adj.

E.S.P. extrasensory perception.

E.S.R. erythrocyte sedimentation rate.

essence (es'ins) 1. the distinctive or individual principle of anything. 2. mixture of alcohol with a volatile oil.

essential (ĭ-sen'shil) 1. constituting the inherent part of a thing; giving a substance its peculiar and necessary qualities. 2. indispensable; required in the diet, as essential fatty acids. 3. idiopathic; having no obvious external cause.

E.S.T. electric shock therapy.

ester (es'ter) a compound formed from an alcohol and an acid by removal of water.

esterase (es'ter-ās) any enzyme which catalyzes the hydrolysis of an ester into its alcohol and acid.

esterify (es-ter'ĭ-fi) to combine with an alcohol with elimination of a molecule of water, forming an ester.

esterolysis (es''ter-ol'ĭ-sis) the hydrolysis of an ester into its alcohol and acid. **esterolyt'ic,** adj.

esthematology (es''them-ah-tol'ah-je) esthesiology.

esthesiology (es-the''ze-ol'ah-je) the scientific study or description of the sense organs and sensations.

esthesioneurosis (es-the''ze-o-nōōr-o'sis) any disorder of the sensory nerves.

esthesodic (es''the-zod'ik) conducting or pertaining to conduction of sensory impulses.

esthetics (es-thet'iks) the branch of philosophy dealing with beauty; in dentistry, a philosophy concerned especially with the appearance of a dental restoration, as achieved through its color or form.

estivation (es''tĭ-va'shin) the dormant state in which certain animals pass the summer.

estolate (es'to-lāt) USAN contraction for propionate lauryl sulfate.

estradiol (es''trah-di'ol, es-tra'de-ol) the most potent estrogen in humans; pharmacologically, it is usually used in the form of its esters (e.g., *e. benzoate, e. cypionate, e. valerate*), or as a semisynthetic derivative (*ethinyl e.*). For properties and uses, see *estrogen.*

estrin (es'trin) estrogen.

estrinization (es''trin-ĭ-za'shin) production of

the cellular changes in the vaginal epithelium characteristic of estrus.

estriol (es'tre-ol) a relatively weak human estrogen, being a metabolic product of estradiol and estrone found in high concentrations in urine; see *estrogen*.

estrogen (es'trah-jen) a generic term for estrus-producing compounds; the female sex hormones, including estradiol, estriol, and estrone. In humans, the estrogens are formed in the ovary, adrenal cortex, testis, and fetoplacental unit, and are responsible for female secondary sex characteristic development, and during the menstrual cycle, act on the female genitalia to produce an environment suitable for fertilization, implantation, and nutrition of the early embryo. Estrogen is used as a palliative in postmenopausal cancer of the breast and in prostatic cancer, as oral contraceptives, for relief of menopausal discomforts, etc. **conjugated e's,** a mixture of the sulfate esters of estrogenic substances, principally estrone and equilin; the uses are those of estrogens. **esterified e's,** a mixture of esters of estrogenic substances, principally estrone; the uses are those of estrogens.

estrogenic (es″trah-jen'ik) estrus-producing; having the properties of, or similar to, an estrogen.

estrone (es'trōn) an estrogen isolated from pregnancy urine, the human placenta, and palm kernel oil, and also prepared synthetically; for properties, see *estrogen*.

estrophilin (es″tro-fil'in) a cell protein that acts as a receptor for estrogen, found in estrogenic target tissue and in estrogen-dependent tumors and metastases.

estrous (es'trus) pertaining to estrus.

estrus (es'trus) the recurrent, restricted period of sexual receptivity in female mammals other than human females, marked by intense sexual urge. **es'trual,** adj.

e.s.u. electrostatic unit.

esylate (es'ĭ-lāt) USAN contraction for ethanesulfonate.

ethacrynate sodium (eth-ah-krin-āt) the sodium salt of ethacrynic acid, $C_{13}H_{11}Cl_2NaO_4$, used intravenously as a diuretic.

ethacrynic acid (eth-ah-krin'ik) a powerful diuretic, $C_{13}H_{12}Cl_2O_4$, administered orally or parenterally, effective in promoting sodium and chloride excretion.

ethanol (eth'ah-nol) alcohol (1).

ethanolamine (eth″ah-nol'ah-mēn) a colorless, moderately viscous liquid with an ammonical odor, $NH_2 \cdot CH_2 \cdot CH_2OH$, contained in cephalins and phospholipids, and derived metabolically by decarboxylation of serine. The oleate is used as a sclerosing agent in the treatment of varicose veins.

ethaverine (eth″ah-vĕ'rēn) an analogue of papaverine, $C_{24}H_{29}NO_4$, used as an antispasmodic and smooth muscle relaxant.

ethchlorvynol (eth-klor'vĭ-nol) a sedative, C_7H_9ClO.

ether (e'ther) 1. diethyl ether: a colorless, transparent, mobile, very volatile, highly inflammable liquid, $C_2H_5 \cdot O \cdot C_2H_5$, with a characteristic odor; given by inhalation to produce general anesthesia. 2. any of a class of organic compounds characterized by the linkage of hydrocarbon groups by an oxygen atom bonded to two carbon atoms. **diethyl e.,** see *ether* (1). **vinyl e.,** a clear colorless liquid used as an inhalation anesthetic to produce general anesthesia.

ethereal (ĭ-thēr'e-il) 1. pertaining to, prepared with, containing, or resembling ether. 2. evanescent; delicate.

ethinamate (ĕ-thin'ah-māt) a short-acting, non-barbiturate sedative, $C_{19}H_{13}NO_2$.

ethmocarditis (eth″mo-kar-dīt'is) inflammation of the connective tissue of the heart.

ethmofrontal (-front'il) pertaining to the ethmoid and frontal bones.

ethmoid (eth'moid) 1. sievelike; cribriform. 2. the ethmoid bone.

ethmoidectomy (eth″moi-dek'tah-me) excision of ethmoidal cells or of a portion of the ethmoid bone.

ethmoidotomy (eth″moi-dot'ah-me) incision into the ethmoid sinus.

ethmomaxillary (-mak'sĭ-lĕ-re) pertaining to the ethmoid and maxillary bones.

ethmoturbinal (-turb'in-il) pertaining to the superior and middle nasal conchae.

ethnic (eth'nik) pertaining to a group sharing cultural bonds or physical characteristics.

ethnobiology (eth″no-bi-ol'ah-je) the scientific study of physical characteristics of different races of mankind.

ethnology (eth-nol'ah-je) the science dealing with the races of men, their descent, relationship, etc.

ethoheptazine (eth″o-hep'tah-zēn) an analgesic, $C_{16}H_{23}NO_2$.

ethology (e-thol'ah-je) the scientific study of animal behavior, particularly in the natural state. **etholog'ical,** adj.

ethopropazine (eth″o-pro'pah-zēn) a homologue of promethazine, $C_{19}H_{24}N_2S$, used as the hydrochloride salt in the treatment of parkinsonism.

ethosuximide (-suk'sĭ-mīd) an anticonvulsant, $C_7H_{11}NO_2$.

ethotoin (e-thōt'o-in) a phenylhydantoin derivative, $C_{11}H_{12}N_2O_2$, used as an anticonvulsant in grand mal epilepsy and psychomotor seizures.

ethoxzolamide (eth″ok-zol'ah-mīd) a carbonic anhydrase inhibitor, $C_9H_{10}N_2O_3S_2$, used as a diuretic and to reduce intraocular pressure in glaucoma.

ethyl (eth'il) the monovalent radical, C_2H_5. **e. acetate,** a flavoring agent and antispasmodic, $CH_3COOC_2H_5$. **e. aminobenzoate,** benzocaine. **e. chloride,** a local anesthetic, C_2H_5Cl, applied topically to intact skin. **e. linoleate,** a lipid occurring on the skin of warm-blooded animals and responsible for its passive water-holding capacity. **e. oleate,** a mobile, colorless liquid, $C_{20}H_{38}O_2$, used as a vehicle for pharmaceutical preparations. **e. vanillin,** a flavoring agent, $C_9H_{10}O_3$.

ethylcellulose (eth″il-sel'ūl-ōs) an ethyl ether of

cellulose; used as a pharmaceutical tablet binder.

ethylene (eth′ĭ-lēn) a colorless flammable gas, $CH_2:CH_2$, with a slightly sweet odor and taste; used as an inhalation anesthetic. **e. oxide,** a bactericidal agent, occurring as a colorless gas with a pleasant ethereal odor; used as a disinfectant, especially for disposable equipment.

ethylenediamine (eth″ĭ-lēn-di′ah-mēn) a solvent, $C_2H_8N_2$, used in pharmaceutical preparations.

ethylenediaminetetraacetic acid (EDTA) (eth″ĭ-lēn-di″ah-mēn-tĕ-trah-ah-sēt′ik) a chelating agent that binds calcium and other metals; used as an anticoagulant for preserving blood specimens; also used medicinally. See *edetate.*

ethylnorepinephrine (eth″il-nor-ep″ĭ-nef′rin) a sympathomimetic, $C_{10}H_{15}NO_3$, used as the hydrochloride salt in treatment of bronchial asthma.

ethynodiol diacetate (ĕ-thi″no-di′ōl) a progestin, $C_{24}H_{32}O_4$, used in combination with an estrogen as an oral contraceptive.

etidocaine (ĕ-te′dah-kān) a local anesthetic of the amide type, $C_{17}H_{28}N_2O$, used for percutaneous infiltration anesthesia, peripheral nerve block, and caudal and epidural block.

etiolation (ēt″e-o-la′shin) 1. blanching or paleness of a plant grown in the dark due to lack of chlorophyll. 2. the process by which the skin becomes pale when deprived of sunlight.

etiology (ēt″e-ol′ah-je) the science dealing with causes of disease. **etiolog′ic, etiolog′ical,** adj.

Eu chemical symbol, *europium.*

eu- word element [Gr.], *normal; good; well; easy.*

Eubacteriales (u″bak-tēr″e-a′lēz) in former taxonomic systems an order of schizomycetes comprising the true bacteria.

Eubacterium (u-bak-tēr′e-im) a genus of bacteria of the family Propionibacteriaceae, found as saprophytes in soil and water, and normal inhabitants of human skin and cavities, occasionally causing infection of soft tissue.

eucalyptol (u″kah-lip′tol) the chief constituent of eucalyptus oil, also obtained from other oils, and used as a flavoring agent, expectorant, and local anesthetic.

Eucaryotae (u-kar″e-ōt′e) a kingdom of organisms that includes higher plants and animals, fungi, protozoa, and most algae (except blue-green algae), which are made of eukaryotic cells.

euchlorhydria (u″klor-hi′dre-ah) the presence of the normal amount of hydrochloric acid in the gastric juice.

eucholia (u-kōl′e-ah) normal condition of the bile.

euchromatin (u-kro′mah-tin) that state of chromatin in which it stains lightly, is genetically active, and is considered to be partially or fully uncoiled.

eucrasia (u-kra′ze-ah) 1. a state of health; proper balance of different factors constituting a healthy state. 2. a state in which the body reacts normally to ingested or injected drugs, proteins, etc.

eugenol (u′jĭ-nol) the chief constituent of clove oil, $C_{10}H_{12}O_2$; used as a dental topical analgesic and antiseptic.

euglobulin (u-glob′ūl-in) one of a class of globulins characterized by being insoluble in water but soluble in saline solutions.

eugonic (u-gon′ik) growing luxuriantly; said of bacterial cultures.

eukaryon (u-kar′e-on) 1. a highly organized nucleus bounded by a nuclear membrane, a characteristic of cells of higher organisms; cf. *prokaryon.* 2. eukaryote.

eukaryosis (u″kar-e-o′sis) the state of having a true nucleus.

Eukaryotae (u-kar″e-ōt′e) Eucaryotae.

eukaryote (u-kar′e-ōt) an organism whose cells have a true nucleus bounded by a nuclear membrane within which lie the chromosomes; eukaryotic cells also contain many membrane-bound organelles in which cellular functions are performed. The cells of higher plants and animals, fungi, protozoa, and most algae are eukaryotic. Cf. *prokaryote.*

eukaryotic (u″kar-e-ot′ik) pertaining to a eukaryon or to a eukaryote.

eulaminate (u-lam′ĭ-nāt) having the normal number of laminae, as certain areas of the cerebral cortex.

eumetria (u-me′tre-ah) a normal condition of nerve impulse, so that a voluntary movement just reaches the intended goal; the proper range of movement.

eunuch (u′nik) a male deprived of the testes or external genitals, especially one castrated before puberty (so that male secondary sex characteristics fail to develop).

eunuchoidism (u′nik-oi-dizm) deficiency of the testes or of their secretion, with impaired sexual power and eunuchoid symptoms. **female e.,** hypogonadism in which the ovaries fail to function at puberty, resulting in infertility, absence of development of secondary sex characteristics, infantile sexual organs, and excessive growth of the long bones. **hypergonadotropic e.,** that associated with high levels of gonadotropins, as in Klinefelter's syndrome. **hypogonadotropic e.,** that due to lack of gonadotropin secretion.

eupepsia (u-pep′se-ah) good digestion; the presence of a normal amount of pepsin in the gastric juice. **eupep′tic,** adj.

euphoria (u-for′e-ah) bodily comfort; well-being; absence of pain or distress. In psychiatry, abnormal or exaggerated sense of well-being. **euphor′ic,** adj.

euploid (u′ploid) 1. having a balanced set or sets of chromosomes, in any number. 2. a euploid individual or cell.

eupnea (ūp-ne′ah) normal respiration. **eup-ne′ic,** adj.

Eurax (ūr′aks) trademark for preparations of crotamiton.

eurhythmia (ūr-ith′me-ah) regularity of the pulse.

europium (ūr-o′pe-um) chemical element (*see table*), at. no. 63, symbol Eu.

Eurotium (ūr-o'she-um) a genus of fungi or molds.

eury- word element [Gr.], *wide; broad.*

eurycephalic (ūr"ĭ-sĭ-fal'ik) having a wide head.

euryon (ūr'e-on) a point on either parietal bone marking either end of the greatest transverse diameter of the skull.

euthanasia (u"thah-na'zhah) 1. an easy or painless death. 2. mercy killing; the deliberate ending of life of a person suffering from an incurable disease.

euthermic (u-therm'ik) characterized by the proper temperature; promoting warmth.

eutocia (u-to'she-ah) normal labor, or childbirth.

Eutrombicula (u"trom-bik'ūl-ah) a subgenus of *Trombicula;* see *chigger.*

eutrophia (u-tro'fe-ah) a state of normal (good) nutrition. **eutroph'ic,** adj.

eutrophication (u"tro-fĭ-ka'shin) the accidental or deliberate promotion of excessive growth (multiplication) of an organism to the disadvantage of other organisms in the same ecosystem by oversupplying it with nutrients.

eV electron volt.

evacuant (ĭ-vak'u-int) 1. promoting evacuation. 2. an agent which promotes evacuation.

evacuation (e-vak"u-a'shin) 1. an emptying, as of the bowels. 2. a dejection or stool; material discharged from the bowels.

eventration (e"ven-tra'shin) 1. protrusion of the bowels through the abdomen. 2. removal of the abdominal viscera. **diaphragmatic e.,** elevation of the dome of the diaphragm, usually due to phrenic nerve paralysis.

eversion (e-ver'zhin) a turning inside out; a turning outward.

evisceration (e-vis"er-a'shin) 1. extrusion of the viscera, or internal organs; disembowelment. 2. removal of the contents of the eyeball, leaving the sclera.

evocation (ev"ah-ka'shin) the calling forth of morphogenetic potentialities through contact with organizer material.

evocator (ev'o-kāt"er) a chemical substance emitted by an organizer that evokes a specific morphogenetic response from competent embryonic tissue in contact with it.

evolution (ev"ol-oo'shin) a developmental process in which an organ or organism becomes more and more complex by differentiation of its parts; a continuous and progressive change according to certain laws and by means of resident forces. **convergent e.,** the appearance of similar forms and/or functions in two or more lines not sufficiently related phylogenetically to account for the similarity. **organic e.,** the origin and development of species; the theory that existing organisms are the result of descent with modification from those of past times.

evulsion (e-vul'shin) extraction by force.

ex- word element [L.], *away from; out of.*

exa- (ek'sah) a word element used in naming units of measurement to designate a quantity 10^{18} (a quintillion, or million million million) times the unit to which it is joined.

examination (eg-zam"ĭ-na'shin) inspection or investigation, especially as a means of diagnosing disease, qualified according to the methods used, as physical, cystoscopic, etc.

exanthem (eg-zan'them) 1. any eruptive disease or fever. 2. an eruption characterizing an eruptive fever. **e. sub'itum,** an acute, mild, viral disease of children, with continuous or remittent fever lasting about 3 days, falling by crisis, and followed by a rash on the trunk.

exanthema (eg"zan-the'mah), pl. *exanthe'mata* [Gr.] exanthem.

exanthematous (eg"zan-them'ah-tis) characterized by or of the nature of an eruption or rash.

exarticulation (eks"ar-tik-ūl-a'shin) amputation at a joint; partial removal of a joint.

excalation (eks"kah-la'shin) absence or exclusion of one member of a normal series, such as a vertebra.

excavatio (eks"kah-va'she-o), pl. *excavatio'nes* [L.] excavation.

excavation (-va'shin) 1. the act of hollowing out. 2. a hollowed-out space, or pouchlike cavity. **atrophic e.,** cupping of the optic disk, due to atrophy of the optic nerve fibers. **dental e.,** removal of carious material from a tooth in preparation for filling. **e. of optic disk, physiologic e.,** a depression in the center of the optic disk. **rectouterine e.,** a sac formed by a fold of peritoneum dipping down between the uterus and rectum. **rectovesical e.,** the space between the rectum and bladder in the peritoneal cavity of the male. **vesicouterine e.,** the space between the bladder and uterus in the peritoneal cavity of the female.

excernent (ek-sern'int) causing an evacuation or discharge.

excess (ek'ses) a surplus, an amount greater than that which is normal or that which is required. **antigen e.,** the presence of more than enough antigen to saturate all available antibody binding sites.

exchange (eks-chānj) 1. the substitution of one thing for another. 2. to substitute one thing for another. **plasma e.,** the removal of plasma from withdrawn blood, with retransfusion of the formed elements into the donor; done for removal of circulating antibodies or abnormal plasma constituents. The plasma removed is replaced by type-specific frozen plasma or by albumin.

exchanger (eks-chānj'er) an apparatus by which something may be exchanged. **heat e.,** a device placed in the circuit of extracorporeal circulation to induce rapid cooling and rewarming of blood.

excipient (ek-sip'e-int) any more or less inert substance added to a drug to give suitable consistency or form to the drug; a vehicle.

excise (ek-sīz') to remove by cutting.

excitation (ek"si-ta'shin) an act of irritation or stimulation; a condition of being excited or of responding to a stimulus; the addition of energy, as the excitation of a molecule by absorption of photons. **direct e.,** electrostimulation of a muscle by placing the electrode on the muscle itself. **indirect e.,** electrostimulation of a muscle by placing the electrode on its nerve.

excitor (ek-si′tor) a nerve which stimulates a part to greater activity.

exclave (eks′klāv) a detached part of an organ.

exclusion (eks-kloo′zhin) a shutting out or elimination; surgical isolation of a part, as of a segment of intestine, without removal from the body.

excochleation (eks″kok-le-a′shin) curettement of a cavity.

excoriation (eks-ko″re-a′shin) any superficial loss of substance, as that produced on the skin by scratching.

excrement (eks′krĭ-mint) fecal matter; matter cast out as waste from the body.

excrescence (eks-kres′ins) an abnormal outgrowth; a projection of morbid origin. **excres′-cent,** adj.

excreta (eks-krēt′ah) excretion products; waste material excreted from the body.

excretion (eks-kre′shin) 1. the act, process, or function of excreting. 2. material that is excreted. **ex′cretory,** adj.

excursion (eks-kur′zhin) a range of movement regularly repeated in performance of a function, e.g., excursion of the jaws in mastication. **excur′sive,** adj.

excyclophoria (eks″si-klo-for′e-ah) cyclophoria in which the upper pole of the visual axis deviates toward the temple.

excyclotropia (-tro′pe-ah) cyclotropia in which the upper pole of the visual axis deviates toward the temple.

excystation (ek″sis-ta′shin) escape from a cyst or envelope, as in that stage in the life cycle of parasites occurring after the cystic form has been swallowed by the host.

exenteration (eks-ent″er-a′shin) surgical removal of the inner organs; evisceration. **pelvic e.,** excision of the organs and adjacent structures of the pelvis.

exenterative (eks-ent′er-ah-tiv) pertaining to or requiring exenteration, as exenterative surgery.

exercise (ek′ser-sīz) performance of physical exertion for improvement of health or correction of physical deformity. **active e.,** motion imparted to a part by voluntary contraction and relaxation of its controlling muscles. **active resistive e.,** motion voluntarily imparted to a part against resistance. **isometric e.,** active exercise performed against stable resistance, without change in the length of the muscle. **isotonic e.,** active exercise without appreciable change in the force of muscular contraction, with shortening of the muscle. **passive e.,** motion imparted to a part by another person or outside force, or produced by voluntary effort of another segment of the patient's own body.

exfetation (eks″fe-ta′shin) ectopic or extrauterine pregnancy.

exflagellation (eks-flaj″il-a′shin) the protrusion or formation of flagelliform microgametes from a microgametocyte in malarial parasites and some related sporozoa.

exfoliation (eks-fo″le-a′shin) a falling off in scales or layers. **exfo′liative,** adj. **lamellar e. of newborn,** a congenital hereditary disorder in which the infant (collodion baby) is born entirely covered with a collodion- or parchment-like membrane that peels off within 24 hours, after which there may be complete healing, or the scales may re-form and the process repeated; in the more severe form, the infant (harlequin fetus) is entirely covered with thick, horny, armor-like scales, and is usually stillborn or dies soon after birth.

exhalation (eks″hah-la′shin) 1. the giving off of watery or other vapor, or of an effluvium. 2. a vapor or other substance exhaled or given off. 3. the act of breathing out.

exhaustion (eg-zaws′chin) 1. privation of energy with consequent inability to respond to stimuli; lassitude. 2. withdrawal. 3. a condition of emptiness caused by withdrawal. 4. emptying by a process of withdrawal. **heat e.,** an effect of excessive exposure to heat, marked by subnormal body temperature with dizziness, headache, nausea, and sometimes delirium and/or collapse.

exhibitionism (ek″sĭ-bish′in-izm) a paraphilia marked by recurrent sexual urges for and fantasies of exposing one's genitals to an unsuspecting stranger.

exhibitionist (ek″sĭ-bish′in-ist) a person who indulges in exhibitionism.

exo- word element [Gr.], *outside; outward.*

exocardial (-kar′de-il) situated, occurring, or developed outside the heart.

exocrine (ek′sah-krin) 1. secreting externally via a duct. 2. denoting such a gland or its secretion.

exocytosis (ek″so-si-to′sis) 1. the discharge from a cell of particles that are too large to diffuse through the wall; the opposite of endocytosis. 2. the aggregation of migrating leukocytes in the epidermis as part of the inflammatory response.

exodeviation (-de″ve-a′shin) a turning outward; in ophthalmology, exotropia.

exodontics (-don′tiks) that branch of dentistry dealing with extraction of teeth.

exoenzyme (-en′zīm) an enzyme which acts outside the cell which secretes it.

exoerythrocytic (-ĕ-rith″ro-sit′ik) occurring outside the erythrocyte; applied to developmental stages of malarial parasites taking place in cells other than erythrocytes.

exogamy (ek-sog′ah-me) 1. protozoan fertilization by union of elements that are not derived from the same cell. 2. marriage outside a particular group.

exogastrula (ek″so-gas′troo-lah) an abnormal gastrula in which invagination is hindered and the mesentoderm bulges outward.

exogenous (ek-soj′in-is) originating outside or caused by factors outside the organism.

exomphalos (eks-om′fah-los) 1. hernia of the abdominal viscera into the umbilical cord. 2. congenital umbilical hernia.

exonuclease (ek″so-noo′kle-ās) a nuclease that

cleaves single mononucleotides from the end of a polynucleotide chain.

exopeptidase (-pep′tĭ-dās) a proteolytic enzyme whose action is limited to terminal peptide linkages.

exophoria (-for′e-ah) deviation of the visual axis of one eye away from that of the other eye in the absence of visual fusional stimuli. **exopho′ric,** adj.

exophthalmometry (ek″sof-thal-mom′ĭ-tre) measurement of the extent of protrusion of the eyeball in exophthalmos. **exophthalmomet′ric,** adj.

exophthalmos (ek″sof-thal′mus) abnormal protrusion of the eye. **exophthal′mic,** adj.

exophytic (ek″so-fit′ik) growing outward; in oncology, proliferating on the exterior or surface epithelium of an organ or other structure in which the growth originated.

exoskeleton (-skel′it-in) a hard structure formed on the outside of the body, as a crustacean's shell; in vertebrates, applied to structures produced by the epidermis, as hair, nails, hoofs, teeth, etc.

exosmosis (ek″sos-mo′sis) osmosis or diffusion from within outward.

exostosis (ek″sos-to′sis), pl. *exosto′ses* [Gr.] a benign growth projecting from a bone surface characteristically covered by cartilage. **exostot′ic,** adj. **e. cartilagi′nea,** a variety of osteoma consisting of a layer of cartilage developing beneath the periosteum of a bone. **multiple exostoses, hereditary,** a dominant condition in which multiple bony excrescences grow out from the cortical surfaces of long bones.

exothermal, exothermic (ek″so-therm′il; -therm′ik) marked or accompanied by evolution of heat; liberating heat and energy.

exotoxin (-tok′sin) a potent toxin formed and excreted by the bacterial cell, and free in the surrounding medium. **exotox′ic,** adj.

exotropia (-tro′pe-ah) strabismus in which there is permanent deviation of the visual axis of one eye away from that of the other, resulting in diplopia. **exotro′pic,** adj.

expectorant (ek-spek′ter-int) 1. promoting expectoration. 2. an agent that promotes expectoration. **liquefying e.,** an expectorant that promotes the ejection of mucus from the respiratory tract by decreasing its viscosity.

expectoration (ek-spek″ter-a′shin) 1. the coughing up and spitting out of material from the lungs, bronchi, and trachea. 2. sputum.

experiment (ek-sper′ĭ-ment) a procedure done in order to discover or demonstrate some fact or general truth. **experimen′tal,** adj. **control e.,** one made under standard conditions, to test the correctness of other observations.

expirate (eks′pĭ-rit) exhaled air or gas. **single e.,** the gas exhaled at a single expiration.

expire (ek-spi′er) 1. to breathe out. 2. to die.

explant 1. (eks-plant′) to take from the body and place in an artificial medium for growth. 2. (eks′plant) tissue taken from the body and grown in an artificial medium.

exploration (eks″plor-a′shin) investigation or examination for diagnostic purposes. **explo′ratory,** adj.

exposure (eks-po′zher) 1. the act of laying open, as surgical exposure. 2. the condition of being subjected to something, as to infectious agents, extremes of weather or radiation, which may have a harmful effect. 3. in radiology, a measure of the amount of ionizing radiation at the surface of the irradiated object, e.g., the body.

expression (eks-presh′in) 1. the aspect or appearance of the face as determined by the physical or emotional state. 2. the act of squeezing out or evacuating by pressure.

expressivity (eks″pres-siv′it-e) the extent to which a heritable trait is manifested by an individual carrying the principal gene or genes that determine it.

exsanguination (ek-sang″gwin-a′shin) extensive loss of blood due to internal or external hemorrhage.

exsiccation (ek″sĭ-ka′shin) the act of drying out; in chemistry, the deprival of a crystalline substance of its water of crystallization.

exsorption (ek-sorp′shin) the movement of substances out of cells, especially the movement of substances out of the blood into the intestinal lumen.

exstrophy (ek′strah-fe) the turning inside out of an organ. **e. of bladder,** congenital absence of a portion of the lower abdominal wall and the anterior vesical wall, with eversion of the posterior vesical wall through the deficit and with an open pubic arch and widely separated ischia connected by a fibrous band. **e. of cloaca, cloacal e.,** a developmental anomaly in which two segments of bladder (hemibladders) are separated by an area of intestine with a mucosal surface, which appears as a large red tumor in the midline of the lower abdomen.

ext. extract.

extender (eks-ten′der) something that enlarges or prolongs. **artificial plasma e.,** a substance that can be transfused to maintain fluid volume of the blood in event of great necessity, supplemental to the use of whole blood and plasma.

extension (eks-ten′shin) 1. the movement by which the two ends of any jointed part are drawn away from each other. 2. a movement bringing the members of a limb into or toward a straight condition. **nail e.,** extension exerted on the distal fragment of a fractured bone by means of a nail or pin (Steinmann pin) driven into the fragment. **Steinmann e.,** nail e.

extensor (eks-ten′ser) [L.] any muscle that extends a joint.

exteriorize (eks-tēr′e-er-īz) 1. to form a correct mental reference of the image of an object seen. 2. in psychiatry, to turn one's interest outward. 3. to transpose an internal organ to the exterior of the body.

extern (eks′tern) a medical student or graduate in medicine who assists in patient care in the hospital but does not reside there.

external (eks-tern′il) situated or occurring on the outside. In anatomy, situated toward or near the outside; lateral.

externus (eks-tern′is) external; in anatomy, denoting a structure farther from the center of the part or cavity.

exteroceptor (eks″ter-o-sep′ter) a sensory nerve ending stimulated by the immediate external environment, such as those in the skin and mucous membranes. **exterocep′tive**, adj.

exterofective (-fek′tiv) responding to external stimuli; a term applied to the cerebrospinal nervous system.

extima (eks′tĭ-mah) outermost; the outermost coat of a blood vessel.

extinction (eks-tink′shin) in psychology, the disappearance of a conditioned response as a result of nonreinforcement; also, the process by which the disappearance is accomplished.

extorsion (eks-tor′shin) the outward rotation of the upper pole of the vertical meridian of each eye.

extra- word element [L.], *outside; beyond the scope of; in addition.*

extract (eks′trakt) a concentrated preparation of a vegetable or animal drug.

extraction (eks-trak′shin) 1. the process or act of pulling or drawing out. 2. the preparation of an extract. **breech e.,** extraction of an infant from the uterus in breech presentation. **flap e.,** extraction of a cataract by an incision which makes a flap of cornea. **serial e.,** the selective extraction of deciduous teeth during an extended period of time to allow autonomous adjustment.

extractive (eks-trak′tiv) any substance present in an organized tissue, or in a mixture in a small quantity, and requiring extraction by a special method.

extractor (eks-trak′ter) an instrument for removing a calculus or foreign body. **vacuum e.,** a device to assist delivery consisting of a metal traction cup that is attached to the fetus' head; negative pressure is applied and traction is made on a chain passed through the suction tube.

extraembryonic (-em″bre-on′ik) external to the embryo proper, as the extraembryonic coelom or extraembryonic membranes.

extramalleolus (-mal-e′ah-lis) the external malleolus.

extramedullary (-med′il-ĕ″re) situated or occurring outside a medulla, especially the medulla oblongata.

extramural (-mūr′il) situated or occurring outside the wall of an organ or structure.

extranuclear (-noo′kle-er) situated or occurring outside a cell nucleus.

extraplacental (-plah-sen′til) outside of or independent of the placenta.

extrapolation (ek-strap″ah-la′shin) inference of a value on the basis of that which is known or has been observed.

extrapulmonary (-pul′min-e″re) not connected with the lungs.

extrapyramidal (-pĭ-ram′id′l) outside the pyramidal tracts; see under *system.*

extrasystole (-sis′tah-le) a premature cardiac contraction that is independent of the normal rhythm and arises in response to an impulse outside the sinoatrial node. **atrial e.,** one in which the stimulus is thought to arise in the atrium elsewhere than at the sinus. **atrioventricular e.,** one in which the stimulus is thought to arise in the atrioventricular node. **infranodal e.,** ventricular e. **interpolated e.,** a contraction taking place between two normal heart beats. **nodal e.,** atrioventricular e. **retrograde e.,** a premature ventricular contraction, followed by a premature atrial contraction, due to transmission of the stimulus backward, usually over the bundle of His. **ventricular e.,** one in which either a pacemaker or re-entry site is in the ventricular structure.

extravasation (eks-trav″ah-za′shin) 1. a discharge or escape, as of blood, from a vessel into the tissues; blood or other substance so discharged. 2. the process of being extravasated.

extraversion (-ver′zhin) extroversion.

extremitas (eks′trem′ĭ-tas), pl. *extremita′tes* [L.] extremity.

extremity (eks-trem′it-e) 1. the distal or terminal portion of elongated or pointed structures. 2. the arm or leg.

extrinsic (eks-trin′sik) of external origin.

extroversion (eks″trah-ver′zhin) 1. a turning inside out; exstrophy. 2. direction of one's energies and attention outward from the self.

extrovert (eks′trah-vert) a person whose interest is turned outward.

extrude (ek-strood′) 1. to force out, or to occupy a position distal to that normally occupied. 2. in dentistry, to occupy a position occlusal to that normally occupied.

extubation (eks″too-ba′shin) removal of a tube used in intubation.

exuberant (eg-zu′ber-int) copious or excessive in production; showing excessive proliferation.

exudate (eks′u-dāt) a fluid with a high content of protein and cellular debris which has escaped from blood vessels and has been deposited in tissues or on tissue surfaces, usually as a result of inflammation.

exumbilication (eks″um-bil″ĭ-ka′shin) 1. marked protrusion of the navel. 2. umbilical hernia.

exuviation (eg-zoo″ve-a′shin) shedding an epithelial structure, e.g., deciduous teeth.

ex vivo (eks″ve′vo) outside the living body; denoting removal of an organ (e.g., the kidney) for reparative surgery, after which it is returned to the original site.

eye (i) the organ of vision; see Plate XIII. **black e.,** a bruise of the tissue around the eye, marked by discoloration, swelling, and pain. **compound e.,** the multifaceted eye of insects. **cross e.,** esotropia. **exciting e.,** the eye that is primarily injured and from which the influences start which involve the other eye in sympathetic ophthalmia. **Klieg e.,** conjunctivitis, edema of the eyelids, lacrimation, and photophobia due to exposure to intense lights (Klieg lights). **pink e.,** acute contagious conjunctivitis. **shipyard e.,** epidemic keratoconjunctivitis. **wall e.,** 1. leukoma of the cornea. 2. exophoria.

eyeball (i′bawl″) the ball or globe of the eye.

eyebrow (i'brow″) 1. supercilium; the transverse elevation at the junction of the forehead and the upper eyelid. 2. supercilia; the hairs growing on this elevation.

eyecup (i'kup″) 1. a small vessel for application of cleansing or medicated solution to the exposed area of the eyeball. 2. physiologic cup.

eyeglass (i'glas″) a lens for aiding the sight.

eyeground (i'grownd″) the fundus of the eye as seen with the ophthalmoscope.

eyelash (i'lash″) cilium; one of the hairs growing on the edge of an eyelid.

eyelid (i'lid″) either of two movable folds (upper and lower) protecting the anterior surface of the eyeball. **third e.**, nictitating membrane.

eyepiece (i'pēs″) the lens or system of lenses of a microscope (or telescope) nearest the user's eye, serving to further magnify the image produced by the objective.

eyestrain (i'strān″) fatigue of the eye from overuse or from uncorrected defect in focus of the eye.

F

F chemical symbol, *fluorine*.

F. Fahrenheit; field of vision; formula; French.

F₁ first filial generation.

F₂ second filial generation.

fabella (fah-bel'ah), pl. *fabel'lae* [L.] see *Table of Bones*.

F.A.C.D. Fellow of American College of Dentists.

face (fās) 1. the anterior, or ventral, aspect of the head from the forehead to the chin, inclusive. 2. any presenting aspect or surface. **fa'cial**, adj. **moon f.**, the peculiar rounded face seen in various conditions, as in Cushing's syndrome, or after administration of adrenal corticoids.

face-bow (fās'bo″) a device used in dentistry to record the positional relations of the maxillary arch to the temporomandibular joints and to orient dental casts in this same relationship to the opening axis of the articulator.

facet (fas'it) a small plane surface on a hard body, as on a bone.

facetectomy (fas″it-ek'tah-me) excision of the articular facet of a vertebra.

faci(o)- word element [L.], *face*.

-facient word element [L.], *making, causing to become*.

facies (fa'she-ēz), pl. *fa'cies* [L.] 1. the face. 2. a specific surface of a body structure, part, or organ. 3. the expression or appearance of the face.

facilitation (fah-sil″ĭ-ta'shin) hastening or assistance of a natural process; the increased excitability of a neuron after stimulation by a subthreshold presynaptic impulse.

facilitative (fah-sil'ĭ-tāt-iv) in pharmacology, denoting a reaction arising as an indirect result of drug action, as development of an infection after the normal microflora has been altered by an antibiotic.

facing (fās'ing) a piece of porcelain cut to represent the outer surface of a tooth.

faciobrachial (fa″she-o-bra'ke-il) pertaining to the face and the arm.

faciolingual (-ling'gwil) pertaining to the face and tongue.

facioplasty (fa'she-o-plas″te) restorative or plastic surgery of the face.

facioplegia (fa″she-o-ple'je-ah) facial paralysis. **faciople'gic**, adj.

F.A.C.O.G. Fellow of the American College of Obstetricians and Gynecologists.

F.A.C.P. Fellow of American College of Physicians.

F.A.C.S. Fellow of American College of Surgeons.

F.A.C.S.M. Fellow of the American College of Sports Medicine.

factitial (fak-tish'il) artificially produced; unintentionally produced.

factor (fak'ter) an agent or element that contributes to the production of a result. **accelerator f.**, coagulation Factor V. **angiogenesis f.**, a substance that causes the growth of new blood vessels, found in tissues with high metabolic requirements and also released by macrophages to initiate revascularization in wound healing. **antihemorrhagic f.**, vitamin K. **antinuclear f. (ANF)**, see under *antibody*. **f. B**, a complement component (C3 proactivator) that participates in the alternate complement pathway. **B cell differentiation f's**, factors derived from T cells that stimulate B cells to differentiate into antibody-secreting cells. **clone-inhibiting f. (CIF)** a lymphokine that exhibits a direct cytostatic effect against actively growing tissue-culture tumor cell lines. **C3 nephritic f.**, a gamma globulin that is not an immunoglobulin in the plasma of some individuals with membranoproliferative glomerulonephritis with hypocomplementemia; it initiates the alternate complement pathway. **coagulation f's**, factors essential to normal blood clotting, whose absence, diminution, or excess may lead to abnormality of the clotting mechanism. Twelve factors, commonly designated by Roman numerals (I to V and VII to XIII) have been described (factor VI is no longer considered to have a clotting function). Platelet factors, designated by Arabic numerals, also play a role in coagulation. *Factor I*, fibrinogen; it is converted to fibrin by the action of thrombin. Deficiency results in afibrinogemia or hypofibrinogenemia. *Factor II*, prothrombin; it is converted to thrombin by extrinsic prothrombin converting principle. Deficiency leads to hypoprothrombinemia. *Factor III*, tissue thromboplastin; it is important in formation of extrinsic prothrombin converting principle. *Factor IV*, calcium.

Factor V, proaccelerin; it functions in both intrinsic and extrinsic pathways of blood coagulation. Deficiency leads to parahemophilia. *Factor VII,* proconvertin; it functions in the extrinsic pathway of blood coagulation. Deficiency, either hereditary or acquired (vitamin K deficiency), leads to hemorrhagic tendency. *Factor VIII,* antihemophilic factor. Deficiency, a sex-linked recessive trait, results in classical hemophilia. *Factor IX,* plasma thromboplastin component; Christmas factor. Deficiency results in hemophilia B. *Factor X,* Stuart factor. Deficiency may result in a systemic coagulation disorder. *Factor XI,* plasma thromboplastin antecedent. Deficiency results in hemophilia C. *Factor XII,* Hageman factor; it initiates the intrinsic process of blood clotting *in vitro. Factor XIII,* fibrin stabilizing factor; it polymerizes fibrin monomers. Deficiency causes a clinical hemorrhagic diathesis. **colony stimulating f.,** a glycoprotein lymphokine produced by blood monocytes, tissue macrophages, and stimulated lymphocytes and required for the differentiation of stem cells into granulocyte and monocyte cell colonies; it may be necessary for granulopoiesis and has been used as an experimental cancer agent. **f. D,** a factor that, when activated, serves as a serine esterase–splitting factor B from C3b in the alternate complement pathway. **extrinsic f.,** cyanocobalamin. **F f., fertility f.,** the plasmid that determines the mating type of conjugating bacteria, being present in the donor (male) bacterium and absent in the recipient (female). **glucose tolerance f.,** a biologically active complex of chromium and nicotinic acid that facilitates the reaction of insulin with receptor sites on tissues. **growth inhibitory f's,** see *clone-inhibiting f.* and *proliferation-inhibiting f.* **Hageman f.,** coagulation Factor XII. **histamine releasing f.,** a lymphokine produced by activated lymphocytes that induces the release of histamine by basophils. **insulin-like growth f's,** insulin-like substances in serum that do not react with insulin antobodies; they are growth hormone–dependent and possess all the growth-promoting properties of the somatomedins. **intrinsic f.,** a glycoprotein secreted by the parietal cells of the gastric glands, necessary for the absorption of vitamin B_{12}. Lack of intrinsic factor, with consequent deficiency of vitamin B_{12}, results in pernicious anemia. **LE f.,** an immunoglobulin (a 7S antibody) that reacts with leukocyte nuclei, found in the serum in systemic lupus erythematosus. **leukocyte inhibitory f., (LIF),** a lymphokine that prevents polymorphonuclear leukocytes from migrating. **leukocyte mitogenic f. (LMF),** a lymphokine causing blast transformation and synthesis of DNA in normal lymphocytes. **lymph node permeability f. (LNPF),** a substance from normal lymph nodes which produces vascular permeability. **lymphocyte transforming f. (LTF),** a lymphokine causing transformation and clonal expansion of nonsensitized lymphocytes. **myocardial depressant f. (MDF),** a peptide formed in response to a fall in systemic blood pressure, which has a negatively inotropic effect on myocardial muscle fibers. **osteoclast activating f.,**

a lymphokine produced by lymphocytes which facilitates bone resorption. **platelet f's,** factors important in hemostasis which are contained in or attached to the platelets: *platelet factor 1* is coagulation Factor V from the plasma; *platelet factor 2* is an accelerator of the thrombin-fibrinogen reaction; *platelet factor 3* plays a role in the generation of intrinsic prothrombin converting principle; *platelet factor 4* is capable of inhibiting the activity of heparin. **platelet-activating f. (PAF),** an immunologically produced substance which leads to clumping and degranulation of blood platelets. **platelet-derived growth f.,** a substance contained in the alpha granules of blood platelets whose action contributes to the repair of damaged blood vessel walls. **proliferation-inhibiting f. (PIF),** a lymphokine that inhibits mitosis in tissue culture cells. **R f.,** the bacterial plasmid (R plasmid) responsible for resistance to antibiotics; it is transmitted to other bacterial cells by conjugation, as well as to the progeny of any cell containing it. **releasing f's,** factors elaborated in one structure (as in the hypothalamus) that effect the release of hormones from another structure (as from the anterior pituitary gland), including corticotropin relasing factor, melanocyte-stimulating hormone releasing factor, and prolactin releasing factor. Applied to substances of unknown chemical structure, while substances of established chemical identity are called *releasing hormones.* **resistance f.,** R f., **Rh f., Rhesus f.,** genetically determined antigens present on the surface of erythrocytes; incompatibility for these antigens between mother and offspring is responsible for erythroblastosis fetalis. **rheumatoid f.,** a protein (IgM) detectable by serological tests, which is found in the serum of most patients with rheumatoid arthritis and in other related and unrelated diseases and sometimes in apparently normal persons. Abbreviated RF. **risk f.,** a clearly defined occurrence or characteristic that has been associated with the increased rate of a subsequently occurring disease. **Stuart f., Stuart-Prower f.,** coagulation Factor X.

facultative (fak′ul-ta″tiv) not obligatory; pertaining to the ability to adjust to particular circumstances or to assume a particular role.

faculty (fak′il-te) 1. a normal power or function, especially of the mind. 2. the teaching staff of an institution of learning.

FAD flavin-adenine dinucleotide.

fae- for words beginning thus, see those beginning *fe-.*

failure (fāl′yer) inability to perform or to function properly. **heart f.,** see under *H.* **kidney f., renal f.,** inability of the kidney to excrete metabolites at normal plasma levels under normal loading, or inability to retain electrolytes when intake is normal; in the acute form, marked by uremia and usually by oliguria, with hyperkalemia and pulmonary edema.

faint (fānt) syncope.

falcate (fal′kāt) falciform.

falcial (-shil) pertaining to a falx.

falciform (-sĭ-form) sickle-shaped.

falcular (-kūl-er) falciform.

fallout (fawl′owt″) the settling to the earth's surface of radioactive fission products from the atmosphere after a nuclear explosion.

false-negative (fawls′neg′ah-tiv) 1. denoting a test result that wrongly excludes an individual from a category. 2. an individual so excluded. 3. an instance of a false-negative result.

false-positive (fawls′pos′it-iv) 1. denoting a test result that wrongly assigns an individual to a category. 2. an individual so categorized. 3. an instance of a false-positive result.

falsification (fawl″sĭ-fĭ-ka′shin) lying. **retrospective f.,** unconscious distortion of past experiences to conform to present emotional needs.

falx (falks), pl. *fal′ces* [L.] a sickle-shaped structure. **f. cerebel′li,** a fold of dura mater separating the cerebellar hemispheres. **f. ce′rebri,** the fold of dura mater in the longitudinal fissure, separating the cerebral hemispheres.

familial (fah-mil′e-il) occurring in more members of a family than would be expected by chance.

family (fam′ĭ-le) 1. a group descended from a common ancestor. 2. a taxonomic subdivision subordinate to an order (or suborder) and superior to a tribe (or subfamily).

F and R force and rhythm (of pulse).

fang (fang) 1. the root of a tooth. 2. a tooth of a carnivore with which it seizes and tears its prey, or the envenomed tooth of a serpent.

Fannia (fan′e-ah) a genus of flies whose larvae cause intestinal and urinary myiasis in man.

fantasy (fan′tah-se) an imaged sequence of events satisfying one's unconscious wishes or expressing one's unconscious conflicts.

F.A.P.H.A. Fellow of the American Public Health Association.

farad (far′ad) the unit of electric capacity; capacity to hold 1 coulomb with a potential of 1 volt.

faraday (far′ah-da) the quantity of electrical charge associated with one gram equivalent of an electrochemical reaction, equal to about 96,510 coulombs.

farcy (far′se) see *glanders.*

farinaceous (far″ĭ-na′shis) 1. of the nature of flour or meal. 2. starchy; containing starch.

farsightedness (far-sīt′id-nis) hyperopia.

fascia (fash′e-ah), pl. *fas′ciae* [L.] a sheet or band of fibrous tissue such as lies deep to the skin or invests muscles and various body organs. **fas′cial,** adj. **f. adhe′rens,** that portion of the junctional complex of the cells of an intercalated disk that is the counterpart of the zonula adherens of epithelial cells. **f. cribro′sa,** the superficial fascia of the thigh covering the saphenous opening. **endothoracic f.,** that beneath the serous lining of the thoracic cavity. **extrapleural f.,** a prolongation of the endothoracic fascia sometimes found at the root of the neck, important as a possible modifier of the auscultatory sounds at the apex of the lung. **necrotizing f.,** a gas-forming, fulminating, necrotic infection of the superficial and deep fascia, resulting in thrombosis of the subcutaneous vessels and gangrene of the underlying tissues. It is usually caused by multiple pathogens and is frequently associated with diabetes mellitus. **f. profun′da,** a dense, firm, fibrous membrane investing the trunk and limbs and giving off sheaths to the various muscles. **Scarpa's f.,** the deep, membranous layer of the subcutaneous abdominal fascia. **Tenon's f.,** see under *capsule.* **thyrolaryngeal f.,** that covering the thyroid body and attached to the cricoid cartilage. **Tyrrell's f.,** that between the bladder and rectum.

fascicle (fas′ĭ-k'l) a small bundle or cluster, especially of nerve or muscle fibers. **fascic′ular,** adj.

fasciculated (fah-sik′ūl-āt-ĕd) clustered together or occurring in bundles, or fasciculi.

fasciculation (fah-sik″ūl-a′shin) 1. the formation of fascicles. 2. a small local involuntary muscular contraction visible under the skin, representing spontaneous discharge of fibers innervated by a single motor nerve filament.

fasciculus (fah-sik′ūl-us), pl. *fasci′culi* [L.] fascicle. **f. cuneatus of medulla oblongata,** the continuation into the medulla oblongata of the fasciculus cuneatus of the spinal cord. **f. cuneatus of spinal cord,** the lateral portion of the posterior funiculus of the spinal cord, composed of ascending fibers that end in the nucleus cuneatus. **f. gracilis of medulla oblongata,** the continuation into the medulla oblongata of the fasciculus gracilis of the spinal cord. **f. gracilis of spinal cord,** the median portion of the posterior funiculus of the spinal cord, composed of ascending fibers that end in the nucleus gracilis.

fasciitis (īt′is) inflammation of a fascia. **nodular f., proliferative f.,** a benign, reactive proliferation of fibroblasts in the subcutaneous tissues, commonly affecting the deep fascia. **pseudosarcomatous f.,** a benign soft tissue tumor occurring subcutaneously and sometimes arising from deep muscle and fascia.

fasciodesis (-od′ĭ-sis) suture of a fascia to skeletal attachment.

Fasciola (fah-si′ol-ah) a genus of flukes, including *F. hepa′tica,* the common liver fluke of herbivores, occasionally found in the human liver.

fasciola (fah-si′ol-ah), pl. *fasci′olae* [L.] 1. a small band of striplike structure. 2. a small bandage. **fasci′olar,** adj.

fascioliasis (fas″e-ol-i′ah-sis) infection with *Fasciola.*

fasciolopsiasis (-op-si′ah-sis) infection with *Fasciolopsis.*

Fasciolopsis (-op′sis) a genus of trematodes, including *F. bus′ki,* the largest of the intestinal flukes, found in the small intestines of residents throughout Asia.

fasciotomy (fas″e-ot′ah-me) incision of a fascia.

fast (fast) 1. immovable, or unchangeable; resistant to the action of a specific drug, stain, or destaining agent. 2. abstention from food.

fastigium (fas-tij′e-um) [L.] 1. the highest point in the roof of the fourth ventricle of the brain. 2. the acme, or highest point. **fastig′ial,** adj.

Fastin (fast′in) trademark for a preparation of phentermine hydrochloride.

fat (fat) 1. adipose tissue. 2. an ester of glycerol with fatty acids, usually palmitic, oleic, or stearic acid. **fat′ty,** adj. **polyunsaturated f.,** one containing fatty acids having more than one double bond in the carbon chain. **saturated f.,** one containing fatty acids having only single bonds in the carbon chain. **unsaturated f.,** one containing fatty acids with double bonds in the carbon chain.

fatigability (fat″ĭ-gah-bil′it-e) easy susceptibility to fatigue.

fatigue (fah-tēg) a state of increased discomfort and decreased efficiency due to prolonged or excessive exertion; loss of power or capacity to respond to stimulation.

fatty acid (fat′e) any monobasic aliphatic acid containing only carbon, hydrogen, and oxygen, which combines with glycerin to form fat. **essential f. a.,** an unsaturated fatty acid that cannot be formed in the body and therefore must be provided by the diet; the most important are linoleic acid, linolenic acid, and arachidonic acid.

fauces (faw′sēz) the passage between the throat and pharynx. **fau′cial,** adj.

fauna (faw′nah) the collective animal organisms of a given locality.

faveolate (fah-ve′o-lāt) honeycombed; alveolate.

favid (fa′vid) a secondary skin eruption due to allergy in favus.

favism (fa′vizm) an acute hemolytic anemia precipitated by fava beans (ingestion, or inhalation of pollen), usually caused by deficiency of glucose-6-phosphate dehydrogenase in the erythrocytes.

favus (fa′vus) a type of tinea capitis, with formation of prominent honeycomb-like masses, due to *Trichophyton schoenleini.* **f. of fowl,** a chronic dermatomycosis affecting the comb of fowl, caused by *Trichophyton megnini.*

Fc fragment, crystallizable; a fragment by papain digestion of immunoglobulin molecules. It contains most of the antigenic determinants.

Fc′ a fragment produced in minute quantities by papain digestion of immunoglobulin molecules. It contains the principal part of the C terminal portion of two Fc fragments.

Fd the heavy chain portion of a Fab fragment produced by papain digestion of an IgG molecule.

FDA Food and Drug Administration.

F.D.I. Fédération Dentaire Internationale (International Dental Association).

Fe chemical symbol, *iron* (L. *ferrum*).

fear (fēr) a normal emotional response, in contrast to anxiety and phobia, to consciously recognized external sources of danger, which is manifested by alarm, apprehension, or disquiet.

febricant (feb′rĭ-kint) causing fever.

febricide (feb′rĭ-sīd) 1. lowering bodily temperature in fever. 2. an agent that lowers fever.

febricity (feb-ris′it-e) feverishness, being febrile.

febrifacient (feb″rĭ-fa′shint) producing fever.

febrific (feb-rif′ik) producing fever.

febrifugal (feb-rif′u-gil) dispelling fever.

febrile (feb′ril) pertaining to fever; feverish.

febris (feb′ris) [L.] fever. **f. meliten′sis, f. un′dulans,** brucellosis.

fecalith (fe′kah-lith) an intestinal concretion formed around a center of fecal matter.

fecaloid (fe′kil-oid) resembling feces.

feces (fe′sēz), pl. of *faex* [L.] excrement discharged from the bowels. **fe′cal,** adj.

fecula (fek′ūl-ah) 1. lees or sediment. 2. starch.

feculent (fek′ūl-int) 1. having dregs or sediment. 2. excrementitious.

fecundation (fe″kin-da′shin) fertilization; impregnation.

fecundity (fĕ-kun′dit-e) the ability to produce offspring frequently and in large numbers. In demography, the physiological ability to reproduce, as opposed to fertility.

feedback (fēd′bak) the return of some of the output of a system as input so as to exert some control in the process; feedback is *negative* when the return exerts an inhibitory control; *positive* when it exerts a stimulatory effect.

feed-forward (fēd-for′wird) the anticipatory effect that one intermediate in a metabolic or endocrine control system exerts on another intermediate further along in the pathway; such effect may be positive or negative.

feeding (fēd′ing) the taking or giving of food. **artificial f.,** feeding of a baby with food other than mother's milk. **breast f.,** see under B. **forced f.,** administration of food by force to those who cannot or will not receive it.

fellatio (fĕ-la′she-o) oral stimulation or manipulation of the penis.

felon (fel′in) a purulent infection involving the pulp of the distal phalanx of a finger.

feltwork (felt′werk) a complex of closely interwoven fibers, as of nerve fibers.

feminism (fem′ĭ-nizm) the appearance or existence of female secondary sex characters in the male.

feminization (fem″ĭ-ni-za′shin) 1. the normal induction or development of female sex characters. 2. the induction or development of female secondary sex characters in the male. **testicular f.,** a condition in which the subject is phenotypically female, but lacks nuclear sex chromatin and is of XY chromosomal sex.

femoral (fem′ah-ril) pertaining to the femur or to the thigh.

femorocele (fem′ah-ro-sēl″) femoral hernia.

femto- (fem′to) a combining form used in naming units of measurement to indicate one-quadrillionth (10^{-15}) of the unit designated by the root with which it is combined.

femur (fe′mer), pl. *fem′ora* [L.] 1. see *Table of Bones.* 2. the thigh.

fenestra (fĭ-nes′trah), pl. *fenes′trae* [L.] a window-like opening. **f. co′chleae,** a round opening in the inner wall of the middle ear covered by the secondary tympanic membrane. **f. ova′lis,** vestibuli. **f. rotun′da,** f. cochleae. **f. vesti′buli,** an oval opening in the inner wall of the middle ear, which is closed by the base of the stapes.

fenestration (fen″is-tra′shin) 1. the act of perforating or condition of being perforated. 2. the surgical creation of a new opening in the labyrinth of the ear for restoration of hearing in otosclerosis. **aortopulmonary f.,** aortic septal defect.

fenfluramine (fen-floor'ah-mēn) an amphetamine derivative, $C_{12}H_{16}F_3N$, used as an anorexic in the form of the hydrochloride salt.

fenoprofen (fen″ah-pro'fen) an anti-inflammatory, analgesic, and antipyretic, $C_{15}H_{14}O_3$.

fentanyl (fen'tah-nil) a piperidine derivative $C_{22}H_{22}N_2O$; the citrate salt is used as a narcotic analgesic and, in combination with droperidol (known as *Innovar*), as a neuroleptanalgesic.

ferment 1. (fer-ment') to undergo fermentation. 2. (ferm'ent) any substance that causes fermentation.

fermentation (ferm″en-ta'shin) the anaerobic enzymatic conversion of organic compounds, especially carbohydrates, to simpler compounds, especially to ethyl alcohol, producing energy in the form of ATP.

fermium (ferm'e-um) chemical element (*see table*), at. no. 100, symbol Fm.

ferning (fern'ing) the appearance of a fernlike pattern in a dried specimen of cervical mucus, an indication of the presence of estrogen.

-ferous word element [L.], *bearing; producing.*

ferredoxin (fĕ″rĭ-dok'sin) a nonheme iron-containing protein having a very low redox potential; the ferredoxins participate in electron transport in photosynthesis, nitrogen fixation, and various other biological processes.

ferric (fĕ'rik) containing iron in its plus-three oxidation state, Fe(III) (also with Fe^{3+}).

ferritin (fĕ'rit-in) the iron-apoferritin complex, which is one of the chief forms in which iron is stored in the body.

ferrokinetics (-ki-net'iks) the turnover or rate of change of iron in the body.

ferroprotein (-pro'te-in) a protein combined with an iron-containing radical; ferroproteins are respiratory carriers.

ferrous (fĕ'ris) containing iron in its plus-two oxidation state, Fe(II) (sometimes designated Fe^{2+}); for ferrous compounds see under the salt, e.g., sulfate.

ferruginous (fah-roo'jin-is) 1. containing iron or iron rust. 2. of the color of iron rust.

ferrum (fĕ'rum) [L.] iron (symbol Fe).

fertility (fer-til'it-e) the capacity to conceive or induce conception. **fer'tile,** adj.

fertilization (fert″il-iz-a'shin) union of male and female elements, leading to development of a new individual. **external f.,** union of the gametes outside the bodies of the originating organisms, as in most fish. **internal f.,** union of the gametes inside the body of the female, the sperm having been transferred from the body of the male by an accessory sex organ or other means.

fervescence (fer-ves'ins) increase of fever or body temperature.

fester (fes'ter) to suppurate superficially.

festination (fes″tĭ-na'shin) an involuntary tendency to take short accelerating steps in walking.

festoon (fes-tōōn') a carving in the base material of a denture that simulates the contours of the natural tissues being replaced.

fetal (fēt'il) of or pertaining to a fetus or the period of its development.

fetalization (fēt″il-iz-a'shin) retention in the adult of characters that at an earlier stage of evolution were only infantile and were rapidly lost as the organism attained maturity.

fetation (fe-ta'shin) 1. development of the fetus. 2. pregnancy.

feticide (fēt'ĭ-sīd) the destruction of the fetus.

fetid (fēt'id, fet'id) having a rank, disagreeable smell.

fetish (fet'ish, fēt'ish) an object symbolically endowed with special meaning; an object or body part charged with special erotic interest.

fetishism (fet'ish-izm, fēt-ish-izm) 1. a primitive religion marked by belief in fetishes. 2. a paraphilia marked by recurrent sexual urges for and fantasies of using fetishes, usually articles of clothing, for sexual arousal or orgasm. **transvestic f.,** recurrent sexual urges for and fantasies of cross-dressing.

fetology (fe-tol'ah-je) that branch of medicine dealing with the fetus *in utero.*

fetometry (fe-tom'ĭ-tre) measurement of the fetus, especially of its head.

α-fetoprotein alpha-fetoprotein.

fetor (fe'tor, fēt'er) stench or offensive odors. **f. o'ris,** halitosis. **hepatic f., f. hepa'ticus,** the peculiar odor of the breath characteristic of hepatic disease.

fetoscope (fēt'ah-skōp) 1. a specially designed stethoscope for listening to the fetal heart beat. 2. an endoscope for viewing the fetus *in utero.*

fetus (fēt'is) [L.] the developing young in the uterus, specifically the unborn offspring in the postembryonic period, in man from seven or eight weeks after fertilization until birth. **harlequin f.,** a newborn infant with the severest form of lamellar exfoliation of the newborn. **mummified f.,** a dried-up and shriveled fetus. **f. papyra'ceus,** a dead fetus pressed flat by the growth of a living twin. **parasitic f.,** an incomplete minor fetus attached to a larger, more completely developed fetus, or autosite.

fever (fe'ver) 1. pyrexia; elevation of body temperature above the normal (98.6° F. or 37° C.). 2. any disease characterized by elevation of body temperature. **blackwater f.,** a dangerous complication of falciparum malaria, with passage of dark red to black urine, severe toxicity, and high mortality. **boutonneuse f.,** a tickborne disease endemic in the Mediterranean area, Crimea, Africa, and India, due to infection with *Rickettsia conorii,* with chills, fever, primary skin lesion (tache noire), and rash appearing on the second to fourth day. **central f.,** sustained fever resulting from damage to the thermoregulatory centers of the hypothalamus. **childbed f.,** puerperal septicemia. **Colorado tick f.,** a tickborne, nonexanthematous, febrile, viral disease occurring in the Rocky Mountain regions of the United States. **continued f.,** one not varying more than 1.0° to 1.5° F. in 24 hours. **drug f.,** febrile reaction to a therapeutic agent, including vaccines, antineoplastics, antimicrobials, etc. **elephantoid f.**, a recurrent acute febrile condition occurring with filariasis; it may be associated with elephantiasis or lymphangitis. **enteric f.**, 1. typhoid f. 2. paratyphoid. **epidemic hemorrhagic f.**, an acute infectious disease characterized by fever, purpura, peripheral vascular collapse, and acute renal failure, caused by a filterable agent thought to be transmitted to man by mites or chiggers. **familial Mediterranean f.**, a hereditary disease usually occurring in Armenians and Sephardic Jews, and marked by short recurrent attacks of fever with pain in the abdomen, chest, or joints and erythema resembling that seen in erysipelas; it is sometimes complicated by amyloidosis. **Haverhill f.**, an acute form of rat-bite fever due to *Streptobacillus moniliformis*, transmitted by the bite of an infected rat, with an erythematous eruption, severe generalized arthritis, adenitis, headache, and vomiting. **hay f.**, a seasonal form of allergic rhinitis, with acute conjunctivitis, lacrimation, itching, swelling of the nasal mucosa, nasal catarrh, sudden attacks of sneezing, and often asthmatic symptoms; regarded as an anaphylactic or allergic condition excited by a specific allergen (e.g., pollen) to which the person is sensitized. **hay f., nonseasonal, hay f. perennial**, nonseasonal allergic rhinitis. **hemorrhagic f's**, a group of viral diseases of diverse etiology but having many similar clinical characteristics: increased capillary permeability, leukopenia, and thrombocytopenia are common to all. They are manifested by sudden onset, fever, headache, generalized myalgia, backache, conjunctivitis, and severe prostration, followed by various hemorrhagic symptoms, which result in focal inflammatory reaction and necrosis, with mild leukocytosis. **intermittent f.**, an attack of malaria or other fever, with recurring paroxysms of elevated temperature separated by intervals during which the temperature is normal. **Katayama f.**, fever associated with severe schistosomal infections, accompanied by hepatosplenomegaly and by eosinophilia. **Lassa f.**, a highly fatal, acute, febrile disease caused by an extremely virulent arenavirus, occurring in West Africa, and characterized by progressively increasing prostration, sore throat, ulcerations of the mouth or throat, rash, and general aches and pains. **mud f.**, leptospiral jaundice. **paratyphoid f.**, paratyphoid. **parenteric f.**, a disease clinically resembling typhoid fever and paratyphoid, but not caused by *Salmonella*. **parrot f.**, psittacosis. **pharyngoconjunctival f.**, an epidemic disease due to an adenovirus, occurring chiefly in school children, with fever, pharyngitis, conjunctivitis, rhinitis, and enlarged cervical lymph nodes. **phlebotomus f.**, a febrile viral disease of short duration, transmitted by the sandfly *Phlebotomus papatasii*, with dengue-like symptoms, occurring in Mediterranean and Middle East countries. **Pontiac f.**, a self-limited disease first noted in an outbreak in Pontiac, Michigan, marked by fever, cough, muscle aches, chills, headache, chest pain, confusion, and pleuritis, caused by a strain of *Legionella pneumophila*. **pretibial f.**, an infection due to *Leptospira autumnalis*, marked by a rash on the pretibial region, with lumbar and postorbital pain, malaise, coryza, and fever. **puerperal f.**, septicemia accompanied by fever, in which the focus of infection is a lesion of the mucous membrane of the parturient canal due to trauma during childbirth; usually due to a streptococcus. **Q f.**, a febrile rickettsial infection, usually respiratory, first described in Australia, caused by *Coxiella burnetii*. **rat-bite f.**, either of two clinically similar acute infectious diseases, usually transmitted through a rat bite, one form (bacillary) of which is caused by *Streptobacillus moniliformis* and the other form (spirillary) by *Spirillum minor*. **recurrent f.**, relapsing f. **relapsing f.**, any of a group of infectious diseases due to various species of *Borrelia*, marked by alternating periods of fever and apyrexia, each lasting from five to seven days. **remittent f.**, one varying 2° F. or more in 24 hours, but without return to normal temperature. **rheumatic f.**, a febrile disease occurring as a sequela to Group A hemolytic streptococcal infections, characterized by multiple focal inflammatory lesions of the connective tissue structures, especially of the heart, blood vessels, and joints, and by the presence of Aschoff bodies in the myocardium and skin. **Rift Valley f.**, a febrile disease with dengue-like symptoms, due to an arbovirus, transmitted by mosquitoes or by contact with diseased animals; first observed in the Rift Valley, Kenya. **Rocky Mountain spotted f.**, infection with *Rickettsia rickettsii*, transmitted by ticks, marked by fever, muscle pain, and weakness followed by a macular petechial eruption that begins on the hands and feet and spreads to the trunk and face, by central nervous system symptoms, etc. **scarlet f.**, an acute disease caused by Group A β-hemolytic streptococci, marked by pharyngotonsillitis and a skin rash caused by an erythrogenic toxin produced by the organism; the rash is a diffuse, bright scarlet erythema with many points of deeper red. Desquamation of the skin begins as a fine scaling with eventual peeling of the palms and soles. **septic f.**, fever due to septicemia. **South African tick-bite f.**, a tickborne infection in South Africa, due to *Rickettsia conorii*, the etiologic agent of boutonneuse fever. **typhoid f.**, infection by *Salmonella typhosa* chiefly involving the lymphoid follicles of the ileum, with chills, fever, headache, cough, prostration, abdominal distention, splenomegaly, and a maculopapular rash; perforation of the bowel occurs in about 5% of untreated cases. **yellow f.**, an acute, infectious, mosquito-borne viral disease, endemic primarily in tropical South America and Africa, marked by fever, jaundice due to necrosis of the liver, and albuminuria.

FFA free fatty acids.

fiber (fi′ber) 1. an elongated, threadlike structure. 2. in nutrition, the sum of the constituents of the diet that are not digested by gastrointestinal enzymes. **A f's**, myelinated fibers of the somatic nervous system having a diameter of 1μ to 22μ and a conduction velocity of 5–120 meters per second. **accelerating f's, accelerator f's**, adrenergic fibers that transmit the impulses which accelerate the heart beat. **adren-**

ergic f's, nerve fibers that liberate epinephrine-like substances at the time of passage of nerve impulses across a synapse. **alpha f's,** motor and proprioceptive fibers of the A type, having conduction velocities of 70–120 meters per second and ranging from 13μ to 22μ in diameter. **alveolar f's,** fibers of the periodontal ligament extending from the cementum of the tooth root to the walls of the alveolus. **arcuate f.,** any of the bow-shaped fibers in the brain, such as those connecting adjacent gyri in the cerebral cortex, or the external or internal arcuate fibers of the medulla oblongata. **association f's,** nerve fibers that interconnect portions of the cerebral cortex within a hemisphere. Short association fibers interconnect neighboring gyri; long fibers interconnect more widely separated gyri and are arranged into bundles or fasciculi. **B f's,** myelinated preganglionic autonomic axons having a fiber diameter of $\leq 3\mu$ and a conduction velocity of 3–15 meters per second. **basilar f's,** those that form the middle layer of the zona arcuata and the zona pectinata of the organ of Corti. **beta f's,** touch and temperature fibers of the A type, having conduction velocities of 30–70 meters per second and ranging from 8μ to 13μ in diameter. **C f's,** unmyelinated postganglionic fibers of the autonomic nervous system, also the unmyelinated fibers at the dorsal roots and at free nerve endings, having a conduction velocity of 0.6–2.3 meters per second and a diameter of 0.3μ to 1.3μ. **collagen f's, collagenic f's, collagenous f's,** the soft, flexible, white fibers which are the most characteristic constituent of all types of connective tissue, consisting of the protein collagen, and composed of bundles of fibrils that are in turn made up of smaller units (microfibrils) which show a characteristic crossbanding with a major periodicity of 65 nm. **dietary f.,** that part of whole grains, vegetables, fruits, and nuts that resists digestion in the gastrointestinal tract; it consists of carbohydrate (cellulose, etc.) and lignin. **elastic f's,** yellowish fibers of elastic quality traversing the intercellular substance of connective tissue. **gamma f's,** A fibers that conduct touch and pressure impulses and innervate the intrafusal fibers of the muscle spindle; they conduct at velocities of 15–40 meters per second and range from 3μ to 7μ in diameter. **Gottstein's f's,** the external cells and the nerve fibers associated with them, forming part of the expansion of the auditory nerve in the cochlea. **gray f's,** unmyelinated nerve fibers found largely in the sympathetic nerves. **medullated f's,** myelinated f's. **motor f's,** nerve fibers that transmit impulses to a muscle fiber. **Müller's f's,** elongated neuroglial cells traversing all the layers of the retina, forming its principal supporting element. **muscle f.,** any of the cells of skeletal or cardiac muscle tissue. Skeletal muscle fibers are cylindrical multinucleate cells containing contracting myofibrils, across which run transverse striations. Cardiac muscle fibers have one or sometimes two nuclei, contain myofibrils, and are separated from one another by an intercalated disk; although striated, cardiac muscle fibers branch to form an interlacing network. See Plate XIV. **nerve f.,** a

slender process of a neuron, especially the prolonged axon which conducts nerve impulses away from the cell; classified on the basis of the presence or absence of a myelin sheath as myelinated or unmyelinated. See Plate XI. **nonmedullated f's,** unmyelinated f's. **osteogenetic f's, osteogenic f's,** precollagenous fibers formed by osteoclasts and becoming the fibrous component of bone matrix. **preganglionic f's,** fibers constituting a preganglionic neuron. **pressor f's,** 1. nerve fibers which, when stimulated reflexly, cause or increase vasomotor tone. 2. cardiac pressor f's. **Purkinje's f's,** modified cardiac muscle fibers in the subendothelial tissue that rapidly transmit impulses in the heart and serve to coordinate contractions of the heart. **radicular f's,** fibers in the roots of the spinal nerves. **reticular f.,** immature connective tissue fibers staining with silver, forming the reticular framework of lymphoid and myeloid tissue, and occurring in interstitial tissue of glandular organs, papillary layer of the skin, and elsewhere. **Sharpey's f's,** 1. collagenous fibers that pass from the periosteum and are embedded in the outer circumferential and interstitial lamellae of bone. 2. terminal portions of principal fibers that insert into the cementum of a tooth. **somatic f's,** nerve fibers, afferent or efferent, that stimulate or activate skeletal muscle and somatic tissues. **spindle f's,** the microtubules radiating from the centrioles during mitosis and forming a spindle-shaped configuration. **traction f's,** spindle f's. **unmyelinated f's,** nerve fibers that lack the myelin sheath. **vasomotor f's,** unmyelinated nerve fibers going chiefly to arteriolar muscles. **white f's,** collagenous f's.

fiber-illuminated   (fi′ber-il-loo″min-a′ted) transmitting light by bundles of glass or plastic fibers, using a lens system to transmit the image; said of endoscopes of such design.

fiberoptics (-op′tiks) the transmission of an image along flexible bundles of glass or plastic fibers, each of which carries an element of the image.

fibr(o)- word element [L.], *fiber; fibrous.*

fibra (fi′brah), pl. *fi′brae* [L.] fiber.

fibril (fi′bril) a minute fiber or filament. **fibril′lar, fib′rillary,** adj. **dentinal f's,** component fibrils of the dentinal matrix.

fibrilla (fi-bril′ah), pl. *fibril′lae* [L.] a fibril.

fibrillation (fi″brĭ-la′shin) 1. a small, local, involuntary, muscular contraction, due to spontaneous activation of single muscle cells or muscle fibers. 2. the quality of being made up of fibrils. 3. the initial degenerative changes in osteoarthritis, marked by softening of the articular cartilage and development of vertical clefts between groups of cartilage cells. **atrial f.,** atrial arrhythmia marked by rapid randomized contractions of the atrial myocardium, causing a totally irregular, and often rapid, ventricular rate. **ventricular f.,** cardiac arrhythmia marked by fibrillary contractions of the ventricular muscle due to rapid repetitive excitation of myocardial fibers without coordinated ventricular contraction.

fibrin (fi′brin) an insoluble protein that is essential to clotting of blood, formed from fibrinogen by action of thrombin.

fibrinase (-ās) coagulation Factor XIII.

fibrinocellular (fi″brĭ-no-sel′ūl-er) made up of fibrin and cells.

fibrinogen (fi-brin′ah-jen) 1. coagulation Factor I. 2. human fibrinogen: a sterile fraction of normal human plasma, administered to increase the coagulability of the blood.

fibrinogenic (fi-brin″ah-jen′ĭk) producing or causing the formation of fibrin.

fibrinogenolysis (fi″brin-o-jin-ol′ĭ-sis) the proteolytic destruction of fibrinogen in circulating blood. **fibrinogenolyt′ic,** adj.

fibrinogenopenia (fi-brin″ah-jen″ah-pe′ne-ah) deficiency of fibrinogen in the blood. **fibrinogenope′nic,** adj.

fibrinoid (fi′brĭ-noid) 1. resembling fibrin. 2. a homogeneous, eosinophilic, relatively acellular refractile substance with some of the staining properties of fibrin.

fibrinolysin (fi″brĭ-nol′ĭ-sin) 1. plasmin. 2. a preparation of proteolytic enzyme formed from profibrinolysin (plasminogen); to promote dissolution of thrombi.

fibrinopenia (fi″brĭ-no-pe′ne-ah) deficiency of fibrinogen in the blood.

fibrinopeptide (-pep′tĭd) either of two peptides (A and B) split off from fibrinogen during coagulation by the action of thrombin.

fibrinopurulent (-pūr′ool-int) characterized by the presence of both fibrin and pus.

fibrinuria (fi″brin-ūr′e-ah) the presence of fibrin in the urine.

fibroadenoma (fi″bro-ad″ĕ-no′mah) adenoma containing fibrous elements.

fibroadipose (-ad′ĭ-pōs) both fibrous and fatty.

fibroareolar (-ah-re′ol-er) both fibrous and areolar.

fibroblast (fi′bro-blast) 1. an immature fiber-producing cell of connective tissue capable of differentiating into chondroblast, collagenoblast, or osteoblast. 2. collagenoblast; the collagen-producing cell. They also proliferate at the site of chronic inflammation. **fibroblas′tic,** adj.

fibroblastoma (fi″bro-blas-to′mah) any tumor arising from fibroblasts, now classified as fibromas or fibrosarcomas.

fibrobronchitis (-brong-kīt′is) croupous bronchitis.

fibrocalcific (-kal-sif′ik) pertaining to or characterized by partially calcified fibrous tissue.

fibrocarcinoma (-kar″sĭ-no′mah) scirrhous carcinoma.

fibrocartilage (-kart′ĭ-lij) cartilage of parallel, thick, compact collagenous bundles, separated by narrow clefts containing the typical cartilage cells (chondrocytes). **fibrocartilag′inous,** adj. **elastic f.,** that containing elastic fibers. **interarticular f.,** any articular disk.

fibrocartilago (-kart″ĭ-la′go), pl. *fibrocartilag′ines* [L.] fibrocartilage.

fibrochondritis (-kon-drīt′is) inflammation of fibrocartilage.

fibrocollagenous (-kol-laj′in-is) both fibrous

and collagenous; pertaining to or composed of fibrous tissue mainly composed of collagen.

fibrocyst (fi′bro-sist) cystic fibroma.

fibrocystic (fi″bro-sist′ik) characterized by an overgrowth of fibrous tissue and development of cystic spaces, especially in a gland.

fibrocyte (fi′bro-sīt) fibroblast.

fibroelastic (-e-last′ik) both fibrous and elastic.

fibroelastosis (-e″las-to′sis) overgrowth of fibroelastic elements. **endocardial f.,** a condition characterized by left ventricular hypertrophy and conversion of the endocardium into a thick fibroelastic coat, with ventricular capacity sometimes reduced, but often increased.

fibroepithelioma (-ep″ĭ-thēl″e-o′mah) a tumor composed of both fibrous and epithelial elements.

fibroid (fi′broid) 1. having a fibrous structure; resembling a fibroma. 2. fibroma. 3. leiomyoma; *fibroids* is a colloquial clinical term for leiomyoma of the uterus.

fibroidectomy (fi″broid-ek′tah-me) excision of a uterine fibroma.

fibrolipoma (fi″bro-lĭ-po′mah) a lipoma with excessive fibrous tissue. **fibrolipo′matous,** adj.

fibroma (fi-bro′mah) a tumor composed mainly of fibrous or fully developed connective tissue. **ameloblastic f.,** an odontogenic fibroma, marked by simultaneous proliferation of both epithelial and mesenchymal tissue, without formation of enamel or dentin. **chondromyxoid f.,** a rare benign, slowly growing tumor of bone of chondroblastic origin, usually affecting the large long bones of the lower extremity. **cystic f.,** one that has undergone cystic degeneration. **nonosteogenic f.,** a degenerative and proliferative lesion of the medullary and cortical tissues of bone. **ossifying f., ossifying f. of bone,** a benign, relatively slow-growing, central bone tumor, usually of the jaws, especially the mandible, which is composed of fibrous connective tissue within which bone is formed.

fibromatosis (fi″bro-mah-to′sis) 1. the presence of multiple fibromas. 2. the formation of a fibrous, tumor-like nodule arising from the deep fascia, with a tendency to local recurrence. **f. gingi′vae, gingival f.,** noninflammatory fibrous hyperplasia of the gingiva manifested as a dense, diffuse, smooth or nodular overgrowth of the gingival tissues. **palmar f.,** fibromatosis involving the palmar fascia, and resulting in Dupuytren's contracture. **plantar f.,** fibromatosis involving the plantar fascia manifested as single or multiple nodular swellings, sometimes accompanied by pain but usually unassociated with contractures.

fibromyitis (-mi-īt′is) inflammation of muscle with fibrous degeneration.

fibromyoma (-mi-o′mah) a myoma containing fibrous elements.

fibromyxoma (-mik-so′mah) myxofibroma.

fibromyxosarcoma (-mik″so-sar-ko′mah) a sarcoma containing fibrous and mucous elements.

fibronectin (-nek′tin) an adhesive glycoprotein: one form circulates in plasma, acting as an opsonin; another is a cell-surface protein which mediates cellular adhesive interactions.

fibropapilloma (-pap″il-o′mah) a papilloma containing much fibrous tissue.

fibroplasia (-pla′ze-ah) the formation of fibrous tissue. **fibroplas′tic,** adj. **retrolental f.,** a condition characterized by retinal vascular proliferation and tortuosity and by fibrous tissue behind the lens, leading to detached retina and arrest of growth of the eye, generally attributed to use of excessively high concentrations of oxygen in the care of premature infants.

fibrosarcoma (-sar-ko′mah) a sarcoma derived from collagen-producing fibroblasts. **odontogenic f.,** a malignant tumor of the jaws, originating from one of the mesenchymal components of the tooth or tooth germ.

fibrosis (fi-bro′sis) formation of fibrous tissue; fibroid degeneration. **fibrot′ic,** adj. **congenital hepatic f.,** a developmental disorder of the liver marked by formation of irregular broad bands of fibrous tissue containing multiple cysts formed by disordered terminal bile ducts, resulting in vascular constriction and portal hypertension. **cystic f., cystic f. of pancreas,** a generalized hereditary disorder of infants, children, and young adults, associated with widespread dysfunction of the exocrine glands, marked by signs of chronic pulmonary disease, obstruction of pancreatic ducts by amorphous eosinophilic concretions with consequent pancreatic enzyme deficiency, by abnormally high electrolyte levels in sweat, and occasionally by biliary cirrhosis. **endomyocardial f.,** idiopathic myocardiopathy occurring endemically in various regions of Africa and rarely in other areas, characterized by cardiomegaly, marked thickening of the endocardium with dense, white fibrous tissue that frequently extends to involve the inner third or half of the myocardium, and congestive heart failure. **idiopathic pulmonary f.,** chronic inflammation and progressive fibrosis of the pulmonary alveolar walls, with steadily progressive dyspnea, resulting in death from lack of oxygen or right heart failure. **mediastinal f.,** development of whitish, hard fibrous tissue in the upper portion of the mediastinum, sometimes obstructing the air passages and large blood vessels.

fibrositis (fi″bro-sīt′is) inflammatory hyperplasia of the white fibrous tissue, especially of the muscle sheaths and facial layers of the locomotor system.

fibrothorax (-thor′aks) adhesion of the two pleural layers, the lung being covered by thick nonexpansible fibrous tissue.

fibula (fib′ūl-ah), pl. *fib′ulae* [L.] see *Table of Bones.* **fib′ular,** adj.

fibulocalcaneal (fib″ūl-o-kal-ka′ne-il) pertaining to fibula and calcaneus.

F.I.C.D. Fellow of the International College of Dentists.

ficin (fi′sin) a highly active, crystallizable proteinase from the sap of fig trees, which catalyzes the hydrolysis of many proteins at acid (4.1) pH, the clotting of milk, and "digestion" of some living worms, e.g., whipworms. Ficin is used as a protein digestant and to enhance the agglutination of red blood cells with IgC antibodies (e.g., Rh antibodies). It also shows esterase ac-

tivity. It has been used in dogs as a trichuricide.

F.I.C.S. Fellow of the International College of Surgeons.

field (fēld) 1. an area or open space, as an operative field or visual field. 2. a range of specialization in knowledge, study, or occupation. 3. in embryology, the developing region within a range of modifying factors. **auditory f.,** the space or range within which stimuli may be perceived as sound. **individuation f.,** a region in which an organizer influences adjacent tissue to become a part of a total embryo. **morphogenetic f.,** an embryonic region out of which definite structures normally develop. **visual f.,** the area within which stimuli will produce the sensation of sight with the eye in a straight-ahead position.

FIGLU formiminoglutamic acid.

figure (fig′yer) 1. an object of particular form. 2. a number, or numeral. **mitotic f's,** stages of chromosome aggregation exhibiting a pattern characteristic of mitosis.

fila (fil′ah) [L.] plural of *filum.*

filament (fil′ah-ment) a delicate fiber or thread. **filamentous** (fil″ah-ment′is) composed of long, threadlike structures.

filamentum (fil″ah-men′tum), pl. *filamen′ta* [L.] filament.

Filaria (fil-a′re-ah) a former generic name for members of the superfamily Filarioidea. **F. bancrof′ti,** *Wuchereria bancrofti.* **F. medinen′sis,** *Dracunculus medinensis.* **F. san′guinis-ho′minis,** *Wuchereria bancrofti.*

filaria (fil-a′re-ah), pl. *fila′riae* [L.] a nematode worm of the superfamily Filarioidea. **fila′rial,** adj.

filaricide (fil-ār′ĭ-sīd) an agent which destroys filariae. **filaricid′al,** adj.

Filarioidea (fil-a″re-oi′de-ah) a superfamily or order of parasitic nematodes, the adults being threadlike worms that invade the tissues and body cavities where the female deposits microfilariae (prelarvae).

filiform (fil′ĭ-form, fīl′ĭ-form) 1. threadlike. 2. an extremely slender bougie.

fillet (fil′it) 1. a loop, as of cord or tape, for making traction. 2. in the nervous system, a long band of nerve fibers.

filling (fil′ing) 1. material inserted in a prepared tooth cavity. 2. restoration of the crown with appropriate material after removal of carious tissue from a tooth. **complex f.,** one for a complex cavity. **composite f.,** one consisting of a composite resin. **compound f.,** one for a cavity that involves two surfaces of a tooth.

film (film) 1. a thin layer or coating. 2. a thin sheet of material (e.g., gelatin, cellulose acetate) specially treated for use in photography or radiography; used also to designate the sheet after exposure to the energy to which it is sensitive. **bite-wing f.,** an x-ray film for radiography of oral structures, with a protruding tab to be held between the upper and lower teeth. **gelatin f., absorbable,** sterile, nonantigenic, absorbable, water-insoluble film used as an aid in surgical closure and repair of defects in dura and pleura and as a local hemostatic. **plain f.,** a radiograph made without the use of a contrast medium. **spot f.**, a radiograph of a small anatomic area obtained (a) by rapid exposure during fluoroscopy to provide a permanent record of a transiently observed abnormality, or (b) by limitation of radiation passing through the area to improve definition and detail of the image produced. **x-ray f.**, film sensitized to roentgen (x-) rays, either before or after exposure.

film badge (film baj) a pack of radiographic film used for the detection and approximate measurement of radiation exposure of personnel.

filopodium (fi″lo-po′de-um), pl. *filopo′dia* [L.] a filamentous pseudopodium of ectoplasm.

filopressure (-presh′er) compression of a blood vessel by a thread.

filter (fil′ter) a device for eliminating certain elements, as (1) particles of certain size from a solution, or (2) rays of certain wavelength from a stream of radiant energy. **Berkefeld's f.**, one composed of diatomaceous earth, impermeable to ordinary bacteria. **Millipore f.**, trademark for a device used to filter nutrient solutions as they are administered intravenously.

filterable (-ah-b'l) capable of passing through the pores of a filter.

filtrate (fil′trāt) a liquid that has passed through a filter.

filtration (fil-tra′shin) passage through a filter or through a material that prevents passage of certain molecules.

filum (fi′lum), pl. *fi′la* [L.] a threadlike structure or part. **f. termina′le**, a slender, threadlike prolongation of the spinal cord from the conus medullaris to the back of the coccyx.

fimbria (fim′bre-ah), pl. *fim′briae* [L.] 1. a fringe, border, or edge; a fringelike structure. 2. pilus (2). **f. hippocam′pi**, the band of white matter along the median edge of the ventricular surface of the hippocampus. **fimbriae of uterine tube**, the numerous divergent fringelike processes on the distal part of the infundibulum of the uterine tube.

fimbriate (fim′bre-āt) fringed.

fimbriocele (fim′bre-o-sēl″) hernia containing the fimbriae of the uterine tube.

finger (fing′ger) one of the five digits of the hand. **baseball f.**, partial permanent flexion of the terminal phalanx of a finger caused by a ball or other object striking the end or back of the finger, resulting in rupture of the attachment of the extensor tendon. **clubbed f.**, one with enlargement of the terminal phalanx without constant osseous changes. **index f.**, the second digit of the hand; the forefinger. **ring f.**, the fourth digit of the hand. **webbed f's**, syndactyly; fingers more or less united by strands of tissue.

fingerprint (-print) 1. an impression of the cutaneous ridges of the fleshy distal portion of a finger. 2. in biochemistry, the characteristic pattern of a peptide after subjection to an analytical technique.

first aid (furst ād) emergency care and treatment of an injured or ill person before complete medical and surgical treatment can be secured.

fission (fish′in) 1. the act of splitting. 2. asexual reproduction in which the cell divides into two (*binary f.*) or more (*multiple f.*) daughter parts, each of which becomes an individual organism. 3. nuclear fission; the splitting of the atomic nucleus, with release of energy.

fissiparous (fi-sip′ah-ris) propagated by fission.

fissula (fis′ūl-ah), pl. *fis′sulae* [L.] a small cleft.

fissura (fish-ūr′ah), pl. *fissu′rae* [L.] fissure. **f. in a′no**, anal fissure.

fissure (fish′er) 1. any cleft or groove, normal or otherwise, especially a deep fold in the cerebral cortex involving its entire thickness. 2. a fault in the enamel surface of a tooth. **abdominal f.**, a congenital cleft in the abdominal wall. **anal f.**, **f. in a′no**, painful lineal ulcer at the margin of the anus. **anterior median f.**, a longitudinal furrow along the midline of the anterior aspect of the spinal cord and medulla oblongata. **basisylvian f.**, the part of the sylvian fissure between the temporal lobe and the orbital surface of the frontal bone. **f. of Bichat**, transverse f. (2). **branchial f.**, see under *cleft.* **calcarine f.**, see under *sulcus.* **central f.**, see under *sulcus.* **collateral f.**, see under *sulcus.* **enamel f.**, fissure (2). **Henle's f's**, spaces filled with connective tissue between the muscular fibers of the heart. **hippocampal f.**, see under *sulcus.* **palpebral f.**, the longitudinal opening between the eyelids. **parieto-occipital f.**, see under *sulcus.* **portal f.**, porta hepatis. **posterior median f.**, see under *sulcus.* **presylvian f.**, the anterior branch of the fissure of Sylvius. **Rolando's f.**, central sulcus. **spheno-occipital f.**, the fissure between the basilar part of the occipital bone and the sphenoid bone. **sylvian f., f. of Sylvius**, one extending laterally between the temporal and frontal lobes, and turning posteriorly between the temporal and parietal lobes. **transverse f.**, 1. porta hepatis. 2. the transverse cerebral fissure between the diencephalon and the cerebral hemispheres.

fistula (fis′chool-ah) an abnormal passage or communication, usually between two internal organs, or leading from an internal organ to the body surface. **anal f.**, one near the anus, which may or may not communicate with the rectum. **arteriovenous f.**, one between an artery and a vein. **blind f.**, one open at one end only, opening on the skin (*external blind f.*) or on an internal mucous surface (*internal blind f.*). **branchial f.**, a persisting branchial cleft. **craniosinus f.**, one between the cerebral space and one of the sinuses, permitting escape of cerebrospinal fluid into the nose. **fecal f.**, a colonic fistula opening on the external body surface, discharging feces. **gastric f.**, an abnormal passage communicating with the stomach; often applied to a surgically created opening from the stomach through the abdominal wall. **incomplete f.**, blind f. **pulmonary arteriovenous f., congenital**, a congenital anomalous communication between the pulmonary arterial and venous systems, allowing unoxygenated blood to enter the systemic circulation. **salivary f.**, an abnormal passage communicating with a salivary duct. **Thiry's f.**, an opening created into the intestine to obtain specimens of intestinal juice.

umbilical f., one communicating with the gut or the urachus at the umbilicus.

fistulatome (-tōm″) an instrument for cutting a fistula.

fistulization (fis″chool-iz-a′shin) 1. the process of becoming fistulous. 2. the surgical creation of fistula.

fistulotomy (fis″chool-ot′ah-me) incision of a fistula.

fit (fit) a convulsion, paroxysm, or sudden attack. **running f.,** cursive epilepsy.

fixation (fik-sa′shun) 1. the process of making or the state of being immovable. 2. in psychiatry: (1) the cessation of psychosexual development before maturity; (2) a close, suffocating attachment to another person, e.g., one's mother or father. 3. in microscopy, the preservation of tissue so that its structure may be examined in detail with minimal alteration of the normal state. 4. in chemistry, the process whereby a substance is removed from the gaseous or solution phase and localized. 5. in ophthalmology, direction of the gaze so that the visual image of the object falls on the fovea centralis. 6. in film processing, the chemical removal of all undeveloped salts of the film emulsion, as on x-ray films. **complement f., f. of complement,** addition of another serum containing an antibody and the corresponding antigen to a hemolytic serum, making the complement incapable of producing hemolysis.

fixative (fik′sit-iv) an agent used in preserving a histologic or pathologic specimen so as to maintain the normal structure of its constituent elements.

flaccid (flak′sid) weak, lax, and soft.

flagellate (flaj′il-āt) 1. any microorganism having flagella. 2. any protozoon of the subphylum Mastigophora. 3. having flagella.

flagellation (flaj″il-a′shin) 1. massage by tapping the part with the fingers. 2. whipping or being whipped to achieve erotic pleasure. 3. exflagellation.

flagellosis (flaj″il-o′sis) infestation with flagellate protozoa.

flagellospore (flah-jel′ah-spōr) zoospore.

flagellum (flah-jel′um), pl. *flagel′la* [L.] a long mobile, whiplike appendage arising from a basal body at the surface of a cell, serving as a locomotor organelle; in eukaryotic cells, flagella contain nine pairs of microtubules arrayed around a central pair; in bacteria, they contain tightly wound strands of flagellin.

Flagyl (flag′′l) trademark for a preparation of metronidazole.

flail (flāl) exhibiting abnormal or pathologic mobility, as flail chest or flail joint.

flame (flām) 1. the luminous, irregular appearance usually accompanying combustion, or an appearance resembling it. 2. to render an object sterile by exposure to a flame.

flange (flanj) a projecting border or edge; in dentistry, that part of the denture base which extends from around the embedded teeth to the border of the denture.

flank (flank) the side of the body between ribs and ilium.

flap (flap) 1. a mass of tissue for grafting, usually including skin, only partially removed from one part of the body so that it retains its own blood supply during transfer to another site. 2. an uncontrolled movement. **free f.,** an island flap detached from the body and reattached at the distant recipient site by microvascular anastomosis. **jump f.,** one cut from the abdomen and attached to a flap of the same size on the forearm; the forearm flap is transferred later to some other part of the body to fill a defect there. **myocutaneous f.,** a compound flap of skin and muscle with adequate vascularity to permit sufficient tissue to be transferred to the recipient site. **rope f.,** one made by elevating a long strip of tissue from its bed except at its two ends, the cut edges then being sutured together to form a tube. **skin f.,** a full-thickness mass or flap of tissue containing epidermis, dermis, and subcutaneous tissue. **sliding f.,** a flap carried to its new position by a sliding technique.

flare (flār) a diffuse area of redness on the skin around the point of application of an irritant, due to a vasomotor reaction.

flask (flask) 1. a laboratory vessel, usually of glass and with a constricted neck. 2. a metal case in which materials used in making artificial dentures are placed for processing. **Erlenmeyer f.,** a conical glass flask with a broad base and narrow neck. **volumetric f.,** a narrow-necked vessel of glass calibrated to contain or deliver an exact volume at a given temperature.

flatfoot (flat′foot) a condition in which one or more arches of the foot have flattened out.

flatness (-nes) a peculiar sound lacking resonance, heard on percussing an abnormally solid part.

flatulence (flä′chool-ins) excessive formation of gases in the stomach or intestine.

flatus (flāt′is) 1. gas or air in the gastrointestinal tract. 2. gas or air expelled through the anus.

flatworm (flat′wurm) an individual organism of the phylum Platyhelminthes.

flav(o)- word element [L.], *yellow*.

flavin (fla′vin) any of a group of water-soluble yellow pigments widely distributed in animals and plants, including riboflavin and yellow enzymes. **f.-adenine dinucleotide (FAD),** a coenzyme that is a condensation product of riboflavin phosphate and adenylic acid; it forms the prosthetic group of certain enzymes, including D-amino acid oxidase and xanthine oxidase, and is important in electron transport in mitochondria. **f. mononucleotide (FMN),** a derivative of riboflavin consisting of a three-ring system (isoalloxazine) attached to an alcohol (ritibol); it acts as a coenzyme for a number of oxidative enzymes, including 1-amino acid oxidase and cytochrome C reductase.

flavivirus (fla″ve-vi′ris) a subcategory of togaviruses; the type species is the yellow fever virus.

Flavobacterium (fla″vo-bak-tēr′e-im) a genus of schizomycetes (family Achromobacteraceae), characteristically producing yellow, orange, red, or yellow-brown pigmentation, found in soil and water; some species are said to be pathogenic.

flavoenzyme (-en′zīm) any enzyme containing a flavin nucleotide (FMN or FAD) as a prosthetic group.

flavonoid (fla′vah-noid) a generic term for a group of compounds widely distributed in higher plants; one subgroup (anthocyanins) accounts for most of the yellow, red, and blue pigmentation, while another (bioflavonoids) are concerned in maintenance of a normal state of capillary walls.

flavoxate (fla-voks′āt) a smooth muscle relaxant, $C_{24}H_{25}NO_4$; the hydrochloride salt is used in treatment of spasms of the urinary tract.

flaxseed (flak′sēd) linseed.

fl.dr. fluid dram.

flea (fle) a small, wingless, bloodsucking insect; many fleas are parasitic and may act as disease carriers.

fleece (flēs) a mass of interlacing fibrils. **f. of Stilling,** the lacework of white fibers surrounding the dentate nucleus.

flesh (flesh) the soft, muscular tissue of the animal body. **goose f.,** cutis anserina. **proud f.,** exuberant amounts of soft, edematous, granulation tissue developing during healing of large surface wounds.

Flexeril (flek′sah-ril) trademark for a preparation of cyclobenzaprine hydrochloride.

flexibilitas (flek″sĭ-bil′ĭ-tas) [L.] flexibility. **f. ce′rea,** waxy flexibility.

flexibility (flek″sĭ-bil′it-e) the state of being unusually pliant. **waxy f.,** a cataleptic state in which the limbs retain any position in which they are placed.

flexion (flek′shin) the act of bending or the condition of being bent.

flexor (flek′ser) any muscle that flexes a joint; see *Table of Muscles.*

flexura (flek-shoōr′ah), pl. *flexu′rae* [L.] flexure.

flexure (flek′sher) a bend or fold; a curvature. **caudal f.,** the bend at the aboral end of the embryo. **cephalic f.,** the curve in the midbrain of the embryo. **cervical f.,** a bend in the neural tube of the embryo at the junction of the brain and spinal cord. **cranial f.,** cephalic f. **dorsal f.,** one of the flexures in the mid-dorsal region of the embryo. **duodenojejunal f.,** the bend at the junction of duodenum and jejunum. **lumbar f.,** the ventral curvature in the lumbar region of the back. **mesencephalic f.,** a bend in the neural tube of the embryo at the level of the mesencephalon. **nuchal f.,** cervical f. **pontine f.,** a flexure of the hindbrain in the embryo. **sacral f.,** caudal f. **sigmoid f.,** see under *colon.*

floaters (flōt′ers) "spots before the eyes"; deposits in the vitreous of the eye, usually moving about and probably representing fine aggregates of vitreous protein occurring as a benign degenerative change.

floccillation (flok″sil-a′shin) carphology.

floccose (flok′ōs) woolly; said of bacterial growth of short, curved chains variously oriented.

flocculation (flok″ūl-a′shin) a colloid phenomena in which the disperse phase separates in discrete, usually visible, particles rather than congealing into a continuous mass, as in coagulation.

flocculus (flok′ūl-is), pl. *floc′culi* [L.] 1. a small tuft or mass, as of wool or other fibrous material. 2. a small mass on the lower side of each cerebral hemisphere, continuous with the nodule of the vermis. **floc′cular,** adj.

flooding (flud′ing) in behavior therapy, the treatment of phobias and anxieties by repeated exposure to aversive stimuli, whether in the imagination or in real life.

flora (flor′ah) the collective plant organisms of a given locality. **intestinal f.,** the bacteria normally within the lumen of the intestine.

flowmeter (flo′mēt-er) an apparatus for measuring the rate of flow of liquids or gases.

floxuridine (floks-ūr′ĭ-dēn) a derivative of fluouracil, $C_9H_{11}FN_2O_5$, used as an antiviral and antineoplastic agent. Abbreviated FUDR.

fl.oz. fluid ounce.

flu (floo) colloquialism for *influenza.*

fluctuation (fluk″choo-a′shin) a variation, as about a fixed value or mass; a wavelike motion.

flucytosine (floo-sīt′ah-sēn″) an antifungal, $C_4H_4FN_3O$, used in the treatment of severe candidal and cryptococcal infections.

fludrocortisone (floo″dro-kort′ĭ-sōn) a synthetic adrenal corticoid with effects similar to those of hydrocortisone and desoxycorticosterone.

fluid (floo′id) 1. a liquid or gas; any liquid of the body. 2. composed of molecules which freely change their relative positions without separation of the mass. **amniotic f.,** the liquid within the amnion that bathes the developing fetus and protects it from mechanical injury. **cerebrospinal f.,** the fluid contained within the ventricles of the brain, the subarachnoid space, and the central canal of the spinal cord. **interstitial f.,** the extracellular fluid bathing most tissues, excluding the fluid within the lymph and blood vessels. **intracellular f.,** the portion of the total body water with its dissolved solutes which are within the cell membranes. **Müller's f.,** a fluid for preserving anatomic specimens. **Scarpa's f.,** endolymph. **seminal f.,** semen.

fluidextract (floo″id-ek′strakt) a liquid preparation of a vegetable drug, containing alcohol as a solvent or preservative, of such strength that each milliliter contains the extraction of 1 gm. of the standard drug it represents.

fluidrachm (floo′ĭ-dram) fluid dram.

fluke (flook) any trematode.

flumen (floo′men), pl. *flu′mina* [L.] a stream. **flu′mina pilo′rum,** the lines along which the hairs of the body are arranged.

flumethasone (floo-meth′ah-sōn) an anti-inflammatory glucocorticoid, $C_{22}H_{28}F_2O_5$, used topically to treat certain dermatoses.

fluocinolone acetonide (floo″ah-sin′ah-lōn) an anti-inflammatory glucocorticoid, $C_{24}H_{30}F_2O_6$, used topically in eczematous dermatoses.

fluocinonide (-sin′ah-nīd) an ester of fluocinolone acetonide; used topically to treat dermatoses.

fluorescein (floor-es′e-in) a fluorescing dye, $C_{20}H_{10}O_5$; its sodium salt is used in solution to reveal corneal lesions and as a test of circulation in the retina and extremities.

239 **fold**

fluorescence (floor-es'ins) the property of emitting light while exposed to light, the wavelength of the emitted light being longer than that of the absorbed light. **fluores'cent,** adj.

fluoridation (floor-ĭ-da'shin) treatment with fluorides; the addition of fluorides to a public water supply as a public health measure to reduce the incidence of dental caries.

fluorimeter (floor-im'it-er) fluorometer.

fluorine (floor'ēn) chemical element (*see table*), at. no. 9, symbol F.

fluorochrome (floor'ah-krōm) a fluorescent compound used as a dye to mark protein with a fluorescent label.

fluorometer (-om'ĭt-er) the instrument used in fluorometry, consisting of an energy source (e.g., a mercury arc lamp or xenon lamp) to induce fluorescence, monochromators for selection of the wavelength, and a detector.

fluorometholone (floor''o-meth'ah-lōn) an anti-inflammatory glucocorticoid, $C_{22}H_{29}FO_4$, used in dermatoses with an allergic or inflammatory basis and associated with pruritus.

fluorometry (floor-om'ĭ-tre) an analytical technique for identifying minute amounts of a substance by detection and measurement of the characteristic wavelength of the light it emits during fluorescence.

fluoronephelometer (-o-nef''il-om'ĭ-ter) an instrument for analysis of a solution by measuring the light scattered or emitted by it.

fluorophotometry (-o-fah-tom'ĭ-tre) the measurement of light given off by fluorescent substances. **vitreous f.,** the measurement of light given off by intravenously injected fluorescein that has leaked through the retinal vessels into the vitreous; done to detect the breakdown of the blood-retinal barrier, an early ocular change in diabetes mellitus.

fluoroscope (floor'-ah-skōp) an instrument for visual observation of the form and motion of the deep structures of the body by means of x-ray shadows projected on a fluorescent screen.

fluorosis (floor-o'sis) 1. a condition due to ingestion of excessive amounts of fluorine. 2. fluoride intoxication, which may be due to such factors as accidental ingestion of fluoride-containing insecticides and rodenticides, chronic inhalation of industrial dusts or gases containing fluorides, or prolonged ingestion of water containing large amounts of fluorides; characterized by skeletal changes, consisting of combined osteosclerosis and osteomalacia (osteofluorosis) and by mottled enamel of the teeth when exposure occurs during enamel formation. **endemic f., chronic,** that due to unusually high concentrations of fluorine in the natural drinking water supply, typically causing dental fluorosis but also combined osteosclerosis and osteomalacia.

fluorouracil (floor''ah-ūr'ah-sil) an antimetabolite, $C_4H_3FN_2O_2$, used as an antineoplastic agent.

Fluothane (floo'ah-thān) trademark for a preparation of halothane.

fluoxymesterone (floo-ok''se-mes'ter-ōn) an androgen, $C_{20}H_{29}FO_3$, used in the treatment of

male hypogonadism and in the palliative therapy of certain breast cancers.

fluphenazine (floo-fen'ah-zēn) a major tranquilizer, $C_{22}H_{26}F_3N_3OS$, used as the enanthate and hydrochloride salts.

flurandrenolide (floor''an-dren'ol-īd) a glucocorticoid, $C_{27}H_{33}FO$, used in dermatoses.

flurazepam (floor-az'ĭ-pam) a hypnotic, $C_{21}H_{23}ClFN_3O$, used as the hydrochloride salt.

flush (flush) redness, usually transient, of the face and neck.

flutter (flut'er) a rapid vibration or pulsation. **atrial f.,** cardiac arrhythmia in which the atrial contractions are rapid (200–320 per minute), but regular. **diaphragmatic f.,** peculiar wavelike fibrillations of the diaphragm of unknown cause. **impure f.,** atrial flutter in which the atrial rhythm is irregular. **mediastinal f.,** abnormal motility of the mediastinum during respiration. **pure f.,** atrial flutter in which the atrial rhythm is regular. **ventricular f.,** a possible transition stage between ventricular tachycardia and ventricular fibrillation, the electrocardiogram showing rapid, uniform, regular oscillations, 250 or more per minute.

flutter-fibrillation (-fi-bril-a'shin) impure flutters constantly varying in their resemblance to flutter or fibrillation, respectively.

flux (fluks) 1. an excessive flow or discharge. 2. matter discharged.

fly (fli) a dipterous, or two-winged, insect which is often the vector of organisms causing disease. **tsetse f.,** see *Glossina.*

Fm chemical symbol, *fermium.*

FMN flavin mononucleotide.

focus (fo'kis), pl. *fo'ci* [L.] 1. the point of convergence of light rays or sound waves. 2. the chief center of a morbid process. **fo'cal,** adj. **Ghon f.,** the primary parenchymal lesion of primary pulmonary tuberculosis in children.

focusing (fo'kis-ing) the act of converging at a point. **isoelectric f.,** electrophoresis in which the protein mixture is subjected to an electric field in a gel medium in which a pH gradient has been established; each protein then migrates until it reaches the site at which the pH is equal to its isoelectric point.

foe- for words beginning thus, see those beginning *fe-.*

fog (fog) a colloid system in which the dispersion medium is a gas and the disperse particles are liquid.

fogging (fog'ing) in ophthalmology, a method of determining refractive error in astigmatism, the patient being first made artificially myopic in order to relax accommodation.

foil (foil) metal in the form of an extremely thin, pliable sheet.

folate (fo'lāt) any of a group of substances whose molecules are made up of a form of pteroic acid conjugated with L-glutamic acid. Folates act as coenzymes that promote one-carbon transfer, and are present in natural foods, including mammalian cells.

fold (fōld) plica; a thin, recurved margin, or doubling. **amniotic f.,** the folded edge of the amnion where it rises over and finally encloses the embryo. **aryepiglottic f.,** a fold of mucous membrane extending on each side between the lateral border of the epiglottis and the summit of the arytenoid cartilage. **costocolic f.,** phrenicocolic ligament. **Douglas' f.,** a crescentic line marking the termination of the posterior layer of the sheath of the rectus abdominis muscle, just below the level of the iliac crest. **gastric f's,** the series of folds in the mucous membrane of the stomach. **gluteal f.,** the crease separating the buttocks from the thigh. **head f.,** a fold of blastoderm at the cephalic end of the developing embryo. **lacrimal f.,** a fold of mucous membrane at the lower opening of the nasolacrimal duct. **Marshall's f.,** vestigial f. **medullary f.,** neural f. **mesonephric f.,** see under *ridge.* **nail f.,** the fold of palmar skin around the base and sides of the nail. **neural f.,** one of the paired folds lying on either side of the neural plate that form the neural tube. **semilunar f. of conjunctiva,** a mucous fold at the medial angle of the eye. **tail f.,** a fold of blastoderm at the caudal end of the developing embryo. **urogenital f.,** see under *ridge.* **ventricular f., vestibular f.,** a false vocal cord. **vestigial f.,** a pericardial fold enclosing the remnant of the embryonic left anterior cardinal vein. **vocal f.,** the true vocal cord.

folic acid (fo′lik) a vitamin of the B group, pteroylglutamic acid, which is involved in the synthesis of amino acids and DNA; its deficiency causes megaloblastic anemia. See *tetrahydrofolic acid* and *folic acid antagonist.*

folie (fo-le′) [Fr.] psychosis; insanity. **f. à deux** (ah duh′) occurrence of an identical psychosis simultaneously in two closely associated persons. **f. circulaire** (ser-ku-lair′) circular psychosis. **f. du doute** (du doot) pathologic inability to make even the most trifling decisions. **f. du pourquoi** (du poor-kwah′) psychopathologic constant questioning. **f. gémellaire** (zha-mĕ-lair′) psychosis occurring simultaneously in twins. **f. raisonnante** (rez-un-nahnt′) the delusional form of any psychosis.

folinic acid (fo-lin′ik) 5-formyltetrahydrofolic acid, a metabolically active derivative of folic acid used to treat folic acid deficiency and as an antidote to folic acid antagonists. Called also *leucovorin.*

folium (fo′le-um), pl. *fo′lia* [L.] a leaflike structure, especially one of the leaflike subdivisions of the cerebellar cortex.

follicle (fol′ĭ-k'l) a sac or pouchlike depression or cavity. **follic′ular,** adj. **atretic f.,** an involuted ovarian follicle. **gastric f's,** lymphoid masses in the gastric mucosa. **graafian f's,** vesicular ovarian f's. **hair f.,** one of the tubular invaginations of the epidermis enclosing the hairs, and from which the hairs grow. **intestinal f's,** see under *gland.* **lingual f's,** nodular masses of lymphoid tissue at the root of the tongue, constituting the lingual tonsil. **lymph f., lymphatic f.,** 1. a small collection of actively proliferating lymphocytes in the cortex of a lymph node. 2. a small collection of lymphoid tissue in the mucous membrane of the gastrointestinal tract, where they occur singly (*solitary lymphatic f.*) or closely packed together (*aggregated lymphatic f's*). **Naboth's f's, nabothian f's,** cystlike formations due to occlusion of the lumina of glands in the mucosa of the uterine cervix, causing them to be distended with retained secretion. **ovarian f.,** the ovum and its encasing cells, at any stage in its development. **ovarian f's, primary,** immature ovarian follicles, each comprising an immature ovum and the few specialized epithelial cells surrounding it. **ovarian f's, primordial,** an ovarian follicle consisting of an egg enclosed by a single layer of cells. **ovarian f's, vesicular,** graafian follicles; maturing ovarian follicles among whose cells fluid has begun to accumulate, leading to the formation of a single cavity and leaving the ovum located in the cumulus oophorous. **sebaceous f.,** a hair follicle with a relatively large sebaceous gland, producing a relatively insignificant hair. **solitary f's,** 1. areas of concentrated lymphatic tissue in the mucosa of the colon. 2. small lymph follicles scattered throughout the mucosa and submucosa of the small intestine.

folliculi (fol-ik′ūl-i) plural of *folliculus.*

folliculitis (fol-ik″ūl-īt′is) inflammation of a follicle. **f. bar′bae,** sycosis vulgaris. **f. decal′vans,** suppurative folliculitis leading to scarring, with permanent hair loss on the involved area. **keloid f., f. keloida′lis,** infection of the hair follicles on the back of the neck, with formation of persistent hard follicular papules, leading to development of typical keloidal plaques. **f. ulerythemato′sa reticula′ta,** a condition in which numerous, closely crowded, small atrophic areas separated by narrow ridges appear on the face, the affected area being erythematous and the skin stretched and hard. **f. variolifor′mis,** see under *acne.*

folliculosis (fol-ik″ūl-o′sis) excessive development of lymph follicles.

folliculus (fol-ik′ūl-is), pl. *follic′uli* [L.] follicle.

fomentation (fo″men-ta′shin) treatment by warm moist applications; also, the substance thus applied.

fomes (fo′mēz), pl. *fo′mites* [L.] an inanimate object or material on which disease-producing agents may be conveyed.

fomite (fo′mīt) fomes.

fontanel, fontanelle (fon″tah-nel′) a soft spot; one of the membrane-covered spaces remaining at the junction of the sutures in the incompletely ossified skull of the fetus or infant.

fonticulus (fon-tik′u-lus), pl. *fontic′uli* [L.] a fontanel.

foot (foot) the extremity of the human leg, consisting of the tarsus, metatarsus, phalanges, and the surrounding tissue. **athlete's f.,** tinea pedis. **club f.,** see *talipes.* **dangle f., drop f.,** a condition in which the foot hangs in a plantar-flexed position, due to lesion of the peroneal nerve. **flat f., flatfoot. immersion f.,** a condition resembling trench foot occurring in persons who have spent long periods in water. **Madura f.,** maduromycosis. **march f.,** painful swelling of the foot, usually with fracture of a metatarsal bone, after excessive foot strain. **perivascular feet,** terminal expansions of the cytoplasmic processes of some astrocytes by which they are attached to blood vessels. **sucker f.,** an expansion of a process of an astrocyte, by which the latter is attached to a small blood vessel. **trench f.,** a condition of the feet resembling frostbite, due to the prolonged action of water on the skin combined with circulatory disturbance due to cold and inaction.

footdrop (foot′drop) dropping of the foot from paralysis of the anterior muscles of the leg.

footplate (foot′plāt) the flat portion of the stapes, which is set into the oval window on the medial wall of the middle ear.

foot-pound (-pownd) the energy necessary to raise 1 pound of mass a distance of 1 foot.

foramen (for-a′men), pl. *foramina* [L.] a natural opening or passage, especially one into or through a bone. **aortic f.,** hiatus aorticus. **apical f.,** an opening at or near the apex of the root of a tooth. **auditory f., external,** external acoustic meatus. **auditory f., internal,** a passage for the auditory and facial nerves in petrous bone. **Botallo's f.,** f. ovale (1). **cecal f., f. ce′cum,** 1. a blind opening between the frontal crest and the crista galli. 2. a depression on the dorsum of the tongue at the median sulcus. **cotyloid f.,** a passage between the margin of the acetabulum and the transverse ligament. **epiploic f.,** an opening connecting the two sacs of the peritoneum, below and behind the porta hepatis. **esophageal f.,** see under *hiatus.* **ethmoidal foramina, fora′mina ethmoida′lia,** small openings in the ethmoid bone at the junction of the medial wall with the roof of the orbit, the *anterior* transmitting the nasal branch of the ophthalmic nerve and the anterior ethmoid vessels, and the *posterior* transmitting the posterior ethmoid vessels. **incisive f.,** one of the openings of the incisive canals into the incisive fossa of the hard palate. **infraorbital f.,** a passage for the infraorbital nerve and artery. **interventricular f.,** a communication between the lateral and third ventricle. **intervertebral f.,** a passage for a spinal nerve and vessels formed by notches on pedicles of adjacent vertebrae. **jugular f.,** an opening formed by the jugular notches on the temporal and occipital bones. **f. of Key and Retzius,** an opening at the end of each lateral recess of the fourth ventricle by which the ventricular cavity communicates with the subarachnoid space. **f. la′cerum, f. la′cerum me′dium,** a gap formed at the junction of the great wing of the sphenoid bone, tip of the petrous part of the temporal bone, and basilar part of the occipital bone. **f. la′cerum poste′rius,** jugular f. **f. of Magendie,** a deficiency in the lower part of the roof of the fourth ventricle through which the ventricular cavity communicates with the subarachnoid space. **f. mag′num,** a large opening in the anterior inferior part of the occipital bone, between the cranial cavity and vertebral canal. **mastoid f.,** an opening in the temporal bone behind the mastoid process. **medullary f.,** vertebral f. (1). **nutrient f.,** any of the passages admitting nutrient vessels to the medullary cavity of bone. **obturator f.,** the large opening between the os pubis and ischium. **olfactory f.,** any of the many openings of the cribriform plate of the ethmoid bone. **optic f.,** see under *canal.* **f. ova′le,** 1. a fetal opening between the heart's atria. 2. an aperture in the great wing of the sphenoid for vessels and nerves. **palatine f., anterior,** incisive f. **palatine f., greater,** the lower opening of the greater palatine canal, found laterally on the horizontal plate of each palatine bone, transmitting a palatine nerve and artery. **pterygopalatine f.,** greater palatine f. **quadrate f.,** vena cava f. **f. rotun′dum,** a round opening in the great wing of sphenoid for the maxillary branch of the trigeminal nerve. **Scarpa's f.,** an opening behind the upper medial incisor, for the nasopalatine nerve. **sciatic f.,** either of two foramina, the greater and the smaller sciatic foramina, formed by the sacrotuberal and sacrospinal ligaments in the sciatic notch of the hip bone. **sphenopalatine f.,** 1. a space between the orbital and sphenoidal processes of the palatine bone, opening into the nasal cavity, and transmitting the sphenopalatine artery and nasal nerves. 2. greater palatine f. **spinous f.,** a hole in the great wing of the sphenoid for the middle meningeal artery. **stylomastoid f.,** an opening between the styloid and mastoid processes, for the facial nerve and the stylomastoid artery. **supraorbital f.,** a passage in the frontal bone for the supraorbital artery and nerve; often present as a notch bridged only by fibrous tissue. **thebesian foramina,** minute openings in the walls of the right atrium through which the smallest cardiac veins empty into the heart. **thyroid f.,** 1. an inconstant opening in the thyroid cartilage, due to incomplete union of the fourth and fifth branchial cartilages. 2. obturator f. **vena cava f.,** an opening in the diaphragm for the inferior vena cava and some branches of the right vagus nerve. **vertebral f.,** 1. the large opening in a vertebra formed by its body and arch. 2. transverse f. **f. of Vesalius,** an occasional opening medial to the foramen ovale of the sphenoid, for passage of a vein from the cavernous sinus. **Weitbrecht's f.,** a foramen in the capsule of the shoulder joint. **f. of Winslow,** epiploic f. **zygomaticotemporal f.,** an opening on the temporal surface of the zygomatic bone.

foramina (for-am′ĭ-nah) plural of *foramen.*

force (fōrs) energy or power; that which originates or arrests motion or other activity. **electromotive f.,** that which gives rise to an electric current. **occlusal f.,** the force exerted on opposing teeth when the jaws are brought into approximation. **reserve f.,** energy above that required for normal functioning; in the heart, the power that will take care of the additional circulatory burden imposed by exertion. **Van der Waals f's,** the relatively weak, short-range forces of attraction existing between atoms and molecules, which results in the attraction of nonpolar organic compounds to each other (hydrophobic bonding).

forceps (fōr′seps), pl. *for′cipes* [L.] 1. a two-bladed instrument with a handle for compressing or grasping tissues in surgical operations, and for handling sterile dressings, etc. 2. any forcipate organ or part. **alligator f.,** strong toothed for-

forcipate
242

ceps having a double clamp. **artery f.,** one for grasping and compressing an artery. **axis-traction f.,** specially jointed obstetrical forceps so made that traction can be applied in the line of the pelvic axis. **bayonet f.,** a forceps whose blades are offset from the axis of the handle. **Chamberlen f.,** the original form of obstetrical forceps. **clamp f.,** a forceps-like clamp with an automatic lock, for compressing arteries, etc. **dental f.,** one for the extraction of teeth. **dressing f.,** one with scissor-like handles for grasping lint, drainage tubes, etc., used in dressing wounds. **fixation f.,** one for holding a part steady during operation. **Hodge's f.,** a form of obstetrical forceps. **Kocher's f.,** a strong forceps for holding tissues during operation or for compressing bleeding tissue. **Laborde's f.,** a flat forceps for making traction on the tongue to stimulate the respiratory center in asphyxiation. **Levret's f.,** an obstetrical forceps curved to correspond with the curve of the parturient canal. **Löwenberg's f.,** one for removing adenoid growth. **f. ma'jor,** the terminal fibers of the corpus callosum that pass from the splenium into the occipital lobes. **f. mi'nor,** the terminal fibers of the corpus callosum that pass from the genu to the frontal lobes. **mousetooth f.,** one with one or more fine teeth at the tip of each blade. **obstetrical f.,** one for extracting the fetal head from the maternal passages. **Péan's f.,** a clamp for hemostasis. **rongeur f.,** one for use in cutting bone. **sequestrum f.,** one with small but strong serrated jaws for removing pieces of bone forming a sequestrum. **speculum f.,** a long, slender forceps for use through a speculum. **tenaculum f.,** one having a sharp hook at the end of each jaw. **torsion f.,** one for making torsion on an artery to arrest hemorrhage. **volsella f., vulsellum f.,** one with teeth for grasping and applying traction. **Willett f.,** a vulsellum for applying scalp traction to control hemorrhage in placenta previa.

forcipate (fŏr'sĭ-pāt) shaped like a forceps.

forearm (fōr'arm) antebrachium; the part of the arm between elbow and wrist.

forebrain (-brān) prosencephalon: 1. the part of the brain developed from the anterior of the three primary brain vesicles, comprising the diencephalon and telencephalon. 2. the most anterior of the primary brain vesicles.

foreconscious (-kon-shis) preconscious.

forefoot (-foot) 1. one of the front feet of a quadruped. 2. the fore part of the foot.

foregut (-gut) the endodermal canal of the embryo cephalic to the junction of the yolk stalk, giving rise to the pharynx, lung, esophagus, stomach, liver, and most of the small intestine.

forehead (-ed) frons; the part of the face above the eyes.

forensic (for-en'zik) pertaining to or applied in legal proceedings.

foreplay (for'pla) the sexually stimulating play preceding intercourse.

foreskin (-skin) the prepuce.

forewaters (-wat-erz) the part of the amniotic sac that pouches into the uterine cervix in front of the presenting part of the fetus.

formaldehyde (for-mal'dĭ-hīd) a powerful disinfectant gas, HCHO, usually used in solution.

formalin (for'mah-lin) a 37% aqueous solution of gaseous formaldehyde used as a fixative.

formamidase (for-mam'ĭ-dās) an enzyme that catalyzes the hydrolysis of formylkynurenine to kynurenine and formate in tryptophan metabolism.

formate (for'māt) a salt of formic acid.

formatio (for-ma'she-o), pl. *formatio'nes* [L.] formation.

formation (for-ma'shin) 1. the process of giving shape or form; the creation of an entity, or of a structure of definite shape. 2. a structure of definite shape. **reaction f.,** the development of mental mechanisms which hold in check and repress the components of forbidden wishes. **reticular f.,** areas of diffuse neurons collectively resembling a network in the spinal cord, brain stem, and thalamus; it controls many of the unconscious motor activities of the body.

forme (form), pl. *formes* [Fr.] form. **f. fruste** (pl. form froost) *formes frustes*) an atypical, especially a mild or incomplete, form, as of a disease. **f. tardive** a form tahr-dēv') a late-occurring form of a disease that usually appears at an earlier age.

formic acid (for'mik) a colorless, pungent liquid with vesicant properties, HCOOH, from nettles and ants and other insects; derivable from oxalic acid and from glycerin and from the oxidation of formaldehyde.

formication (for″mĭ-ka'shin) a sensation as if small insects were crawling on the skin.

formiminoglutamic acid (FIGLU) (for-mim″ĭ-no-gloo-tam'ik) a product of histidine metabolism. The urine FIGLU concentration is elevated in some individuals with folic acid deficiency.

formol (for'mol) formaldehyde solution.

formula (for'mūl-ah), pl. *for'mulae, for'mulas* [L.] an expression, using numbers or symbols, of the composition of, or of directions for preparing, a compound, such as a medicine, or of a procedure to follow to obtain a desired result, or of a single concept. **chemical f.,** a combination of symbols used to express the chemical composition of a substance. **dental f.,** an expression in symbols of the number and arrangement of teeth in the jaws. Letters represent the various types of teeth: I, *incisor;* C, *canine;* P, *premolar,* M, *molar.* Each letter is followed by a horizontal line. Numbers above the line represent maxillary teeth; those below, mandibular teeth. The human dental formula is $I\frac{2}{2}C\frac{1}{1}M\frac{2}{2} = 10$ (one side only) for deciduous teeth, and $I\frac{2}{2}C\frac{1}{1}P\frac{2}{2}M\frac{3}{3} = 16$ (one side only) for permanent teeth. **empirical f.,** a chemical formula which expresses the proportions of the elements present in a substance. **molecular f.,** a chemical formula expressing the number of atoms of each element present in a molecule of a substance, without indicating how they are linked. **spatial f., stereochemical f.,** a chemical formula giving the numbers of atoms of each element present in a molecule of a substance, which atom is linked to which, the types of linkages involved, and the relative positions of the atoms in space. **structural f.,** a chemical formula showing the spatial arrangement of the atoms and the linkage of every atom. **vertebral f.,** an expression of the number of vertebrae in each region of the spinal column; the human vertebral formula is $C_7T_{12}L_5$-$S_5Cd_4 = 33$.

formulary (for'mūl-er''e) a collection of formulae. **National F.,** see under *N.*

formulate (for'mūl-āt) 1. to state in the form of a formula. 2. to prepare in accordance with a prescribed or specified method.

formulation (for''mūl-a'shin) the act or product of formulating. **American Law Institute f.,** a section of the American Law Institute's Model Penal Code which states that "a person is not responsible for criminal conduct if at the time of such conduct as a result of mental disease or defect he lacks substantial capacity either to appreciate the wrongfulness of his conduct or to conform his conduct to the requirement of the law."

formyl (for'mil) the radical, HCO or H·C:O—, of formic acid.

fornix (for'niks), pl. *for'nices* [L.] 1. an archlike structure or the vaultlike space created by such a structure. 2. fornix of cerebrum; either of a pair of arched fiber tracts that unite under the corpus callosum, so that together they comprise two columns, a body, and two crura.

fossa (fos'ah), pl. *fos'sae* [L.] a trench or channel; in anatomy, a hollow or depressed area. **acetabular f.,** a nonarticular area in the floor of the acetabulum. **adipose fossae,** spaces in the female breast which contain fat. **canine f.,** a depression on the external surface of the maxilla. **cerebral f.,** any of the depressions on the floor of the cranial cavity. **condylar f., condyloid f.,** either of two pits on the lateral part of the occipital bone. **coronoid f.,** a depression in the humerus for the coronoid process of the ulna. **cranial f.,** any one of three hollows (anterior, middle, and posterior) in the base of the cranium for the lobes of the brain. **digastric f.,** a depression on the inner surface of the mandible, giving attachment to the anterior belly of the digastric muscle. **digital f.,** trochanteric f. **duodenojejunal f.,** either of two peritoneal pockets, one behind the inferior and the other behind the superior duodenal fold. **ethmoid f.,** the groove in the cribriform plate of the ethmoid bones, for the olfactory bulb. **hyaloid f.,** a depression in the front of the vitreous body, lodging the lens. **hypophyseal f.,** a depression in the sphenoid, lodging the pituitary gland. **iliac f.,** a concave area occupying much of the inner surface of the ala of the ilium, especially anteriorly; from it arises the iliacus muscle. **incisive f.,** a slight depression on the anterior surface of the maxilla above the incisor teeth. **infratemporal f.,** an irregularly shaped cavity medial or deep to the zygomatic arch. **ischiorectal f.,** a potential space between the pelvic diaphragm and the skin below it; an anterior recess extends a variable distance between the pelvic and urogenital diaphragms. **Jobert's f.,** a fossa in the popliteal region bounded by the adductor magnus and the gracilis and sartorius.

lacrimal f., a shallow depression in the roof of the orbit, lodging the lacrimal gland. **mandibular f.,** a depression in the temporal bone in which the condyle of the mandible rests. **mastoid f.,** a small triangular area between the posterior wall of the external acoustic meatus and the posterior root of the zygomatic process of the temporal bone. **nasal f.,** the portion of the nasal cavity anterior to the middle meatus. **navicular f.,** 1. the vaginal vestibule between the vaginal orifice and the frenulum of the pudendal labia. 2. the lateral expansion of the urethra of the glans penis. 3. a depression on the internal pterygoid process of the sphenoid, giving attachment to the tensor veli palatini muscle. **f. ova'lis cor'dis,** a fossa in the right atrium of the heart; remains of the fetal foramen ovale. **ovarian f.,** a shallow pouch on the posterior surface of the broad ligament in which the ovary is located. **rhomboid f.,** the floor of the fourth ventricle, made up of the dorsal surfaces of the medulla oblongata and pons. **Rosenmüller's f.,** see under *cavity.* **subarcuate f.,** a depression in the posterior inner surface of the petrous portion of the temporal bone. **subsigmoid f.,** a fossa between the mesentery of the sigmoid flexure and that of the descending colon. **supraspinous f.,** a depression above the spine of the scapula. **sylvian f.,** fissure of Sylvius. **tibiofemoral f.,** a space between the articular surfaces of the tibia and femur mesial or lateral to the inferior pole of the patella. **trochanteric f.,** a depression on the medial surface of the greater trochanter, receiving the tendon of the obturator externus muscle. **urachal f.,** one on the inner abdominal wall, between the urachus and the hypogastric artery. **Waldeyer's f.,** the two duodenal fossae regarded as one. **zygomatic f.,** infratemporal f.

fossette (fŏ-set') 1. a small depression. 2. a small, deep corneal ulcer.

fossula (fos'ūl-ah), pl. *fos'sulae* [L.] a small fossa.

foulage (foo-lahzh') [Fr.] kneading and pressing of the muscles in massage.

foundation (fown-da'shin) the structure or basis on which something is built. **denture f.,** the portion of the structures and tissues of the mouth available to support a denture.

fovea (fo've-ah), pl. *fo'veae* [L.] a small pit or depression. Often used alone to indicate the central fovea of the retina. **central f., f. centralis,** a small pit in the center of the macula lutea, the area of clearest vision, where the retinal layers are spread aside, and light falls directly on the cones. **submandibular f.,** a depression on the medial aspect of the mandible, lodging part of the submandibular gland.

foveation (fo''ve-a'shin) formation of pits on a surface as on the skin; a pitted condition.

foveola (fo-ve'ah-lah), pl. *fove'olae* [L.] a minute pit or depression.

Fr chemical symbol, *francium.*

fractionation (frak''shin-a'shin) 1. in radiology, division of the total dose of radiation into small doses administered at intervals. 2. in chemistry, separation of a substance into components, as by distillation or crystallization. 3. in histology, isolation of components of living cells by differential centrifugation.

fracture (frak′cher) 1. the breaking of a part, especially a bone. 2. a break or rupture in a bone. **avulsion f.,** separation of a small fragment of bone cortex at the site of attachment of a ligament or tendon. **Barton's f.,** fracture of the distal end of the radius into the wrist joint. **Bennett's f.,** fracture of the base of the first metacarpal bone running into the carpometacarpal joint, complicated by subluxation. **blow-out f.,** fracture of the orbital floor caused by a sudden increase of intraorbital pressure due to traumatic force; the orbital contents herniate into the maxillary sinus so that the inferior rectus or inferior oblique muscle may become incarcerated in the fracture site, producing diplopia on looking up. **capillary f.,** one that appears on a radiogram as a fine, hairlike line, the segments of bone not being separated; sometimes seen in fractures of the skull. **Colles' f.,** fracture of the lower end of the radius, the lower fragment being displaced backward; if the lower fragment is displaced forward, it is a *reversed Colles' fracture.* **comminuted f.,** one in which the bone is splintered or crushed. **complete f.,** one involving the entire cross section of the bone. **compound f.,** open f. **depressed f.,** fracture of the skull in which a fragment is depressed. **direct f.,** one at the site of injury. **dislocation f.,** fracture of a bone near an articulation with concomitant dislocation of that joint. **Dupuytren's f.,** Pott's f. **Duverney's f.,** fracture of the ilium just below the anterior inferior spine. **fissure f.,** a crack extending from a surface into, but not through, a long bone. **greenstick f.,** one in which one side of a bone is broken, the other being bent. **hangman's f.,** fracture through the pedicles of the axis (C2) with or without subluxation of the second cervical vertebra or the third. **impacted f.,** one in which one fragment is firmly driven into the other. **incomplete f.,** one which does not involve the complete cross section of the bone. **interperiosteal f.,** incomplete or greenstick fracture. **intrauterine f.,** fracture of a fetal bone incurred *in utero.* **Jefferson f.,** fracture of the atlas (first cervical vertebra). **lead pipe f.,** one in which the bone cortex is slightly compressed and bulged on one side with a slight crack on the other side of the bone. **Le Fort's f.,** bilateral horizontal fracture of the maxilla. Le Fort fractures are classified as follows: *Le Fort I f.,* a horizontal segmented fracture of the alveolar process of the maxilla, in which the teeth are usually contained in the detached portion of the bone. *Le Fort II f.,* unilateral or bilateral fracture of the maxilla, in which the body of the maxilla is separated from the facial skeleton and the separated portion is pyramidal in shape; the fracture may extend through the body of the maxilla down the midline of the hard palate, through the floor of the orbit, and into the nasal cavity. *Le Fort III f.,* a fracture in which the entire maxilla and one or more facial bones are completely separated from the craniofacial skelton; such fractures are almost always accompanied by multiple fractures of the

facial bones. **Monteggia's f.,** one in the proximal half of the shaft of the ulna, with dislocation of the head of the radius. **open f.,** one in which a wound through the adjacent or overlying soft tissues communicates with the site of the break. **parry f.,** Monteggia's f. **pathologic f.,** one due to weakening of the bone structure by pathologic processes, such as neoplasia, osteomalacia, or osteomyelitis. **ping-pong f.,** an indented fracture of the skull, resembling the indentation that can be produced with the finger in a ping-pong ball; when elevated it resumes and retains its normal position. **pyramidal f. (of maxilla),** Le Fort II f. **silver-fork f.,** Colles' f. **simple f.,** closed f. **Smith's f.,** reversed Colles' f. **spiral f.,** one in which the bone has been twisted apart. **spontaneous f.,** pathologic f. **sprain f.,** the separation of a tendon from its insertion, taking with it a piece of bone. **Stieda's f.,** fracture of the internal condyle of the femur. **transverse facial f.,** Le Fort III f. **transverse maxillary f.,** a term sometimes used for horizontal maxillary fracture (Le Fort I f.). **trophic f.,** one due to nutritional (trophic) disturbance.

frae- for words beginning thus, see those beginning *fre-*.

fragilitas (frah-jil″ĭ-tas) [L.] fragility. **f. crin′ium,** a brittleness of the hair. **f. os′sium,** osteogenesis imperfecta. **f. un′guium,** abnormal brittleness of the nails.

fragility (frah-jil′it-e) susceptibility, or lack of resistance, to influences capable of causing disruption of continuity or integrity. **f. of blood,** erythrocyte f. **capillary f.,** abnormal susceptibility of capillary walls to rupture. **erythrocyte f.,** susceptibility of erythrocytes to hemolysis when exposed to increasingly hypotonic saline solutions (*osmotic f.*) or when subjected to mechanical trauma (*mechanical f.*).

fragmentography, mass (frag″men-tog′rah-fe) an instrumental method in which samples are separated by gas chromatography and the components are identified by mass spectrometry.

frambesia (fram-be′ze-ah) yaws. **f. tro′pica,** yaws.

frambesioma (fram-be″ze-o′mah) mother yaw.

frame (frām) a rigid structure for giving support to or for immobilizing a part. **Balkan f.,** an apparatus for continuous extension in treatment of fractures of the femur, consisting of an overhead bar, with pulleys attached, by which the leg is supported in a sling. **Bradford f.,** a canvas-covered, rectangular frame of pipe; used as a bed frame in disease of the spine or thigh. **quadriplegic standing f.,** a device for supporting in the upright position a patient whose four limbs are paralyzed. **Stryker f.,** one consisting of canvas stretched on anterior and posterior frames, on which the patient can be rotated around his longitudinal axis. **trial f.,** an eyeglass frame designed to permit insertion of different lenses used in correcting refractive errors of vision.

Francisella (fran″sĭ-sel′ah) a genus of microorganisms, including *F.* (*Pasteurella*) *tularen′sis,* the etiologic agent of tularemia.

francium (fran′se-um) chemical element (*see table*), at. no. 87, symbol Fr.

F.R.C.P. Fellow of the Royal College of Physicians.

F.R.C.S. Fellow of the Royal College of Surgeons.

freckle (frek′'l) a pigmented spot on the skin due to accumulation of melanin resulting from exposure to sunlight. **melanotic f. of Hutchinson,** a noninvasive malignant melanoma occurring most often on the face of women during the fourth decade.

freemartin (fre′mart-in) a sexually maldeveloped female calf born as a twin to a normal male calf; it is usually sterile and intersexual as a result of male hormone reaching it through anastomosed placental vessels.

freeze-drying (frēz-dri′ing) a method of tissue preparation in which the tissue specimen is frozen and then dehydrated at low temperature in a high vacuum.

freeze-etching (-ech′ing) a method used to study unfixed cells by electron microscopy, in which the object to be studied is placed in 20% glycerol, frozen at −100° C., and then mounted on a chilled holder.

freeze-fracturing (-frak′cher-ing) a method of preparing cells for electron-microscopical examination: a tissue specimen is frozen at −150° C., inserted into a vacuum chamber, and fractured by a microtome; a platinum carbon replica of the exposed surfaces is made, freed of the underlying specimen, and then examined.

freeze-substitution (-sub-stĭ-too′shin) a modification of freeze-drying in which the ice within the frozen tissue is replaced by alcohol or other solvents at a very low temperature.

fremitus (frem′it-us) a vibration perceptible on palpation. **friction f.,** the vibration caused by the rubbing together of two dry body surfaces. **hydatid f.,** see under *thrill*. **rhonchal f.,** palpable vibrations produced by passage of air through a mucus-filled, large bronchial tube. **tactile f.,** vibration, as in the chest wall, felt on the thorax while the patient is speaking. **tussive f.,** one felt on the chest when the patient coughs. **vocal f.,** one caused by speaking, perceived on auscultation.

frenoplasty (fre′no-plas″te) the correction of an abnormally attached frenum by surgically repositioning it.

frenulum (fren′ūl-um), pl. *fren′ula* [L.] a small fold of integument or mucous membrane that limits the movements of an organ or part. **f. of clitoris,** a fold formed by union of the labia minora with the clitoris. **f. of ileocecal valve,** a fold formed by the joined extremities of the ileocecal valve, partially encircling the lumen of the colon. **f. of lip,** a median fold of mucous membrane connecting the inside of each lip to the corresponding gum. **f. of prepuce of penis,** the fold under the penis connecting it with the prepuce. **f. of superior medullary velum,** a band lying in the superior medullary velum at its attachment to the inferior colliculi. **f. of tongue,** the vertical fold of mucous membrane under the tongue, attaching it to the floor of the

mouth. **f. val′vulae co′li,** f. of ileocecal valve. **f. ve′li,** f. of superior medullary velum.

frenum (fre′num), pl. *fre′na* [L.] a restraining structure or part; see *frenulum*. **fre′nal,** adj.

frequency (fre′kwin-se) 1. the number of occurrences of a periodic process in a unit of time. 2. in statistics, the number of occurrences of a determinable entity per unit of time or of population. **urinary f.,** urination at short intervals without increase in daily volume or urinary output, due to reduced bladder capacity.

freudian (froi′de-in) pertaining to Sigmund Freud, the founder of psychoanalysis, and to his doctrines regarding the causes and treatment of neuroses and psychoses.

friable (fri′ah-b'l) easily pulverized or crumbled.

friction (frik′shin) the act of rubbing.

frigidity (frĭ-jid′it-e) coldness; especially, sexual unresponsiveness of the female to physical stimulation.

frigolabile (frig″o-la′bīl) easily affected or destroyed by cold.

frigostable (-sta′b'l) resistant to cold or low temperatures.

frit (frit) imperfectly fused material used as a basis for making glass and in the formation of porcelain teeth.

frolement (frōl-maw′) [Fr.] 1. a rustling sound heard on auscultation in pericardial disease. 2. a brushing movement in massage.

frons (fronz) [L.] the forehead.

frontad (frunt′ad) toward a front, or frontal aspect.

frontal (frunt′il) 1. pertaining to the forehead. 2. denoting a longitudinal plane of the body.

frontalis (fron-ta′lis) [L.] frontal.

frontomaxillary (-mak′sil-ĕ″re) pertaining to the frontal bone and maxilla.

frontotemporal (-tem′por-il) pertaining to the frontal and temporal bones.

frost (frost) a deposit resembling frozen dew or vapor. **urea f.,** the appearance on the skin of salt crystals left by evaporation of the sweat in urhidrosis.

frostbite (frost′bīt″) injury to tissues due to exposure to cold.

frottage (fro-tahzh′) [Fr.] 1. rubbing movement in massage. 2. sexual gratification by rubbing against a person of the opposite sex.

frotteur (fro-tur′) one who practices frottage (2).

fructivorous (fruk-tiv′er-is) subsisting on or eating fruit.

fructofuranose (fruk″to-fūr′ah-nōs) the combining and more reactive form of fructose.

β-fructofuranosidase (-fūr″ah-no′sĭ-dās) an enzyme occurring in yeasts and other organisms that catalyzes the hydrolysis of sugars with a terminal unsubstituted β-D-fructofuranosyl residue.

fructokinase (-ki′nās) an enzyme that catalyzes the transfer of a high-energy phosphate group to D-fructose.

fructose (fruk′tōs) a sugar, $C_6H_{12}O_6$, found in honey and many sweet fruits; used as a fluid and nutrient replenisher.

fructosemia (fruk″tōs-ēm′e-ah) the presence of

fructose in the blood, as in fructose intolerance.

fructoside (fruk'tah-sīd) a compound that bears the same relation to fructose as a glucoside does to glucose.

fructosuria (fruk″tōs-ūr'e-ah) the presence of fructose in the urine. **essential f.,** a benign hereditary disorder of carbohydrate metabolism due to a defect in fructokinase and manifested only by fructose in the blood and urine.

fructosyl (fruk'tah-sil) a radical of fructose.

frustration (frus-tra'shin) increased emotional tension due to failure to achieve sought gratifications or satisfactions.

FSH follicle-stimulating hormone.

FSH/LH-RH follicle-stimulating hormone and luteinizing hormone releasing hormone.

FSH-RH follicle-stimulating hormone releasing hormone.

fuchsin (fook'sin) any of several red to purple dyes. **acid f.,** a mixture of sulfonated fuchsins; used in various complex stains. **basic f.,** a histologic stain, a mixture of pararosaniline, rosaniline, and magenta II. Also, a mixture of rosaniline and pararosaniline hydrochlorides used as a local anti-infective.

fuchsinophilia (fook″sin-o-fil'e-ah) the property of staining readily with fuchsin dyes. **fuchsinophil'ic,** adj.

fucose (fu'kōs) a monosaccharide occurring as L-fucose in a number of mucopolysaccharides and mucoproteins.

fucosidase (fu-ko'sĭ-dās) an enzyme occurring in two forms that catalyzes the hydrolysis of fucoside to an alcohol and fucose.

fucosidosis (fu″ko-sĭ-do'sis) a hereditary neurovisceral disease due to deficient enzymatic activity of fucosidase and resulting in accumulation of fucose in all tissues; it is marked by progressive cerebral degeneration, muscle weakness with eventual spasticity, emaciation, cardiomegaly, thick skin, and excessive sweating.

fugacity (fu-gas'it-e) a measure of the escaping tendency of a substance from one phase to another phase, or from one part of a phase to another part of the same phase.

-fugal word element [L.], *driving away; fleeing from; repelling.*

fugue (fūg) a dissociative reaction in which amnesia is accompanied by physical flight from customary surroundings.

fulgurate (ful'gūr-āt) 1. to come and go like a flash of lightning. 2. to destroy by contact with electric sparks generated by a high-frequency current.

fulminate (ful'mĭ-nāt) to occur suddenly with great intensity. **ful'minant,** adj.

fumagillin (fu″mah-jil'in) an antibiotic, $C_{26}H_{34}$-O_7, elaborated by strains of *Aspergillus fumigatus.*

fumarase (fu'mah-rās) an enzyme that catalyzes the interconversion of fumarate and malate.

fumarate (fu'mar-āt) a salt of fumaric acid.

fumaric acid (fu-mar'ik) an unsaturated dibasic acid, $C_4H_4O_4$; it is the trans-isomer of maleic acid and an intermediate in the tricarboxylic acid cycle.

fumigation (fu″mĭ-ga'shin) exposure to disinfecting fumes.

fuming (fūm'ing) emitting a visible vapor.

functio (funk'she-o) [L.] function. **f. lae'sa,** loss of function; one of the cardinal signs of inflammation.

functional (funk'shin'l) pertaining to a function; affecting the function but not the structure.

fundament (fun'dah-ment) 1. a base or foundation, as the breech or rump. 2. the anus and parts adjacent to it.

fundiform (fun'dĭ-form) shaped like a loop or sling.

fundoplication (fun″do-pli-ka'shin) mobilization of the lower end of the esophagus and plication of the fundus of the stomach up around it.

fundus (fun'dis), pl. *fun'di* [L.] the bottom or base of anything; the bottom or base of an organ, or the part of a hollow organ farthest from its mouth. **fun'dal, fun'dic,** adj. **f. of eye,** the back portion of the interior of the eyeball, visible through the pupil by use of the ophthalmoscope. **f. of gallbladder,** the inferior, dilated portion of the gallbladder. **f. of stomach,** the part of the stomach to the left and above the level of the opening of the esophagus. **f. tym'pani,** the floor of the tympanic cavity. **f. of urinary bladder,** the base or posterior surface of the urinary bladder. **f. of uterus,** the part of the uterus above the orifices of the uterine tubes.

funduscope (fun'dah-skōp) ophthalmoscope. **funduscop'ic,** adj.

fungal (fung'g'l) pertaining to or caused by a fungus.

fungate (fung'gāt) to produce fungus-like growths; to grow rapidly, like a fungus.

fungi (fun'ji) plural of *fungus.*

fungicide (fun'jĭ-sīd) an agent that destroys fungi. **fungici'dal,** adj.

fungistasis (fun″jĭ-sta'sis) inhibition of the growth of fungi. **fungistat'ic,** adj.

fungitoxic (fun″jĭ-tok'sik) exerting a toxic effect upon fungi.

fungoid (fung'goid) resembling a fungus.

fungosity (fung-gos'it-e) a fungoid growth or excrescence.

fungus (fung'gis), pl. *fun'gi* [L.] a general term for a group of eukaryotic protists (mushrooms, yeasts, molds, etc.) marked by the absence of chlorophyll and the presence of a rigid cell wall. **cerebral f.,** hernia cerebri. **imperfect f.,** a fungus whose perfect (sexual) stage is unknown. **mycelial f.,** any fungus that forms mycelia, in contrast to a yeast fungus. **perfect f.,** a fungus for which both sexual and asexual types of spore formation are known.

funicle (fu'nĭ-k'l) funiculus.

funiculitis (fu-nik″ūl-īt'is) 1. inflammation of the spermatic cord. 2. inflammation of that portion of a spinal nerve root lying within the intervertebral canal.

funiculoepididymitis (fu-nik″ūl-o-ep″ĭ-did″i-mīt′is) inflammation of the spermatic cord and the epididymis.

funiculus (fu-nik′ūl-is), pl. *funi′culi* [L.] a cord; a cordlike structure or part. **funic′ular**, adj. **anterior f.**, the white substance of the spinal cord lying on either side between the anterior median fissure and the ventral root. **cuneate f.**, see under *fasciculus.* **lateral f.**, 1. the white substance of the spinal cord lying on either side between the dorsal and ventral roots. 2. the continuation into the medulla oblongata of all the fiber tracts of the lateral funiculus of the spinal cord with exception of the lateral pyramidal tract. **posterior f.**, the white substance of the spinal cord lying on either side between the posterior median sulcus and the dorsal root. **f. sperma′ticus**, the spermatic cord.

funiform (fu′nĭ-form) resembling a rope or cord.

funis (fu′nis) any cordlike structure, particularly the umbilical cord.

furazolidone (fū″rah-zol′ĭ-dōn) an antibacterial and antiprotozoal, $C_8H_7N_3O_5$.

furcation (fur-ka′shin) the anatomical area of a multirooted tooth where the roots divide.

furfuraceous (fer″fūr-a′shis) fine and loose; said of scales resembling bran or dandruff.

furfural, furfurol (fur′fūr-al; -rol) an aromatic compound from the distillation of bran, sawdust, etc., which causes convulsions in animals.

furor (fūr′or) fury; rage. **f. epilep′ticus**, an attack of intense anger occurring in epilepsy.

furosemide (fūr-o′sĭ-mīd) a sulfonamide, $C_{12}H_{11}ClN_2O_5S$, used as a diuretic in the treatment of edema and hypertension.

furrow (fur′o) a groove or trench. **atrioventricular f.**, the transverse groove marking off the atria of the heart from the ventricles. **digital f.**, any one of the transverse folds across the joints on the palmar surface of a finger. **genital f.**, a groove that appears on the genital tubercle of the fetus at the end of the second month. **gluteal f.**, the furrow which separates the buttocks. **mentolabial f.**, the hollow just above the chin. **nympholabial f.**, a groove separating the labium majus and labium minus on each side. **primitive f.**, see under *groove.* **scleral f.**, see under *sulcus.*

furuncle (fūr′ung-k'l) a boil; a painful nodule formed in the skin by circumscribed inflammation of the corium and subcutaneous tissue, enclosing a central slough or "core"; due to staphylococci entering the skin through hair follicles. **furun′cular**, adj.

furunculosis (fūr-ung″kūl-o′sis) 1. the persistent sequential occurrence of furuncles over a period of weeks or months. 2. the simultaneous occurrence of a number of furuncles.

furunculus (fūr-ung′kū-lis) [L.] furuncle.

Fusarium (fu-sa′re-um) a genus of fungi; some species are plant pathogens and some are opportunistic infectious agents of man and animals.

fuscin (fu′sin) a brown pigment of the retinal epithelium.

fusible (fu′zĭ-b'l) capable of being melted.

fusimotor (fu″sĭ-mōt′er) denoting motor nerve fibers (of gamma motoneurons) that innervate intrafusal fibers of the muscle spindle.

fusion (fu′zhin) 1. the act or process of melting. 2. the merging or coherence of adjacent parts or bodies. 3. the coordination of separate images of the same object in the two eyes into one. 4. the operative formation of an ankylosis or arthrosis. **diaphyseal-epiphyseal f.**, operative establishment of bony union between the epiphysis and diaphysis of a bone. **nuclear f.**, the fusion of two atomic nuclei to form a single heavier nucleus, resulting in the release of enormous amounts of energy. **spinal f.**, spondylosyndesis.

Fusobacterium (fu″zo-bak-tēr′e-um) a genus of anaerobic gram-negative bacteria found as normal flora in the mouth and large bowel, and often in necrotic tissue, probably as secondary invaders. *F. plautivincen′ti* is found in necrotizing ulcerative gingivitis (trench mouth) and necrotizing ulcerative stomatitis. *F. necroph′orum* is found in abscesses of the liver, lungs, and other tissues and in chronic ulcer of the colon.

fusocellular (-sel′u-ler) having spindle-shaped cells.

fusospirillosis (-spi″ril-o′sis) necrotizing ulcerative gingivitis.

fusospirochetosis (-ke-to′sis) infection with fusiform bacilli and spirochetes.

G

G conductance; gauss; Gibbs free energy; giga-; gravitational constant; glycine, glucose, and guanidine or guanosine.

g gram; standard gravity.

g. gram (or grams).

Ga chemical symbol, *gallium*.

gadolinium (gad″ah-lin′e-um) chemical element (*see table*), at. no. 64, symbol Gd.

gag (gag) 1. a surgical device for holding the mouth open. 2. to retch, or to strive to vomit.

gain (gān) to acquire, obtain, or increase. **antigen g.**, the acquisition by cells of new antigenic determinants not normally present or not normally accessible in the parent tissue. **secondary g.**, external and incidental advantage derived from an illness, such as rest, gifts, personal attention, release from responsibility, and disability benefits.

gait (gāt) the manner or style of walking. **antalgic g.**, a limp adopted so as to avoid pain on weight-bearing structures, characterized by a very short stance phase. **ataxic g.**, an unsteady, uncoordinated walk, employing a wide base. **festinating g.**, a gait in which the patient involuntarily moves with short, accelerating steps, often on tiptoe, as in paralysis agitans; festination. **helicopod g.**, a gait in which the feet describe half circles, as in some hysterical disorders. **spastic g.**, a gait in which the legs are held together and move in a stiff manner, the toes seeming to drag and catch. **steppage g.**, the gait in drop foot in which the advancing leg is lifted high so that the toes can clear the ground. **tabetic g.**, an ataxic gait in which the feet slap the ground. **waddling g.**, a gait suggesting that of a duck, characteristic of progressive muscular dystrophy.

galact(o)- word element [Gr.], *milk*.

galactacrasia (gah-lak″tah-kra′ze-ah) abnormal condition of the breast milk.

galactagogue (gah-lak′tah-gog) promoting milk flow; an agent that so acts.

galactan (gah-lak′tin) a carbohydrate which yields galactose upon hydrolysis.

galactischia (gal″ak-tisk′e-ah) suppression of milk secretion.

galactoblast (gah-lak′tah-blast) a colostrum corpuscle in the acini of the mammary gland.

galactocele (gah-lak′tah-sēl) 1. a milk-containing, cystic enlargement of the mammary gland. 2. hydrocele filled with milky fluid.

galactography (gal″ak-tog′rah-fe) radiography of the mammary ducts after injection of a radiopaque substance into the duct system.

galactokinase (gah-lak″to-ki′nās) an enzyme that catalyzes the transfer of a high-energy phosphate group from a donor to D-galactose, producing D-galactose-1-phosphate.

galactolipid, galactolipin (-lip′id; -lip′in) a cerebroside which yields galactose on hydrolysis.

galactophagous (gal″ak-tof′ah-gus) subsisting upon milk.

galactophlysis (gal″ak-tof′lĭ-sis) a vesicular eruption containing milky fluid.

galactophore (gah-lak′tah-for) 1. galactophorous. 2. a milk duct.

galactophorous (gal″ak-tof′er-is) conveying milk.

galactophygous (gal″ak-tof′ĭ-gis) arresting the flow of milk.

galactoplania (gah-lak″to-pla′ne-ah) secretion of milk in some abnormal part.

galactopoietic (-poi-et′ik) 1. pertaining to, marked by, or promoting milk production. 2. an agent that promotes milk flow.

galactorrhea (-re′ah) excessive or spontaneous milk flow; persistent secretion of milk irrespective of nursing.

galactose (gah-lak′tōs) a monosaccharide, $C_6H_{12}O_6$. D-galactose is found in lactose, cerebrosides of the brain, raffinose of the sugar beet, and in many gums and seaweeds; L-galactose in flaxseed mucilage.

galactosemia (gah-lak″tōs-ēm′e-ah) any of three recessive disorders of galactose metabolism: the classic form, due to deficiency of the enzyme galactose-1-phosphate uridyl transferase, is marked by hepatomegaly, cataracts, and mental retardation.

galactosidase (-si′dās) an enzyme that catalyzes the conversion of galactoside to galactose; it occurs in two forms: α-galactosidase (melibiase) and β-galactosidase (lactase).

galactoside (gah-lak′tah-sīd) a glycoside containing galactose.

galactosis (gal″ak-to′sis) the formation of milk by the lacteal glands.

galactostasis (gal″ak-tos′tah-sis) 1. cessation of milk secretion. 2. abnormal collection of milk in the mammary glands.

galactotoxism, galactoxism (-tok′sizm; gal″-ak-tok′sizm) poisoning by milk.

galacturia (gal″ak-tūr′e-ah) chyluria.

galea (ga′le-ah), pl. *ga′leae* [L.] a helmet-shaped structure. **g. aponeuro′tica**, the aponeurosis connecting the two bellies of the occipitofrontalis muscle.

galenicals, galenics (ga-len′ik′lz; -iks) medicines prepared according to Galen's formulas; now used to denote standard preparations containing one or several organic ingredients, as contrasted with pure chemical substances.

gall (gawl) the bile.

gallbladder (gawl′blad-er) the reservoir for bile on the posteroinferior surface of the liver.

gallium (gal′e-im) chemical element (*see table*), at. no. 31, symbol Ga. **g.-67**, a radioisotope of gallium having a half-life of 78.1 hours; used in the imaging of soft tissue tumors of Hodgkin's disease and bronchogenic carcinoma.

gallon (gal′n) a unit of liquid measure (4 quarts, 3.785 liters, or 3785 ml.).

gallop (gal′ip) a disordered rhythm of the heart; see under *rhythm*.

gallsickness (gawl-sik′nis) anaplasmosis.

gallstone (gawl′stōn) a calculus formed in the gallbladder or bile duct.

GALT gut-associated lymphoid tissue.

galvanocontractility (gal″vah-no-kon″trak-til′it-e) contractility in response to a galvanic stimulus.

galvanometer (gal″vah-nom′it-er) an instrument for measuring current by electromagnetic action.

galvanonervous (gal″vah-no-nurv′is) produced by application of galvanic current to a nerve.

galvanopalpation (-pal-pa′shin) testing of nerves of the skin by galvanic current.

gamete (gam′ēt) 1. one of two cells, male (*spermatozoon*) and female (*ovum*), whose union is necessary in sexual reproduction to initiate the development of a new individual. 2. the malarial parasite in its sexual form in a mosquito's stomach, either male (*microgamete*) or female (*macrogamete*); the latter is fertilized by the former to develop into an ookinete. **gamet′ic**, adj.

gametocide (gam′it-ah-sīd″) an agent that destroys gametes or gametocytes. **gametoci′dal**, adj.

gametocyte (gah-mēt′ah-sīt) 1. an oocyte or spermatocyte; a cell that produces gametes. 2. the sexual form, male or female, of certain sporozoa, such as malarial plasmodia, found in the erythrocytes, which may produce gametes when ingested by the secondary host. See also *macrogametocyte* and *microgametocyte*.

gametogony (gam″i-tog′ah-ne) 1. the development of merozoites of malarial plasmodia and other sporozoa into male and female gametes, which later fuse to form a zygote. 2. reproduction by means of gametes.

gamma (gam′ah) third letter of the Greek alphabet, γ; used in names of chemical compounds to distinguish one of three or more isomers or to indicate position of substituting atoms or groups.

gamma-aminobutyric acid (GABA) (ahme″no-bu-tir′ik) an amino acid that is one of the principal inhibitory neurotransmitters in the central nervous system.

gamma benzene hexachloride (gam′ah ben′zēn hek″sah-klor′īd) lindane.

gamma globulin see under *globulin*.

gammaglobulinopathy (gam″ah-glob″ūl-in-op′ah-the) gammopathy.

gammopathy (gam-op′ah-the) abnormal proliferation of the lymphoid cells producing immunoglobulins; the gammopathies include multiple myeloma, macroglobulinemia, and Hodgkin's disease.

gamogenesis (gam″ah-jen′ĭ-sis) sexual reproduction. **gamogenet′ic**, adj.

gangli(o)- word element [Gr.], *ganglion*.

ganglia (gang′gle-ah) plural of *ganglion*.

gangliform (gang′glĭ-form) having the form of a ganglion.

gangliitis (gang″gle-īt′is) ganglionitis.

ganglioblast (gang″gle-o-blast″) an embryonic cell of the cerebrospinal ganglia.

gangliocytoma (gang″gle-o-si-to′mah) ganglioneuroma.

ganglioform (gang′gle-ah-form″) gangliform.

ganglioglioma (gang″gle-o-gli-o′mah) a glioma rich in mature neurons or ganglion cells.

ganglioglioneuroma (-gli″o-nōōr-o′mah) ganglioneuroma.

ganglioma (gang″gle-o′mah) ganglioneuroma.

ganglion (gang′gle-in), pl. *gan′glia, ganglions* [Gr.] 1. a knot, or knotlike mass; in anatomy, a group of nerve cell bodies, located outside the central nervous system; occasionally applied to certain nuclear groups within the brain or spinal cord, e.g., basal ganglia. 2. a form of cystic tumor on an aponeurosis or a tendon. **gan′glial, ganglion′ic**, adj. **Acrel's g.**, a cystic tumor on an extensor tendon of the wrist. **Andersch's g.**, inferior g. (1). **autonomic ganglia,** aggregations of cell bodies of neurons of the autonomic nervous system. **basal ganglia,** specific interconnected gray masses deep in the cerebral hemispheres and in the upper brainstem, which are involved in motor coordination. **Bochdalek's g.,** superior dental plexus. **cardiac ganglia,** ganglia of the cardiac plexus near the arterial ligament. **carotid g.,** an occasional small enlargement in the internal carotid plexus. **celiac ganglia,** two irregularly shaped ganglia, one on each crus of the diaphragm within the celiac plexus. **cephalic ganglia,** parasympathetic ganglia in the head, consisting of the ciliary, otic, pterygopalatine, and submandibular ganglia. **cerebrospinal ganglia,** those associated with the cranial and spinal nerves. **cervical g.,** 1. any of the three ganglia (inferior, middle, and superior) of the sympathetic trunk in the neck region. 2. one near the cervix uteri. **cervicothoracic g.,** one formed by fusion of the inferior cervical and the first thoracic ganglia. **cervicouterine g.,** cervical g. (2). **ciliary g.,** a parasympathetic ganglion in the posterior part of the orbit. **Cloquet's g.,** a swelling of nasopalatine nerve in anterior palatine canal. **Corti's g.,** spiral g. **dorsal root g.,** spinal g. **Ehrenritter's g.,** superior g. (1). **false g.,** an enlargement on a nerve that does not have a true ganglionic structure. **gasserian g.,** trigeminal g. **geniculate g.,** the sensory ganglion of the facial nerve, on the geniculum of the facial nerve. **g. im′par,** the ganglion commonly found in front of the coccyx, where the sympathetic trunks of the two sides unite. **jugular g.,** superior g. (1 and 2). **Lee's g.,** cervical g. (2). **Ludwig's g.,** one near the right atrium of the heart, connected with the cardiac plexus. **lumbar ganglia,** the ganglia on the sympathetic trunk, usually four or five on either side. **Meckel's g.,** pterygopalatine g. **Meissner's g.,** one of the small groups of nerve cells in Meissner's plexus. **mesenteric g., inferior,** a sympathetic ganglion near the origin of the inferior mesenteric artery. **mesenteric g., superior,** one or more sympathetic ganglia at the sides of, or just below, the superior mesenteric artery. **otic g.,** a parasympathetic ganglion immediately below the foramen ovale; its postganglionic fibers supply the parotid gland. **parasympathetic ganglia,** aggregations of

F
G
H

cell bodies of cholinergic neurons of the parasympathetic nervous system; they are located near to or within the wall of the organs being innervated. **phrenic g.,** a sympathetic ganglion often found within the phrenic plexus at its junction with the cardiac plexus. **Remak's g.,** a sympathetic ganglion in the heart wall near the superior vena cava. **Ribes' g.,** the alleged ganglion in the termination of the internal carotid plexus around the anterior communicating artery of the brain. **sacral ganglia,** those of the sacral part of the sympathetic trunk, usually three or four on either side. **Scarpa's g.,** vestibular g. **semilunar g.,** 1. trigeminal g. 2. [pl.] celiac ganglia. **sensory g.,** any of the ganglia of the peripheral nervous system that transmit sensory impulses; also, the collective masses of nerve cell bodies in the brain subserving sensory functions. **simple g.,** a cystic tumor in a tendon sheath. **sphenopalatine g.,** pterygopalatine g. **spinal g.,** one on the dorsal root of each spinal nerve. **spiral g.,** the ganglion on the cochlear nerve, located within the modiolus, sending fibers peripherally to the organ of Corti and centrally to the cochlear nuclei of the brain stem. **splanchnic g.,** 1. one on the greater splanchnic nerve near the twelfth thoracic vertebra. 2. celiac plexus. **submandibular g., submaxillary g.,** a parasympathetic ganglion located superior to the deep part of the submandibular gland, on the lateral surface of the hyoglossal muscle. **superior g.,** 1. the upper of two ganglia on the glossopharyngeal nerve as it passes through the jugular foramen. 2. the upper of two ganglia of the vagus nerve just as it passes through the jugular foramen. **sympathetic ganglia,** aggregations of cell bodies of adrenergic neurons of the sympathetic nervous system; they are arranged in chainlike fashion on either side of the spinal cord. **trigeminal g.,** one on the sensory root of the fifth cranial nerve in a cleft in the dura mater on the anterior surface of the petrous part of the temporal bone, giving off the ophthalmic and maxillary and part of the mandibular nerve. **tympanic g.,** an enlargement on the tympanic branch of the glossopharyngeal nerve. **vagal g.,** 1. inferior g. (2). 2. superior g. (2). **ventricular ganglia,** Bidder's ganglia. **vestibular g.,** the sensory ganglion of the vestibular part of the eighth cranial nerve, located in the upper part of the lateral end of the internal acoustic meatus. **Wrisberg's g.,** cardiac g. **wrist g.,** cystic enlargement of a tendon sheath on the back of the wrist.

ganglionectomy (gang″gle-ah-nek′tah-me) excision of a ganglion.

ganglioneuroma (-nōōr-o′mah) a benign neoplasm composed of nerve fibers and mature ganglion cells.

ganglionostomy (-nos′tah-me) surgical creation of an opening into a cystic tumor on a tendon sheath or aponeurosis.

ganglioplegic (-ple′jik) blocking transmission of impulses through the sympathetic and parasympathetic ganglia; an agent that so acts.

ganglioside (gang′gle-ah-sīd) a class of galactose-containing cerebrosides found in central nervous system tissues; they are glycolipids of the basic composition ceramide-glucose-galactose-N-acetyl neuraminic acid. The form GM_1 accumulates in tissues in generalized gangliosidosis, the form GM_2 in Tay-Sachs disease.

gangliosidosis (gang″gle-o-si-do′sis) a group of lipid storage disorders marked by accumulation of gangliosides in tissues due to an enzyme defect and by progressive psychomotor deterioration usually beginning in infancy or childhood and usually fatal.

gangrene (gang′grēn) death of tissue, usually in considerable mass, generally with loss of vascular (nutritive) supply and followed by bacterial invasion and putrefaction. **diabetic g.,** moist gangrene associated with diabetes. **dry g.,** that occurring without subsequent bacterial decomposition, the tissues becoming dry and shriveled. **embolic g.,** a condition following cutting off of blood supply by embolism. **gas g.,** an acute, severe, painful condition in which the muscles and subcutaneous tissues become filled with gas and a serosanguineous exudate; due to infection of wounds by anaerobic bacteria, among which are various species of *Clostridium*. **moist g.,** that associated with proteolytic decomposition resulting from bacterial action. **symmetric g.,** gangrene of corresponding digits on both sides, due to vasomotor disturbances.

gangrenosis (gang″grin-o′sis) the development of gangrene.

ganoblast (gan′ah-blast) ameloblast.

Gantrisin (gan′trĭ-sin) trademark for preparations of sulfisoxazole.

gap (gap) an unoccupied interval in time; an opening or hiatus. **air-bone g.,** the lag between the audiographic curves for air- and bone-conducted stimuli, as an indication of loss of bone conduction of the ear. **auscultatory g.,** a period in which sound is not heard in the auscultatory method of sphygmomanometry. **interocclusal g.,** see under *distance*.

gargle (gar′g'l) 1. a solution for rinsing mouth and throat. 2. to rinse the mouth and throat by holding a solution in the open mouth and agitating it by expulsion of air from the lungs.

gargoylism (gar′goil-izm) Hurler's syndrome.

gas (gas) any elastic aeriform fluid in which the molecules are separated from one another and so have free paths. **gas′eous,** adj. **alveolar g.,** the gas in the alveoli of the lungs, where gaseous exchange with the capillary blood takes place. **coal g.,** a gas, poisonous because it contains carbon monoxide, produced by destructive distillation of coal; much used for domestic cooking. **laughing g.,** nitrous oxide. **tear g.,** one which produces severe lacrimation by irritating the conjunctivae.

gaskin (gas′kin) the thigh of a horse.

gaster (gas′ter) [Gr.] stomach.

Gasterophilus (-of′il-is) a genus of botflies the larvae of which develop in the gastrointestinal tract of horses and may sometimes infect man.

gastr(o)- word element [Gr.], *stomach.*

gastradenitis (gas″trad-in-īt′is) inflammation of the stomach glands.

gastralgia (gas-tral′je-ah) gastric colic.

gastrectomy (gas-trek′tah-me) excision of the stomach (*total g.*) or of a portion of it (*partial or subtotal g.*).

gastricsin (gas-trik′sin) a proteolytic enzyme isolated from gastric juice; its precursor is pepsinogen but it differs from pepsin in molecular weight and in the amino acids at the N terminal.

gastrin (gas′trin) a polypeptide hormone secreted by certain cells of the pyloric glands, which strongly stimulates secretion of gastric acid and pepsin, and weakly stimulates secretion of pancreatic enzymes and gallbladder contraction.

gastrinoma (gas″trin-o′mah) a gastrin-secreting, non-beta islet cell tumor of the pancreas, associated with Zollinger-Ellison syndrome.

gastritis (gas-trīt′is) inflammation of the stomach. **atrophic g.,** chronic gastritis with atrophy of the mucous membrane and glands. **catarrhal g.,** inflammation and hypertrophy of the gastric mucosa, with excessive secretion of mucus. **erosive g., exfoliative g.,** that in which the gastric surface epithelium is eroded. **giant hypertrophic g.,** excessive proliferation of the gastric mucosa, producing diffuse thickening of the stomach wall. **hypertrophic g.,** gastritis with infiltration and enlargement of the glands. **polypous g.,** hypertrophic gastritis with polypoid projections of the mucosa. **pseudomembranous g.,** that in which a false membrane occurs in patches within the stomach. **toxic g.,** that due to action of a poison or corrosive agent.

gastroanastomosis (-ah-nas″tah-mo′sis) gastrogastrostomy.

gastrocele (gas′tro-sēl) hernial protrusion of the stomach or of a gastric pouch.

gastrocnemius (gas″trok-ne′me-us) see *Table of Muscles.*

gastrocoele (gas′trah-sēl) archenteron.

gastrocolitis (-ko-līt′is) inflammation of the stomach and colon.

gastrocolostomy (-kol-os′tah-me) surgical anastomosis of the stomach to the colon.

gastrocutaneous (-ku-tān′e-us) pertaining to the stomach and skin, or communicating with the stomach and the cutaneous surface of the body, as a gastrocutaneous fistula.

gastrodiaphany (-di-af′ah-ne) examination of the stomach by transillumination of its walls with a small electric lamp.

Gastrodiscoides (-dis-koi′dēz) a genus of trematodes parasitic in the intestinal tract.

gastroduodenitis (-doo-od″in-īt′is) inflammation of the stomach and duodenum.

gastroduodenostomy (-doo″od-in-os′tah-me) surgical anastomosis of the stomach to a formerly remote part of the duodenum.

gastrodynia (-din′e-ah) pain in the stomach.

gastroenteralgia (-en″ter-al′je-ah) pain in the stomach and intestine.

gastroenteritis (-en″ter-īt′is) inflammation of the stomach and intestine. **eosinophilic g.,** a disorder, commonly associated with intolerance to specific foods, marked by infiltration of the mucosa of the small intestine by eosinophils,

with edema but without vasculitis and by eosinophilia of the peripheral blood. Symptoms depend on the site and extent of the disorder. The stomach is also frequently involved. **Norwalk g.,** gastroenteritis caused by the Norwalk virus.

gastroenteroanastomosis (-en″ter-o-ah-nas″-tah-mo′sis) anastomosis between the stomach and small intestine.

gastroenterology (-en″ter-ol′ah-je) the study of the stomach and intestine and their diseases.

gastroenteroptosis (-en″ter-op-to′sis) downward displacement or prolapse of the stomach and intestine.

gastroenterotomy (-en″ter-ot′ah-me) incision into the stomach and intestine.

gastroepiploic (-ep″ĭ-plo′ik) pertaining to the stomach and epiploon (omentum).

gastroesophagitis (-ĕ-sof″ah-jīt′is) inflammation of the stomach and esophagus.

gastrofiberscope (-fi′ber-skōp) a fiberscope for viewing the stomach.

gastrogastrostomy (-gas-tros′tah-me) surgical anastomosis of two previously remote portions of the stomach.

gastrogavage (-gah-vahzh′) artificial feeding through a tube passed into the stomach.

gastrohepatitis (-hep″ah-tīt′is) inflammation of the stomach and liver.

gastroileitis (-il″e-īt′is) inflammation of the stomach and ileum.

gastroileostomy (-il″e-os′tah-me) surgical anastomosis of the stomach to the ileum.

gastrojejunocolic (-je-joo″no-kol′ik) pertaining to the stomach, jejunum, and colon.

gastrolienal (-li′in-il) gastrosplenic.

gastrolithiasis (gas″tro-lĭ-thi′ah-sis) the presence or formation of calculi in the stomach.

gastrolysis (gas-trol′ĭ-sis) surgical division of perigastric adhesions to mobilize the stomach.

gastromalacia (gas″tro-mah-la′she-ah) softening of the wall of the stomach.

gastromegaly (-meg′ah-le) enlargement of the stomach.

gastromycosis (gas″tro-mi-ko′sis) fungal infection of the stomach.

gastromyxorrhea (-mik″so-re′ah) excessive secretion of mucus by the stomach.

gastropathy (gas-trop′ah-the) any disease of the stomach.

gastropexy (gas′trah-pek″se) surgical fixation of the stomach.

Gastrophilus (gas-trof′ĭ-lus) *Gasterophilus.*

gastrophrenic (gas″trah-fren′ik) pertaining to the stomach and diaphragm.

gastroplication (-plĭ-ka′shin) treatment of gastric dilatation by stitching a fold in the stomach wall.

gastroptosis (gas″trop-to′sis) downward displacement of the stomach.

gastropylorectomy (-pi″lo-rek′tah-me) excision of the pyloric part of the stomach.

gastrorrhagia (-ra′je-ah) hemorrhage from the stomach.

gastrorrhea (gas″tro-re′ah) excessive secretion by the glands of the stomach.

gastroschisis (gas-tros′kĭ-sis) congenital fissure of the abdominal wall.

gastroscope (gas′trah-skōp) an endoscope for inspecting the interior of the stomach. **gastroscop′ic**, adj.

gastroselective (gas″tro-sĭ-lek′tiv) having an affinity for receptors involved in regulation of gastric activities.

gastrospasm (gas′trah-spazm) spasm of the stomach.

gastrostaxis (-stak′sis) the oozing of blood from the stomach mucosa.

gastrostogavage (gas-tros″to-gah-vahzh′) feeding through a gastric fistula.

gastrostolavage (-lah-vahzh′) irrigation of the stomach through a gastric fistula.

gastrostomy (gas-tros′tah-me) creation of an artificial opening into the stomach.

gastrotomy (gas-trot′ah-me) incision into the stomach.

gastrotonometer (gas″tro-to-nom′it-er) an instrument for measuring intragastric pressure.

gastrotropic (-trop′ik) having an affinity for or exerting a special effect on the stomach.

gastrotympanities (-tim″pah-ni′tēz) tympanitic distention of the stomach.

gastrula (gas′troo-lah) the embryonic state following the blastula; the simplest type consists of two layers (ectoderm and endoderm) which have invaginated to form the archenteron and an opening, the blastopore.

gauntlet (gawnt′let) a bandage covering the hand and fingers like a glove.

gauss (gows) the unit of magnetic flux density.

gauze (gawz) a light, open-meshed fabric of muslin or similar material. **absorbable g.**, gauze made from oxidized cellulose. **absorbent g.**, white cotton cloth of various thread counts and weights, supplied in various lengths and widths and in different forms (rolls or folds). **petrolatum g.**, a sterile material produced by saturation of sterile absorbent gauze with sterile white petrolatum. **zinc gelatin impregnated g.**, absorbent gauze impregnated with zinc gelatin.

gavage (gah-vahzh′) [Fr.] 1. forced feeding, especially through a tube passed into the stomach. 2. superalimentation.

gaze (gāz) to look steadily in one direction.

Gd chemical symbol, *gadolinium*.

Ge chemical symbol, *germanium*.

gegenhalten (ga″gin-halt′in) [Ger.] an involuntary resistance to passive movement, as may occur in cerebral cortical disorders.

gel (jel) a firm colloid although containing much liquid; a colloid in gelatinous form. **aluminum hydroxide g.**, a suspension of aluminum hydroxide and hydrated oxide used as a gastric antacid, especially in the treatment of peptic ulcer. **aluminum phosphate g.**, a water suspension of aluminum phosphate and some flavoring agents, used as a gastric antacid, especially in the treatment of gastric ulcer. **basic aluminum carbonate g.**, an aluminum hydroxide-aluminum carbonate gel, used as a phosphorus-binding agent in prevention of re-

current phosphatic calculi and as a gastric antacid. **sodium fluoride and orthophosphoric acid g.**, an aqueous suspension containing fluoride and carboxymethylcellulose; used as a topical dental caries prophylactic.

gelasmus (ji-laz′mis) hysterical laughter.

gelatin (jel′ah-tin) a substance obtained by partial hydrolysis of collagen derived from skin, white connective tissue, and bones of animals; used as a suspending agent and in the manufacture of capsules and suppositories; suggested for use as a plasma substitute, and has been used as an adjuvant protein food. **zinc g.**, a preparation of zinc oxide, gelatin, glycerin, and purified water, applied topically as a protective.

gelation (jĭ-la′shin) conversion of a sol into a gel.

geld (geld) to remove the testes, especially of the horse.

gelosis (je-lo′sis) a hard lump in a tissue, especially in muscle.

Gemella (jĕ-mel′ah) a genus of aerobic or facultatively anaerobic cocci (family Streptococcaceae), occurring singly or in pairs with adjacent sides flattened; they are found as parasites of mammals.

gemellology (jem″el-ol′ah-je) the scientific study of twins and twinning.

geminate (jem′ĭ-nāt) paired; occurring in twos.

gemmation (jĕ-ma′shin) budding; asexual reproduction in which a portion of the cell body is thrust out and then becomes separated, forming a new individual.

gemmule (jem′ūl) 1. a reproductive bud; the immediate product of gemmation. 2. one of the many little spinelike processes on the dendrites of a nerve cell.

-gen word element [Gr.], *an agent that produces*.

genal (je′nil) pertaining to the cheek; buccal.

gender (jen′der) sex; the category to which an individual is assigned on the basis of sex.

gene (jēn) the biologic unit of heredity, self-reproducing and located at a definite position (locus) on a particular chromosome. **allelic g's**, genes situated at corresponding loci in a pair of chromosomes. **complementary g's**, two independent pairs of nonallelic genes, neither of which will produce its effect in the absence of the other. **dominant g.**, one that is phenotypically expressed when present in homozygotes or heterozygotes. **Hg., histocompatibility g.**, one that determines the specificity of tissue antigenicity (HLA antigens), and thus the compatibility of donor and recipient in tissue transplantation and blood transfusion. **holandric g's**, genes in the nonhomologous region of the Y chromosome. **immune response (Ir) g's**, genes of the major histocompatibility complex (MHC) that govern the immune response to individual immunogens. **Is g's**, genes that govern the formation of suppressor T-lymphocytes. **lethal g.**, one whose presence brings about the death of the organism or permits survival only under certain conditions. **mutant g.**, one that has undergone a detectable mutation. **operator g.**, one serving as a starting point for reading the genetic code, and which, through interaction with a repressor, controls the activity of structural genes associated with it in the operon. **recessive g.,** one that produces an effect in the organism only when it is homozygous. **regulator g., repressor g.,** one that synthesizes repressor, a substance which, through interaction with the operator gene, switches off the activity of the structural genes associated with it in the operon. **sex-linked g.,** one carried on a sex chromosome, especially on an X chromosome. **structural g.,** one that specifies the amino acid sequence of a polypeptide chain.

genera (jen′er-ah) plural of *genus.*

generation (jen″ĕ-ra′shin) 1. the process of reproduction. 2. a class composed of all individuals removed by the same number of successive ancestors from a common predecessor, or occupying positions on the same level in a genealogical (pedigree) chart. **alternate g.,** the alternate generation by asexual and sexual means in an animal or plant species. **asexual g.,** production of a new organism not originating from union of gametes. **filial g., first,** the first-generation offspring of two parents; symbol F_1. **filial g., second,** all of the offspring produced by two individuals of the first filial generation; symbol F_2. **parental g.,** the generation with which a particular genetic study is begun; symbol P_1. **sexual g.,** production of a new organism from the zygote formed by the union of gametes. **spontaneous g.,** the discredited concept of continuous generation of living organisms from nonliving matter.

generator (jen′er-āt-er) something that produces or causes to exist; a machine that converts mechanical to electrical energy. **pulse g.,** the power source for a cardiac pacemaker system, usually powered by a lithium battery, supplying impulses to the implanted electrodes, either at a fixed rate or in some programmed pattern.

generic (jǐ-nĕ′rik) 1. pertaining to a genus. 2. nonproprietary; denoting a drug name not protected by a trademark, usually descriptive of the drug's chemical structure.

genesis (jen′ĕ-sis) creation; origination; used as a word termination joined to an element indicating the thing created, e.g., carcinogenesis.

genetic (jǐ-net′ik) 1. pertaining to reproduction or to birth or origin. 2. inherited.

genetics (jǐ-net′iks) the study of heredity. **biochemical g.,** the science concerned with the chemical and physical nature of genes and the mechanism by which they control the development and maintenance of the organism. **clinical g.,** the study of genetic factors influencing the occurrence of a pathologic condition.

genetotrophic (jǐ-net″ah-trof′ik) pertaining to genetics and nutrition; relating to problems of nutrition that are hereditary in nature, or transmitted through the genes.

genial (jǐ-ni′il) pertaining to the chin.

genic (jen′ik) pertaining to or caused by the genes.

-genic word element [Gr.], *giving rise to; causing.*

genicular (jǐ-nik′ūl-er) pertaining to the knee.

geniculate (jǐ-nik′ūl-āt) bent, like a knee.

geniculum (jǐ-nik′ūl-im), pl. *geni′cula* [L.] a little

knee; used in anatomic nomenclature to designate a sharp kneelike bend in a small structure or organ.

genion (jǐ-ni′on) apex of lower genial tubercle.

genital (jen′i-t′l) 1. pertaining to reproduction, or to the reproductive organs. 2. [pl.] the reproductive organs.

genitalia (jen″ĭ-tāl′e-ah) the reproductive organs. **external g.,** the reproductive organs external to the body, including pudendum, clitoris, and female urethra in the female, and scrotum, penis, and male urethra in the male. **indifferent g.,** the reproductive organs of the embryo prior to the establishment of definitive sex.

genito- word element [L.], *the organs of reproduction.*

genitography (jen″ĭ-tog′rah-fe) radiography of the urogenital sinus and internal duct structures after injection of a contrast medium through the sinus opening.

genitourinary (jen″it-o-ūr′in-e″re) urogenital.

genodermatosis (je″no-der″mah-to′sis) a genetic disorder of the skin, usually generalized.

genome (je′nōm) the complete set of hereditary factors contained in the haploid set of chromosomes. **genom′ic,** adj.

genotype (jen″ah-tīp) 1. the entire genetic constitution of an individual; also, the alleles present at one or more specific loci. 2. the type species of a genus. **genotyp′ic,** adj.

-genous word element [Gr.], *arising or resulting from; produced by.*

gentamicin (jen″tah-mi′sin) an antibiotic complex isolated from the actinomycetes of the genus *Micromonospora,* effective against many gram-negative bacteria, especially *Pseudomonas* species, as well as certain gram-positive species, especially *Staphylococcus aureus.*

gentian (jen′shin) the dried rhizome and roots of *Gentiana lutea;* has been used as a bitter tonic. **g. violet,** an antibacterial, antifungal, and anthelmintic dye, applied topically in the treatment of infections of the skin and mucous membranes associated with gram-positive bacteria and molds, and administered orally in pinworm and liver fluke infections.

gentianophilic (jen″shan-ah-fil′ik) staining readily with gentian violet.

gentianophobic (-fo′bik) not staining with gentian violet.

genu (je′nu), pl. *ge′nua* [L.] the knee; any kneelike structure. **g. extror′sum,** bowleg. **g. intror′sum,** knock-knee. **g. recurva′tum,** hyperextensibility of the knee joint. **g. val′gum,** knock-knee. **g. va′rum,** bowleg.

genus (je′nus), pl. *ge′nera* [L.] a taxonomic category (taxon) subordinate to a tribe (or subtribe) and superior to a species (or subgenus).

geo- word element [Gr.], *the earth; the soil.*

geode (je′ōd) a dilated lymph space.

geomedicine (je″o-med′ĭ-sin) the branch of medicine dealing with the influence of climatic and environmental conditions on health.

geophagia, geophagism (je″o-fa′je-ah; je-of′-ah-jizm) the eating of earth (soil) or clay.

geotrichosis (-trĭ-ko′sis) a candidiasis-like infection due to *Geotrichum candidum*, which may attack the bronchi, lungs, mouth, or intestinal tract.

Geotrichum (je-ah′trĭ-kum) a genus of yeastlike fungi, including *G. can′didum*, found in the feces and in dairy products.

geotropism (je-ah′trah-pizm) a tendency of growth or movement toward or away from the earth; the influence of gravity on growth.

ger-, gero-, geronto- word element [Gr.], *old age; the aged.*

geratic (jĭ-rat′ik) pertaining to old age.

geratology (jĕ″rah-tol′ah-je) gereology.

geriatrics (jer″e-ă′triks) the department of medicine dealing especially with the problems of aging and diseases of the elderly. **dental g.,** gerodontics. **geriat′ric,** adj.

geriodontics (-o-don′tiks) gerodontics.

germ (jurm) 1. a pathogenic microorganism. 2. a living substance capable of developing into an organ, part, or organism as a whole; a primordium. **dental g.,** collective tissues from which a tooth is formed. **enamel g.,** the epithelial rudiment of the enamel organ.

germanium (jer-ma′ne-um) chemical element (*see table*), at. no. 32, symbol Ge.

germicidal (jurm″ĭ-si′d′l) lethal to pathogenic microorganisms.

germinal (jurm′ĭ-nil) pertaining to or of the nature of a germ cell or the primitive stage of development.

germination (jurm″ĭ-na′shin) the sprouting of a seed or spore or of a plant embryo.

germinoma (jurm″ĭ-no′mah) a neoplasm of germ tissue (testis or ovum), e.g., a seminoma.

geroderma, gerodermia (-der′mah; -der′me-ah) dystrophy of the skin and genitals, giving the appearance of old age.

gerodontics (-don′tiks) dentistry dealing with the dental problems of older people. **gerodon′tic,** adj.

geromarasmus (-mah-raz′mis) the emaciation sometimes characteristic of old age.

geromorphism (-mor′fizm) premature senility.

gerontology (jer″on-tol′ah-je) the scientific study of the problems of aging in all its aspects.

gerontopia (-to′pe-ah) senopia.

gerontotherapeutics (je-ron″to-thĕ″rah-pūt′iks) the science of retarding and preventing many of the aspects of senescence.

gerontoxon (jĕ″ron-tok′son) arcus senilis.

geropsychiatry (jer″o-si-ki′ah-tre) a subspecialty of psychiatry dealing with mental illness in the elderly.

gestagen (jes′tah-jen) any hormone with progestational activity.

gestaltism (gah-shtahlt′izm) the theory in psychology that the objects of mind, as immediately presented to direct experience, come as complete unanalyzable wholes or forms (Gestalten) which cannot be split up into parts.

gestation (jes-ta′shin) the period of development of the young in viviparous animals, from the time of fertilization of the ovum until birth; see also *pregnancy.*

gestosis (jes-to′sis) any toxemic manifestation in pregnancy.

GeV gigaelectron volt.

GFR glomerular filtration rate.

ghost (gōst) a faint or shadowy figure lacking the customary substance of reality. **red cell g.,** an erythrocyte membrane that remains intact after hemolysis.

GH-RH growth hormone releasing hormone.

G.I. gastrointestinal; globin insulin.

giantism (ji′int-izm) 1. gigantism. 2. excessive size, as of cells or nuclei.

Giardia (je-ar′de-ah) a genus of flagellate protozoa parasitic in the intestinal tract of man and animals, which may cause protracted, intermittent diarrhea with symptoms suggesting malabsorption; *G. lam′blia* (*G. intestina′lis*) is the species found in man.

gibberellin (gib″er-el′in) any of a class of phytohormones whose most striking activity is the promotion of lateral bud development in decapitated plant stems; first isolated from fungi of the genus *Gibberella.*

gibbosity (gĭ-bos′it-e) the condition of being humped; kyphosis.

gibbus (gib′is) a hump.

gid (gid) a disease of the brain and spinal cord of domestic animals, especially sheep, due to *Coenurus cerebralis*, and marked by unsteadiness of gait.

giga- word element [Gr.], *huge;* used in naming units of measurement to designate an amount 10^9 (one billion) times the size of the unit to which it is joined, e.g., gigameter (10^9 meters); symbol G.

gigantism (ji-gin′tizm) abnormal overgrowth; excessive size and stature. **cerebral g.,** gigantism in the absence of increased levels of growth hormone, attributed to a cerebral defect; infants are large, and accelerated growth continues for the first 4 or 5 years, the rate being normal thereafter. The hands and feet are large, the head large and dolichocephalic, the eyes have an antimongoloid slant, with hypertelorism. The child is clumsy, and mental retardation of varying degree is usually present. **pituitary g.,** Launois' syndrome.

gigantomastia (ji-gan′to-mas′te-ah) extreme hypertrophy of the breast.

ginger (jin′jer) the dried rhizome of the tropical plant *Zingiber officinale;* used as a flavoring.

gingiva (jin-ji′vah, jin′jĭ-vah), pl. *gingi′vae* [L.] the gum; the mucous membrane, with supporting fibrous tissue, covering the tooth-bearing border of the jaw. **gingi′val, gin′gival,** adj. **alveolar g.,** the portion covering the alveolar process. **areolar g.,** the portion attached to the alveolar process by loose areolar connective tissue. **free g.,** the portion of the gingiva that surrounds the tooth and is not directly attached to the tooth surface. **marginal g.,** the portion of the free gingiva localized at the labial, buccal, lingual, and palatal aspects of the teeth; gingival margin.

gingivally (jin-ji′val-e) toward the gingiva.

gingivectomy (jin″ji-vek′tah-me) surgical excision of all loose infected and diseased gingival tissue.

gingivitis (jin″ji-vit′is) inflammation of the gingiva. **atrophic g., senile,** a condition characterized by hyperkeratinization and areas of desquamation in the gingiva. **fusospirochetal g.,** necrotizing ulcerative g. **herpetic g.,** infection of the gingivae by the herpes simplex virus. **necrotizing ulcerative g.,** trench mouth; a gingival infection marked by redness and swelling, necrosis, pain, hemorrhage, a necrotic odor, and often a pseudomembrane; see also under *gingivostomatitis.* **pregnancy g.,** any of various gingival changes ranging from gingivitis to the so-called pregnancy tumor. **Vincent's g.,** necrotizing ulcerative g.

gingivo- word element [L.], *gingival.*

gingivosis (jin″ji-vo′sis) a chronic, diffuse inflammation of the gingivae, with desquamation of papillary epithelium and mucous membrane.

gingivostomatitis (jin″ji-vo-sto″mah-tit′is) inflammation of the gingivae and oral mucosa. **herpetic g.,** that due to infection with herpes simplex virus, with redness of the oral tissues, formation of multiple vesicles and painful ulcers, and fever. **necrotizing ulcerative g.,** that due to extension of necrotizing ulcerative gingivitis to other areas of the oral mucosa.

ginglymoid (jing′gli-moid) resembling a hinge; pertaining to a ginglymus.

ginglymus (jing′gli-mus) a joint that allows movement in but one plane, forward and backward, as does a door hinge.

girdle (gur′d'l) cingulum; an encircling structure or part; anything encircling the body. **pectoral g.,** shoulder g. **pelvic g.,** the encircling bony structure supporting the lower limbs. **shoulder g., thoracic g.,** the encircling bony structure supporting the upper limbs.

gitalin (jit′ah-lin) amorphous gitalin; a mixture of digitalis glycosides used as a cardiotonic in congestive heart failure and cardiac arrhythmias.

gizzard (giz′erd) the muscular second stomach of a bird.

glabella (glah-bel′ah) the area on the frontal bone above the nasion and between the eyebrows.

glabrous (gla′brus) smooth and bare.

gladiolus (glah-di′o-lus) corpus sterni.

glairy (glār′e) resembling egg white.

gland (gland) an aggregation of cells specialized to secrete or excrete materials not related to their ordinary metabolic needs. **accessory g.,** a minor mass of glandular tissue near or at some distance from a gland of similar structure. **adrenal g.,** a flattened body above either kidney, consisting of a cortex and a medulla, the former elaborating steroid hormones, and the latter epinephrine and norepinephrine. **aggregate g's, agminated g's,** Peyer's patches. **apocrine g.,** one whose discharged secretion contains part of the secreting cells. **axillary g's,** lymph nodes situated in the axilla. **Bartholin's g.,** one of two small bodies on either side of the vaginal orifice. **Blandin's g's,** anterior

lingual g's. **bronchial g's,** seromucous glands in the mucosa and submucosa of bronchial walls. **Bruch's g's,** lymph follicles in the conjunctiva of lower lid. **Brunner's g's,** duodenal g's. **bulbocavernous g., bulbourethral g.,** one of two glands embedded in the substance of the sphincter of the urethra, posterior to the membranous part of the urethra. **cardiac g's,** mucin-secreting glands of the cardiac part (cardia) of the stomach. **celiac g's,** lymph nodes anterior to the abdominal aorta. **ceruminous g's,** cerumen-secreting glands in the skin of the external auditory canal. **cervical g's,** 1. the lymph nodes of the neck. 2. compound clefts in the wall of the uterine cervix. **ciliary g's,** sweat glands that have become arrested in their development, situated at the edges of the eyelids. **circumanal g's,** specialized sweat and sebaceous glands around the anus. **closed g.,** endocrine g. **coccygeal g.,** glomus coccygeum. **compound g.,** one made up of a number of smaller units whose excretory ducts combine to form ducts of progressively higher order. **conglobate g.,** a lymph node. **Cowper's g.,** bulbourethral g. **ductless g's,** endocrine g's. **duodenal g's,** glands in the submucosa of the duodenum, opening into the glands of the small intestine. **Ebner's g's,** serous glands at the back of the tongue near the taste buds. **eccrine g.,** one of the ordinary, or simple, sweat glands, which is of the merocrine type. **endocrine g's,** organs whose secretions (hormones) are released directly into the circulatory system; they include the pituitary, thyroid, parathyroid, and adrenal glands, the pineal body, and the gonads. **exocrine g.,** one whose secretion is discharged through a duct opening on an internal or external surface of the body. **fundic g's, fundus g's,** tubular glands in the mucosa of the fundus and body of the stomach, containing acid- and pepsin-secreting cells. **Galeati's g's,** duodenal g's. **gastric g's,** the secreting glands of the stomach, including the fundic, cardiac, and pyloric glands. **gastric g's, proper,** fundic g's. **Gay's g's,** circumanal g's. **glossopalatine g's,** mucous glands at the posterior end of the smaller sublingual glands. **guttural g.,** one of the mucous glands of the pharynx. **Harder's g's, harderian g's,** accessory lacrimal glands at the inner corner of the eye in animals that have nictitating membranes. **haversian g's,** synovial villi. **hematopoietic g's,** glandlike bodies that take part in blood formation, e.g., the spleen. **hemolymph g's,** see under *node.* **holocrine g.,** one whose discharged secretion contains the entire secreting cells. **intestinal g's,** straight tubular glands in the mucous membrane of the intestine, opening, in the small intestine, between the bases of the villi, and containing argentaffin cells. **jugular g.,** accessory lacrimal glands deep in the conjunctival connective tissue, mainly near the upper fornix. **lacrimal g's,** the glands which secrete tears. **g's of Lieberkühn,** intestinal g's. **lingual g's,** the seromucous glands on the surface of the tongue. **lingual g's, anterior,** the seromucous glands near the apex of the tongue. **Littre's g's,** 1. preputial g's. 2. urethral g's (male). **lymph g.,** see under *node.* **mammary g.,** the specialized gland of the skin of female mammals, which secretes milk for nourishment of the young. **meibomian g's,** sebaceous follicles between the cartilage and conjunctiva of eyelids. **merocrine g.,** one in which the secretory cells maintain their integrity throughout the secretory cycle. **mixed g's,** 1. seromucous g's. 2. glands that have both exocrine and endocrine portions. **monoptychic g.,** one in which the tubules or alveoli are lined with a single layer of secreting cells. **Morgagni's g's,** urethral g's (male). **mucous g's,** glands which secrete mucus. **nabothian g's,** see under *follicle.* **Nuhn's g's,** anterior lingual g's. **olfactory g's,** small mucous glands in the olfactory mucosa. **parathyroid g's,** small bodies in the region of the thyroid gland, developed from the entoderm of the branchial clefts, occurring in a variable number of pairs, commonly two; they secrete parathyroid hormone and are concerned chiefly with the metabolism of calcium and phosphorus. **paraurethral g's,** see under *duct.* **parotid g.,** the largest of the three paired salivary glands, located in front of the ear. **Peyer's g's,** see under *patch.* **pineal g.,** see under *body.* **pituitary g.,** the hypophysis; the epithelial body of dual origin at the base of the brain in the sella turcica, attached by a stalk to the hypothalamus; it consists of two main lobes, the *anterior lobe,* secreting several important hormones which regulate the proper functioning of the thyroids, gonads, adrenal cortex, and other endocrine organs, and the *posterior lobe,* whose cells serve as a reservoir for hormones having antidiuretic and oxytocic action, releasing them as needed. **preen g.,** a large, compound alveolar structure on the back of birds, above the base of the tail, which secretes an oily "water-proofing" material that the bird applies to its feathers and skin by preening. **preputial g's,** small sebaceous glands of the corona of the penis and the inner surface of the prepuce, which secrete smegma. **prostate g.,** see *prostate.* **pyloric g's,** the mucin-secreting glands of the pyloric part of the stomach. **racemose g's,** glands composed of acini arranged like grapes on a stem. **saccular g.,** one consisting of a sac or sacs, lined with glandular epithelium. **salivary g's,** glands of the oral cavity whose combined secretion constitutes the saliva, including the parotid, sublingual, and submandibular glands and numerous small glands in the tongue, lips, cheeks, and palate. **sebaceous g's,** holocrine glands in the corium that secrete an oily substance and sebum. **serous g.,** a gland that secretes a watery albuminous material, commonly but not always containing enzymes. **sex g's, sexual g's,** see *testis* and *ovary.* **simple g.,** one with a nonbranching duct. **Skene's g's,** paraurethral ducts. **solitary g's,** see under *follicle.* **submandibular g., submaxillary g.,** a salivary gland on the inner side of each ramus of the lower jaw. **suprarenal g.,** adrenal g. **Susanne's g.,** a mucous gland of the mouth, beneath the alveolingual groove. **sweat g's,** glands that secrete sweat, situated in the corium or subcutaneous tissue, opening by a duct on the body surface. The ordinary or *eccrine sweat g's* are distributed over most of the body surface, and promote cooling by evaporation of the secretion; the *apocrine sweat g's* empty into the upper portion of a hair follicle instead of directly onto the skin, and are found only in certain body areas, as around the anus and in the axilla. **target g.,** one specifically affected by a pituitary hormone. **tarsal g's,** meibomian g's. **thymus g.,** see *thymus.* **thyroid g.,** an endocrine gland consisting of two lobes, one on each side of the trachea, joined by a narrow isthmus, producing hormones (thyroxine and triiodothyronine), which require iodine for their elaboration and which are concerned in regulating metabolic rate; it also secretes calcitonin. **Tyson's g's,** preputial g's. **unicellular g.,** a single cell that functions as a gland, e.g., a goblet cell. **urethral g's,** mucous glands in the wall of the urethra. **Virchow's g.,** sentinel node. **vulvovaginal g.,** Bartholin g. **Waldeyer's g's,** glands in the attached edge of the eyelid. **Weber's g's,** the tubular mucous glands of the tongue. **Zeis' g's,** modified rudimentary sebaceous glands attached directly to the eyelash follicles. **Zuckerkandl's g's,** para-aortic bodies.

glanders (glan'derz) a contagious disease of horses, communicable to man, due to *Pseudomonas mallei,* and marked by purulent inflammation of the mucous membranes and cutaneous eruption of nodules that coalesce and break down, forming deep ulcers, which may end in necrosis of cartilage and bone; the more chronic and constitutional form is known as *farcy.*

glandilemma (glan″dĭ-lem′ah) the capsule or outer envelope of a gland.

glandula (glan′dül-ah) pl. *glan′dulae* [L.] a gland.

glandule (glan′dül) a small gland.

glans (glanz), pl. *glan′des* [L.] a small, rounded mass or glandlike body. **g. clito′ridis,** erectile tissue on the free end of the clitoris. **g. pe′nis,** the cap-shaped expansion of the corpus spongiosum at the end of the penis.

glanular (glan′ül-er) pertaining to the glans penis or to the glans clitoris.

glass (glas) 1. a hard, brittle, often transparent material, usually consisting of the fused amorphous silicates of potassium or sodium, and of calcium, with silica in excess. 2. a container, usually cylindrical, made from glass. 3. (pl.) lenses worn to aid or improve vision; see also *glasses* and *lens.*

glasses (glas′iz) spectacles; lenses arranged in a frame holding them in the proper position before the eyes, as an aid to vision. **bifocal g.,** those with lenses having two different refracting powers, one for distant and one for near vision. **trifocal g.,** glasses with lenses having three different refractive powers, one for distant, one for intermediate, and one for near vision.

glaucoma (glaw-ko′mah) a group of eye diseases characterized by an increase in intraocular pressure, causing pathological changes in the optic disk and typical visual field defects. **congenital g.,** that due to defective development of the structures in and around the anterior chamber of the eye and resulting in impairment of aqueous humor; see *infantile g.*

Donders' g., g. simplex. **infantile g.**, buphthalmos; hydrophthalmos; congenital glaucoma that may be fully developed at birth with enlarged eyes and hazy corneas, or may develop at any time up to two or three years of age. **narrow-angle g.**, a form of primary glaucoma in an eye characterized by a shallow anterior chamber and a narrow angle, in which filtration is compromised as a result of the iris blocking the angle. **open-angle g.**, a form of primary glaucoma in an eye in which the angle of the anterior chamber remains open, but filtration is gradually diminished because of the tissues of the angle. **primary g.**, increased intraocular pressure occurring in an eye without previous disease.

glaze (glāz) in dentistry, a ceramic veneer added to a porcelain restoration, to simulate enamel.

gleet (glēt) 1. chronic gonorrheal urethritis. 2. a urethral discharge, especially one that is mucous or purulent.

glenoid (gle′noid) resembling a pit or socket.

glia (gli′ah) neuroglia.

gliacyte (-sīt) a cell of the neuroglia.

gliadin (-din) a protein present in wheat; it contains the toxic factor associated with celiac disease.

glial (gli′il) of or pertaining to the neuroglia.

glioblastoma (-blas-to′mah) any malignant astrocytoma. **g. multifor′me**, astrocytoma Grade III or IV; a rapidly growing tumor, usually of the cerebral hemispheres, composed of spongioblasts, astroblasts, and astrocytes.

glioma (gli-o′mah) a tumor composed of neuroglia in any of its states of development; sometimes extended to include all intrinsic neoplasms of the brain and spinal cord, as astrocytomas, ependymomas, etc. **glio′matous**, adj. **g. re′tinae**, retinoblastoma.

gliomatosis (gli″o-mah-to′sis) excessive development of the neuroglia, especially of the spinal cord, in certain cases of syringomyelia.

gliosis (gli-o′sis) an excess of astroglia in damaged areas of the central nervous system.

glissade (glis-ād′) [Fr.] a gliding involuntary movement of the eye in changing the point of fixation; it is a slower, smoother movement than is a saccade. **glissad′ic**, adj.

glissonitis (glis″ah-nīt′is) inflammation of Glisson's capsule.

globi (glo′bi) 1. plural of *globus*. 2. encapsulated globular masses containing bacilli; seen in smears of lepromatous leprosy lesions.

globin (glo′bin) the protein constituent of hemoglobin; also, any member of a group of proteins similar to the typical globin.

globoside (glob′ah-sīd) a sphingoglycolipid containing acetylated amino sugars and simple hexoses, occurring in human serum, spleen, liver, and erythrocytes, and accumulating in tissues in Sandhoff's disease.

globule (glob′ūl) a small spherical mass; a little globe or pellet, as of medicine. **glob′ular**, adj.

globulin (glob′ūl-in) a class of proteins insoluble in water, but soluble in saline solutions (euglobulins), or water-soluble proteins (pseudoglobulins); their other physical properties resemble true globulins; see *serum g*. **accelerator g.**, coagulation Factor V. **alpha g's**, globulins in plasma which, in neutral or alkaline solutions, have the greatest electrophoretic mobility, in this respect most nearly resembling the albumins. **antihemophilic g.**, coagulation Factor VIII. **beta g's**, globulins in plasma which, in neutral or alkaline solutions, have an electrophoretic mobility between that of the alpha and that of the gamma globulins. **gamma g's**, a group of plasma globulins which, in neutral or alkaline solutions, have the slowest electrophoretic mobility and which have sites of antibody activity; see *immunoglobulin*. **hepatitis B immune g.**, a sterile nonpyrogenic solution consisting of globulins derived from blood plasma of human donors who have high titers of antibodies against hepatitis B surface antigen; used as a passive immunizing agent. **immune g.**, a sterile solution containing many antibodies normally present in adult human blood, derived from donor plasma or serum; used for passive immunization against infectious hepatitis, poliomyelitis, rubella, rubeola, and varicella, and in the treatment of gamma globulin deficiency. **pertussis immune g.**, a sterile solution of globulins derived from the blood plasma of human donors immunized with pertussis vaccine; used for the prophylaxis and treatment of pertussis. **rabies immune g.**, a sterile nonpyrogenic solution of globulins from blood plasma or serum of human donors who have been immunized with rabies vaccine and have high titers of rabies antibody; used as a passive immunizing agent. **Rh₀(D) immune g.**, a sterile solution of globulins derived from human blood plasma containing antibody to the erythrocyte factor $Rh_o(D)$; used to suppress formation of active Rh_o antibodies in Rh_o-negative mothers after delivery or miscarriage of a Rh_o-positive baby or fetus, and thus to prevent erythroblastosis fetalis in the next pregnancy if the child is Rh_o-positive. **tetanus immune g.**, a sterile solution of gamma globulins derived from the blood plasma of human donors who have been immunized with tetanus toxoid; used in the prophylaxis and treatment of tetanus. **vaccinia immune human g.**, a sterile solution of globulins derived from the blood plasma of human donors who have been immunized against vaccinia with vaccinia virus smallpox vaccine; used as a passive immunizing agent.

globus (glo′bus), pl. *glo′bi* [L.] 1. a sphere or ball; a spherical structure. 2. a subjective sensation as of a lump or mass. 3. see *globi* (2). **g. hyste′ricus**, subjective sensation of a lump in the throat. **g. pal′lidus**, the smaller and more medial part of the lentiform nucleus of the brain.

glomangioma (glo-man″je-o′mah) a benign, often painful tumor derived from a glomus, usually occurring on the distal portion of the fingers or toes, in the skin, or in deeper structures.

glomera (glom′er-ah) plural of *glomus*.

glomerular (glo-mer′ūl-er) pertaining to or of the nature of a glomerulus, especially a renal glomerulus.

glomeruli (glo-mer′ūl-i) plural of *glomerulus*.

glomerulonephritis (glo-mer″ūl-o-nef-rīt′is)

nephritis with inflammation of the capillary loops in the renal glomeruli. **IgA g.,** a chronic form marked by a hematuria and proteinuria and by deposits of immunoglobulin A in the mesangial areas of the renal glomeruli, with subsequent reactive hyperplasia of mesangial cells. **lobular g.,** a form in which all glomeruli are affected, with accentuation of the lobulation of the glomerular tufts; it is marked by constant proteinuria and microscopic hematuria. **membranoproliferative g., mesangiocapillary g.,** a chronic, slowly progressive glomerulonephritis in which the glomeruli are enlarged as a result of proliferation of mesangial cells and irregular thickening of the capillary walls which narrows the capillary lumina; the onset is sudden, with hematuria, proteinuria, or nephrotic syndrome and a persistent reduction in serum complement levels and deposition of activated complement components in the glomerular capillaries.

glomerulopathy (glo-mer″ūl-op′ah-the) any disease of the renal glomeruli. **diabetic g.,** intercapillary glomerulosclerosis.

glomerulosclerosis (glo-mer″ūl-o-sklĕ-ro′sis) fibrosis and scarring resulting in senescence of the renal glomeruli. **intercapillary g.,** a degenerative complication of diabetes, manifested as albuminuria, nephrotic edema, hypertension, renal insufficiency, and retinopathy.

glomerulus (glo-mer′ūl-us), pl. *glomer′uli* [L.] a small tuft or cluster, as of blood vessels or nerve fibers; often used alone to designate one of the renal glomeruli. **olfactory g.,** one of the small globular masses of dense neuropil in the olfactory bulb containing the first synapse in the olfactory pathway. **renal glomeruli,** globular tufts of capillaries, one projecting into the expanded end or capsule of each of the uriniferous tubules, which together with the glomerular capsule constitute the renal corpuscle.

glomus (glo′mus), pl. *glo′mera* [L.] a small histologically recognizable body composed of fine arterioles connecting directly with veins, and having a rich nerve supply. **glo′mera aor′tica,** aortic bodies. **g. caro′ticum,** carotid body. **g. choroi′deum,** an enlargement of the choroid plexus of the lateral ventricle. **g. coccy′geum,** a collection of arteriovenous anastomoses near the tip of the coccyx formed by the middle sacral artery. **g. jugula′re,** an aggregation of chemoreceptors in the bulb of the jugular vein.

gloss(o)- word element [Gr.], *tongue.*

glossectomy (glos-ek′tah-me) excision of all or a portion of the tongue.

Glossina (glos-i′nah) a genus of biting flies, the tsetse flies, which serve as vectors of trypanosomes causing various forms of trypanosomiasis in man and animals.

glossitis (glos-īt′is) inflammation of the tongue. **g. area′ta exfoliati′va,** geographic tongue. **rhomboid g., median,** a congenital anomaly of the tongue, with a reddish patch or plaque on the midline of the dorsal surface.

glossocele (glos′ah-sēl) swelling and protrusion of the tongue.

glossograph (glos′ah-graf) an apparatus for registering tongue movements in speech.

glossology (glos-ol′ah-je) 1. sum of knowledge regarding the tongue. 2. treatise on nomenclature.

glossoplasty (glos′ah-plas″te) plastic surgery of the tongue.

glossorrhaphy (glos-or′ah-fe) suture of the tongue.

glossotrichia (glos″ah-trik′e-ah) hairy tongue.

glottic (glot′ik) pertaining to the glottis or to the tongue.

glottis (glot′is), pl. *glot′tides* [Gr.] the vocal apparatus of the larynx, consisting of the true vocal cords and the opening between them. **glot′tal,** adj.

Glu glutamic acid or glutamyl.

glucagon (gloo′kah-gon) a polypeptide hormone secreted by the alpha cells of the islets of Langerhans in response to hypoglycemia or to stimulation by growth hormone, which stimulates glycogenolysis in the liver; used as an antihypoglycemic.

glucagonoma (gloo″kah-gon-o′mah) a glucagon-secreting tumor of the alpha cells of the islets of Langerhans.

glucan (gloo′kan) any polysaccharide composed only of recurring units of glucose; a homopolymer of glucose.

gluceptate (glu-sep′tāt) USAN contraction for glucoheptonate.

glucocerebroside (gloo″ko-sĕ′rĕ-bro-sīd) a cerebroside with a glucose sugar.

glucocorticoid (-kor″tĭ-koid) 1. any of the group of corticosteroids predominantly involved in carbohydrate metabolism, and also in fat and protein metabolism and many other activities (e.g., alteration of connective tissue response to injury and inhibition of inflammatory and allergic reactions); some also exhibit varying degrees of mineralocorticoid activity. In man, the most important glucocorticoids are cortisol (hydrocortisone) and cortisone. 2. of, pertaining to, or resembling a glucocorticoid.

glucofuranose (-fūr″ah-nōs) a form of glucose in which carbon atoms 1 and 4 are bridged by an oxygen atom.

glucokinase (-ki′nās) an enzyme that in the presence of ATP catalyzes glucose to glucose 6-phosphate.

glucokinetic (-ki-net′ik) activating sugar so as to maintain the sugar level of the body.

gluconate (gloo′ko-nāt) a salt of gluconic acid, containing the $HOCH_2(CHOH)_5COO-$ radical.

gluconeogenesis (gloo″ko-ne″o-jen′ĭ-sis) the synthesis of glucose by the liver and kidney from noncarbohydrate sources, such as amino and fatty acids.

gluconic acid (gloo-kon′ik) $CH_2OH(CHOH)_4-COOH$, an intermediate product formed in biosynthesis of pentoses.

glucophore (gloo′ko-for) the group of atoms in a molecule which gives the compound a sweet taste.

glucopyranose (-pi′rah-nōs) a form of glucose in

which carbon atoms 1 and 5 are bridged by an oxygen atom.

glucoregulation (-reg″ūl-a′shin) regulation of glucose metabolism.

glucosamine (-sam′in) an amino derivative of glucose, $C_6H_{13}NO_5$, occurring in many polysaccharides.

glucosan (gloo′ko-san) a polymer yielding glucose on hydrolysis.

glucose (gloo′kōs) D-glucose, a monosaccharide (hexose), $C_6H_{12}O_6$, also known as *dextrose*, found in certain foodstuffs, especially fruits. It is the end product of carbohydrate metabolism, and is the chief source of energy for living organisms, its utilization being controlled by insulin. Excess glucose is converted to glycogen and stored in the liver and muscles for use as needed, and, beyond that, is converted to fat and stored as adipose tissue. Glucose appears in the urine in diabetes mellitus. **liquid g.,** a thick syrupy, sweet liquid, consisting chiefly of dextrose, with dextrins, maltose, and water, obtained by incomplete hydrolysis of starch; used as a flavoring agent, as a food, and in the treatment of dehydration. **g. 1-phosphate,** an intermediate in carbohydrate metabolism. **g. 6-phosphate,** an intermediate in carbohydrate metabolism.

glucosidase (gloo-kōs′ĭ-dās) an enzyme of the hydrolase class that splits a glucoside, occurring as α-, β-, and α-1,3-glucosidase; α-g. (maltase) occurs in the intestinal juice, and β-g. (cellobiase) in the kidney, liver, and intestinal mucosa.

glucoside (gloo′kos-īd) a glycoside in which the sugar constituent is glucose.

glucuronic acid (gloo-ku-ron′ik) a uronic acid formed by oxidation of C-6 of glucose to a carboxy group; it occurs in proteoglycans (mucopolysaccharides) and is conjugated to many poisons and drugs by the liver, forming glucuronides, which are excreted in the urine.

β-**glucuronidase** (gloo″ku-ron′ĭ-dās) an enzyme that attacks glycosidic linkages in natural and synthetic glucuronides and has been implicated in estrogen metabolism and cell division; occurs in the spleen, liver, and endocrine glands.

glucuronide (gloo-kūr′on-īd) any glycosidic compound of glucuronic acid; glucuronides, which are generally inactive, constitute the major proportion of metabolites of many phenols, alcohols, and carboxylic acids.

glutamate (glōōt′ah-māt) a salt of glutamic acid; in biochemistry, the term is often used interchangeably with glutamic acid.

glutamic acid (gloo-tam′ik) a crystalline dibasic nonessential amino acid, $C_5H_9NO_4$, widely distributed in proteins, and thought to be a neurotransmitter that inhibits neural excitation in the central nervous system; its hydrochloride salt is used as a gastric acidifier. The monosodium salt of L-glutamic acid (*sodium glutamate*) is used in treating encephalopathies associated with hepatic disease, and to enhance the flavor of foods and tobacco.

glutaminase (gloo-tam′ĭ-nās) an enzyme that catalyzes the splitting of glutamine into glutamic acid and ammonia.

glutamine (glōōt′ah-mēn) the monoamide of glutamic acid, $C_5H_{10}N_2O_3$, an amino acid occurring in proteins; it is an important carrier of urinary ammonia and is broken down in the kidney by the enzyme glutaminase.

glutaraldehyde (glōōt″ah-ral′dĕ-hīd) a disinfectant, $C_5H_8O_2$, used in aqueous solution for sterilization of non-heat–resistant equipment; also used topically as an anhidrotic and as a tissue fixative for light and electron microscopy.

glutaric acid (gloo-tar′ik) pentanedioic acid, $C_5H_8O_4$, an intermediate in the metabolism of tryptophan and lysine.

glutathione (glōōt″ah-thi′ōn) reduced glutathione (GSH), a tripeptide of glutamic acid, cysteine, and glycine, which serves as a reducing agent in many biochemical reactions being converted to oxidized glutathione (GSSG) in which the cysteine residues of two glutathione molecules are connected by a disulfide bridge. Reduced glutathione is important in protecting erythrocytes from oxidation and hemolysis; deficiency causes sensitivity to oxidant drugs.

gluteal (glōōt′e-il) pertaining to the buttocks.

gluten (glōōt′n) the protein of wheat and other grains that gives to the dough its tough elastic character.

glutethimide (gloo-teth′ĭ-mīd) a hypnotic and sedative, $C_{13}H_{15}NO_2$.

glutinous (glōōt′in-is) adhesive; sticky.

Gly glycine.

glycan (gli′kan) polysaccharide.

glycemia (gli-sēm′e-ah) the presence of glucose in the blood.

glyceraldehyde (glis″er-al′dĕ-hīd) a compound, glyceric aldehyde, $CH_2OHCHOHCHO$, formed by the oxidation of glycerol.

glyceric acid (glĭ-sēr′ik) $CH_2OH \cdot CHOH \cdot COOH$, an intermediate product in the transformation in the body of carbohydrate to lactic acid, formed by oxidation of glycerol.

glyceride (glis′er-īd) an organic acid ester of glycerol, designated, according to the number of ester linkages, as mono-, di-, or triglyceride.

glycerin (glis′er-in) glycerol; a clear, colorless, syrupy liquid, $C_3H_8O_3$, used as a humectant and solvent for drugs; it is a trihydric sugar alcohol, being the alcoholic component of fats.

glycerol (glis′er-ol) a water- and alcohol-soluble trihydric sugar alcohol, $CH_2OH \cdot CHOH \cdot CH_2OH$, being the alcoholic component of the fats. It is an intermediate in the metabolism of fatty acids and serves as a phosphate acceptor. Pharmaceutical preparations are called *glycerin*.

glycerolize (glis′er-ol-īz) to treat with or preserve in glycerol, as in the exposure of red blood cells to glycerol solution so that glycerol diffuses into the cells before they are frozen for preservation.

glyceryl (glis′er-il) the mono-, di-, or trivalent radical formed by the removal of hydrogen from one, two, or three of the hydroxy groups of glycerol. **g. monostearate,** an emulsifying agent. **g. trinitrate,** nitroglycerin.

glycine (gli′sēn) a nonessential amino acid, H_2-NCH_2COOH, occurring as a constituent of proteins and functioning as an inhibitory neurotransmitter in the central nervous system; used as a gastric antacid and dietary supplement, and in the treatment of various myopathies.

glycocalyx (gli″ko-kal′iks) the glycoprotein-polysaccharide covering that surrounds many cells.

glycocholate (-ko′lāt) a salt of glycocholic acid.

glycocholic acid (gli″ko-ko′lik) cholyglycine.

glycogen (gli′kah-jen) a polysaccharide, the chief carbohydrate storage material in animals, formed by and largely stored in the liver and to a lesser extent in muscles; it is depolymerized to glucose and liberated as needed. **glycogen′ic,** adj.

glycogenase (-jĭ-nās″) an enzyme which splits glycogen into dextrin and maltose.

glycogenesis (gli″ko-jen′ĭ-sis) the conversion of glucose to glycogen for storage in the liver. **glycogenet′ic,** adj.

glycogenolysis (-jĭ-nol′ĭ-sis) the splitting up of glycogen in the liver, yielding glucose. **glycogenolyt′ic,** adj.

glycogenosis (-jĭ-no′sis), pl. *glycogeno′ses.* glycogen storage disease.

glycogeusia (gli″ko-gūs′e-ah) a sweet taste in the mouth.

glycohemoglobin (-he″mo-glo′bin) glycosylated hemoglobin.

glycol (gli′kol) any of a group of aliphatic dihydric alcohols, having marked hygroscopic properties and useful as solvents and plasticizers.

glycolic acid (gli-kol′ik) $CH_2OH \cdot COOH$, formed by electrolytic reduction of oxalic acid or by the action of sodium hydroxide on monochloroacetic acid; used in pH control. Also produced in the body as an intermediate product in the conversion of serine to glycine.

glycolipid (gli″ko-lip′id) a lipid containing carbohydrate groups, usually galactose but also glucose, inositol, or others; the glycolipids include the cerebrosides.

glycolysis (gli-kol′ĭ-sis) the anaerobic enzymatic conversion of glucose to the simpler compounds lactate or pyruvate, resulting in energy stored in the form of ATP, as occurs in muscle. **glycolyt′ic,** adj.

glyconeogenesis (gli″ko-ne″o-jen′ĭ-sis) gluconeogenesis.

glycopenia (-pe′ne-ah) a deficiency of sugar in the tissues.

glycopeptide (-pep′tīd) any of a class of peptides that contain carbohydrates, including those that contain amino sugars.

glycophilia (-fil′e-ah) a condition in which a small amount of glucose produces hyperglycemia.

glycophorin (-for′in) a protein that projects through the thickness of the cell membrane of erythrocytes; it is attached to oligosaccharides at the outer cell membrane surface and to contractile proteins (spectrin and actin) at the cytoplasmic surface.

glycoprotein (-prōt′e-in) any of a class of conjugated proteins consisting of a compound of protein with a carbohydrate group.

glycopyrrolate (-pir′ol-āt) an anticholinergic, $C_{19}H_{28}BrNO_3$, used in gastrointestinal disorders.

glycorrhea (-re′ah) any sugary discharge from the body.

glycosaminoglycan (gli″kos-ah-me″no-gli′kan) any of the carbohydrates containing amino sugars occurring in proteoglycans, e.g., hyaluronic acid or chondroitin sulfate.

glycosecretory (-se-krēt′er-e) concerned in secretion of glycogen.

glycosemia (-sēm′e-ah) glycemia.

glycosialia (-si-a′le-ah) sugar in the saliva.

glycosialorrhea (-si″ah-lo-re′ah) excessive flow of saliva containing glucose.

glycosidase (gli-ko′sĭ-dās) any hydrolytic enzyme acting on glycosyl compounds.

glycoside (gli′kah-sīd) any compound containing a carbohydrate molecule (sugar), particularly any such natural product in plants, convertible, by hydrolytic cleavage, into a sugar and a nonsugar component (aglycone), and named specifically for the sugar contained, as glucoside (glucose), pentoside (pentose), fructoside (fructose), etc. **cardiac g.,** any of a group of glycosides occurring in certain plants (e.g., *Digitalis, Strophanthus, Urginea*), acting on the contractile force of cardiac muscle.

glycosphingolipid (gli″ko-sfing″go-lip′id) a sphingolipid containing the sugar glucose or galactose.

glycostatic (-stat′ik) tending to maintain a constant sugar level.

glycosuria (-ōs-ūr′e-ah) the presence of glucose in the urine. **renal g.,** that due to inherited inability of the renal tubules to reabsorb glucose completely.

glycosyl (gli′ko-sil) a radical derived from a carbohydrate.

glycosylation (gli″ko-sī-la′shin) the formation of linkages with glycosyl groups.

glycotropic (gli″ko-trop′ik) having an affinity for sugar; causing hyperglycemia.

glycuresis (gli″kūr-e′sis) the normal increase in glucose content of the urine which follows an ordinary carbohydrate meal.

glycyrrhiza (glis″ĭ-ri′zah) licorice; the dried rhizome and roots of the legume *Glycyrrhiza glabra*, used as a flavored vehicle for drugs.

glyoxylic acid (gli-ok-sil′ik) $CHO \cdot COOH$, formed in the oxidative deamination of glycine.

gm gram.

GMP guanosine monophosphate.

gnat (nat) a small dipterous insect. In Great Britain the term is applied to mosquitoes; in America to insects smaller than mosquitoes.

gnath(o)- word element [Gr.], *jaw.*

gnathion (na′the-on) the most outward and everted point on the profile curvature of the chin.

gnathitis (na-thīt′is) inflammation of the jaw.

gnathodynamometer (-di″nah-mom′it-er) an instrument for measuring the force exerted in closing the jaws.

gnathology (nah-thol′ah-je) a science dealing with the masticatory apparatus as a whole, including morphology, anatomy, histology, physiology, pathology, and therapeutics. **gnatholog′ic,** adj.

gnathoschisis (nah-thos′kĭ-sis) congenital cleft of the upper jaw, as in cleft palate.

Gnathostoma (nah-thos′tah-mah) a genus of nematodes parasitic in cats, swine, cattle, and sometimes man.

gnathostomiasis (nah-thos″to-mi′ah-sis) infection with the nematode *Gnathostoma spinigerum,* acquired from eating undercooked fish infected with the larvae.

gnosia (no′se-ah) the faculty of perceiving and recognizing. **gnos′tic,** adj.

gnotobiology (nōt″ah-bi-ol′ah-je) gnotobiotics.

gnotobiota (-bi-ōt′ah) the specifically and entirely known microfauna and microflora of a specially reared laboratory animal.

gnotobiote (-bi′ōt) a specially reared laboratory animal whose microflora and microfauna are specifically known in their entirety. **gnotobiot′ic,** adj.

Gn-RH gonadotropin-releasing hormone.

goiter (goit′er) enlargement of the thyroid gland, causing a swelling in the front part of the neck. **goi′trous,** adj. **aberrant g.,** goiter of a supernumerary thyroid gland. **adenomatous g.,** that caused by adenoma or multiple colloid nodules of the thyroid gland. **Basedow's g.,** a colloid goiter which has become hyperfunctioning after administration of iodine. **colloid g.,** a large, soft thyroid gland with distended spaces filled with colloid. **diving g.,** a movable goiter, located sometimes above and sometimes below the sternal notch. **exophthalmic g.,** goiter characterized by exophthalmos; see *Graves' disease.* **fibrous g.,** goiter in which the capsule and the stroma of the thyroid gland are hyperplastic. **follicular g.,** parenchymatous g. **intrathoracic g.,** one in which a portion of the enlarged gland is in the thoracic cavity. **iodide g.,** that occurring in reaction to iodides at high concentrations, due to inhibition of iodide organification. **lingual g.,** enlargement of the upper end of the thyroglossal duct, forming a tumor at the posterior part of the dorsum of the tongue. **lymphadenoid g.,** struma lymphomatosa. **nodular g.,** goiter with circumscribed nodules within the gland. **nontoxic g.,** that occurring sporadically and not associated with hyperthyroidism or hypothyroidism. **parenchymatous g.,** one marked by increase in follicles and proliferation of epithelium. **simple g.,** simple hyperplasia of the thyroid gland. **suffocative g.,** one which causes dyspnea by pressure. **toxic g.,** Graves' disease. **wandering g.,** diving g.

goitrin (goi′trin) a goitrogenic substance isolated from rutabagas and turnips.

gold (gōld) chemical element (*see table*), at. no. 79, symbol Au; gold compounds (all of which are poisonous) are used in medicine, chiefly in treating arthritis. **g.-198,** a radioisotope of gold having a half life of 2.7 days and emitting gamma and beta radiation. Symbol ^{198}Au. **cohesive g.,** chemically pure gold that forms a solid mass when properly condensed into a tooth cavity. **g. sodium thiomalate,** $C_4H_3Au\text{-}Na_2O_4S\cdot H_2O$; used in treatment of rheumatoid arthritis and nondisseminated lupus erythematosus. **g. thioglucose,** aurothioglucose.

gomitoli (go-mit′o-li) a network of capillaries in the upper infundibular stem (of the hypothalamus) that surround terminal arterioles of the superior hypophyseal arteries and that lead into portal veins to the adenohypophysis.

gomphosis (gom-fo′sis) a type of fibrous joint in which a conical process is inserted into a socket-like portion.

gon- word element [Gr.], 1. *seed; semen.* 2. *knee.*

gonad (go′nad, gon′ad) a gamete-producing gland; an ovary or testis. **gonad′al, gonad′ial,** adj. **indifferent g.,** the sexually undifferentiated gonad of the early embryo.

gonadorelin (go″nad-o-rel′in) gonadotropin releasing hormone.

gonadotrope (go-nad′ah-trōp) a basophilic cell of the anterior pituitary specialized to secrete follicle-stimulating hormone or luteinizing hormone.

gonadotroph (go-nad′ah-trōf) gonadotrope.

gonadotrophic (gon″ah-do-trōf′ik) gonadotropic.

gonadotropic (-trop′ik) stimulating the gonads; applied to hormones of the anterior pituitary which influence the gonads.

gonadotropin (-trōp′in) any hormone that stimulates the gonads. Two such hormones are secreted by the anterior pituitary: follicle-stimulating hormone and luteinizing hormone, both of which are active, but with differing effects, in both sexes. **chorionic g.,** a gonad-stimulating principle produced by the cytotrophoblastic cells of the placenta and excreted through the kidneys; used to treat certain cases of cryptorchidism and male hypogonadism, and to induce ovulation and pregnancy in certain infertile, anovulatory women.

gonagra (go-nag′rah) gout in the knee.

gonalgia (go-nal′je-ah) pain in the knee.

gonarthritis (gon″ar-thrīt′is) inflammation of the knee joint.

gonarthrocace (-ar-throk′ah-se) tuberculous arthritis of the knee.

gonecystis (gon″e-sis′tis) a seminal vesicle.

gonecystitis (-sis-tīt′is) inflammation of a seminal vesicle.

gonecystopyosis (-sis″to-pi-o′sis) suppuration in a seminal vesicle.

gonidium (go-nid′e-um), pl. *gonid′ia* [Gr.] 1. the algal component of the thallus of a lichen. 2. a motile reproductive unit of certain nitrogen-fixing bacteria.

goniometer (go″ne-om′it-er) an instrument for measuring angles. **finger g.,** one for measuring the limits of flexion and extension of the interphalangeal joints of the fingers.

gonion (go′ne-on), pl. *go′nia* [Gr.] the most inferior, posterior, and lateral point on the external angle of the mandible. **go′nial,** adj.

goniopuncture (go″ne-o-punk′cher) insertion of a knife blade through the clear cornea, just within the limbus, across the anterior chamber of the eye and through the opposite corneoscleral wall, in treatment of glaucoma.

gonioscope (go′ne-ah-skōp″) an optical instrument for examining the anterior chamber of the eye and for demonstrating ocular motility and rotation.

goniotomy (-ot′ah-me) an operation for glaucoma; it consists in opening Schlemm's canal under direct vision.

gono- word element [Gr.], *seed; semen.*

gonocele (gon′ah-sēl) spermatocele.

gonococcemia (gon″ah-kok-sēm′e-ah) the presence of gonococci in the blood.

gonococcus (-kok′us), pl. *gonococ′ci* [L.] an individual of the species *Neisseria gonorrhoeae*, the etiologic agent of gonorrhea. **gonococ′cal, gonococ′cic,** adj.

gonocyte (gon′ah-sīt) the primitive reproductive cell of the embryo.

gonophore (-fōr) an accessory generative organ, such as the oviduct.

gonorrhea (gon″ah-re′ah) infection with *Neisseria gonorrhoeae*, most often transmitted venereally, marked in males by urethritis with pain and purulent discharge; commonly asymptomatic in females, but may extend to produce salpingitis, oophoritis, tubo-ovarian abscess, and peritonitis. Bacteremia may occur in both sexes, causing skin lesions, arthritis, and rarely meningitis or endocarditis. **gonorrhe′al,** adj.

Gonyaulax (gon″e-aw′laks) a genus of dinoflagellates found in fresh, salt, or brackish waters, having yellow to brown chromatophores; it includes *G. catanel′la,* a poisonous species, which helps to form the destructive red tide in the ocean; see also under *poison.*

gonycampsis (gon″ĭ-kamp′sis) abnormal curvature of the knee.

gonyocele (gon′e-o-sēl″) synovitis or tuberculous arthritis of the knee.

gonyoncus (gon″e-ong′kus) tumor of the knee.

gorget (gor′jet) a wide-grooved lithotome director.

GOT glutamic-oxaloacetic transaminase; see *aspartate aminotransferase.*

gouge (gowj) a hollow chisel for cutting and removing bone.

goundou (gōōn′doo) a sequel of yaws and endemic syphilis, marked by headache, purulent nasal discharge, and formation of bony exostoses at the side of the nose.

gout (gowt) a group of disorders of purine and pyrimidine metabolism, characterized by typhi causing recurrent paroxysmal attacks of acute inflammatory arthritis usually affecting a single peripheral joint, usually responsive to colchicine, and usually followed by complete remission; hyperuricemia and uric acid urolithiasis are also present in fully developed cases. **gout′y,** adj. **latent g., masked g.,** lithemia without the typical features of gout. **rheumatic g.,** rheumatoid arthritis.

G.P. general practitioner; general paresis (see *dementia paralytica*).

G6PD glucose-6-phosphate dehydrogenase.

GPT glutamic-pyruvic transaminase; see *alanine aminotransferase.*

gr. grain.

gradient (gra′de-int) rate of increase or decrease of a variable value, or its representative curve.

graduated (graj′oo-āt″id) marked by a succession of lines, steps, or degrees.

graft (graft) any tissue or organ for implantation or transplantation; to implant or transplant such tissue. See also *flap.* **accordion g.,** a full-thickness graft in which slits have been made so that it may be stretched to cover a larger area. **autodermic g., autoepidermic g.,** a skin graft taken from the patient's own body. **avascular g.,** a graft of tissue in which not even transient vascularization is achieved. **Blair-Brown g.,** a split-skin graft of intermediate thickness. **bone g.,** a piece of bone used to take the place of a removed bone or bony defect. **cable g.,** a nerve graft made up of several sections of nerve in the manner of a cable. **delayed g.,** a skin graft sutured back into its bed and subsequently shifted to a new recipient site. **dermal g., dermic g.,** skin from which epidermis and subcutaneous fat have been removed; used instead of fascia in various plastic procedures. **epidermic g.,** a piece of epidermis implanted on a raw surface. **fascia g.,** one taken from the fascia lata or the lumbar fascia. **fascicular g.,** a nerve graft in which bundles of nerve fibers are approximated and sutured separately. **full-thickness g.,** a skin graft consisting of the full thickness of the skin, with little or none of the subcutaneous tissue. **heterodermic g.,** a skin graft taken from a donor of another species. **heterologous g., heteroplastic g.,** xenograft. **homologous g., homoplastic g.,** allograft. **isologous g., isoplastic g.,** isograft. **Krause-Wolfe g.,** full-thickness g. **lamellar g.,** replacement of the superficial layers of an opaque cornea by a thin layer of clear cornea from a donor eye. **nerve g.,** replacement of an area of defective nerve with a segment from a sound one. **omental g's,** free or attached segments of omentum used to cover suture lines following gastrointestinal or colonic surgery. **pedicle g.,** see under *flap.* **penetrating g.,** a full-thickness corneal transplant. **periosteal g.,** a piece of periosteum to cover a denuded bone. **pinch g.,** a piece of skin graft about ¼ inch in diameter, obtained by elevating the skin with a needle and slicing it off with a knife. **Reverdin g.,** epidermic g. **sieve g.,** a skin graft from which tiny circular islands of skin are removed so that a larger denuded area can be covered, the sievelike portion being placed over one area, and the individual islands over surrounding or other denuded areas. **split-skin g.,** a skin graft consisting of only a portion of the skin thickness. **thick-split g.,** a skin graft cut in pieces, often including about two thirds of the full thickness of the skin. **Thiersch's g.,** Ollier-Thiersch g. **white g.,** avascular g.

grain (grān) 1. a seed, especially of a cereal plant. 2. the twentieth part of a scruple: 0.065 gm.; abbreviated gr.

gram (gram) the basic unit of mass (weight) of

the metric system, being the equivalent of 15.432 grains; abbreviated g. or gm.

-gram word element [Gr.], *written; recorded.*

gram-equivalent (gram″e-kwiv′ah-lint) see *chemical equivalent.*

gramicidin (gram″ĭ-si′din) gramicidin D; an antibacterial polypeptide produced by *Bacillus brevis* and one of the two main components of tyrothricin. *Gramicidin S* is a closely related substance produced by a strain of *B. brevis.*

graminivorous (-niv′er-is) eating or subsisting on cereal grains.

gram-molecule (gram-mol″ĭ-kūl) see *mole* (3).

gram-negative (-neg′ah-tiv) losing the stain or decolorized by alcohol in Gram's method of staining, characteristic of bacteria having a cell wall surface more complex in chemical composition than the gram-positive bacteria.

gram-positive (-poz′it-iv) retaining the stain or resisting decolorization by alcohol in Gram's method of staining, a primary characteristic of bacteria whose cell wall is composed of peptidoglycan and teichoic acid.

grana (gra′nah) dense green, chlorophyll-containing bodies in chloroplasts of plant cells.

grandiose (gran′dĭ-ōs) in psychiatry, pertaining to exaggerated belief or claims of one's importance or identity, often manifested by delusions of great wealth, power, or fame.

grand mal (grahn mal) [Fr.] see under *epilepsy.*

granulatio (gran″la′she-o), pl. *granulatio′nes* [L.] a granule, or granular mass.

granulation (-a′shin) 1. the division of a hard substance into small particles. 2. the formation in wounds of small, rounded masses of tissue during healing; also the mass so formed. **arachnoid g's,** enlarged arachnoid villi projecting into the venous sinuses and creating slight depressions on the inner surface of the cranium. **exuberant g's,** excessive proliferation of granulation tissue in healing wounds.

granule (gran′ūl) 1. a small particle or grain. 2. a small pill made from sucrose. **acidophil g's,** granules staining with acid dyes. **acrosomal g.,** a large globule contained within a membrane-bounded acrosomal vesicle, which enlarges further to become the cap of the acrosome of a spermatozoon. **alpha g's,** 1. oval granules found in blood platelets; they are lysosomes containing acid phosphatase. 2. large granules in the alpha cells of the islets of Langerhans; they secrete glucagon. 3. acidophilic granules in the alpha cells of the adenohypophysis. **amphophil g's,** those that stain with both acid and basic dyes. **azure g's, azurophil g's,** those staining easily with azure dyes; they are coarse reddish granules seen in many lymphocytes. **basal g.,** see under *body.* **basophil g's,** granules staining with basic dyes, such as those of the beta cells of the adenohypophysis. **beta g's,** 1. granules in the beta cells of the islets of Langerhans; they secrete insulin. 2. basophilic granules in the beta cells of the adenohypophysis. **elementary g's,** hemoconia. **eosinophil g's,** those staining with eosin; see *alpha g's* (1). **iodophil g's,** granules staining brown with iodine, seen in polymorphonuclear leukocytes in

various acute infectious diseases. **keratohyalin g's,** irregularly shaped granules, representing deposits of keratohyalin on tonofibrils in the granular layer of the epidermis. **Langerhans' g's,** peculiar rod-shaped, membrane-bound structures with a central linear density, found in the Langerhans cells of the epidermis. **membrane-coating g's,** granules in the uppermost cells of the prickle-cell layer of the epidermis, which may deposit dense material on the inner aspect of the cell membrane; they contain the enzyme acid phosphatase, and may be involved in the desquamation of the horny layer of the epidermis. **metachromatic g's,** granules present in many bacterial cells, having an avidity for basic dyes and causing irregular staining of the cell. **Nissl g's,** see under *body.* **oxyphil g's,** acidophil g's. **pigment g's,** small masses of coloring matter in pigment cells. **proacrosomal g.,** one of the small, dense bodies found inside one of the vacuoles of the Golgi body, which fuse to form an acrosomal granule. **Schüffner's g's,** see under *dot.* **seminal g's,** the small granular bodies in the spermatic fluid. **specific atrial g's,** membrane-bound spherical granules with a dense homogeneous interior concentrated in the core of sarcoplasm of the atrial cardiac muscle, extending in either direction from the poles of the nucleus, usually near the Golgi complex; they also may be in limited numbers in other regions of the cell.

granuloadipose (gran″ūl-o-ad′ĭ-pōs) showing fatty degeneration containing granules of fat.

granuloblast (gran″ūl-o-blast″) myeloblast.

granuloblastosis (gran″ūl-o-blas-to′sis) avian leukosis with increase in immature, granular blood cells in the circulating blood; there may be infiltration of the liver and spleen.

granulocyte (gran′ūl-o-sīt″) any cell containing granules, especially a granular leukocyte. **granulocyt′ic,** adj. **band-form g.,** band cell.

granulocytopenia (-sīt″-o-pe′ne-ah) agranulocytosis.

granulocytopoiesis (-sīt″o-poi-e′sis) the production of granulocytes. **granulocytopoiet′ic,** adj.

granulocytosis (-si-to′sis) an excess of granulocytes in the blood.

granuloma (gran″ūl-o′mah) a tumor-like mass or nodule of granulation tissue, with actively growing fibroblasts and capillary buds, consisting of a collection of modified macrophages resembling epithelial cells surrounded by a rim of mononuclear cells, chiefly lymphocytes, and sometimes a center of giant multinucleate cells; it is due to a chronic inflammatory process associated with infectious disease or invasion by a foreign body. **apical g.,** modified granulation tissue containing elements of chronic inflammation located adjacent to the root apex of a tooth with infected necrotic pulp. **benign g. of thyroid,** chronic inflammation of the thyroid gland, converting it into a bulky tumor which later becomes extremely hard. **coccidioidal g.,** coccidioidomycosis. **eosinophilic g.,** 1. a form of xanthomatosis marked by the presence of rarefactions of cysts in one or more bones, sometimes associated with eosinophilia. 2. a disorder similar to eosinophilic gastroenteritis, characterized by localized nodular or pedunculated lesions of the submucosa and muscle walls, especially of the pyloric area of the stomach, caused by infiltration of eosinophils, but without peripheral eosinophilia and allergic symptoms. 3. anisakiasis. **g. fissura′tum,** a firm, reddish, fissured, fibrotic granuloma of the gum and buccal mucosa, occurring on an edentulous alveolar ridge between the ridge and cheek. **infectious g.,** one due to a specific microorganism, as the tubercle bacilli. **g. inguina′le,** a granulomatous venereal disease, usually seen in dark-skinned people, marked by purulent ulceration of the external genitals, caused by *Calymmatobacterium granulomatis.* **lethal midline g.,** a rare, destructive necrotizing granuloma that results in destruction of the midface and invariably in death. It is nearly always preceded by longstanding nonspecific inflammation of the nose or nasal sinuses, with purulent, often bloody discharge. **lipoid g.,** one containing lipoid cells; xanthoma. **lipophagic g.,** a granuloma attended by the loss of subcutaneous fat. **midline g.,** lethal midline g. **paracoccidioidal g.,** paracoccidioidomycosis. **peripheral giant cell reparative g.,** a pedunculated or sessile lesion of the gingivae or alveolar ridge, apparently rising from the periodontal ligament or mucoperiosteum, and usually due to trauma. **pyogenic g.,** a benign, solitary nodule resembling granulation tissue, found anywhere on the body, commonly intraorally, usually at the site of trauma as a response of the tissues to a nonspecific infection. **swimming pool g.,** a granulomatous lesion that complicates injuries sustained in swimming pools, attributed to *Mycobacterium balnei;* it tends to heal spontaneously in a few months or years. **trichophytic g.,** a form of tinea corporis, occurring chiefly on the lower legs, due to *Trichophyton* infecting hairs at the site of involvement, marked by raised, circumscribed, rather boggy granulomas, disseminated or arranged in chains; the lesions are slowly absorbed, or undergo necrosis, leaving depressed scars. **g. tro′picum,** yaws.

granulomatosis (gran″ūl-o″mah-to′sis) the formation of multiple granulomas. **g. sidero′tica,** a condition in which brownish nodules are seen in the enlarged spleen. **Wegener's g.,** a progressive disease, with granulomatous lesions of the respiratory tract, focal necrotizing arteriolitis and, finally, widespread inflammation of all organs of the body.

granulomere (gran′ūl-o-mēr″) the center portion of a platelet in a dry, stained blood smear, apparently filled with fine, red granules.

granulopenia (gran″ūl-o-pe′ne-ah) agranulocytosis.

granuloplastic (gran′ūl-o-plas″tik) forming granules.

granulopoiesis (gran″ūl-o-poi-e′sis) the formation of granulocytes. **granulopoiet′ic,** adj.

granulosa (gran″ūl-o′sah) pertaining to cells of the cumulus oophorus.

granulosis (gran″ūl-o′sis) the formation of granules. **g. r′ubra na′si,** redness and marked

sweating confined to the nose and surrounding area of the face, with red papules and sometimes many small vesicles, seen most often in children, and usually clearing up at puberty.

granum (gra′num) [L.] grain.

graph (graf) a diagram or curve representing varying relationships between sets of data. Often used as a word ending denoting a recording instrument.

-graphy word element [Gr.], *writing or recording; a method of recording.* **-graph′ic,** adj.

grattage (grah-tahzh′) [Fr.] removal of granulations by scraping.

gravedo (grah-ve′do) head cold; nasal catarrh.

gravel (grav′l) calculi occurring in small particles.

gravid (grav′id) pregnant.

gravida (grav′ĭ-dah) a pregnant woman; called *g. I* (*primigravida*) during the first pregnancy, *g. II* (*secundigravida*) during the second, and so on.

gravidocardiac (grav″ĭ-do-kar′de-ak) pertaining to heart disease in pregnancy.

gravimetric (grav″ĭ-mĕ′trik) pertaining to measurement by weight; performed by weight, as the gravimetric method of drug assay.

gravity (grav′it-e) weight; tendency toward the center of the earth. **specific g.,** the weight of a substance compared with that of another taken as a standard.

gray (gra) the SI unit of absorbed radiation dose, defined as the transfer of 1 joule of energy per kilogram of absorbing material (1 J/kg); 1 gray equals 100 rads.

grease (grēs) an inflammatory swelling in a horse's leg, with formation of cracks in the skin and excretion of oily matter.

green (grēn) 1. the color of grass or of an emerald. 2. a green dye. **brilliant g.,** a basic dye having powerful bacteriostatic properties for gram-positive organisms; used topically as an anesthetic. **indocyanine g.,** a tricarbocyanine dye used intravenously in determination of blood volume, cardiac output, and hepatic function. **malachite g.,** a triphenylmethane dye used as a stain for bacteria and as an antiseptic for wounds.

Gregarina (greg″ah-ri′nah) a genus of sporozoa, species of which are parasitic in insects.

GRH growth hormone releasing hormone.

grid (grid) 1. a grating; in radiology, a device consisting of a series of narrow lead strips closely spaced on their edges and separated by spacers of low density material; used to reduce the amount of scattered radiation reaching the x-ray film. 2. a chart with horizontal and perpendicular lines for plotting curves. **baby g.,** a direct-reading chart on infant growth. **Wetzel g.,** a direct-reading chart for evaluating physical fitness in terms of body build, developmental level, and basal metabolism.

grip (grip) grippe. **devil's g.,** epidemic pleurodynia.

grippe (grip) influenza.

griseofulvin (gris″e-o-ful′vin) an antibiotic, $C_{17}H_{17}ClO_6$, isolated from *Penicillium griseoful-*

vum and other *Penicillium* species; used as a fungistatic in dermatophytoses.

groove (grōōv) a narrow, linear hollow or depression. **branchial g.**, an external furrow lined with ectoderm, occurring in the embryo between two branchial arches. **Harrison's g.**, a horizontal groove along the lower border of the thorax corresponding to the costal insertion of the diaphragm; seen in advanced rickets in children. **medullary g., neural g.**, that formed by beginning invagination of the neural plate of the embryo to form the neural tube.

group (grōōp) 1. an assemblage of objects having certain things in common. 2. a number of atoms forming a recognizable and usually transferable portion of a molecule. **azo g.**, a bivalent chemical group composed of two nitrogen atoms, —N:N—. **blood g.**, see under *B*. **diagnosis-related g's**, groupings of diagnostic categories used as a basis for hospital payment schedules by Medicare and other third party payment plans. **encounter g.**, a sensitivity group in which the members strive to gain emotional rather than intellectual insight, with emphasis on the expression of interpersonal feelings in the group situation. **prosthetic g.**, 1. an organic radical, nonprotein in nature, which together with a protein carrier forms an enzyme. 2. a cofactor tightly bound to an enzyme, i.e., it is an integral part of the enzyme and not readily dissociated from it. 3. a cofactor that may reversibly dissociate from the protein component of an enzyme; a coenzyme. **sensitivity g., sensitivity training g., T g., training g.**, a nonclinical group not intended for persons with severe emotional problems, which, in an effort to develop the assets of leadership, management, counseling, or other roles, focuses on self-awareness and understanding and on interpersonal interactions.

group-transfer (grōōp'trans'fer) denoting a chemical reaction (excluding oxidation and reduction) in which molecules exchange functional groups, a process catalyzed by enzymes called transferases.

growth (grōth) 1. a normal process of increase in size of an organism as a result of accretion of tissue similar to that originally present. 2. an abnormal formation, such as a tumor. 3. the proliferation of cells, as in a bacterial culture. **appositional g.**, growth by addition at the periphery of a particular part. **interstitial g.**, that occurring in the interior of structures already formed. **new g.**, neoplasm.

grumous (groo'mis) lumpy or clotted.

gryposis (grĭ-po'sis) abnormal curvature, as of the nails.

GSH reduced glutathione.

GSSG oxidized glutathione.

gt. [L.] *gutta* (drop).

GTP guanosine triphosphate.

gtt. [L.] *guttae* (drops).

GU genitourinary.

guaiac (gwi'ak) a resin from the wood of trees of the genus *Guajacum*, used as a reagent and formerly in treatment of rheumatism.

guaifenesin (gwi-fen'ĕ-sin) the glyceryl ester of guaiacol, $C_{10}H_{14}O_4$, used as an expectorant.

guaithylline (gwi'thĭ-lin) a bronchodilator and expectorant, $C_7H_8N_4O_2 \cdot C_{10}H_{14}O_4$.

guanase (gwan'ās) guanine deaminase.

guanethidine (gwan-eth'ĭ-dēn) an adrenergic blocking agent, $C_{10}H_{22}N_4$; the sulfate salt is used as an antihypertensive.

guanidinoacetic acid (gwan''ĭ-din''o-ah-sēt'ik) an intermediate product in the synthesis of creatine.

guanine (gwan'ēn) a purine base, $C_5H_5N_5O$, one of the fundamental components of nucleic acids (DNA and RNA).

guanosine (gwan'o-sēn) a nucleoside, guanine riboside, one of the major constituents of RNA. **g. monophosphate (GMP)**, a nucleotide important in metabolism and RNA synthesis. **g. triphosphate (GTP)**, an energy-rich compound involved in several metabolic reactions.

gubernaculum (goo''ber-nak'ŭl-um), pl. *guberna'cula* [L.] a guiding structure. **g. tes'tis**, the fetal ligament attached at one end to the lower end of the epididymis and testis and, at its other end, to the bottom of the scrotum; it is present during the descent of the testis into the scrotum and then atrophies.

guillotine (gil'ah-tēn) an instrument with a sliding blade for excising a tonsil or the uvula.

gullet (gul'it) the esophagus.

gum (gum) 1. mucilaginous excretion of various plants. 2. gingiva. **g. arabic**, acacia. **karaya g.**, the dried gummy exudation from *Sterculia* species, which becomes gelatinous when moisture is added; used as a bulk laxative. Because of its adhesive properties, products containing karaya gum are used as dental adhesives and as skin adhesives and protective skin barriers in the fitting and care of colostomy appliances and in other conditions in which there is a stoma. **sterculia g.**, karaya g.

gumboil (gum'boil) gingival abscess.

gumma (gum'ah) a soft, gummy tumor, such as that occurring in tertiary syphilis.

gurney (gur'ne) a wheeled cot used in hospitals.

gustation (gus-ta'shin) the act of tasting or the sense of taste. **gus'tatory**, adj.

gustin (gus'tin) a polypeptide present in saliva and containing two zinc atoms; it is necessary for normal development of the taste buds.

gut (gut) 1. the intestine or bowel. 2. the primitive digestive tube, consisting of the fore-, mid-, and hindgut. 3. catgut. **blind g.**, cecum. **head g.**, foregut. **postanal g.**, an extension of the embryonic gut caudal to the cloaca. **preoral g.**, Seessel's pouch. **primitive g.**, archenteron. **tail g.**, postanal g.

gutta (gut'ah), pl. *gut'tae* [L.] a drop.

gutta-percha (gut''ah-pur'chah) the coagulated latex of a number of trees of the family Sapotaceae; used as a dental cement and in splints.

guttat. [L.] *guttatim* (drop by drop).

guttatim (gah-tāt'im) [L.] drop by drop.

guttural (gut'er-il) pertaining to the throat.

Gy gray.

gymnastics (jim-nas'tiks) systematic muscular

exercise. **Swedish g.,** a system following a rigid pattern of movement, utilizing little equipment and stressing correct body posture.

Gymnodinium (jim''no-din′e-um) a genus of dinoflagellates, most species of which have many colored chromatophores, found in water; when present in great numbers, they help to form the destructive red tide in the ocean.

gyn-, gyne-, gyneco-, gyno- word element [Gr.], *woman*.

gynaeco- for words beginning thus, see those beginning *gyneco-*.

gynandrism (jin-an′drizm) 1. hermaphroditism. 2. female pseudohermaphroditism.

gynandroblastoma (jĭ-nan''dro-blas-to′mah) an ovarian tumor containing elements of both arrhenoblastoma and granulosa cell tumor.

gynandromorphism (jĭ-nan''drah-mor′fizm) the presence of chromosomes of both sexes in different tissues of the body, producing a mosaic of male and female sex characteristics. **gynandromorph′ous,** adj.

gynecic (jĭ-ne′sik) pertaining to women.

gynecogenic (jin''ĭ-ko-jen′ik) producing female characteristics.

gynecoid (jin′ĭ-koid) woman-like.

gynecology (jin''ĭ-kol′ah-je, gi''nĭ-) the branch of medicine dealing with diseases of the genital tract in women. **gynecolog′ic,** adj.

gynecomania (jin''ĭ-ko-ma′ne-ah) satyriasis.

gynecomastia (-mas''te-ah) excessive development of the male mammary glands, even to the functional state.

Gyne-Lotrimin (gi''nĭ-lo′trĭ-min) trademark for a preparation of clotrimazole.

gynephobia (jin''ĭ-fo′be-ah) morbid aversion to women.

gynogenesis (jin''o-jen′ĭ-sis) development of an egg that is stimulated by a sperm in the absence of any participation of the sperm nucleus.

gynoplastics (jin′o-plas''tiks) the plastic or reconstructive surgery of female reproductive organs. **gynoplas′tic,** adj.

gypsum (jip′sum) native calcium sulfate dihydrate; when calcined, it becomes *plaster of Paris*, much used in making permanent dressings for fractures and in dentistry for taking dental impressions.

gyration (ji-ra′shin) revolution about a fixed center.

gyre (ji′er) gyrus.

gyrectomy (ji-rek′tah-me) excision or resection of a cerebral gyrus, or a portion of the cerebral cortex.

Gyrencephala (ji''ren-sef′ah-lah) a group of higher mammals, including man, having a brain marked by convolutions.

gyri (ji′rī) plural of *gyrus*.

gyrose (ji′rōs) marked by curved lines or circles.

gyrospasm (ji′rah-spazm) rotatory spasm of the head.

gyrous (ji′ris) gyrose.

gyrus (ji′ris), pl. *gy′ri* [L.] one of the many well developed folds in the white medullary layer of the cerebral cortex, separated by fissures or sulci. **angular g.,** one continuous anteriorly with the supramarginal gyrus. **gy′ri bre′ves in′sulae,** the short, rostrally placed gyri on the surface of the insula. **Broca's g.,** inferior frontal gyrus. **central g., anterior,** precentral g. **central g., posterior,** postcentral g. **cerebral gyri,** the tortuous elevations (convolutions) on the surface of the cerebral hemisphere, caused by infolding of the cortex and separated by fissures or sulci. **cingulate g.,** an arch-shaped convolution situated just above the corpus callosum. **g. fornica′tus,** the marginal portion of the cerebral cortex on the medial aspect of the hemisphere, including the cingulate gyrus, parahippocampal gyrus, and others. **fusiform g.,** one on the inferior surface of the hemisphere between the inferior temporal and parahippocampal gyri, consisting of a lateral (*lateral occipitotemporal g.*) and a medial (*medial occipitotemporal g.*) part. **g. geni′culi,** a vestigial gyrus at the anterior end of the corpus callosum. **infracalcarine g.,** lingual g. **lingual g.,** one on the occipital lobe forming the inferior lip of the calcarine sulcus and, with the cuneus, the visual cortex. **g. lon′gus in′sulae,** the long, occipitally directed gyrus on the surface of the insula. **occipital g.,** any of the three (superior, middle, and inferior) gyri of the occipital lobe. **occipitotemporal g., lateral,** the lateral portion of the fusiform gyrus. **occipitotemporal g., medial,** the medial portion of the fusiform gyrus. **g. olfacto′rius media′lis** of Retzius, area subcallosa. **orbital gyri,** irregular gyri on the orbital surface of the frontal lobe. **parahippocampal g.,** one between the hippocampal and collateral sulci. **postcentral g.,** the convolution of the frontal lobe immediately behind the central sulcus; the primary sensory area of the cerebral cortex. **precentral g.,** the convolution of the frontal lobe immdiately in front of the central sulcus; the primary motor area of the cerebral cortex. **gy′ri profun′di ce′rebri,** the deeply placed cerebral gyri. **g. rec′tus,** one on the orbital surface of the frontal lobe. **supracallosal g.,** indusium griseum. **supramarginal g.,** that part of the inferior parietal convolution which curves around the upper end of the sylvian fissure. **temporal g.,** any of the gyri of the temporal lobe, including the inferior, middle, superior, and transverse temporal gyri; the more prominent of the latter (*anterior transverse temporal g.*) represents the cortical center for hearing. **gyri transiti′vi,** various small folds on the cerebral surface that are too inconstant to bear special names.

H

H chemical symbol, *hydrogen.*

H. [L.] *ho'ra* (hour); horizontal; hyperopia.

H⁺ symbol, *hydrogen ion.*

Ha chemical symbol, *hahnium.*

HAA hepatitis-associated antigen.

habena (hah-be'nah) habenula (2). **habe'nal, habe'nar,** adj.

habenula (hah-ben'ūl-ah), pl. *habe'nulae* [L.] 1. a frenulum, or reinlike structure, such as one of a set of structures in the cochlea. 2. a small eminence on the dorsomesial eminence of the thalamus, just in front of the posterior commissure. **haben'ular,** adj.

habit (hab'it) 1. an action which has become automatic or characteristic by repetition. 2. predisposition; bodily temperament.

habitat (hab'ĭ-tat) the natural abode of an animal or plant species.

habituation (hah-bich"u-a'shin) 1. the gradual adaptation to a stimulus or to the environment. 2. a condition due to repeated consumption of a drug, with a desire to continue its use, but with little or no tendency to increase the dose.

habitus (hab'it-is) [L.] 1. attitude (2). 2. physique.

Habronema (hab"ro-ne'mah) a genus of nematodes parasitic in the stomach of horses; their larvae may be transmitted to the horse's skin, where they may cause dermatitis and a type of granuloma; in the conjunctiva, they cause worm-containing granulomas.

hachement (ahsh-maw') [Fr.] hacking or chopping stroke in massage.

hae- for words beginning thus, see also those beginning *he-*.

Haemadipsa (he"mah-dip'sah) a genus of leeches.

Haemaphysalis (hem"ah-fis'ah-lis) a genus of hard-bodied ticks, species of which are important vectors of disease.

Haemobartonella (he"mo-bar"to-nel'ah) a genus of microorganisms of the family Bartonellaceae, species of which are parasitic in various lower animals.

Haemophilus (he-mof'il-is) a genus of hemophilic gram-negative bacteria (family Pasteurellaceae) including *H. aegyp'ticus,* the cause of acute contagious conjunctivitis; *H. ducrey'i,* the cause of chancroid; *H. influen'zae* (once thought to be the cause of epidemic influenza), the cause of lethal meningitis in infants; and *H. vagina'lis,* associated with, and possibly the cause of, human vaginitis.

hafnium (haf'ne-um) chemical element (*see table*), at. no. 72, symbol Hf.

hahnium (hah'ne-um) a transuranic element, at. no. 105, symbol Ha.

hair (hār) pilus; a threadlike structure, especially the specialized epidermal structure composed of keratin and developing from a papilla sunk in the corium, produced only by mammals and characteristic of that group of animals. Also, the aggregate of such hairs. **auditory h's,** hairlike attachments of the epithelial cells of the inner ear. **bamboo h.,** trichorrhexis nodosa. **beaded h.,** hair marked with alternate swellings and constrictions, as in monilethrix. **burrowing h.,** one that grows horizontally beneath the surface of the skin. **club h.,** one whose root is surrounded by a bulbous enlargement composed of keratinized cells, preliminary to normal loss of the hair from the follicle. **ingrown h.,** one that emerges from the skin but curves and reenters it. **lanugo h.,** the fine hair on the body of the fetus, constituting the lanugo. **resting h.,** see *telogen.* **sensory h's,** hairlike projections on the surface of sensory epithelial cells. **tactile h's,** hairs sensitive to touch. **taste h's,** short hairlike processes projecting freely into the lumen of the pit of a taste bud from the peripheral ends of the taste cells. **terminal h.,** the coarse hair on various areas of the body during adult years. **twisted h.,** one which at spaced intervals is twisted through an axis of 180 degrees, being abnormally flattened at the site of twisting.

hairball (hār'bawl) trichobezoar.

halation (hal-a'shin) indistinctness of the image caused by illumination coming from the same direction as the object being viewed.

halazone (hal'ah-zōn) a disinfectant for water supplies, $C_7H_5Cl_2NO_4S$.

halcinonide (hal-sin'ah-nīd) a synthetic glucocorticoid, $C_{24}H_{32}ClFO_5$; used as a topical anti-inflammatory.

Haldol (hal'dol) trademark for a preparation of haloperidol.

half-life (haf'līf) the time in which the radioactivity originally associated with a particular isotope is reduced by half through radioactive decay. **antibody h.,** a measure of the mean survival time of antibody molecules following their formation, usually expressed as the time required to eliminate 50 per cent of a known quantity of immunoglobulin from the animal body. Half-life varies from one immunoglobulin class to another. **biological h.,** the time required for a living tissue, organ, or organism to eliminate one-half of a radioactive substance which has been introduced into it.

half-value (haf-val'u) see under *layer.*

halfway house (haf'wa hows") a residence for patients (e.g., mental patients, drug addicts, alcoholics) who do not require hospitalization but who need an intermediate degree of care until they can return to the community.

halisteresis (hah-lis"ter-e'sis) osteomalacia. **halisteret'ic,** adj.

halitosis (hal"ĭ-to'sis) offensive odor of the breath.

halitus (hal'it-is) an exhalation of vapor; an expired breath.

hallucination (hah-loo"sin-a'shin) a sense perception (sight, touch, sound, smell, or taste) that has no basis in external stimulation. **hallu'cinatory,** adj. **haptic h.,** tactile h. **hypna-**

267

hallucinogen

gogic h., one occurring between sleeping and awakening. **olfactory h.,** a hallucination of smell. **tactile h.,** a hallucination of touch.

hallucinogen (hah-loo′sin-ah-jen″) an agent that is capable of producing hallucinations. **hallucinogen′ic,** adj.

hallucinosis (hah-loo″sin-o′sis) a psychosis marked by hallucinations. **acute h.,** **alcoholic h.,** alcoholic psychosis marked by auditory hallucinations and delusions of persecution. **organic h.,** an organic brain syndrome characterized by the presence of hallucinations caused by a specific organic factor and not associated with delirium.

hallux (hal′uks) the great toe. **h. doloro′sa,** a painful disease of the great toe, usually associated with flatfoot. **h. flex′us,** **h. rigidus.** **h. mal′leus,** hammer toe affecting the great toe. **h. ri′gidus,** painful flexion deformity of the great toe with limitation of motion at the metatarsophalangeal joint. **h. val′gus,** angulation of the great toe toward the other toes of the foot. **h. va′rus,** angulation of the great toe away from the other toes of the foot.

halmatogenesis (hal″mah-to-jen′ĭ-sis) a sudden alteration of type from one generation to another.

halo (ha′lo) 1. a luminous or colored circle, as the colored circle seen around a light in glaucoma. 2. a ring seen around the macula lutea in ophthalmoscopic examinations. 3. the imprint of the ciliary processes on the vitreous body. **Fick's, h.,** a colored circle appearing around a light, due to the wearing of contact lenses. **h. glaucomato′sus, glaucomatous h.,** peripapillary atrophy seen in severe or chronic glaucoma. **senile h.,** a zone of variable width around the optic papilla, due to exposure of various elements of the choroid as a result of senile atrophy of the pigmented epithelium.

haloduric (hal″o-du′rik) capable of existing in a medium containing a high concentration of salt.

halogen (hal′ah-jen) a nonmetallic element of the seventh group of the periodic system: chlorine, iodine, bromine, fluorine, and astatine.

haloid acid (hal′oid) one containing no oxygen, but composed of hydrogen and a halogen element.

halometer (hah-lom′ĭt-er) 1. an instrument for measuring ocular halos. 2. an instrument for estimating the size of erythrocytes by measuring the diffraction halos which they produce.

haloperidol (hal″o-per′ĭ-dol) a tranquilizer, C_{21}-$H_{23}ClFNO_2$, with antiemetic, hypotensive, and hypothermic actions; used especially in the management of psychoses and to control vocal utterances and tics of Gilles de la Tourette's syndrome.

halophilic (hal″ah-fil′ik) pertaining to or characterized by an affinity for salt; requiring a high concentration of salt for optimal growth.

haloprogin (-pro′jin) a synthetic topical antifungal, $C_9H_4Cl_3IO$; used in the treatment of tinea.

halothane (hal′ah-thān) a general inhalation anesthetic, $C_2HBrClF_3$.

hamartia (ham-ar′she-ah) defect in tissue combination during development.

hamartoma (ham″ar-to′mah) a benign tumor-like nodule composed of an overgrowth of mature cells and tissues normally present in the affected part, but often with one element predominating.

hamate (ham′āt) hooked, as the hamate bone.

hammer (ham′er) 1. an instrument with a head designed for striking blows. 2. malleus (1).

hamster (ham′ster) a small rodent, used extensively in laboratory experiments.

hamstring (ham′string) one of the tendons bounding the popliteal space laterally and medially. **inner h's,** tendons of gracilis, sartorius, and two other muscles of leg. **outer h.,** tendon of biceps flexor femoris.

hamulus (hă′mu-lis), pl. *ha′muli* [L.] any hook-shaped process. **ham′ular,** adj.

hand (hand) the extremity of the arm, consisting of the carpus, metacarpus, and fingers. **ape h.,** one with the thumb permanently extended. **claw h.,** see *clawhand.* **cleft h.,** a malformation in which the division between the fingers extends into the metacarpus; also, a hand with the middle digits absent. **club h.,** see *clubhand.* **drop h.,** wristdrop. **lobster-claw h.,** cleft h. **writing h.,** in paralysis agitans, assumption of the position by which a pen is commonly held.

H and E hematoxylin and eosin (stain).

handedness (hand′id-nis) the preferential use of the hand of one side in voluntary motor acts.

handicap (han′dĭ-kap) any physical or mental defect, congenital or acquired, preventing or restricting a person from participating in normal life or limiting his capacity to work.

handpiece (-pēs) that part of a dental engine held in the operator's hand and engaging the bur or working point while it is being revolved.

hangnail (hang′nāl) a shred of eponychium on a proximal or lateral nail fold.

haploid (hap′loid) having half the number of chromosomes characteristically found in the somatic (diploid) cells of an organism; typical of the gametes of a species whose union restores the diploid number.

haploidentity (hap″lo-i-den′tit-e) the condition of having the same antigenic phenotype at certain specified loci; said of donor-recipient combinations in transplantation studies.

haploscope (hap′lah-skōp) a stereoscope for testing the visual axis.

haplotype (-tīp) the group of alleles of linked genes, e.g., the HLA complex, contributed by either parent; the haploid genetic constitution contributed by either parent.

hapten (hap′ten) partial antigen; a specific nonprotein substance which does not itself elicit antibody formation, but does elicit the immune response when coupled with a carrier protein. **hapten′ic,** adj.

haptics (hap′tiks) the science of the sense of touch.

haptoglobin (hap″to-glo′bin) a group of serum $α_2$-globulin glycoproteins that bind free hemoglobin; different types, genetically determined, are distinguished electrophoretically.

harelip (hār′lip) a congenital cleft of the upper lip.

harvest (har′vist) to remove tissues or cells from a donor and preserve them for transplantation.

hashish (hash-ēsh′) a preparation of the unadulterated resin scraped from the flowering tops of female hemp plants (*Cannabis sativa*), smoked or chewed for its intoxicating effects. It is far more potent than marihuana.

haustellum (haw-stel′im), pl. *haustel′la*. a hollow tube with an eversible set of five stylets, by which certain ectoparasites, e.g., bedbugs and lice, attach themselves to the host and through which blood is drawn up.

haustration (hos-tra′shin) 1. the formation of a haustrum. 2. a haustrum.

haustrum (hos′trum), pl. *haus′tra* [L.] a recess. **haus′tral,** adj. **haus′tra co′li,** sacculations in the wall of the colon produced by adaptation of its length to the tenia coli, or by the arrangement of the circular muscle fibers.

HAV hepatitis A virus.

HB hepatitis B.

Hb hemoglobin.

HB$_c$Ag hepatitis B core antigen.

HB$_e$Ag hepatitis B e antigen.

HB$_s$Ag hepatitis B surface antigen.

HBV hepatitis B virus.

H.C. Hospital Corps.

HDL high-density lipoprotein.

He chemical symbol, *helium.*

head (hed) caput; the upper, anterior, or proximal extremity of a structure, especially the part of an organism containing the brain and organs of special sense. **big h.,** see *bighead.*

headache (hed′āk) pain in the head. **cluster h.,** a migraine-like disorder marked by attacks of unilateral intense pain over the eye and forehead, with flushing and watering of the eyes and nose; attacks last about an hour and occur in clusters. **histamine h.,** cluster h. **migraine h.,** see *migraine.* **sick h.,** migraine. **tension h.,** a type due to prolonged overwork, emotional strain or both, affecting especially the occipital region.

healing (hēl′ing) a process of cure; the restoration of integrity to injured tissue. **h. by first intention,** that in which union or restoration of continuity occurs directly without intervention of granulations. **h. by second intention,** union by closure of a wound with granulations.

health (helth) a state of physical, mental, and social well-being. **public h.,** the field of medicine concerned with safeguarding and improving the health of the community as a whole.

health maintenance organization (HMO) a broad term encompassing a variety of health care delivery systems utilizing group practice and providing alternatives to the fee-for-service private practice of medicine and allied health professions.

hearing loss (hēr′ing los′) partial or complete loss of hearing; see also *deafness.* **Alexander's h. l.,** congenital deafness due to cochlear aplasia

involving chiefly the organ of Corti and adjacent ganglion cells of the basal coil of the cochlea; high-frequency hearing loss results. **conductive h. l.,** that due to a defect of the sound-conducting apparatus, i.e., of the external auditory canal or middle ear. **pagetoid h. l.,** that occurring in osteitis deformans of the bones of the skull. **paradoxic h. l.,** that in which the hearing is better during loud noise. **sensorineural h. l.,** that due to a defect in the inner ear or the acoustic nerve. **transmission h.l.,** conductive h.l.

heart (hart) cor; the viscus of cardiac muscle that maintains the circulation of the blood; see Plate VI. **athletic h.,** hypertrophy of the heart without valvular disease, sometimes seen in athletes. **fatty h.,** 1. one that has undergone fatty degeneration. 2. a condition in which fat has accumulated about and in the heart muscle. **fibroid h.,** one affected with chronic myocarditis, in which fibrous tissue replaces portions of the myocardium. **horizontal h.,** a counterclockwise rotation of the electrical axis (deviation to the left) of the heart. **irritable h.,** neurocirculatory asthenia. **left h.,** the left atrium and ventricle, which propel the blood through the systemic circulation. **right h.,** the right atrium and ventricle, which propel the venous blood into the pulmonary circulation. **soldier's h.,** neurocirculatory asthenia. **three-chambered h.,** congenital absence of the ventricular or atrial septum so that the heart has a single ventricle with two atria or a single atrium with two ventricles. **tobacco h.,** one showing irregularity of action attributed to excessive use of tobacco.

heart beat (hart′bēt″) see *beat.*

heart block (-blok″) impairment of conduction in heart excitation; often applied specifically to atrioventricular heart block. **atrioventricular (A-V) h.b.,** a form in which the blocking is at the atrioventricular junction. It is *first degree* when A-V conduction time is prolonged; *second degree (partial h.b.)* when some but not all atrial impulses reach the ventricle; *third degree (complete h.b.)* when no atrial impulses at all reach the ventricle, and the atria and ventricles act independently of each other. **bundle-branch h.b.,** a form in which one ventricle is excited before the other because of absence of conduction in one of the branches of the bundle of His. **complete h.b.,** see *atrioventricular h.b.* **interventricular h.b.,** bundle-branch h.b. **Mobitz type I h.b.,** second degree A-V heart block in which the P-R interval increases progressively until an atrial impulse is blocked. **Mobitz type II h.b.,** second degree A-V heart block in which the P-R interval is fixed, with periodic blocking of an atrial impulse. **sinoatrial h.b.,** partial or complete impairment of conduction from the sinoatrial node to the atria, resulting in delay or absence of an atrial beat.

heartburn (-burn″) pyrosis; a retrosternal sensation of burning occurring in waves and rising toward the neck; it may be accompanied by a reflux of fluid into the mouth, and is often associated with gastroesophageal reflux.

heart failure (-fāl-yer) inability of the heart to

maintain a circulation sufficient to meet the body's needs; most often applied to myocardial failure affecting the right or left ventricle. **backward h.f.,** a concept of heart failure emphasizing the contribution of passive engorgement of the systemic venous system as a cause. **congestive h.f.,** that marked by breathlessness and abnormal retention of sodium and water, resulting in edema, with congestion of the lungs or peripheral circulation, or both. **forward h.f.,** a concept of heart failure emphasizing the inadequacy of cardiac output as the primary cause and considering venous distention to be secondary. **high output h.f.,** that in which cardiac output remains high, associated with hyperthyroidism, anemia, emphysema, etc. **left-sided h.f., left ventricular h.f.,** failure of adequate output by the left ventricle, marked by pulmonary congestion and edema. **low output h.f.,** that in which cardiac output is diminished, associated with cardiovascular diseases. **right-sided h.f., right ventricular h.f.,** failure of adequate output by the right ventricle, marked by venous engorgement, hepatic enlargement, and pitting edema.

heartwater (-wot″er) a fatal rickettsial disease of cattle, sheep, and goats marked by fluid accumulation in the pericardium and pleural cavity.

heartworm (-wurm″) an individual of the species *Dirofilaria immitis.*

heat (hēt) 1. the sensation of an increase in temperature; the energy producing such a sensation. 2. energy transferred as a result of a gradient in temperature. 3. estrus. **conductive h.,** heat transmitted by direct contact, as with a hot water bottle. **convective h.,** heat conveyed by currents of a warm medium, such as air or water. **conversive h.,** heat developed in tissues by resistance to passage of high-energy radiations. **prickly h.,** miliaria rubra.

heatstroke (hēt′strōk″) see under *stroke.*

heaves (hēvz) chronic pulmonary emphysema of horses.

hebetic (hĕ-bet′ik) pertaining to puberty.

hebetude (heb′ĕ-tōōd) dullness; apathy.

hecto- word element [Fr.], *hundred;* used in naming units of measurements to designate an amount 100 times (10²) the size of the unit to which it joined; symbol h.

hedonism (he′din-izm) excessive devotion to pleasure.

heel (hēl) calx; the hindmost part of the foot. **cracked h.,** pitted keratolysis.

height (hīt) the vertical measurement of an object or body. **h. of contour,** 1. a line encircling a tooth representing its greatest circumference. 2. the line encircling a tooth in a more or less horizontal plane and passing through the surface point of greatest radius. 3. the line encircling a tooth at its greatest bulge or diameter with respect to a selected path of insertion.

helcoid (hel′koid) like an ulcer.

heli(o)- word element [Gr.], *sun.*

helical (hel′ĭ-k′l) shaped like a helix.

helicine (hel′ĭ-sin) 1. of spiral form. 2. of or pertaining to a helix.

helicopodia (hel″ĭ-ko-po′de-ah) helicopod gait.

helicotrema (hel″ĭ-ko-tre′mah) a foramen between the scala tympani and scala vestibuli.

heliencephalitis (hē″le-en-sef″ah-lit′is) encephalitis from exposure to the sun (sunstroke).

helium (hēl′e-im) chemical element (*see table*), at. no. 2, symbol He. It is obtained from natural gas. Used as a diluent for other gases, being especially useful with oxygen in the treatment of certain cases of respiratory obstruction, and as a vehicle for general anesthetics.

helix (hēl′iks) 1. a coiled structure. 2. the superior and posterior free margin of the pinna of the ear. **α-h., alpha h.,** the structural arrangement of parts of protein molecules in which a single polypeptide chain forms a right-handed helix. **double h., Watson-Crick h.,** a representation of the structure of DNA, consisting of two coiled chains, each containing information completely specifying the other chain.

helminth (hel′minth) a parasitic worm.

helminthagogue (hel-min′thah-gog) anthelmintic.

helminthemesis (hel″min-them′ĭ-sis) the vomiting of worms.

helminthology (hel″min-thol′ah-je) the scientific study of parasitic worms.

heloma (hēl-o′mah) a corn. **h. du′rum,** hard corn. **h. mol′le,** soft corn.

helotomy (hēl-ot′ah-me) the excision or the paring of corns or calluses.

hemacytometer (he″mah-si-tom′ĭ-ter) hemocytometer.

hemadsorption (hem″ad-sorp′shin) the adherence of red cells to other cells, particles, or surfaces. **hemadsor′bent,** adj.

hemagglutinin (-glōōt′in-in) an antibody that causes agglutination of erythrocytes. **cold h.,** one which acts only at temperatures near 4° C. **warm h.,** one which acts only at temperatures near 37° C.

hemal (he′m′l) 1. pertaining to the blood or the blood vessels. 2. ventral to the spinal axis, where the heart and great vessels are located, as, e.g., the hemal arches.

hemalum (hem-al′im) a mixture of hematoxylin and alum used as a nuclear stain.

hemanalysis (he″mah-nal′ĭ-sis) analysis of the blood.

hemangioameloblastoma (he-man″je-o-ah-mel″o-blas-to′mah) a highly vascular ameloblastoma.

hemangioblast (he-man′je-ah-blast) a mesodermal cell which gives rise to both vascular endothelium and hemocytoblasts.

hemangioblastoma (he-man″je-o-blas-to′mah) a capillary hemangioma of the brain consisting of proliferated blood vessel cells or angioblasts.

hemangioendothelioblastoma (-en″do-thēl′e-o-blas-to′mah) a tumor of mesenchymal origin of which the cells tend to form endothelial cells and line blood vessels.

hemangioendothelioma (-en″do-thēl″e-o′mah) a hemangioma in which endothelial cells are the most prominent component.

hemangioendotheliosarcoma (-en″do-thēl″e-o-sar-ko′mah) hemangiosarcoma.

hemangioma (he-man″je-o′mah) a benign tumor made up of newly formed blood vessels. **ameloblastic h.,** a highly vascular ameloblastoma. **cavernous h.,** a red-blue spongy tumor made up of a connective tissue framework enclosing large, cavernous, vascular spaces containing blood. **sclerosing h.,** a solidly cellular lesion purportedly developing from a hemangioma by proliferation of endothelial cells and connective tissue stroma.

hemangiopericytoma (-per″ĭ-si-to′mah) a tumor composed of spindle cells with a rich vascular network, which apparently arises from pericytes.

hemangiosarcoma (-sar-ko′mah) a malignant tumor formed of endothelial and fibroblastic tissue.

hemapheresis (hem″ah-fĕ′rĭ-sis) any procedure in which blood is withdrawn, a portion (plasma, leukocytes, platelets, etc.) is separated and retained, and the remainder is retransfused into the donor.

hemarthrosis (hem″ar-thro′sis) extravasation of blood into a joint or its synovial cavity.

hemat(o)- word element [Gr.], *blood.* See also words beginning *hem-* and *hemo-*.

hematemesis (hem″ah-tem′ĭ-sis) the vomiting of blood.

hemathermous (hem″ah-therm′is) warm-blooded.

hematic (he-mat′ik) 1. pertaining to or containing blood. 2. hematinic.

hematidrosis (hem″it-ĭ-dro′sis) excretion of bloody sweat.

hematin (hem′it-in) 1. the hydroxide of heme, $C_{34}H_{33}FeN_4O_5$; used as a reagent. 2. heme.

hematinic (hem″ah-tin′ik) 1. pertaining to hematin (heme). 2. an agent that improves the quality of blood, increasing the hemoglobin level and the number of erythrocytes.

hematinuria (hem″it-in-ūr′e-ah) the presence of hematin (heme) in the urine.

hematocele (hem′ah-to-sēl″) an effusion of blood into a cavity, especially into the tunica vaginalis testis. **parametric h., pelvic h., retrouterine h.,** a tumor formed by effusion of blood into the pouch of Douglas.

hematochezia (hem″it-o-ke′ze-ah) the passage of bloody stools.

hematochyluria (hem″it-o-ke′ze-ah) the discharge of blood and chyle with the urine, due to *Wuchereria bancrofti.*

hematocoelia (-sēl′e-ah) effusion of blood into the peritoneal cavity.

hematocolpometra (-kol″po-me′trah) accumulation of menstrual blood in the vagina and uterus.

hematocolpos (-kol′pos) accumulation of blood in the vagina.

hematocrit (he-mat′ah-krit) the volume percentage of erythrocytes in whole blood; also, the apparatus or procedure used in its determination.

hematocyturia (hem″it-o-si-tūr′e-ah) the presence of erythrocytes in the urine.

hematogenic (-jen′ik) 1. hematopoietic. 2. hematogenous.

hematogenous (hem″ah-toj′ĭ-nus) produced by or derived from the blood; disseminated through the blood stream.

hematoidin (hem″ah-toi′din) a substance apparently chemically identical with bilirubin but formed in the tissues from hemoglobin, particularly under conditions of reduced oxygen tension.

hematology (-tol′ah-je) the science dealing with the morphology of blood and blood-forming tissues, and with their physiology and pathology.

hematolymphangioma (hem″it-o-lim-fan″je-o′mah) a tumor that is composed of blood and lymph vessels.

hematolysis (hem″ah-tol′ĭ-sis) hemolysis. **hematolyt′ic,** adj.

hematoma (he″mah-to′mah) a localized collection of extravasated blood, usually clotted, in an organ, space, or tissue. **subdural h.,** a massive blood clot beneath the dura mater that causes neurologic symptoms by pressure on the brain.

hematomediastinum (hem″it-o-me″de-as-ti′-num) hemomediastinum.

hematometra (-me′trah) an accumulation of blood in the uterus.

hematometry (he″mah-tom′ĭ-tre) measurement of hemoglobin and estimation of the percentage of various cells in the blood.

hematomyelia (hem″ah-to-mi-e′le-ah) hemorrhage into the substance of the spinal cord.

hematomyelitis (-mi″il-īt′is) acute myelitis with bloody effusion into the spinal cord.

hematomyelopore (-mi″il-o-por) formation of canals in the spinal cord due to hemorrhage.

hematopathology (hem″it-o-pah-thol′ah-je) the study of diseases of the blood.

hematophagia (-fa′je-ah) 1. blood drinking. 2. subsisting on blood. 3. hemocytophagia. **hematoph′agous,** adj.

hematopoiesis (-poi-e′sis) the formation and development of blood cells. **extramedullary h.,** that occurring outside the bone marrow, as in the spleen, liver, and lymph nodes.

hematopoietic (-poi-et′ik) 1. pertaining to or affecting the formation of blood cells. 2. an agent that promotes the formation of blood cells.

hematoporphyrin (-por′fĭ-rin) an iron-free derivative of heme, a product of the decomposition of hemoglobin.

hematorrhachis (hem″it-ōr′ah-kis) hematomyelia.

hematorrhea (hem″it-ah-re′ah) copious hemorrhage.

hematosalpinx (-sal′pinks) an accumulation of blood in the uterine tube.

hematospermatocele (hem″it-o-sper-mat′ah-sēl) a spermatocele containing blood.

hematosteon (hem″ah-tos′te-on) hemorrhage into the medullary cavity of a bone.

hematotoxic (hem″it-o-tok′sik) 1. pertaining to blood poisoning. 2. poisonous to the blood and hematopoietic system.

hematotropic (-trop′ik) having a specific affinity for or exerting a specific effect on the blood or blood cells.

hematoxylin (hem″ah-tok′sil-in) an acid coloring matter from the heartwood of *Haematoxylon campechianum;* used as a histologic stain and also as an indicator.

hematuria (hem″ah-tūr′e-ah) the presence of blood in the urine. **endemic h.,** urinary schistosomiasis. **enzootic bovine h.,** a disease of cattle marked by blood in the urine, anemia, and debilitation. **essential h.,** that for which no cause has been determined. **false h.,** redness of the urine due to ingestion of food or drugs containing pigment. **renal h.,** that in which the blood comes from the kidney. **urethral h.,** that in which the blood comes from the urethra. **vesical h.,** that in which the blood comes from the bladder.

heme (hēm) an iron compound of protoporphyrin which constitutes the pigment portion or protein-free part of the hemoglobin molecule and is responsible for its oxygen-carrying properties.

hemeralopia (hem″er-ah-lo′pe-ah) day blindness.

hemi- word element [Gr.], *half.*

hemiachromatopsia (-a″kro-mah-top′se-ah) color blindness in half, or in corresponding halves, of the visual field.

hemiamyosthenia (-ah-mi″os-the′ne-ah) lack of muscular power on one side of the body.

hemianalgesia (-an″al-je′ze-ah) analgesia on one side of the body.

hemianesthesia (-an″es-the′ze-ah) anesthesia of one side of the body. **crossed h., h. crucia′ta,** loss of sensation on one side of the face and loss of pain and temperature sense on the opposite side of the body.

hemianopia (hem″e-an-o′pe-ah) defective vision or blindness in half of the visual field of one or both eyes; loosely, scotoma in less than half of the visual field of one or both eyes. **absolute h.,** blindness to light, color, and form in half of the visual field. **binasal h.,** that in which the defect is in the nasal half of the visual field in each eye. **binocular h.,** true h. **bitemporal h.,** that in which the defect is in the temporal half of the visual field in each eye. **complete h.,** that affecting an entire half of the visual field in each eye. **congruous h.,** that in which the defect is approximately the same in each eye. **crossed h.,** heteronymous h. **heteronymous h.,** that affecting both nasal or both temporal halves of the field of vision. **homonymous h.,** that affecting the nasal half of the field of vision of one eye and the temporal half of the other. **nasal h.,** that affecting the medial half of the visual field, i.e., the half nearest the nose. **quadrant h., quadrantic h.,** quadrantanopia. **temporal h.,** that affecting the lateral vertical half of the visual field, i.e., the half nearest the temple.

hemiapraxia (-ah-prak′se-ah) apraxia on one side of the body only.

hemiataxia (-ah-tak′se-ah) ataxia on one side of the body.

hemiathetosis (-ath″ĭ-to′sis) athetosis of one side of the body.

hemiatrophy (-ă′trah-fe) atrophy of one side of the body or one half of an organ or part.

hemiaxial (-aks′e-il) at any oblique angle to the long axis of the body or a part.

hemiballism, hemiballismus (-bal′izm; -bah-liz′mus) ballismus involving one side of the body, most marked in the upper limb.

hemibladder (-blad′er) a half bladder; a developmental anomaly in which the bladder is formed as two physically separated parts, each with its own ureter.

hemiblock (-blok) failure in conduction of cardiac impulse in either of the two main divisions of the left branch of the bundle of His; the interruption may occur in either the anterior (superior) or posterior (inferior) division.

hemic (he′mik, hem′ik) pertaining to blood.

hemicardia (hem″e-kar′de-ah) the presence of only one side of a four-chambered heart.

hemicentrum (-sen′trum) either lateral half of a vertebral centrum.

hemichorea (-ko-re′ah) chorea affecting only one side of the body.

hemichromatopsia (-kro″mah-top′se-ah) color blindness in half of the visual field.

hemicrania (-kra′ne-ah) 1. unilateral headache. 2. incomplete anencephaly.

hemicraniosis (-kra″ne-o′sis) hyperostosis of one side of the cranium and face.

hemidesmosome (-des″mah-sōm) a structure representing half of a desmosome, found on the basal surface of some epithelial cells, forming the site of attachment between the basal surface of the cell and the basement membrane.

hemidiaphoresis (-di″ah-for-e′sis) hemihyperhidrosis.

hemidysesthesia (-dis″es-the′ze-ah) disorder of sensation on one side of the body.

hemiepilepsy (-ep″il-ep″se) epilepsy affecting one side of the body.

hemifacial (-fa′shil) pertaining to or affecting half of the face.

hemigastrectomy (-gas-trek′tah-me) excision of half of the stomach.

hemigeusia (-gu′ze-ah) absence of the sense of taste on one side of the tongue.

hemiglossectomy (-glos-ek′tah-me) excision of one side of the tongue.

hemiglossitis (-glos-īt′is) inflammation of one half of the tongue.

hemihidrosis (-hĭ-dro′sis) sweating on one side of the body only.

hemihypalgesia (-hīp″al-je′ze-ah) diminished sensitivity to pain on one side of the body.

hemihyperesthesia (-hi″per-es-the′ze-ah) increased sensitiveness of one side of the body.

hemihyperhidrosis (-hĭ-dro′sis) excessive perspiration on one side of the body.

hemihypertrophy (hem″e-hi-pur′trah-fe) overgrowth of one side of the body or of a part.

hemihypesthesia (-hīp″es-thēz′e-ah) diminished sensitiveness of one side of the body.

hemihypotonia (-hi″po-to′ne-ah) diminished muscle tone of one side of the body.

hemilaminectomy (-lam″in-ek′tah-me) removal of a vertebral lamina on one side only.

hemilaryngectomy (-lar″in-jek′tah-me) excision of one lateral half of the larynx.

hemilateral (-lat′er-il) affecting one lateral half of the body only.

heminephrectomy (hem″e-ně-frek′tah-me) excision of part (half) of a kidney.

hemiopia (-o′pe-ah) hemianopia. **hemiop′ic,** adj.

hemiparanesthesia (hem″e-par″an-es-the′ze-ah) anesthesia of the lower half of one side.

hemiparaplegia (-par″ah-ple′je-ah) paralysis of the lower half of one side.

hemiparesis (-pah-re′sis, -par′is-is) paresis affecting one side of the body.

hemiparetic (-pah-ret′ik) 1. pertaining to hemiparesis. 2. one affected with hemiparesis.

hemiplacenta (-plah-sen′tah) an organ composed of the chorion, yolk sac, and, usually, allantois, which puts marsupial embryos into temporary relation with the maternal uterus.

hemiplegia (-ple′je-ah) paralysis of one side of the body. **hemiple′gic,** adj. **alternate h.,** paralysis of one side of the face and the opposite side of the body. **cerebral h.,** that due to a brain lesion. **crossed h.,** alternate h. **facial h.,** paralysis of one side of the face. **spastic h.,** hemiplegia with spasticity of the affected muscles and increased tendon reflexes. **spinal h.,** that due to lesion of spinal cord.

Hemiptera (hem-ip′ter-ah) an order of insects, winged or wingless, including ordinary bugs and lice, having mouth parts adapted to piercing and sucking.

hemirachischisis (hem″e-rah-kis′kĭ-sis) rachischisis without prolapse of the spinal cord.

hemisection (-sek′shin) 1. bisection. 2. division into two equal parts.

hemispasm (hem′e-spazm) spasm affecting one side only.

hemisphere (hem′ĭ-sfēr) half of a spherical or roughly spherical structure or organ. **cerebellar h.,** either of two lobes of the cerebellum lateral to the vermis. **cerebral h.,** one of the paired structures forming the bulk of the human brain, which together comprise the cerebral cortex, centrum semiovale, basal ganglia, and rhinencephalon, and contain the lateral ventricles. **dominant h.,** that cerebral hemisphere which is more concerned than the other in the integration of sensations and the control of voluntary functions.

hemispherium (hem″ĭ-sfēr′e-um), pl. *hemisphe′ria* [L.] either cerebral hemisphere.

hemivertebra (-vurt′ĭ-brah) a developmental anomaly in which one side of a vertebra is incompletely developed.

hemizygosity (-zi-gos′it-e) the state of having only one of a pair of alleles transmitting a specific character. **hemizy′gous,** adj.

hemo- word element [Gr.], *blood.* See also words beginning *hem-* and *hemato-.*

hemoblast (he′mo-blast) hemocytoblast. **lymphoid h. of Pappenheim,** pronormoblast.

hemoblastosis (he″mo-blas-to′sis) general term for proliferative disorders of the blood-forming tissues.

hemocatheresis (-kah-ther′ĭ-sis) the destruction of red blood cells. **hemocatheret′ic,** adj.

Hemoccult (he′mo-kult) trademark for a guaiac reagent strip test for occult blood.

hemochorial (he″mo-kor′e-il) denoting a type of placenta in which maternal blood comes in direct contact with the chorion.

hemochromatosis (-kro″mah-to′sis) a disorder of iron metabolism with excess deposition of iron in the tissues, bronze skin pigmentation, hepatic cirrhosis, and diabetes mellitus. **hemochromatot′ic,** adj.

hemoconcentration (he″mo-kon″sen-tra′shin) decrease of the fluid content of the blood, with resulting increase in concentration of its formed elements.

hemoconia (-ko′ne-ah), pl. *hemoco′niae* [L.] small, round or dumbbell-shaped bodies exhibiting brownian movement, observed in blood platelets in darkfield microscopy of a wet film of blood.

hemocyanin (-si′ah-nin) a blue copper-containing respiratory pigment occurring in the blood of mollusks and arthropods.

hemocyte (he′mo-sīt) a blood cell.

hemocytoblast (he″mo-sīt′ah-blast) the free stem cell from which, according to some theorists, all other blood cells are derived.

hemocytoblastoma (-si″to-blas-to′mah) a tumor containing all the cells typical of bone marrow.

hemocytocatheresis (-kah-ther′ĭ-sis) hemolysis.

hemocytometer (-si-tom′it-er) an instrument used in counting blood cells.

hemocytotripsis (-sīt″ah-trip′sis) disintegration of blood cells by pressure.

hemodiagnosis (-di″ig-no′sis) diagnosis by examination of the blood.

hemodialysis (-di-al′ĭ-sis) removal of certain elements from the blood by virtue of differences in rates of their diffusion through a semipermeable membrane while being circulated outside the body.

hemodialyzer (-di′ah-līz″er) an apparatus for performing hemodialysis.

hemodilution (-di-loo′shin) increase in fluid content of blood, resulting in diminution in the concentration of formed elements.

hemodynamics (-di-nam′iks) the study of the movements of the blood and of the forces concerned therein. **hemodynam′ic,** adj.

hemoendothelial (-en-do-thēl′e-il) denoting a type of placenta in which maternal blood comes in contact with the endothelium of chorionic vessels.

hemofiltration (-fil-tra′shin) the removal of waste products from the blood by passing the blood through extracorporeal filters.

hemoflagellate (-flaj′ě-lāt) any flagellate protozoan parasite of the blood; the term includes the genera *Trypanosoma* and *Leishmania.*

hemofuscin (-fūs′in) a brownish-yellow pigment

resulting from hemoglobin decomposition; it gives urine a deep ruddy color.

hemoglobin (-glo′bin) the oxygen-carrying pigment of the erythrocytes, formed by the developing erythrocyte in the bone marrow, made up of four different globin polypeptide chains, each composed of several hundred amino acids. Hemoglobin A is normal adult hemoglobin. Many abnormal hemoglobins have been reported, including hemoglobin E, H, M, and S; homozygosity for hemoglobin S results in sickle cell anemia, heterozygosity in sickle cell trait. Symbol Hb. **fetal h.,** that forming more than half of the hemoglobin of the fetus, present in minimal amounts in adults and abnormally elevated in certain blood disorders. **muscle h.,** myoglobin. **reduced h.,** that not combined with oxygen.

hemoglobinemia (-glo″bin-ēm′e-ah) the presence of excessive hemoglobin in the blood plasma.

hemoglobinolysis (-glo″bin-ol′ĭ-sis) the splitting up of hemoglobin.

hemoglobinometer (-glo″bin-om′it-er) a laboratory instrument for colorimetric determination of the hemoglobin content of the blood.

hemoglobinopathy (-glo″bin-op′ah-the) a hematologic disorder due to alteration in the genetically determined molecular structure of the hemoglobin, with characteristic clinical and laboratory abnormalities and often overt anemia.

hemoglobinuria (-glo″bin-ūr′e-ah) the presence of free hemoglobin in the urine. **hemoglobinu′ric,** adj. **bacillary h.,** an infectious toxemic disease due to *Clostridium haemolyticum,* affecting primarily cattle; symptoms include fever, bloody diarrhea, dark red urine, anemia, and hemoglobinuria. **march h.,** that occurring after prolonged exercise. **toxic h.,** that which is consequent upon the ingestion of various poisons.

hemohistioblast (he″mo-his′te-ah-blast″) the hypothetical stem cell from which all blood cells are derived.

hemoid (he′moid) resembling blood.

hemokinesis (he″mo-ki-ne′sis) the flow of blood in the body. **hemokinet′ic,** adj.

hemolymph (he′mo-limf) 1. blood and lymph. 2. the bloodlike fluid of those invertebrates having open blood-vascular systems.

hemolysin (he-mol′ĭ-sin) a substance that liberates hemoglobin from erythrocytes by interrupting their structural integrity.

hemolysis (he-mol′ĭ-sis) the liberation of hemoglobin, consisting in separation of the hemoglobin from the red cells and its appearance in the plasma. **hemolyt′ic,** adj. **immune h.,** lysis by complement of erythrocytes sensitized as a consequence of interaction with specific antibody to the erythrocytes.

hemolysoid (he-mol′ĭ-soid) a hemolysin so altered that it still combines with erythrocytes but does not cause hemolysis.

hemolyze (he′mah-līz) to subject to or to undergo hemolysis.

hemomediastinum (he″mo-me″de-as-ti′num) an effusion of blood into the mediastinum.

hemometra (-me′trah) hematometra.

hemopathology (-pah-thol′ah-je) the study of diseases of the blood.

hemopathy (he-mop′ah-the) any disease of the blood. **hemopath′ic,** adj.

hemopericardium (-pě″ri-kar′de-um) an effusion of blood within the pericardium.

hemopexin (-pek′sin) a heme-binding serum glycoprotein.

hemopexis (-pek′sis) coagulation of blood.

hemophagocyte (-fag′ah-sīt) a phagocyte that destroys blood cells.

hemophil (hēm′ah-fil) 1. thriving on blood. 2. a microorganism which grows best in media containing hemoglobin.

hemophilia (hēm″ah-fil′e-ah) a hereditary hemorrhagic diathesis due to deficiency of a blood coagulation factor. **h. A,** classical hemophilia; an X-linked recessive form affecting males, due to deficiency of coagulation Factor VIII. **h. B,** Factor IX deficiency; see *coagulation factors.* **h. C,** Factor XI deficiency; see *coagulation factors.* **classical h.,** h. A. **vascular h.,** von Willebrand's disease.

hemophilic (-fil′ik) 1. having an affinity for blood; in bacteriology, growing well in culture media containing blood or having a nutritional affinity for constituents of fresh blood. 2. pertaining to or characterized by hemophilia.

hemophilioid (-fil′e-oid) resembling classical hemophilia clinically; applied to a number of hereditary or acquired hemorrhagic disorders not due solely to coagulation Factor VIII deficiency.

Hemophilus (he-mof′il-is) Haemofilus.

hemoplastic (he′mo-plas″tik) hematopoietic.

hemopneumopericardium (-noo″mo-pe″rĭ-kar′de-um) effused blood and air in the pericardium.

hemopneumothorax (-noo″mo-thor′aks) pneumothorax with hemorrhagic effusion.

hemoprecipitin (-pre-sip′it-in) a blood precipitin.

hemoprotein (-pro′tēn) a conjugated protein containing heme as the prosthetic group.

hemopsonin (he″mop-so′nin) an opsonin making erythrocytes more liable to phagocytosis.

hemoptysis (he-mop′tĭ-sis) the spitting of blood or of blood-stained sputum. **parasitic h.,** a disease due to infection of the lungs with lung flukes of the genus *Paragonimus,* with cough and spitting of blood and gradual deterioration of health.

hemorrhage (hem′ah-rij) the escape of blood from the vessels; bleeding. **hemorrhag′ic,** adj. **capillary h.,** the oozing of blood from the minute vessels. **cerebral h.,** hemorrhage into the cerebrum; see *stroke syndrome.* **concealed h.,** internal h. **fibrinolytic h.,** that due to abnormalities in the fibrinolytic system. **internal h.,** that in which the extravasated blood remains within the body. **nasal h.,** epistaxis. **petechial h.,** subcutaneous hemorrhage occurring in minute spots. **postpartum h.,** that which follows soon after labor or childbirth. **primary h.,** that occurring immediately after injury. **secondary h.,** bleeding which follows an injury after a lapse of time. **unavoidable h.,** that caused by detachment of a placenta previa. **uterine h., essential,** hemorrhage from the uterus, usually with hypertrophy of the uterine mucosa and cystic disease of the ovary.

hemorrhagin (-ra′jin) a cytolysin in certain venoms and poisons which is destructive to endothelial cells and blood vessels.

hemorrhea (-re′ah) hematorrhea.

hemorrheology (he″mo-re-ol′ah-je) the study of the deformation and flow properties of cellular and plasmatic components of blood in macroscopic, microscopic, and submicroscopic dimensions, and the rheological properties of vessel structure with which the blood comes in direct contact.

hemorrhoid (hem′ah-roid) a varicose dilatation of a vein of the superior or inferior hemorrhoidal plexus. **hemorrhoi′dal,** adj. **external h.,** varicose dilatation of a vein of the inferior hemorrhoidal plexus, distal to the pectinate line and covered with modified anal skin. **internal h.,** a varicose dilatation of a vein of the superior hemorrhoidal plexus, originating above the pectinate line and covered by mucous membrane. **prolapsed h.,** an internal hemorrhoid which has descended below the pectinate line and protruded outside the anal sphincter. **strangulated h.,** an internal hemorrhoid which has been prolapsed sufficiently and for long enough time for its blood supply to become occluded by the constricting action of the anal sphincter. **thrombosed h.,** one containing clotted blood.

hemorrhoidectomy (hem″ah-roi-dek′tah-me) excision of hemorrhoids.

hemosiderin (he″mo-sid′er-in) an insoluble form of tissue storage iron, visible microscopically both with and without the use of special stains.

hemosiderosis (-sid″er-o′sis) a focal or general increase in tissue iron stores without associated tissue damage. **pulmonary h.,** the deposition of abnormal amounts of hemosiderin in the lungs, due to bleeding into the lung interstitium.

hemostasis (he″mah-sta′sis, he-mos′tah-sis) 1. the arrest of bleeding by the physiological properties of vasoconstriction and coagulation or by surgical means. 2. interruption of blood flow through any vessel or to any anatomical area.

hemostat (he′mah-stat) 1. a small surgical clamp for constricting bleeding blood vessels. 2. an antihemorrhagic agent.

hemotherapy (-thĕ′rah-pe) the use of blood or its products in treating disease.

hemothorax (-thor′aks) collection of blood in the pleural cavity.

hemotoxic (-tok′sik) hematotoxic.

hemotoxin (-tok′sin) an exotoxin characterized by hemolytic activity.

hemotroph (he′mah-trōf) the sum total of nutritive substances supplied to the embryo from the maternal blood. **hemotroph′ic,** adj.

henry (hen′re) the unit of electrical inductance.

hepar (he′par) [Gr.] the liver.

heparan sulfate (hep′ah-ran) a sulfated mucopolysaccharide structurally related to heparin, which occurs normally in the liver, aorta, and lung; it is an accumulation product in several mucopolysaccharidoses.

heparin (hep′ah-rin) an acidic mucopolysaccharide present in many tissues, especially the liver and lungs, and having potent anticoagulant properties. It also has lipotrophic properties, promoting transfer of fat from blood to the fat depots by activation of lipoprotein lipase. Also, a mixture of active principles capable of prolonging blood clotting time, obtained from domestic animals; used in the prophylaxis and treatment of disorders in which there is excessive or undesirable clotting and as a preservative for blood specimens.

heparinize (hep′er-in-īz″) to render blood incoagulable with heparin.

hepat(o)- word element [Gr.], *liver.*

hepatatrophia (hep″it-ah-tro′fe-ah) atrophy of the liver.

hepatic (hĕ-pat′ik) pertaining to the liver.

hepatic(o)- word element [Gr.], *hepatic duct.*

hepaticoduodenostomy (hĕ-pat″ĭ-ko-doo″o-dĕ-nos′tah-me) anastomosis of the hepatic duct to the duodenum.

hepaticogastrostomy (-gas-tros′tah-me) anastomosis of the hepatic duct to the stomach.

hepaticolithotomy (-lĭ-thot′ah-me) incision of the hepatic duct, with removal of calculi.

hepaticostomy (hĕ-pat″ĭ-kos′tah-me) fistulization of the hepatic duct.

hepatitis (hep″ah-tīt′is) inflammation of the liver. **h. A,** a self-limited viral disease of worldwide distribution, usually transmitted by oral ingestion of infected material, but it may also be transmitted parenterally. It usually begins abruptly with fever, malaise, and nonspecific gastrointestinal symptoms, followed by jaundice, pruritus, dark urine, pale stools, and hepatomegaly with tenderness; malaise, tiredness, and minor abnormalities of hepatic function may persist during convalescence. **anicteric h.,** a mild viral hepatitis without jaundice. **h. B,** an acute viral illness transmitted parenterally or by oral ingestion of contaminated material. Prodromal symptoms include urticarial skin lesions and arthritis, and the acute illness tends to be more prolonged and more variable than in viral hepatitis type A; otherwise, the clinical and pathological symptoms are similar. **cholangiolitic h., cholestatic h.,** inflammation of the bile ducts of the liver associated with obstructive jaundice. **delta h.,** infection with hepatitis delta virus, occurring either simultaneously with or as a superinfection in hepatitis B, whose severity it may increase. **infectious h.,** h. A. **infectious necrotic h. of sheep,** black disease. **lupoid h.,** chronic active hepatitis characterized by the presence of LE cells in the peripheral blood. **neonatal h.,** hepatitis of uncertain etiology occurring soon after birth and marked by prolonged persistent jaundice, which may progress to cirrhosis. **non-A, non-B h.,** a clinical syndrome of acute viral hepatitis occurring without the serologic markers of hepatitis A or B. It is the major cause of post-transfusion hepatitis and occurs commonly following parenteral drug abuse. **post-transfusion h.,** viral hepatitis, now primarily non-A, non-B hepatitis, transmitted via transfusion of blood or blood products, especially multiple pooled donor products such as clotting factor concentrates. **serum h.,** h. B. **transfusion h.,** post-transfusion h. **viral h.,** h. A., h. B., delta h., and non-A, non-B. h.

hepatization (hep″it-iz-a′shin) transformation into a liver-like mass, especially the solidified state of the lung in lobar pneumonia. The early stage, in which the pulmonary exudate is blood stained, is called *red h.* The later stage, in which the red cells disintegrate and a fibrinosuppurative exudate persists, is called *gray h.*

hepatoblastoma (hep″it-o-blas-to′mah) a malignant intrahepatic tumor consisting chiefly of embryonic tissue, occurring in infants and young children.

hepatocarcinoma (-kar″sin-o-′mah) hepatocellular carcinoma.

hepatocele (hep′it-o-sēl) hernia of the liver.

hepatocholangiocarcinoma (-ko-lan″je-o-kar″sin-o′mah) cholangiohepatoma.

hepatocirrhosis (-sī-ro′sis) cirrhosis of the liver.

hepatocyte (hep′it-o-sīt″) a hepatic cell.

hepatogastric (-gas′trik) pertaining to the liver and stomach.

hepatogram (hep′it-ah-gram″) 1. a tracing of the liver pulse in the sphygmogram. 2. a roentgenogram of the liver.

hepatoid (hep′ah-toid) resembling the liver.

hepatojugular (hep″it-o-jug′ūl-er) pertaining to the liver and jugular vein; see under *reflux.*

hepatolith (hep′it-o-lith″) a biliary calculus in the liver.

hepatolithiasis (-lī-thi′ah-sis) the presence of calculi in the biliary ducts of the liver.

hepatology (hep″ah-tol′ah-je) the scientific study of the liver and its diseases.

hepatolysin (-tol′ĭ-sin) a cytolysin destructive to liver cells.

hepatolysis (hep″ah-tol′ĭ-sis) destruction of the liver cells. **hepatolyt′ic,** adj.

hepatoma (hep″ah-to′mah) a tumor of the liver, especially hepatocellular carcinoma (malignant h.).

hepatomegaly (-meg′ah-le) enlargement of the liver.

hepatomelanosis (-mel″ah-no′sis) melanosis of the liver.

hepatomphalocele (hep″ah-tom′fah-lo-sēl″) umbilical hernia with liver involvement in the hernial sac.

hepatopexy (hep′it-o-pek″se) surgical fixation of a displaced liver.

hepatopneumonic (hep″it-o-noo-mon′ik) pertaining to, affecting, or communicating with the liver and lungs.

hepatoportal (-port′il) pertaining to the portal system of the liver.

hepatorenal (-rēn′il) pertaining to the liver and kidneys.

hepatorrhexis (hep″it-o-rek′sis) rupture of the liver.

hepatosis (hep″ah-to′sis) any functional disorder of the liver. **serous h.,** veno-occlusive disease of the liver.

hepatosplenitis (hep″it-o-splen-īt′is) inflammation of the liver and spleen.

hepatosplenomegaly (-splen″o-meg′ah-le) enlargement of the liver and spleen.

hepatotoxemia (hep″it-o-tok-sēm′e-ah) blood poisoning originating in the liver.

hepatotoxin (-tok′sin) a toxin that destroys liver cells. **hepatotox′ic,** adj.

hept-, hepta- word element [Gr.], *seven.*

heptachromic (hep″tah-kro′mik) 1. pertaining to or exhibiting seven colors. 2. able to distinguish all seven colors of the spectrum.

heptose (hep′tōs) a sugar whose molecule contains seven carbon atoms.

herb (erb, herb) any leafy plant without a woody stem, especially one used as a household remedy or as a flavor.

herbivorous (her-biv′ah-ris) subsisting upon plants.

heredity (hĕ-red′it-e) 1. the genetic transmission of a particular quality or trait from parent to offspring. 2. the genetic constitution of an individual.

heredofamilial (hĕ″rid-o-fah-mil′e-il) occurring in certain families under circumstances that implicate a hereditary basis.

Herellea (hĕ-rel′e-ah) in former systems of classification, a genus of bacteria whose species are now included in the genus *Acinetobacter.* **H. vagini′cola,** Acinetobacter calcoaceticus.

heritability (her″it-ah-bil′it-e) the quality of being heritable; a measure of the extent to which a phenotype is influenced by the genotype.

hermaphroditism (her-maf′rah-dīt-izm) a state characterized by the presence of both ovarian and testicular tissues and of ambiguous morphologic criteria of sex; see also *pseudohermaphroditism.* **bilateral h.,** that in which gonadal tissue typical of both sexes occurs on each side of the body. **false h.,** pseudohermaphroditism. **lateral h.,** presence of gonadal tissue typical of one sex on one side of the body and tissue typical of the other sex on the opposite side. **transverse h.,** that in which the external genital organs are typical of one sex and the gonads typical of the other sex. **true h.,** see *hermaphroditism.*

hermetic (her-met′ik) impervious to air.

hernia (hern′e-ah) protrusion of a portion of an organ or tissue through an abnormal opening. **her′nial,** adj. **abdominal h.,** one through the abdominal wall. **Barth's h.,** one between the serosa of the abdominal wall and that of a persistent vitelline duct. **Béclard's h.,** femoral hernia at the saphenous opening. **Bochdalek's h.,** congenital posterolateral diaphragmatic hernia, with extrusion of bowel and other abdominal viscera into the thorax; due to failure of closure of the pleuroperitoneal hiatus. **h. ce′rebri,** protrusion of brain substance through the skull. **Cloquet's h.,** crural h., pectineal. **complete h.,** one in which the sac and its contents have passed through the hernial orifice. **diaphragmatic h.,** hernia through the diaphragm. **diverticular h.,** protrusion of a congenital diverticulum of the gut. **epigastric h.,** a hernia through the linea alba above the navel. **extrasaccular h.,** sliding h. **fat h.,** hernial protrusion of peritoneal fat through the abdominal wall. **femoral h.,** protrusion of a loop of intestine into the femoral canal. **gastroesophageal h.,** hiatal hernia in which the distal esophagus and part of the stomach protrude into the thorax. **Hesselbach's h.,** femoral hernia with a pouch through the cribriform fascia. **hiatal h., hiatus h.,** protrusion of any structure through the esophageal hiatus of the diaphragm. **Holthouse's h.,** an inguinal hernia that has turned outward into the groin. **incarcerated h.,** a hernia so occluded that it cannot be returned by manipulation; it may or may not be strangulated. **incisional h.,** one occurring through an old abdominal incision. **inguinal h.,** hernia into the inguinal canal. **intermuscular h., interparietal h.,** an interstitial hernia lying between one or another of the fascial or muscular planes of the abdomen. **interstitial h.,** one in which a knuckle of intestine lies between two layers of the abdominal wall. **ischiatic h.,** hernia through the sacrosciatic foramen. **labial h.,** one into a labium majus. **obturator h.,** a protrusion through obturator foramen. **paraesophageal h.,** hiatal hernia in which part or almost all of the stomach protrudes through the hiatus into the thorax to the left of the esophagus, with the gastroesophageal junction remaining in place. **properitoneal h.,** an interstitial hernia lying between the parietal peritoneum and the transverse fascia. **reducible h.,** one that can be returned by manipulation. **retrograde h.,** herniation of two loops of intestine, the portion between the loops lying within the abdominal wall. **Richter's h.,** incarcerated or strangulated hernia in which only a portion of the circumference of the bowel wall is involved. **scrotal h.,** inguinal hernia which has passed into the scrotum. **sliding h.,** hernia of the cecum (on the right) or the sigmoid colon (on the left) in which the wall of the viscus forms a portion of the hernial sac, the remainder of the sac being formed by the parietal peritoneum. **sliding hiatal h.,** hiatal hernia in which the upper stomach and the cardioesophageal junction protrude upward into the posterior mediastinum; the protrusion, which may be fixed or intermittent, is partially covered by a peritoneal sac. **strangulated h.,** incarcerated hernia so tightly constricted as to compromise the blood supply of the hernial sac, leading to gangrene of the sac and its contents. **synovial h.,** protrusion of the inner lining membrane through the stratum fibrosum of a joint capsule. **umbilical h.,** herniation of part of the umbilicus, the defect in the abdominal wall and protruding bowel being covered with skin and subcutaneous tissue. **h. u'teri inguina'le,** see *persistent müllerian duct syndrome.* **vaginal h.,** hernia into the vagina; colpocele. **ventral h.,** hernia through the abdominal wall.

herniation (hern"e-a'shin) abnormal protrusion of an organ or other body structure through a defect or natural opening in a covering membrane, muscle, or bone. **h. of nucleus pul-**

posus, rupture or prolapse of the nucleus pulposus into the spinal cord.

hernioplasty (hern'e-o-plas"te) operation for the repair of hernia.

herniorrhaphy (hern"e-or'ah-fe) surgical repair of hernia, with suturing.

herniotomy (hern"e-ot'ah-me) a cutting operation for the repair of hernia.

heroin (hĕr'ro-in) diacetylmorphine; a highly addictive morphine derivative, $C_{21}H_{23}NO_5$; the importation of heroin and its salts into the United States, as well as its use in medicine, is illegal.

herpangina (her"pan-ji'nah) an infectious febrile disease due to a coxsackievirus, marked by vesicular or ulcerated lesions on the fauces or soft palate.

herpes (her'pēz) any inflammatory skin disease marked by the formation of small vesicles in clusters; the term is usually restricted to such diseases caused by herpesviruses and is used alone to refer to *herpes simplex* or to *herpes zoster.* **herpet'ic,** adj. **h. febri'lis,** see *h. simplex.* **genital h., h. genita'lis,** herpes simplex of the genitals; in women, the vesicular stage may give rise to confluent painful ulcerations and may be accompanied by neurologic symptoms. **h. gestatio'nis,** a variant of dermatitis herpetiformis peculiar to pregnant women, and clearing upon termination of pregnancy. **h. progenita'lis,** genital h. **h. sim'plex,** an acute viral disease marked by groups of vesicles on the skin, often on the borders of the lips or nares (*cold sores*), or on the genitals (*genital h.*); it often accompanies fever (*fever blisters, h. febrilis*). **h. zos'ter,** shingles; an acute, unilateral, self-limited inflammatory disease of cerebral ganglia and the ganglia of posterior nerve roots and peripheral nerves in a segmented distribution, caused by the chickenpox virus, and characterized by groups of small vesicles in the cutaneous areas along the course of affected nerves, and associated with neuralgic pain. **h. zos'ter ophthal'micus,** herpes zoster involving the ophthalmic nerve, with a vesicular erythematous rash along the nerve path (forehead, eyelid, and cornea) preceded by lancinating pain; there is iridocyclitis, and corneal involvement may lead to keratitis and corneal anesthesia. **h. zos'ter o'ticus,** Ramsey Hunt syndrome.

herpesvirus (her"pēz-vi'ris) any of a group of DNA viruses which includes the etiologic agents of herpes simplex, herpes zoster, chickenpox, and cytomegalic inclusion disease in humans, and of pseudorabies and other animal diseases.

Herpesvirus hominis (hom'ĭ-nis) the herpesvirus that causes herpes simplex, occurring in two immunological types: type I (primarily nongenital infections) and type II (primarily genital infections).

hersage (ār-sahzh') [Fr.] surgical separation of the fibers of a peripheral nerve.

hertz (hurts) a unit of frequency, equal to one cycle per second. Symbol, Hz.

hesperidin (hes-per'ĭ-din) a flavone glycoside, $C_{28}H_{34}O_{15}$, isolated from the rind of certain citrus fruits; used to reduce capillary permeability.

hetacillin (het″ah-sil′in) a semisynthetic penicillin, $C_{19}H_{23}N_3O_4S$, which is converted in the body to ampicillin, and has actions and uses similar to those of ampicillin.

heter(o)- word element [Gr.], *other; dissimilar.*

heterecious (-e′shis) parasitic on different hosts in various stages of its existence.

heteresthesia (-es-the′ze-ah) variation of cutaneous sensibility on adjoining areas.

heterergic (het″er-ur′jik) having different effects; said of two drugs one of which produces a particular effect and the other does not.

heteroagglutination (het″er-o-ah-gloot″in-a′-shin) agglutination of particulate antigens of one species by agglutinins derived from another species.

heteroantibody (-an″tĭ-bod′e) an antibody combining with antigens originating from a species foreign to the antibody producer.

heteroantigen (-an′tĭ-jin) an antigen originating from a species foreign to the antibody producer.

heteroblastic (-blas′tik) originating in a different kind of tissue.

heterocellular (-sel′ūl-er) composed of cells of different kinds.

heterochromatin (-kro′mah-tin) that state of chromatin in which it is dark-staining, genetically inactive, and tightly coiled.

heterochromia (-kro′me-ah) diversity of color in a part normally of one color. **h. i′ridis,** difference of color in the two irides, or in different areas in the same iris.

heterocrine (het′er-o-krin) secreting more than one kind of matter.

heterocyclic (het″er-o-si′klik) having a closed chain or ring formation including atoms of different elements.

heterocytotropic (-si″to-trop′ik) having an affinity for cells from different species.

heterodermic (-derm′ik) denoting a skin graft from an individual of another species.

heterodont (het′er-o-dont″) having teeth of different shapes, as molars, incisors, etc.

heterodromous (het″er-ah′drah-mis) moving, acting, or arranged in the opposite direction.

heteroerotism (het″er-o-ĕ′rah-tizm) sexual feeling directed toward another person.

heterogamety (-gam′it-e) production by an individual of one sex (as the human male) of unlike gametes with respect to the sex chromosomes. **heterogamet′ic,** adj.

heterogamy (het″er-og′ah-me) reproduction resulting from the union of gametes differing in size and structure. **heterog′amous,** adj.

heterogeneous (-je′ne-is) not of uniform composition, quality, or structure.

heterogenesis (-jen′ĭ-sis) 1. alternation of generations; reproduction differing in character in successive generations. 2. asexual generation. 3. spontaneous generation. **heterogenet′ic,** adj.

heterogony (het″er-og′ah-ne) heterogenesis.

heterograft (het′er-o-graft″) xenograft.

heterohemagglutination (het″er-o-hem″ah-gloot″in-a′shin) agglutination of erythrocytes of one species by a hemagglutinin derived from an individual of a different species.

heterohemolysin (-he-mol′ĭ-sin) a hemolysin which destroys red blood cells of animals of species other than that of the animal in which it is formed; it may occur naturally or be induced by immunization.

heteroimmunity (-im-mūn′it-e) 1. an immune state induced in an individual by immunization with cells of an animal of another species. 2. a state in which an immune response to exogenous antigen (e.g., drugs or pathogens) results in immunopathological changes. **heteroimmune′,** adj.

heterokeratoplasty (-ker′it-o-plas″te) grafting of corneal tissue taken from an individual of another species.

heterokinesis (-ki-ne′sis) differential distribution of sex chromosomes in the developing gametes of a heterogametic organism.

heterologous (het″er-ol′ah-gus) 1. made up of tissue not normal to the part. 2. xenogeneic.

heterolysis (het″er-ol′ĭ-sis) lysis of the cells of one species by lysin from a different species. **heterolyt′ic,** adj.

heteromeric (het″er-o-mĕ′rik) sending processes through one of the commissures to the white matter of the opposite side of the spinal cord; said of neurons.

heterometaplasia (-met″ah-pla′ze-ah) formation of tissue foreign to the part where it is formed.

heterometropia (-mĭ-tro′pe-ah) the state in which the refraction in the two eyes differs.

heteromorphosis (-mor-fo′sis) the development, in regeneration, of an organ or structure different from the one that was lost.

heteromorphous (-mor′fis) of abnormal shape or structure.

heteronomous (het″er-on′ĭ-mis) 1. in biology, subject to different laws of growth; specialized along different lines. 2. in psychology, subject to another's will.

heteronymous (het″er-on′ĭ-mis) standing in opposite relations.

hetero-osteoplasty (het″er-o-os′te-ah-plas″te) osteoplasty with bone taken from an individual of another species.

heterophagosome (het″er-o-fag′ah-sōm) an intracytoplasmic vacuole formed by phagocytosis or pinocytosis, which becomes fused with a lysosome, subjecting its contents to enzymatic digestion.

heterophagy (het″er-of′ah-je) the taking into a cell of exogenous material by phagocytosis or pinocytosis and the digestion of the ingested material after fusion of the newly formed vacuole with a lysosome.

heterophil (het′er-ah-fil″) 1. a granular leukocyte represented by neutrophils in man, but characterized in other mammals by granules which have variable sizes and staining characteristics. 2. heterophilic.

heterophilic (het″er-ah-fil′ik) 1. having affinity for antigens or antibodies other than the one for which it is specific. 2. staining with a type of stain other than the usual one.

heterophoria (-for'e-ah) failure of the visual axes to remain parallel after elimination of visual fusional stimuli. **heterophor'ic,** adj.

heterophthalmia (het″er-of-thal'me-ah) difference in the direction of the visual axes, or in the color, of the two eyes.

Heterophyes (het″er-of'ĭ-ēz) a genus of minute trematode worms parasitic in the intestine of fish-eating mammals.

heteroplasia (-pla'ze-ah) replacement of normal by abnormal tissue; malposition of normal cells. **heteroplas'tic,** adj.

heteroplasty (het'er-ah-plas″te) heterotransplantation.

heteroploidy (-ploi″de) the state of having an abnormal number of chromosomes.

heteropsia (het″er-op'se-ah) unequal vision in the two eyes.

heteropyknosis (het″er-o-pik-no'sis) 1. the quality of showing variations in density throughout. 2. a state of differential condensation observed in different chromosomes, or in different regions of the same chromosome; it may be attenuated (*negative h.*) or accentuated (*positive h.*). **heteropyknot'ic,** adj.

heterosexual (-sek'shoo-il) 1. pertaining to, characteristic of, or directed toward the opposite sex. 2. one who is sexually attracted to persons of the opposite sex.

heterosis (het″er-o'sis) the existence, in the first generation hybrid, of greater vigor than is shown by either parent strain.

heterosporous (het″er-os'per-is) having two kinds of spores, which reproduce asexually.

heterosuggestion (het″er-o-sug-jes'chin) suggestion received from another person, as opposed to autosuggestion.

heterotonia (het″er-o-to'ne-ah) a state characterized by variations in tension or tone. **heteroton'ic,** adj.

heterotopia (-to'pe-ah) displacement or misplacement of parts; the presence of a tissue in an abnormal location. **heterotop'ic,** adj.

heterotransplantation (-trans″plan-ta'shin) transplantation of tissues or cells from one individual to another of a different species (a xenograft).

heterotrophic (het″er-o-trōf'ik) not self-sustaining; said of microorganisms requiring a reduced form of carbon for energy and synthesis.

heterotropia (-tro'pe-ah) strabismus.

heterotypic (-tip'ik) pertaining to, characteristic of, or belonging to a different type. **heterotyp'ical,** adj.

heteroxenous (het″er-ok'sin-is) requiring more than one host to complete the life cycle.

heterozygosity (het″er-o-zi-gos'it-e) the state of having different alleles in regard to a given character. **heterozy'gous,** adj.

heuristic (hūr-is'tik) encouraging or promoting investigation; conducive to discovery.

hex(a)- word element [Gr.], *six.*

hexachlorophene (-klor'ah-fēn) a local antiseptic and detergent for application to the skin,

$C_{13}H_6Cl_6O_2$; also used to combat flukes in ruminants.

hexad (hek'sad) 1. a group or combination of six similar or related entities. 2. an element with a valence of six.

hexadactyly (hek″sah-dak'til-e) the occurrence of six digits on one limb.

hexafluorenium bromide (-flur-en'ĭ-um) a neuromuscular blocking agent, $C_{36}H_{42}Br_2N_2$, used in anesthesiology to prolong and potentiate the skeletal muscle relaxing action of succinylcholine during surgery.

hexamethonium (hek″sah-mĕ-thōn'e-um) a ganglionic blocking agent, $C_{12}H_{30}N_2$, used in the form of salts to produce hypotension.

hexane (hek'sān) a saturated hydrogen obtained by distillation from petroleum.

hexavitamin (-vīt'ah-min) a preparation of vitamins A and D, ascorbic acid, thiamine hydrochloride, riboflavin, and niacinamide.

hexobarbital (hek″so-bar'bit-awl) an ultrashort-acting sedative and hypnotic, $C_{12}H_{16}N_2$-O_3; also used as the sodium salt to induce general anesthesia.

hexocyclium methylsulfate (-si'kle-um) an anticholinergic, $C_{21}H_{36}N_2O_5S$, having antisecretory and antispasmodic activities; used in the management of peptic ulcer and other gastrointestinal disorders accompanied by hyperacidity, hypermotility, and spasm.

hexokinase (-ki'nās) an enzyme that catalyzes the transfer of a high-energy phosphate group of a donor to D-glucose, producing D-glucose-6-phosphate.

hexosamine (hek'sōs-am″in) a nitrogenous sugar in which an amino group replaces a hydroxyl group.

hexose (hek'sōs) a monosaccharide containing six carbon atoms in a molecule.

hexosephosphate (hek″sōs-fos'fāt) an ester of glucose with phosphoric acid, which aids in the absorption of sugar and is important in carbohydrate metabolism.

hexylcaine (hek'sil-kān) a local anesthetic, C_{18}-$H_{23}NO_2$, used as the hydrochloride salt.

hexylresorcinol (hek″sil-rĭ-zor'sĭ-nawl) an anthelmintic for intestinal roundworms and trematodes, $C_{12}H_{18}O_2$.

HF Hageman factor (coagulation Factor XII).

Hf chemical symbol, *hafnium.*

Hg chemical symbol, *mercury* (L., *hydrargyrum*).

Hgb hemoglobin.

HGH human growth hormone.

H.H.S. Department of Health and Human Services; formerly Department of Health, Education, and Welfare (H.E.W.).

hiatus (hi-a'tis), pl. *hia'tus* [L.] a gap, cleft, or opening. **hia'tal,** adj. **aortic h.,** the opening in the diaphragm through which the aorta and thoracic duct pass. **esophageal h.,** the opening in the diaphragm for the passage of the esophagus and the vagus nerves. **saphenous h.,** the depression in the fascia lata bridged by the cribriform fascia and perforated by the great saphenous vein. **semilunar h.,** the groove in the ethmoid bone through which the anterior ethmoidal air cells, the maxillary sinus, and sometimes the frontonasal duct drain via the ethmoid infundibulum.

hibernation (hi″ber-na′shin) the dormant state in which certain animals pass the winter, marked by narcosis and by sharp reduction in body temperature and metabolism. **artificial h.,** a state of reduced metabolism, muscle relaxation, and a twilight sleep resembling narcosis, produced by controlled inhibition of the sympathetic nervous system and causing attenuation of the homeostatic reactions of the organism.

hibernoma (hi″ber-no′mah) a rare benign tumor made up of large polyhedral cells with a coarsely granular cytoplasm, occurring on the back or around the hips; so called because it resembles the dorsal fat pads of hibernating animals.

hiccough, hiccup (hik′up) sharp inspiratory sound with spasm of the glottis and diaphragm.

hidr(o)- word element [Gr.], *sweat.*

hidradenitis (hi″drad-in-īt′is) inflammation of the sweat glands. **h. suppurati′va,** a severe, chronic, recurrent suppurative infection of the apocrine sweat glands.

hidradenoid (hi-drad′in-oid) resembling a sweat gland; having components resembling elements of a sweat gland.

hidradenoma (hi″drad-in-o′mah) a general term for tumors of the skin the components of which resemble epithelial elements of sweat glands; they may be nodular (solid) or papillary.

hidrocystoma (hi″dro-sis-to′mah) a retention cyst of a sweat gland.

hidropoiesis (-poi-e′sis) the formation of sweat. **hidropoiet′ic,** adj.

hidroschesis (hi-dros′kis-is) anhidrosis.

hidrotic (hi-drot′ik, hi-drot′ik) pertaining to, characterized by, or causing sweating.

hilitis (hi-līt′is) inflammation of a hilus.

hilum (hi′lum) hilus.

hilus (hi′lus), pl. *hi′li* [L.] a depression or pit on an organ, giving entrance and exit to vessels and nerves. **hi′lar,** adj.

hindbrain (hīnd′brān) rhombencephalon: 1. the part of the brain developed from the posterior of the three primary brain vesicles, comprising the metencephalon and myelencephalon. 2. the most caudal of the three primary brain vesicles.

hindfoot (-foot) the back of the foot, comprising the region of the talus and calcaneus.

hindgut (-gut) the embryonic structure from which the caudal intestine, chiefly the colon, is formed.

hip (hip) coxa; the area lateral to and including the hip joint; loosely, the hip joint. **snapping h.,** slipping of the hip joint, sometimes with an audible snap, due to slipping of a tendinous band over the greater trochanter.

hippo (hip′o) ipecac.

hippocampus (hip″o-kam′pus), pl. *hippocam′pi* [L.] a curved elevation in the floor of the inferior horn of the lateral ventricle; a functional component of the limbic system, its efferent projections form the fornix. **hippocam′pal,** adj. **h. ma′jor,** hippocampus. **h. mi′nor,** calcar avis.

Hippocrates (hip-pok′rah-tēz) the Greek physician (5th century B.C.) regarded as the "Father of Medicine." Many of his writings and those of his school have survived, among which appears the Hippocratic oath, the ethical guide of the medical profession. **hippocrat′ic,** adj.

hippuria (hĭ-pūr′e-ah) an excess of hippuric acid in the urine.

hippuric acid (hĭ-pūr′ik) $C_6H_5 \cdot CO \cdot NH \cdot CH_2 \cdot$- COOH, formed by conjugation of benzoic acid and glycine.

hippus (hip′us) abnormal exaggeration of the rhythmic contraction and dilation of the pupil, independent of changes in illumination or in fixation of the eyes.

hirci (hir′si), sing. *hir′cus* [L.] the hairs growing in the axilla.

hircus (her′kus) see *hirci.*

hirsutism (-izm) abnormal hairiness, especially in women.

hirudicide (hĭ-rōōd′is-īd) an agent that is destructive to leeches. **hirudici′dal,** adj.

hirudin (hĭ-rōōd′in) the active principle of the buccal secretion of leeches; it prevents coagulation by acting as an antithrombin.

Hirudinea (hir″u-din′e-ah) a class of annelids, the leeches.

Hirudo (hĭ-rōōd′o) a genus of leeches, including *H. medicina′lis,* formerly used extensively for drawing blood.

hist(io)(o)- word element [Gr.], *tissue.*

histamine (his′tah-mēn, -min) an amine, C_5H_9-N_3, produced by decarboxylation of histidine, found in all body tissues. It induces capillary dilation, which increases capillary permeability and lowers blood pressure; contraction of most smooth muscle tissue; increased gastric acid secretion; and acceleration of the heart rate. It is also a mediator of immediate hypersensitivity. There are two types of cellular receptors of histamine: H_1 receptors, which mediate contraction of smooth muscle and capillary dilation; and H_2 receptors, which mediate acceleration of heart rate and promotion of gastric acid secretion. Both H_1 and H_2 receptors mediate the contraction of vascular smooth muscle. Histamine may also be a neurotransmitter in the central nervous system. It is used as a diagnostic aid in testing gastric secretion and in the diagnosis of pheochromocytoma. **histamin′ic,** adj.

histaminergic (-ur′jic) pertaining to the effects of histamine at histamine receptors of target tissues.

histidase (his′tĭ-dās) an enzyme of the liver that converts histidine to urocanic acid.

histidine (his′tĭ-din, -dēn) an amino acid obtainable from many proteins by the action of sulfuric acid and water; it is essential for optimal growth in infants. Its decarboxylation results in formation of histamine.

histidinemia (his″tĭ-din-ēm′e-ah) a hereditary metabolic defect marked by excessive histidine in the blood and urine due to deficient histidase activity; many affected persons show mild mental retardation and disordered speech development.

histidinuria (his″tĭ-din-ūr′e-ah) an excess of histidine in the urine; see *histidinemia*.

histiocyte (his′te-ah-sīt″) a large phagocytic interstitial cell of the reticuloendothelial system; macrophage. **histiocyt′ic,** adj.

histiocytosis (-si-to′sis) a condition marked by an abnormal appearance of histiocytes in the blood. **h. X,** a generic term that embraces eosinophilic granuloma, Letterer-Siwe disease, and Hand-Schüller-Christian disease.

histiogenic (-jen′ik) histogenous.

histoblast (his′tah-blast) a tissue-forming cell.

histochemistry (his″to-kem′is-tre) that branch of histology dealing with the identification of chemical components in cells and tissues. **histochem′ical,** adj.

histoclinical (-klin′ĭ-k'l) combining histological and clinical evaluation.

histocompatibility (-kom-pat″ĭ-bil′it-e) that quality of being accepted and remaining functional; said of that relationship between the genotypes of donor and host in which a graft generally will not be rejected, a relationship determined by the presence of compatible HLA antigens. **histocompat′ible,** adj.

histodifferentiation (-dif″er-en″she-a′shin) the acquisition of tissue characteristics by cell groups.

histogenesis (-jen′is-is) the formation or development of tissues from the undifferentiated cells of the germ layer of the embryo. **histogenet′ic,** adj.

histogenous (his-toj′in-is) formed by the tissues.

histogram (his′tah-gram) a graph in which values found in a statistical study are represented by vertical bars or rectangles.

histoid (his′toid) 1. developed from but one kind of tissue. 2. like one of the tissues of the body.

histoincompatibility (his″to-in″kom-pat″ĭ-bil′it-e) the quality of not being accepted or not remaining functional; said of that relationship between the genotypes of donor and host in which a graft generally will be rejected. **histoincompat′ible,** adj.

histokinesis (-ki-ne′sis) movement in the tissues of the body.

histology (his-tol′ah-je) that department of anatomy dealing with the minute structure, composition, and function of tissues. **histolog′ic, histolog′ical,** adj. **pathologic h.,** the science of diseased tissues.

histolysis (his-tol′ĭ-sis) dissolution or breaking down of tissues. **histolyt′ic,** adj.

histoma (his-to′mah) any tissue tumor.

Histomonas (his-tom′o-nas) a genus of protozoa parasitic in the cecum, liver, and other tissues of various fowl.

histomoniasis (his″to-mon-i′ah-sis) infection with *Histomonas.* **h. of turkeys,** blackhead; an infectious disease of turkeys due to *Histomonas meleagridis,* with intestinal and hepatic lesions and dark discoloration of the comb.

histone (his′tōn) a simple protein, soluble in water and insoluble in dilute ammonia, found combined as salts with acidic substances, e.g., the protein combined with nucleic acid or the globin of hemoglobin.

histophysiology (-fiz″e-ol′ah-je) the correlation of function with the microscopic structure of cells and tissues.

Histoplasma (-plaz′mah) a genus of fungi, including *H. capsula′tum,* the cause of histoplasmosis in man.

histoplasmin (-plaz′min) a preparation of growth products of *Histoplasma capsulatum,* injected intracutaneously as a test for histoplasmosis.

histoplasmoma (-plaz-mo′mah) a rounded granulomatous density of the lung due to infection with *Histoplasma capsulatum;* seen radiographically as a coin-shaped lesion.

histoplasmosis (-plaz-mo′sis) infection with *Histoplasma capsulatum;* it is usually asymptomatic but may cause acute pneumonia, or disseminated reticuloendothelial hyperplasia with hepatosplenomegaly and anemia, or an influenza-like illness with joint effusion and erythema nodosum. Reactivated infection involves the lungs, meninges, heart, peritoneum, and adrenals. **ocular h.,** disseminated choroiditis resulting in scars in the periphery of the fundus near the optic nerve, and characteristic disciform macular lesions; *Histoplasma capsulatum* is implicated strongly as the causative agent.

histothrombin (-throm′bin) thrombin derived from connective tissue.

histotomy (his-tot′ah-me) dissection of tissues; microtomy.

histotoxic (his″tah-tok′sik) poisonous to tissue.

histotroph (his′tah-trōf) the sum total of nutritive substances supplied to the embryo in viviparous animals from sources other than the maternal blood.

histotrophic (his″tah-trōf′ik) 1. encouraging formation of tissue. 2. pertaining to histotroph.

histotropic (-trop′ik) having affinity for tissue cells.

histrionism (his′tre-in-izm″) a morbid or hysterical adoption of an exaggerated manner and gestures. **histrion′ic,** adj.

HIV human immunodeficiency virus.

hives (hīvz) urticaria.

Hl latent hyperopia.

HLA see under *antigen.*

Hm manifest hyperopia.

HMO health maintenance organization.

Ho chemical symbol, *holmium.*

hock (hok) the tarsal joint or region of the hind leg of the horse and ox.

hodoneuromere (ho″do-nōōr′ah-mēr) a segment of the embryonic trunk with its pair of nerves and their branches.

hol(o)- word element [Gr.], *entire; whole.*

holandric (hol-an′drik) inherited exclusively through the male descent; transmitted through genes located on the Y chromosome.

holism (hol′izm) the conception of man as a functioning whole. **holis′tic,** adj.

holmium (hol′me-um) chemical element (*see table*), at. no. 67, symbol Ho.

holoblastic (-blas′tik) undergoing cleavage in

which the entire ovum participates; dividing completely.

holocrine (ho'lah-krin) exhibiting glandular secretion in which the entire secretory cell laden with its secretory products is cast off.

holodiastolic (hol″o-di″ah-stol′ik) pertaining to the entire diastole.

holoendemic (-en-dem′ik) affecting practically all the residents of a particular region.

holoenzyme (-en′zīm) the active compound formed by combination of a coenzyme and an apoenzyme.

holography (hol-og′rah-fe) the lensless recording of three-dimensional images on film by means of laser beams.

holophytic (-fit′ik) obtaining food like a plant; said of certain protozoa.

holoprosencephaly (-pros″en-sef′ah-le) developmental failure of cleavage of the prosencephalon with a deficit in midline facial development and with cyclopia in the severe form; sometimes due to trisomy 13–15.

holorachischisis (-rah-kis′kĭ-sis) fissure of the entire vertebral column with prolapse of the entire spinal cord.

holozoic (-zo′ik) having the nutritional characters of an animal, i.e., digesting protein.

homaluria (hom″il-ūr′e-ah) production and excretion of urine at a normal, even rate.

homatropine (ho-mă′trah-pin) the tropine ester of mandelic acid, $C_{16}H_{21}NO_3$, having anticholinergic effects similar to but weaker than those of atropine; used as a mydriatic, cycloplegic, and as an inhibitor of gastric spasm and secretion.

homaxial (ho-mak′se-il) having axes of the same length.

home(o)-, homoe(o)-, homoi(o)- word element [Gr.], *similar; same; unchanging.*

homeopathy (ho″me-op′ah-the) a system of therapeutics based on the administration of minute doses of drugs which are capable of producing in healthy persons symptoms like those of the disease treated. **homeopath′ic**, adj.

homeoplasia (ho″me-o-pla′ze-ah) formation of new tissue like that normal to the part. **homeoplas′tic**, adj.

homeostasis (-sta′sis) a tendency to stability in the normal physiological states of the organism. **homeostat′ic**, adj.

homeotherapy (-thĕ′rah-pe) treatment or prevention of disease with a substance similar to the causative agent of the disease.

homergic (hōm-ur′jik) having the same effect; said of two drugs each of which produces the same overt effect.

Homo (ho′mo) [L.] the genus of primates containing the single species *H. sapiens* (man).

hom(o)- 1. word element [Gr.], *same.* 2. chemical prefix indicating addition of one CH_2 group to the main compound.

homobiotin (ho″mo-bi′it-in) a homologue of biotin having an additional CH_2 group in the side chain and acting as a biotin antagonist.

homocarnosine (-kar′nah-sēn) a dipeptide consisting of γ-aminobutyric acid and histidine; it is a normal constituent of the human brain.

homocysteine (-sis-te′in) a transmethylation product of methionine; it is an intermediate in the synthesis of cystine.

homocystine (-sis-tēn) a homologue of cystine from demethylation of methionine.

homocystinuria (-sis″tin-ūr′e-ah) an inborn error of sulfur amino acid metabolism due to lack of cystathionine synthase; it is characterized by homocystine in the urine and by mental retardation, hepatomegaly, ectopia lentis, and cardiovascular and skeletal disorders.

homocytotropic (-sīt″ah-trop′ik) having an affinity for cells of the same species.

homodromous (ho-mah′drah-mis) moving or acting in the same or in the usual direction.

homogametic (ho″mo-gah-met′ik) having only one kind of gametes with respect to the sex chromosomes, as in the human female.

homogenate (ho-moj′in-āt) material obtained by homogenization.

homogeneous (-je′ne-is) of uniform quality, composition, or structure throughout.

homogenesis (-jen′ĭ-sis) reproduction by the same process in each generation. **homogenet′ic**, adj.

homogenize (ho-moj′in-īz) to render homogeneous.

homogentisic acid (ho″mo-jen-tis′ik) 2,5-dihydyroxyphenyl acetic acid, an intermediate product of the metabolism of tyrosine and phenylalanine, which is ultimately metabolized to acetone; see also *alkapton bodies* and *alkaptonuria.*

homograft (ho′mah-graft) allograft.

homologous (hah-mol′ah-gus) 1. corresponding in structure, position, origin, etc. 2. allogeneic.

homologue (hom′ah-log) 1. any homologous organ or part. 2. in chemistry, one of a series of compounds distinguished by addition of a CH_2 group in successive members.

homolysin (hah-mol′ĭ-sin) a lysin produced by injection into the body of an antigen derived from an individual of the same species.

homonomous (hah-mon′im-is) designating homologous serial parts, such as somites.

homonymous (hah-mon′im-is) standing in the same relation.

homophilic (ho″mo-fil′ik) reacting only with a specific antigen.

homoplastic (-plas′tik) 1. pertaining to homoplasty. 2. denoting organs or parts, as the wings of birds and insects, that resemble one another in structure and function but not in origin or development.

homopolysaccharide (ho″mo-pol″e-sak′ah-rīd) a polysaccharide consisting of a single recurring monosaccharide unit.

homorganic (hom″or-gan′ik) produced by the same or by homologous organs.

homosexual (ho″mo-sek′shoo-il) 1. sexually attracted by persons of the same sex. 2. a homosexual individual.

homotopic (ho″mo-top′ik) occurring at the same place upon the body.

homotype (ho′mo-tīp) a part having reversed symmetry with its mate, as the hand. **homotyp′ic,** adj.

homovanillic acid (ho″mo-vah-nil′ik) a major terminal urinary metabolite, converted from dopa, dopamine, and norepinephrine.

homozygosis (ho″mo-zi-go′sis) the formation of a zygote by the union of gametes that have one or more identical alleles.

hoof-bound (hoof′bownd) dryness and contraction of a horse's hoof, causing lameness.

hook (hook) a curved instrument for traction or holding. **Braun's h.,** an instrument used in fetal decapitation. **palate h., posterior h.,** one for raising the palate in rhinoscopy. **Tyrrell's h.,** a slender hook used in eye surgery.

hookworm (hook′wurm) a nematode parasitic in the intestines of man and other vertebrates; two important species are *Necator americanus* (American, or New World, h.) and *Ancylostoma duodenale* (Old World h.). Infection may cause serious illness; see under *disease,* and see *ground itch.*

hoose (hooz) a bronchopulmonary disease of cattle, sheep, and swine caused by nematodes.

hordeolum (hor-de′ah-lum) stye; a localized, purulent, inflammatory infection of a sebaceous gland (meibomian or zeisian) of the eyelid; *external h.* occurs on the skin surface at the edge of the lid, *internal h.* on the conjunctival surface.

horizon (hah-ri′zin) a specific anatomic stage of embryonic development, of which 23 have been defined, beginning with fertilization and ending with the fetal stage.

hormion (hor′me-on) point of union of the sphenoid bone with the posterior border of vomer.

hormone (hor′mōn) a chemical substance produced in the body which has a specific regulatory effect on the activity of certain cells or a certain organ or organs. **hormo′nal,** adj. **adrenocortical h.,** any of the corticosteroids elaborated by the adrenal cortex, the major ones being the glucocorticoids and mineralocorticoids, and including some androgens, progesterone, and perhaps estrogens. **adrenocorticotropic h. (ACTH),** corticotropin. **adrenomedullary h's,** substances secreted by the adrenal medulla, including epinephrine and norepinephrine. **androgenic h's,** the masculinizing hormones: androsterone and testosterone. **antidiuretic h. (ADH),** vasopressin. **corpus luteum h.,** progesterone. **cortical h.,** adrenocortical h. **follicle-stimulating h. (FSH),** one of the gonadotropic hormones of the anterior pituitary, which stimulates the growth and maturation of graafian follicles in the ovary, and stimulates spermatogenesis in the male. See also *menotropins.* **follicle-stimulating hormone releasing h., (FSH-RH),** gonadotropin releasing h. **gonadotropic h.,** gonadotropin. **gonadotropin releasing h. (Gn-RH),** a decapeptide hormone of the hypothalamus, which stimulates the release of follicle-stimulating hormone and luteinizing hormone from the pituitary gland; used in the differential diagnosis of hypothalamic, pituitary, and gonadal dysfunction. **growth h.**

(GH), a substance that stimulates growth, especially a secretion of the anterior pituitary, that directly influences protein, carbohydrate, and lipid metabolism and controls the rate of skeletal and visceral growth. **growth hormone release inhibiting h.,** somatostatin. **growth hormone releasing h. (GH-RH),** one elaborated by the hypothalamus, which stimulates the release of growth hormone from the pituitary gland. **interstitial cell-stimulating h.,** luteinizing h. **lactation h., lactogenic h.,** prolactin. **luteinizing h.,** a gonadotropic hormone of the anterior pituitary gland, acting with follicle-stimulating hormone, to cause ovulation of mature follicles and secretion of estrogen by thecal and granulosa cells of the ovary; it is also concerned with corpus luteum formation. In the male, it stimulates development of the interstitial cells of the testes and their secretion of testosterone. **luteinizing hormone releasing h. (LH-RH),** gonadotropin releasing h. **luteotropic h.,** luteotropin. **melanocyte-stimulating h. (MSH),** a peptide secreted by the adenohypophysis in man and in the rhomboid fossa in lower vertebrates, influencing melanin formation and deposition in the body, and causing color changes in the skin of amphibians, fishes, and reptiles. **neurohypophyseal h's,** those stored and released by the neurohypophysis, i.e., oxytocin and vasopressin. **ovarian h's,** those secreted by the ovary, including the estrogens and gestagens. **parathyroid h.,** a polypeptide hormone secreted by the parathyroid glands, which influences calcium and phosphorus metabolism and bone formation. **placental h.,** one secreted by the placenta, including chorionic gonadotropin, relaxin, and other substances having estrogenic, progestational, or adrenocorticoid activity. **plant h.,** phytohormone. **progestational h.,** 1. progesterone. 2. [pl.] see under *agent.* **sex h's,** hormones having estrogenic *(female sex h's)* or androgenic *(male sex h's)* activity. **somatotrophic h., somatotropic h.,** growth h. **somatotropin release inhibiting h.,** somatostatin. **somatotropin releasing h. (SRH),** growth hormone releasing h. **thyroid h's,** thyroxine, calcitonin, and triiodothyronine; or in the singular, thyroxine and/or triiodothyronine. **thyrotropic h.,** thyrotropin. **thyrotropin releasing h. (TRH),** a tripeptide hormone of the hypothalamus, which stimulates release of thyrotropin from the pituitary gland. In humans, it also acts as a prolactin releasing factor. It is used in the diagnosis of mild hyperthyroidism and Graves' disease, and in differentiating between primary, secondary, and tertiary hypothyroidism.

hormonogen (hor′mon-ah-jen″) prohormone.

horn (horn) cornu; a pointed projection such as the paired processes on the head of various animals; any horn-shaped structure. **horn′y,** adj. **cicatricial h.,** a hard, dry outgrowth from a cicatrix, commonly scaly and rarely osseus. **cutaneous h.,** a horny excrescence on the skin, commonly on the face or scalp. **h. of pulp,** an extension of the pulp into an accentuation of the roof of the pulp chamber directly under a cusp or a developmental lobe of the tooth.

h. of spinal cord, the horn-shaped structure, anterior or posterior, seen in transverse section of the spinal cord; the anterior horn is formed by the anterior column of the cord, the posterior by the posterior column.

horopter (hor-op'ter) the sum of all points seen in binocular vision with the eyes fixed.

horror (hor'er) dread; terror. **h. autotox'icus,** self-tolerance.

horsepox (hors'poks) a mild form of smallpox affecting horses.

hospice (hos'pis) a facility that provides palliative and supportive care for terminally ill patients and their families, either directly or on consulting basis.

hospital (hos'pit'l) an institute for the treatment of the sick. **lying-in h., maternity h.,** one for the care of obstetric patients. **open h.,** 1. a mental hospital, or section of a hospital, without locked doors or other forms of physical restraint. 2. one to which physicians who are not staff members may send their own patients and supervise their treatment. **teaching h.,** one that conducts formal educational programs or courses of instruction that lead to granting of recognized certificates, diplomas, or degrees, or that are required for professional certification or licensure.

hospitalization (hos''pit'l-iz-a'shin) 1. the placing of a patient in a hospital for treatment. 2. the term of confinement in a hospital. **partial h.,** a psychiatric treatment program for patients who do not need full-time hospitalization, involving a special facility or an arrangement within a hospital setting to which the patient may come for treatment during the day only, overnight, or over the weekend.

host (hōst) 1. an organism that harbors or nourishes another organism (the parasite). 2. the recipient of an organ or other tissue derived from another organism (the donor). **accidental h.,** one that accidentally harbors an organism that is not ordinarily parasitic in the particular species. **definitive h., final h.,** the organism in which a parasite passes its adult and sexual existence. **intermediate h.,** the organism in which a parasite passes its natural or nonsexual existence. **paratenic h.,** an animal acting as a substitute intermediate host of a parasite, usually having acquired the parasite by ingestion of the original host. **primary h.,** definitive h. **reservoir h.,** an animal (or species) that is infected by a parasite and which serves as a source of infection for man or another species.

hot line (hot līn) round-the-clock telephone assistance for those in need of crisis intervention, and staffed by nonprofessionals with mental health professionals serving as advisors or in a back-up capacity.

H.P. house physician.

HTLV human T-cell leukemia/lymphoma virus.

hum (hum) a low, steady, prolonged sound. **venous h.,** a continuous blowing, singing, or humming murmur heard on auscultation over the right jugular vein in the sitting or erect position; it is an innocent sign that is obliter-ated on assumption of the recumbent position or on exerting pressure over the vein.

humectant (hu-mek'tint) 1. moistening. 2. a moistening or diluent medicine.

humerus (hu'mer-is), pl. *hu'meri* [L.] see *Table of Bones.*

humor (hu'mer), pl. *humo'res, humors* [L.] any fluid or semifluid of the body. **hu'moral,** adj. **aqueous h.,** the fluid produced in the eye and filling the spaces (anterior and posterior chambers) in front of the lens and its attachments. **ocular h.,** either of the humors (aqueous or vitreous) of the eye. **vitreous h.,** 1. the fluid portion of the vitreous body. 2. vitreous body.

humpback (hump'bak) kyphosis.

hunchback (hunch'bak) 1. kyphosis. 2. a person with kyphosis.

hunger (hung'ger) a craving, as for food. **air h.,** a distressing dyspnea occurring in paroxysms.

HVL half-value layer.

hyal(o)- word element [Gr.], *glassy.*

hyalin (hi'ah-lin) a translucent albuminoid product of amyloid degeneration.

hyaline (hi'ah-lin) glassy and transparent or nearly so.

hyalinosis (hi''ah-lin-o'sis) hyaline degeneration.

hyalitis (hi''ah-līt'is) inflammation of the vitreous body or the vitreous (hyaloid) membrane. **asteroid h.,** see under *hyalosis.* **suppurative h.,** purulent inflammation of the vitreous body.

hyalogen (hi-al'ah-jen) an albuminous substance occurring in cartilage, vitreous body, etc., and convertible into hyalin.

hyalomere (hi'ah-lo-mēr'') the pale, homogeneous portion of a blood platelet.

Hyalomma (hi''ah-lom'ah) a genus of ticks of Africa, Asia, and Europe; ectoparasites of animals and man, they may transmit disease and cause serious injury by their bite.

hyalomucoid (hi''ah-lo-mu'koid) the mucoid of the vitreous body.

hyalonyxis (-nik'sis) puncturing of the vitreous body.

hyalophagia (-fa'je-ah) the eating of glass.

hyaloplasm (hi'ah-lo-plazm'') 1. the more fluid, finely granular substance of the cytoplasm of a cell. 2. axoplasm. **nuclear h.,** karyolymph.

hyaloserositis (hi''ah-lo-sēr''ah-sīt'is) inflammation of serous membranes, with hyalinization of the serous exudate into a pearly investment of the affected organ. **progressive multiple h.,** Concato's disease.

hyalosis (hi''ah-lo'sis) degenerative changes in the vitreous humor. **asteroid h.,** the presence of spherical or star-shaped opacities in the vitreous humor.

hyalosome (hi-al'o-sōm) a structure resembling the nucleolus of a cell, but staining only slightly.

hyaluronate (hi''ah-lōōr'ah-nāt) a salt or ester of hyaluronic acid.

hyaluronic acid (hi''ah-lōōr-on'ik) a sulfate-free mucopolysaccharide in the intercellular substance of various tissue, especially the skin;

also isolated from the vitreous humor, synovial fluid, umbilical cord., etc.

hyaluronidase (hi″ah-loōr-on′ĭ-dās) an enzyme that catalyzes the hydrolysis of hyaluronic acid, found in leeches, snake and spider venom, and in testes, and produced by various pathogenic bacteria, enabling them to spread through tissues; a preparation from mammalian testes is used to promote absorption and diffusion of solutions injected subcutaneously.

hybenzate (hi-ben′zāt) USAN contraction for o-(4-hydroxybenzoyl)benzoate.

hybrid (hi′brid) an offspring of parents of different strains, varieties, or species.

hybridoma (hi″brid-o′mah) a cell culture consisting of a clone of a hybrid cell formed by fusing cells of different kinds.

hyclate (hi′klāt) USAN contraction for monohydrochloride hemiethanolate hemihydrate.

hydatid (hi′dah-tid) 1. hydatid cyst. 2. any cystlike structure. **h. of Morgagni,** a cystlike remnant of the müllerian duct attached to a testis or to the oviduct. **sessile h.,** the hydatid of Morgagni connected with a testis.

hydatidiform (hi″dah-tid′ĭ-form) resembling a hydatid cyst; see under *mole.*

hydatidosis (hi″dah-tĭ-do′sis) hydatid disease.

hydatidostomy (hi″dah-tĭ-dos′tah-me) incision and drainage of a hydatid cyst.

Hydergine (hi′der-jēn) trademark for a preparation of dihydrogenated ergot alkaloids used for the treatment of mood depression and confusion in the elderly.

hydr(o)- word element [Gr.], *hydrogen; water.*

hydragogue (hi′drah-gog) 1. producing watery discharge, especially from the bowels. 2. a cathartic that causes watery purgation.

hydralazine (hi-dral′ah-zēn) an antihypertensive, $C_8H_8N_4$, used as the hydrochloride salt.

hydranencephaly (hi″dran-en-sef′ah-le) absence of the cerebral hemispheres, their normal site being occupied by cerebrospinal fluid. **hydranencephal′ic,** adj.

hydrargyria, hydrargyrism (hi″drar-jir′e-ah; hi-drar′jĭ-rizm) mercury poisoning; see *mercury.*

hydrargyrum (hi-drar′jĭ-rum) [L.] mercury.

hydrarthrosis (hi″drar-thro′sis) an accumulation of effused watery fluid in a joint cavity. **hydrarthro′dial,** adj.

hydratase (hi′drah-tās) any enzyme that catalyzes the hydration or dehydration of C—O linkages.

hydrate (hi′drāt) 1. any compound of a radical with water. 2. any salt or other compound containing water of crystallization.

hydration (hi-dra′shin) the absorption of or combination with water.

hydraulics (hi-draw′liks) the science dealing with the mechanics of liquids.

hydrazine (hi′drah-zin) a gaseous diamine, H_4N_2, or any of its substitution derivatives.

hydrencephalomeningocele (hi″dren-sef″ah-lo-mah-ning′go-sēl) hernial protrusion through a cranial defect of meninges containing cerebrospinal fluid and brain substance.

hydriodic acid (hi″dri-od′ik) a gaseous haloid acid, HI; its aqueous solution and syrup have been used as alteratives.

hydroa (hi-dro′ah) a vesicular eruption, with intense itching and burning, occurring on skin surfaces exposed to sunlight.

hydrobromic acid (hi″dro-bro′mik) a gaseous haloid acid, HBr.

hydrocalycosis (hi″dro-kal″ĭ-ko′sis) a usually asymptomatic cystic dilatation of a major renal calix, lined by transitional epithelium and due to obstruction of the infundibulum.

hydrocarbon (-kar′bin) an organic compound that contains carbon and hydrogen only. **alicyclic h.,** one that has cyclic structure and aliphatic properties. **aliphatic h.,** one that does not contain an aromatic ring. **aromatic h.,** one that has cyclic structure and a closed conjugated system of double bonds.

hydrocele (hi′drah-sēl) a circumscribed collection of fluid, especially in the tunica vaginalis of the testis or along the spermatic cord.

hydrocephalocele (-sef′ah-lo-sēl″) encephalocystocele.

hydrocephalus (-sef′ah-lus) a congenital or acquired condition marked by dilatation of the cerebral ventricles, usually occurring secondarily to obstruction of the cerebrospinal fluid pathways, and accompanied by an accumulation of cerebrospinal fluid within the skull; typically, there is enlargement of the head, prominence of the forehead, brain atrophy, mental deterioration, and convulsions. **hydrocephal′ic,** adj. **communicating h.,** that in which there is free access of fluid between the ventricles of the brain and the spinal canal. **h. ex va′cuo,** compensatory replacement by cerebrospinal fluid of the volume of tissue lost in atrophy of the brain. **noncommunicating h.,** that due to obstruction of the flow of cerebrospinal fluid within the brain ventricles or through their exit foramina. **normal-pressure h., normal-pressure occult h.,** dementia, ataxia, and urinary incontinence with enlarged ventricles associated with inadequacy of the subarachnoid spaces, but with normal cerebrospinal fluid pressure. **obstructive h.,** noncommunicating h. **otitic h.,** that caused by spread of inflammation of otitis media to the cranial cavity.

hydrochloric acid (hi″dro-klor′-ik) hydrogen chloride is aqueous solution, HCl, a highly corrosive mineral acid; it is used as a laboratory reagent and is a constituent of gastric juice, secreted by the gastric parietal cells.

hydrochloride (-klor′īd) a salt of hydrochloric acid.

hydrochlorothiazide (-klor″o-thi′ah-zīd) an orally effective diuretic and antihypertensive, $C_7H_8ClN_3O_4S_2$.

hydrocholecystis (-ko″le-sis′tis) distention of the gallbladder with watery fluid.

hydrocholeresis (-ko″lĕ-re′sis) choleresis marked by increased water output, or induction of excretion of bile relatively low in specific gravity, viscosity, and total solid content.

hydrocirsocele (-sir′sah-sēl) hydrocele combined with varicocele.

hydrocodone (-ko′dōn) a semisynthetic product of codeine, $C_{18}H_{21}NO$, having narcotic analgesic effects similar to but more active than those of codeine; used as an antitussive.

hydrocolloid (-kol′oid) a colloid system in which water is the dispersion medium.

hydrocortisone (-kor′tĭ-sōn) the major glucocorticoid, $C_{21}H_{30}O_5$, elaborated by the human adrenal cortex (or *cortisol*, as it is usually referred to by biochemists); it has life-maintaining properties and appreciable mineralocorticoid activity. A synthetic preparation is used in treatment of inflammations, allergies, pruritus, collagen diseases, adrenocortical deficiency, severe status asthmaticus, shock, and certain neoplasms.

hydrocyanic acid (-si-an′ik) hydrogen cyanide; see under *hydrogen.*

HydroDiuril (hi″dro-di′ūr-il) trademark for a preparation of hydrochlorothiazide.

hydroencephalocele (-en-sef′ah-lo-sēl) encephalocystocele.

hydroflumethiazide (-floo″mah-thi′ah-zīd) an antihypertensive and diuretic, $C_8H_8F_3N_3O_4S_2$.

hydrofluoric acid (-flōōr-ik) a gaseous haloid acid, HF, extremely poisonous and corrosive.

hydrogen (hi′dro-jen) chemical element (*see table*), at. no. 1, symbol H; it exists as the mass 1 isotope (*protium, light,* or *ordinary, h.*), mass 2 isotope (*deuterium, heavy h.*), and mass 3 isotope (*tritium*). **h. cyanide,** an extremely poisonous liquid or gas, HCN, used as a rodenticide and insecticide. **h. peroxide,** a strongly disinfectant cleansing and bleaching liquid, H_2O_2, used in dilute solution in water. **h sulfide,** an ill-smelling, colorless, poisonous gas, H_2S.

hydrogenase (-ās″) an enzyme that catalyzes the reduction of various substances by combining them with molecular hydrogen.

hydrokinetic (-ki-net′ik) relating to movement of water or other fluid, as in a whirlpool bath.

hydrokinetics (-ki-net′iks) the science treating of fluids in motion.

hydrolase (hi′drah-lās) one of the six main classes of enzymes, comprising those that catalyze the hydrolytic cleavage of a compound.

hydro-lyase (hi″dro-li′ās) any lyase that removes water from a compound in the form of the water molecule.

hydrolymph (hi′drah-limf) the thin, watery nutritive fluid of certain lower animals.

hydrolysate (hi-drol′ĭ-sāt) any compound produced by hydrolysis. **protein h.,** a sterile solution of amino acids and short-chain peptides; used as a fluid and nutrient replenisher.

hydrolysis (hi-drol′ĭ-sis) the cleavage of a compound by the addition of water, the hydroxyl group being incorporated in one fragment and the hydrogen atom in the other. **hydrolyt′ic,** adj.

hydroma (hi-dro′mah) hygroma.

hydromeningocele (hi″dro-mah-ning′go-sēl) protrusion of the meninges, containing fluid, through a defect in the skull or vertebral column.

hydrometer (hi-drom′it-er) an instrument for determining the specific gravity of a fluid.

hydrometrocolpos (-me″tro-kol′pos) a collection of watery fluid in the uterus and vagina.

hydrometry (hi-drom′ĭ-tre) measurement of specific gravity with a hydrometer.

hydromicrocephaly (hi″dro-mi″krah-sef′ah-le) smallness of the head with an abnormal amount of cerebrospinal fluid.

hydromorphone (-mor′fōn) a morphine alkaloid, $C_{17}H_{19}NO_3$, having narcotic analgesic effects similar to but greater and of shorter duration than those of morphine.

hydromyelia (hi″dro-mi-ēl′e-ah) dilatation of the central canal of the spinal cord with an abnormal accumulation of fluid.

hydromyelomeningocele (-mi″il-o-mĕ-ning′-go-sēl) a defect of the spine marked by protrusion of the membranes and tissue of the spinal cord, forming a fluid-filled sac.

hydromyoma (-mi-o′mah) uterine leiomyoma with cystic degeneration.

hydronephrosis (-nĕ-fro′sis) distention of the renal pelvis and calices with urine, due to obstruction of the ureter, with atrophy of the kidney parenchyma. **hydronephrot′ic,** adj.

hydronium (hi-dro′ne-im) the hydrated proton H_3O^+; it is the form in which the proton (hydrogen ion, H^+) exists in aqueous solution, a combination of H^+ and H_2O.

hydropericarditis (hi″dro-per″ĭ-kar-dīt′is) pericarditis with watery effusion.

hydroperitoneum (-per″it-o-ne′im) ascites.

hydrophilic (-fil′ik) readily absorbing moisture; hygroscopic; having strongly polar groups that readily interact with water.

hydrophobia (hi″drah-fo′be-ah) rabies.

hydrophobic (-fo′bik) 1. pertaining to hydrophobia (rabies). 2. not readily absorbing water, or being adversely affected by water. 3. lacking polar groups and therefore insoluble in water.

hydrophthalmos (hi″drof-thal′mos) distention of eyeball in infantile glaucoma.

hydropic (hi-drop′ik) pertaining to or affected with dropsy.

hydropneumatosis (hi″dro-noo″mah-to′sis) a collection of fluid and gas in the tissues.

hydropneumogony (-noo-mo′go-ne) injection of air into a joint to detect the presence of effusion.

hydropneumoperitoneum (-per″it-o-ne′im) a collection of fluid and gas in the peritoneal cavity.

hydropneumothorax (-thor′aks) a collection of fluid and gas within the pleural cavity.

Hydropres (hi′dro-pres) trademark for a fixed combination preparation of hydrochlorothiazide and reserpine.

hydrops (hi′drops) [L.] abnormal accumulation of serous fluid in the tissues or in a body cavity; dropsy. **fetal h., h. feta′lis,** gross edema of the entire body, associated with severe anemia, occurring in hemolytic disease of the newborn.

hydroquinone (-kwin′ōn) a skin depigmenting agent, $C_6H_6O_2$.

hydrorrhea (-re′ah) a copious watery discharge.

h. gravida′rum, watery discharge from the vagina during pregnancy.

hydrosarcocele (-sar′ko-sēl) hydrocele and sarcocele together.

hydrosol (hi′drah-sawl) a sol in which the dispersion medium is water.

hydrostatics (hi″dro-stat′iks) science of equilibrium of fluids and the pressures they exert. **hydrostat′ic,** adj.

hydrotaxis (-tak′sis) taxis in response to the influence of water or moisture.

hydrothionemia (thi″on-ēm′e-ah) hydrogen sulfide in the blood.

hydrothorax (-thor′aks) a collection of serous fluid within the pleural cavity.

hydrotropism (hi-drah′trah-pizm) a growth response of a nonmotile organism to the presence of water or moisture.

hydrotubation (hi″dro-too-ba′shin) introduction into the uterine tube of hydrocortisone in saline solution followed by chymotrypsin in saline solution to maintain its patency.

hydroureter (-ūr-ēt′er) distention of the ureter with urine or watery fluid, due to obstruction.

hydroxide (hi-drok′sīd) any compound containing a hydroxyl group.

hydroxocobalamin (hi-drok″so-kah-bal′ah-min) an analogue of cyanocobalamin having exceptionally long-acting hematopoietic activity.

hydroxy- chemical prefix indicating the presence of the univalent radical OH.

hydroxyamphetamine (hi-drok″se-am-fet′ah-min) a sympathomimetic amine, $C_9H_{13}NO$; its hydrobromide salt is used as a nasal decongestant, pressor, and mydriatic.

hydroxyapatite (-ap′ah-tīt) an inorganic constituent of bone matrix and teeth, imparting rigidity to these structures.

β-hydroxybutyric acid (hi-drok″se-bu-tir′ik) beta-hydroxybutyric acid.

hydroxychloroquine (-klor′ah-kwin) a drug, $C_{18}H_{26}ClN_3O$, used as the sulfate salt in the treatment of malaria, lupus erythematosus, rheumatoid arthritis, and symptomatic giardiasis.

25-hydroxycholecalciferol (-ko″le-kal-sif′er-ol) a metabolically activated form of cholecalciferol synthesized in the liver.

hydroxyindoleacetic acid (in″dōl-ah-sēt′ik) a product of serotonin metabolism present in cerebrospinal fluid and in increased amount in the urine in carcinoid.

hydroxyl (hi-drok′sil) the univalent radical OH.

hydroxylase (hi-drok′sĭ-lās) any enzyme causing the coupled oxidation of two donors, with incorporation of oxygen into one of them.

hydroxyprogesterone (hi-drok″se-pro-jes′ter-ōn) a synthetic progestin, $C_{27}H_{40}O_4$; used in the treatment of functional uterine bleeding, menstrual abnormalities, threatened abortion, and uterine cancer.

hydroxyproline (-pro′lēn) an amino acid produced in the digestion of hydrolytic decomposition of proteins, especially of collagens.

hydroxyprolinemia (-pro″lin-ēm′e-ah) a disorder of amino acid metabolism characterized by an excess of free hydroxyproline in the plasma and urine, due to a defect in the enzyme hydroxyproline oxidase.

hydroxypropyl methylcellulose (-pro′pil) the propylene glycol ether of methylcellulose; used as a suspending and viscosity-increasing agent and tablet excipient in pharmaceuticals, and applied topically to the conjunctiva to protect the cornea during certain ophthalmic procedures and to lubricate the cornea.

5-hydroxytryptamine (-trip′tah-mēn) serotonin.

hydroxyurea (-ūr-e′ah) an antineoplastic, CH_4-N_2O_2, which is an inhibitor of ribonucleotide reductase; used in the treatment of melanoma, resistant chronic myelocytic leukemia, and recurrent, metastatic, or inoperable ovarian carcinoma.

hydroxyzine (hi-drok′sĭ-zēn) a central nervous system depressant, $C_{21}H_{27}ClN_2O_2$, having antispasmodic, antihistaminic, and antifibrillatory actions; used as the hydrochloride or pamoate salt.

hydruria (hi-droōr′e-ah) excretion of urine of low osmolality or low specific gravity.

hygiene (hi′jēn) science of health and its preservation. **hygien′ic,** adj. **mental h.,** the science dealing with development of healthy mental and emotional reactions and habits. **oral h.,** proper care of the mouth and teeth.

hygienist (hi′je-en″ist) a specialist in hygiene. **dental h.,** an auxiliary member of the dental profession, trained in the art of removing calcareous deposits and stains from surfaces of teeth and in providing additional services and information on prevention of oral disease.

hygro- word element [Gr.], *moisture.*

hygroma (hi-gro′mah) an accumulation of fluid in a sac, cyst, or bursa. **hygrom′atous,** adj. **h. col′li,** a watery tumor of the neck. **cystic h., h. cys′ticum,** see under *lymphangioma.*

hygrometry (hi-grom′ĭ-tre) measurement of moisture in atmosphere.

hygroscopic (hi″gro-skop′ik) readily absorbing moisture.

Hygroton (hi′gro-ton) trademark for a preparation of chlorthalidone.

hymen (hi′min) the membranous fold partially or wholly occluding the external vaginal orifice. **hy′menal,** adj.

hymenolepiasis (-o-lep-i′ah-sis) infection with *Hymenolepis.*

Hymenolepis (-ol′ĭ-pis) a genus of tapeworms, including *H. na′na,* found in rodents, rats, and man, especially children.

hymenology (-ol′ah-je) the science dealing with the membranes of the body.

Hymenoptera (-op′ter-ah) an order of insects with two pairs of well developed membranous wings, like bees and wasps.

hyoepiglottic, hyoepiglottidean (hi″o-ep″ĭ-glot′ik; -ep″ĭ-go-tid′e-in) pertaining to the hyoid bone and epiglottis.

hyoglossal (-glah′s′l) pertaining to the hyoid bone and tongue or to the hyoglossus muscle.

hyoid (hi′oid) shaped like Greek letter upsilon (ʋ); pertaining to the hyoid bone.

hyoscine (hi′ah-sīn) scopolamine.

hyoscyamine (hi″ah-si′ah-mēn) an anticholinergic alkaloid, $C_{17}H_{23}NO_3$, usually obtained from species of *Hyoscyamus* and other solanaceous plants; it is the levorotatory component of racemic atropine with actions and uses similar to those of atropine but with more potent central and peripheral effects.

hyp- see *hypo-*.

hypalgesia (hi″pal-je′ze-ah) diminished sensibility to pain. **hypalge′sic,** adj.

hypamnios (hīp-am′ne-os) deficiency of amniotic fluid.

hypanakinesis (hīp″an-ah-ki-ne′sis) hypokinesia.

hyparterial (hīp″ar-tēr′e-il) beneath an artery.

hypaxial (hi-pak″se-al) ventral to the long axis of the body.

hyper- word element [Gr.], *abnormally increased; excessive.*

hyperacid (-as′id) abnormally or excessively acid.

hyperactivity (-ak-tiv′it-e) excessive activity; hyperkinesia. See *attention-deficit hyperactivity disorder.*

hyperacusis (-ah-ku′sis) an exceptionally acute sense of hearing.

hyperadenosis (-ad″in-o′sis) enlargement of glands.

hyperadiposis (-ad″ĭ-po′sis) extreme fatness.

hyperadrenalism (-ah-drēn′ah-lizm) overactivity of the adrenal glands.

hyperadrenocorticism (-ah-drēn″o-kort′ĭ-sizm) hypersecretion of the adrenal cortex.

hyperaldosteronism (-al″do-stēr′ōn-izm) aldosteronism.

hyperalgesia (-al-je′ze-ah) excessive sensitiveness to pain. **hyperalge′sic,** adj.

hyperalimentation (-al″ĭ-min-ta′shin) the ingestion or administration of a greater than optimal amount of nutrients. **parenteral h.,** intravenous administration of the total nutrient requirements of patients with gastrointestinal dysfunction.

hyperalphalipoproteinemia (-al″fah-lip″o-prōt″e-in-ēm′e-ah) the presence of abnormally high levels of α-lipoproteins in the serum.

hyperammonemia (-ah″mōn-ēm′e-ah) a metabolic disturbance marked by elevated levels of ammonia in the blood.

hyperanakinesia (-an″ah-ki-ne′ze-ah) excessive motor activity. See *attention-deficit hyperactivity disorder.*

hyperaphia (-a′fe-ah) tactile hyperesthesia. **hyperaph′ic,** adj.

hyperarousal (-ah-row′z'l) a state of increased psychological and physiological tension marked by such effects as reduced pain tolerance, insomnia, fatigue, and accentuation of personality traits.

hyperazotemia (-az″o-tēm′e-ah) an excess of nitrogenous matter in the blood.

hyperbaric (-bār′ik) characterized by greater than normal weight; applied to gases under greater than atmospheric pressure, or to a solution of greater specific gravity than another taken as a reference standard.

hyperbarism (-bar′izm) a condition due to exposure to ambient gas pressure or atmospheric pressures exceeding the pressure within the body.

hyperbetalipoproteinemia (-bāt″ah-lip″o-prōt″e-in-ēm′e-ah) increased accumulation of β-lipoproteins in the blood.

hyperbilirubinemia (-bil″ĭ-roo″bin-ēm′e-ah) excess of bilirubin in the blood; classified as conjugated or unconjugated, according to the predominant form of bilirubin present.

hyperbradykininism (-brad″ĭ-ki′nin-izm) a syndrome in which bradykininemia is associated with a fall in systolic blood pressure on standing, increased diastolic pressure and heart rate, and purplish discoloration and ecchymoses over the legs.

hypercalcemia (-kal-sēm′e-ah) an excess of calcium in the blood. **idiopathic h.,** a condition of infants, associated with vitamin D intoxication, characterized by elevated serum calcium levels, increased density of the skeleton, mental deterioration, and nephrocalcinosis.

hypercapnia (-kap′ne-ah) an excess of carbon dioxide in the blood. **hypercap′nic,** adj.

hypercarbia (-kar′be-ah) hypercapnia.

hypercatharsis (-kah-thar′sis) excessive purgation. **hypercathar′tic,** adj.

hypercellularity (-sel″ūl-ar′it-e) abnormal increase in the number of cells present, as in bone marrow. **hypercell′ular,** adj.

hyperchloremia (-klor-ēm′e-ah) an excess of chlorides in the blood. **hyperchlore′mic,** adj.

hyperchlorhydria (-klōr-hi′dre-ah) an excess of hydrochloric acid in the gastric juice.

hypercholesterolemia (-kol-es″ter-ol-ēm′e-ah) an excess of cholesterol in the blood. **hypercholesterole′mic,** adj. **familial h.,** hyperlipoproteinemia (type II).

hyperchromasia (-kro-ma′ze-ah) hyperchromatism.

hyperchromatism (-kro′mit-izm) 1. excessive pigmentation. 2. degeneration of cell nuclei, which become filled with particles of pigment (chromatin). 3. increased staining capacity. **hyperchromat′ic,** adj.

hyperchromia (-kro′me-ah) 1. hyperchromatism. 2. abnormal increase in the hemoglobin content of erythrocytes.

hyperchylia (-kīl′e-ah) excessive secretion of gastric juice.

hyperchylomicronemia (-kīl″o-mi″kro-nēm′e-ah) presence in the blood of an excessive number of particles of fat (chylomicrons).

hypercorticism (-kort″ĭ-sizm) hyperadrenocorticism.

hypercryalgesia (-kri″al-je′ze-ah) excessive sensitiveness to cold.

hypercupremia (-ku-prēm′e-ah) an excess of copper in the blood.

hypercyanotic (-si″ah-not′ik) extremely cyanotic.

hypercythemia (-si-thēm′e-ah) an excess of red blood cells in the blood.

hypercytosis (-si-to′sis) abnormally increased number of cells, especially of leukocytes.

hyperdicrotic (-di-krot′ik) markedly dicrotic.

hyperdistention (-dis-ten′shin) excessive distention.

hyperdynamia (-di-nām′e-ah) excessive muscular activity. **hyperdynam′ic**, adj.

hyperechema (-e-kēm′ah) exaggeration of auditory sensations.

hyperemesis (-em′ĭ-sis) excessive vomiting. **hyperemet′ic**, adj. **h. gravida′rum,** the pernicious vomiting of pregnancy. **h. lacten′tium,** excessive vomiting in nursing babies.

hyperemia (-ēm′e-ah) an excess of blood in a part. **hypere′mic**, adj. **active h., arterial h.,** that due to local or general relaxation of arterioles. **fluxionary h.,** active h. **leptomeningeal h.,** congestion of the pia-arachnoid. **passive h.,** that due to obstruction to flow of blood from the area. **reactive h.,** that due to increase in blood flow after its temporary interruption. **venous h.,** passive h.

hypereosinophilia (-e″ah-sin″ah-fil′e-ah) eosinophilia (2).

hyperequilibrium (-e″kwĭ-lib′re-um) excessive tendency to vertigo.

hyperergasia (-er-ga′ze-ah) excessive functional activity.

hyperesophoria (-es″o-for′e-ah) deviation of the visual axes upward and inward.

hyperesthesia (-es-the′ze-ah) increased sensitivity to stimulation. **hyperesthet′ic**, adj. **acoustic h., auditory h.,** hyperacusia. **cerebral h.,** that which is due to a cerebral lesion. **gustatory h.,** hypergeusesthesia. **muscular h.,** muscular oversensitivity to pain or fatigue. **olfactory h.,** hyperosmia. **oneiric h.,** increased sensitivity or pain during sleep and dreams. **optic h.,** abnormal sensitivity of the eye to light. **tactile h.,** excessive tactile sensibility.

hyperexophoria (-ek″so-for′e-ah) deviation of the visual axes upward and outward.

hyperferremia (-fĕ-rēm′e-ah) an excess of iron in the blood. **hyperferre′mic**, adj.

hyperfibrinogenemia (-fi-brin″ah-jin-ēm′e-ah) excessive fibrinogen in the blood.

hyperfunction (-funk′shin) excessive functioning of a part or organ.

hypergalactia, hypergalactosis (-gah-lak′she-ah; gal″ak-to′sis) excessive secretion of milk. **hypergalac′tous**, adj.

hypergammaglobulinemia (-gam″ah-glob″ūl-in-ēm′e-ah) increased gamma globulins in the blood. **hypergammaglobuline′mic**, adj. **monoclonal h.,** an excess of homogeneous immunoglobulin molecules of a single specificity in the blood following proliferation of a clone of immunoglobulin-producing cells.

hypergenesis (-jen′ĭ-sis) excessive development. **hypergenet′ic**, adj.

hypergeusesthesia, hypergeusia (-gūs″es-the′ze-ah; -gu′ze-ah) abnormal acuteness of the sense of taste.

hypergia (hi-purj′e-ah) 1. hypoergasia. 2. diminished sensitivity in allergy.

hyperglobulia (-glo-būl′e-ah) polycythemia.

hyperglucagonemia (-gloo″kah-gon-ēm′e-ah) abnormally high levels of glucagon in the blood.

hyperglycemic (-gli-sēm′ik) 1. pertaining to, characterized by, or causing hyperglycemia. 2. an agent that increases the glucose level of the blood.

hyperglyceridemia (-glis″er-ĭ-dēm′e-ah) excess of glycerides in the blood.

hyperglycinemia (-gli″sin-ēm′e-ah) a hereditary metabolic disorder involving excessive glycine in the blood and urine. One form is characterized by episodic vomiting, lethargy, dehydration, ketosis, and increased susceptibility to infection; a second form by generalized hypotonia, lethargy, absence of reflexes, and periodic myoclonic jerks.

hyperglycinuria (-gli′sin-ūr′e-ah) an excess of glycine in the urine; see *hyperglycinemia.*

hyperglycogenolysis (-gli″ko-jin-ol′ĭ-sis) excessive glycogenolysis, resulting in excessive dextrose in the body.

hyperglycorrhachia (-or-a′ke-ah) excessive sugar in the cerebrospinal fluid.

hypergonadism (hi″per-go′nad-izm) abnormally increased functional activity of the gonads, with excessive growth and precocious sexual development.

hyperhedonia (-he-dōn′e-ah) morbid increase of the feeling of pleasure in agreeable acts.

hyperhidrosis (-hĭ-dro′sis) excessive perspiration. **hyperhidrot′ic**, adj.

hyperhydration (-hi-dra′shin) abnormally increased water content of the body.

hyperimmune (-im-mūn′) possessing very large quantities of specific antibodies in the serum.

hyperimmunoglobulinemia (-im″ūn-o-glob″u-lin-ēm′e-ah) abnormally high levels of immunoglobulins in the serum.

hyperinsulinism (-in′sūl-in-izm″) 1. excessive secretion of insulin. 2. insulin shock.

hyperirritability (-ir″it-ah-bil′it-e) pathological responsiveness to slight stimuli.

hyperisotonic (-i″so-ton′ik) denoting a solution containing more than 0.45% salt, in which erythrocytes become crenated as a result of exosmosis.

hyperkalemia (-kal-ēm′e-ah) an excess of potassium in the blood; hyperpotassemia. **hyperkale′mic**, adj.

hyperkeratinization (-ker″it-in-i-za′shin) excessive development or retention of keratin in the epidermis.

hyperkeratosis (-kĕ″rah-to′sis) 1. hypertrophy of the horny layer of the skin, or any disease characterized by it. 2. hypertrophy of the cornea. 3. thickening of the horny layer of the skin in cattle, due to ingestion of grease containing high levels of chlorinated hydrocarbons. **hyperkeratot′ic**, adj. **epidermolytic h.,** a hereditary disease, with hyperkeratosis, blisters, and erythema; at birth, the skin is entirely covered with thick, horny, armor-like plates that are soon shed, leaving a raw surface on which the scales re-form. **h. follicula′ris in cu′tem pe′netrans,** a disease marked by keratotic pegs that develop in hair follicles and eccrine ducts, penetrating the epidermis and extending down into the corium, causing foreign-body reaction and pain.

hyperketonemia (-ke″tōn-ēm′e-ah) abnormally increased concentration of ketone bodies in the blood.

hyperkinemia (-ki-nēm′e-ah) abnormally high cardiac output. **hyperkine′mic,** adj.

hyperkinesia (-ki-ne′ze-ah) abnormally increased motor function or activity; see *hyperkinetic syndrome.* **hyperkinet′ic,** adj.

hyperlactation (-lak-ta′shin) lactation in greater than normal amount or for a longer than normal period.

hyperlipemia (-li-pēm′e-ah) elevated concentration of triglycerides in the plasma. **carbohydrate-induced h.,** hyperlipoproteinemia (type IV). **fat-induced h.,** hyperlipoproteinemia (type I).

hyperlipidemia (-lip″i-dēm′e-ah) a general term for elevated concentrations of any or all of the lipids in the plasma.

hyperlipoproteinemia (-lip″o-prōt″e-in-ēm′e-ah) an excess of lipoproteins in the blood, due to a disorder of lipoprotein metabolism. The acquired form occurs secondarily to another disorder or as a result of environmental factors (e.g., diet). The hereditary form is classified into five major phenotypes based on clinical features, enzymatic abnormalities, and serum lipoprotein electrophoretic patterns. *Type I* may be manifested clinically by repeated bouts of abdominal pain and vomiting, recurrent acute pancreatitis, eruptive xanthomas, hepatosplenomegaly, and lipemia retinalis; *Type II* by tendinous and tuberous xanthomas, xanthelasmas, early onset of corneal arcus, and accelerated atherosclerosis; *Type III* chiefly by planar xanthomas; *Type IV* by increased incidence of vascular disease, abnormal glucose tolerance, and family history of diabetes mellitus; and *Type V* by diabetes mellitus, eruptive xanthomas, and recurrent acute pancreatitis.

hyperlithuria (-lĭ-thūr′e-ah) excess of lithic (uric) acid in the urine.

hyperlucency (-loo′sin-se) excessive radiolucency.

hypermagnesemia (-mag″nis-ēm′e-ah) an abnormally large magnesium content of the blood plasma.

hypermastia (-mas′te-ah) 1. the presence of one or more supernumerary mammary glands. 2. hypertrophy of the mammary gland.

hypermenorrhea (-men″or-e′ah) excessive menstrual bleeding, but occurring at regular intervals and being of usual duration.

hypermetabolism (-mĕ-tab′ol-izm) increased metabolism. **extrathyroidal m.,** abnormally elevated basal metabolism unassociated with thyroid disease.

hypermetria (-me′tre-ah) ataxia in which movements overreach the intended goal.

hypermetrope (-mĕ′trōp) hyperope.

hypermetropia (-mĕ-tro′pe-ah) hyperopia.

hypermorph (hi′per-morf) 1. a person who is tall but of low sitting height. 2. in genetics, a mutant gene that shows an increase in the activity it influences. **hypermor′phic,** adj.

hypermotility (hi″per-mo-til′it-e) abnormally increased motility, as of the gastrointestinal tract.

hypermyotrophy (-mi-ah′trah-fe) excessive development of muscular tissue.

hypernasality (-na-zal′it-e) a quality of voice in which the emission of air through the nose is excessive due to velopharyngeal incompetence; it causes deterioration of intelligibility of speech.

hypernatremia (-na-tre′me-ah) an excess of sodium in the blood. **hypernatre′mic,** adj.

hyperneocytosis (-ne″o-si-to′sis) leukocytosis with an excessive number of immature forms of leukocytes.

hypernephroma (-nĕ-fro′mah) renal cell carcinoma whose structure resembles that of adrenocortical tissue.

hypernutrition (-noo-trish′in) overfeeding and its ill effects.

hyperopia (hi″per-o′pe-ah) farsightedness; a visual defect in which parallel light rays reaching the eye come to a focus behind the retina, vision being better for far objects than for near. **hypero′pic,** adj. **absolute h.,** that which cannot be corrected by accommodation. **axial h.,** that due to shortness of the anteroposterior diameter of the eye. **facultative h.,** that which can be entirely corrected by accommodation. **latent h.,** that degree of the total hyperopia corrected by the physiologic tone of the ciliary muscle, revealed by cycloplegic examination. **manifest h.,** that degree of the total hyperopia not corrected by the physiologic tone of the ciliary muscle, revealed by cycloplegic examination. **relative h.,** facultative h. **total h.,** manifest and latent hyperopia combined.

hyperorchidism (-or′kid-izm) excessive functional activity of the testes.

hyperorexia (-or-ek′se-ah) excessive appetite.

hyperorthocytosis (-or″tho-si-to′sis) leukocytosis with a normal proportion of the various forms of leukocytes.

hyperosmolality (-oz″mol-al′it-e) an increase in the osmolality of the body fluids.

hyperosmolarity (-oz″mol-ar′it-e) abnormally increased osmolar concentration.

hyperostosis (-os-to′sis) hypertrophy of bone. **hyperostot′ic,** adj. **h. cra′nii,** hyperostosis involving the cranial bones. **frontal internal h.,** thickening of the inner table of the frontal bone, which may be associated with hypertrichosis and obesity, and most commonly affecting women near menopause. **general cortical h.,** a hereditary disorder beginning during puberty, marked chiefly by osteosclerosis of the skull, mandible, clavicles, ribs, and diaphyses of long bones, associated with elevated blood alkaline phosphatase. **infantile cortical h.,** a disease of young infants, with soft tissue swelling over affected bones, fever, irritability, and periods of remission and exacerbation. **Morgagni's h.,** frontal internal h.

hyperoxaluria (-ok″sil-ūr′e-ah) an excess of oxalate in the urine. **enteric h.,** formation of calcium oxalate calculi in the urinary tract, occurring after extensive resection or disease of the ileum, due to excessive absorption of oxalate from the colon. **primary h.,** an inborn error of metabolism, with excessive urinary excretion of oxalate, nephrolithiasis, nephrocalcinosis, early onset of renal failure, and often a generalized deposit of calcium oxalate.

hyperoxia (-ok′se-ah) an excess of oxygen in the system. **hyperox′ic,** adj.

hyperparasite (-par′ah-sīt) a parasite that preys on a parasite. **hyperparasit′ic,** adj.

hyperparathyroidism (-par″ah-thi′roid-izm) excessive activity of the parathyroid glands. *Primary h.* is associated with neoplasia or hyperplasia; the excess of parathyroid hormone leads to alteration in function of bone cells, renal tubules, and gastrointestinal mucosa. *Secondary h.* occurs when the serum calcium tends to fall below normal, as in chronic renal disease, etc. *Tertiary h.* refers to that due to a parathyroid adenoma arising from secondary hyperplasia caused by chronic renal failure.

hyperperistalsis (-per″ĭ-stal′sis) excessively active peristalsis.

hyperphalangism (-fal′an-jizm) the presence of a supernumerary phalanx on a digit.

hyperphenylalaninemia (-fen″il-al″ah-nin-ēm′e-ah) an excess of phenylalanine in the blood, as in phenylketonuria.

hyperphonesis (-fōn-e′sis) intensification of the sound in auscultation or percussion.

hyperphoria (-for′e-ah) upward deviation of the visual axis of one eye in the absence of visual fusional stimuli.

hyperphosphatasemia (-fos″fit-ās-ēm′e-ah) high levels of alkaline phosphatase in the blood; see *hyperphosphatasia.*

hyperphosphatasia (-fos″fah-ta′ze-ah) a hereditary condition marked by abnormally high alkaline phosphatase levels in the serum and by macrocranium, short neck and thorax, lateral bowing of the femurs, and anterior bowing of the tibias.

hyperphosphaturia (-fos″fah-tōōr′e-ah) an excess of phosphates in the urine.

hyperphrenia (-frēn′e-ah) 1. extreme mental excitement. 2. accelerated mental activity.

hyperpigmentation (-pig″min-ta′shin) abnormally increased pigmentation.

hyperpituitarism (-pĭ-tu′it-er-izm″) a condition due to pathologically increased activity of the pituitary gland, either of the basophilic cells, resulting in basophil adenoma causing compression of the pituitary gland, or of the eosinophilic cells, producing overgrowth, acromegaly, and gigantism (*true h.*).

hyperplasia (-pla′ze-ah) abnormal increase in the number of normal cells in normal arrangement in an organ or tissue, which increases its volume. **hyperplas′tic,** adj.

hyperplasmia (-plaz′me-ah) 1. excess in the proportion of blood plasma to corpuscles. 2. increase in size of erythrocytes due to absorption of plasma.

hyperploidy (hi′per-ploid″e) the state of having more than the typical number of chromosomes in unbalanced sets, as in Down's syndrome.

hyperpnea (hi″purp-ne′ah) abnormal increase in depth and rate of respiration. **hyperpne′ic,** adj.

hyperpolarization (hi″per-pōl″er-iz-a′shin) any increase in the amount of electrical charge separated by the cell membrane, and hence in the strength of the transmembrane potential.

hyperponesis (-pon-e′sis) excessive action-potential output from the motor and premotor areas of the cortex. **hyperponet′ic,** adj.

hyperposia (-po′ze-ah) abnormally increased ingestion of fluids for relatively brief periods.

hyperpotassemia (-pot″ah-se′me-ah) hyperkalemia.

hyperpraxia (-prak′se-ah) abnormal mental activity; restlessness.

hyperprebetalipoproteinemia (-pre-bāt″ah-lip″o-prōt″e-in-ēm′e-ah) an excess of prebetalipoproteins in the blood.

hyperproinsulinemia (-pro-in″sūl-in-ēm′e-ah) elevated levels of proinsulin or proinsulin-like material in the blood.

hyperprolinemia (-pro″lin-ēm′e-ah) a disorder of amino acid metabolism marked by an excess of proline in the body fluids.

hyperprosexia (-pro-sek′se-ah) preoccupation with one idea to the exclusion of all others.

hyperproteosis (-prōt″e-o′sis) a condition due to an excess of protein in the diet.

hyperpsychosis (-si-ko′sis) exaggeration of mental activity with abnormal rapidity of the flow of thought.

hyperpyrexia (-pi-rek′se-ah) excessively high body temperature; hyperthermia. **hyperpyrex′ial, hyperpyret′ic,** adj. **malignant h.,** see under *hyperthermia.*

hyperreactive (-re-ak′tiv) showing a greater than normal response to stimuli.

hyperreninemia (-re″nin-ēm′e-ah) elevated levels of renin in the blood.

hyperresonance (-rez′in-ins) exaggerated resonance on percussion.

hypersalivation (-sal″ĭ-va′shin) ptyalism.

hypersarcosinemia (-sar″ko-sēn-ēm′e-ah) an inborn error of metabolism due to a defect of sarcosine dehydrogenase and marked by elevated levels of sarcosine in the blood.

hypersecretion (-se-kre′shin) excessive secretion.

hypersensitivity (-sen″sĭ-tiv′it-e) a state of altered reactivity in which the body reacts with an exaggerated immune response to a foreign agent. **hypersen′sitive,** adj. **contact h.,** that produced by contact of the skin with a chemical substance having the properties of an antigen or hapten; it includes contact dermatitis. **delayed h.,** a slowly developing increase in cell-mediated (T-lymphocyte) immune response to a specific antigen, as occurs in graft rejection, autoimmune disease, etc. **immediate h.,** antibody-mediated hypersensitivity characterized by release of mediators from reagin-sensitized mast cells, causing increased vascular permeability, edema, and smooth muscle contraction; it includes anaphylaxis and atopy.

hypersomnia (-som′ne-ah) pathologically excessive sleep or drowsiness.

hypersomnolence (hi″per-som′no-lens) a sleep disorder that includes excessive amounts of sleep and excessive daytime sleepiness.

hypersplenism (-splen′izm) a condition characterized by exaggeration of the hemolytic function of the spleen, resulting in deficiency of peripheral blood elements, and by hypercellularity of the bone marrow and splenomegaly.

hypersthenia (-sthēn′e-ah) great strength or tonicity. **hypersthen′ic**, adj.

hypertelorism (-tēl′er-izm) abnormally increased distance between two organs or parts. **ocular h., orbital h.,** increase in the interorbital distance, often associated with cleidocranial or craniofacial dysostosis and sometimes with mental deficiency.

hypertension (-ten′shin) persistently high arterial blood pressure; it may have no known cause (*essential, idiopathic,* or *primary h.*) or be associated with other diseases (*secondary h.*). **accelerated h.,** progressive hypertension with the funduscopic vascular changes of malignant hypertension but without papilledema. **adrenal h.,** that associated with an adrenal tumor which secretes mineral corticosteroids. **borderline h.,** a condition in which the arterial blood pressure is sometimes within the normotensive range and sometimes within the hypertensive range. **Goldblatt h.,** see under *kidney*. **labile h.,** borderline h. **malignant h.,** a severe hypertensive state with papilledema of the ocular fundus and vascular hemorrhagic lesions, thickening of the small arteries and arterioles, left ventricular hypertrophy, and poor prognosis. **ocular h.,** persistently elevated intraocular pressure in the absence of any other signs of glaucoma; it may or may not progress to chronic simple glaucoma. **pale h.,** malignant h. **portal h.,** abnormally increased pressure in the portal circulation. **pulmonary h.,** abnormally increased pressure in the pulmonary circulation. **red h.,** benign h. **renal h.,** that associated with or due to renal disease with a factor of parenchymatous ischemia. **renovascular h.,** that due to occlusive disease of the renal arteries. **systemic venous h.,** elevation of systemic venous pressure, usually detected by inspection of the jugular veins.

hypertensive (-ten′siv) 1. marked by increased blood pressure. 2. an individual with abnormally increased blood pressure.

hyperthecosis (-the-ko′sis) hyperplasia and excessive luteinization of the cells of the inner stromal layer of the ovary.

hyperthelia (-thēl′e-ah) the presence of supernumerary nipples.

hyperthermalgesia (-thurm″il-je′ze-ah) abnormal sensitivity to heat.

hyperthermia (-thurm′e-ah) greatly increased body temperature. **hyperther′mal, hyperther′mic,** adj. **malignant h.,** an autosomal dominant inherited condition affecting patients undergoing general anesthesia, marked by sudden, rapid rise in body temperature, associated with signs of increased muscle metabolism, and, usually, muscle rigidity.

hyperthymia (-thi′me-ah) excessive emotionalism.

hyperthymism (-thi′mizm) excessive activity of the thymus gland.

hyperthyroidism (-thi′roid-izm) excessive thyroid gland activity, marked by increased metabolic rate, goiter, and disturbances in the autonomic nervous system and in creatine metabolism; sometimes used to refer to *Graves′ disease*. **hyperthy′roid,** adj.

hypertonia (-tōn′e-ah) a condition of excessive tone of the skeletal muscles; increased resistance of muscle to passive stretching.

hypertonic (-ton′ik) 1. denoting increased tone or tension. 2. denoting a solution having greater osmotic pressure than the solution with which it is compared.

hypertonicity (-to-nis′it-e) the state or quality of being hypertonic.

hypertrichosis (-trĭ-ko′sis) excessive growth of hair. Cf. *hirsutism*.

hypertriglyceridemia (-tri-glis″er-i-dēm′e-ah) an excess of triglycerides in the blood; a familial form occurs in hyperlipoproteinemia types I and IV.

hypertrophy (hi-pur′trah-fe) enlargement or overgrowth of an organ or part due to increase in size of its constituent cells. **hypertroph′ic,** adj. **ventricular h.,** hypertrophy of the myocardium of a ventricle.

hypertropia (hi″per-tro′pe-ah) strabismus in which there is permanent upward deviation of the visual axis of an eye.

hyperuricemia (-ūr″is-ēm′e-ah) an excess of uric acid in the blood. **hyperurice′mic,** adj.

hypervalinemia (-val″in-ēm′e-ah) an inborn error of metabolism characterized by elevated levels of serum valine, valinuria, and failure to thrive.

hyperventilation (-ven″til-a′shin) abnormally increased pulmonary ventilation, resulting in reduction of carbon dioxide tension, which, if prolonged, may lead to alkalosis.

hyperviscosity (-vis-kos′it-e) excessive viscosity, as of the blood.

hypervitaminosis (-vīt″ah-min-o′sis) a condition due to ingestion of an excess of one or more vitamins; symptom complexes are associated with excessive intake of vitamins A and D. **hypervitaminot′ic,** adj.

hypervolemia (-vol-ēm′e-ah) abnormal increase in the plasma volume in the body.

hypesthesia (hi″pes-the′ze-ah) hypoesthesia.

hypha (hi′fah), pl. *hy′phae* [L.] one of the filaments composing the mycelium of a fungus. **hy′phal,** adj.

hyphedonia (hīp″he-dōn′e-ah) diminution of power of enjoyment.

hyphema (hi-fēm′ah) hemorrhage within the anterior chamber of the eye.

hyphemia (hi-fēm′e-ah) 1. oligemia, or deficiency of blood. 2. hyphema.

hyphidrosis (hip″hĭ-dro′sis) too scanty perspiration.

Hyphomyces (hi″fōm-i′sēz) a genus of phycomycetous fungi. *H. des′truens* causes hyphomycosis destruens equi.

Hyphomycetes (-mi-sēt′ēz) the mycelial (hyphal) fungi, i.e., the molds.

hyphomycosis (-mi-ko′sis) infections with *Hyphomyces.* **h. des′truens e′qui,** a disease of horses and mules caused by *Hyphomyces destruens,* marked by subcutaneous abscesses that eventually break through the skin, leaving large raw surfaces.

hypn(o)- word element [Gr.], *sleep; hypnosis.*

hypnagogue (hip′nah-gog) 1. hypnotic; pertaining to drowsiness. 2. an agent that induces sleep or drowsiness.

hypnalgia (hip-nal′je-ah) pain during sleep.

hypnoanalysis (hip″no-ah-nal′ĭ-sis) a method of psychotherapy combining psychoanalysis with hypnosis.

hypnodontics (-don′tiks) the application of hypnosis and controlled suggestion in the practice of dentistry.

hypnogenic (-jen′ik) inducing sleep or a hypnotic state.

hypnoid (hip′noid) resembling hypnosis.

hypnolepsy (hip′nol-ep″se) narcolepsy.

hypnology (hip-nol′ah-je) scientific study of sleep or of hypnotism.

hypnosis (hip-no′sis) an artificially induced passive state in which there is increased amenability and responsiveness to suggestions and commands. **hypnot′ic,** adj.

hypnotic (hip-not′ik) 1. inducing sleep; also, an agent that so acts. 2. pertaining to or of the nature of hypnotism.

hypnotism (hip′nah-tizm) 1. the method or practice of inducing hypnosis. 2. hypnosis.

hypnotize (-tīz) to put into a condition of hypnosis.

hypo (hi′po) 1. colloquialism for a hypodermic inoculation or syringe. 2. sodium thiosulfite.

hypo-, hyp- word element [Gr.], *beneath; under; deficient.*

hypoacusia, hypoacusis (-ah-ku′ze-ah; -ah-ku′sis) slightly diminished auditory sensitivity.

hypoadrenalism (-ah-drēn′il-izm) deficiency of adrenal activity, as in Addison's disease.

hypoadrenocorticism (-ah-drēn″o-kort′is-izm) deficient activity of the adrenal cortex.

hypoalbuminosis (-al-bu-min-o′sis) abnormally low level of albumin.

hypoalimentation (-al″ĭ-men-ta′shin) insufficient nourishment.

hypoazoturia (-az″o-tu′re-ah) diminished nitrogenous material in the urine.

hypobaric (-bār′ik) characterized by less than normal pressure or weight; applied to gases under less than atmospheric pressure, or to solutions of lower specific gravity than another taken as a standard of reference.

hypobarism (-bar′izm) the condition resulting when ambient gas or atmospheric pressure is below that within the body tissues.

hypobaropathy (-bār-op′ah-the) the disturbances experienced at high altitudes due to reduced air pressure.

hypoblast (hi′po-blast) the entoderm. **hypoblas′tic,** adj.

hypocapnia (-kap′ne-ah) deficiency of carbon dioxide in the blood. **hypocap′nic,** adj.

hypocarbia (-kar″be-ah) hypocapnia.

hypochloremia (-klor-ēm′e-ah) abnormally diminished levels of chloride in the blood. **hypochlore′mic,** adj.

hypochlorhydria (-klōr-hi′dre-ah) lack of hydrochloric acid in the gastric juice.

hypochlorization (-klōr″iz-a′shin) reduction of sodium chloride salt in the diet.

hypochlorous acid (-klor′is) an unstable compound, HClO, with disinfectant and bleaching action; its sodium salt (*sodium hypochlorite*) is used in solution as a disinfectant.

hypocholesteremia (-kol-es″ter-ēm′e-ah) hypocholesterolemia.

hypocholesterolemia (-kol-es″ter-ol-ēm′e-ah) abnormally low levels of cholesterol in the blood. **hypocholesterole′mic,** adj.

hypochondria (-kon′dre-ah) 1. plural of *hypochondrium.* 2. hypochondriasis.

hypochondriac (-kon′dre-ak) 1. pertaining to the hypochondrium or to hypochondriasis. 2. a person affected with hypochondriasis.

hypochondriasis (-kon-dri′ah-sis) morbid anxiety about one's health, with numerous and varying symptoms that cannot be attributed to organic disease. **hypochondri′acal,** adj.

hypochondrium (-kon′dre-um), pl. *hypochon′dria.* The upper lateral abdominal region, overlying the costal cartilages, on either side of the epigastrium. **hypochon′drial,** adj.

hypochromasia (-kro-ma′ze-ah) 1. staining less intensely than normal. 2. decrease of hemoglobin in erythrocytes so that they are abnormally pale. **hypochromat′ic,** adj.

hypochromatism (-kro′mit-izm) abnormally deficient pigmentation, especially deficiency of chromatin in a cell nucleus.

hypochromatosis (-kro″mah-to′sis) the gradual fading and disappearance of the cell nucleus (chromatin).

hypochromia (-kro′me-ah) 1. hypochromasia (2). 2. hypochromatism. **hypochro′mic,** adj.

hypocomplementemia (-kom″plē-men-te′me-ah) diminution of complement levels in the blood.

hypocorticism (-kort′is-izm) hypoadrenocorticism.

hypocyclosis (-si-klo′sis) insufficient accommodation in the eye.

hypocythemia (-si-thēm′e-ah) deficiency in the number of erythrocytes in the blood.

Hypoderma (-durm′ah) a genus of ox-warble or heel flies whose larvae cause warbles in cattle and a form of larva migrans in man.

hypodermiasis (-der-mi′ah-sis) a creeping eruption of the skin in man and cattle caused by the larvae of *Hypoderma.*

hypodermic (-durm′ik) applied or administered beneath the skin.

hypodermis (-durm′is) 1. subcutaneous tissue. 2. the outer cellular layer of invertebrates that secretes the cuticular exoskeleton.

hypodermoclysis (-der-mok′lĭ-sis) subcutaneous injection of fluids, e.g., saline solution.

hypodipsia (-dip′se-ah) abnormally diminished thirst.

hypodontia (-don′she-ah) partial anodontia.

hypodynamia (-di-nām′e-ah) abnormally diminished power. **hypodynam′ic,** adj.

hypoeccrisia (-e-kriz′e-ah) abnormally diminished excretion. **hypoeccrit′ic,** adj.

hypoechoic (-ĕ-ko′ik) in ultrasonography, giving off few echoes; said of tissues or structures that reflect relatively few of the ultrasound waves directed at them.

hypoergia, hypoergy (-urj′e-ah; -urj′e) hyposensitivity. **hypoer′gic,** adj.

hypoesophoria (-es″o-for′e-ah) deviation of the visual axes downward and inward.

hypoesthesia (-es-the′ze-ah) abnormally decreased sensitivity to stimulation. **hypoesthet′ic,** adj.

hypoexophoria (-ek″so-for′e-ah) deviation of the visual axes downward and laterally.

hypoferremia (-fĕ-rēm′e-ah) deficiency of iron in the blood.

hypofertility (-fer-til′it-e) diminished reproductive capacity. **hypofer′tile,** adj.

hypofibrinogenemia (-fi-brin″o-jin-ēm′e-ah) deficiency of fibrinogen in the blood.

hypogalactia (-gah-lak′she-ah) deficiency of milk secretion. **hypogalac′tous,** adj.

hypogammaglobulinemia (-gam″ah-glob″u-lin-ēm′e-ah) an immunological deficiency state marked by abnormally low levels of generally all classes of serum gamma globulins, with heightened susceptibility to infectious diseases. It may be congenital or secondary, or it may be physiological, which occurs in normal infants and which, when prolonged, is called *transient h.* **hypogammaglobuline′mic,** adj. **common variable h.,** see under *immunodeficiency.*

hypoganglionosis (-gang″gle-on-o′sis) deficiency in the number of myenteric ganglion cells in the distal segment of the large bowel, resulting in constipation; a variant of congenital megacolon.

hypogastrium (-gas′tre-um) the pubic region, the lowest middle abdominal region.

hypogastroschisis (-gas-tros′kĭ-sis) congenital fissure of the hypogastrium.

hypogenesis (-jen′ĭ-sis) defective embryonic development. **hypogenet′ic,** adj.

hypogenitalism (-jen′it′l-izm″) hypogonadism.

hypogeusesthesia, hypogeusia (-gūs″es-the′-ze-ah; -gu′ze-ah) abnormally diminished sense of taste.

hypoglucagonemia (-gloo″kah-gon-ēm′e-ah) abnormally reduced levels of glucagon in the blood.

hypoglycemia (-gli-sēm′e-ah) deficiency of glucose concentration in the blood, which may lead to nervousness, hypothermia, headache, confusion, and sometimes convulsions and coma.

hypoglycemic (-gli-sēm′ik) 1. pertaining to,

characterized by, or causing hypoglycemia. 2. an agent that lowers blood glucose levels.

hypoglycorrhachia (-ra′ke-ah) abnormally low sugar content in the cerebrospinal fluid.

hypogonadism (hi″po-go′nad-izm) decreased functional activity of the gonads, with retardation of growth and sexual development.

hypogonadotropic (-gon″ah-do-trop′ik) relating to or caused by deficiency of gonadotropin.

hypohidrosis (-hĭ-dro′sis) abnormally diminished secretion of sweat. **hypohidrot′ic,** adj.

hypokalemia (-kah-lēm′e-ah) abnormally low potassium levels in the blood, which may lead to neuromuscular and renal disorders and to electrocardiographic abnormalities; hypopotassemia.

hypokalemic (-kah-lēm′ik) 1. pertaining to or characterized by hypokalemia. 2. an agent that lowers blood potassium levels.

hypokinesia (-ki-ne′ze-ah) abnormally diminished motor activity. **hypokinet′ic,** adj.

hypolactasia (-lak-ta′ze-ah) deficiency of lactase activity in the intestines.

hypoleydigism (-līd″ig-izm) abnormally diminished secretion of androgens by Leydig's cells.

hypolipidemic (-lip″id-ēm′ik) promoting the reduction of lipid concentrations in the serum.

hypomagnesemia (-mag″nis-ēm′e-ah) abnormally low magnesium content of the blood, manifested chiefly by neuromuscular hyperirritability.

hypomania (-mān′e-ah) mania of a moderate type. **hypoman′ic,** adj.

hypomenorrhea (-men″er-e′ah) diminution of menstrual flow or duration.

hypomere (hi′po-mēr) 1. the ventrolateral portion of a myotome, innervated by an anterior ramus of a spinal nerve. 2. the lateral plate of mesoderm that develops into the walls of the body cavities.

hypometria (-me′tre-ah) ataxia in which movements fall short of reaching the intended goal.

hypomnesia (hi″pom-ne′ze-ah) defective memory.

hypomorph (-hi′po-morf) 1. a person who is short in standing height as compared with his sitting height. 2. in genetics, a mutant gene that shows only a partial reduction in the activity it influences. **hypomor′phic,** adj.

hypomyotonia (-mi″ah-tōn′e-ah) deficient muscular tonicity.

hypomyxia (-mik′se-ah) decreased secretion of mucus.

hyponasality (-na-zal′it-e) a quality of voice in which there is a complete lack of nasal emission of air and nasal resonance, so that the speaker sounds as if he has a cold.

hyponatremia (-na-trēm′e-ah) deficiency of sodium in the blood; salt depletion.

hyponeocytosis (-ne″o-si-to′sis) leukopenia with the presence of immature leukocytes in the blood.

hyponoia (-noi′ah) sluggish mental activity.

hyponychium (-nik′e-um) the thickened epidermis beneath the free distal end of the nail. **hyponych′ial,** adj.

hypo-orthocytosis (-or″tho-si-to′sis) leukopenia with a normal proportion of the various forms of leukocytes.

hypoparathyroidism (-par″ah-thi′roid-izm) the condition produced by greatly reduced function of or removal of the parathyroid glands, with hypocalcemia, which may lead to tetany; hyperphosphatemia, with decreased bone resorption; and other symptoms.

hypoperfusion (-per-fu′zhin) decreased blood flow through an organ, as in circulatory shock; if prolonged, it may result in permanent cellular dysfunction and death.

hypopharynx (hi″po-fǎ′rinks) laryngopharynx.

hypophonesis (-fon-e′sis) diminution of the sound in auscultation or percussion.

hypophonia (-fōn′e-ah) a weak voice due to incoordination of the vocal muscles.

hypophoria (-for′e-ah) downward deviation of the visual axis of one eye in the absence of visual fusional stimuli.

hypophosphatasia (-fos″fah-ta′ze-ah) an inborn error of metabolism marked by abnormally low serum alkaline phosphatase activity and excretion of phosphoethanolamine in the urine. It is manifested by rickets in infants and children and by osteomalacia in adults. It is most severe in babies under six months of age.

hypophosphatemia (-fos″fah-tēm′e-ah) deficiency of phosphates in the blood, as may occur in rickets and osteomalacia. See also *hypophosphatasia.* **hypophosphate′mic,** adj.

hypophosphoric acid (hi″po-fos-for′ik) H_2PO_3; its salts are hypophosphates.

hypophosphorous acid (hi″po-fos-for′us) a toxic, monobasic acid with strong reducing properties, H_3PO_2, which forms hypophosphites; used in 30 to 32% and 50% solutions.

hypophrenia (-fre′ne-ah) mental retardation. **hypophren′ic,** adj.

hypophysectomy (hi-pof″ǐ-sek′tah-me) excision of the pituitary gland (hypophysis).

hypophyseoportal (hi″po-fiz″e-o-port′′l) denoting the portal system of the pituitary gland, in which hypothalamic venules connect with capillaries of the anterior pituitary.

hypophyseoprivic, hypophysioprivic (-priv′ik) deficient in hormonal secretion of the pituitary gland (hypophysis).

hypophysis (hi-pof′ǐ-sis), pl. *hypoph′yses* [Gr.] pituitary gland. **hypophys′eal,** adj. **h. ce′rebri,** pituitary gland. **pharyngeal h.,** a mass in the pharyngeal wall with structure similar to that of the pituitary gland.

hypopiesis (hi″po-pi-e′sis) abnormally low pressure, as low blood pressure. **hypopiet′ic,** adj.

hypopituitarism (-pǐ-tu′it-er-izm″) the condition resulting from diminution or cessation of hormonal secretion by the pituitary gland, especially the anterior pituitary.

hypoplasia (-pla′ze-ah) incomplete development or underdevelopment of an organ or tissue. **hypoplas′tic,** adj. **enamel h.,** incomplete or defective development of the enamel of the teeth; it may be hereditary or acquired. **oligomeganephronic renal h.,** oligomeganephronia.

hypopnea (hi-pop′ne-ah) abnormal decrease in depth and rate of respiration. **hypopne′ic,** adj.

hypoporosis (hi″po-por-o′sis) deficient callus formation after bone fracture.

hypopotassemia (-pot″is-ēm′e-ah) hypokalemia.

hypoprosody (-pros′ah-de) diminution of the normal variation of stress, pitch, and rhythm of speech.

hypopselaphesia (hi″po-sel″ah-fe′ze-ah) dullness of the tactile sense.

hypoptyalism (-ti′ah-lizm) abnormally decreased secretion of saliva.

hypopyon (hi-po′pe-on) an accumulation of pus in the anterior chamber of the eye.

hyposalivation (-sal″ǐ-va′shin) hypoptyalism.

hyposecretion (-se-kre′shin) diminished secretion, as by a gland.

hyposensitive (-sen′sit-iv) 1. exhibiting abnormally decreased sensitivity. 2. being less sensitive to a specific allergen after repeated and gradually increasing doses of the offending substance.

hyposmia (hi-poz′me-ah) diminished acuteness of the sense of smell.

hyposomatotropism (hi″po-so″mat-ah-tro′-pizm) deficient secretion of somatotropin (growth hormone) or of inadequate secretion of somatotropin, resulting in short stature.

hyposomnia (-som′ne-ah) insomnia.

hypospadias (-spa′de-is) a developmental anomaly in which the male urethra opens on the underside of the penis or on the perineum. **female h.,** a developmental anomaly in the female in which the urethra opens into the vagina.

hyposplenism (-splen′izm) diminished functioning of the spleen, resulting in an increase in peripheral blood elements.

hypostasis (hi-pos′tah-sis) poor or stagnant circulation in a dependent part of the body or an organ.

hypostatic (hi″pah-stat′ik) 1. pertaining to, due to, or associated with hypostasis. 2. abnormally static; said of certain inherited traits that are liable to be suppressed by other traits.

hyposthenia (hi″pos-the′ne-ah) an enfeebled state; weakness. **hyposthen′ic,** adj.

hypostypsis (-stip′sis) moderate astringency. **hypostyp′tic,** adj.

hyposynergia (-sin-urj′e-ah) defective coordination.

hypotelorism (-tēl′er-izm) abnormally decreased distance between two organs or parts. **ocular h., orbital h.,** abnormal decrease in the intraorbital distance.

hypotension (-ten′shin) abnormally low blood pressure. **orthostatic h., postural h.,** a fall in blood pressure occurring upon standing or when standing motionless in a fixed position.

hypotensive (-ten′siv) marked by low blood pressure or serving to reduce blood pressure.

hypothalamus (-thal′ah-mus) the part of the diencephalon forming the floor and part of the lateral wall of the third ventricle; anatomically, it includes the optic chiasm, mamillary bodies, tuber cinereum, infundibulum, and pituitary gland, but for physiological purposes the pituitary gland is considered a distinct structure. The hypothalamic nuclei serve to activate, control, and integrate the peripheral autonomic mechanisms, endocrine activities, and many somatic functions. **hypothalam′ic,** adj.

hypothenar (hi-poth′in-ar) 1. the fleshy eminence on the palm along the ulnar margin. 2. relating to this eminence.

hypothermia (hi″po-thurm′e-ah) low body temperature, as that due to exposure to cold weather or such a state induced as a means of decreasing metabolism and thereby the need for oxygen, as used in various surgical procedures. **hypother′mal, hypother′mic,** adj.

hypothesis (hi-poth′ĭ-sis) a supposition that appears to explain a group of phenomena and is assumed as a basis of reasoning and experimentation. **lattice h.,** a theory of the nature of the antigen-antibody reaction which postulates reaction between multivalent antigen and divalent antibody to give an antigen-antibody complex of a lattice-like structure. **Lyon h.,** the random and fixed inactivation (in the form of sex chromatin) of one X chromosome in mammalian cells at an early stage of embryogenesis, leading to mosaicism of paternal and maternal X chromosomes in the female.

hypothymia (-thi′me-ah) abnormally diminished emotionalism.

hypothymism (-thi′mizm) diminished thymus activity.

hypothyroidism (-thi′roid-izm) deficiency of thyroid activity. In adults, it is marked by decreased metabolic rate, tiredness, and lethargy. See also *cretinism* and *myxedema.* **hypothy′roid,** adj.

hypotonia (-tōn′e-ah) diminished tone of the skeletal muscles.

hypotonic (-ton′ik) 1. denoting decreased tone or tension. 2. denoting a solution having less osmotic pressure than one with which it is compared.

hypotransferrinemia (-trans-fer″in-ēm′e-ah) deficiency of transferrin in the blood.

hypotrichosis (-trĭ-ko′sis) presence of less than the normal amount of hair.

hypotrophy (hi-pah′trah-fe) abiotrophy.

hypotropia (hi″po-tro′pe-ah) strabismus in which there is permanent downward deviation of the visual axis of one eye.

hypotympanotomy (-tim″pah-not′ah-me) surgical opening of the hypotympanum.

hypotympanum (-tim′pah-num) the lower part of the cavity of the middle ear, in the temporal bone.

hypouricemia (-ur″is-ēm′e-ah) deficiency of uric acid in the blood, along with xanthinuria, due to deficiency of xanthine oxidase, the enzyme required for conversion of hypoxanthine to xanthine and of xanthine to uric acid.

hypoventilation (-vent″il-a′shin) reduction in the amount of air entering the pulmonary alveoli.

hypovolemia (-vōl-ēm′e-ah) abnormally decreased volume of circulating fluid (plasma) in the body. **hypovole′mic,** adj.

hypovolia (-vōl′e-ah) diminished water content or volume, as of extracellular fluid.

hypoxanthine (-zan′thēn) an intermediate product of uric acid synthesis, formed from adenylic acid and itself a precursor of xanthine.

hypoxemia (hi″pok-sēm′e-ah) deficient oxygenation of the blood.

hypoxia (hi-pok′se-ah) reduction of oxygen supply to a tissue below physiological levels despite adequate perfusion of the tissue by blood. **hypox′ic,** adj. **anemic h.,** that due to reduction of the oxygen-carrying capacity of the blood as a result of a decrease in the total hemoglobin or an alteration of the hemoglobin constituents. **histotoxic h.,** that due to impaired utilization of oxygen by tissues. **hypoxic h.,** that due to insufficient oxygen reaching the blood. **stagnant h.,** that due to failure to transport sufficient oxygen because of inadequate blood flow.

hypsarrhythmia (hip″sah-rith′me-ah) an electroencephalographic abnormality commonly associated with infantile spasms, with random, high-voltage slow waves and spikes spreading to all cortical areas.

hypsokinesis (hip″so-ki-ne′sis) a backward swaying or falling when in erect posture; seen in paralysis agitans and other forms of the amyostatic syndrome.

hyster(o)- word element [Gr.], *uterus; hysteria.*

hysterectomy (his″ter-ek′tah-me) excision of the uterus. **abdominal h.,** that performed through the abdominal wall. **cesarean h.,** cesarean section followed by removal of the uterus. **complete h.,** total h. **partial h.,** subtotal h. **radical h.,** excision of the uterus, upper vagina, and parametrium. **subtotal h.,** that in which the cervix is left in place. **total h.,** that in which the uterus and cervix are completely excised. **vaginal h.,** that performed through the vagina.

hysteresis (his″ter-e′sis) a time lag in the occurrence of two associated phenomena, as between cause and effect.

hystereurynter (his″ter-ūr-in′ter) an instrument for dilating the os uteri.

hystereurysis (-ūr′is-is) dilation of the os uteri.

hysteria (his-tě′re-ah) a neurosis with symptoms based on conversion, characterized by lack of control over acts and emotions, by morbid self-consciousness, by anxiety, by exaggeration of the effect of sensory impressions, and by simulation of various disorders. **hyster′ical,** adj. **anxiety h.,** that with recurring attacks of anxiety. **conversion h., dissociative h.,** see *hysterical neurosis.* **fixation h.,** that with symptoms based on those of an organic disease. **h. ma′jor,** that with sudden onset of dream states, stupors, and paralyses. **h. mi′nor,** that with mild convulsions in which consciousness is not lost.

hysterics (his-tě′riks) popular term for an uncontrollable emotional outburst.

hysterocele (his′ter-ah-sēl″) metrocele.

hysterocleisis (his″ter-o-kli′sis) surgical closure of the os uteri.

hysteroepilepsy (-ep'il-ep''se) severe hysteria with epileptiform convulsions.

hysterography (his''ter-og'rah-fe) 1. the graphic recording of the strength of uterine contractions in labor. 2. radiography of the uterus after instillation of a contrast medium.

hysteroid (his'ter-oid) resembling hysteria.

hysterolith (his'ter-o-lith'') a uterine calculus.

hysterolysis (his''ter-ol'ĭ-sis) freeing of the uterus from adhesions.

hysteromyoma (his''ter-o-mi-o'mah) leiomyoma of the uterus.

hysteromyomectomy (-mi''o-mek'tah-me) excision of a leiomyoma of the uterus.

hysteromyotomy (-mi-ot'ah-me) incision of the uterus for removal of a solid tumor.

hysteropexy (his'ter-o-pek''se) surgical fixation of a displaced uterus.

hysteroptosis (his''ter-op-to'sis) metroptosis.

hysterorrhaphy (his''ter-or'ah-fe) 1. suture of the uterus. 2. hysteropexy.

hysterorrhexis (his''ter-o-rek'sis) metrorrhexis.

hysterosalpingectomy (-sal''pin-jek'tah-me) excision of the uterus and uterine tubes.

hysterosalpingography (-sal''ping-gog'rah-fe) radiography of the uterus and uterine tubes.

hysterosalpingo-oophorectomy (-sal''ping-go-o''of-ah-rek'tah-me) excision of the uterus, uterine tubes, and ovaries.

hysterosalpingostomy (-sal''ping-gos'tah-me) anastomosis of a uterine tube to the uterus.

hysteroscope (his'ter-ah-skōp'') an endoscope for direct visual examination of the cervical canal and uterine cavity.

hysterospasm (-spazm'') spasm of the uterus.

hysterotomy (his''ter-ot'ah-me) incision of the uterus, performed either transabdominally (*abdominal h.*) or vaginally (*vaginal h.*).

hysterotrachelorrhaphy (his''ter-o-tra''kel-or'rah-fe) suture of the uterine cervix.

hysterotrachelotomy (-tra''kel-ot'ah-me) incision of the uterine cervix.

hysterotubography (-too-bog'rah-fe) hysterosalpingography.

Hz hertz.

I

I chemical symbol, *iodine*.

-ia word element, *state; condition*.

IAEA International Atomic Energy Agency.

-iasis word element [Gr.], *condition; state*.

iatr(o)- word element [Gr.], *medicine; physician*.

iatric (i-ă'trik) pertaining to medicine or to a physician.

-iatrics word element [Gr.], *medical treatment*.

iatrogenic (-jen'ik) resulting from the activity of physicians; said of any adverse condition in a patient resulting from treatment by a physician or surgeon.

-iatry word element [Gr.], *medical treatment*.

ibuprofen (i-bu'pro-fen) an anti-inflammatory agent, $C_{13}H_{18}O_2$, also having analgesic and antipyretic actions; used in the treatment of rheumatoid arthritis and osteoarthritis.

IC inspiratory capacity; irritable colon.

ICD International Classification of Diseases (of the World Health Organization); intrauterine contraceptive device.

ichor (i'kor) watery discharge from wounds or sores. **i'chorous**, adj.

ichorrhea (i''kor-e'ah) copious discharge of ichor.

ichthammol (ik-tham'ol) a reddish brown to brownish black viscous fluid obtained by destructive distillation of certain bituminous schists, sulfonated and neutralized with ammonia; used as a local skin anti-infective.

ichthy(o)- word element [Gr.], *fish*.

ichthyoid (ik'the-oid) fishlike.

ichthyology (ik''the-ol'ah-je) the study of fishes.

ichthyosarcotoxin (ik''the-o-sar''ko-tok'sin) a toxin found in the flesh of poisonous fishes.

ichthyosarcotoxism (-sar''ko-tok'sizm) poisoning from eating of poisonous fish, marked by gastrointestinal and neurological disturbances.

ichthyosis (ik''the-o'sis) 1. any of several generalized skin disorders marked by dryness, roughness, and scaliness, due to hypertrophy of the horny layer resulting from excessive production or retention of keratin, or a molecular defect in the keratin. 2. i. vulgaris. **ichthyot'ic**, adj. **i. hys'trix**, a rare form of epidermolytic hyperkeratosis, marked by generalized, dark brown, linear verrucoid ridges somewhat like porcupine skin. **lamellar i.**, a hereditary disease present at or soon after birth, with large, quadrilateral, grayish brown scales; it may be associated with short stature, oligophrenia, spastic paralysis, genital hypoplasia, hypotrichia, and shortened life-span. **i. sim'plex**, i. vulgaris. **i. u'teri**, transformation of the columnar epithelium of the endometrium into stratified squamous epithelium. **i. vulga'ris**, hereditary ichthyosis present at or shortly after birth, with large, thick, dry scales on the neck, ears, scalp, face, and flexural surfaces.

I.C.N. International Council of Nurses.

I.C.S. International College of Surgeons.

ICSH interstitial cell-stimulating hormone.

ictal (ik't'l) pertaining to, marked by, or due to a stroke or an acute epileptic seizure.

icterogenic (ik''ter-o-jen'ik) causing jaundice.

icterohepatitis (-hep''ah-tīt'is) inflammation of the liver with marked jaundice.

icterus (ik'ter-is) [L.] jaundice. **icter'ic**, adj. **i. gra'vis**, acute yellow atrophy. **i. neonato'rum**, jaundice in newborn children.

ictus (ik'tis) a seizure, stroke, blow, or sudden attack. **ic'tal,** adj.

ICU intensive care unit.

ID₅₀ median infective dose.

id¹ (id) in psychoanalytic theory, the innate, unconscious, primitive aspect of the personality dominated by the pleasure principle.

id² (id) a sterile cutaneous eruption occurring as an allergic reaction to an agent causing a primary infection elsewhere; also used as a word termination attached to a root specifying the causative factor.

IDD insulin-dependent diabetes.

-ide (īd) a suffix indicating a binary chemical compound.

idea (i-de'ah) a mental impression or conception. **autochthonous i.,** a strange idea which comes into the mind in some unaccountable way, but is not a hallucination. **compulsive i.,** one that persists despite reason and will, and impels toward some inappropriate act. **dominant i.,** a morbid impression that controls or colors every action and thought. **fixed i.,** a persistent morbid impression or belief that cannot be changed by reason. **i. of reference,** the incorrect idea that words and actions of others refer to one's self or the projection of the causes of one's own imaginary difficulties upon someone else.

ideal (i-de'il) a pattern or concept of perfection. **ego i.,** the standard of perfection unconsciously created by a person for himself.

idealization (i-de''il-iz-a'shin) a conscious or unconscious mental mechanism, in which the individual overestimates an admired aspect or attribute of another person.

ideation (i''de-a'shin) the formation of ideas or images. **idea'tional,** adj.

idée fixe (e-da' fēks') [Fr.] fixed idea.

identification (i-den''ti-fi-ka'shin) an unconscious defense mechanism by which one person patterns himself after another.

identity (i-den'tit-e) the aggregate of characteristics by which an individual is recognized by himself and others. **gender i.,** a person's concept of himself as being male and masculine or female and feminine, or ambivalent.

ideogenetic, ideogenous (i''de-o-jin-net'ik; i''-de-oj'in-is) related to vague sense impressions rather than organized images.

ideology (i''de-ol'ah-je, id''e-) 1. the science of the development of ideas. 2. the body of ideas characteristic of an individual or of a social unit.

ideomotion (i''de-o-mo'shin) muscular action induced by a dominant idea.

ideomotor (-mōt'er) aroused by an idea or thought; said of involuntary motion so aroused.

idio- word element [Gr.], *self; peculiar to a substance or organism.*

idiocy (id'e-ah-se) severe mental retardation. **amaurotic i., amaurotic familial i.,** a general term for several genetic lipidoses of diverse biochemical and clinical characteristics, including Batten disease, Jansky-Bielschowsky disease, Sandhoff disease, Tay-Sachs disease, Vogt-Spielmeyer disease, and neuronal ceroid lipofuscinosis. **cretinoid i.,** cretinism. **epileptic i.,**

that combined with epilepsy. **microcephalic i.,** that associated with microcephaly. **mongolian i.,** Down's syndrome.

idioglossia (id''e-o-glos'e-ah) imperfect articulation, with the utterance of meaningless vocal sounds. **idioglot'tic,** adj.

idiogram (id'e-ah-gram) a drawing or photograph of the chromosomes of a particular cell.

idiopathic (id''e-o-path'ik) self-originated; occurring without known cause.

idiosyncrasy (id''e-o-sing'krah-se) 1. a habit peculiar to an individual. 2. an abnormal susceptibility to an agent (e.g., a drug) peculiar to an individual. **idiosyncrat'ic,** adj.

idiot (id'e-it) a person afflicted with severe mental retardation. **i.-savant,** a mentally retarded person with a particular mental faculty developed to an unusually high degree, as for mathematics, music, etc.

idiotrophic (id''e-o-trof'ik) capable of selecting its own nourishment.

idioventricular (-ven-trik'ūl-er) pertaining to the cardiac ventricle alone.

idoxuridine (i''doks-ūr'ĭ-dēn) an analogue of pyrimidine, $C_9H_{11}IN_2O_5$, which inhibits viral DNA synthesis; used as an antiviral agent in the treatment of herpes simplex keratitis.

IDU idoxuridine.

Ig immunoglobulin of any of the five classes: IgA, IgD, IgE, IgG, and IgM.

ile(o)- word element [L.], *ileum.*

ileac (il'e-ak) 1. of the nature of ileus. 2. pertaining to the ileum.

ileitis (-īt'is) inflammation of the ileum. **distal i., regional i.,** Crohn's disease affecting the ileum.

ileocecostomy (-se-kos'tah-me) surgical anastomosis of the ileum to the cecum.

ileocolitis (-ko-līt'is) inflammation of the ileum and colon. **i. ulcero'sa chro'nica,** chronic ileocolitis with fever, rapid pulse, anemia, diarrhea, and right iliac pain.

ileocolostomy (-kol-os'tah-me) surgical anastomosis of the ileum to the colon.

ileocystoplasty (-sis'tah-plas''te) repair of the wall of the urinary bladder with an isolated segment of the wall of the ileum.

ileocystostomy (-sis-tos'tah-me) use of an isolated segment of ileum to create a passage from the urinary bladder to an opening in the abdominal wall.

ileoileostomy (-il''e-os'tah-me) surgical anastomosis between two parts of the ileum.

ileorrhaphy (il''e-or'ah-fe) suture of the ileum.

ileosigmoidostomy (il''e-o-sig''moi-dos'tah-me) surgical anastomosis of the ileum to the sigmoid colon.

ileostomy (il''e-os'tah-me) surgical creation of an opening into the ileum, with a stoma on the abdominal wall.

ileotomy (-ot'ah-me) incision of the ileum.

ileum (il'e-im) the distal portion of the small intestine, extending from the jejunum to the cecum. **duplex i.,** congenital duplication of the ileum.

ileus (il'e-us) intestinal obstruction. **adynamic i.,** that due to inhibition of bowel motility.

dynamic i., hyperdynamic i., spastic i. **mechanical i.,** that due to mechanical causes, such as hernia, adhesions, volvulus, etc. **meconium i.,** ileus in the newborn due to blocking of the bowel with thick meconium. **occlusive i.,** mechanical i. **paralytic i., i. paraly′ticus,** adynamic i. **spastic i.,** mechanical ileus due to persistent contracture of a bowel segment. **i. subpar′ta,** that due to pressure of the gravid uterus on the pelvic colon.

ili(o)- word element [L.], *ilium.*

iliofemoral (-fem′er-il) pertaining to the ilium and femur.

iliolumbar (-lum′bar) pertaining to the iliac and lumbar regions.

iliopectineal (il″e-o-pek-tin′e-il) pertaining to the ilium and pubes.

ilium (il′e-im), pl. *i′lia* [L.] see *Table of Bones.*

ill (il) 1. not well; sick. 2. a disease or disorder. **colt i.,** navel ill in colts. **louping i.,** a tickborne viral encephalomyelitis of sheep. **navel i.,** septicemia affecting foals, calves, and lambs with omphalophlebitis and abscesses in the joints causing polyarthritis; due to infection through the open navel by various organisms.

illness (il′nis) a condition marked by deviation from the normal state; sickness. **emotional i., mental i.,** see under *disorder.*

illumination (il-oo″min-a′shin) the lighting up of a part, organ, or object for inspection. **darkfield i., dark-ground i.,** the casting of peripheral light rays upon a microscopical object from the side, the center rays being blocked out; the object appears bright on a dark background.

illusion (il-oo′zhin) a mental impression derived from misinterpretation of an actual experience. **illu′sional,** adj.

Ilosone (il′o-sōn) trademark for preparations of erythromycin estolate.

im- a prefix, replacing *in-* before words beginning *b, m,* and *p.*

I.M. intramuscularly.

image (im′ij) a picture or concept with likeness to an objective reality. **body i.,** the three-dimensional concept of one's self, recorded in the cortex by perception of everchanging body postures, and constantly changing with them. **false i.,** that formed by the deviating eye in strabismus. **mirror i.,** one with right and left relations reversed, as in the reflection of an object in a mirror. **motor i.,** the organized cerebral model of the possible movements of the body. **Purkinje's i's, Purkinje-Sanson i's,** three reflected images of an object seen in observing the pupil of the eye: two on the posterior and anterior surfaces of the lens, one on the anterior surface of the cornea. **real i.,** one formed where the emanating rays are collected, in which the object is pictured as being inverted. **virtual i.,** a picture from projected light rays that are intercepted before focusing.

imaging (im′ah-jing) the production of diagnostic images, e.g., radiography, ultrasonography, or scintillation photography. **electrostatic i.,** a method of visualizing deep structures of the body, in which an electron beam is passed through the patient and the emerging beam strikes an electrostatically charged plate, dissipating the charge according to the strength of the beam. A film is then made from the plate. **magnetic resonance i. (MRI),** a method of visualizing soft tissues of the body by applying an external magnetic field that makes it possible to distinguish between hydrogen atoms in different environments.

imago (ĭ-ma′go), pl. *ima′goes,* or *ima′gines* [L.] 1. the adult or definitive form of an insect. 2. a childhood memory or fantasy of a loved person which persists in adult life.

imbalance (im-bal′ins) lack of balance, especially between muscles, as in insufficiency of ocular muscles. **autonomic i.,** defective coordination between the sympathetic and parasympathetic nervous systems, especially with respect to vasomotor activities. **sympathetic i.,** vagotonia. **vasomotor i.,** autonomic i.

imbecility (im″bĭ-sil′lit-e) mental retardation less severe than in idiocy but more severe than in moronity.

imbibition (im″bĭ-bish′in) absorption of a liquid.

imbricated (im′brĭ-kāt″id) overlapping like shingles.

ImD₅₀ the immunizing dose of vaccine or antigen sufficient to protect 50 percent of the animals in a particular test group.

imidazole (im″id-az′ōl) a base found combined with alanine in histidine.

imide (im′īd) any compound containing the bivalent group, $>$NH, to which are attached only acid radicals.

iminoglycinuria (ĭ-me″no-gli″sin-ūr′e-ah) a benign hereditary disorder of renal tubular reabsorption of glycine and imino acids (proline and hydroxyproline), marked by excessive levels of all three substances in the urine.

imipramine (ĭ-mip′rah-mēn) an antidepressant, $C_{19}H_{24}N_2$, used as the hydrochloride salt.

immersion (ĭ-mer′shin) 1. the plunging of a body into a liquid. 2. the use of the microscope with the object and object glass both covered with a liquid.

immiscible (ĭ-mis′ĭ-b'l) not susceptible to being mixed.

immobilization (im-mo″bil-iz-a′shin) the rendering of a part incapable of being moved.

immune (ĭ-mūn′) 1. resistant to a disease because of the formation of humoral antibodies or the development of cellular immunity, or both, or from some other mechanism, as interferon activity in viral infections. 2. characterized by the development of humoral antibodies or cellular immunity, or both, following antigenic challenge. 3. produced in response to antigenic challenge, as immune serum globulin.

immunity (ĭ-mūn′it-e) 1. the condition of being immune; security against a particular disease; nonsusceptibility to the invasive or pathogenic effects of foreign microorganisms or to the toxic effect of antigenic substances. See also *active i., nonspecific i.,* and *passive i.* 2. heightened responsiveness to antigenic challenge that leads to more rapid binding or elimination of antigen than in the nonimmune state. 3. the capacity to distinguish foreign material from self, and to neutralize, eliminate, or metabolize that which is foreign by the physiologic mechanisms of the immune response. **acquired i.,** that occurring as a result of prior exposure to an infectious agent or its antigens (*active i.*), or of passive transfer of antibody or immune lymphoid cells (*passive i.*). **active i.,** see *acquired i.* **artificial i.,** acquired (active or passive) immunity produced by deliberate exposure to an antigen, as in vaccination. **cell-mediated i. (CMI), cellular i.,** acquired immunity in which the role of T-lymphocytes is predominant. **genetic i.,** innate i. **herd i.,** the resistance of a group to attack by a disease to which a large proportion of the members are immune. **humoral i.,** acquired immunity in which the role of circulating antibodies is predominant. **inherent i., innate i.,** that determined by the genetic constitution of the individual. **maternal i.,** humoral immunity passively transferred across the placenta from mother to fetus. **natural i.,** the resistance of the normal animal to infection. **nonspecific i.,** that which does not involve humoral or cell-mediated immunity, but includes lysozyme and interferon activity, etc. **passive i.,** see *acquired i.* **specific i.,** immunity against a particular disease or antigen.

immunization (im″ūn-iz-a′shin) the process of rendering a subject immune, or of becoming immune. **active i.,** stimulation with a specific antigen to induce an immune response. **passive i.,** the conferral of specific immune reactivity on previously nonimmune individuals by administration of sensitized lymphoid cells or serum from immune individuals.

immunoadjuvant (-aj′ah-vint, -ad-joo′vint) a nonspecific stimulator of the immune response, e.g., BCG vaccine or Freund's complete and incomplete adjuvants.

immunoadsorbent (-ad-sor′bint) a preparation of antigen attached to a solid support or antigen in an insoluble form, which adsorbs homologous antibodies from a mixture of immunoglobulins.

immunoassay (-as′a) quantitative determination of antigenic substances (e.g., hormones, drugs, vitamins) by serological means, as by immunofluorescent techniques, radioimmunoassay, etc.

immunobiology (-bi-ol′ah-je) that branch of biology dealing with immunologic effects on such phenomena as infectious disease, growth and development, recognition phenomena, hypersensitivity, heredity, aging, cancer, and transplantation.

immunoblastic (-blas′tik) pertaining to or involving the stem cells (immunoblasts) of lymphoid tissue.

immunochemistry (-kem′is-tre) the study of the physical chemical basis of immune phenomena and their interactions.

immunochemotherapy (-ke″mo-the′rah-pe) a combination of immunotherapy and chemotherapy.

immunocompetence (-kom′pit-ins) the capacity to develop an immune response following exposure to antigen. **immunocom′petent,** adj.

immunocomplex (-kom′pleks) antibody combined with its specific antigen; deposition of immunocomplexes that fix complement in tissues may lead to inflammation and tissue injury, as in immune complex glomerulonephritis.

immunocompromised (-kom′prom-īzd) having the immune response attenuated by administration of immunosuppressive drugs, by irradiation, by malnutrition, and by certain disease processes (e.g., cancer).

immunoconglutinin (-kon-glōōt′in-in) antibody formed against complement components that are part of an antigen-antibody complex, especially C3.

immunocyte (im′ūn-ah-sīt″) any cell of the lymphoid series which can react with antigen to produce antibody or to participate in cell-mediated reactions.

immunocytoadherence (im″ūn-o-sīt″o-ad-hēr′ins) the aggregation of red cells to form rosettes around lymphocytes with surface immunoglobulins.

immunodeficiency (-dĕ-fish′in-se) a deficiency of the immune response due to hypoactivity or decreased numbers of lymphoid cells. **immunodefi′cient,** adj. **common variable i.,** hypogammaglobulinemia of late onset marked by increased incidence of recurrent pyogenic infections, especially pneumococcal pneumonia; cellular immune dysfunction occurs in some individuals. **severe combined i. (SCID),** a group of genetic disorders marked by defective humoral and cell-mediated immunity, and manifested by lack of antibody formation and of delayed hypersensitivity and by inability to reject foreign tissue transplants.

immunodermatology (-durm″ah-tol′ah-ge) the study of immunologic phenomena as they affect skin disorders and their treatment or prophylaxis.

immunodiffusion (-dĭ-fu′zhin) the diffusion of antigen and antibody from separate reservoirs to form decreasing concentration gradients in hydrophilic gels.

immunodominance (-dom′in-ins) the degree to which a subunit of an antigenic determinant is involved in binding or reacting with antibody.

immunoelectrophoresis (-e-lek″tro-for-e′sis) a method of distinguishing proteins and other materials on the basis of their electrophoretic mobility and antigenic specificities. **rocket i.,** electrophoresis in which antigen migrates from a well through agar gel containing antiserum, forming cone-shaped (rocket) precepitin bands.

immunofluorescence (-floo″or-es′ins) a method of determining the location of antigen (or antibody) in a tissue section or smear by the pattern of fluorescence resulting when the specimen is exposed to the specific antibody (or antigen) labeled with a fluorochrome.

immunogen (im′ūn-ah-jen) any substance capable of eliciting an immune response.

immunogenetics (im″ūn-o-jin-et′iks) the study of the genetic factors controlling the individual's immune response and the transmission of those factors from generation to generation. **immunogenet′ic,** adj.

immunogenicity (-jin-is′it-e) the property enabling a substance to provoke an immune response, or the degree to which a substance possesses this property. **immunogen′ic**, adj.

immunoglobulin (-glob′ūl-in) a protein of animal origin with known antibody activity, synthesized by lymphocytes and plasma cells and found in serum and in other body fluids and tissues; abbreviated Ig. There are five distinct classes based on structural and antigenic properties: IgA, IgD, IgE, IgG, and IgM. **secretory i′s**, IgA immunoglobulins in which two IgA molecules are linked by a polypeptide (secretory piece) and by a J chain; they are present in nonvascular fluids.

immunohematology (-hem″ah-tol′ah-je) the study of antigen-antibody reactions as they relate to blood disorders.

immunohistochemical (-his″to-kem′ĭ-k'l) denoting the application of antigen-antibody interactions to histochemical techniques, as in the use of immunofluorescence.

immunoincompetent (-in-kom′pit-int) lacking the ability or capacity to develop an immune response to antigenic challenge.

immunology (im″ū-nol′ah-je) that branch of biomedical science concerned with the response of the organism to antigenic challenge, the recognition of self and not self, and all the biological, serological, and physical chemical effects of immune phenomena. **immunolog′ic**, adj.

immunomodulation (im″ūn-o-mod″ūl-a′shin) adjustment of the immune response to a desired level, as in immunopotentiation, immunosuppression, or induction of immunologic tolerance.

immunopathogenesis (-path″o-jen′ĭ-sis) the process of development of a disease in which an immune response or the products of an immune reaction are involved.

immunopathology (im″ūn-o-pah-thol′ah-je) 1. that branch of biomedical science concerned with immune reactions associated with disease, whether the reactions be beneficial, without ef-

fect, or harmful. 2. the structural and functional manifestations associated with immune responses to disease. **immunopatholog′ic**, adj.

immunopotency (-pōt′′n-se) the immunogenic capacity of an individual antigenic determinant on an antigen molecule to initiate antibody synthesis.

immunopotentiation (-pah-ten″she-a′shin) accentuation of the response to an immunogen by administration of another substance.

immunoprecipitation (-pre-sip″ĭ-ta′shin) precipitation resulting from interaction of specific antibody and antigen.

immunoproliferative (-pro-lif′er-it-iv) characterized by the proliferation of the lymphoid cells producing immunoglobulins, as in the gammopathies.

immunoradiometry (-ra″de-om′ĭ-tre) the use of radiolabelled antibody (in the place of radiolabelled antigen) in radioimmunoassay techniques. **immunoradiomet′ric**, adj.

immunoregulation (-reg″ūl-a′shin) the control of specific immune responses and interactions between B- and T-lymphocytes and macrophages.

immunoresponsiveness (-re-spon′siv-nis) the capacity to react immunologically.

immunosorbent (-sor′bint) an insoluble support for antigen or antibody used to absorb homologous antibodies or antigens, respectively, from a mixture; the antibodies or antigens so removed may then be eluted in pure form.

immunostimulation (-stim″ūl-a′shin) stimulation of an immune response, e.g., by use of BCG vaccine.

immunosuppression (-sah-presh′ĭn) the artificial prevention of the immune response, as by use of radiation, antimetabolites, etc.

immunosuppressive (-sah-pres′iv) 1. pertaining to or inducing immunosuppression. 2. an agent that induces immunosuppression.

immunotherapy (-thĕ′rah-pe) passive immunization of an individual by administration of

THE HUMAN IMMUNOGLOBULINS

	MOL. WT.	NO. OF SUBCLASSES	FUNCTION
IgM	900,000	2	Activation of classic complement pathway; opsonization
IgG	150,000	4	Activation of classic and alternative complement pathways; opsonization (IgG1 and IgG3 only); only class transferred across placenta, thus providing fetus and neonate with protection against infection
IgA	155,000 (serum IgA) 325,000 (secretory IgA)	2	Activation of alternative complement pathway; secretory IgA is the predominant immunoglobulin in secretions
IgD	180,000	—	Not yet determined
IgE	190,000	—	Mediation of immediate hypersensitivity reactions

preformed antibodies (serum or gamma globulin) actively produced in another individual; by extension, the term has come to include the use of immunopotentiators, replacement of immunocompetent lymphoid tissue (e.g., bone marrow or thymus), etc.

immunotoxin (-tok′sin) any antitoxin.

immunotransfusion (-trans-fu′zhin) transfusion of blood from a donor previously rendered immune to the disease affecting the patient.

impacted (im-pak′tid) firmly wedged in firmly. In obstetrics, denoting twins so situated during delivery that pressure of one against the other prevents complete engagement of either.

impaction (im-pak′shin) the condition of being impacted. **dental i.,** prevention of eruption, normal occlusion, or routine removal of a tooth because of its being locked in position by bone, dental restoration, or surfaces of adjacent teeth. **fecal i.,** a collection of hardened feces in the rectum or sigmoid.

impalpable (im-pal′pah-b'l) not detectable by touch.

impedance (im-pēd′ins) obstruction or opposition to passage or flow, as of an electric current or other form of energy. **acoustic i.,** an expression of the opposition to passage of sound waves, being the product of the density of a substance and the velocity of sound in it.

imperforate (im-pur′for-āt) not open; abnormally closed.

impermeable (im-purm′e-ah-b'l) not permitting passage, as of fluid.

impetigo (im″pĭ-ti′go) impetigo contagiosa; a streptococcal or staphylococcal skin infection marked by vesicles or bullae that become pustular, rupture and form yellow crusts. **impetig′inous,** adj. **i. bullo′sa, bullous i.,** impetigo in which the developing vesicles progress to form bullae, which collapse and become covered with crusts. **i. contagio′sa,** impetigo. **i. herpetifor′mis,** a very rare, acute dermatitis with symmetrically ringed, pustular lesions, occurring chiefly in pregnant women and associated with severe constitutional symptoms. **neonatal i., i. neonato′rum,** bulbous impetigo of newborn infants. **i. vulga′ris,** impetigo.

implant 1. (im-plant′) to insert or to graft (tissue, or inert or radioactive material) into intact tissues or a body cavity. 2. (im′plant) any material so inserted or grafted into the body.

implantation (im″plan-ta′shin) 1. attachment of the blastocyst to the epithelial lining of the uterus, its penetration through the epithelium, and, in humans, its embedding in the compact layer of the endometrium, occurring six or seven days after fertilization of the ovum. 2. the insertion of an organ or tissue in a new site in the body. 3. the insertion or grafting into the body of biological, living, inert, or radioactive material.

implosion (im-plo′zhin) in behavior therapy, the treatment of phobias by repeated exposure to the worst possible phobic situations. The patient is instructed to imagine or is presented with the most fearful and anxiety-producing objects until the anxiety does not occur.

impotence (im′pit-ins) lack of power, chiefly of copulative power in the male due to failure to initiate an erection or maintain an erection until ejaculation.

impregnation (im″preg-na′shin) 1. the act of fertilizing. 2. saturation.

impressio (im-pres′e-o), pl. *impressio′nes* [L.] impression (1).

impression (im-presh′in) 1. a slight indentation, as one produced in the surface of one organ by pressure exerted by another. 2. a negative imprint of an object made in some plastic material that later solidifies. 3. an effect produced upon the mind, body, or senses by some external stimulus or agent. **basilar i.,** a developmental deformity of the occipital bone and upper cervical spine, in which the latter seems to have pushed the floor of the occipital bone upward. **cardiac i.,** an impression made by the heart on another organ. **dental i.,** one made of the jaw and/or teeth in some plastic material, which is later filled in with plaster of Paris to produce a facsimile of the oral structures present.

imprinting (im′print-ing) a species-specific, rapid kind of learning during a critical period of early life in which social attachment and identification are established.

impulse (im′puls) 1. a sudden pushing force. 2. a sudden uncontrollable determination to act. 3. nerve i. **cardiac i.,** movement of the chest wall caused by the heart beat. **nerve i.,** the electrochemical process propagated along nerve fibers.

impulsion (im-pul′shin) blind obedience to internal drives, without regard for acceptance by others or pressure from the superego; seen in children and in adults with weak psychic organization.

In chemical symbol, *indium.*

in- 1. a prefix, *in, within,* or *into.* 2. an intensive prefix. 3. an antonymous prefix.

I.N.A. International Neurological Association.

inactivation (in-ak″tĭ-va′shin) the destruction of biological activity, as of a virus, by the action of heat or other agent.

inanimate (-an′im-it) 1. without life. 2. lacking in animation.

inanition (in″ah-nish′in) the exhausted state due to prolonged undernutrition; starvation.

inappetence (in-ap′it-ins) lack of appetite or desire.

inarticulate (in″ar-tik′ūl-it) 1. not having joints; disjointed. 2. uttered so as to be unintelligible; incapable of articulate speech.

in articulo mortis (in ar-tik′ūl-o mor′tis) [L.] at the moment of death.

inborn (in′born″) congenital; formed or acquired during intrauterine life.

inbreeding (-brēd-ing) the mating of closely related individuals or of individuals having closely similar genetic constitutions.

incarceration (in-kar″ser-a′shun) unnatural retention or confinement of a part.

incest (in′sest″) sexual activity between persons so closely related that marriage between them is legally or culturally prohibited.

incidence (-sid-ins) the rate at which a certain

event occurs, as the number of new cases of a specific disease occurring during a certain period.

incident (-sid-int) impinging upon, as incident radiation.

incision (-sizh′in) 1. a cut or a wound made by cutting with a sharp instrument. 2. the act of cutting.

incisor (-si′zer) 1. adapted for cutting. 2. any of the four front teeth in either jaw.

incisura (in″si-su′rah), pl. *incisu′rae* [L.] incisure.

incisure (in-si′zher) a cut, incision, or notch. **i's of Lanterman, i's of Lanterman-Schmidt,** oblique slashes or lines on the sheath of the medullated nerve fibers. **Rivinus′ i.,** tympanic notch; a defect in the upper tympanic part of the temporal bone, filled by the upper portion of the tympanic membrane.

inclinatio (in″klĭ-na′she-o), pl. *inclinatio′nes* [L.] inclination.

inclination (-klĭ-na′shin) a sloping or leaning; the angle of deviation from a particular line or plane of reference; in dentistry, the deviation of a tooth from the vertical. **pelvic i.,** the angle between the plane of the pelvic inlet and the horizontal plane.

inclusion (in-kloo′zhin) 1. the act of enclosing or the condition of being enclosed. 2. anything that is enclosed; a cell inclusion. **cell i.,** a usually lifeless, often temporary, constituent in the cytoplasm of a cell. **dental i.,** 1. a tooth so surrounded with bony tissue that it is unable to erupt. 2. a cyst of oral soft tissue or bone.

incompatible (-kom-pat′ĭ-b'l) not suitable for combination, simultaneous administration, or transplantation; mutually repellent.

incompetent (-kom′pit-int) 1. unable to function properly. 2. a person determined by the courts to be unable to manage his own affairs.

incontinence (-kon′tĭ-nens) 1. inability to control excretory functions. 2. immoderation or excess. **incon′tinent,** adj. **fecal i.,** involuntary passage of feces and flatus. **stress i.,** involuntary escape of urine due to strain on the orifice of the bladder, as in coughing or sneezing. **urinary i.,** inability to control the voiding of urine.

incontinentia (-kon″tĭ-nen′she-ah) [L.] incontinence. **i. al′vi,** fecal incontinence. **i. pigmen′ti,** a hereditary disorder in which early vesicular and later verrucous and bizarrely pigmented skin lesions are associated with eye, bone, and central nervous system defects. **i. uri′nae,** urinary incontinence.

incoordination (in″ko-or″din-a′shin) lack of normal adjustment of muscular motions.

incorporation (in-kor″por-a′shin) 1. the union of a substance with another, or with others, in a composite mass. 2. the unconscious mental mechanism by which attitudes of another person are taken into the mind of an individual.

increment (in′kri-mint) increase or addition; the amount by which a value or quantity is increased. **incremen′tal,** adj.

incrustation (in″krus-ta′shin) 1. the formation of a crust. 2. a crust, scab, or scale.

incubate (in′ku-bāt) 1. to subject to or to undergo incubation. 2. material that has undergone incubation.

incubation (in″ku-ba′shin) 1. the provision of proper conditions for growth and development, as for bacterial or tissue cultures. 2. the development of an infectious disease from time of the entrance of the pathogen to the appearance of clinical symptoms. 3. the development of the embryo in the eggs of oviparous animals. 4. the maintenance of an artificial environment for an infant, especially a premature infant.

incubator (in′ku-bāt-er) an apparatus for maintaining optimal conditions (temperature, humidity, etc.) for growth and development, as one used in the early care of premature infants, or one used for cultures.

incubus (in′ku-bis) 1. nightmare. 2. a heavy mental burden.

incudal (-ku-dil) pertaining to the incus.

incudomalleal (in″ku-do-mal′e-il) pertaining to the incus and malleus.

incudostapedial (-stah-pe′de-il) pertaining to the incus and stapes.

incurable (in-kūr′ah-b'l) 1. not susceptible of being cured. 2. a person with a disease which cannot be cured.

incus (ing′kus) [L.] see *Table of Bones.*

incyclophoria (in″si-klo-for′e-ah) cyclophoria in which the upper pole of the visual axis deviates toward the nose.

incyclotropia (-tro′pe-ah) cyclotropia in which the upper pole of the vertical axis deviates toward the nose.

indanedione (in″dān-di′ōn) any of a group of synthetic anticoagulants derived from 1,3-indanedione, e.g., pheninindione, which impair the hepatic synthesis of the vitamin K–dependent coagulation factors (prothrombin, Factors VII, IX, and X).

Inderal (in′der-al) trademark for a preparation of propranolol hydrochloride.

index (in′deks), pl. *indexes* or *in′dices* [L.] 1. the second digit of the hand, the forefinger. 2. the numerical ratio of measurement of any part in comparison with a fixed standard. **Colour I.,** a publication of the Society of Dyers and Colourists and the American Association of Textile Chemists and Colorists containing an extensive list of dyes and dye intermediates. Each chemically distinct compound is identified by a specific number, the C.I. number, avoiding the confusion of trivial names used for dyes in the dye industry. **I. Medicus,** a monthly publication of the National Library of Medicine in which the world's leading biomedical literature is indexed by author and subject. **mitotic i.,** the ratio of the number of cells in a population undergoing mitosis to the number not undergoing mitosis. **opsonic i.,** a measure of opsonic activity determined by the ratio of the number of microorganisms phagocytized by normal leukocytes in the presence of serum from an individual infected by the microorganism, to the number phagocytized from a normal individual. **phagocytic i.,** the average number of bacteria ingested per leukocyte of the patient's blood. **refractive i.,** the refractive power of a medium compared with that of air (assumed to be 1). **short increment sensitivity i. (SISI),** a hearing test in which randomly spaced, 0.5-second tone bursts are superimposed at 1- to 5-decibel increments in intensity on a carrier tone having the same frequency and an intensity of 20 decibels above the speech recognition threshold. **therapeutic i.,** originally, the ratio of the maximum tolerated dose to the minimum curative dose; now defined as the ratio of the median lethal dose (LD_{50}) to the median effective dose (ED_{50}). It is used in assessing the safety of a drug. **vital i.,** the ratio of births to deaths within a given time in a population.

indican (in'dĭ-kan) 1. a yellow glycoside, $C_{14}H_{17}NO_6$, from indigo plants, which yields glucose and indoxyl on hydrolysis. 2. potassium indoxyl sulfate, $C_8H_6NSO_4K$, formed by decomposition of tryptophan in the intestines and excreted in the urine.

indicator (in'dĭ-kāt"er) 1. the index finger, or the extensor muscle of the index finger. 2. any substance that indicates the appearance or disappearance of a chemical by a color change or attainment of a certain pH.

indigestion (in"dĭ-jes'chin) lack or failure of digestion; commonly used to denote vague abdominal discomfort after meals. **acid i.,** hyperchlorhydria. **fat i.,** steatorrhea. **gastric i.,** that taking place in, or due to a disorder of, the stomach. **intestinal i.,** disorder of the digestive function of the intestine. **sugar i.,** defective ability to digest sugar, resulting in fermental diarrhea.

indigitation (in-dij"ĭ-ta'shin) intussusception (1).

indigo (in'dĭ-go) a blue dyeing material from various leguminous and other plants, being the aglycone of indican and also made synthetically; sometimes found in the sweat and urine.

indigotin (in"dĭ-gōt'in) a neutral tasteless, insoluble, dark blue powder, $C_{16}H_{10}N_2O_2$, the principal ingredient of commercial indigo.

indigotindisulfonate sodium (in"dĭ-go"tin-di-sul'fon-āt) a dye, $C_{16}H_8N_2Na_2O_8S$, used as a diagnostic aid in cystoscopy.

indium (in'de-um) chemical element (*see table*), at. no. 49, symbol In.

individuation (in"dĭ-vij"oo-a'shin) 1. the process of developing individual characteristics. 2. differential regional activity in the embryo occurring in response to organizer influence.

Indocin (in'do-sin) trademark for a preparation of indomethacin.

indole (in'dōl) a compound obtained from coal tar and indigo and produced by decomposition of tryptophan in the intestine, where it contributes to the peculiar odor of feces. It is excreted in the urine in the form of indican.

indolent (in'dah-lint) causing little pain; slow growing.

indomethacin (in"do-meth'ah-sin) an anti-inflammatory, antipyretic, and analgesic agent, $C_{19}H_{16}ClNO_4$, used in arthritic disorders and degenerative joint disease.

indoxyl (in-dok'sil) an oxidation product of in-

dole, C_8H_7NO, formed in tryptophan decomposition, and excreted in the urine as indican.

inducer (in-dūs'er) in biosynthesis, a compound that induces synthesis of a specific enzyme or sequence of enzymes, by antagonizing the corresponding repressor.

induction (-duk'shin) 1. the process or act of inducing, or causing to occur, especially the production of a specific morphogenetic effect in the embryo through evocators or organizers, or the production of anesthesia or unconsciousness by use of appropriate agents. 2. the generation of an electric current or magnetic properties in a body because of its proximity to an electrified or magnetized object.

inductor (-duk'ter) a tissue elaborating a chemical substance that acts to determine growth and differentiation of embryonic parts.

induration (in"dūr-a'shin) quality of being hard; process of hardening; an abnormally hard spot or place. **in'durative,** adj. **black i.,** the hardening and pigmentation of lung tissue, as in pneumonia. **brown i.,** 1. a deposit of altered blood pigment in the lung in pneumonia. 2. increase of pulmonary connective tissue and excessive pigmentation, due to chronic congestion from valvular heart disease or to anthracosis. **cyanotic i.,** hardening of an organ from chronic venous congestion. **granular i.,** cirrhosis. **gray i.,** induration of lung tissue in or after pneumonia, without pigmentation. **red i.,** interstitial pneumonia in which the lung is red and congested.

indusium griseum (in-du'ze-um gris'e-um) [L.] a thin layer of gray matter on the dorsal surface of the corpus callosum.

inebriation (-e"bre-a'shin) the condition of being drunk.

inert (in-ert') inactive.

inertia (-ur'shah) [L.] inactivity; inability to move spontaneously. **colonic i.,** weak muscular activity of the colon, leading to distention of the organ and constipation. **uterine i.,** sluggishness of uterine contractions in labor.

in extremis (in ek-stre'mis) [L.] at the point of death.

infant (-fint) the human young from the time of birth to two years of age. **floppy i.,** see under *syndrome.* **immature i.,** one weighing between 17 ounces and 2.2 lbs. (500–999 gm.) at birth, with little chance of survival. **mature i.,** one weighing 5½ lbs. (2500 gm.) or more at birth, with optimal chance of survival. **newborn i.,** the human young during the first two to four weeks after birth. **postmature i., post-term i.,** one born at any time after the beginning of the forty-second week (288 days) of gestation. **premature i.,** one weighing between 2½ and 5½ lbs. (1000–2499 gm.) at birth, with poor to good chance of survival. **preterm i.,** one born at any time before the thirty-seventh completed week (259 days) of gestation. **term i.,** one born any time from the beginning of the thirty-eighth week (260 days) to the end of the forty-first week (287 days) of gestation.

infantilism (in'fin-til-izm, in-fan'til-izm) persistence of childhood characters into adult life, marked by mental retardation, underdevelopment of sex organs, and often dwarfism. **cachectic i.,** that due to chronic infection or poisoning. **sexual i.,** continuance of prepubertal sex characters and behavior after the usual age of puberty. **universal i.,** general dwarfishness in stature, with absence of secondary sex characteristics.

infarct (in′farkt) a localized area of ischemic necrosis produced by occlusion of the arterial supply or the venous drainage of the part. **anemic i.,** one due to the sudden arrest of circulation in a vessel, or to decoloration of hemorrhagic blood. **hemorrhagic i.,** one that is red owing to oozing of erythrocytes into the injured area.

infarction (in-fark′shin) 1. the formation of an infarct. 2. an infarct. **cardiac i.,** myocardial i. **cerebral i.,** an ischemic condition of the brain, causing a persistent focal neurologic deficit in the area affected. **mesenteric i.,** coagulation necrosis of the intestines due to a decrease in blood flow in the mesenteric vasculature. **myocardial i.,** gross necrosis of the myocardium, due to interruption of the blood supply to the area. **pulmonary i.,** localized necrosis of lung tissue, due to obstruction of the arterial blood supply.

infection (-fek′shin) 1. invasion and multiplication of microorganisms in body tissues, especially that causing local cellular injury due to competitive metabolism, toxins, intracellular replication, or antigen-antibody response. 2. an infectious disease. **droplet i.,** infection due to inhalation of respiratory pathogens suspended on liquid particles exhaled by someone already infected. **endogenous i.,** that due to reactivation of organisms present in a dormant focus, as occurs in tuberculosis, etc.

inferior (in-fēr′e-er) situated below, or directed downward; used in anatomy, used in reference to the lower surface of a structure, or to the lower of two (or more) similar structures.

infertility (in″fer-til′it-e) diminution or absence of ability to produce offspring. **infer′tile,** adj.

infestation (-fes-ta′shin) parasitic attack or subsistence on the skin and/or its appendages, as by insects, mites, or ticks; sometimes used to denote parasitic invasion of the organs and tissues, as by helminths.

infiltration (in″fil-tra′shun) the diffusion or accumulation in a tissue or cells of substances not normal to it or in amounts in excess of the normal; also, the material so accumulated. **adipose i.,** fatty i. **calcareous i.,** deposit of lime and magnesium salts in the tissues. **cellular i.,** the migration and accumulation of cells within the tissues. **fatty i.,** 1. a deposit of fat in tissues, especially between cells. 2. the presence of fat vacuoles in the cell cytoplasm.

infirm (in-furm′) weak; feeble, as from disease or old age.

infirmary (-furm′ah-re) a hospital or place where the sick or infirm are maintained or treated.

inflammagen (in-flam′ah-jen) an irritant that elicits both edema and the cellular response of inflammation.

inflammation (in″flah-ma′shin) a protective tissue response to injury or destruction of tissues, which serves to destroy, dilute, or wall off both the injurious agent and the injured tissues. The classical signs of acute inflammation are pain (dolor), heat (calor), redness (rubor), swelling (tumor), and loss of function (functio laesa). **inflam′matory,** adj. **acute i.,** inflammation, usually of sudden onset, marked by the classical signs (see *inflammation*), in which vascular and exudative processes predominate. **catarrhal i.,** a form affecting mainly a mucous surface, marked by a copious discharge of mucus and epithelial debris. **chronic i.,** prolonged and persistent inflammation marked chiefly by new connective tissue formation; it may be a continuation of an acute form or a prolonged low-grade form. **exudative i.,** one in which the prominent feature is an exudate. **fibrinous i.,** one marked by an exudate of coagulated fibrin. **granulomatous i.,** a form, usually chronic, marked by granuloma formation. **hyperplastic i.,** proliferative i. **interstitial i.,** one affecting chiefly the stroma of an organ. **parenchymatous i.,** one affecting chiefly the essential tissue elements of an organ. **productive i., proliferative i.,** one leading to the production of new connective tissue fibers. **pseudomembranous i.,** an acute inflammatory response to a powerful necrotizing toxin, e.g., diphtheria toxin, with formation, on a mucosal surface, of a false membrane composed of precipitated fibrin, necrotic epithelium, and inflammatory white cells. **purulent i.,** suppurative i. **serous i.,** one producing a serous exudate. **subacute i.,** a condition intermediate between chronic and acute inflammation, exhibiting some of the characteristics of each. **suppurative i.,** one marked by pus formation. **ulcerative i.,** that in which necrosis on or near the surface leads to loss of tissue and creation of a local defect (ulcer).

inflation (in-fla′shin) distention, or the act of distending, with air, gas, or fluid.

inflection, inflexion (-flek′shin) the act of bending inward, or the state of being bent inward.

influenza (in″floo-en′zah) an acute viral infection of the respiratory tract, occurring in isolated cases, epidemics, and pandemics, with inflammation of the nasal mucosa, pharynx, and conjunctiva, headache, and severe, often generalized, myalgia. **influen′zal,** adj.

infolding (in-fold′ing) 1. the folding inward of a layer of tissue, as in the formation of the neural tube in the embryo. 2. the enclosing of redundant tissue by suturing together the walls of an organ on either side of it.

infra- word element [L.], *beneath.*

infrabulge (in′frah-bulj) the surfaces of a tooth gingival to the height of contour, or sloping cervically.

infraclusion (-kloo′zhin) a condition in which the occluding surface of a tooth does not reach the normal occlusal plane and is out of contact with the opposing tooth.

infraction (in-frak′shin) incomplete bone fracture without displacement.

infradentale (in″frah-den-ta′le) a cephalometric landmark, being the highest anterior point on the gingiva between the mandibular medial (central) incisors.

infradian (-de′in) pertaining to a period longer than 24 hours; applied to the cyclic behavior of certain phenomena in living organisms (infradian rhythm).

infraduction (in-frah-duk′shin) the downward rotation of an eye around its horizontal axis.

infraocclusion (-ah-kloo′zhin) infraclusion.

infrared (-red′) denoting electromagnetic radiation of wavelength greater than that of the red end of the spectrum, having wavelengths of 0.75–1000 μ; sometimes subdivided into *long-wave* or *far i.* (about 3.0–1000 μ) and *short-wave* or *near i.* (about 0.75–3.0 μ).

infrasonic (-son′ik) below the frequency range of sound waves.

infraspinous (-spi′nis) beneath the spine of the scapula.

infraversion (-ver′zhin) 1. infraclusion. 2. the downward deviation of one eye. 3. conjugate downward rotation of both eyes.

infundibuliform (in″fun-dib′ūl-ĭ-form″) shaped like a funnel.

infundibuloma (in″fun-dib″ūl-o′mah) a tumor of the stalk (infundibulum) of the hypophysis.

infundibulum (in″fun-dib′ūl-um), pl. *infundi′bula* [L.] 1. any funnel-shaped passage. 2. conus arteriosus. **infundib′ular, adj. ethmoidal i.,** 1. a passage connecting the nasal cavity with anterior ethmoidal cells and frontal sinus. 2. a sinuous passage connecting the middle nasal meatus with the anterior ethmoidal cells and often with the frontal sinus. **i. of hypothalamus,** a hollow, funnel-shaped mass in front of the tuber cinereum, extending to the posterior lobe of the pituitary gland. **i. of uterine tube,** the distal, funnel-shaped portion of the uterine tube.

infusion (in-fu′zhin) 1. the steeping of a substance in water to obtain its soluble principles. 2. the product obtained by this process. 3. the slow therapeutic introduction of fluid other than blood into a vein.

ingestant (-jes′tint) a substance that is or may be taken into the body by mouth or through the digestive system.

ingestion (-jes′chin) the taking of food, drugs, etc., into the body by mouth.

ingravescent (in″grah-ves′int) gradually becoming more severe.

inguen (in′gwen), pl. *in′guina* [L.] the groin.

inguinal (in′gwĭn-il) pertaining to the groin.

inhalant (in-hāl′int) a substance that is or may be taken into the body by way of the nose and trachea (through the respiratory system). **antifoaming i.,** an agent that is inhaled as a vapor to prevent the formation of foam in the respiratory passages of a patient with pulmonary edema.

inhalation (in″hah-la′shin) 1. the drawing of air or other substances into the lungs. 2. any drug or solution of drugs administered (as by means of nebulizers or aerosols) by the nasal or oral respiratory route.

inheritance (-her′it-ins) 1. the acquisition of characters or qualities by transmission from parent to offspring. 2. that which is transmitted from parent to offspring. **cytoplasmic i.,** extrachromosomal i. **dominant i.,** see under *gene.* **extrachromosomal i.,** the inheritance of traits controlled by genes on the DNA of mitochondria in the ooplasm. **intermediate i.,** inheritance in which the phenotype of the heterozygote falls between that of either homozygote. **maternal i.,** extrachromosomal i. **recessive i.,** see under *gene.* **sex-linked i., X-linked i.,** see under *gene.*

inhibition (in″ĭ-bish′in, -hĭ-bish′in) arrest or restraint of a process; in psychiatry, the unconscious restraining of an instinctual drive. **inhib′itory,** adj. **competitive i.,** inhibition of enzyme activity in which the inhibitor (a substrate analogue) competes with the substrate for binding sites on the enzymes. **contact i.,** inhibition of cell division and cell motility in normal animal cells when in close contact with each other. **end-product i.,** inhibition of an activity resulting from the effect of the end product of a biosynthetic process on an earlier step in the process. **noncompetitive i.,** inhibition of enzyme activity by substances that combine with the enzyme at a site other than that utilized by the substrate.

inhibitor (in-hib′it-er) 1. any substance that interferes with a chemical reaction, growth, or other biologic activity. 2. a chemical substance that inhibits or checks the action of a tissue organizer or the growth of microorganisms. 3. an effector that reduces the catalytic activity of an enzyme. **monoamine oxygenase i.,** any of a group of antidepressant drugs that act by blocking the action of monoamine oxygenase, the enzyme that catalyzes the deamination of monoamines.

inion (in′e-on) the external occipital protuberance. **in′ial,** adj.

initis (ĭ-nīt′is) inflammation of the substance of a muscle.

injection (-jek′shin) 1. the forcing of a liquid into a part, as into the subcutaneous tissues, the vascular tree, or an organ. 2. a substance so forced or administered; in pharmacy, a solution of a medicament suitable for injection. 3. congestion. **hypodermic i.,** injection into the subcutaneous tissues. **intracutaneous i., intradermal i.,** one made into the corium or substance of the skin. **intramuscular i.,** one made into the substance of a muscle. **intravenous i.,** one made into a vein. **Ringer's i.,** a sterile solution of sodium chloride, potassium chloride, and calcium chloride in water for injection; used as a fluid and electrolyte replenisher. **sodium chloride i.,** a sterile isotonic solution of sodium chloride in water for injection; used as a fluid and electrolyte replenisher, as an irrigating solution, and as a vehicle for drugs. **subcutaneous i.,** hypodermic i.

injury (in′jer-e) harm or hurt; a wound or maim; usually applied to damage inflicted on the body by an external force. **birth i.,** impairment of body function or structure due to adverse influences to which the infant has been subjected at birth. **Goyrand's i.,** pulled elbow. **whiplash i.,** a nonspecific term applied to injury to the spine and spinal cord due to sudden extension of the neck.

inlay (in'la) material laid into a defect in tissue; in dentistry, a filling made outside the tooth to correspond with the cavity form and then cemented into the tooth.

inlet (-let) a means or route of entrance. **pelvic i.,** the upper limit of the pelvic cavity.

I.N.N. International Nonproprietary Names, the designations recommended by the World Health Organization for pharmaceuticals.

innate (in'āt) inborn; hereditary; congenital.

innervation (in"er-va'shin) 1. the distribution or supply of nerves to a part. 2. the supply of nervous energy or of nerve stimulation sent to a part.

inniidiation (ĭ-nid"e-a'shin) development of cells in a part to which they have been carried by metastasis.

innominate (ĭ-nom'ĭ-nāt) nameless.

inochondritis (in"o-kon-drīt'is) inflammation of a fibrocartilage.

inoculable (ĭ-nok'ūl-ah-b'l) 1. susceptible of being inoculated; transmissible by inoculation. 2. not immune against a disease transmissible by inoculation.

inoculation (ĭ-nok"ūl-a'shin) introduction of microorganisms, infective material, serum, or other substances into tissues of living organisms, or culture media; introduction of a disease agent into a healthy individual to produce a mild form of the disease followed by immunity.

inoculum (ĭ-nok'ūl-um), pl. *ino'cula* [L.] material used in inoculation.

inoperable (in-op'er-ah-b'l) not susceptible to treatment by surgery.

inorganic (in"or-gan'ik) 1. having no organs. 2. not of organic origin.

inorganic acid any acid containing no carbon atoms.

inoscopy (in-os'kah-pe) the diagnosis of disease by artificial digestion and examination of the fibers or fibrinous matter of sputum, blood, effusions, etc.

inosemia (in"o-se'me-ah) 1. the presence of inositol in the blood. 2. an excess of fibrin in the blood.

inosine (in'ah-sin) a purine nucleoside containing the base hypoxanthine and the sugar ribose, which occurs in transfer RNAs. **i. monophosphate (IMP),** a nucleotide produced by the deamination of adenosine monophosphate (AMP) in the metabolism of purine nucleotides.

inositol (in-o'sĭ-tol) a cyclic sugar alcohol, $C_6H_{12}O_6$; usually referring to the most abundant isomer, *myo*-inositol, which is found in many plant and animal tissues.

inotropic (in'o-trop"ik) affecting the force of muscular contractions.

inquest (in'kwest) a legal inquiry before a coroner or medical examiner, and usually a jury, into the manner of death.

insalubrious (in"sah-loo'bre-is) injurious to health.

insanity (in-san'it-e) a legal term for mental illness, roughly equivalent to psychosis and implying inability to be responsible for one's acts. **insane',** adj.

inscriptio (in-skrip'she-o) [L.] inscription. **i. tendi'nea,** see under *intersectio*.

inscription (-skrip'shin) 1. a mark, or line. 2. that part of a prescription containing the names and amounts of the ingredients.

Insecta (in-sek'tah) a class of arthropods whose members are characterized by division into three parts: head, thorax, and abdomen.

insemination (-sem"in-a'shin) the deposit of seminal fluid within the vagina or cervix. **artificial i.,** that done by artificial means.

insensible (-sen'sĭ-b'l) 1. devoid of sensibility or consciousness. 2. not perceptible to the senses.

insertion (-ser'shin) 1. the act of implanting, or condition of being implanted. 2. the site of attachment, as of a muscle to the bone that it moves. **velamentous i.,** attachment of the umbilical cord to the membranes.

insidious (-sid'e-is) coming on stealthily; of gradual and subtle development.

insight (in'sīt") self-understanding; in psychiatry, referring to the extent to which the patient is aware of his illness and understands its nature.

in situ (in sĭ'too) [L.] in its normal place; confined to the site of origin.

insoluble (in-sol'u-b'l) not susceptible of being dissolved.

insomnia (in-som'ne-ah) inability to sleep; abnormal wakefulness.

insonate (-so'nāt) to expose to ultrasound waves.

insorption (-sorp'shin) movement of a substance into the blood, especially from the gastrointestinal tract into the circulating blood.

inspersion (-sper'shin) sprinkling, as with powder.

inspiration (in"spĭ-ra'shin) the drawing of air into the lungs. **inspi'ratory,** adj.

inspissated (in-spis'āt-id) being thickened, dried, or made less fluid by evaporation.

instar (in'stahr) any stage of an arthropod between molts.

instep (-step) the dorsal part of the arch of the foot.

instillation (in"stil-a'shin) administration of a liquid drop by drop.

instinct (in'stinkt) a complex of unlearned responses characteristic of a species. **death i.,** in psychoanalysis, the latent instinctive impulse toward death. **herd i.,** the instinct or urge to be one of a group and to conform to its standards of conduct and opinion.

instrumentation (in"stroo-men-ta'shin) the use of instruments; work performed with instruments.

insudation (-su-da'shin) 1. the accumulation, as in the kidney, of a substance derived from the blood. 2. the substance so accumulated.

insufficiency (-sah-fish'in-se) inability to perform properly an allotted function. **adrenal i.,** hypoadrenalism. **aortic i.,** see under *regurgitation*. **cardiac i.,** heart failure. **coronary i.,** decrease in flow of blood through the coronary blood vessels. **i. of the externi,** deficient power in the externi muscles of the eye, resulting in esophoria. **ileocecal i.,** inability of the ileocecal valve to prevent backflow of contents from the cecum into the ileum. **i. of the interni,** deficient power in the interni muscles of the eye, resulting in exophoria. **mitral i.,** see under *regurgitation.* **pulmonary i.,** see under *regurgitation.* **thyroid i.,** hypothyroidism. **tricuspid i.,** see under *regurgitation.* **valvular i.,** see under *regurgitation.* **velopharyngeal i.,** failure of velopharyngeal closure due to cleft palate, muscular dysfunction, etc., resulting in defective speech. **venous i.,** inadequacy of the venous valves with impairment of venous drainage, resulting in edema. **vertebrobasilar i.,** transient ischemia of the brain stem and cerebellum due to stenosis of the vertebral or basilar artery.

insufflation (-sah-fla′shin) 1. blowing of a powder, vapor, or gas into a body cavity. 2. finely powdered or liquid drugs carried into the respiratory passages by such devices as aerosols. **perirenal i.,** injection of air around the kidney for roentgen examination of the adrenal glands. **tubal i.,** see *Rubin's test.*

insula (in′sūl-ah), pl. *in′sulae* [L.] a triangular area of the cerebral cortex forming the floor of the lateral cerebral fossa.

insular (in′sūl-er) pertaining to the insula or to an island, as the islands of Langerhans.

insulation (in″sūl-a′shin) 1. the surrounding of a space or body with material designed to prevent the entrance or escape of radiant or electrical energy. 2. the material so used.

insulin (in′sūl-in) a double-chain protein hormone formed from proinsulin in the beta cells of the pancreatic islets of Langerhans. The major fuel-regulating hormone, it is secreted into the blood in response to a rise in concentration of blood glucose or amino acids. Insulin promotes the storage of glucose and the uptake of amino acids, increases protein and lipid synthesis, and inhibits lipolysis and gluconeogenesis. A sterile solution of insulin is used in the treatment of diabetes mellitus. **globin zinc i.,** an intermediate-acting insulin consisting of insulin modified by the addition of zinc chloride and globin. **isophane i., NPH i.,** a neutral, crystalline protamine zinc insulin. **protamine zinc i.,** insulin modified by addition of zinc chloride and protamine. **regular i.,** the active principle of the pancreas of slaughter-house animals (cattle or swine), used in sterile acidified solution.

insulinogenesis (in″sūl-in″o-jen′ĭ-sis) the formation and release of insulin by the islands of Langerhans.

insulinoma (in″sūl-in-o′mah) a tumor of the beta cells of the islets of Langerhans; although usually benign, it is one of the chief causes of hypoglycemia.

insulitis (in″sūl-īt′is) cellular infiltration of the islands of Langerhans, possibly in response to invasion by an infectious agent.

insulopenic (in″sūl-o-pe′nik) diminishing, or pertaining to a decrease in, the level of circulating insulin.

insusceptibility (in″sah-sep″tĭ-bil′ĭt-e) the state of being unaffected; immunity.

intake (in′tāk″) the substances, or the quantities thereof, taken in and utilized by the body.

integration (in″tĭ-gra′shin) harmonious assimilation into a common body or activity; anabolic activity.

integumentary (in-teg″u-men′tĕ-re) 1. pertaining to or composed of skin. 2. serving as a covering.

integumentum (in-teg″u-men′tum) [L.] integument.

intellect (in′tĭ-lekt) the mind, thinking faculty, or understanding.

intellectualization (in″tĭ-lek″choo-il-ĭ-za′shin) the mental process in which reasoning is used as a defense against confronting unconscious conflict and its stressful emotions.

intention (in-ten′shin) a manner of healing; see under *healing.*

inter- word element [L.], *between.*

interaction (in″ter-ak′shin) the quality, state, or process of (two or more things) acting on each other. **drug i.,** the action of one drug upon the effectiveness or toxicity of another (or others).

interbrain (in′ter-brān″) 1. thalamencephalon. 2. diencephalon.

intercalary (in-turk′ah-lĕ″re) inserted between; interposed.

intercartilaginous (in″ter-kart″il-aj′ĭ-nis) between, or connecting, cartilages.

intercostal (-kos′t′l) between two ribs.

intercourse (in′ter-kors) mutual exchange. **sexual i.,** coitus.

intercricothyrotomy (in″ter-krĭk″o-thi-rot′ah-me) incision of the larynx through the cricothyroid membrane; inferior laryngotomy.

intercritical (-krit′ĭ-k′l) denoting the period between attacks, as of gout.

intercurrent (-kur′int) occurring during and modifying the course of another disease.

intercusping (-kusp′ing) the occlusion of the cusps of the teeth of one jaw with the depressions in the teeth of the other jaw.

interdental (-den′t′l) between the proximal surfaces of adjacent teeth in the same arch.

interdentium (-den′she-um) the interproximal space.

interdigitation (-dij″ĭ-ta′shin) 1. an interlocking of parts by finger-like processes. 2. one of a set of finger-like processes.

interface (in′ter-fās) the boundary between two systems or phases.

interfascicular (in″ter-fah-sik′ūl-er) between adjacent fascicles.

interfemoral (-fem′er-il) between the thighs.

interferon (-fēr′on) any of a family of glycoproteins, production of which can be stimulated by viral infection, by intracellular parasites, and by bacteria and bacterial endotoxins, that exert antiviral activity and have immunoregulatory functions; they also inhibit the growth of nonviral intracellular parasites. Interferons are designated α, β, and γ on the basis of association with certain producer cells and functions; all animal cells, however, can produce interferons and some cells can produce more than one type. Interferon α has been used in the experimental treatment of some types of neoplasia.

interictal (-ik′t′l) occurring between attacks or paroxysms.

interkinesis (-ki-ne′sis) the period between the first and second divisions in meiosis.

interleukin (in-ter-look′in) a generic term for a group of protein factors produced by macrophages and T cells in response to antigenic or mitogenic stimulation and affecting primarily T cells. Three types of interleukins are distinguished, designated 1, 2, and 3; interleukin-2 is used as an anticancer drug in the treatment of a wide variety of solid tumors.

interlobitis (-lo-bīt′is) interlobular pleurisy.

interlobular (-lob′ūl-er) between lobules.

intermediate (-me′de-it) 1. between; intervening; resembling, in part, each of two extremes. 2. a substance formed in a chemical process that is essential to formation of the end product of the process.

intermedin (-mēd′in) melanocyte-stimulating hormone.

intermedius (-mēd′e-is) [L.] intermediate; in anatomy, denoting a structure lying between a lateral and a medial structure.

intermittent (-mit′int) marked by alternating periods of activity and inactivity.

intern (in′turn″) a medical graduate serving and residing in a hospital preparatory to being licensed to practice medicine.

internal (in-turn′′l) situated or occurring on the inside; in anatomy, many structures formerly called internal are now termed medial.

internalization (in-turn′′′l-iz-a′shin) a mental mechanism whereby certain external attributes, attitudes, or standards of others are unconsciously taken as one's own.

internatal (in″ter-nāt′′l) between the nates, or buttocks.

interneuron (-noōr′on) a neuron between the primary afferent neuron and the final motoneuron. Also, any neuron whose processes are entirely confined within a specific area, as within the olfactory lobe.

internist (in-turn′ist) a specialist in internal medicine.

internship (in′turn-ship) the position or term of service of an intern in a hospital.

internuclear (in″ter-noōk′le-er) situated between nuclei or between nuclear layers of the retina.

internuncial (-nun′shil) transmitting impulses between two different parts.

internus (in-turn′us) [L.] internal; in anatomy, denoting a structure nearer to the center of an organ or part.

interocclusal (in″ter-ah-kloōz′′l) situated between the occlusal surfaces of opposing teeth in the two dental arches.

interoceptor (-sep′ter) a sensory nerve ending that is located in and transmits impulses from the viscera. **interocep′tive,** adj.

interofective (-fek′tiv) affecting the interior of

the organism—a term applied to the autonomic nervous system.

interparietal (-pah-ri′it′l) 1. intermural. 2. between the parietal bones.

interphase (in′ter-fāz) the interval between two successive cell divisions, during which the chromosomes are not individually distinguishable.

interplant (-plant) an embryonic part isolated by transference to an indifferent environment provided by another embryo.

interpolation (in-tur″pil-a′shin) 1. surgical implantation of tissue. 2. the determination of intermediate values in a series on the basis of observed values.

interpretation (-prĭ-ta′shin) in psychotherapy, the therapist's explanation to the patient of the latent or hidden meanings of what he says, does, or experiences.

interproximal (in″ter-prok′sĭ-mil) between two adjoining surfaces.

intersectio (-sek′she-o), pl. *intersectio′nes* [L.] intersection. **i. tendin′ea,** a fibrous band traversing the belly of a muscle, dividing it into two parts.

intersection (-sek′shin) a site at which one structure crosses another.

intersex (in′ter-seks) 1. intersexuality. 2. an individual who exhibits intersexuality. **female i.,** a female pseudohermaprodite. **male i.,** a male pseudohermaphrodite. **true i.,** a true hermaphrodite.

intersexuality (in″ter-sek″shoo-al′it-e) an intermingling, in varying degrees, of the characters of each sex, including physical form, reproductive tissue, and sexual behavior, in one individual, as a result of some flaw in embryonic development; see *hermaphroditism* and *pseudohermaphroditism.* **intersex′ual,** adj.

interspace (in′ter-spās) a space between similar structures.

interstice (in-turs′tis) a small interval, space, or gap in a tissue or structure.

interstitial (in″ter-stish′′l) pertaining to parts or interspaces of a tissue.

interstitium (-stish′ĭ-um) 1. interstice. 2. interstitial tissue.

intertransverse (-tranz-vers′) between transverse processes of the vertebrae.

intertrigo (-tri′go) an erythematous skin eruption occurring on apposed skin surfaces.

interureteral (-ūr-ēt′er-il) interureteric.

interureteric (-ūr-ĭ-ter′ik) between ureters.

intervaginal (-vaj′ĭ-nil) between sheaths.

interval (in′ter-vil) the space between two objects or parts; the lapse of time between two events. **atrioventricular i., A–V i.,** P–R i. **c.-a. i., cardioarterial i.,** the time between the apex beat and arterial pulsation. **lucid i.,** a brief period of remission of symptoms in a psychosis. **postsphygmic i.,** see under *period.* **P–R i.,** the time between the onset of the P wave (atrial activity) and the QRS complex (ventricular activity). **presphygmic i.,** see under *period.* **QRST i., Q–T i.,** the duration of ventricular electrical activity.

intervention (-ven′shin) the act or fact of interfering so as to modify. **crisis i.,** 1. an immediate, short-term, psychotherapeutic approach, the goal of which is to help resolve a personal crisis within the individual's immediate environment. 2. the procedures involved in responding to an emergency.

intervillous (-vil′is) between or among villi.

intestine (in-tes′tin) the part of the alimentary canal extending from the pyloric opening of the stomach to the anus. See Plates *IV, V,* and *XV.* **intes′tinal,** adj. **large i.,** the distal portion of the intestine, about 5 feet long, extending from its junction with the small intestine to the anus and comprising the cecum, colon, rectum, and anal canal. **small i.,** the proximal portion of the intestine about 20 feet long, smaller in caliber than the large intestine, extending from the pylorus to the cecum and comprising the duodenum, jejunum, and ileum.

intestinum (in″tes-ti′nim), pl. *intesti′na* [L.] intestine.

intima (in′tĭ-mah) an innermost structure; see *tunica intima.* **in′timal,** adj.

intimitis (in″tĭ-mīt′is) endarteritis.

intolerance (in-tol′er-ins) inability to withstand or consume; inability to absorb or metabolize nutrients. **drug i.,** the state of reacting to the normal pharmacologic doses of a drug with the symptoms of overdosage.

intorsion (-tor′shin) inward rotation of the upper pole of the vertical meridian of each eye toward the midline of the face.

intoxication (-tok″sĭ-ka′shin) 1. poisoning; the state of being poisoned. 2. the condition caused from the excessive use of alcohol; simple drunkenness. 3. an organic brain syndrome marked by the presence in the body of an exogenous psychoactive substance producing a substance-specific syndrome of effects on the central nervous system, and leading to maladaptive behavior or impaired social or occupational functioning. **alcohol idiosyncratic i.,** maladaptive behavioral change, usually belligerence, from consuming alcohol insufficient to cause intoxication in most people. **pathological i.,** alcohol idiosyncratic i.

intra- word element [L.], *inside; within.*

intracanalicular (-kan″al-ik′ūl-er) within canaliculi.

intracardiac (-kar′de-ak) within the heart.

intracellular (-sel′ūl-er) within a cell or cells.

intracervical (-ser′vik′l) within the canal of the cervix uteri.

intractable (in-trakt′ah-b′l) resistant to cure, relief, or control.

intracystic (-sis′tik) within the bladder or a cyst.

intradural (-dūr′l) within or beneath the dura mater.

intrafat (-fat′) situated in or introduced into fatty tissue, as the subcutaneous tissue.

intrafusal (-fu′z′l) pertaining to the striated fibers within a muscle spindle.

Intralipid (-lip′id) trademark for an intravenous fat emulsion used to prevent or correct deficiency of essential fatty acids and to provide calories in high density form during total parenteral nutrition.

intralobular (-lob′ūl-er) within a lobule.

intramedullary (-med′il-ĕ″re, mĭ-dul′ah-re) within (1) the spinal cord, (2) the medulla oblongata, or (3) the marrow cavity of a bone.

intramuscular (-mus′kūl-er) within the muscular substance.

intraoperative (-op′er-āt″iv) occurring during a surgical operation.

intraparietal (-pah-ri′it′l) 1. intramural. 2. within the parietal region of the brain.

intrapartum (-part′um) occurring during childbirth or during delivery.

intrapsychic (-si′kik) taking place within the mind.

intraspinal (-spīn′′l) within the spinal column.

intrathecal (-the′k′l) within a sheath; through the theca of the spinal cord into the subarachnoid space.

intratracheal (-tra′ke-il) endotracheal.

intratympanic (-tim-pan′ik) within the tympanic cavity.

intravasation (in-tră″vah-sa′shin) the entrance of foreign material into vessels.

intravital (-vīt′′l) occurring during life.

intra vitam (in′trah vīt′am) [L.] during life.

intrinsic (in-trin′sik) situated entirely within or pertaining exclusively to a part.

introitus (-tro′it-is), pl. *intro′itus* [L.] the entrance to a cavity or space.

introjection (in″trah-jek′shin) a mental mechanism in which loved or hated external objects are unconsciously and symbolically taken within oneself.

intromission (-mish′in) the entrance of one part or object into another.

introspection (-spek′shin) contemplation or observation of one's own thoughts and feelings; self-analysis. **introspec′tive,** adj.

introsusception (-sah-sep′shin) intussusception.

introversion (-vur′zhin) 1. the turning outside in, more or less completely, of an organ. 2. preoccupation with oneself, with reduction of interest in the outside world.

intubation (in″too-ba′shin) the insertion of a tube into a body canal or hollow organ, as into the trachea. **endotracheal i.,** insertion of a tube into the trachea for administration of anesthesia, maintenance of an airway, aspiration of secretions, ventilation of the lungs, or prevention of entrance of foreign material into the tracheobronchial tree. The tube may be inserted through the nose (*nasotracheal i.*) or mouth (*orotracheal i.*). **nasal i.,** insertion of a tube into the respiratory or gastrointestinal tract through the nose. **oral i.,** insertion of a tube into the respiratory or gastrointestinal tract through the mouth.

intumescence (in″too-mes′ins) 1. a swelling, normal or abnormal. 2. the process of swelling. **intumes′cent,** adj.

intumescentia (in-too″mis-en′she-ah) intumescence.

intussusception (in″tah-sah-sep′shin) 1. prolapse of one part of the intestine into the lumen of an immediately adjacent part. 2. the reception into an organism of matter, such as food, and its transformation into new protoplasm.

intussusceptum (-sep′tum) the portion of intestine that has prolapsed in intussusception.

intussuscipiens (-sip′e-ens) the portion of intestine containing the intussusceptum.

inulin (in′ūl-in) a starch occurring in the rhizome of certain plants, yielding fructose on hydrolysis, and used in tests of renal function.

inunction (in-unk′shin) 1. the act of anointing or applying an ointment by friction. 2. an ointment made with lanolin as a menstruum.

in utero (in ūt′er-o) [L.] within the uterus.

in vacuo (in vak′u-o) [L.] in a vacuum.

invagination (-vaj″in-a′shin) 1. the infolding of one part within another part of a structure, as of the blastula during gastrulation. 2. intussusception.

invasion (in-va′zhin) 1. the attack or onset of a disease. 2. the simple, harmless entrance of bacteria into the body or their deposition in tissue, as opposed to infection. 3. the infiltration and destruction of surrounding tissue, characteristic of malignant tumors.

invasive (-va′siv) 1. having the quality of invasiveness. 2. involving puncture of the skin or insertion of an instrument or foreign material into the body; said of diagnostic techniques.

invasiveness (-va′siv-nis) 1. the ability of microorganisms to enter the body and spread in the tissues. 2. the ability to infiltrate and actively destroy surrounding tissue, a property of malignant tumors. **inva′sive**, adj.

inversion (-vur′zhin) 1. a turning inward, inside out, or other reversal of the normal relation of a part. 2. homosexuality. 3. a chromosomal aberration due to the inverted reunion of the middle segment after breakage of a chromosome at two points, resulting in a change in sequence of genes or nucleotides. **i. of uterus,** a turning of the uterus whereby the fundus is forced through the cervix, protruding into or completely outside of the vagina. **visceral i.,** the more or less complete right and left transposition of the viscera.

invert (in′vurt) a homosexual.

invertebrate (-vert′ĭ-brāt) 1. having no spinal column. 2. any animal having no spinal column.

investment (-vest′mint) material in which a denture, tooth, crown, or model for a dental restoration is enclosed for curing, soldering, or casting, or the process of such enclosure.

inveterate (-vet′er-āt) confirmed and chronic; long-established and difficult to cure.

in vitro (in ve′tro) [L.] within a glass; observable in a test tube; in an artificial environment.

in vivo (in ve′vo) [L.] within the living body.

involucrum (in″vol-oo′krum), pl. *involu′cra* [L.] a covering or sheath, as of a sequestrum.

involution (-oo′shin) 1. a rolling or turning inward. 2. one of the movements in the gastrulation of many animals. 3. a retrograde change of the body or of an organ, as the retrograde changes in the female genital organs that result

in normal size after delivery. 4. the progressive degeneration occurring naturally with age, resulting in shriveling of organs or tissues. **involu′tional,** adj.

Io chemical symbol, *ionium.*

iocetamic acid (i″o-se-tam′ik) a water-soluble iodinated radiopaque x-ray contrast medium, $C_{12}H_{13}I_3N_2O_3$.

iodic acid (i-od′ik) a monobasic acid, HIO_3, formed by oxidation of iodine with nitric acid or chlorates, which has strong acid and reducing properties.

iodide (-dīd) a binary compound of iodine.

iodination (i″ah-din-a′shin) the incorporation or addition of iodine in a compound.

iodine (i′ah-dīn) chemical element (*see table*), at. no. 53, symbol I; it is essential in nutrition, being necessary for synthesis of the thyroid hormones thyroxine and triiodothyronine. Iodine solution is used as a topical anti-infective. **protein-bound i.,** iodine firmly bound to protein in the serum, determination of which constitutes one test of thyroid function. **radioactive i.,** radioiodine.

iodinophilous (i″ah-din-of′ĭ-lis) easily stainable with iodine.

iodipamide (i″ah-dip′ah-mīd) a radiopaque medium, $C_{20}H_{14}I_6N_2O_6$, used in the form of its meglumine and sodium salts in cholecystography.

iodism (i′ah-dizm) chronic poisoning by iodine or iodides, with coryza, ptyalism, frontal headache, emaciation, weakness, and skin eruptions.

iodochlorhydroxyquin (i-o″do-klor″r″hi-drok′-sĭ-kwin) an anti-infective, C_9H_5ClINO, used topically in the treatment of amebiasis, *Trichomonas vaginalis* infection, and eczema.

iododerma (-durm′ah) any skin lesion resulting from iodism.

iodoform (i-o′dah-form) a local anti-infective, CHI_3.

iodohippurate sodium (i″ah-do-hip′ūr-āt) an iodine-containing compound, $C_9H_7INNaO_3$, administered as a radiopaque medium in pyelography. When labeled with radioactive iodine, it may be used as a diagnostic aid in determination of renal function.

iodophilia (-fil′e-ah) a reaction shown by leukocytes in certain pathologic conditions, as in toxemia and severe anemia, in which the polymorphonuclears show diffuse brownish coloration when treated with iodine or iodides.

iodopsin (i″ah-dop′sin) a photosensitive violet pigment found in the retinal cones of some animals and important for color vision.

iodoquinol (i-o″dah-kwin′ol) an amebicide, $C_{15}H_{13}I_2NO_4$, used in the treatment of intestinal amebiasis and *Trichomonas* vaginitis.

iodum (i-o′dum) [L.] iodine.

ion (i′on) an atom or molecule that has gained or lost one or more electrons and acquired a positive charge (a cation) or negative charge (an anion). **ion′ic,** adj. **dipolar i.,** zwitterion.

Ionamin (i-o′nah-min) trademark for a preparation of phentermine.

ionization (i″in-iz-a′shin) 1. the dissociation of a substance in solution into ions. 2. iontophoresis.

ionophore (i′on-ah-for″) any molecule, as of a drug, that increases the permeability of cell membranes to a specific ion.

iontophoresis (i-on″to-for-e′sis) the introduction of ions of soluble salts into the body by means of electric current. **iontophoret′ic**, adj.

iopanoic acid (i″o-pah-no′ik) $C_{11}H_{12}I_3NO_3$; used as a radiopaque medium in cholecystography.

iophendylate (i″o-fen′dĭ-lāt) a radiopaque medium, $C_{19}H_{29}IO_2$, used in myelography.

iothalamate (-thal′ah-māt) a radiopaque medium for angiography and urography.

I.P. intraperitoneally; isoelectric point.

I.P.A.A. International Psychoanalytical Association.

ipecac (ip′ĕ-kak) the dried rhizome and roots of *Cephaelis ipecacuanha* or *Cephaelis acuminata;* used as an emetic or expectorant.

ipodate (i′po-dāt) a radiopaque contrast medium, $C_{12}H_{13}I_3N_2O_2$, used in cholecystography.

IPPB intermittent positive pressure breathing.

ipsi- word element [L.], *same; self.*

ipsilateral (ip″sĭ-lat′er-il) situated on or affecting the same side.

I.Q. intelligence quotient.

Ir chemical symbol, *iridium.*

irid(o)- word element [Gr.], *iris of the eye; a colored circle.*

iridauxesis (ir″id-awk-se′sis) thickening of the iris.

iridectomesodialysis (ir″ĭ-dek″to-me″so-di-al′ĭ-sis) excision and separation of adhesions around the inner edge of the iris.

iridectomy (ir″ĭ-dek′tah-me) excision of part of the iris.

iridectropium (ir″ĭ-dek-tro′pe-um) eversion of the iris.

iridemia (ir″ĭ-dēm′e-ah) hemorrhage from the iris.

iridencleisis (ir″ĭ-den-kli′sis) surgical incarceration of a slip of the iris within a corneal or limbal incision to act as a wick for aqueous drainage in glaucoma.

iridentropium (ir″ĭ-den-tro′pe-um) inversion of the iris.

irideremia (ir″ĭ-der-e′me-ah) congenital absence of the iris.

irides (ir′ĭ-dēz) [Gr.] plural of *iris.*

iridescence (ir″ĭ-des′ins) the condition of gleaming with bright and changing colors. **irides′cent,** adj.

iridesis (i-rid′ĭ-sis) repositioning of the pupil by fixation of a sector of iris in a corneal or limbal incision.

iridic (i-rid′ik) pertaining to the iris.

iridium (ĭ-rid′e-um, i-rid′e-um) chemical element (*see table*), at. no. 77, symbol Ir.

iridoavulsion (ir″ĭ-do-ah-vul′shin) complete tearing away of the iris from its periphery.

iridocele (i-rid′ah-sēl) hernial protrusion of part of the iris through the cornea.

iridocoloboma (-kol″ah-bo′mah) congenital fissure or coloboma of the iris.

iridoconstrictor (-kon-strik′ter) a muscle element or an agent which acts to constrict the pupil of the eye.

iridocyclitis (-si-klīt′is) inflammation of the iris and ciliary body. **heterochromic i.,** a unilateral low-grade form leading to depigmentation of the iris of the affected eye.

iridocystectomy (-sis-tek′tah-me) excision of part of the iris to form an artificial pupil.

iridodesis (ir″ĭ-dod′ĭ-sis) iridesis.

iridodialysis (ir″ĭ-do-di-al′ĭ-sis) the separation or loosening of the iris from its attachments.

iridodilator (-di-lāt′er) a muscle element or an agent which acts to dilate the pupil of the eye.

iridodonesis (-do-ne′sis) tremulousness of the iris on movement of the eye, occurring in subluxation of the lens.

iridokeratitis (-ker″ah-tīt′is) inflammation of the iris and cornea.

iridokinesia, iridokinesis (-ki-ne′ze-ah; -kine′sis) contraction and expansion of the iris. **iridokinet′ic,** adj.

iridoleptynsis (-lep-tin′sis) thinning or atrophy of the iris.

iridomalacia (ir″i-do-mah-la′she-ah) softening of the iris.

iridomesodialysis (-me″so-di-al′ĭ-sis) surgical loosening of adhesions around the inner edge of the iris.

iridomotor (-mōt′er) pertaining to movements of the iris.

iridoncus (ir″id-ong′kus) tumor or swelling of the eye.

iridoperiphakitis (-per″ĭ-fah-kīt′is) inflammation of the lens capsule.

iridoplegia (-ple′je-ah) paralysis of the sphincter of the iris.

iridoptosis (ir″id-op-to′sis) prolapse of the iris.

iridorhexis (-rek′sis) 1. rupture of the iris. 2. the tearing away of the iris.

iridoschisis (ir″ĭ-dos′kĭ-sis) splitting of the mesodermal stroma of the iris into two layers, with fibrils of the anterior layer floating in the aqueous.

iridosteresis (-stĕ-re′sis) removal of all or part of the iris.

iridotasis (ir″ĭ-dot′ah-sis) surgical stretching of the iris for glaucoma.

iridotomy (ir″ĭ-dot′o-me) incision of the iris.

iris (i′ris) the circular pigmented membrane behind the cornea, perforated by the pupil. See Plate XIII.

iritis (i-rīt′is) inflammation of the iris. **irit′ic,** adj. **serous i.,** iritis with a serous exudate.

iritoectomy (ir″it-o-ek′tah-me) surgical excision of deposits of after-cataract on the iris, together with iridectomy, to form an artificial pupil.

iritomy (i-rit′ah-me) iridotomy.

iron (i′ern) chemical element (*see table*), at. no. 26, symbol Fe; it is an essential constituent of hemoglobin, cytochrome, and other components of respiratory enzyme systems. Depletion of iron stores may result in iron-deficiency anemia. **i.-59,** a radioisotope or iron having a half-life of 45 days; used in ferrokinetics tests to determine the rate at which iron is cleared from the plasma and incorporated in red cells. Symbol ^{59}Fe.

irotomy (i-rot'ah-me) iridotomy.

irradiate (ĭ-rād'e-āt) to treat with radiant energy.

irreducible (ir''ĭ-doo'sĭ-b'l) not susceptible to reduction, as a fracture, hernia, or chemical substance.

irrigation (ir''ĭ-ga'shin) washing by a stream of water or other fluid.

irritability (ir''it-ah-bil'ĭt-e) the quality of being irritable. **myotatic i.**, the ability of a muscle to contract in response to stretching.

irritable (ir''it-ah-b'l) 1. capable of reacting to a stimulus. 2. abnormally sensitive to stimuli.

irritation (ir''ĭ-ta'shin) 1. the act of stimulating. 2. a state of overexcitation and undue sensitivity. **ir'ritative,** adj.

IRV inspiratory reserve volume.

ischemia (is-ke'me-ah) deficiency of blood in a part, due to functional constriction or actual obstruction of a blood vessel. **ische'mic,** adj.

ischi(o)- word element [Gr.], *ischium.*

ischial (is'ke-il) ischiatic.

ischiatic (is''ke-at'ik) pertaining to the ischium.

ischidrosis (is''kĭ-dro'sis) anhidrosis.

ischiocapsular (-kap'sūl-er) pertaining to the ischium and the capsular ligament of the hip joint.

ischiococcygeal (is''ke-o-kok-sij'e-il) pertaining to the ischium and coccyx.

ischiodynia (-din'e-ah) pain in the ischium.

ischiopubic (is''ke-o-pu'bik) pertaining to the ischium and pubes.

ischium (is'ke-um), pl. *is'chia* [L.] see *Table of Bones* and Plate II.

ischuria (is-kūr'e-ah) retention or suppression of the urine. **ischuret'ic,** adj.

iseikonia (is''i-kōn'e-ah) iso-iconia. **iseikon'ic,** adj.

isethionate (is''eth-i'ah-nāt) USAN contraction for 2-hydroxyethanesulfonate.

island (i'lind) a cluster of cells or isolated piece of tissue. **blood i's,** aggregations of mesenchymal cells in the angioblast of the embryo, developing into vascular endothelium and blood cells. **i's of Langerhans,** see under *islet.* **i's of pancreas,** islets of Langerhans. **i. of Reil,** insula.

islet (i'lit) an island. **i's of Langerhans,** irregular microscopic structures scattered throughout the pancreas and comprising its endocrine portion. They contain the *alpha cells,* which secrete the hyperglycemic factor glucagon; the *beta cells,* which secrete insulin; and the *delta cells,* which secrete somatostatin. Degeneration of the beta cells is one of the causes of diabetes mellitus. **i's of pancreas,** i's of Langerhans.

iso- word element [Gr.], *equal; alike; same.*

isoagglutinin (i''so-ah-glōōt'in-in) an isoantigen that acts as an agglutinin.

isoallele (-ah-lēl') an allelic gene that is considered as being normal but can be distinguished from another allele by its differing phenotypic expression when in combination with a dominant mutant allele.

isoantibody (-an'tĭ-bod''e) an antibody produced by one individual that reacts with isoantigens of another individual of the same species.

isoantigen (-an'tĭ-jin) an antigen existing in alternative (allelic) forms thus inducing an immune response when one form is transferred to members who lack it; typical isoantigens are the blood group antigens.

isobar (i'so-bar) 1. one of two or more chemical species with the same atomic weight but different atomic numbers. 2. a line on a map or chart depicting the boundaries of an area of constant atmospheric pressure.

isocarboxazid (i''so-kar-bok''sah-zid) an antidepressant, $C_{12}H_{13}N_3O_2$.

isocellular (-sel'ūl-er) made up of identical cells.

isochromatic (-kro-mat'ik) of the same color throughout.

isochromosome (-kro'mah-sōm) an abnormal chromosome having a median centromere and two identical arms, formed by transverse, rather than normal longitudinal, splitting of a replicating chromosome.

isochronic, isochronous (-kron'ik; i-sok'rah-nis) performed in equal times; said of motions and vibrations occurring at the same time and being equal in duration.

isocitrate (i''so-si'trāt) a salt of isocitric acid.

isocitric acid (i-so-si'trik) HOOC—CH₂—CH(COOH)-CH(OH)—COOH, an intermediate in the tricarboxylic acid cycle, formed from oxaloacetic acid and converted to ketoglutaric acid.

isocoria (-kor'e-ah) equality of size of the pupils of the two eyes.

isocortex (-kor'teks) neopallium.

isocytolysin (-si-tol'ĭ-sin) an isoantigen that acts as a cytolysin.

isocytosis (-si-to'sis) equality of size of cells, especially of erythrocytes.

isodactylism (-dak'tĭ-lizm) relatively even length of the fingers.

isodose (i'so-dōs) a radiation dose of equal intensity to more than one body area.

isoelectric (i''so-e-lek'trik) showing no variation in electric potential.

isoenergetic (-en''er-jet'ik) exhibiting equal energy.

isoenzyme (-en'zīm) isozyme.

isoflurophate (-flōōr'ah-fāt) diisopropyl fluorophosphate or diisopropyl phosphorofluoridate: an anticholinesterase, $C_6H_{14}FO_3P$, used topically as a miotic in glaucoma.

isogamety (-gam'ĭt-e) production by an individual of one sex of gametes identical with respect to the sex chromosome. **isogamet'ic,** adj.

isogamy (i-sog'ah-me) reproduction resulting from union of two gametes identical in size and structure, as in protozoa. **isog'amous,** adj.

isogeneic (i''so-jĭ-ne'ik) syngeneic.

isogenesis (-jen'ĭ-sis) similarity in the processes of development.

isograft (i'sah-graft) a graft between genetically identical individuals.

isohemagglutinin (-hem''ah-glōōt'in-in) an isoantigen that agglutinates erythrocytes.

isohemolysin (-he-mol′ĭ-sin) an isoantigen that causes hemolysis.

isohypercytosis (-hi″per-si-to′sis) increase in the number of leukocytes with normal proportions of neutrophil cells.

isohypocytosis (-hi″po-si-to′sis) decrease in the number of leukocytes, with normal relation between the number of various forms.

iso-iconia (-i-kōn′e-ah) a condition in which the image of an object is the same in both eyes. **iso-icon′ic,** adj.

isoimmunization (-im″ūn-iz-a′shin) development of antibodies in response to isoantigens.

isolate (i′sah-lāt) 1. to separate from others. 2. a group of individuals prevented by geographic, genetic, ecologic, social, or artificial barriers from interbreeding with others of their kind.

isolation (i″sah-la′shin) the act of isolating or state of being isolated, such as (a) the physiologic separation of a part, as by tissue culture or by interposition of inert material; (b) the segregation of patients with a communicable disease; (c) the successive propagation of a growth of microorganisms until a pure culture is obtained; (d) the chemical extraction of an unknown substance in pure form from a tissue; (e) an unconscious mental mechanism in which there is defensive failure to connect behavior with motives, or contradictory attitudes and behavior with each other.

isolecithal (-les′ĭ-thil) having yolk evenly distributed throughout the cytoplasm of the ovum.

isoleucine (-loo′sēn) an amino acid produced by hydrolysis of fibrin and other proteins; essential for optimal infant growth and for nitrogen equilibrium in adults.

isologous (i-sol′ah-gis) characterized by an identical genotype.

isolysin (i-sol′ĭ-sin) a lysin acting on cells of animals of the same species as that from which it is derived.

isomer (i′sah-mer) any compound exhibiting, or capable of exhibiting isomerism. **isomer′ic,** adj.

isomerase (i-som′er-ās) a major class of enzymes comprising those that catalyze the process of isomerization.

isomerism (i-som′ah-rizm) the possession by two or more distinct compounds of the same molecular formula, each molecule having the same number of atoms of each element, but in different arrangement. **geometric i.,** stereoisomerism said to be dependent upon some form of restricted rotation, enabling the molecular components to occupy different spatial positions. **optical i.,** stereoisomerism in which an appreciable number of molecules exhibit different effects on polarized light. **structural i.,** isomerism in which the compounds have the same molecular but different structural formulas, the linkages of the atoms being different.

isomerization (i-som″er-i-za′shin) the process whereby any isomer is converted into another isomer, usually requiring special conditions of temperature, pressure, or catalysts.

isometric (-mĕ′trik) maintaining, or pertaining to, the same measure of length; of equal dimensions.

isometropia (-mĭ-tro′pe-ah) equality in refraction of the two eyes.

isomorphism (-mor′fizm) identity in form; in genetics, referring to genotypes of polyploid organisms which produce similar gametes even though containing genes in different combinations on homologous chromosomes. **isomor′phous,** adj.

isoniazid (-ni′ah-zid) a tuberculostatic, $C_6H_7N_3O$.

isophoria (i″so-for′e-ah) equality in the tension of the vertical muscles of each eye.

isoprecipitin (i″so-pre-sip′it-in) an isoantigen that acts as a precipitin.

isopropamide iodide (-pro′pah-mīd) an anticholinergic, $C_{23}H_{33}IN_2O$, used as an antisecretory and antispasmodic in gastrointestinal disorders.

isopropanol (-pro′pah-nol) isopropyl alcohol.

isoproterenol (-pro″tah-re′nol) a sympathomimetic, $C_{11}H_{17}NO_3$, used chiefly, in the form of the hydrochloride and sulfate salts, as a bronchodilator and cardiac stimulant.

isopter (i-sop′ter) a curve representing areas of equal visual acuity in the field of vision.

Isopto-Carpine (i-sop′to-kar″pēn) trademark for a preparation of pilocarpine hydrochloride.

isopyknosis (i″so-pik-no′sis) the quality of showing uniform density throughout, especially the uniformity of condensation observed in comparison of different chromosomes or in different areas of the same chromosome. **isopyknot′ic,** adj.

Isordil (i′sor-dil) trademark for preparations of isosorbide dinitrate.

isorrhea (i″sor-e′ah) an equilibrium between the intake and output, by the body, of water and solutes. **isorrhe′ic,** adj.

isosensitization (-sen″sit-iz-a′shin) allosensitization.

isosexual (-sek′shoo-il) pertaining to or characteristic of the same sex.

isosmotic (i″soz-mot′ik) having the same osmotic pressure.

isosorbide (i″so-sor′bīd) an osmotic diuretic, $C_6H_{10}O_4$; the dinitrate of isosorbide is used as a coronary vasodilator in coronary insufficiency and angina pectoris.

Isospora (i-sos′por-ah) a genus of sporozoan parasites (order Coccidia), found in birds, amphibians, reptiles, and various mammals, including man; *I. bel′li* and *I. hom′inis* cause coccidiosis in man.

isospore (i′so-spor) 1. an isogamete of organisms that reproduce by spores. 2. an asexual spore produced by a homosporous organism.

isosthenuria (i″sos-thin-ūr′e-ah) maintenance of a constant osmolality of the urine, regardless of changes in osmotic pressure of the blood.

isotherm (i′sah-therm) a line on a map or chart depicting the boundaries of an area in which the temperature is the same.

isotone (i′sah-tōn) one of several nuclides having the same number of neutrons, but differing in number of protons in their nuclei.

isotonia (i″sah-tōn′e-ah) 1. a condition of equal

tone, tension, or activity. **2.** equality of osmotic pressure between two elements of a solution or between two different solutions.

isotonic (-ton′ik) **1.** of equal tension. **2.** denoting a solution in which body cells can be bathed without net flow of water across the semipermeable cell membrane; also, denoting a solution having the same tonicity as another solution with which it is compared.

isotope (i′sah-tōp) a chemical element having the same atomic number as another (i.e., the same number of nuclear protons), but having a different atomic mass (i.e., a different number of nuclear neutrons).

isotretinoin (i″sah-tret′in-o-in) a synthetic form of retinoic acid, used orally to clear cystic and conglobate acne.

isotropic (i″sah-trop′ik) **1.** having the same value of a property, e.g., refractive index, in all directions. **2.** being singly refractive.

isoxsuprine (i-sok′su-prēn) a vasodilator, C_{18}-$H_{23}NO_3$, used as the hydrochloride salt.

isozyme (i′sah-zīm) one of the multiple forms in which an enzyme may exist in an organism or in different species, the various forms differing chemically, physically, or immunologically, but catalyzing the same reaction.

issue (ish′oo) a discharge of pus, blood, or other matter; a suppurating lesion emitting such a discharge.

isthmectomy (is-mek′tah-me) excision of an isthmus, especially the isthmus of the thyroid.

isthmoparalysis (is″mo-pah-ral′ĭ-sis) isthmoplegia.

isthmus (is′mis) a narrow connection between two larger bodies or parts. **is′thmian,** adj. **i. of auditory tube, i. of eustachian tube,** the narrowest part of the auditory tube at the junction of its bony and cartilaginous parts. **i. of fauces,** the constricted aperture between the cavity of the mouth and the pharynx. **i. of rhombencephalon,** the narrow segment of the fetal brain, forming the plane of separation between the rhombencephalon and cerebrum. **i. of thyroid,** the band of tissue joining the lobes of the thyroid. **i. of uterine tube,** the narrower, thicker-walled portion of the uterine tube closest to the uterus. **i. of uterus,** the constricted part of the uterus between the cervix and the body of the uterus.

itch (ich) a skin disorder attended with itching. **bakers' i.,** any of several inflammatory dermatoses of the hands, especially chronic monilial paronychia, seen with special frequency in bakers. **barbers' i.,** **1.** tinea barbae. **2.** sycosis vulgaris. **grain i.,** itching dermatitis due to a mite, *Pyemotes ventricosus,* which preys on certain insect larvae which live on straw, grain, and other plants. **grocers' i.,** a vesicular dermatitis caused by certain mites found in stored hides, dried fruits, grain, copra, and cheese. **ground i.,** the itching eruption caused by the entrance into the skin of the larvae of *Ancylostoma duodenale* or *Necator americanus;* see *hookworm disease.* **jock i.,** tinea cruris. **swimmers' i.,** an itching dermatitis due to penetration into the skin of larval forms (cercaria) of schistosomes, occurring in bathers in waters infested with these organisms.

itching (ich′ing) pruritus; an unpleasant cutaneous sensation, provoking the desire to scratch or rub the skin.

iter (it′er) a tubular passage. **i′teral,** adj. **i. ad infundi′bulum,** the passage from the third ventricle of the brain to the infundibulum (1). **i. chor′dae ante′rius,** the opening through which the chorda tympani nerve exits the tympanic cavity. **i. chor′dae poste′rius,** the opening through which the chorda tympani nerve enters the tympanic cavity. **i. den′tium,** the passage through which a permanent tooth erupts through the gums. **i. eter′tio ad quar′tum ventri′culum,** cerebral aqueduct.

-itis, pl. *i′tides.* Word element [Gr.], *inflammation.*

I.U. immunizing unit; international unit.

IUCD intrauterine contraceptive device.

IUD intrauterine contraceptive device.

I.V. intravenously.

Ixodes (iks-o′dēz) a genus of parasitic ticks (family Ixodidae); some species are disease vectors.

ixodiasis (ik″sah-di′ah-sis) any disease or lesion due to tick bites; infestation with ticks.

Ixodidae (iks-od′ĭ-de) a family of ticks (superfamily Ixodoidea), comprising the hard-bodied ticks.

Ixodides (iks-od′ĭ-dēz) the ticks, a suborder of Acarina, including the superfamily Ixodoidea.

Ixodoidea (iks″o-doid′e-ah) a superfamily of arthropods (suborder Ixodides), comprising both the hard- and soft-bodied ticks.

J

J symbol for *joule*.

jacket (jak′it) an enveloping structure or garment for the trunk or upper part of the body. **plaster-of-Paris j.**, a casing of plaster of Paris enveloping the body, to support or correct deformities. **strait j.**, see *straitjacket*.

jackscrew (jak′skroo) a screw-turned device to expand the dental arch and move individual teeth.

jactitation (jak″tĭ-ta′shin) restless tossing to and fro in acute illness.

jaundice (jawn′dis) icterus; yellowness of the skin, scleras, mucous membranes, and excretions due to hyperbilirubinemia and deposition of bile pigments. **acholuric j.**, jaundice without bilirubinemia, associated with elevated unconjugated bilirubin that is not excreted by the kidney. **acholuric familial j.**, hereditary spherocytosis. **breast milk j.**, elevated unconjugated bilirubin in some breast-fed infants due to the presence of 5-β-pregnane-3-α-20-β-diol, which inhibits glucuronyl transferase conjugating activity. **cholestatic j.**, that resulting from abnormal bile flow in the liver. **hematogenous j.**, **hemolytic j.**, that associated with hemolytic anemia. **hepatocellular j.**, that due to injury to or disease of liver cells. **hepatogenic j.**, **hepatogenous j.**, that due to disease or disorder of the liver. **leptospiral j.**, severe leptospirosis with fever, jaundice, myalgia, and occasionally meningitis and nephritis. **malignant j.**, acute yellow atrophy. **mechanical j.**, obstructive j. **j. of the newborn**, icterus neonatorum. **nuclear j.**, kernicterus. **obstructive j.**, that due to blocking of bile flow. **physiologic j.**, mild icterus neonatorum lasting the first few days of life. **retention j.**, that due to inability of the liver to dispose of the bilirubin provided by the circulating blood.

jaw (jaw) either of the two bony tooth-bearing structures (mandible and maxilla) in the head of dentate vertebrates. **Hapsburg j.**, a mandibular prognathous jaw, often accompanied by Hapsburg lip. **lumpy j.**, actinomycosis of cattle. **phossy j.**, phosphonecrosis. **rubber j.**, a softening of the jaw in animals, due to resorption and replacement of the bone by fibrous tissue, occurring with renal osteodystrophy.

jejunectomy (jĕ″joon-ek′tah-me) excision of the jejunum.

jejunocecostomy (jĕ-joon″o-se-kos′tah-me) anastomosis of the jejunum to the cecum.

jejunoileitis (-il″e-it′is) inflammation of the jejunum and ileum.

jejunojejunostomy (-jĕ″joon-os′tah-me) anastomosis between two portions of the jejunum.

jejunostomy (-nos′tah-me) the creation of a permanent opening between the jejunum and the surface of the abdominal wall.

jejunotomy (-not′ah-me) incision of the jejunum.

jejunum (jĕ-joon′im) that part of the small intestine extending from the duodenum to the ileum. **jeju′nal**, adj.

jelly (jel′e) a soft, resilient substance; generally, a colloidal semisolid mass. **cardiac j.**, a substance present between the endothelium and myocardium of the embryonic heart that transforms into the connective tissue of the endocardium. **contraceptive j.**, a nongreasy jelly used in the vagina for prevention of conception. **petroleum j.**, petrolatum. **Wharton's j.**, the intracellular substance of the umbilical cord.

jerk (jurk) a sudden reflex or involuntary movement. **Achilles j.**, **ankle j.**, triceps surae j. **biceps j.**, see under *reflex*. **elbow j.**, involuntary flexion of the elbow on striking the tendon of the biceps or triceps muscle. **jaw j.**, see under *reflex*. **knee j.**, a kick reflex produced by sharply tapping the patellar ligament. **tendon j.**, see under *reflex*. **triceps surae j.**, plantar flexion elicited by a tap on the Achilles tendon, preferably while the patient kneels on a bed or chair, the feet hanging free over the edge.

joint (joint) the site of junction or union between two or more bones, especially one that admits of motion of one or more bones. **amphidiarthrodial j.**, amphidiarthrosis. **arthrodial j.**, plane j. **ball-and-socket j.**, spheroidal j. **biaxial j.**, one with two chief axes of movement, at right angles to each other. **bilocular j.**, one with two synovial compartments separated by an interarticular cartilage. **cartilaginous j.**, one in which the bones are united by cartilage. **Charcot's j.**, see under *arthropathy*. **Chopart's j.**, one between the calcaneus and the cuboid bone and the talus and navicular bone. **cochlear j.**, a hinge joint which permits of some rotation or lateral motion. **composite j.**, **compound j.**, one in which several bones articulate. **condyloid j.**, one in which an ovoid head of one bone moves in an elliptical cavity of another, permitting all movements except axial rotation. **diarthrodial j.**, synovial j. **elbow j.**, the articulation between the humerus, ulna, and radius. **ellipsoidal j.**, one resembling a spheroidal joint, but having an ellipsoidal articular surface. **enarthrodial j.**, spheroidal j. **facet j's**, the articulations of the vertebral column. **false j.**, pseudarthrosis. **fibrocartilaginous j.**, symphysis. **fibrous j.**, one in which the bones are united by fibrous tissue. **flail j.**, an unusually mobile joint. **ginglymoid j.**, ginglymus. **gliding j.**, plane j. **hinge j.**, ginglymus. **hip j.**, the spheroidal joint between the head of the femur and the acetabulum of the hip bone. **immovable j.**, fibrous j. **intercarpal j's**, the articulations between the carpal bones. **knee j.**, the compound joint between the femur, patella, and tibia. **Lisfranc's j.**, the articulation between the tarsal and metatarsal bones. **mixed j.**, one combining features of different types of joints. **multiaxial j.**, spheroidal j. **peg and socket j.**, gomphosis. **pivot j.**, a uniaxial joint in which one bone pivots within a bony or an osseoligamentous ring. **plane j.**, a synovial joint in which the opposed surfaces are flat or only slightly curved. **polyaxial j.,** spheroidal j. **rotary j.,** pivot j. **saddle j.,** one having two saddle-shaped surfaces at right angles to each other. **simple j.,** one in which only two bones articulate. **spheroidal j.,** a synovial joint in which a spheroidal surface on one bone ("ball") moves within a concavity ("socket") on the other bone. **spiral j.,** cochlear j. **stifle j.,** the articulation in quadrupeds corresponding with the knee joint of man, consisting of two joints, one between the femur and tibia and one between the femur and patella. **synarthrodial j.,** fibrous j. **synovial j.,** an articulation permitting more or less free motion, the union of the bony elements being surrounded by an articular capsule enclosing a cavity lined by synovial membrane. **trochoid j.,** pivot j. **uniaxial j.,** one which permits movement in one axis only. **unilocular j.,** a synovial joint having only one cavity.

joule (jōōl) the SI unit of energy, being the work done by a force of one newton acting over a distance of one meter. Symbol J.

jugal (joo′g′l) pertaining to the cheek.

jugale (joo-ga′le) jugal point.

jugular (jug′ūl-er) 1. pertaining to the neck. 2. the jugular vein.

jugum (joo′gum), pl. *ju′ga* [L.] a depression or ridge connecting two structures.

juice (jōōs) any fluid from animal or plant tissue. **gastric j.,** the secretion of the gastric glands. **intestinal j.,** the secretion of glands in the intestinal lining. **pancreatic j.,** the enzyme-containing secretion of the pancreas, conducted through its ducts to the duodenum. **prostatic j.,** the secretion of the prostate, which contributes to semen formation.

jumping (jump′ing) Gilles de la Tourette's syndrome.

junction (junk′shin) the place of meeting or coming together. **junc′tional,** adj. **amelodentinal j.,** dentinoenamel j. **dentinocemental j.,** the line of meeting of the dentin and cementum

on the root of a tooth. **dentinoenamel j.,** the plane of meeting between dentin and enamel on the crown of a tooth. **esophagogastric j.,** the site of transition from the stratified squamous epithelium of the esophagus to the simple columnar epithelium of the cardia of the stomach. **gap j.,** a narrowed portion of the intercellular space in such tissues as that of the myocardium, containing channels linking adjacent cells and through which pass ions, most sugars, amino acids, nucleotides, vitamins, hormones, and cyclic AMP. **gastroesophageal j.,** esophagogastric j. **ileocecal j.,** the junction of the ileum and cecum, located at the lower right side of the abdomen and fixed to the posterior abdominal wall. **mucocutaneous j.,** the site of transition between skin and mucous membrane. **mucogingival j.,** the histologically distinct line marking the separation of the gingival tissue from the oral mucosa. **myoneural j.,** the site of apposition between a nerve fiber and the motor endplate of the skeletal muscle which it innervates. **sclerocorneal j.,** the line of union of the sclera and cornea. **tight j.,** an intercellular junction at which adjacent plasma membranes are joined tightly together by interlinked rows of integral membrane proteins, creating a seal impermeable to intercellular passage of molecules.

junctura (junk-tōōr′ah), pl. *junctu′rae* [L.] a junction or joint.

jurisprudence (jōōr″is-prōōd′ins) the science of the law. **medical j.,** the science of the law as applied to the practice of medicine.

juvenile (ju′vin-īl) 1. pertaining to youth or childhood. 2. a youth or child; a young animal. 3. a cell or organism intermediate between immature and mature forms.

juxta- word element [L.] *situated near; adjoining.*

juxtaglomerular (-glo-mer′ūl-er) near to or adjoining a glomerulus of the kidney.

juxtaposition (-pah-zish′in) apposition.

K

K chemical symbol, *potassium* (L. *kalium*); symbol for *kelvin.*

kak- for words beginning thus, see those beginning *cac-*.

kala-azar (kah″lah-ah-zar′) a fatal infectious disease endemic in the tropics and subtropics, caused by *Leishmania donovani,* and marked by fever, anemia, wasting, splenomegaly, and hepatomegaly.

kaliopenia (ka″le-o-pe′ne-ah) hypokalemia. **kaliope′nic,** adj.

kalium (ka′le-um) [L.] potassium (symbol K).

kallidin (kal′id-in) a kinin liberated by the action of kallikrein on a plasma globulin. Kallidin I is the same as bradykinin.

kallikrein (kal″ĭ-kre′in) one of a group of enzymes present in plasma, various glands, urine, and lymph, the major action of which is liberation of kinins from α-2-globulins.

kallikreinogen (-kri′nah-jen) the inactive precursor of kallikrein normally present in blood.

kanamycin (kan″ah-mi′sin) a water-soluble antibiotic derived from *Streptomyces kanamyceticus,* effective against some gram-positive, many gram-negative, and some acid-fast bacteria; used as the sulfate salt.

kaolin (ka′ah-lin) native hydrated aluminum silicate, powdered and freed from gritty particles by elutriation; used as an adsorbent and in kaolin mixture with pectin.

kaolinosis (ka″ōl-in-o′sis) pneumonoconiosis from inhaling particles of kaolin.

karyo- word element [Gr.], *nucleus.*

karyogamy (kar″e-ah-me) cell conjugation with union of nuclei.

karyokinesis (-ki-ne′sis) division of the nucleus, usually an early stage in the process of cell division, or mitosis. **karyokinet′ic,** adj.

karyolymph (kar′e-ah-limf″) the liquid portion of the nucleus of a cell, in which the other elements are dispersed.

karyolysis (kar″e-ol′ĭ-sis) the dissolution of the nucleus of a cell. **karyolyt′ic,** adj.

karyomorphism (kar″e-ah-mor′fizm) the shape of a cell nucleus.

karyon (kar′e-on) the nucleus of a cell.

karyophage (kar′e-o-fāj″) a protozoon that phagocytizes the nucleus of the cell it infects.

karyoplasm (-plazm″) nucleoplasm.

karyopyknosis (kar″e-o-pik-no′sis) shrinkage of a cell nucleus, with condensation of the chromatin. **karyopyknot′ic,** adj.

karyorrhexis (-rek′sis) rupture of the cell nucleus in which the chromatin disintegrates into formless granules that are extruded from the cell. **karyorrhec′tic,** adj.

karyosome (kar′e-ah-sōm″) any of the condensed irregular clumps of chromatin dispersed in the chromatin network of a cell.

karyotype (kar′e-ah-tīp″) the chromosomal constitution of the cell nucleus; by extension, the photomicrograph of chromosomes arranged according to the Denver classification.

kat katal.

kat(a)- word element [Gr.], *down; against.* See also words beginning *cat(a*)-.

katal (kat′al) a unit of measurement proposed to express activities of all catalysts, being that amount of a catalyst that catalyzes a reaction rate of 1 mole of substrate per second. Symbol kat.

katolysis (kah-tol′ĭ-sis) the incomplete or intermediate conversion of complex chemical bodies into simpler compounds; applied especially to digestive processes.

kcal kilocalorie.

Keflex (kef′leks) trademark for a preparation of cephalexin.

keloid (ke′loid) a sharply elevated, irregularly shaped, progressively enlarging scar due to excessive collagen formation in the corium during connective tissue repair. **keloid′al,** adj.

kelosomus (ke″lo-so′mus) celosomus.

kelvin (kel′vin) the SI unit of thermodynamic temperature, equal to 1/273.15 of the absolute temperature of the triple point of water. Symbol K.

Kenalog (-ah-log) trademark for preparations of triamcinolone acetonide.

keno- word element [Gr.], *empty.*

Kepone (ke′pōn) trademark for a polychlorinated ketone, $C_{10}Cl_{10}O$, used as an insecticide; workers exposed to this nonbiodegradable compound have suffered neurologic symptoms, such as tremors and slurred speech.

kerasin (ker′ah-sin) a cerebroside from brain tissue, yielding galactose, sphingosine, and lignoceric acid on hydrolysis.

kerat(o)- word element [Gr.], *horny tissue; cornea.*

keratan sulfate (ker′ah-tan) either of two sulfated mucopolysaccharides (I and II), containing N-acetyl glucosamine and galactose instead of uronic acid; II also contains D-acetylgalactosamine. It is an important component of the proteoglycan of cartilage, and occurs in the cornea and the nucleus pulposus; also an accumulation product in Morquio's syndrome.

keratectasia (ker″ah-tek-ta′ze-ah) protrusion of a thinned, scarred cornea.

keratic (ker-at′ik) 1. pertaining to keratin. 2. pertaining to the cornea.

keratin (ker′ah-tin) a scleroprotein that is the main constituent of epidermis, hair, nails, horny tissues, and the organic matrix of tooth enamel.

keratinase (-ās″) a proteolytic enzyme that hydrolyzes keratin.

keratinocyte (ker-at′in-o-sīt) the epidermal cell that synthesizes keratin, known in its successive stages in the layers of the skin as basal cell, prickle cell, and granular cell.

keratinoid (ker′ah-tin-oid) a form of keratin-coated tablet insoluble in the stomach but readily soluble in the intestine.

keratinosome (-sōm) a cellular membrane-coating granule.

keratitis (ker″ah-tīt′is) inflammation of the cornea. **k. bullo′sa,** presence of blebs upon the cornea. **dendritic k.,** herpetic keratitis which results in a branching ulceration of the cornea. **herpetic k.,** 1. that, commonly with dendritic ulceration (*dendriform* or *dendritic* k.), due to infection with herpes simplex virus. 2. that occurring in herpes zoster ophthalmicus. **interstitial k.,** chronic keratitis with deep deposits in the cornea, which becomes hazy. **lattice k.,** bilateral hereditary corneal dystrophy with formation of interwoven filamentous lesions. **neuroparalytic k.,** that due to injury to the trifacial nerve which prevents closing of the eyelids, marked by dryness and fissuring of the corneal epithelium. **phlyctenular k.,** see under *keratoconjunctivitis.* **punctate k.,** that marked by discrete punctate opacities. **sclerosing k.,** keratitis with scleritis. **trachomatous k.,** pannus trachomatosus.

keratoacanthoma (ker″ah-to-ak″an-tho′mah) a rapidly growing benign papular lesion, with a crater filled with a keratin plug; it resolves spontaneously.

keratocele (ker′ah-to-sēl″) hernial protrusion of Descemet's membrane.

keratocentesis (ker″ah-to-sen-te′sis) puncture of the cornea.

keratoconjunctivitis (-kon-junk″tĭ-vīt′is) inflammation of the cornea and conjunctiva. **epidemic k.,** a highly infectious form, commonly with regional lymph node involvement, occurring in epidemics; an adenovirus has been repeatedly isolated from affected patients. **phlyctenular k.,** a form marked by formation of a small, gray, circumscribed lesion at the corneal limbus. **k. sic′ca,** a condition marked by hyperemia of the conjunctiva, thickening and drying of the corneal epithelium, itching and burning of the eye and, often, reduced visual acuity. **viral k.**, epidemic k.

keratoconus (-ko′nis) conical protrusion of the central part of the cornea.

keratoderma (-durm′ah) hypertrophy of the horny layer of the skin. **k. blennorrha′gicum,** pustular psoriasis associated with gonorrhea. **k. climacte′ricum, endocrine k.,** circumscribed hyperkeratosis of palms and soles, occurring in menopausal women.

keratogenous (ker″ah-toj′ĭ-nus) giving rise to a growth of horny material.

keratoglobus (ker″ah-to-glo′bus) a bilateral anomaly in which the cornea is enlarged and globular in shape.

keratohelcosis (-hel-ko′sis) ulceration of the cornea.

keratohyalin (-hi′ah-lin) 1. a substance in the granules in the granular layer of the epidermis, which may be involved in keratinization. 2. a substance found in granules in Hassall corpuscles of the thymus.

keratohyaline (-hi′ah-līn) 1. both horny and hyaline. 2. pertaining to keratohyalin or to the keratohyalin granules or the granular layer of the epidermis (keratohyaline layer). 3. keratohyalin.

keratoiritis (ker″ah-to-i-rīt′is) inflammation of the cornea and iris.

keratoleptynsis (-lep-tin′sis) removal of the anterior portion of the cornea and replacement with bulbar conjunctiva.

keratoleukoma (-loo-ko′mah) a white opacity of the cornea.

keratolysis (ker″ah-tol′ĭ-sis) loosening or separation of the horny layer of the epidermis. **pitted k., k. planta′re sulca′tum,** a tropical disease marked by thickening and deep fissuring of the skin of the soles, occurring during the rainy season.

keratoma (ker″ah-to′mah) keratosis.

keratomalacia (ker″ah-to-mah-la′she-ah) softening and necrosis of the cornea associated with vitamin A deficiency.

keratome (ker′ah-tōm) a knife for incising the cornea.

keratometry (ker″ah-tom′ĭ-tre) measurement of corneal curves. **keratomet′ric,** adj.

keratomileusis (ker″ah-to-mĭ-loo′sis) keratoplasty in which a slice of the patient's cornea is removed, shaped to the desired curvature, and then sutured back on the remaining cornea to correct optical error.

keratomycosis (-mi-ko′sis) fungal infection of the cornea. **k. lin′guae,** black tongue.

keratonyxis (-nik′sis) keratocentesis.

keratopathy (ker″ah-top′ah-the) noninflammatory disease of the cornea. **band k.,** a condition characterized by an abnormal gray circumcorneal band.

keratophakia (ker″ah-to-fa′ke-ah) keratoplasty in which a slice of donor's cornea is shaped to a desired curvature and inserted between layers of the recipient's cornea to change its curvature.

keratoplasty (ker′ah-to-plas″te) plastic surgery of the cornea; corneal grafting. **optic k.,** transplantation of corneal material to replace scar tissue which interferes with vision. **refractive k.,** removal of a section of cornea from a patient or donor, which is shaped to the desired curvature and inserted either between (keratophakia) layers of or on (keratomileusis) the patient's cornea to change its curvature and correct optical errors. **tectonic k.,** transplantation of corneal material to replace tissue which has been lost.

keratorhexis, keratorrhexis (ker″ah-to-rek′-sis) rupture of the cornea.

keratoscopy (ker″ah-tos′ko-pe) inspection of the cornea.

keratosis (ker″ah-to′sis) any horny growth, such as a wart or callosity. **keratot′ic,** adj. **actinic k.,** a sharply outlined verrucous or keratotic growth, which may develop into a cutaneous horn, and may become malignant; it usually occurs in the middle-aged or elderly and is due to excessive exposure to the sun. **k. blennor-rha′gica,** keratoderma blennorrhagicum. **k. follicula′ris,** a hereditary form marked by areas of crusting, itching, verrucous papular growths. **k. lin′guae,** leukoplakia of the tongue. **k. palma′ris et planta′ris,** congenital, hereditary thickening of the skin of the palms and soles, sometimes with painful lesions resulting from fissuring; often associated with other anomalies. **k. pila′ris,** hyperkeratosis limited to the hair follicles. **k. pharyn′gea,** horny projections from the tonsils and pharyngeal walls. **k. puncta′ta,** a hereditary hyperkeratosis in which the lesions are localized in multiple points on the palms and soles. **sebor-rheic k., k. seborrhe′ica,** a benign tumor of epidermal origin, marked by numerous yellow or brown, sharply marginated, oval, raised lesions. **senile k., solar k.,** actinic k.

keratosulfate (ker″ah-to-sul′fāt) keratan sulfate.

keratotomy (ker″ah-tot′ah-me) incision of the cornea. **radial k.,** a series of incisions made in the cornea from its outer edge toward its center in spokelike fashion; done to flatten the cornea and thus to correct myopia.

keratotorus (ker″ah-to-tor′is) a vaultlike protrusion of the cornea.

kerion (kēr′e-on) a boggy, exudative tumefaction covered with pustules; associated with tinea infections.

kernicterus (kurn-ik′ter-is) a condition with severe neural symptoms, associated with high levels of bilirubin in the blood.

ketamine (kēt′ah-mēn) a rapid-acting general anesthetic, $C_{13}H_{16}ClNO$.

keto- word element, *ketone group.*

ketoacidosis (kēt″o-as″id-o′sis) acidosis due to accumulation of ketone bodies.

keto acids (kēt′o) compounds containing the groups CO and COOH.

ketoaciduria (-as″id-ūr′e-ah) the presence of keto acids in the urine. **branched-chain k.,** maple syrup urine disease.

ketoaminoacidemia (-ah-me″no-as″id-ēm′e-ah) maple syrup urine disease.

ketogenesis (-jen′i-sis) the production of ketone bodies. **ketogenet′ic,** adj.

α-ketoglutarate (glōōt′ah-rāt) a salt or anion of α-ketoglutaric acid.

α-ketoglutaric acid (kēt″o-gloo-tar′ik) HOOC-(CH₂)₂COCOOH, a metabolic intermediate involved in the tricarboxylic acid cycle, in amino acid metabolism, and in transamination reactions as an amino group acceptor.

ketolysis (ke-tol′ĭ-sis) the splitting up of ketone bodies. **ketolyt′ic,** adj.

ketone (ke′tōn) any of a class of organic compounds containing the carbonyl group, C=O, whose carbon atom is joined to two other carbon atoms, i.e., with the carbonyl group occurring within the carbon chain.

ketonuria (nūr″e-ah) an excess of ketone bodies in the urine.

ketose (ke′tōs) any sugar that contains a ketone group.

ketosis (ke-to′sis) accumulation of excessive amounts of ketone bodies in body tissues and fluids. **ketot′ic,** adj.

ketosteroid (ke″to-stē′roid) a steroid having ketone groups on functional carbon atoms. The *17-ketosteroids* found in normal urine and in excess in certain tumors, have a ketone group on the 17th carbon atom, and include certain androgenic and adrenocortical hormones.

keV kiloelectron volt.

kg. kilogram.

kHz kilohertz.

kidney (kid′ne) either of the two organs in the lumbar region that filter the blood, excreting the end-products of body metabolism in the form of urine, and regulating the concentrations of hydrogen, sodium, potassium, phosphate, and other ions in the extracellular fluid. **abdominal k.,** an ectopic kidney situated above the iliac crest with the hilus adjacent to the second lumbar vertebra. **amyloid k.,** one marked by deposition of amyloid. **artificial k.,** an extracorporeal device through which blood may be circulated for removal of elements that normally are excreted in the urine; a hemodialyzer. **cake k.,** a solid, irregularly lobed organ of bizarre shape, formed by fusion of the two renal anlagen. **cicatricial k.,** a shriveled, irregular, and scarred kidney due to suppurative pyelonephritis. **contracted k.,** an atrophic kidney which may be scarred and granular. **fatty k.,** one affected with fatty degeneration. **flea-bitten k.,** one with small, randomly scattered petechiae on its surface. **floating k.,** hypermobile k. **fused k.,** a single anomalous organ developed as a result of fusion of the renal anlagen. **Goldblatt k.,** one with obstruction of its blood flow, resulting in renal hypertension. **head k.,** pronephros. **horseshoe k.,** an anomalous organ resulting from fusion of the corresponding poles of the renal anlagen. **hypermobile k.,** one that is freely movable. **lumbar k.,** an ectopic kidney situated opposite the sacral promontory in the iliac fossa, anterior to the iliac vessels. **lump k.,** cake k. **middle k.,** mesonephros. **pelvic k.,** an ectopic kidney situated opposite the sacrum and below the aortic bifurcation. **polycystic k.,** see *polycystic disease of kidney,* under *disease.* **primordial k.,** pronephros. **sigmoid k.,** a deformed and fused kidney, the upper pole of one kidney being fused with the lower pole of the other. **sponge k.,** a usually asymptomatic, congenital condition in which multiple small cystic dilatations of the collecting tubules of the medullary portion of the renal pyramids give the organ a spongy, porous feeling and appearance. **thoracic k.,** an ectopic kidney partially or completely protruding above the diaphragm into the posterior mediastinum. **wandering k.,** hypermobile k. **waxy k.,** amyloid k.

kilo- word element [Gr.], *one thousand* (10³), used in naming units of measurement. Symbol, k.

kilocalorie (kil′ah-kal″er-e) a unit of heat equal to 1000 calories. Abbreviated, kcal.

kilogram (kil′ah-gram) a unit of mass (weight) of the metric system, 1000 grams; equivalent to 15,432 grains, or 2.205 pounds (avoirdupois) or 2.679 pounds (apothecaries' weight). Abbreviated kg.

kilohertz (-hurts) one thousand (10³) hertz; abbreviated kHz.

kilometer (kil′ah-mēt″er, kil-om′it-er) 1000 meters; 3280.83 feet; five-eighths of a mile. Abbreviated km.

kilovolt (kil′ah-volt) 1000 volts. Symbol, kV.

kinanesthesia (kin″an-es-the′ze-ah) loss of power of perceiving sensations of movement.

kinase (ki′nās) 1. a subclass of the transferases, comprising the enzymes that catalyze the transfer of a high-energy group from a donor (usually ATP) to an acceptor, and named, according to the acceptor, as *creatine kinase, fructokinase,* etc. 2. an enzyme that activates a zymogen, and named, according to its source, as *enterokinase, streptokinase,* etc.

kine- word element [Gr.], *movement.* See also words beginning *cine-*.

kineplasty (kin′ĭ-plas″te) utilization of the stump of an amputated extremity for producing motion of the prosthesis.

kinescope (kin′ĭ-skōp) an instrument for ascertaining ocular refraction.

kinesi(o)- word element [Gr.], *movement.*

kinesia (ki-ne′se-ah) motion sickness.

kinesiatrics (-ă′triks) kinesitherapy.

kinesics (ki-ne′siks) the study of body movement as a part of the process of communication.

kinesimeter (kin″ĕ-sim′it-er) 1. an instrument for quantitative measurement of motions. 2. an instrument for exploring the body surface to test cutaneous sensibility.

kinesiology (ki-ne″se-ol′ah-je) scientific study of movement of body parts.

kinesioneurosis (ki-ne″se-o-nōōr-o′sis) a functional nervous disorder marked by motor disturbances.

kinesis (ki-ne′sis) [Gr.] 1. movement, e.g., the activity of an organism in response to a stimulus; the direction of the response is not controlled by the direction of the stimulus (in contrast to a taxis). 2. word termination denoting movement or motion, e.g., cytokinesis.

kinesthesia (kin″es-the′ze-ah) the sense by which position, weight, and movement are perceived. **kinesthet′ic**, adj.

kinesthesis (kin″es-the′sis) kinesthesia.

kinetics (kĭ-net′iks, ki-net′iks) the scientific study of the turnover, or rate of change, or a specific factor in the body, commonly expressed as units of amount per unit time. **chemical k.**, the study of the rates and mechanisms of chemical reactions.

kinetocardiography (-kar″de-og′rah-fe) the graphic recording of slow vibrations of the anterior chest wall in the region of the heart, the vibrations representing the absolute motion at a given point on the chest.

kinetochore (ki-nēt′ah-kōr) centromere.

kinetogenic (ki-ne″tah-jen′ik) causing or producing movement.

kinetoplast (ki-nēt′ah-plast) a structure associated with the basal body in many protozoa, primarily the Mastigophora; it is rich in DNA and, like the basal body, it replicates independently.

kinetosis (ki″nĭ-to′sis) any disorder due to unaccustomed motions; see *motion sickness*.

kingdom (king′dim) one of the three major categories into which natural objects are usually classified: the animal (including all animals), plant (including all plants), and mineral (including all substance and objects without life). A fourth, the Protista, includes all single-celled organisms.

kinin (ki′nin) any of a group of endogenous peptides that increase vascular permeability, cause hypotension, and induce contraction of smooth muscle.

kininase II (-ās) an enzyme that catalyzes the cleavage of C-terminal peptides from substrates, including bradykinin and angiotensin I (converting it to angiotensin II).

kininogen (ki-nin′ah-jen) an α_2-globulin of plasma that is a precursor of the kinins.

kinocilium (ki″no-sil′e-um), pl. *kinocil′ia*. A motile, protoplasmic filament on the free surface of a cell.

kinship (kin′ship) a group of individuals of varying degrees of descent from a common ancestor.

Klebsiella (kleb″se-el′ah) a genus of gram-negative bacteria (tribe Escherichieae), including *K. pneumo′niae* (*K. friedlän′deri*), the etiologic agent of Friedländer's pneumonia and other respiratory infections.

kleeblattschädel (kla′blot-shäd′l) [Gr.] cloverleaf skull; a congenital anomaly in which there is intrauterine synostosis of multiple or all cranial sutures. See under *syndrome*.

kleptomania (klep″tah-ma′ne-ah) compulsive stealing, the objects taken usually having a symbolic value of which the subject is unconscious, rather than an intrinsic value.

km. kilometer.

knee (ne) genu; the point of articulation of the femur with the tibia. Also, any kneelike structure. **housemaid's k.**, inflammation of the bursa of the patella, with fluid accumulating

within it. **knock k.**, knock-knee. **trick k.**, a popular term for a knee joint susceptible to locking in position, most often due to longitudinal splitting of the medial meniscus.

knock-knee (nok′ne) genu valgum; a deformity of the thigh or leg, or both, in which the knees are abnormally close together and the space between the ankles is increased.

knot (not) 1. an intertwining of the ends or parts of one or more threads, sutures, or strip of cloth. 2. in anatomy, a knoblike swelling or protuberance. **primitive k.**, a mass of cells at the cranial end of the primitive streak in the early embryo. **surgeon's k., surgical k.**, a knot in which the thread is passed twice through the first loop.

knuckle (nuk″l) the dorsal aspect of any phalangeal joint, or any similarly bent structure.

knuckling (nuk′ling) upward and forward displacement of the fetlock joint of a horse.

koilo- word element [Gr.], *hollowed; concave.*

koilonychia (koi″lo-nik′e-ah) dystrophy of the fingernails in which they are thinned and concave, with raised edges.

koilorrhachic (-rak′ik) having a vertebral column in which the lumbar curvature is anteriorly concave.

koilosternia (-sturn′e-ah) funnel chest.

kolp- for words beginning thus, see those beginning *colp-*.

kolypeptic (ko″le-pep′tik) hindering or checking digestion.

Kr chemical symbol, *krypton.*

kraurosis (kraw-ro′sis) a dried, shriveled condition. **k. vul′vae**, atrophy of the female external genitalia, resulting in drying and shriveling, with leukoplakic patches on the mucosa and intense itching.

kreo- for words beginning thus, see also those beginning *creo-.*

krypto- for words beginning thus, see also those beginning *crypto-.*

krypton (krip′ton) chemical element (*see table*), at. no. 36, symbol Kr.

kuru (koo′roo) a progressive, fatal central nervous system disorder due to a slow virus and transmissible to subhuman primates. It is seen only in New Guinea and thought to be associated with cannibalism.

kV. kilovolt.

kVp kilovolts peak.

kwashiorkor (kwash″e-or′kor) a syndrome due to severe protein deficiency; symptoms include retarded growth, changes in skin and hair pigment, edema, and pathologic changes in the liver. **marasmic k.**, a condition in which there is a deficiency of both calories and protein, with severe tissue wasting, loss of subcutaneous fat, and usually dehydration.

Kwell (kwel) trademark for a preparation of lindane.

kymatism (ki′mah-tizm) myokymia.

kymograph (-graf) an instrument for recording variations and undulations, arterial or other.

kynurenic acid (kin″ūr-ēn′ik) a crystalline acid, $C_9H_5N(OH)COOH$, metabolite of tryptophan found in microorganisms and in mammalian urine.

kynurenine (kin″u-re′nin) a metabolite of tryptophan found in microorganisms and in the urine of normal animals; it is a precursor of kynurenic acid and an intermediate in the conversion of tryptophan to niacin.

kyphos (ki′fos) the hump in the spine in kyphosis.

kyphoscoliosis (ki″fo-skōl″e-o′sis) backward and lateral curvature of the spinal column.

kyphosis (ki-fo′sis) abnormally increased convexity in the curvature of the thoracic spine as viewed from the side. **kyphot′ic,** adj. **k. dorsa′-lis juveni′lis, juvenile k., Scheuermann's k.,** osteochondrosis of the vertebrae.

kyrtorrhachic (kurt″o-rak′ik) having a vertebral column in which the lumbar curvature is convex anteriorly.

kyto- for words beginning thus, see those beginning cyto-.

L

L. Lactobacillus; Latin; left; length; libra (*pound, balance*), licentiate; light sense; limes (*boundary*), liter; lumbar; coefficient of induction.

L- chemical prefix (small capital) specifying that the substance corresponds in chemical composition to the standard substance L-glyceraldehyde. Opposed to D-.

l liter.

l- chemical abbreviation, *levo-* (i.e., left or counterclockwise).

λ lambda, the eleventh letter of the Greek alphabet; symbol for *wavelength* and *decay constant.*

La chemical symbol, *lanthanum.*

labia (la′be-ah) plural of *labium.*

labially (la′be-il-e) toward the lips.

labile (la′bīl) 1. gliding; moving from point to point over the surface; unstable; fluctuating. 2. chemically unstable.

lability (lah-bil′it-e) the quality of being labile; in psychiatry, emotional instability.

labio- word element [L.], *lip.*

labioalveolar (la″be-o-al-ve′ah-ler) 1. pertaining to the lip and dental alveoli. 2. pertaining to the labial side of a dental alveolus.

labiocervical (-serv′ik′l) 1. pertaining to the labial surface of the neck of an anterior tooth. 2. labiogingival.

labiochorea (-kor-e′ah) a choreic affection of the lips in speech, with stammering.

labioclination (-kli-na′shin) deviation of an anterior tooth from the vertical, in the direction of the lips.

labiogingival (-jin-ji′vil, -jin′jĭ-vil) pertaining to or formed by the labial and gingival walls of a tooth cavity.

labiograph (la′be-o-graf″) an instrument for recording lip motions in speaking.

labiomental (la″be-o-ment′l) pertaining to the lip and chin.

labioplacement (-plās′mint) displacement of a tooth toward the lip.

labioversion (la″be-o-ver′zhin) labial displacement of a tooth from the line of occlusion.

labium (la′be-um), pl. *la′bia* [L.] a fleshy border or edge; a lip. **la′bial,** adj. **l. ma′jus** (pl. *la′bia majo′ra*), an elongated fold in the female, one on either side of the rima pudendi. **l. mi′nus** (pl.

la′bia mino′ra), a small skin fold on either side, between the labium majus and the vaginal opening. **la′bia o′ris,** the lips of the mouth.

labor (la′ber) the function of the female by which the infant is expelled through the vagina to the outside world: the *first stage* begins with onset of regular uterine contractions and ends when the os is completely dilated and flush with the vagina; the *second* extends from the end of the first stage until the expulsion of the infant is completed; the *third* extends from expulsion of the infant until the placenta and membranes are expelled; the *fourth* denotes the hour or two after delivery, when uterine tone is established. **artificial l.,** induced l. **dry l.,** that in which the amniotic fluid escapes before the onset of uterine contractions. **false l.,** see under *pain.* **induced l.,** that brought on by mechanical or other extraneous means, usually by the intravenous infusion of oxytocin. **missed l.,** that in which contractions begin and then cease, the fetus being retained for weeks or months. **postmature l., postponed l.,** that occurring two weeks or more after the expected date of confinement. **precipitate l.,** that occurring with undue rapidity. **premature l.,** expulsion of a viable infant before the normal end of gestation; usually applied to interruption of pregnancy between the twenty-eighth and thirty-seventh week.

laboratory (lab′rĭ-tor″e) a place equipped for making tests or doing experimental work. **clinical l.,** one for examination of materials derived from the human body for the purpose of providing information on diagnosis, prevention, or treatment of disease.

labrum (la′brum), pl. *la′bra* [L.] an edge, rim, or lip.

labyrinth (lab′ĭ-rinth) the internal ear, made up of the vestibule, cochlea, and canals. See Plate XII. **labyrin′thine,** adj. **bony l.,** the bony part of the internal ear. **cochlear l.,** the part of the membranous labyrinth that includes the perilymphatic space and the cochlear duct. **endolymphatic l.,** membranous l. **ethmoid l.,** either of the paired lateral masses of the ethmoid bone, consisting of many thin-walled cellular cavities, the ethmoidal cells. **membranous l.,** a system of communicating epithelial sacs and ducts within the bony labyrinth, containing the endolymph. **osseous l.,** bony l. **perilymphatic l.,** perilymphatic space. **vestibular l.,** the part of the membranous labyrinth that includes the utricle and saccule and the semicircular ducts.

labyrinthitis (lab″ĭ-rin-thīt′is) inflammation of the labyrinth; otitis interna. **circumscribed l.,** that due to erosion of the bony wall of a semicircular canal with exposure of the membranous labyrinth.

labyrinthus (lab″ĭ-rin′thus), pl. *labyrin′thi* [L.] labyrinth.

lac (lak), gen. *lac′tis,* pl. *lacta* [L.] 1. milk. 2. any milklike medicinal preparation.

laceration (las″er-a′shin) 1. the act of tearing. 2. a torn, ragged, mangled wound.

lacertus (lah-ser′tus), pl. *lacer′ti* [L.] a name given certain fibrous attachments of muscles.

lacrimation (lak″rĭ-ma′shin) secretion and discharge of tears.

lacrimator (lak′rĭ-māt″er) an agent, as a gas, that induces the flow of tears.

lacrimotomy (lak″rĭ-mot″ah-me) incision of the lacrimal gland, duct, or sac.

lact(o)- word element [L.], *milk.*

lactacidemia (lak-tas″id-ēm′e-ah) an excess of lactic acid in the blood.

lactagogue (lak′tah-gog) galactagogue.

lactam (lak′tam) a cyclic amide formed from aminocarboxylic acids by elimination of water; lactams are isomeric with lactims, which are enol forms of lactams.

β-lactamase (ba″tah-lak′tah-mās) a generic term for a group of enzymes produced by certain species of *Staphylococcus, Bacillus,* and *Clostridium* that hydrolyze the β-lactam ring of penicillins and cephalosporins, destroying their antibiotic activity.

lactase (lak′tās) β-galactosidase.

lactate (lak′tāt) 1. any salt or ester of lactic acid. 2. to secrete milk.

lactation (lak-ta′shin) 1. the secretion of milk. 2. the period of milk secretion.

lacteal (lak′te-il) 1. pertaining to milk. 2. any of the intestinal lymphatics that transport chyle.

lactescence (lak-tes′ins) resemblance to milk.

lactic (lak′tik) pertaining to milk.

lactic acid (lak′tik) CH₃CHOHCOOH, a compound formed in the body in anaerobic metabolism of carbohydrate and also produced by bacterial action in milk. The sodium salt of racemic or inactive lactic acid (*sodium lactate*) is used as an electrolyte and fluid replenisher.

lacticemia (lak″tĭ-sēm′e-ah) lactacidemia.

lactiferous (lak-tif′er-is) conveying milk.

lactifuge (lak′tĭ-fūj) checking or stopping milk secretion; also an agent that so acts.

lactigenous (lak-tij′in-is) producing milk.

lactigerous (lak-tij′er-us) lactiferous.

lactim (lak′tim) see *lactam.*

lactivorous (lak-tiv′er-is) feeding or subsisting upon milk.

Lactobacillaceae (lak″to-bas″il-a′se-e) a family of bacteria (order Eubacteriales).

Lactobacilleae (-bah-sil′e-e) a tribe of bacteria (family Lactobacillaceae).

Lactobacillus (-bah-sil′is) a genus of the tribe Lactobacilleae, some of which are considered to be etiologically related to dental caries, but are otherwise nonpathogenic; they produce lactic acid by fermentation.

lactobacillus (-bah-sil′is), pl. *lactobacil′li* [L.] an organism of the genus *Lactobacillus.*

lactocele (lak′tah-sēl) galactocele.

lactogen (lak′tah-jen) any substance that enhances lactation. **human placental l.,** a hormone secreted by the placenta; it has lactogenic, luteotropic, and growth-promoting activity, and inhibits maternal insulin activity.

lactoglobulin (lak″tah-glob′ūl-in) a globulin occurring in milk.

lactone (lak′tōn) 1. an aromatic liquid from lactic acid. 2. a cyclic organic compound in which the chain is closer by ester formation between a carboxyl and a hydroxyl group in the same molecule.

lactorrhea (lak-tor-e′ah) galactorrhea.

lactose (lak′tōs) a sugar derived from milk, $C_{12}H_{22}O_{11}$, which on hydrolysis yields glucose and galactose.

lactoside (lak′to-sīd) glycoside in which the sugar constituent is lactose.

lactosidosis (lak″to-sĭ-do′sis) accumulation of lactoside in tissues. **ceramide l.,** lactosylceramidosis.

lactosuria (-tōs-ūr′e-ah) lactose in the urine.

lactosylceramidosis (lak-to″sil-ser″ah-mĭd-ōs′is) a sphingolipidosis in which lactosylceramide accumulates in neural and visceral tissue because of defective β-galactosidase.

lactotrope (lak′to-trōp) an acidophilic cell of the anterior pituitary that secretes prolactin.

lactotroph (-trōf) lactotrope.

lactotrophin, lactotropin (lak″to-tro′fin, -tro′-pin) prolactin.

lactovegetarian (-vej″ĭ-tār′e-in) 1. a person who subsists on a diet of milk (or milk products) and vegetables. 2. pertaining to such a diet.

lactulose (lak′tūl-ōs) a synthetic disaccharide, $C_{12}H_{22}O_{11}$; used as a cathartic and to enhance excretion or formation of ammonia in the treatment of portosystemic encephalopathy, including hepatic precoma and coma.

lacuna (lah-ku′nah), pl. *lacu′nae* [L.] 1. a small pit or hollow cavity. 2. a defect or gap, as in the field of vision (scotoma). **lacu′nar,** adj. **absorption l.,** a pit or groove in developing bone that is undergoing resorption; frequently found to contain osteoclasts. **bone l.,** a small cavity within the bone matrix, containing an osteocyte and from which slender canaliculi radiate and penetrate the adjacent lamellae to anastomose with the canaliculi of neighboring lacunae, thus forming a system of cavities interconnected by minute canals. **cartilage l.,** any of the small cavities within the cartilage matrix, containing a chondrocyte. **Howship's l.,** absorption l. **intervillous l.,** one of the blood spaces of the placenta in which the fetal villi are found. **l. mag′na,** navicular fossa (2). **osseous l.,** bone l. **l. pharyn′gis,** a depression at the pharyngeal end of the eustachian tube. **trophoblastic l.,** intervillous l.

lacunule (lah-kūn'ūl) a minute lacuna.

lacus (la'kus), pl. *la'cus* [L.] lake. **l. lacrima'lis,** lacrimal lake.

lae- for words beginning thus, see those beginning *le-*.

Laetrile (la'ĕ-tril) trademark for *l*-mandelonitrile-β-glucuronic acid, derived by hydrolysis of amygdalin and oxidation of the resulting *l*-mandelonitrile-β-glucoside; alleged to have antineoplastic properties. Sometimes used interchangeably with *amygdalin*.

laeve (le've) [L.] nonvillous.

lag (lag) 1. the time between application of a stimulus and the reaction. 2. the period after inoculation of bacteria into a culture medium, in which growth or cell division is slow.

lagena (lah-je'nah) 1. a part of the upper extremity of the cochlear duct. 2. the organ of hearing in nonmammalian vertebrates.

lageniform (lah-jen'ĭ-form) flask-shaped.

lagophthalmos (lag''of-thal'mos) inability to shut the eyes completely.

lake (lāk) 1. to undergo separation of hemoglobin from erythrocytes. 2. a circumscribed collection of fluid in a hollow or depressed cavity. See also *lacuna*. **lacrimal l.,** the triangular space at the medial angle of the eye, where the tears collect. **marginal l's,** discontinuous venous lacunae, relatively free of villi, near the edge of the placenta, formed by merging of the marginal portions of the intervillous space with the subchorial lake. **subchorial l.,** the portion of the placenta, relatively free of villi, just beneath the chorionic plate; at the edge of the placenta it becomes continuous with irregular channels to form the marginal lakes.

lal(o)- word element [Gr.], *speech; babbling.*

lallation (lah-la'shin) a babbling, infantile form of speech.

laloplegia (lal''o-ple'je-ah) paralysis of the organs of speech.

lalorrhea (-re'ah) excessive flow of words.

lambda (lam'dah) point of union of the lambdoid and sagittal sutures.

lambdoid (lam'doid) shaped like the Greek letter lambda, Λ or λ.

Lamblia (lam'ble-ah) *Giardia.*

lambliasis (lam-bli'ah-sis) giardiasis.

lame (lām) incapable of normal locomotion; deviation from normal gait.

lamella (lah-mel'ah), gen. and pl. *lamel'lae* [L.] 1. a thin leaf or plate, as of bone. 2. a medicated disk or wafer to be inserted under the eyelid. **lamel'lar,** adj. **circumferential l.,** one of the layers of bone that underlie the periosteum and endosteum. **concentric l.,** haversian l. **endosteal l.,** one of the bony plates lying beneath the endosteum. **ground l.,** interstitial l. **haversian l.,** one of the concentric bony plates surrounding a haversian canal. **intermediate l., interstitial l.,** one of the bony plates that fill in between the haversian systems. **vitreous l.,** lamina basalis.

lamellipodia (lah-mel''ĭ-pōd'ē-ah), sing. *lamel-*

lipodium. Delicate sheetlike extensions of cytoplasm which form transient adhesions with the cell substrate and wave gently, enabling the cell to move along the substrate.

lamina (lam'ĭ-nah), gen. and pl. *la'minae* [L.] a thin, flat plate or layer, used in anatomic nomenclature to designate such a structure, or a layer of a composite structure. Often used alone to mean the vertebral lamina. **l. basa'lis,** one of the pair of longitudinal zones of the embryonic neural tube, from which develop the ventral gray columns of the spinal cord and the motor centers of the brain. **l. basila'ris,** the posterior wall of the cochlear duct, separating it from the scala tympani. Bowman's l., see under *membrane.* **l. choroidocapilla'ris,** the inner layer of the choroid, composed of a single-layered network of small capillaries. **l. cribro'sa,** 1. fascia cribrosa. 2. (of *ethmoid bone*) the horizontal plate of ethmoid bone forming the roof of the nasal cavity, and perforated by many foramina for passage of olfactory nerves. 3. (*of sclera*) the perforated part of the sclera through which pass the axons of the retinal ganglion cells. **elastic l.,** 1. Bowman's membrane. 2. Descemet's membrane. **epithelial l.,** the layer of ependymal cells covering the choroid plexus. **l. pro'pria,** 1. the connective tissue layer of mucous membrane. 2. the middle fibrous layer of the tympanic membrane. **l. reticula'ris,** the perforated hyaline membrane covering the organ of Corti. **l. spira'lis,** 1. a double plate of bone winding spirally around the modiolus, dividing the spiral canal of the cochlea into the scala tympani and scali vestibuli. 2. a bony projection on the outer wall of the cochlea in the lower part of the first turn. **terminal l. of hypothalamus,** the thin plate derived from the telencephalon, forming the anterior wall of the third ventricle of the cerebrum. **vertebral l., l. of vertebral arch,** either of the pair of broad plates of bone flaring out from the pedicles of the vertebral arches and fusing together at the midline to complete the dorsal part of the arch and provide a base for the spinous process.

laminagraphy (lam''ĭ-nag'rah-fe) see *body-section roentgenography.*

laminectomy (lam''ĭ-nek'tah-me) excision of the posterior arch of a vertebra.

laminotomy (lam''ĭ-not'ah-me) transection of a lamina of a vertebra.

lamp (lamp) an apparatus for furnishing heat or light. **annealing l.,** an alcohol lamp for heating gold leaf for tooth fillings. **mercury vapor l.,** one in which the arc is in mercury vapor, enclosed in a quartz burner; used in light therapy; it may be air or water-cooled. **quartz l.,** a mercury vacuum lamp made of melted quartz glass embedded in a running water bath; used for applying ultraviolet light treatment.

lamziekte (lam'zēk-te) a disease of cattle in South Africa, characterized by motor paralysis and due to ingestion by phosphorus-deficient animals of bones, contaminated by toxin produced by *Clostridium botulinum.*

lanatoside C (lah-nat'ah-sīd) a cardiotonic glycoside, $C_{49}H_{76}O_{20}$, from the leaves of *Digitalis lanata;* used like digitalis.

lance (lans) 1. lancet. 2. to cut or incise with a lancet.

lancet (lan′set) a small, pointed, two-edged surgical knife.

lancinating (lan′sĭ-nāt″ing) tearing, darting, or sharply cutting; said of pain.

lanolin (lan′ah-lin) a purified, fatlike substance from the wool of sheep, *Ovis aries*, mixed with 25 to 30% water; used as a water-in-oil ointment base. **anhydrous l.**, lanolin containing not more than 0.25% water; used as an absorbent ointment base.

Lanoxin (lah-nok′sin) trademark for preparations of digoxin.

lanthanum (lan′thah-num) chemical element (*see table*), at. no. 57, symbol La.

lanugo (lah-nu′go) the fine hair on the body of the fetus.

laparo- word element [Gr.], *loin or flank; abdomen* (loosely).

laparoscope (lap′ah-rah-skōp″) an endoscope for examining the peritoneal cavity.

laparotomy (lap″ah-rot′o-me) incision through the flank or, more generally, through any part of the abdominal wall.

laparotrachelotomy (lap″ah-ro-tra″kah-lot′ah-me) low cervical cesarean section, with incision into the lower uterine segment.

lapinization (lap″in-i-za′shin) serial passage of a virus or vaccine through rabbits to modify its characteristics.

lapis (la′pis, lap′is) [L.] stone.

lard (lard) purified internal fat of the abdomen of the hog.

Larotid (lar′ot-id) trademark for preparations of amoxicillin.

larva (lar′vah), pl. *lar′vae* [L.] an independent, immature stage in the life cycle of an animal in which it is unlike the parent and must undergo changes in form and size to reach the adult stage. **l. cur′rens,** a variant of larva migrans caused by *Strongyloides stercoralis*, in which the progression of the linear lesion is much more rapid. **l. mi′grans,** creeping eruption; a convoluted threadlike skin eruption that appears to migrate, caused by the burrowing beneath the skin of roundworm larvae, particularly *Ancylostoma* larvae. Similar lesions are caused by the larvae of botflies. **l. migrans, ocular,** infection of the eye with larvae of *Toxocara canis* or *T. cati*, which may lodge in the choroid or retina or migrate to the vitreous; on the death of the larvae, a granulomatous inflammation occurs, the lesion varying from a translucent elevation of the retina to massive retinal detachment and pseudoglioma. **l. mi′grans, visceral,** a condition due to prolonged migration of nematode larvae in human tissue other than skin; commonly caused by the larvae of *Toxocara canis* or *T. cati*, which do not complete their life cycle in humans.

larvate (lar′vāt) masked; concealed; said of a disease or symptom of disease.

laryng(o)- word element [Gr.], *larynx*.

laryngeal (lah-rin′je-il) pertaining to the larynx.

laryngemphraxis (lar″in-jem-frak′sis) obstruction or closure of the larynx.

laryngismus (-jiz′mis) spasm of the larynx. **laryngis′mal,** adj. **l. paraly′ticus,** roaring. **l. stri′dulus,** sudden laryngeal spasm with crowing inspiration.

laryngitis (-jīt′is) inflammation of the larynx. **laryngit′ic,** adj. **atrophic l.,** an extreme form of chronic catarrhal laryngitis. **chronic catarrhal l.,** a form marked by atrophy of the glands of the mucous membrane. **subglottic l.,** inflammation of the under surface of the vocal cords.

laryngocele (lah-ring′gah-sēl) a congenital anomalous air sac communicating with the cavity of the larynx, which may bulge outward on the neck.

laryngofissure (-fish′er) median laryngotomy.

laryngography (lar″ing-gog′rah-fe) radiography of the larynx.

laryngology (-gol′ah-je) that branch of medicine having to do with the throat, pharynx, larynx, nasopharynx, and tracheobronchial tree.

laryngopathy (-gop′ah-the) any disorder of the larynx.

laryngopharyngectomy (-far″in-jek′tah-me) excision of the larynx and pharynx.

laryngopharynx (-far′inks) the portion of the pharynx below the upper edge of the epiglottis, opening into the larynx and esophagus.

laryngophony (lar″ing-gof′ah-ne) the vocal sound heard in auscultating the larynx.

laryngoplasty (lah-ring′go-plas″te) plastic repair of the larynx.

laryngoplegia (lah-ring″go-ple′je-ah) paralysis of the larynx.

laryngoptosis (-to′sis) lowering and mobilization of the larynx as sometimes seen in the aged.

laryngorhinology (-ri-nol′ah-je) the branch of medicine that deals with the larynx and nose.

laryngoscopy (lar″ing-gos′kah-pe) visual examination of the interior larynx. **laryngoscop′ic,** adj.

laryngostenosis (lah-ring″go-stĕ-no′sis) narrowing or stricture of the larynx.

laryngostomy (lar″ing-gos′tah-me) surgical fistulization of the larynx.

laryngotomy (-got′ah-me) incision of the larynx. **inferior l.,** laryngotomy through the cricothyroid membrane. **median l.,** laryngotomy through the thyroid cartilage. **superior l., subhyoid l.,** laryngotomy through the thyrohyoid membrane.

laryngotracheitis (-tra″ke-īt′is) inflammation of the larynx and trachea. **avian l., infectious l.,** a viral disease of poultry characterized by respiratory distress, gasping, and expectoration of bloody exudate.

laryngotracheotomy (-tra″ke-ot′ah-me) incision of the larynx and trachea.

laryngoxerosis (-zēr-o′sis) dryness of the larynx.

larynx (lar′inks), pl. *laryn′ges* [Gr.] the organ of voice; the air passage between the lower pharynx and the trachea, containing the vocal cords and formed by nine cartilages: the thyroid, cricoid, and epiglottis and the paired arytenoid, corniculate, and cuneiform cartilages. See Plates VI and VII.

laser (la′zer) a device that transfers light of various frequencies into an extremely intense, small, and nearly nondivergent beam of monochromatic radiation in the visible region, with all the waves in phase; capable of mobilizing immense heat and power when focused at close range, it is used as a tool in surgery, in diagnosis, and in physiologic studies. **argon l.,** a laser with ionized argon as the active medium, whose beam is in the blue and green visible light spectrum; used for photocoagulation. **carbon dioxide l.,** a laser with carbon dioxide gas as the active medium, which produces infrared radiation at 10,600 nm; used to excise and incise tissue and to vaporize. **helium-neon l.,** a laser with a mixture of ionized helium and neon gases as the active medium, whose beam is in the red visible light spectrum; used as a guiding beam for lasers operating at nonvisible wavelengths. **krypton l.,** a laser with krypton ionized by electric current as the active medium, whose beam is in the yellow-red visible light spectrum; used for photocoagulation. **neodymium:yttrium-aluminum-garnet (Nd:YAG) l.,** a laser whose active medium is a crystal of yttrium, aluminum, and garnet doped with neodymium ions, and whose beam is in the near infrared spectrum at 1060 nm; used for photocoagulation and photoablation.

Lasix (la′siks) trademark for preparations of furosemide.

lassitude (las″ĭ-tōōd) weakness; exhaustion.

latentiation (la-ten″she-a′shin) the process of making latent; in pharmacology, chemical modification of a biologically active compound to affect its absorption, distribution, etc., the modified compound being transformed after administration to the active compound by biological processes.

laterad (lat′er-ad) toward the lateral aspect.

lateral (lat′er-il) 1. denoting a position farther from the median plane or midline of the body or a structure. 2. pertaining to a side.

lateralis (lat″er-a′lis) [L.] lateral.

laterality (lat″er-al′ĭt-e) a tendency to use preferentially the organs (hand, foot, ear, eye) of the same side in voluntary motor acts. **crossed l.,** the preferential use of contralateral members of the different pairs of organs in voluntary motor acts, e.g., right eye and left hand. **dominant l.** the preferential use of ipsilateral members of the different pairs of organs in voluntary motor acts, e.g., right eye and hand (dextrality) or left eye and hand (sinistrality).

lateroduction (lat″er-o-duk′shin) movement of an eye to either side.

lateroflexion (-flek′shin) flexion to one side.

laterotorsion (-tor′shin) twisting of the vertical meridian of the eye to either side.

lateroversion (-vur′zhin) abnormal turning to one side.

latex (la′teks) a viscid, milky juice secreted by some seed plants.

lathyrism (lath″ĭ-rizm) a morbid condition marked by spastic paraplegia, pain, hyperesthesia, and paresthesia, due to ingestion of the seeds of leguminous plants of the genus *Lathyrus,* which includes many kinds of peas. **lathyrit′ic,** adj.

latissimus (lah-tis″ĭ-mus) [L.] widest; in anatomy, denoting a broad structure.

latrodectism (lă″tro-dek′tizm) intoxication due to venom of spiders of the genus *Latrodectus.*

Latrodectus (-dek′tus) a genus of poisonous spiders, including *L. mac′tans,* the black widow spider, whose bite may cause severe symptoms or even death.

LATS long-acting thyroid stimulator.

latus (la′tus) [L.] 1. broad, wide. 2. the side or flank.

lauric acid (lawr′ik) $C_{12}H_{24}O_2$, found in many vegetable oils, especially laurel seed oil and coconut oil, and in milk fat.

lavage (lah-vahzh′) 1. the irrigation or washing out of an organ, as of the stomach or bowel. 2. to wash out, or irrigate.

law (law) a uniform or constant fact or principle. **all-or-none l.,** see *all-or-none.* **Allen's paradoxic l.,** the more sugar a normal person is given the more is utilized; the reverse is true in diabetics. **Beer's l.,** in spectrophotometry, the absorbance of a solution is proportional to the concentration of the absorbing solute and to the path length of the light beam through the solution. **Bell's l.,** the anterior roots of spinal nerves are motor roots, the posterior are sensory. **Boyle's l.,** at a constant temperature the volume of a perfect gas varies inversely as the pressure, and the pressure varies inversely as the volume. **Charles' l.,** at a constant pressure the volume of a given mass of a perfect gas varies directly with the absolute temperature. **l. of conservation of energy,** in any given system the amount of energy is constant; energy is neither created nor destroyed, but only transformed from one form to another. **l. of conservation of matter,** in any chemical reaction atoms are neither created nor destroyed; the total mass of the system remains constant. **Dalton's l.,** the pressure exerted by a mixture of nonreacting gases is equal to the sum of the partial pressures of the separate components. **Fechner's l.,** the sensation produced by a stimulus varies as the logarithm of the stimulus. **Hellin's l.,** one in about 89 pregnancies ends in the birth of twins; one in 89 × 89 (7921), of triplets; one in 89 × 89 × 89 (704,969), of quadruplets. **Henry's l.,** the solubility of a gas in a liquid solution is proportionate to the partial pressure of the gas. **l. of independent assortment,** the members of gene pairs segregate independently during meiosis **Mendel's l., mendelian l.,** in the inheritance of certain traits or characters, offspring are not intermediate in type between the parents, but inherit from one or the other parent in this respect. Thus, if a plant with the factor tallness (TT) is mated with one with the factor shortness (SS), then the offspring will inherit these factors in the ratio TT, 2TS, SS. This law is usually expressed as the *law of independent assortment* and the *law of*

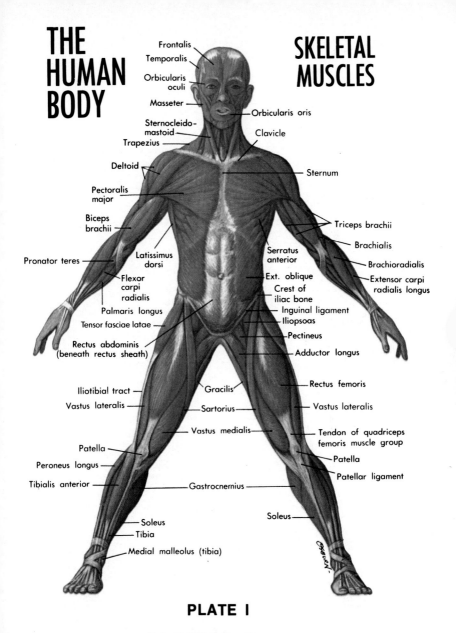

THE HUMAN BODY

SKELETAL MUSCLES

Frontalis
Temporalis
Orbicularis oculi
Masseter
Orbicularis oris
Sternocleido-mastoid
Clavicle
Trapezius
Deltoid
Sternum
Pectoralis major
Biceps brachii
Triceps brachii
Brachialis
Pronator teres
Serratus anterior
Brachioradialis
Latissimus dorsi
Ext. oblique
Extensor carpi radialis longus
Flexor carpi radialis
Crest of iliac bone
Palmaris longus
Inguinal ligament
Tensor fasciae latae
Iliopsoas
Pectineus
Rectus abdominis (beneath rectus sheath)
Adductor longus
Iliotibial tract
Gracilis
Rectus femoris
Vastus lateralis
Sartorius
Vastus lateralis
Vastus medialis
Tendon of quadriceps femoris muscle group
Patella
Peroneus longus
Patella
Patellar ligament
Tibialis anterior
Gastrocnemius
Soleus
Soleus
Tibia
Medial malleolus (tibia)

PLATE I

BONES

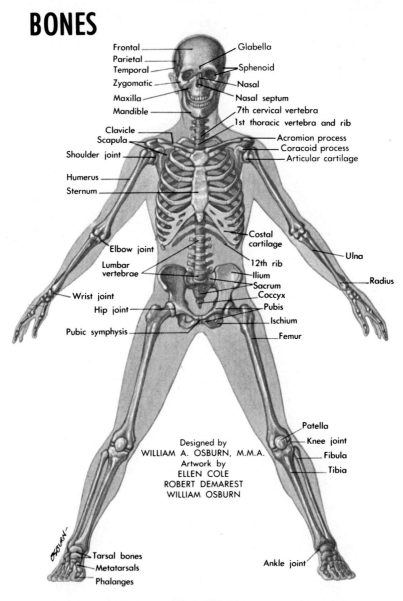

Frontal — Glabella
Parietal — Sphenoid
Temporal — Nasal
Zygomatic — Nasal
Maxilla — Nasal septum
Mandible — 7th cervical vertebra
— 1st thoracic vertebra and rib
Clavicle — Acromion process
Scapula — Coracoid process
Shoulder joint — Articular cartilage
Humerus
Sternum
— Costal cartilage
Elbow joint — Ulna
Lumbar vertebrae — 12th rib
— Ilium
— Sacrum
Wrist joint — Coccyx — Radius
Hip joint — Pubis
Pubic symphysis — Ischium
— Femur

Patella
Knee joint
Fibula
Tibia

Designed by
WILLIAM A. OSBURN, M.M.A.
Artwork by
ELLEN COLE
ROBERT DEMAREST
WILLIAM OSBURN

Tarsal bones
Metatarsals — Ankle joint
Phalanges

PLATE II

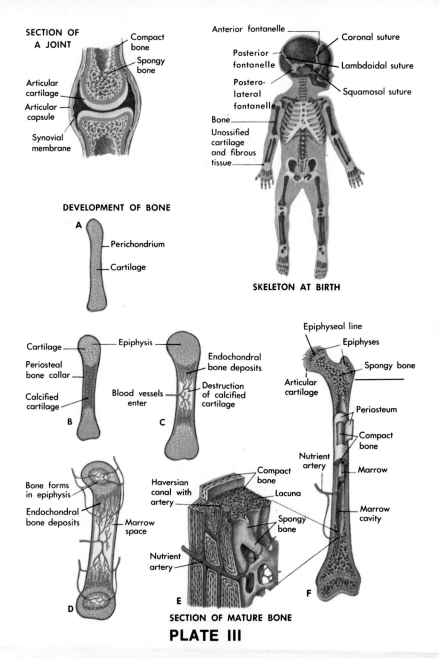

SECTION OF A JOINT

Compact bone
Spongy bone
Articular cartilage
Articular capsule
Synovial membrane

Anterior fontanelle
Coronal suture
Posterior fontanelle
Lambdoidal suture
Postero-lateral fontanelle
Squamosal suture
Bone
Unossified cartilage and fibrous tissue

SKELETON AT BIRTH

DEVELOPMENT OF BONE

A
Perichondrium
Cartilage

B
Cartilage
Epiphysis
Periosteal bone collar
Calcified cartilage

C
Endochondral bone deposits
Blood vessels enter
Destruction of calcified cartilage

D
Bone forms in epiphysis
Endochondral bone deposits
Marrow space

E
Haversian canal with artery
Compact bone
Lacuna
Spongy bone
Nutrient artery

SECTION OF MATURE BONE

F
Epiphyseal line
Epiphyses
Spongy bone
Articular cartilage
Periosteum
Compact bone
Nutrient artery
Marrow
Marrow cavity

PLATE III

THE ORGANS OF DIGESTION

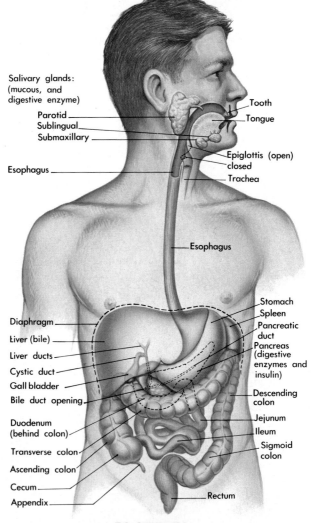

Salivary glands:
(mucous, and
digestive enzyme)

Parotid
Sublingual
Submaxillary

Esophagus

Tooth
Tongue

Epiglottis (open)
closed
Trachea

Esophagus

Stomach
Spleen
Pancreatic
duct
Pancreas
(digestive
enzymes and
insulin)

Diaphragm
Liver (bile)
Liver ducts
Cystic duct
Gall bladder
Bile duct opening

Duodenum
(behind colon)

Transverse colon
Ascending colon
Cecum
Appendix

Descending
colon
Jejunum
Ileum
Sigmoid
colon

Rectum

PLATE IV

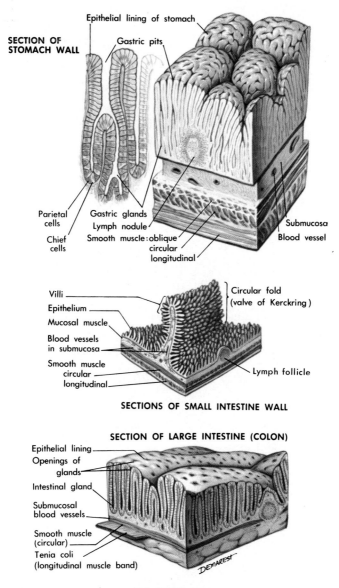

SECTION OF STOMACH WALL

Epithelial lining of stomach

Gastric pits

Parietal cells

Chief cells

Gastric glands

Lymph nodule

Smooth muscle: oblique
circular
longitudinal

Submucosa

Blood vessel

Villi

Epithelium

Mucosal muscle

Blood vessels in submucosa

Smooth muscle
circular
longitudinal

Circular fold (valve of Kerckring)

Lymph follicle

SECTIONS OF SMALL INTESTINE WALL

SECTION OF LARGE INTESTINE (COLON)

Epithelial lining

Openings of glands

Intestinal gland

Submucosal blood vessels

Smooth muscle (circular)

Tenia coli (longitudinal muscle band)

DEMAREST

PLATE V

THE ORGANS OF RESPIRATION AND THE HEART

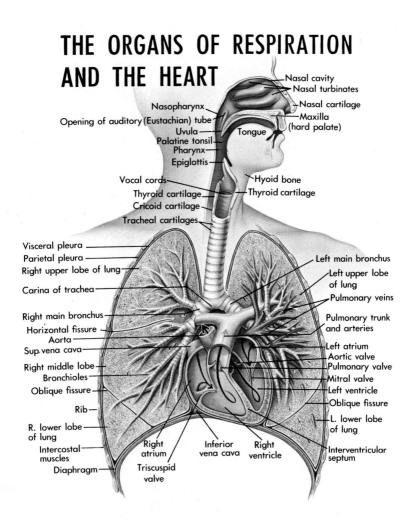

Nasal cavity
Nasal turbinates
Nasal cartilage
Maxilla (hard palate)
Nasopharynx
Opening of auditory (Eustachian) tube
Uvula
Tongue
Palatine tonsil
Pharynx
Epiglottis
Vocal cords
Hyoid bone
Thyroid cartilage
Thyroid cartilage
Cricoid cartilage
Tracheal cartilages
Visceral pleura
Parietal pleura
Left main bronchus
Right upper lobe of lung
Left upper lobe of lung
Carina of trachea
Pulmonary veins
Right main bronchus
Pulmonary trunk and arteries
Horizontal fissure
Aorta
Left atrium
Sup. vena cava
Aortic valve
Right middle lobe
Pulmonary valve
Bronchioles
Mitral valve
Oblique fissure
Left ventricle
Oblique fissure
Rib
L. lower lobe of lung
R. lower lobe of lung
Intercostal muscles
Right atrium
Inferior vena cava
Right ventricle
Interventricular septum
Diaphragm
Triscuspid valve

PLATE VI

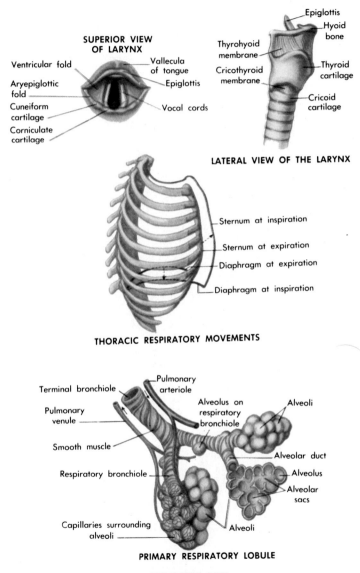

SUPERIOR VIEW OF LARYNX

Ventricular fold
Aryepiglottic fold
Cuneiform cartilage
Corniculate cartilage
Vallecula of tongue
Epiglottis
Vocal cords

Epiglottis
Hyoid bone
Thyrohyoid membrane
Cricothyroid membrane
Thyroid cartilage
Cricoid cartilage

LATERAL VIEW OF THE LARYNX

Sternum at inspiration
Sternum at expiration
Diaphragm at expiration
Diaphragm at inspiration

THORACIC RESPIRATORY MOVEMENTS

Terminal bronchiole
Pulmonary arteriole
Pulmonary venule
Alveolus on respiratory bronchiole
Alveoli
Smooth muscle
Respiratory bronchiole
Alveolar duct
Alveolus
Alveolar sacs
Capillaries surrounding alveoli
Alveoli

PRIMARY RESPIRATORY LOBULE

PLATE VII

THE MAJOR BLOOD VESSELS

VEINS   **ARTERIES**

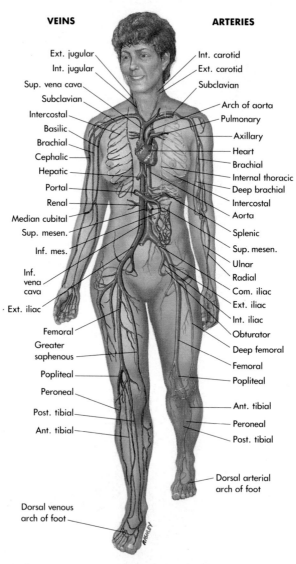

Ext. jugular
Int. jugular
Sup. vena cava
Subclavian
Intercostal
Basilic
Brachial
Cephalic
Hepatic
Portal
Renal
Median cubital
Sup. mesen.
Inf. mes.
Inf.
vena
cava
Ext. iliac
Femoral
Greater
saphenous
Popliteal
Peroneal
Post. tibial
Ant. tibial
Dorsal venous
arch of foot

Int. carotid
Ext. carotid
Subclavian
Arch of aorta
Pulmonary
Axillary
Heart
Brachial
Internal thoracic
Deep brachial
Intercostal
Aorta
Splenic
Sup. mesen.
Ulnar
Radial
Com. iliac
Ext. iliac
Int. iliac
Obturator
Deep femoral
Femoral
Popliteal
Ant. tibial
Peroneal
Post. tibial
Dorsal arterial
arch of foot

PLATE VIII

DETAILS OF CIRCULATORY STRUCTURES

A VEIN

A LARGE ARTERY

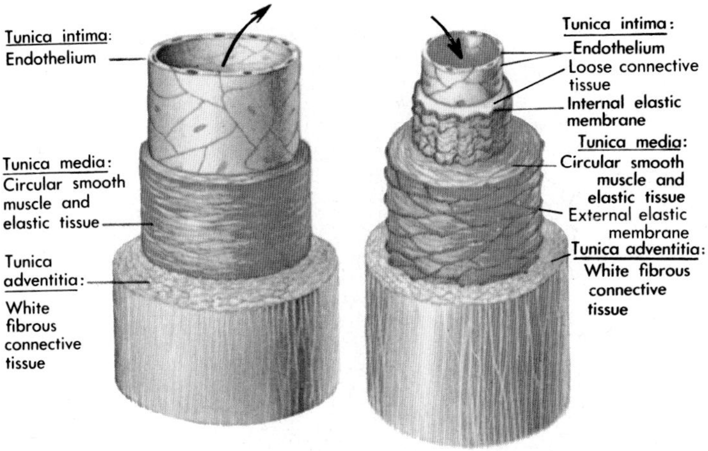

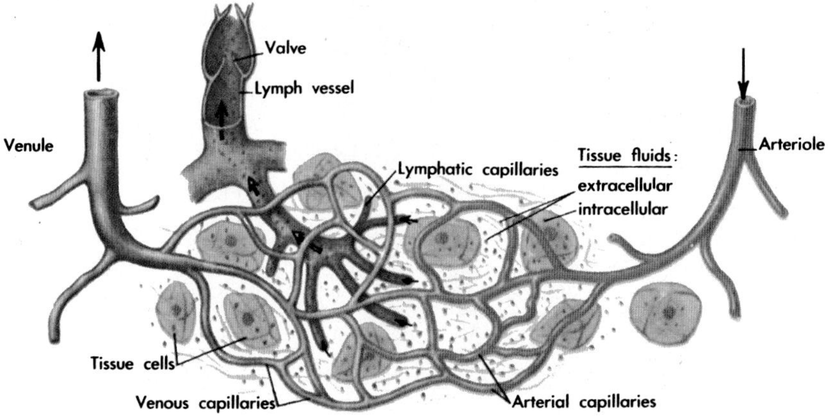

Tunica intima:
Endothelium

Tunica media:
Circular smooth
muscle and
elastic tissue

Tunica
adventitia:

White
fibrous
connective
tissue

Tunica intima:
Endothelium
Loose connective
tissue
Internal elastic
membrane
Tunica media:
Circular smooth
muscle and
elastic tissue
External elastic
membrane
Tunica adventitia:
White fibrous
connective
tissue

Valve

Lymph vessel

Venule

Lymphatic capillaries

Tissue fluids:
extracellular
intracellular

Arteriole

Tissue cells

Venous capillaries

Arterial capillaries

A CAPILLARY BED

PLATE IX

THE BRAIN AND SPINAL NERVES

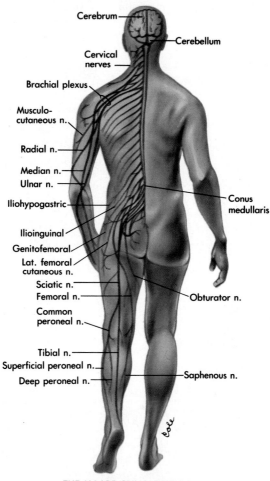

Cerebrum

Cerebellum

Cervical nerves

Brachial plexus

Musculo-cutaneous n.

Radial n.

Median n.

Ulnar n.

Iliohypogastric

Ilioinguinal

Genitofemoral

Lat. femoral cutaneous n.

Sciatic n.

Femoral n.

Common peroneal n.

Tibial n.

Superficial peroneal n.

Deep peroneal n.

Conus medullaris

Obturator n.

Saphenous n.

THE MAJOR SPINAL NERVES

PLATE X

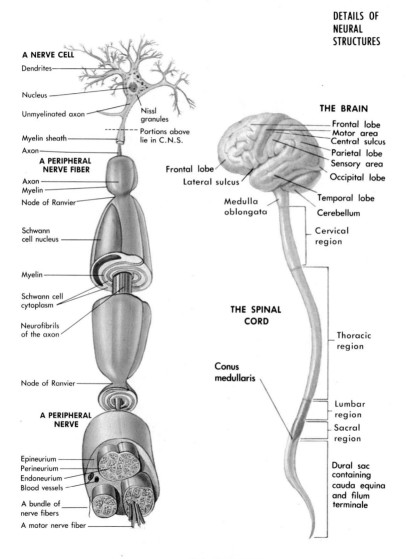

DETAILS OF
NEURAL
STRUCTURES

A NERVE CELL

Dendrites

Nucleus

Unmyelinated axon

Nissl
granules

Portions above
lie in C.N.S.

Myelin sheath

Axon

**A PERIPHERAL
NERVE FIBER**

Axon

Myelin

Node of Ranvier

Schwann
cell nucleus

Myelin

Schwann cell
cytoplasm

Neurofibrils
of the axon

Node of Ranvier

**A PERIPHERAL
NERVE**

Epineurium
Perineurium
Endoneurium
Blood vessels

A bundle of
nerve fibers

A motor nerve fiber

THE BRAIN

Frontal lobe
Motor area
Central sulcus
Parietal lobe
Sensory area
Occipital lobe

Frontal lobe
Lateral sulcus

Temporal lobe

Medulla
oblongata

Cerebellum

Cervical
region

**THE SPINAL
CORD**

Thoracic
region

**Conus
medullaris**

Lumbar
region

Sacral
region

Dural sac
containing
cauda equina
and filum
terminale

PLATE XI

ORGANS OF SPECIAL SENSE

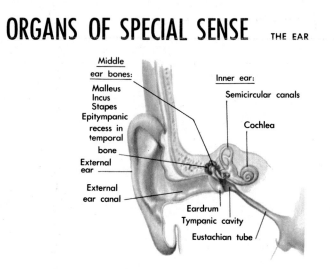

Middle
ear bones:
Malleus
Incus
Stapes
Epitympanic
recess in
temporal
bone
External
ear
External
ear canal

Inner ear:
Semicircular canals
Cochlea

Eardrum
Tympanic cavity
Eustachian tube

THE ORGAN OF HEARING

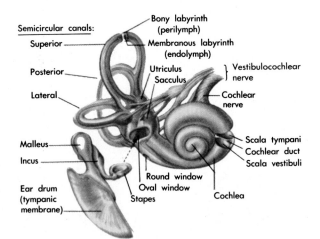

Semicircular canals:
Superior
Posterior
Lateral
Malleus
Incus
Ear drum
(tympanic
membrane)

Bony labyrinth
(perilymph)
Membranous labyrinth
(endolymph)
Utriculus
Sacculus } Vestibulocochlear
nerve
Cochlear
nerve

Scala tympani
Cochlear duct
Scala vestibuli

Round window
Oval window
Stapes
Cochlea

THE MIDDLE EAR AND INNER EAR

PLATE XII

THE LACRIMAL APPARATUS AND THE EYE

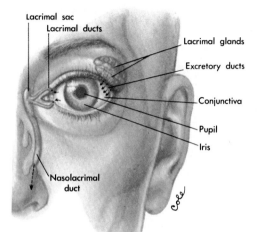

Lacrimal sac

Lacrimal ducts

Lacrimal glands

Excretory ducts

Conjunctiva

Pupil

Iris

Nasolacrimal duct

THE LACRIMAL APPARATUS

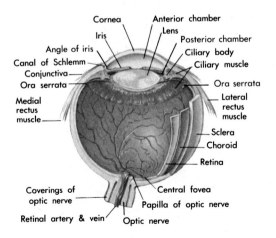

Cornea

Anterior chamber

Iris

Lens

Posterior chamber

Angle of iris

Ciliary body

Canal of Schlemm

Ciliary muscle

Conjunctiva

Ora serrata

Ora serrata

Medial rectus muscle

Lateral rectus muscle

Sclera

Choroid

Retina

Coverings of optic nerve

Central fovea

Papilla of optic nerve

Retinal artery & vein

Optic nerve

HORIZONTAL SECTION OF THE EYE

PLATE XIII

STRUCTURAL DETAILS

SKELETAL MUSCLE

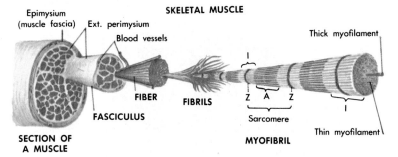

Epimysium (muscle fascia)
Ext. perimysium
Blood vessels
Thick myofilament
FIBER
FIBRILS
FASCICULUS
Z   A   Z
Sarcomere
I
Thin myofilament
SECTION OF A MUSCLE
MYOFIBRIL

BRAIN

Sensory cortex
Thalamus
Motor cortex
Pons
Ascending sensory tracts
Medulla
Descending motor tract
Fibers cross to opposite side
Dorsal root
Spinal ganglion
SIMPLE REFLEX ARC
Ventral root
SPINAL CORD

PLATE XIV

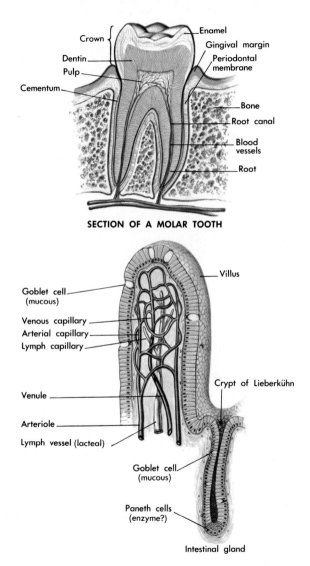

SECTION OF A MOLAR TOOTH

Crown
Enamel
Gingival margin
Dentin
Periodontal membrane
Pulp
Cementum
Bone
Root canal
Blood vessels
Root

Villus
Goblet cell (mucous)
Venous capillary
Arterial capillary
Lymph capillary
Crypt of Lieberkühn
Venule
Arteriole
Lymph vessel (lacteal)
Goblet cell (mucous)
Paneth cells (enzyme?)
Intestinal gland

SECTIONS OF SMALL INTESTINE WALL

PLATE XV

THE PARANASAL SINUSES

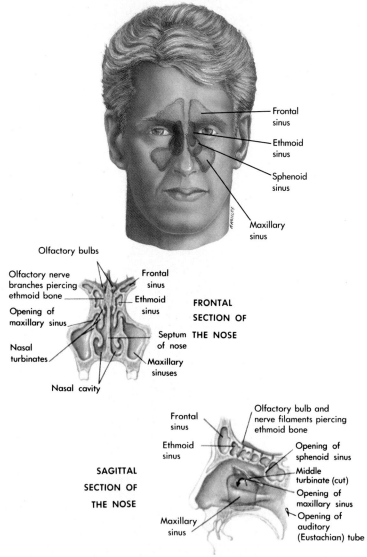

Frontal sinus

Ethmoid sinus

Sphenoid sinus

Maxillary sinus

Olfactory bulbs

Olfactory nerve branches piercing ethmoid bone

Opening of maxillary sinus

Nasal turbinates

Nasal cavity

Frontal sinus

Ethmoid sinus

Septum of nose

Maxillary sinuses

FRONTAL SECTION OF THE NOSE

Olfactory bulb and nerve filaments piercing ethmoid bone

Frontal sinus

Ethmoid sinus

Opening of sphenoid sinus

Middle turbinate (cut)

Opening of maxillary sinus

Opening of auditory (Eustachian) tube

SAGITTAL SECTION OF THE NOSE

Maxillary sinus

PLATE XVI

segregation. **Nysten's l.,** rigor mortis affects first the muscles of mastication, next those of the face and neck, then those of the trunk and arms, and last those of the legs and feet. **Ohm's l.,** the strength of an electric current varies directly as the electromotive force and inversely as the resistance. **Raoult's l.,** 1. *(for freezing points)* the depression of the freezing point for the same type of electrolyte dissolved in a given solvent is proportional to the molecular concentration of the solute. 2. *(for vapor pressures)* (a), the vapor pressure of a volatile substance from a liquid solution is equal to the mole fraction of that substance times its vapor pressure in the pure state. (b), when a nonvolatile nonelectrolyte is dissolved in a solvent, the decrease in vapor pressure of that solvent is equal to the mole fraction of the solute times the vapor pressure of the pure solvent. **l. of segregation,** in each generation the ratio of (a) pure dominants, (b) dominants giving descendants in the proportion of three dominants to one recessive, and (c) pure recessives is 1 : 2 : 1. This ratio follows from the fact that the two alleles of a gene cannot be a part of a single gamete, but must segregate to different gametes. **Weber's l.,** the variation of stimulus which causes the smallest appreciable change in sensation maintains an approximately fixed ratio to the whole stimulus. **Weber-Fechner l.,** for a sensation to increase by arithmetical progression, the stimulus must increase by geometrical progression.

lawrencium (law-ren'se-um) chemical element *(see table),* at. no. 103, symbol Lw.

laxative (lak'sit-iv) 1. aperient; mildly cathartic. 2. a cathartic or purgative. **bulk l.,** one promoting bowel evacuation by increasing fecal volume.

laxator (lak-sāt'er) that which slackens or relaxes.

layer (la'er) stratum; a sheetlike mass of tissue of nearly uniform thickness, several of which may be superimposed, one above the other, as in the epidermis. **bacillary l.,** l. of rods and cones. **basal l.,** 1. the deepest layer of the epidermis. 2. the deepest layer of the uterine mucosa. **blastodermic l.,** germ l. **clear l.,** the clear translucent layer of the epidermis, just beneath the horny layer. **columnar l.,** mantle l. **compact l.,** the layer of the endometrium nearest the surface, containing the necks of the uterine glands. **enamel l.,** the outermost layer of cells of the enamel organ. **functional l.,** the compact and spongy layers of the endometrium considered together, the cells of which are cast off at menstruation and parturition; known as the *decidua* during pregnancy. **ganglionic l. of cerebellum,** the thin middle gray layer of the cerebral cortex, consisting of a single layer of Purkinje cells. **germ l.,** any of the three primary layers of cells of the embryo (ectoderm, entoderm, and mesoderm), from which the tissues and organs develop. **germinative l.,** 1. malpighian l. 2. basal l. (1). **granular l.,** 1. the layer of epidermis between the clear and prickle-cell layers. 2. the deep layer of the cortex of the cerebellum. 3. the layer of follicle cells lining the theca of the vesicular ovarian follicle.

Henle's l., the outermost layer of the inner root sheath of the hair follicle. **horny l.,** 1. stratum corneum; the outermost layer of the epidermis, consisting of dead and desquamating cells. 2. the outer, compact layer of the nail. **malpighian l.,** the basal layer and prickle-cell layer of the epidermis considered together. **mantle l.,** the middle layer of the wall of the primitive neural tube, containing primitive nerve cells and later forming the gray substance of the central nervous system. **odontoblastic l.,** the epithelioid layer of odontoblasts in contact with the dentin of teeth. **prickle-cell l.,** stratum spinosum; the layer of the epidermis between the granular and basal layers, marked by the presence of prickle cells. **Rauber's l.,** the most external of the three layers forming the blastodisc in the early embryo. **l. of rods and cones,** a layer of the retina immediately beneath the pigment epithelium, between it and external limiting membrane, containing the rods and cones. **spongy l.,** the middle layer of the endometrium, containing the tortuous portions of the uterine glands; see also *functional l.* **subendocardial l.,** the layer of loose fibrous tissue uniting the endocardium and myocardium.

lb. [L.] *li'bra* (pound).

LD₅₀ median lethal dose.

LDL low-density lipoprotein.

L-dopa see *dopa.*

LE lupus erythematosus; left eye.

lead¹ (led) chemical element *(see table),* at. no. 82, symbol Pb. Poisoning is caused by absorption or ingestion of lead, and affects the brain, nervous and digestive systems, and blood.

lead² (lēd) any of the conductors connected to the electrocardiograph; also any of the records made by the electrocardiograph, varying with the part of the body from which the current is led off. Usually, three peripheral leads are used: lead I, right arm and left arm; lead II, right arm and left leg; lead III, left arm and left leg. **aV_F l.,** a unipolar lead in which the positive lead is on the left leg. **aV_L l.,** a unipolar lead in which the positive terminal is on the left arm. **bipolar l.,** an array involving two electrodes placed at different body sites. **limb l's,** any of the three leads customarily used in electrocardiography. **precordial l's,** leads in which the exploring electrode is placed on the chest and the other is connected to one or more extremities, indicated as follows: CR = chest + right arm; CL = chest + left arm; CF = chest + left leg; V = chest + junction of leads from right and left arms and left leg. Subscript numbers 1 to 6 indicate at which points on the chest the lead is taken. **unipolar l.,** an array of two electrodes, only one of which transmits potential variation.

learning (lern'ing) a long-lasting adaptive behavioral change due to experience. **latent l.,** that which occurs without reinforcement, becoming apparent only when a reinforcement or reward is introduced.

lecithal (les'ĭ-thil) having a yolk; used especially as a word termination (*isolecithal,* etc.).

lecithin (les'ĭ-thin) any of a group of phospholipids found in animal tissues, especially nerve tissue, the liver, semen, and egg yolk, consisting of esters of glycerol with two molecules of long-chain aliphatic acids and one of phosphoric acid, the latter being esterified with the alcohol group of choline.

lecithinase (-ās) phospholipase.

lecitho- word element [Gr.], *the yolk of an egg or ovum.*

lecithoblast (les'ĭ-tho-blast″) the primitive entoderm of a two-layered blastodisc.

lectin (lek'tin) any of a group of hemagglutinating proteins found primarily in plant seeds, which bind specifically to the branching sugar molecules of glycoproteins and glycolipids on the surface of cells.

leech (lēch) any of the annelids of the class Hirudinea, especially *Hirudo medicinalis;* some species are bloodsuckers and were formerly used for drawing blood.

leg (leg) the lower limb, especially the part from knee to foot. **bandy l.,** bowleg. **bayonet l.,** ankylosis of the knee after backward displacement of the tibia and fibula. **bow l.,** see *bowleg.* **milk l.,** phlegmasia alba dolens. **restless l's,** a disagreeable, creeping, irritating sensation in the legs, usually the lower legs, relieved only by walking or keeping the legs moving. **scissor l.,** deformity with crossing of the legs in walking.

Legionella (le″jah-nel'ah) a genus of gram-negative, aerobic, rod-shaped bacteria which normally inhabit lakes, streams, and moist soil; organisms have frequently been isolated from cooling-tower water, evaporative condensers, tap water, shower heads, and treated sewage. **L. micda'dei,** a species that is the causative agent of Pittsburgh pneumonia. **L. pneumo'phila,** a species that is the causative agent of legionnaires' disease.

legionellosis (le″jin-el-o'sis) disease caused by infection with *Legionella pneumophila;* see *legionnaires' disease* and *Pontiac fever.*

legume (lĕ'gūm) the pod or fruit of a leguminous plant, such as peas or beans.

leiodermia (li″ah-derm′e-ah) abnormal smoothness and glossiness of the skin.

leiomyofibroma (-mi″o-fi-bro′mah) epithelioid leiomyoma.

leiomyoma (-mi-o′mah) a benign tumor derived from smooth muscle, most often of the uterus. **epithelioid l.,** leiomyoma, usually of the stomach, in which the cells are polygonal rather than spindle shaped.

leiomyosarcoma (-mi″o-sar-ko′mah) a sarcoma containing cells of smooth muscle.

Leishmania (lēsh-ma′ne-ah) a genus of parasitic protozoa, including several species pathogenic for humans. In some classifications, organisms are placed in four complexes comprising species and subspecies: *L. donova'ni* (causing visceral leishmaniasis or kala-azar), *L. tro'pica* (causing the Old World form of cutaneous leishmaniasis), *L. mexica'na* (causing the New World form of cutaneous leishmaniasis), and *L. brazilien'sis* (causing mucocutaneous leishmaniasis).

leishmaniasis (lēsh″mah-ni′ah-sis) infection with *Leishmania.* **American l.,** mucocutaneous l. **cutaneous l.,** an endemic granulomatous disease, divided into two forms: an Old World form caused by *Leishmania tropica* and a New World form caused by *L. mexicana* or *L. braziliensis.* **diffuse cutaneous l.,** chronic generalized cutaneous leishmaniasis, in which the lesions resemble those of lepromatous leprosy. **lupoid l.,** l. recidivans. **mucocutaneous l.,** cutaneous leishmaniasis endemic in Central and South America, caused by *Leishmania braziliensis,* characterized by ulceration of mucous membranes of the nose, mouth, and pharynx, causing widespread destruction of tissue with marked deformity. **l. reci'divans,** a prolonged, relapsing form of cutaneous leishmaniasis resembling tuberculosis of the skin. **l. tegmenta'ria diffu'sa,** diffuse cutaneous l. **visceral l.,** kala-azar.

lemmoblastic (lem″o-blas'tik) forming or developing into neurilemma tissue.

lemniscus (lem-nis′kus), pl. *lemnis'ci* [L.] a ribbon or band; in anatomy, a band or bundle of fibers in the central nervous system.

length (lenkth) the longest dimension of an object, or of the measurement between the two ends. **crown-heel l.,** the distance from the crown of the head to the heel in embryos, fetuses, and infants; the equivalent of standing height in older persons. **crown-rump l.,** the distance from the crown of the head to the breech in embryos, fetuses, and infants; the equivalent of sitting height in older persons. **focal l.,** the distance between a lens and an object from which all rays of light are brought to a focus.

lens (lenz) 1. a piece of glass or other transparent material so shaped as to converge or scatter light rays; see also *glasses.* 2. crystalline lens; the transparent, biconvex body separating the posterior chamber and vitreous body, and constituting part of the refracting mechanism of the eye; see Plate XIII. **achromatic l.,** one corrected for chromatic aberration. **aplanatic l.,** one that serves to correct spherical aberrations. **biconcave l.,** one concave on both faces. **biconvex l.,** one convex on both faces. **bifocal l.,** see under *glasses.* **concavoconvex l.,** one with one concave and one convex face. **contact l.,** a curved shell of glass or plastic applied directly over the globe or cornea to correct refractive errors. **convexoconcave l.,** one having one convex and one concave face. **crystalline l.,** lens (2). **decentered l.,** one in which the optical axis does not pass through the center. **honeybee l.,** a magnifying eyeglass lens designed to resemble the multifaceted eye of the honeybee. It consists of three or six small telescopes mounted in the upper portion of the spectacles and directed toward the center and right and left visual fields. Prisms are included to provide a continuous, unbroken magnified field of view. **omnifocal l.,** one whose power increases continuously and regularly in a downward direction, avoiding the discontinuity in field and power inherent in bifocal and trifocal lenses. **planoconvex l.,** a lens with one plane and one convex side. **spherical l.,** one that is a segment of a sphere. **trial l's,** lenses used in determining visual acuity. **trifocal l.,** see under *glasses.*

lenticonus (len″tĭ-ko′nus) a congenital conical bulging, anteriorly or posteriorly, of the lens of the eye.

lenticular (len-tik′ūl-er) 1. pertaining to or shaped like a lens. 2. pertaining to the lens of the eye. 3. pertaining to the lenticular nucleus.

lentiform (len′tĭ-fŏrm) lens-shaped.

lentigines (len-tij′ĭ-nēz) plural of *lentigo*.

lentiginosis (len-tĭj″ĭ-no′sis) a condition marked by multiple lentigines. **progressive cardiomyopathic l.**, multiple symmetrical lentigines, hypertrophic obstructive cardiomyopathy, and retarded growth, sometimes with mental retardation.

lentiglobus (len″tĭ-glo′bus) exaggerated curvature of the lens of the eye, producing an anterior spherical bulging.

lentigo (len-ti′go), pl. *lentig′ines* [L.] a flat brownish pigmented spot on the skin due to increased deposition of melanin and an increased number of melanocytes. **l. malig′na, malignant l.**, melanotic freckle of Hutchinson.

leontiasis (le″on-ti′ah-sis) the leonine facies of lepromatous leprosy, due to nodular invasion of the subcutaneous tissue. **l. os′sea**, hypertrophy of the bones of the cranium and face, giving it a vaguely leonine appearance.

leper (lep′er) a person with leprosy; a term now in disfavor.

lepidic (lĕ-pid′ik) pertaining to scales.

lepra (lep′rah) leprosy; before about 1850, psoriasis.

leprechaunism (lep′rĕ-kon″izm) a lethal familial congenital condition in which the infant is small and has elfin facies and severe endocrine disorders, as indicated by enlarged clitoris and breasts.

leprid (lep′rid) cutaneous lesion or lesions of tuberculoid leprosy: hypopigmented or erythematous nodules or plaques, lacking bacilli.

leproma (lep-ro′mah) a superficial granulomatous nodule rich in leprosy bacilli, the characteristic lesion of lepromatous leprosy.

lepromatous (-tus) pertaining to lepromas; see under *leprosy*.

lepromin (lep′rah-min) a repeatedly boiled, autoclaved, gauze-filtered suspension of finely triturated lepromatous tissue and leprosy bacilli, used in the skin test for tissue resistance to leprosy.

leprostatic (-stat′ik) inhibiting the growth of *Mycobacterium leprae;* an agent that so acts.

leprosy (lep′rah-se) a chronic communicable disease caused by *Mycobacterium leprae* and characterized by the production of granulomatous lesions of the skin, mucous membranes, and peripheral nervous system. Two principal, or polar, types are recognized: lepromatous and tuberculoid. **lepromatous l.,** that form marked by the development of lepromas and by an abundance of leprosy bacilli from the onset; nerve damage occurs only slowly, and the skin reaction to lepromin is negative. It is the only form which may regularly serve as a source of infection. **tuberculoid l.,** the form in which leprosy bacilli are few or lacking and nerve damage occurs early, so that all skin lesions are

denervated from the onset, often with dissociation of sensation; the skin reaction to lepromin is positive, and the patient is rarely a source of infection to others.

lepto- word element [Gr.], *slender; delicate.*

leptocephalus (lep″to-sef′ah-lus) a person with an abnormally tall, narrow skull.

leptocyte (lep′tah-sīt) an erythrocyte characterized by a hemoglobinated border surrounding a clear area containing a center of pigment.

leptomeninges (-mĕ-nin′jēz) the pia mater and arachnoid taken together; the pia-arachnoid. **leptomenin′geal,** adj.

leptomeningitis (-men″in-jīt′is) inflammation of the leptomeninges.

leptomeningopathy (-men″ing-gop′ah-the) any disease of the leptomeninges.

leptomonad (-mo′nad) 1. of or pertaining to *Leptomonas.* 2. denoting the leptomonad form; see *promastigote.* 3. a protozoon exhibiting the leptomonad (promastigote) form.

Leptomonas (-mo′nis) a genus of protozoa of the family Trypanosomatidae, parasitic in the digestive track of insects.

leptopellic (-pel′ik) having a narrow pelvis.

Leptospira (lep′to-spi′rah) a genus of aerobic bacteria (family Leptospiraceae); all pathogenic strains (i.e., those that cause leptospirosis) are contained in the species *L. inter′rogans,* which is divided into several serogroups, which are in turn divided into serotypes.

Leptospiraceae (lep″to-spi-ra′se-e) a family of bacteria (order Spirochaetales) consisting of flexible helical cells that are aerobic; it consists of one genus, *Leptospira.*

leptospirosis (lep″to-spi-ro′sis) any infectious disease due to certain serotypes of *Leptospira,* manifested by lymphocytic meningitis, hepatitis, and nephritis, separately or in combination.

leptotene (lep′to-tēn) the stage of meiosis in which the chromosomes are threadlike in shape.

leptothricosis (lep″to-thrĭ-ko′sis) leptotrichosis. **l. conjuncti′vae,** Parinaud's oculoglandular syndrome caused by *Leptothrix.*

Leptothrix (lep′tah-thriks) a genus of schizomycetes (family Chlamydobacteriaceae), widely distributed and usually found in fresh water.

leptotrichosis (lep″to-trĭ-ko′sis) any infection with *Leptothrix.*

lesbianism (lez′be-in-izm″) homosexuality between women.

lesion (le′zhin) any pathological or traumatic discontinuity of tissue or loss of function of a part. **Armanni-Ebstein l.,** vacuolization of the renal tubular epithelium in diabetes. **Blumenthal l.,** a proliferative vascular lesion in the smaller arteries in diabetes. **central l.,** any lesion of the central nervous system. **Ghon's primary l.,** Ghon focus. **Janeway l.,** a small erythematous or hemorrhagic lesion, usually on the palms or soles, in bacterial endocarditis. **primary l.,** the original lesion manifesting a disease, as a chancre.

lethargy (leth′er-je) a condition of drowsiness or indifference.

leucine (loo'sēn) an amino acid, $C_6H_{13}NO_2$, essential for optimal growth in infants and for nitrogen equilibrium in adults.

leuco- for words beginning thus, see also those beginning *leuko-*.

Leuconostoc (loo″ko-nos'tok) a genus of slime-forming saprophytic bacteria (tribe Streptococceae) found in milk and fruit juices, including *L. citro'vorum*, *L. dextran'icum*, and *L. mesenteroi'des*.

leucovorin (-vor'in) folinic acid, $C_{20}H_{23}N_7O_7$; used as an antidote for folic acid antagonists, e.g., methotrexate, and in the treatment of megaloblastic anemias due to folic acid deficiency.

leuk(o)- word element [Gr.], *white; leukocyte.*

leukapheresis (loo″kah-fĕ-re'sis) the selective separation and removal of leukocytes from withdrawn blood, the remainder of the blood then being retransfused into the donor.

leukemia (loo-kēm'e-ah) a progressive, malignant disease of the blood-forming organs, marked by distorted proliferation and development of leukocytes and their precursors in the blood and bone marrow. **leuke'mic**, adj. **acute nonlymphocytic l.**, leukemia occurring primarily after treatment with alkylating agents, marked by pancytopenia, megaloblastic bone marrow, nucleated red cells in the peripheral marrow, and resistance to treatment; survival time is usually short. **adult T-cell l.**, a form of leukemia associated with human T-cell leukemia/lymphoma virus, characterized by adult onset, leukemic cells with T cell properties, frequent dermal involvement, lymphadenopathy, and hepatosplenomegaly; the course may be subacute or chronic. **basophilic l.**, leukemia in which the basophilic leukocytes predominate. **l. cu'tis**, leukemia with leukocytic invasion of the skin marked by pink, reddish brown, or purple macules, papules, and tumors. **eosinophilic l.**, a form in which eosinophils are the predominating cells. **hairy-cell l.**, leukemic reticuloendotheliosis. **histiocytic l.**, monocytic l. **lymphatic l., lymphoblastic l., lymphocytic l., lymphogenous l., lymphoid l.**, a form associated with hyperplasia and overactivity of the lymphoid tissue, in which the leukocytes are lymphocytes or lymphoblasts. **lymphosarcoma cell l.**, a form marked by large numbers of lymphosarcoma cells in the peripheral blood; depending on degree of bone marrow involvement, it may be a variant of lymphosarcoma. **mast cell l.**, a form marked by overwhelming numbers of tissue mast cells in the peripheral blood. **micromyeloblastic l.**, a form marked by the presence of large numbers of micromyeloblasts. **monocytic l.**, that in which the predominating leukocytes are monocytes. **myeloblastic l.**, leukemia in which myeloblasts predominate. **myelocytic l., myelogenous l., myeloid granulocytic l.**, a form arising from myeloid tissue in which the granular polymorphonuclear leukocytes and their precursors predominate. **plasma cell l., plasmacytic l.**, a form in which the predominating cell in the peripheral blood is the plasma cell. **promyelocytic l.**, a form in which the predominant cells are promyeloblasts, rather than myeloblasts, often associated with abnormal bleeding secondary to thrombocytopenia, hypofibrinogenemia, and decreased levels of coagulation Factor V. **Rieder cell l.**, myeloblastic leukemia in which the blood contains asynchronously developed cells with immature cytoplasm and a lobulated, relatively more mature nucleus. **stem cell l.**, a form in which the predominating cell is so immature and primitive that its classification is difficult.

leukemid (loo-kēm'id) any of the polymorphic skin eruptions associated with leukemia; clinically, they may be nonspecific, i.e., papular, macular, purpuric, etc., but histopathologically they may represent true leukemic infiltrations.

leukemogen (loo-kēm'ah-jen) any substance which produces leukemia. **leukemogen'ic**, adj.

leukemoid (loo-kēm'oid) exhibiting blood and sometimes clinical findings resembling those of true leukemia, but due to some other cause.

leukin (loo'kin) a bactericidal substance from leukocyte extract.

leukoagglutinin (loo″ko-ah-glōōt'in-in) an agglutinin which acts upon leukocytes.

leukoblast (loo'ko-blast) an immature granular leukocyte. **granular l.**, promyelocyte.

leukoblastosis (loo″ko-blas-to'sis) a general term for proliferation of leukocytes.

leukocidin (-si'din) a substance produced by some pathogenic bacteria that is toxic to polymorphonuclear leukocytes (neutrophils).

leukocrit (loo'ko-krit) the volume percentage of leukocytes in whole blood.

leukocyte (-sīt) white cell; a colorless blood corpuscle capable of ameboid movement, whose chief function is to protect the body against microorganisms causing disease and which may be classified in two main groups: *granular* and *nongranular*. **leukocyt'ic**, adj. **agranular l's**, nongranular l's. **basophilic l.**, basophil (2). **endothelial l.**, Mallory's name for the large wandering cells of the circulating blood and the tissues which have notable phagocytic properties; see *endotheliocyte.* **eosinophilic l.**, eosinophil (2). **granular l's**, granulocytes; leukocytes containing abundant granules in their cytoplasm, including neutrophils, eosinophils, and basophils. **hyaline l.**, monocyte. **lymphoid l's**, nongranular l's. **neutrophilic l.**, neutrophil (2). **nongranular l's**, leukocytes without specific granules in their cytoplasm, including lymphocytes and monocytes.

leukocythemia (loo″ko-si-thēm'e-ah) leukemia.

leukocytoblast (-sīt'ah-blast) leukoblast.

leukocytogenesis (-sīt″ah-jen'ĭ-sis) the formation of leukocytes.

leukocytolysis (-si-tol'ĭ-sis) disintegration of leukocytes. **leukocytolyt'ic**, adj.

leukocytoma (-si-to'mah) a tumor-like mass of leukocytes.

leukocytopenia (-sīt″ah-pēn'e-ah) leukopenia.

leukocytoplania (-sīt″ah-plān'e-ah) wandering of leukocytes; passage of leukocytes through a membrane.

leukocytopoiesis (-sīt″ah-poi-e'sis) leukopoiesis.

leukocytosis (-si-to′sis) a transient increase in the number of leukocytes in the blood, due to various causes. **basophilic l.**, increase in number of basophilic leukocytes in the blood. **mononuclear l.**, mononucleosis. **pathologic l.**, that due to some morbid reaction, e.g., infection or trauma.

leukocytotaxis (-sīt″ah-tak′sis) leukotaxis.

leukocytotoxicity (-sīt″ah-tok-sis″it-e) lymphocytotoxicity.

leukoderma (-derm′ah) an acquired condition with localized loss of pigmentation of the skin. **l. acquisi′tum centrif′ugum,** halo nevus. **syphilitic l.**, indistinct coarsely mottled hypopigmentation, usually on the sides of the neck, in late secondary syphilis.

leukodystrophy (-dis′tro-fe) disturbance of the white substance of the brain; see *leukoencephalopathy*. **metachromatic l.**, a hereditary leukoencephalopathy, marked by accumulation of sulfatide in tissues, with diffuse loss of myelin in the central nervous system and progressive dementia and paralysis; classified according to age of onset as infantile, juvenile, and adult.

leukoedema (-ě-de′mah) an abnormality of the buccal mucosa, consisting of an increase in thickness of the epithelium and intracellular edema of the spinous or malpighian layer.

leukoencephalitis (-en-sef″il-īt′is) 1. inflammation of the white substance of the brain. 2. forage poisoning, a contagious disease of horses.

leukoencephalopathy (-en-sef″il-lop′ah-the) any of a group of diseases affecting the white substance of the brain. The term *leukodystrophy* is used to denote such disorders due to defective formation and maintenance of myelin in infants and children.

leukoerythroblastosis (-ě-rith″ro-blas-to′sis) an anemic condition associated with space-occupying lesions of the bone marrow, marked by a variable number of immature erythroid and myeloid cells in the circulation.

leukokeratosis (-ker″ah-to′sis) leukoplakia.

leukokoria (-kor′e-ah) any condition marked by the appearance of a whitish reflex or mass in the pupillary area behind the lens.

leukokraurosis (-kraw-ro′sis) kraurosis vulvae.

leukolymphosarcoma (-lim″fo-sar-ko′mah) lymphosarcoma cell leukemia.

leukoma (loo-ko′mah) 1. a dense, white corneal opacity. 2. leukoplakia of the buccal mucosa. **leukom′atous,** adj. **l. adhae′rens,** a white tumor of the cornea enclosing a prolapsed adherent iris.

leukomyelitis (loo″ko-mi″il-īt′is) inflammation of the white substance of the spinal cord.

leukomyoma (-mi-o′mah) lipomyoma.

leukonecrosis (-ně-kro′sis) gangrene with formation of a white slough.

leukonychia (-nik′e-ah) abnormal whiteness of the nails, either total or in spots or streaks.

leukopathia (-path′e-ah) 1. leukoderma. 2. disease of the leukocytes. **l. un′guium,** leukonychia.

leukopedesis (-pě-de′sis) diapedesis of leukocytes through blood vessel walls.

leukopenia (-pēn′e-ah) reduction of the number of leukocytes in the blood, the count being 5000 or less. **leukope′nic,** adj. **basophilic l.**, abnormal reduction of number of basophilic leukocytes in the blood. **malignant l., pernicious l.**, agranulocytosis.

leukoplakia (-pla′ke-ah) a disease marked by the development on the mucous membranes of the cheeks (*l. buccalis*), gums, or tongue (*l. lingualis*) of white thickened patches which sometimes show a tendency to fissure and to become malignant. **l. vul′vae,** the presence of hypertrophic grayish-white infiltrated patches on the vulvar mucosa.

leukopoietin (-poi-ēt″n) a hypothetical substance believed to serve as the humoral regulator of leukopoiesis; granulopoietin.

leukorrhea (-re′ah) a whitish, viscid discharge from the vagina and uterine cavity.

leukosarcoma (-sar-ko′mah) the development of leukemia in patients originally having a well-differentiated, lymphocytic type of malignant lymphoma.

leukosarcomatosis (-sar-ko″mah-to′sis) the development of multiple sarcomas composed of leukemic cells.

leukosis (loo-ko′sis) proliferation of leukocyte-forming tissue. **avian l., fowl l.**, a group of transmissible, viral diseases of chickens, marked by proliferation of immature erythroid, myeloid, and lymphoid cells.

leukotaxine (loo″ko-tak′sin) a polypeptide that appears in injured tissue and inflammatory exudates; it promotes leukocytosis and leukotaxis and increases capillary permeability.

leukotaxis (-tak′sis) cytotaxis of leukocytes; the tendency of leukocytes to collect in regions of injury and inflammation. **leukotac′tic,** adj.

leukotoxin (-tok′sin) a cytotoxin destructive to leukocytes.

leukotrichia (-trik′e-ah) whiteness of the hair.

leukotriene (loo″ko-tri′ēn) any of a group of biologically active compounds derived from arachidonic acid that function as regulators of allergic and inflammatory reactions. They are identified by the letters A, B, C, D, and E, with subscript numerals indicating the number of double bonds in each molecule.

levallorphan (lev″al-or′fan) an analogue of levorphanol, $C_{19}H_{25}NO$, which acts as an antagonist to analgesic narcotics; used in the treatment of respiratory depression produced by narcotic analgesics.

levamfetamine (lēv″am-fet′ah-mēn) the levorotatory form of amphetamine; used in the treatment of narcolepsy and hyperkinetic behavior disorders, and as an anorexic.

levarterenol (lev″ar-tě-re′nol) norepinephrine.

levator (lě-vāt′er), pl. *levato′res* [L.] 1. a muscle that elevates an organ or structure. 2. an instrument for raising depressed osseous fragments in fractures.

levigation (lev″ĭ-ga′shin) the grinding to a powder of a moist or hard substance.

levo- word element [L.], *left*.

levocardia (le"vo-kar'de-ah) a term denoting normal position of the heart associated with transposition of other viscera (situs inversus).

levoclination (-kli-na'shin) rotation of the upper poles of the vertical meridians of the two eyes to the left.

levodopa (-do'pah) the levorotatory isomer of dopa, $C_9H_{11}NO_4$, used as an antiparkinsonian agent.

levopropoxyphene (-pro-pok'sĭ-fēn) the levo isomer of propoxyphene, $C_{32}H_{37}NO_5$; used as an antitussive.

levorotatory (-rōt'ah-tor"e) turning the plane of polarization of polarized light to the left.

levorphanol (lēv-or'fah-nol) a narcotic analgesic, $C_{17}H_{23}NO$; used as the bitartrate salt.

levothyroxine (le"vo-thi-rok'sin) the levorotatory isomer of thyroxine, $C_{15}H_{10}I_4NO_4$; used as the sodium salt in thyroid replacement therapy.

levotorsion (-tor'shin) levoclination.

levoversion (-ver'zhin) a turning toward the left.

levulose (lev'ūl-ōs) fructose.

L.F.A. left frontoanterior (position of the fetus).

L.F.P. left frontoposterior (position of the fetus).

L.F.T. left frontotransverse (position of the fetus).

LH luteinizing hormone.

LH-RH luteinizing hormone releasing hormone; see *gonadotropin releasing hormone.*

Li chemical symbol, *lithium.*

libido (lĭ-be'do, lĭ-bi'do), pl. *libid'ines* [L.] 1. sexual desire. 2. the energy derived from the primitive impulses. In psychoanalysis the term is applied to the motive power of the sex life; in freudian psychology to psychic energy in general. **libid'inal,** adj.

libra (li'brah) [L.] 1. pound. 2. balance.

Librax (lib'raks) trademark for a fixed combination preparation of chlordiazepoxide hydrochloride and clidinium bromide.

Librium (lib're-um) trademark for preparations of chlordiazepoxide.

lice (līs) plural of *louse.*

licentiate (li-sen'she-āt) one holding a license from an authorized agency entitling him to practice a particular profession.

lichen (līk'n) 1. any of certain plants formed by the mutualistic combination of an alga and a fungus. 2. any of various papular skin diseases in which the lesions are typically small, firm papules set very close together, the specific kind being indicated by a modifying term. **l. amyloido'sus,** a condition characterized by localized cutaneous amyloidosis. **l. fibromucinoido'sus, l. myxedemato'sus,** a condition resembling myxedema but unassociated with hypothyroidism, marked by mucinosis and a widespread eruption of asymptomatic, soft, pale red or yellowish, discrete papules. **l. ni'tidus,** a skin eruption consisting of many, pinhead-sized pale, flat, sharply marginated, glistening, discrete papules, scarcely raised above the skin level. **l. planopila'ris,** a variant of lichen planus characterized by formation of acuminate

horny papules around the hair follicles, in addition to the typical lesions of ordinary lichen planus. **l. pla'nus,** an inflammatory skin disease with wide, flat, violaceous, shiny papules in circumscribed patches; it may involve the hair follicles, nails, and buccal mucosa. **l. ru'ber monilifor'mis,** a variant of lichen simplex chronicus with papules arranged in linear beaded bands. **l. ru'ber pla'nus,** l. planus. **l. sclero'sus et atro'phicus,** a chronic atrophic skin disease marked by white papules with an erythematous halo and keratotic plugging. It sometimes affects the vulva (*kraurosis vulvae*) or penis (*balanitis xerotica obliterans*). **l. scrofuloso'rum, l. scrofulo'sus,** any eruption of minute reddish lichenoid follicular papules in children and young adults with tuberculosis. **l. sim'plex chro'nicus,** a dermatosis of psychogenic origin, marked by a pruritic discrete or, more often, confluent papular eruption, usually confined to a localized area. **l. spinulo'sus,** a condition in which there is a horn or spine in the center of each hair follicle. **l. stria'tus,** a self-limited condition characterized by a linear lichenoid eruption, usually in children.

lichenification (li-ken"ĭ-fĭ-ka'shin) thickening and hardening of the skin, with exaggeration of its normal markings.

Lidex (li'deks) trademark for preparations of fluocinonide.

lidocaine (li'do-kān) a local anesthetic, $C_{14}H_{22}$-N_2O; used as a cardiac antiarrhythmic and to produce infiltration anesthesia and epidural and peripheral nerve blocks.

lie (li) the situation of the long axis of the fetus with respect to that of the mother; see *presentation.* **transverse l.,** the situation during labor when the long axis of the fetus crosses the long axis of the mother; see table under *position.*

lien (li'en) [L.] spleen. **lie'nal,** adj. **l. accesso'rius,** an accessory spleen. **l. mo'bilis,** floating spleen.

lien(o)- word element [L.], *spleen;* see also words beginning *splen(o)-.*

lienocele (li-e'nah-sēl) hernia of the spleen.

lienotoxin (-tok'sin) splenotoxin.

lientery (li'en-tē"re) diarrhea with passage of undigested food. **lienter'ic,** adj.

lienunculus (li"en-ung'kūl-us) accessory spleen.

LIF left iliac fossa; leukocyte inhibitory factor.

life (līf) the aggregate of vital phenomena; the quality or principle by which living things are distinguished from inorganic matter, as manifested by such phenomena as metabolism, growth, reproduction, adaptation, etc.

ligament (lig'ah-mint) 1. a band of fibrous tissue connecting bones or cartilages, serving to support and strengthen joints. 2. a double layer of peritoneum extending from one visceral organ to another. 3. cordlike remnants of fetal tubular structures that are nonfunctional after birth. **ligamen'tous,** adj. **accessory l.,** one that strengthens or supports another. **alar l's,** 1. two bands passing from the apex of the dens to the medial side of each occipital condyle. 2. a pair of folds of the synovial membrane of the knee joint. **arcuate l's,** the arched ligaments which connect the diaphragm with the lowest ribs and the first lumbar vertebra. **Bérard's l.,** the suspensory ligament of the pericardium. **Bertin's l., Bigelow's l.,** iliofemoral l. **Botallo's l.,** a strong thick fibromuscular cord extending from the pulmonary artery to the aortic arch; it is the remains of the ductus arteriosus. **Bourgery's l.,** oblique popliteal ligament; a broad band of fibers extending from the medial condyle of the tibia across the back of the knee joint to the lateral epicondyle of the femur. **broad l.,** a broad fold of peritoneum supporting the uterus, extending from the uterus to the wall of the pelvis on either side. **Brodie's l.,** transverse humeral l. **Burns' l.,** falciform process (1). **Campbell's l.,** suspensory l. (2). **Camper's l.,** urogenital diaphragm. **cardinal l.,** part of a thickening of the visceral pelvic fascia beside the cervix and vagina, passing laterally to merge with the upper fascia of the pelvic diaphragm. **Colles' l.,** a triangular band of fibers arising from the lacunar ligament and pubic bone and passing to the linea alba. **conoid l.,** the posteromedial portion of the coracoclavicular ligament, extending from the coracoid process to the inferior surface of the clavicle. **Cooper's l.,** pectineal l. **coracoclavicular l.,** a band joining the coracoid process of the scapula and the acromial extremity of the clavicle, consisting of two ligaments, the conoid and trapezoid. **cotyloid l.,** a ring of fibrocartilage connected with the rim of the acetabulum. **cruciate l's of knee,** more or less cross-shaped ligaments, one anterior and one posterior, which arise from the femur and pass through the intercondylar space to attach to the tibia. **cysticoduodenal l.,** an anomalous fold of peritoneum extending between the gallbladder and the duodenum. **diaphragmatic l.,** the involuting urogenital ridge that becomes the suspensory ligament of the ovary. **falciform l.,** a sickle-shaped sagittal fold of peritoneum that helps attach the liver to the diaphragm. **Flood's l.,** superior glenohumeral l. **glenohumeral l's,** bands, usually three, on the inner surface of the articular capsule of the humerus, extending from the glenoid lip to the anatomical neck of the humerus. **glenoid l.,** 1. a ring of fibrocartilage connected with the rim of the mandibular fossa. 2. (pl.) dense bands on the plantar surfaces of the metacarpophalangeal joints. 3. see under *lip.* **Henle's l.,** a lateral expansion of the lateral edge of the rectus abdominis which attaches to the pubic bone. **Hey's l's,** falciform process (1). **iliofemoral l.,** a very strong triangular or inverted Y-shaped band covering the anterior and superior portions of the hip joint. **iliotrochanteric l.,** a portion of the articular capsule of the hip joint. **inguinal l.,** a fibrous band running from the anterior superior spine of the ilium to the spine of the pubis. **lacunar l.,** a membrane with its base just medial to the femoral ring, one side attached to the inguinal ligament and the other to the pectineal line of the pubis. **Lisfranc's l.,** a fibrous band extending from the medial cuneiform bone to the second metatarsal. **Lockwood's l.,** a suspensory sheath supporting the eyeball. **medial l.,** a large fan-shaped ligament

on the medial side of the ankle. **meniscofemoral l's,** two small fibrous bands of the knee joint attached to the lateral meniscus, one (the anterior) extending to the anterior cruciate ligament and the other (the posterior) to the medial femoral condyle. **nephrocolic l.,** fasciculi from the fatty capsule of the kidney passing down on the right side to the posterior wall of the ascending colon and on the left side to the posterior wall of the descending colon. **nuchal l.,** a broad, fibrous, roughly triangular sagittal septum in the back of the neck, separating the right and left sides. **patellar l.,** the continuation of the central portion of the tendon of the quadriceps femoris muscle distal to the patella, extending from the patella to the tuberosity of the tibia. **pectineal l.,** a strong aponeurotic lateral continuation of the lacunar ligament along the pectineal line of the pubis. **phrenicocolic l.,** a peritoneal fold passing from the left colic flexure to the adjacent part of the diaphragm. **Poupart's l.,** inguinal l. **pulmonary l.,** a vertical fold extending from the hilus to the base of the lung. **rhomboid l.,** a ligament connecting cartilage of the first rib to the undersurface of the clavicle. **Robert's l.,** anterior meniscofemoral l. **round l.,** 1. (of *femur*) a broad ligament arising from the fatty cushion of the acetabulum and inserted on the head of the femur. 2. (of *liver*) a fibrous cord from the navel to anterior border of the liver. 3. (of *uterus*) a fibromuscular band attached to the uterus near the uterine tube, passing through the inguinal ring to the labium majus. **Schlemm's l's,** two ligamentous bands of the capsule of the shoulder joint. **subflaval l.,** any of a series of bands of yellow elastic tissue between the ventral portions of the laminae of two adjacent vertebrae. **suspensory l.,** 1. (of *lens*) ciliary zonule. 2. (of *axilla*) a layer ascending from the axillary fascia and ensheathing the pectoralis minor muscle. 3. (of *ovary*) the portion of the broad ligament lateral to and above the ovary. **synovial l.,** a large synovial fold. **tendinotrochanteric l.,** a portion of the capsule of the hip joint. **transverse humeral l.,** a band of fibers bridging the intertubercular groove of the humerus and holding the tendon in the groove. **trapezoid l.,** the anterolateral portion of the coracoclavicular ligament, extending from the upper surface of the coracoid process to the trapezoid line of the clavicle. **umbilical l., medial,** a fibrous cord, the remains of the obliterated umbilical artery, running cranialward beside the bladder to the umbilicus. **uteropelvic l's,** expansions of muscular tissue in the broad ligament, radiating from the fascia over the obturator internus to the side of the uterus and the vagina. **ventricular l.,** vestibular l. **vesicoumbilical l.,** medial umbilical l. **vesicouterine l.,** a ligament that extends from the anterior aspect of the uterus to the bladder. **vestibular l.,** the membrane extending from the thyroid cartilage in front to the anterolateral surface of the arytenoid cartilage behind. **vocal l.,** the elastic tissue membrane extending from the thyroid cartilage in front to the vocal process of the arytenoid cartilage behind. **Weitbrecht's l.,** a small ligamentous band extending from the ulnar tuberosity to the radius. **Wrisberg's l.,** posterior meniscofemoral l. **Y l.,** iliofemoral l.

ligamentopexy (lig″ah-men′tah-pek″se) fixation of the uterus by shortening the round ligament.

ligamentum (lig″ah-men′tum), pl. *ligamen′ta* [L.] ligament.

ligand (li′gind, lig′ind) an organic molecule that donates the necessary electrons to form coordinate covalent bonds with metallic ions. Also, an ion or molecule that reacts to form a complex with another molecule.

ligase (li′gās, lig′ās) any of a class of enzymes that catalyze the joining together of two molecules coupled with the breakdown of a pyrophosphate bond in ATP or a similar triphosphate.

ligature (lig′ah-cher) any material, such as thread or wire, used for tying a vessel or to constrict a part.

light (līt) electromagnetic radiation with a range of wavelength between 3900 (violet) and 7700 (red) angstroms, capable of stimulating the subjective sensation of sight; sometimes considered to include ultraviolet and infrared radiation as well. **idioretinal l., intrinsic l.,** the sensation of light in the complete absence of external stimuli. **polarized l.,** light of which the vibrations are made over one plane or in circles or ellipses. **Wood's l.,** ultraviolet radiation from a mercury vapor source, transmitted through a nickel-oxide filter (Wood's filter, or glass), which holds back all but a few violet rays and passes ultraviolet wavelengths of about 365 nm; used in diagnosis of fungal infections of the scalp and erythrasma, and to reveal the presence of porphyrins and fluorescent minerals.

lightening (līt′en-ing) the sensation of decreased abdominal distention produced by the descent of the uterus into the pelvic cavity, two to three weeks before labor begins.

lignoceric acid (lig″no-ser′ik) a saturated fatty acid, $C_{23}H_{47}COOH$, found in wood tar, various cerebrosides, and in small amounts in most natural fats.

limb (lim) 1. one of the paired appendages of the body used in locomotion or grasping; in man, an arm or leg with all its component parts. 2. a structure or part resembling an arm or leg. **anacrotic l.,** the ascending portion of an arterial pulse tracing. **catacrotic l.,** the descending portion of an arterial pulse tracing. **pectoral l.,** the arm, or a homologous part. **pelvic l.,** the leg, or a homologous part. **phantom l.,** the sensation, after amputation of a limb, that the absent part is still present; there may also be paresthesias, transient aches, and intermittent or continuous pain perceived as originating in the absent limb. **thoracic l.,** pectoral l.

limbic (lim′bik) pertaining to a limbus, or margin; see also under *system*.

limbus (lim′bus), pl. *lim′bi* [L.] an edge, fringe, or border. **l. cor′neae,** the edge of the cornea where it joins the sclera. **l. la′minae spira′lis,** the thickened periosteum of the osseous spiral lamina of the cochlea.

lime (līm) 1. calcium oxide. 2. the acid fruit of the tropical tree, *Citrus aurontifolia;* its juice contains ascorbic acid.

limen (li′men), pl. *li′mina* [L.] a threshold or boundary. **l. of insula, l. in′sulae,** the point at which the cortex of the insula is continuous with the cortex of the frontal lobe. **l. na′si,** the ridge marking the boundary between the vestibule of the nose and the nasal cavity proper.

liminal (lim′ĭ-nil) barely perceptible; pertaining to a threshold.

liminometer (lim″ĭ-nom′it-er) an instrument for measuring the strength of a stimulus that just induces a tendon reflex.

limitans (lim′ĭ-tanz) [L.] limiting.

lincomycin (lin″ko-mi″sin) an antibiotic, $C_{18}H_{34}N_2O_6S$, primarily a gram-positive specific antibacterial, produced by a variant of *Streptomyces lincolnensis.*

lindane (lin′dān) the gamma isomer of benzene hexachloride, $C_6H_6Cl_6$; used as a topical pediculicide and scabicide.

line (līn) a stripe, streak, mark, or narrow ridge; often an imaginary line connecting different anatomic landmarks. **lin′ear,** adj. **absorption l's,** dark lines in the spectrum due to absorption of light by the substance through which the light has passed. **base l.,** 1. one from the infraorbital ridge to the external auditory meatus and to the middle line of occiput. 2. a known quantity or a set of known quantities used as a reference point in evaluating similar data. **Beau's l's,** transverse furrows on the fingernails, usually a sign of a systemic disease but also due to other causes. **bismuth l.,** a thin blue-black line along the gingival margin in bismuth poisoning. **blood l.,** a line of direct descent through several generations. **cement l.,** a line visible in microscopic examination of bone in cross section, marking the boundary of an osteon (haversian system). **cleavage l's,** linear clefts in the skin indicative of direction of the fibers. **costoclavicular l.,** parasternal l. **l. of Douglas,** a crescentic line marking the termination of the posterior layer of the sheath of the rectus abdominis muscle. **epiphyseal l.,** one on the surface of an adult long bone, marking the junction of the epiphysis and diaphysis. **l's of expression,** the natural skin lines and creases of the face and neck; the preferred lines of incision in facial and cervical surgery. **gingival l.,** 1. a line determined by the level to which the gingiva extends on a tooth. 2. any linear mark visible on the surface of the gingiva. **gluteal l.,** any of the three rough curved lines (anterior, inferior, and posterior) on the gluteal surface of the ala of the ilium. **Harris l's,** lines of retarded growth seen radiographically at the epiphyses of long bones. **hot l.,** see under H. **iliopectineal l.,** a ridge on the ilium and pubes showing the brim of the true pelvis. **intertrochanteric l.,** a line running obliquely from the greater to the lesser trochanter on the anterior surface of the femur. **lead l.,** a gray or bluish black line at the gingival margin in lead poisoning. **mamillary l.,** an imaginary vertical line passing through the center of the nipple. **median l.,** an imaginary line dividing the body surface equally into right and left sides. **milk l.,** a ridge of thickened epithelium from axilla to groin in the mammalian embryo along which nipples and mammary glands develop; all but one disappear in the human. **mylohyoid l.,** a ridge on inner surface of lower jaw from the base of the symphysis to the ascending rami behind the last molar tooth. **nasobasilar l.,** one through the basion and nasion. **Nélaton's l.,** one from the anterior superior spine of the ilium to the most prominent part of tuberosity of the ischium. **nuchal l's,** three lines (inferior, superior, highest) on the outer surface of the occipital bone; see also *external occipital crest.* **parasternal l.,** an imaginary line midway between the mamillary line and the border of the sternum. **pectinate l.,** one marking the junction of the zone of the anal canal lined with stratified squamous epithelium and the zone lined with columnar epithelium. **pectineal l.,** 1. a line running down the posterior surface of the shaft of the femur, giving attachment to the pectineus muscle. 2. the anterior border of the superior ramus of the pubis. **Retzius' l's,** incremental l's. **semilunar l.,** a curved line along the lateral border of each rectus abdominis muscle, marking the meeting of the aponeuroses of the internal oblique and transverse abdominal muscles. **Shenton's l.,** a curved line seen in radiographs of the normal hip, formed by the top of the obturator foramen. **sternal l.,** an imaginary vertical line on the anterior body surface, corresponding to the lateral border of the sternum. **subcostal l.,** a transverse line on the surface of the abdomen at the level of the lower edge of the tenth costal cartilage. **temporal l's,** curved ridges, inferior and superior, on the outside of the parietal bone, continuous with the temporal line of the frontal bone, a ridge extending upward and backward from the zygomatic process of the frontal bone. **terminal l.,** one on the inner surface of each pelvic bone, from the sacroiliac joint to the iliopubic eminence anteriorly, separating the false from the true pelvis. **trapezoid l.,** a ridge on the inferior surface of the clavicle for attachment of the trapezoid ligament. **Voigt's l's,** a dorsoventral pigmented line of demarcation on the skin along the lateral edge of the biceps muscle; seen in 20–26% of blacks and rarely in whites.

linea (lin′e-ah), pl. *lin′eae* [L.] line; in anatomy, a narrow ridge or streak on the surface of a structure. **l. al′ba,** white line; the tendinous median line on the anterior abdominal wall between the two rectus muscles. **li′neae albican′tes,** see *atrophic striae.* **l. as′pera,** a rough longitudinal line on the back of the femur for muscle attachments. **li′neae atro′phicae,** atrophic striae. **l. epiphysia′lis,** epiphyseal line. **l. glu′tea,** gluteal line. **l. ni′gra,** the linea alba when it has become pigmented in pregnancy. **l. splen′dens,** the sheath for the anterior spinal artery formed by the pia mater in the anterior median fissure of the spinal cord.

liner (līn′er) material applied to the inside of the walls of a cavity or container for protection or insulation of the surface.

lingua (ling′gwah), pl. *lin′guae* [L.] tongue. **lin′gual,** adj. **l. geogra′phica,** geographic tongue. **l. ni′gra,** black tongue. **l. plica′ta,** fissured tongue.

lingual (ling′gwil) pertaining to or near the tongue.

Linguatula (lin-gwah′chil-ah) a genus of wormlike arthropods, the adults of which inhabit the respiratory tract of vertebrates; the larvae are found in the lungs and other internal organs. It includes *L. serra′ta* (*L. rhina′ria*), which parasitizes dogs and cats and sometimes man.

lingula (ling′gūl-ah), pl. *lin′gulae* [L.] a small, tonguelike structure, such as the projection from the lower portion of the upper lobe of the left lung (*l. pulmonis sin′istri*), or the bony ridge between the body and great wing of the sphenoid (*l. sphenoida′lis*). **ling′ular,** adj.

lingulectomy (ling″gūl-ek′tah-me) excision of the lingula of the left lung.

linguo- word element [L.], *tongue.*

linguodistal (-dis′til) pertaining to the lingual and distal surfaces of a tooth, or the lingual and distal walls of a tooth cavity.

linguopapillitis (-pap″ĭ-lit′is) inflammation or ulceration of the papillae of the edges of the tongue.

linguoversion (-ver′zhin) displacement of a tooth lingually from the line of occlusion.

liniment (lin′ĭ-mint) a medicinal preparation in an oily, soapy, or alcoholic vehicle, intended to be rubbed on the skin as a counterirritant or anodyne.

linitis (lĭ-nīt′is) inflammation of gastric cellular tissue. **l. pla′stica,** diffuse fibrous proliferation of the submucous connective tissue of the stomach, resulting in thickening and fibrosis so that the organ is constricted, inelastic, and rigid (like a leather bottle).

linkage (lingk′ij) 1. the connection between different atoms in a chemical compound, or the symbol representing it in structural formulas; see also *bond.* 2. in genetics, the association of genes having loci on the same chromosome, which results in the tendency of a group of such nonallelic genes to be associated in inheritance. 3. in psychology, the connection between a stimulus and its response.

linoleic acid (lin″ol-e′ik) a doubly unsaturated fatty acid, $C_{18}H_{32}O_2$, the most abundant such acid in various vegetable oils.

lint (lint) an absorbent surgical dressing material.

liothyronine (li″o-thī′rah-nēn) the levorotatory isomer of triiodothyronine, $C_{15}H_{12}I_3NO_4$; used as the sodium salt in treatment of hypothyroidism.

liotrix (li′o-triks) a mixture of liothyronine sodium and levothyroxine sodium in a ratio of 1:4 in terms of weight; used for replacement therapy in hypothyroidism.

lip (lip) 1. the upper or lower fleshy margin of the mouth. 2. any liplike part; labium. **cleft l.,** harelip. **glenoid l.,** a ring of fibrocartilage joined to the rim of the glenoid cavity. **Hapsburg l.,** a thick, overdeveloped lower lip that often accompanies Hapsburg jaw.

lip(o)- word element [Gr.], *fat; lipid.*

lipaciduria (-id-ūr′e-ah) fatty acids in the urine.

lipase (li′pās, lip′ās) fat-splitting enzyme; any enzyme that catalyzes the splitting of fats into glycerol and fatty acids.

lipectomy (li-pek′tah-me) excision of a mass of subcutaneous adipose tissue.

lipedema (lip″ĕ-de′mah) an accumulation of excess fat and fluid in subcutaneous tissues.

lipemia (li-pēm′e-ah) an excess of lipids in the blood; hyperlipemia. **alimentary l.,** that occurring after ingestion of food. **l. retina′lis,** that manifested by a milky appearance of the veins and arteries of the retina.

lipid (lip′id) any of a heterogeneous group of fats and fatlike substances, including fatty acids, neutral fats, waxes, and steroids, which are water-insoluble and soluble in nonpolar solvents. Lipids, which are easily stored in the body, serve as a source of fuel, are an important constituent of cell structure, and serve other biological functions. Compound lipids comprise the glycolipids, lipoproteins, and phospholipids.

lipidemia (lip″ĭ-dēm′e-ah) hyperlipidemia.

lipidosis (lip″ĭ-do′sis) any disorder of lipid metabolism involving abnormal accumulation of lipids, including Hand-Schüller-Christian disease, Niemann-Pick disease, Tay-Sachs disease, Gaucher's disease, etc.

lipoarthritis (lip″o-ar-thrīt′is) inflammation of fatty tissue of a joint.

lipoatrophy (-ă′trah-fe) atrophy of subcutaneous fatty tissues of the body.

lipoblast (lip′ah-blast) a connective tissue cell which develops into a fat cell.

lipocardiac (lip″o-kar′de-ak) relating to a fatty heart.

lipochondroma (-kon-dro′mah) a tumor composed of mature lipomatous and cartilaginous elements.

lipochrome (lip′ah-krōm) any of a group of fat-soluble hydrocarbon pigments, such as carotene, xanthophyll, lutein, chromophane, and the natural coloring material of butter, egg yolk, and yellow corn.

lipocyte (-sīt) 1. a fat cell. 2. a fat-storing cell of the liver.

lipodystrophia (lip″ah-dis-tro′fe-ah) lipodystrophy. **l. progressi′va,** progressive lipodystrophy.

lipodystrophy (-dis′trah-fe) any disturbance of fat metabolism. **congenital progressive l.,** total l. **generalized l.,** total l. **intestinal l.,** Whipple's disease. **partial l., progressive l.,** progressive and symmetrical loss of subcutaneous fat from the parts above the pelvis, facial emaciation, and abnormal accumulation of fat about the thighs and buttocks. **total l.,** a recessive condition marked by the virtual absence of subcutaneous adipose tissue, macrosomia, visceromegaly, hypertrichosis, acanthosis nigricans, and reduced glucose tolerance in the presence of high insulin levels.

lipofibroma (-fi-bro′mah) a lipoma containing areas of fibrosis.

lipofuscin (-fu′sin) any of a class of fatty pigments formed by the solution of a pigment in fat.

lipofuscinosis (-fu″sin-o′sis) any disorder due to abnormal storage of lipofuscins. **neuronal ceroid l.,** a type· of amaurotic idiocy marked by accumulation in neurons and other tissues of ceroid and lipofuscin; clinically, there is central nervous deterioration, optic atrophy, macular degeneration, retinitis pigmentosa, and seizures.

lipogenesis (-jen′ĭ-sis) the formation of fat; the transformation of nonfat food materials into body fat. **lipogenet′ic,** adj.

lipogranuloma (lip″o-gran″u-lo′mah) a nodule of lipoid material associated with granulomatous inflammation.

lipogranulomatosis (-gran″ul-o″mah-to′sis) a condition of faulty lipid metabolism in which yellow nodules of lipoid material are deposited in the skin and mucosae, giving rise to granulomatous reactions.

lipoic acid (lĭ-po′ik) $C_8H_{14}O_2S_2$, a bacterial growth factor present in the water-soluble fraction of liver and yeast, necessary for the oxidative decarboxylation of pyruvic acid by *Streptococcus fecalis* and for the growth of *Tetrahymena gelii,* and replacing acetate for the growth of *Lactobacillus casei.*

lipoid (lip′oid) 1. fatlike. 2. lipid.

lipoidemia (lip″oi-dēm′e-ah) lipemia.

lipoidosis (-do′sis) a disturbance of lipid metabolism with abnormal deposit of lipids in the cells.

lipoiduria (-ūr′e-ah) lipiduria.

lipolysis (lĭ-pol′ĭ-sis) the splitting up or decomposition of fat. **lipolyt′ic,** adj.

lipoma (lĭ-po′mah) a benign fatty tumor usually composed of mature fat cells.

lipomatosis (lip″o-mah-to′sis) a condition marked by abnormal localized, or tumor-like, accumulations of fat in the tissues. **renal l., replacement l. of kidney,** partial replacement of the renal parenchyma by adipose tissue.

lipomeningocele (lip″o-men-ing′go-sēl) meningocele associated with an overlying lipoma, as in spina bifida.

lipomyoma (-mi-o′mah) a benign mesenchymoma composed of leiomyomatous and lipomatous tissues.

lipomyxoma (-mik-so′mah) a myxoma containing fatty elements.

lipopenia (-pēn′e-ah) deficiency of lipids in the body.

lipophage (lip′ah-fāj) a cell which absorbs or ingests fat.

lipophagia (lip″ah-fa′je-ah) lipophagy. **l. granulomato′sis,** intestinal lipodystrophy.

lipophagy (lĭ-pof′ah-je) the absorption of fat; lipolysis. **lipopha′gic,** adj.

lipophilia (lip″ah-fil′e-ah) affinity for fat. **lipophil′ic,** adj.

lipopolysaccharide (-pol″e-sak′ah-rīd) a molecule in which lipids and polysaccharides are linked.

lipoprotein (-prō′tēn, -prōt′e-in) a complex of lipids and apolipoproteins, the form in which lipids are transported in the blood. **high-density l. (HDL),** a plasma lipoprotein containing high levels of protein, little triglycerides, moderate levels of phospholipids, and relatively little cholesterol. **low-density l. (LDL),** a plasma lipoprotein containing a low percentage of triglycerides, high levels of cholesterol, and moderate levels of phospholipids and protein. **very low-density l., (VLDL),** a plasma lipoprotein containing high concentrations of triglycerides, moderate concentrations of phospholipids and cholesterol, and little protein.

liposarcoma (lip″o-sar-ko′mah) a malignant tumor characterized by large anaplastic lipoblasts, sometimes with foci of normal fat cells.

liposis (lĭ-po′sis) lipomatosis.

liposoluble (lip″o-sol′yah-b'l) soluble in fats.

lipothymia (-thi′me-ah) syncope.

lipotrophy (li-pah′trah-fe) increase of bodily fat.

lipotroph′ic, adj.

lipotropic (lip″o-trop′ik) acting on fat metabolism by hastening removal or decreasing the deposit of fat in the liver; also, an agent having such effects.

β-lipotropin (-tro′pin) a polypeptide synthesized by cells of the adenohypophysis, which promotes fat mobilization and skin darkening by stimulation of melanocytes. It contains β-endorphin and methionine enkephalin.

lipovaccine (-vak′sēn) a vaccine in a vegetable oil vehicle.

lipoxidase (lĭ-pok′sĭ-dās) lipoxygenase.

lipoxygenase (lĭ-poks′ĭ-jĕ-nās) an enzyme that catalyzes the oxidation of polyunsaturated fatty acids to form a peroxide of the acid.

lipping (lip′ing) 1. a wedge-shaped shadow in the roentgenogram of chondrosarcoma between the cortex and the elevated periosteum. 2. bony overgrowth in osteoarthritis.

liquefacient (lik″wĭ-fa′shint) 1. producing or pertaining to liquefaction. 2. an agent that produces liquefaction.

liquefaction (-fak′shin) conversion into a liquid form.

liquid (lik′wid) 1. a substance that flows readily in its natural state. 2. flowing readily; neither solid nor gaseous.

liquor (lik′er, li′kwor) 1. a liquid, especially an aqueous solution containing a medicinal substance. 2. a term applied to certain body fluids. **l. am′nii,** amniotic fluid. **l. cerebrospina′lis,** cerebrospinal fluid. **l. cotun′nii,** perilymph. **l. folli′culi,** the fluid in a developing ovarian follicle.

lissencephaly (lis″en-sef′ah-le) agyria. **lissencephal′ic,** adj.

Listerella (lis″ter-el′ah) *Listeria.*

Listeria (lis-tēr′e-ah) a genus of gram-positive bacteria (family Corynebacterium); the single species, *L. monocyto′genes,* is found chiefly in lower animals. In man, it produces upper respiratory disease, septicemia, and encephalitic disease.

listerism (lis′ter-izm) the principles and practice of antiseptic and aseptic surgery.

liter (lēt′er) the unit of volume in the metric system, equal to 1000 cubic centimeters or 1 cubic decimeter, or to 1.0567 quarts liquid measure. Abbreviated L. or l.

lith(o)- word element [Gr.], *stone; calculus.*

lithectasy (lĭ-thek′tah-se) extraction of calculi through the mechanically dilated urethra.

lithiasis (lĭ-thi′ah-sis) 1. a condition marked by formation of calculi and concretions. 2. gouty diathesis.

lithium (lith′e-um) chemical element (*see table*), at. no. 3, symbol Li. Its salts, especially *l. carbonate,* are used in the treatment of manic and other psychiatric disorders.

lithoclast (lith′ah-klast) a lithotrite.

lithocystotomy (lith″o-sis-tot′ah-me) incision of the bladder for removal of stone.

lithodialysis (-di-al′ĭ-sis) 1. the solution of calculi in the bladder by injected solvents. 2. litholapaxy.

lithogenesis (-jen′ĭ-sis) formation of calculi. **lithogen′ic, lithog′enous,** adj.

litholapaxy (lĭ-thol″ah-pak′se) the crushing of a stone in the bladder and washing out of the fragments.

litholysis (lĭ-thol′ĭ-sis) dissolution of calculi. **litholyt′ic,** adj.

lithonephritis (lith″o-nĕ-frīt′is) inflammation of the kidney due to irritation by calculi.

lithoscope (-skōp) an instrument for detecting calculi in the bladder.

lithotomy (lĭ-thot′ah-me) incision of a duct or organ for removal of calculi.

lithotripsy (lith′ah-trip″se) litholapaxy. **extracorporeal shock wave l.,** a procedure for treating upper urinary tract stones: the patient is immersed in a large tub of water and a high-energy shock wave generated by a high-voltage spark is focused on the stone by an ellipsoid reflector. The stone disintegrates into particles, which are passed in the urine.

lithotriptic (-trip″tik) dissolving vesical calculi; also, an agent that so acts.

lithotrity (lĭ-thah′trit-e) lithotripsy.

lithous (lith′is) pertaining to or of the nature of a calculus.

lithuresis (lith″ūr-e′sis) the passage of gravel in the urine.

litmus (lit′mis) a pigment prepared from *Rocella tinctoria* and other lichens; used as an acid-base (pH) indicator.

litter (lit′er) 1. a stretcher for carrying sick or wounded. 2. the offspring produced at one birth by a multiparous animal.

livedo (lĭ-ve′do) a discolored patch on the skin. **l. annula′ris, l. racemo′sa, l. reticula′ris,** a reddish blue, netlike mottling of the skin.

livedoid (liv′id-oid) pertaining to livedo.

liver (liv′er) the large, dark-red gland in the upper part of the abdomen on the right side, just beneath the diaphragm. See Plate IV. Its manifold functions include storage and filtration of blood, secretion of bile, conversion of sugars into glycogen, and many other metabolic activities. **fatty l.,** one affected with fatty infiltration. **hobnail l.,** a liver whose surface is marked with nail-like points from cirrhosis.

livid (liv′id) discolored, as from a contusion or bruise; black and blue.

livor (li′vor) discoloration. **l. mor′tis,** discoloration of dependent parts of the body after death.

lixiviation (liks″iv-e-a′shun) separation of soluble from insoluble material by use of an appropriate solvent, and drawing off the solution.

L.M. Licentiate in Midwifery.

L.M.A. left mentoanterior (position of fetus).

L.M.P. left mentoposterior (position of fetus).

L.M.T. left mentotransverse (position of fetus).

LNPF lymph node permeability factor.

L.O.A. left occipitoanterior (position of fetus).

Loa (lo′ah) a genus of filarial nematodes, including *L. lo′a*, a West African species that migrates freely throughout the subcutaneous connective tissue, seen especially about the orbit and even under the conjunctiva, and occasionally causing edematous swellings.

loading (lōd′ing) administering sufficient quantities of a substance to test a subject's ability to metabolize or absorb it.

lobate (lo′bāt) divided into lobes.

lobation (lo-ba′shin) the formation of lobes; the state of having lobes. **renal l.,** the appearance on x-ray films of small notches along the surface of the kidney, indicating the location of renal lobes.

lobe (lōb) 1. a more or less well-defined portion of an organ or gland. 2. one of the main divisions of a tooth crown. **lo′bar,** adj. **caudate l.,** a small lobe of the liver between the inferior vena cava on the right and the left lobe. **ear l.,** the lower fleshy part of the external ear. **frontal l.,** the rostral (anterior) portion of the cerebral hemisphere. **hepatic l.,** one of the lobes of the liver, designated the right and left and the caudate and quadrate. **occipital l.,** the most posterior portion of the cerebral hemisphere, forming a small part of its dorsolateral surface. **parietal l.,** the upper central portion of the cerebral hemisphere, between the frontal and occipital lobes, and above the temporal lobe. **polyalveolar l.,** a congenital disorder characterized in early infancy by the presence of far more than the normal number of alveoli in a lobe of the lungs; thereafter, normal multiplication of alveoli does not take place and they become enlarged, i.e., emphysematous. **prefrontal l.,** the part of the frontal lobe of the brain anterior to the ascending convolution. **quadrate l.,** 1. precuneus. 2. a small lobe of the liver, between the gallbladder on the right, and the left lobe. **spigelian l.,** caudate l. **temporal l.,** the lower lateral lobe of the cerebral hemisphere.

lobectomy (lo-bek′tah-me) excision of a lobe, as of the lung, brain, or liver.

lobopodium (lo″bo-po′de-um), pl. *lobopo′dia* [Gr.] a blunt pseudopodium composed of ectoplasm or of ectoplasm and endoplasm.

lobotomy (lo-bot′ah-me) incision of a lobe; in psychosurgery, section of the central core of white matter in the frontal lobe of the brain.

lobulated (lob′ūl-āt-id) made up of lobules.

lobule (lob′ūl) a small segment or lobe, especially one of the smaller divisions making up a lobe. **lob′ular,** adj. **l's of epididymis,** the wedge-shaped parts of the head of the epididymis, each comprising an efferent ductule of the

testis. **hepatic l's,** the small vascular units comprising the substance of the liver. **l's of lung,** bronchopulmonary segments. **paracentral l.,** a lobe on the medial surface of the cerebral hemisphere, continuous with the pre- and postcentral gyri, limited below by the cingulate sulcus. **parietal l.,** one of the two divisions, inferior and superior, of the parietal lobe of the lung. **portal l.,** a polygonal mass of liver tissue containing portions of three adjacent hepatic lobules, and having a portal vein at its center and a central vein peripherally at each corner. **primary l. of lung, respiratory l.,** the functional unit of the lung, including a respiratory bronchiole, alveolar ducts and sacs, and alveoli. See Plate VII.

lobulus (lob′ūl-us), pl. *lob′uli* [L.] lobule.

lobus (lo′bus), pl. *lo′bi* [L.] lobe.

localization (lo″kil-iz-a′shin) 1. restriction to a circumscribed or limited area. 2. the determination of the site or place of any process or lesion. **cerebral l.,** determination of areas of the cortex involved in performance of certain functions. **germinal l.,** the location on a blastoderm of prospective organs.

locator (lo′kāt-er) a device for determining the site of foreign objects within the body. **electroacoustic l.,** a device which amplifies into an audible click the contact of the probe with a solid object in tissue.

lochia (lo′ke-ah) a vaginal discharge occurring during the first week or two after childbirth. **lo′chial,** adj. **l. al′ba,** the final vaginal discharge after childbirth, when the amount of blood is decreased and the leukocytes are increased. **l. cruen′ta,** l. rubra. **l. purulen′ta,** l. alba. **l. ru′bra,** that occurring immediately after childbirth, consisting almost entirely of blood. **l. sanguinolen′ta,** l. serosa. **l. sero′sa,** the serous vaginal discharge occurring four or five days after childbirth.

lochiometra (-me′trah) distention of the uterus by retained lochia.

lochiometritis (-me-trīt′is) puerperal metritis.

lochiorrhagia (-ra′je-ah) lochiorrhea.

lochiorrhea (-re′ah) an abnormally profuse lochia.

lochioschesis (lo″ke-os′kĕ-sis) retention of the lochia.

lockjaw (lok′jaw) 1. tetanus. 2. trismus.

loco (lo′ko) [Sp.] 1. any of various leguminous plants of the genera *Astragalus, Hosackia, Sophora,* and *Oxytropis,* poisonous to livestock in arid regions because of the selenium they contain.

locomotion (lo″kah-mo′shin) movement, or the ability to move, from one place to another. **locomo′tive,** adj. **brachial l.,** brachiation.

loculus (lok′ūl-us), pl. *lo′culi* [L.] 1. a small space or cavity. 2. an enlargement in the uterus in some mammals, containing an embryo. **loc′ular,** adj.

locum (lo′kum) [L.] place. **l. ten′ens, l. ten′ent,** a practitioner who temporarily takes the place of another.

locus (lo′kus), pl. *lo′ci* [L.] place; site; in genetics, the specific site of a gene on a chromosome.

l. ceru′leus, a pigmented eminence in the superior angle of the floor of the fourth ventricle of the brain.

löffleria (lef-le′re-ah) presence of the diphtheria bacillus without the ordinary symptoms of diphtheria.

log(o)- word element [Gr.], *words; speech.*

logadectomy (log″ah-dek′tah-me) excision of a portion of the conjunctiva.

logamnesia (-am-ne′ze-ah) receptive aphasia.

logaphasia (-ah-fa′ze-ah) expressive aphasia.

logokophosis (-ko-fo′sis) word deafness.

logomania (-ma′ne-ah) overtalkativeness.

logopathy (log-op′ah-the) any disorder of speech due to derangement of the central nervous system.

logopedics (-pe′diks) the study and treatment of speech defects.

logorrhea (-re′ah) excessive or abnormal volubility.

logospasm (log′ah-spazm) the spasmodic utterance of words.

-logy word element [Gr.], *science; treatise; sum of knowledge in a particular subject.*

loiasis (lo-i′ah-sis) infection with nematodes of the genus *Loa.*

loin (loin) the part of the back between the thorax and pelvis.

Lomotil (lo′mo-til) trademark for preparations of diphenoxylate.

lomustine (lo-mus′tēn) CCNU; a nitrosourea, $C_9H_{16}ClN_3O_2$, used as an antineoplastic in the treatment of Hodgkin's disease and brain tumors.

longissimus (lon-jis′ĭ-mus) [L.] longest.

longitudinalis (lon″jĭ-tōōd″in-a′lis) [L.] lengthwise.

longus (long′gus) [L.] long.

loop (lōōp) a turn or sharp curve in a cordlike structure. **capillary l's,** minute endothelial tubes that carry blood in the papillae of the skin. **closed l.,** a system in which the input to one or more of the subsystems is affected by its own output. **Henle's l.,** the U-shaped loop of the uriniferous tubule of the kidney. **open l.,** a system in which an input alters the output, but the output has no effect on the input.

loosening (lōōs″n-ing) in psychiatry, a disorder of thinking in which associations of ideas become so shortened, fragmented, and disturbed as to lack logical relationship.

Lo/Ovral (lo-o′vral) trademark for a preparation of norgestrel with ethinyl estradiol; used as an oral contraceptive.

L.O.P. left occipitoposterior (position of fetus).

loperamide (lo-per′ah-mīd) an antiperistaltic, $C_{29}H_{33}ClN_2O_2$, used as an antidiarrheal and to reduce the volume of discharge from ileostomies.

lophotrichous (lo-fah′trĭ-kus) having two or more flagella at one end (of a bacterial cell).

Lopressor (lo-pres′or) trademark for preparations of metoprolol tartrate.

lorazepam (lor-az′ah-pam) a benzodiazepine derivative, $C_{15}H_{10}Cl_2O_2$, used as an antianxiety agent.

lordosis (lor-do′sis) forward curvature of the lumbar spine. **lordot′ic,** adj.

L.O.T. left occipitotransverse (position of fetus).

lotio (lo′she-o) [L.] lotion.

lotion (lo′shin) a liquid suspension or dispersion for external application to the body.

Lotrimin (lo-trim′in) trademark for preparations of clotrimazole.

loupe (lōōp) [Fr.] a magnifying lens.

louse (lows), pl. *lice* [L.] any of various parasitic insects; species parasitic upon man are *Pediculus humanus capitis* (head l.), *P. humanus corporis* (body, or clothes, l.), and *Phthirus pubis* (crab, or pubic, l.). Lice are major vectors of typhus, relapsing fever, and trench fever.

loxapine (loks′ah-pēn) a tricyclic antipsychotic agent, $C_{18}H_{18}ClN_3O.$

loxoscelism (lok-sos′sil-izm) a morbid condition due to the bite of the spiders *Loxosceles laeta* and *L. reclusa,* beginning with a painful erythematous vesicle and progressing to a gangrenous slough of the affected area.

loxotomy (lok-sot′ah-me) oval amputation.

lozenge (loz′inj) 1. a medicated tablet or disk; a troche. 2. a triangular area of tissue marked for excision in plastic surgery.

L.P.N. Licensed Practical Nurse.

L.S.A. left sacroanterior (position of fetus).

L.Sc.A. left scapuloanterior (position of fetus).

L.Sc.P. left scapuloposterior (position of fetus).

LSD lysergic acid diethylamide.

L.S.P. left sacroposterior (position of fetus).

L.S.T. left sacrotransverse (position of fetus).

LTF lymphocyte transforming factor.

LTH luteotropic hormone.

Lu chemical symbol, *lutetium.*

lucidity (loo-sid′it-e) clearness of mind. **lu′cid,** adj.

lues (loo′ēz) syphilis. **luet′ic,** adj.

lumb(o)- word element [L.], *loin.*

lumbago (lum-ba′go) pain in the lumbar region.

lumbar (lum′bar) pertaining to the loins.

lumbarization (lum″bar-iz-a′shun) nonfusion of the first and second segments of the sacrum so that there is one additional articulated vertebra, the sacrum consisting of only four segments.

lumbodynia (-din′e-ah) lumbago.

lumboinguinal (-ing′gwĭ-nil) pertaining to the loin and groin.

lumbricide (lum′brĭ-sīd) an agent that kills lumbrici (ascarides).

lumbricoid (lum′brĭ-koid) resembling the earthworm; designating the ascaris.

lumbricosis (lum″brĭ-ko′sis) infection with lumbrici (ascarides).

lumbricus (lum-bri′kus), pl. *lumbri′ci* [L.] 1. the earthworm. 2. ascaris.

lumbus (lum′bus) [L.] loin.

lumen (loo′men), pl. *lu′mina* [L.] 1. the cavity or channel within a tube or tubular organ. 2. the unit of light flux; it is the flux emitted in a unit solid angle by a uniform point source of one candela. **lu'minal,** adj. **residual l.,** the remains of Rathke's pouch, between the pars distalis and pars intermedia of the hypophysis.

luminescence (loo"mĭ-nes'ins) the property of giving off light without a corresponding degree of heat.

luminophore (loo'mĭ-nah-for") a chemical group which gives the property of luminescence to organic compounds.

lumirhodopsin (loo"mĭ-rah-dop'sin) an intermediate product of exposure of rhodopsin to light.

lumpectomy (lum-pek'tah-me) 1. surgical excision of only the palpable lesion in carcinoma of the breast. 2. surgical removal of a mass.

lunate (loon'āt) 1. moon-shaped or crescentic. 2. lunate bone; see *Table of Bones.*

lung (lung) the organ of respiration; either of the pair of organs that effect aeration of blood, lying on either side of the heart within the chest cavity. See Plates VI and VII. **black l.,** pneumoconiosis of coal workers. **brown l.,** byssinosis. **farmer's l.,** a morbid condition due to inhalation of moldy hay dust. **iron l.,** popular name for the Drinker respirator. **white l.,** pneumonia alba.

lungworm (-wurm") any parasitic worm that invades the lungs, e.g., *Paragonimus westermani* in man.

lunula (-loon'ŭl-ah), pl. *lu'nulae* [L.] a small, crescentic or moon-shaped area or structure, e.g., the white area at the base of the nail of a finger or toe, or one of the segments of the semilunar valves of the heart.

lupoid (loo'poid) 1. pertaining to lupus vulgaris. 2. a variant of sarcoidosis marked by small papular lesions.

lupus (loo'pus) any of a group of skin diseases in which the lesions are characteristically eroded. **discoid l. erythemato'sus (DLE),** a chronic superficial inflammation of the skin marked by red macules covered with scanty adherent scales which fall off, leaving scars; the lesions typically form a butterfly pattern over the bridge of the nose and cheeks, but other areas may be involved. **drug-induced l.,** a syndrome closely resembling systemic lupus erythematosus, precipitated by prolonged use of certain drugs, most commonly hydralazine, isoniazid, various anticonvulsants, and procainamide. **l. erythemato'sus,** a chronic connective tissue disease manifested in two main types; see *discoid l. erythematosus* and *systemic l. erythematosus.* **l. erythemato'sus profun'dus,** a form in which deep brawny indurations or subcutaneous nodules occur under normal or less often involved skin; the overlying skin may be erythematous, atrophic, and ulcerated and on healing may leave a depressed scar. **l. hypertro'phicus** a variant of lupus vulgaris in which the lesions consist of a warty vegetative growth, often crusted or slightly exudative, usually occurring on moist areas near body orifices. **l. milia'ris dissemina'tus fa'ciei,** a form marked by multiple, discrete, superficial nodules on the face, particularly on the eyelids, upper lip, chin, and nares. **l. per'nio,** 1. soft,

violaceous skin lesions on the cheeks, forehead, nose, ears, and digits, frequently associated with bone cysts, which may be the first manifestation of sarcoidosis or occur in the chronic stage of the disease. 2. a form of discoid lupus erythematosus aggravated by cold, initially resembling chilblains, in which the lesions consist of erythematous infiltrated patches on the exposed areas of the body, especially the finger knuckles. **systemic l. erythemato'sus (S.L.E.),** a chronic generalized connective tissue disorder, ranging from mild to fulminating, marked by skin eruptions, arthralgia, arthritis, leukopenia, anemia, visceral lesions, neurologic manifestations, lymphadenopathy, fever, and other constitutional symptoms. Typically, there are many abnormal immunologic phenomena, including hypergammaglobulinemia and hypocomplementemia, deposition of antigen-antibody complexes, and the presence of antinuclear antibodies and LE cells. **l. vulga'ris,** the most common and severe form of tuberculosis of the skin, most often affecting the face, marked by the formation of reddish brown patches of nodules in the corium, which progressively spread peripherally with central atrophy, causing ulceration and scarring and destruction of cartilage in involved sites.

luteal (loot'e-il) pertaining to or having the properties of the corpus luteum or its active principle.

lutein (loot'e-in) 1. a lipochrome from the corpus luteum, fat cells, and egg yolk. 2. any lipochrome.

luteinization (loot"e-in"iz-a'shin) the process by which a postovulatory ovarian follicle transforms into a corpus luteum through vascularization, follicular cell hypertrophy, and lipid accumulation, the latter in some species giving the yellow color indicated by the term.

luteohormone (loot"e-o-hor'mōn) progesterone.

luteoma (loot"e-o'mah) 1. a luteinized granulosa-theca cell tumor. 2. nodular hyperplasia of ovarian lutein cells sometimes occurring in the last trimester of pregnancy.

luteotrope (loot'e-ah-trōp") lactotrope.

luteotrophic (loot"e-o-trof'ik) luteotropic.

luteotropic (-trop'ik) stimulating formation of the corpus luteum.

luteotropin (-trop'in) prolactin.

lutetium (loo-te'she-um) chemical element (*see table*), at. no. 71, symbol Lu.

Lutzomyia (loot"zo-mi'ah) a genus of sandflies of the family Psychodidae, the females of which suck blood.

lux (luks) the SI unit of illumination, being 1 lumen per meter squared.

luxation (luk-sa'shin) dislocation.

luxus (luk'sus) [L.] excess.

L.V.N. licensed vocational nurse.

Lw chemical symbol, *lawrencium.*

lyase (li'ās) any of a class of enzymes that remove groups from their substrates (other than by hydrolysis), leaving double bonds, or that conversely add groups to double bonds.

lycanthropy (li-kan'thrah-pe) delusion in which the patient believes himself a wolf.

lycopene (li′ko-pēn) the red carotenoid pigment of tomatoes and various berries and fruits.

lycoperdonosis (li″ko-per″do-no′sis) a respiratory disease due to inhalation of spores of the puffball fungus, *Lycoperdon.*

lying-in (li′ing-in) 1. puerperal. 2. puerperium.

lymph (limf) 1. a transparent, usually slightly yellow, often opalescent liquid found within the lymphatic vessels, and collected from tissues in all parts of the body and returned to the blood via the lymphatic system. Its cellular component consists chiefly of lymphocytes. **aplastic l., corpuscular l.,** lymph that contains an excess of leukocytes and does not tend to become organized. **euplastic l.,** that which tends to coagulate and become organized. **inflammatory l.,** lymph produced by inflammation, as in wounds. **plastic l.,** inflammatory lymph having a tendency to become organized. **tissue l.,** lymph derived from body tissues and not from the blood. **vaccine l.,** material containing vaccinia virus collected from vaccinial vesicles of calves; used for active immunization against smallpox.

lymph(o)- word element [L.] *lymph; lymphoid tissue; lymphatics; lymphocytes.*

lympha (lim′fah) [L.] lymph.

lymphadenectasis (lim-fad″in-nek′tah-sis) enlargement of a lymph node.

lymphadenia (lim″fah-de′ne-ah) hypertrophy of lymph nodes.

lymphadenocele (lim-fad′in-o-sēl) a cyst of a lymph node.

lymphadenography (lim″fad-in-og′rah-fe) radiography of lymph nodes after injection of a contrast medium in a lymphatic vessel.

lymphadenoid (lim-fad′in-oid) resembling the tissue of lymph nodes; see under *tissue.*

lymphadenoma (lim-fad″in-o′mah) lymphoma.

lymphadenopathy (-op′ah-the) disease of the lymph nodes. **angioimmunoblastic l., immunoblastic l. dermatopathic l.,** regional lymph node enlargement associated with melanoderma and other dermatoses marked by chronic erythroderma. **giant follicular l.,** see under *lymphoma.* **immunoblastic l.,** a hyperimmune disorder resembling Hodgkin's disease, characterized by malaise, and generalized lymphadenopathy, constitutional symptoms, and proliferation of immunoblasts and small vessels.

lymphadenosis (-o′sis) hypertrophy or proliferation of lymphoid tissue. **l. benig′na cu′tis,** a benign inflammatory hyperplasia of lymphocytes in the skin, principally on the face or ears, in the form of solitary or disseminated yellowish brown to bluish red nodules that usually involute spontaneously.

lymphagogue (lim′fah-gog) an agent promoting the production of lymph.

lymphangiectasia, lymphangiectasis (lim-fan″je-ek-ta′ze-ah; -ek′tah-sis) dilatation of the lymphatic vessels. **lymphangiectat′ic,** adj.

lymphangioendothelioma (lim-fan″je-o-en″do-thēl″e-o′mah) lymphangioma in which endothelial cells are the main component.

lymphangiography (lim-fan″je-og′rah-fe) radi-

ography of lymphatic channels after introduction of a contrast medium.

lymphangiology (lim-fan″je-ol′ah-je) the scientific study of the lymphatic system.

lymphangioma (lim-fan″je-o′mah) a tumor composed of new-formed lymph spaces and channels. **cavernous l.,** dilatation of the lymphatic vessels resulting in cavities filled with lymph. **cystic l., l. cys′ticum,** a cystic growth usually found in the neck or groin, thought to originate from a developmental anomaly of the primitive lymphatic spaces; symptoms are largely due to compression of adjoining structures by the mass.

lymphangiomyomatosis (lim-fan″je-o-mi″o-mah-to′sis) a progressive disorder of women of child-bearing age, marked by nodular and diffuse interstitial proliferation of smooth muscle in the lungs, lymph nodes, and thoracic duct.

lymphangiophlebitis (lim-fan″je-o-flĕ-bīt′is) inflammation of the lymphatic vessels and the veins.

lymphangiosarcoma (lim-fan″je-o-sar-ko′mah) a malignant tumor of lymphatic vessels, usually arising in a limb that is the site of chronic lymphedema.

lymphangitis (lim″fan-jīt′is) inflammation of a lymphatic vessel or vessels.

lymphapheresis (lim″fah-fĕ′rĭ-sis) lymphocytapheresis.

lymphatic (lim-fat′ik) 1. pertaining to lymph or to a lymphatic vessel. 2. a lymphatic vessel.

lymphatism (lim′fah-tizm) a morbid condition due to excessive production or growth of lymphoid tissues, resulting in impaired development and lowered vitality.

lymphatitis (lim″fah-tīt′is) inflammation of some part of the lymphatic system.

lymphatolysis (-tol′ĭ-sis) destruction of lymphatic tissue. **lymphatolyt′ic,** adj.

lymphectasia (lim″fek-ta′ze-ah) distention with lymph.

lymphedema (lim″fah-de′mah) chronic swelling of a part due to accumulation of interstitial fluid (edema) secondary to obstruction of lymphatic vessels or lymph nodes. **congenital l.,** Milroy's disease.

lymphnoditis (limf″nōd-īt′is) inflammation of a lymph node.

lymphoblast (lim′fo-blast) the immature, nucleolated precursor of the mature lymphocyte. **lymphoblas′tic,** adj.

lymphoblastoma (lim″fo-blas-to′mah) poorly differentiated lymphocytic malignant lymphoma.

lymphoblastosis (-blas-to′sis) an excess of lymphoblasts in the blood.

lymphocytapheresis (-si″tah-fĕ′rĭ-sis) the selective removal of lymphocytes from withdrawn blood, which is then retransfused into the donor.

lymphocyte (lim′fo-sīt) a mononuclear, nongranular leukocyte having a deeply staining nucleus containing dense chromatin and a pale-blue–staining cytoplasm. Chiefly a product of lymphoid tissue, it participates in immunity. **lymphocyt′ic,** adj. **B-l′s,** bursa-equivalent lymphocytes; those that migrate to tissues without passing through or being influenced by the thymus; they mature into plasma cells that synthesize humoral antibody. **T-l′s,** thymus-dependent lymphocytes; those that pass through or are influenced by the thymus before migrating to tissues; they are responsible for cell-mediated immunity and delayed hypersensitivity.

lymphocytoblast (-sīt′ah-blast) a lymphoblast.

lymphocytoma (-si-to′mah) well-differentiated lymphocytic malignant lymphoma.

lymphocytopenia (-sīt″o-pēn′e-ah) reduction of the number of lymphocytes in the blood.

lymphocytopheresis (-sīt″ah-fē′rĭ-sis) lymphocytapheresis.

lymphocytosis (-si-to′sis) an excess of normal lymphocytes in the blood or an effusion.

lymphocytotoxicity (-sīt″o-tok-sis′it-e) the quality or capability of lysing lymphocytes, as in procedures in which lymphocytes having a specific cell surface antigen are lysed when incubated with antisera and complement.

lymphoduct (lim′fah-dukt) a lymphatic vessel.

lymphoepithelioma (lim″fo-ep″ĭ-thēl″e-o′mah) a pleomorphic, poorly differentiated carcinoma arising from modified epithelium overlying lymphoid tissue of the nasopharynx.

lymphogenous (lim-foj′in-is) 1. producing lymph. 2. produced from lymph or in the lymphatics.

lymphoglandula (lim″fo-glan′dūl-ah), pl. *lymphoglan′dulae* [L.] a lymph node.

lymphogonia (-gōn′e-ah) large lymphocytes having a large nucleus, little chromatin, and nongranular cytoplasm.

lymphogranuloma (lim″fo-gran″ūl-o′mah) Hodgkin's disease. **l. inguina′le, venereal l., l. vene′reum,** a venereal infection due to a strain of *Chlamydia trachomatis,* marked by a primary transient ulcerative lesion of the genitals, followed by swelling of the regional lymph nodes; later, lymphatic obstruction may result in elephantiasis of the external genitals, while scarring accounts for rectal stricture.

lymphogranulomatosis (-gran″ūl-o″mah-to′-sis) 1. infectious granuloma of the lymphatic system. 2. Hodgkin's disease.

lymphography (lim-fog′rah-fe) roentgenography of the lymphatic channels and lymph nodes after injection of radiopaque material.

lymphokine (lim′fo-kīn) a general term for soluble protein mediators postulated to be released by sensitized lymphocytes on contact with antigen, and believed to play a role in macrophage activation, lymphocyte transformation, and cell-mediated immunity.

lymphokinesis (lim″fo-kīn-e′sis) 1. movement of endolymph in the semicircular canals. 2. the circulation of lymph in the body.

lympholytic (lim″fol-it′ik) causing destruction of lymphocytes.

lymphoma (lim-fo′mah) any neoplastic disorder of lymphoid tissue. Often used to denote *malignant l.,* classifications of which are based on predominant cell type and degree of differentiation; various categories may be subdivided into nodular and diffuse types depending on the predominant pattern of cell arrangement. **Burkitt's l.,** a form of undifferentiated malignant lymphoma, usually occurring in Africa, manifested usually as a large osteolytic lesion in the jaw or as an abdominal mass; the Epstein-Barr virus has been implicated as a causative agent. **diffuse l.,** a malignancy in which the neoplastic cells diffusely infiltrate the entire lymph node, without any definite organized pattern. **follicular center cell l.,** B-cell lymphoma comprising four cytologic subtypes classified by the similarity of the cell size and nuclear characteristics to those of normal follicular center cells. **giant follicular l.,** nodular l. **granulomatous l.,** Hodgkin's disease. **histiocytic l.,** a malignancy characterized by the presence of large tumor cells resembling histiocytes morphologically but considered to be of lymphoid origin. **Lennert's l.,** a malignancy with a high content of epithelioid histiocytes. **lymphoblastic l.,** a malignancy composed of a diffuse, relatively uniform proliferation of cells with round or convoluted nuclei and scanty cytoplasm. **lymphocytic l., plasmacytoid,** B-cell lymphoma presumably representing a tumor of differentiated, possibly functional interfollicular B lymphocytes. **lymphocytic l., poorly differentiated,** malignant lymphoma in which the neoplastic cells are variable in size, configuration, and degree of differentiation; may present a nodular or diffuse histologic pattern; and have distinctive nuclei irregularly shaped, markedly indented, and angular. **lymphocytic l., well-differentiated,** a diffuse malignant neoplasm affecting well-differentiated B lymphocytes, with the predominant cell type consisting of compact, small, normal-appearing lymphocytes with dark-staining round nuclei, scanty cytoplasm, and little size variation. **malignant l.,** a group of malignancies characterized by the proliferation of cells native to the lymphoid tissues, i.e., lymphocytes, histiocytes, and their precursors and derivatives; the group is divided into two major clinicopathologic categories: Hodgkin's disease and non-Hodgkin's lymphoma. **mixed lymphocytic-histiocytic l.,** malignant lymphoma characterized by a mixed population of cells, the smaller cells resembling lymphocytes and the larger ones histiocytes. **nodular l.,** a malignancy in which the lymphomatous cells are clustered into identifiable nodules within the lymph nodes. **non-Hodgkin's l's,** a heterogeneous group of malignancies, the only common feature being an absence of the giant Reed-Sternberg cells characteristic of Hodgkin's disease. **small B-cell l.,** a neoplasm affecting the small B cells of the follicular mantle, which are blocked from further differentiation and therefore fail to form follicles or plasma cells. **T-cell l's,** a heterogeneous group of lymphoid neoplasms affecting the T lymphocytes. **T-cell l., convoluted,** T-cell lymphoma nearly identical to the lymphoblastic type, composed of immature intrathymic cells with marked convoluted nuclei. **T-cell l., cutaneous,** a group of lymphomas exhibiting (1) clonal expansion of malignant T lymphocytes arrested at varying stages of differentiation of cells committed to the series of helper T cells, and (2) malignant infiltration of the skin, which may be the chief or only manifestation of disease. **T-cell l., small lymphocytic,** a rare T-cell lymphoma arising from cells that cannot be easily differentiated morphologically from B lymphocytes and may be associated with T-cell chronic lymphocytic leukemia. **U-cell (undefined) l.,** a group of T-cell lymphomas that cannot be classified into a definite type by either morphologic or known immunocytochemical markers. **undifferentiated l.,** malignant lymphoma composed of undifferentiated cells, i.e., cells that do not show morphologic evidence of maturization toward lymphocytes or histiocytes, vary in size, and may include bizarre giant forms.

lymphomatosis (lim″fo-mah-to′sis) the formation of multiple lymphomas in the body. **avian l., l. of fowl,** avian leukosis involving chiefly the lymphocytes.

lymphomyxoma (lim-fo-mik-so′mah) any benign growth consisting of adenoid tissue.

lymphonodus (lim″fo-no′dus) lymph node.

lymphopathia (-path′e-ah) lymphopathy. **l. vene′reum,** see under *lymphogranuloma*.

lymphopenia (lim″fo-pēn′e-ah) decrease in the number of lymphocytes of the blood.

lymphoplasmapheresis (lim-fo-plaz-mah-fē′-ris-is) selective separation and removal of plasma and lymphocytes from withdrawn blood, the remainder of the blood then being retransfused to the donor.

lymphoplasmia (-plaz′me-ah) absence of hemoglobin from red blood cells.

lymphoproliferative (-pro-lif′er-ah″tiv) pertaining to or characterized by proliferation of lymphoid tissue.

lymphoreticular (-rĕ-tik′ūl-er) pertaining to reticuloendothelial cells of lymph nodes.

lymphoreticulosis (-re-tik″ūl-o′sis) proliferation of the reticuloendothelial cells of the lymph nodes. **benign l.,** cat-scratch fever.

lymphorrhagia (-ra′je-ah) lymphorrhea.

lymphorrhea (-re′ah) flow of lymph from cut or ruptured lymph vessels.

lymphorrhoid (lim′fah-roid) a localized dilatation of a perianal lymph channel, resembling a hemorrhoid.

lymphosarcoma (lim″fo-sar-ko′mah) a general term applied to malignant neoplastic disorders of lymphoid tissue, but not including Hodgkin's disease; see *lymphoma*.

lymphostasis (lim-fos′tah-sis) stoppage of lymph flow.

lymphotaxis (lim″fo-tak′sis) the property of attracting or repulsing lymphocytes.

lymphotoxin (-tok′sin) a chemical mediator released by sensitized lymphocytes and involved in target-cell injury and inhibition of cell division.

lyonization (li″in-ĭ-za′shin) the process by which or the condition in which all X chromosomes of the cells in excess of one are inactivated on a random basis.

lyophilic (li″o-fil′ik) having an affinity for, or stable in, solution.

lyophilization (li-of″ĭ-lĭ-za′shin) the creation of a stable preparation of a biological substance by rapid freezing and dehydration of the frozen product under high vacuum.

lyophobic (li″ah-fo′bik) not having an affinity for, or unstable in, solution.

lyotropic (-trop′ik) readily soluble.

lypressin (li-pres′in) a synthetic preparation of lysine vasopressin used as an antidiuretic and vasoconstrictor in the treatment of diabetes insipidus due to deficiency of endogenous posterior pituitary antidiuretic hormone (vasopressin).

lyse (līz) 1. to cause or produce disintegration of a compound, substance, or cell. 2. to undergo lysis.

lysemia (li-sēm′e-ah) disintegration of the blood.

lysergic acid diethylamide (LSD), (li-sur′jik, di-eth″il-am′īd) a hallucinogenic compound, $C_{20}H_{25}N_3O$, derived from lysergic acid, which has been used experimentally in the study and treatment of mental disorders and has been found to be antagonistic to serotonin in its action on smooth muscle. The side effects include bizarre behavior and psychosis.

lysergide (li′ser-jīd) lysergic acid diethylamide.

lysin (li′sin) an antibody capable of causing dissolution of cells, including hemolysin, bacteriolysin, etc.

lysine (li′sēn) a naturally occurring amino acid, essential for optimal growth in human infants and for maintenance of nitrogen equilibrium in adults.

lysinogen (li-sin′ah-jen) lysogen.

lysis (li′sis) 1. destruction or decomposition, as of a cell or other substance, under influence of a specific agent. 2. mobilization of an organ by division of restraining adhesions. 3. gradual abatement of the symptoms of a disease.

-lysis (li′sis) word element [Gr.], *dissolution*. **-lyt′ic,** adj.

lysogen (li′sah-jen) an antigen inducing the formation of lysin.

lysogenicity (-jin-is′it-e) 1. the ability to produce lysins or cause lysis. 2. the potentiality of a bacterium to produce phage. 3. the specific association of the phage genome (prophage) with the bacterial genome in such a way that only a few, if any, phage genes are transcribed.

lysokinase (-ki′nās) general term for substances of the fibrinolytic system that activates plasma proactivators.

lysosome (li′sah-sōm) one of the minute bodies occurring in many types of cells, containing various hydrolytic enzymes and normally involved in the process of localized intracellular digestion. **lysoso′mal,** adj. **secondary l.,** one that has fused with a phagosome (or pinosome), bringing hydrolases in contact with the ingested material and resulting in digestion of the material.

lysozyme (li′sah-zīm) a basic enzyme present in saliva, tears, egg white, and animal fluids, which functions as an antibacterial agent.

lyssa (lis′ah) rabies. **lys′sic,** adj.
lyssophobia (lis″ah-fo′be-ah) morbid fear of rabies.

lytic (lit′ik) 1. pertaining to lysis or to a lysin. 2. producing lysis.
lyze (līz) lyse.

M

M symbol for *molar* (solution) and for *mega*.

m median; meter; milli-.

m- meta-.

μ symbol for *micro* and for *micron*.

M.A. Master of Arts; meter angle; mental age.

mA milliampere.

macerate (mas′er-āt) to soften by wetting or soaking.

machine (mah-shēn′) a mechanical contrivance for doing work or generating energy. **heartlung m.,** a combination blood pump (artificial heart) and blood oxygenator (artificial lung) used in open-heart surgery.

macr(o)- word element [Gr.], *large; abnormal size.*

Macracanthorhynchus (mak″rah-kan″thoring′kus) a genus of parasitic worms (phylum Acanthocephala), including *M. hirudina′ceus*, found in swine.

macrencephaly (mak″ren-sef′ah-le) hypertrophy of the brain.

macroamylase (mak″ro-am′ĭ-lās) a complex in which normal serum amylase is bound to a variety of specific binding proteins, forming a complex too large for renal excretion.

macrobiota (-bi-ōt′ah) the macroscopic living organisms of a region. **macrobiot′ic,** adj.

macroblast (mak′ro-blast) an abnormally large, nucleated red blood cell; a large young normoblast with megaloblastic features.

macroblepharia (mak′ro-blĕ-fār′e-ah) abnormal largeness of the eyelid.

macrocephaly (-sef′ah-le) excessive size of the head.

macrocheilia (-ki′le-ah) excessive size of lip.

macrocheiria (-ki′re-ah) megalocheiria.

macrocolon (-ko′lon) megacolon.

macrocrania (-kra′ne-ah) excessive size of the skull in relation to the face.

macrocyte (mak′ro-sīt) an abnormally large erythrocyte. **macrocyt′ic,** adj.

macrocythemia (mak″ro-si-thēm′e-ah) the presence of macrocytes in the blood.

macrocytosis (-si-to′sis) macrocythemia.

macrodactyly (-dak′tĭ-le) megalodactyly.

Macrodantin (-dan′tin) trademark for a preparation of nitrofurantoin.

macroelement (-el′ĭ-mint) a chemical element, such as sodium or potassium, that is essential in nutrition and is distributed throughout the tissues in relatively large amounts, as opposed to trace elements.

macrofauna (-faw′nah) the macroscopic animal organisms of a region.

macroflora (-flor′ah) the macroscopic vegetable organisms of a region.

macrogamete (-gam′ēt) the larger, less active female gamete in anisogamy, which is fertilized by the smaller male gamete (microgamete).

macrogametocyte (-gah-mēt′ah-sīt) 1. a cell that produces macrogametes. 2. the female gametocyte of certain Sporozoa, such as malarial plasmodia, which matures into a macrogamete.

macrogenitosomia (-jen″it-ah-so′me-ah) excessive bodily development, with unusual enlargement of the genital organs. **m. pre′cox,** macrogenitosomia occurring at an early age.

macroglia (mah-krog′le-ah) neuroglial cells of ectodermal origin, i.e., the astrocytes and oligodendrocytes considered together.

macroglobulin (mak″ro-glob′ūl-in) a globulin of unusually high molecular weight, in the range of 1,000,000.

macroglobulinemia (-glob″ūl-in-ēm′e-ah) increased levels of macroglobulins in the blood. **Waldenström's m.,** a progressive syndrome of the endothelial system seen chiefly in males past age 50, associated with macroglobulinemia, adenopathy, hepatosplenomegaly, hemorrhagic phenomena, anemia, and lymphocytosis and plasmacytosis of bone marrow.

macrognathia (-nath′e-ah) enlargment of the jaw. **macrognath′ic,** adj.

macrogyria (-ji′re-ah) moderate reduction in the number of sulci of the cerebrum, sometimes with increase in the brain substance, resulting in excessive size of the gyri.

macrolide (mak′ro-līd) any antibiotic with molecules having many-membered lactone rings.

macromastia (mak″ro-mas′te-ah) excessive size of the breasts.

macromelia (-mēl′e-ah) enlargement of one or more limbs.

macromethod (mak′ro-meth″id) a chemical method using customary (not minute) quantities of the substance being analyzed.

macromolecule (mak″ro-mol′ĭ-kūl) a very large molecule having a polymeric chain structure, as in proteins, polysaccharides, etc. **macromolec′ular,** adj.

macromonocyte (-mon′ah-sīt) a giant monocyte.

macromyeloblast (-mi′ĭ-lo-blast″) a large myeloblast.

macronormoblast (-nor′mah-blast) macroblast.

macronucleus (-noo′kle-us) in ciliate protozoa, the larger of two types of nucleus in each cell, which governs cell metabolism and growth.

macronychia (-nik′e-ah) abnormal length of the fingernails.

macrophage (mak′rah-fāj) any of the large,

mononuclear, highly phagocytic cells derived from monocytes that occur in the walls of blood vessels (adventitial cells) and in loose connective tissue (histiocytes, phagocytic reticular cells). They are components of the reticuloendothelial system. Macrophages are usually immobile but become actively mobile when stimulated by inflammation; they also interact with lymphocytes to facilitate antibody production. **alveolar m's,** rounded, granular, mononuclear phagocytes within the alveoli of the lungs that ingest inhaled particulate matter. **armed m's,** those capable of inducing cytotoxicity as a consequence of antigen-binding by cytophilic antibodies on their surfaces or by factors derived from T-lymphocytes.

macrophthalmia (mak″rof-thal′me-ah) abnormal enlargement of the eyeball.

macropolycyte (mak″ro-pol′ĭ-sīt) a hypersegmented polymorphonuclear leukocyte of greater than normal size.

macropsia (mah-krop′se-ah) a disorder of visual perception in which objects appear larger than their actual size.

macroscopic (-skop′ik) of large size; visible to the unaided eye.

macrosomatia (-so-ma′she-ah) great bodily size.

macrostomia (-sto′me-ah) greatly exaggerated width of the mouth.

macrotia (mak-ro′she-ah) abnormal enlargement of the pinna of the ear.

macula (mak′ūlah), pl. *ma′culae* [L.] 1. a stain, spot, or thickening; in anatomy, an area distinguishable by color or otherwise from its surroundings. Often used alone to refer to the macula retinae. 2. a macule: a discolored spot on the skin that is not raised above the surface. 3. a corneal scar, appreciated as a gray spot. 4. macula lutea. **mac′ular, mac′ulate,** adj. **ma′culae acus′ticae,** the macula sacculi and macula utriculi considered together. **m. adhe′rens,** desmosome. **ma′culae atro′phicae,** white scarlike patches formed on the skin by atrophy. **ma′culae caeru′leae,** faint grayish blue spots, sometimes found peripheral to the axilla or groin in pediculosis corporis or pubis. **cerebral m.,** tache cérébrale. **m. cribro′sa,** one of three perforated areas (inferior, medial, and superior) on the vestibular wall through which branches of the vestibulocochlear nerve pass to the saccule, utricle, and semicircular canals. **m. den′sa,** a zone of heavily nucleated cells in the distal renal tubule. **m. fla′va,** a yellow nodule at one end of a vocal cord. **m. folli′culi,** follicular stigma. **m. germinati′va,** germinal area. **m. lu′tea, m. re′tinae,** an irregular yellowish depression on the retina, lateral to and slightly below the optic disk. **m. sac′culi,** a thickening on the wall of the saccule where the epithelium contains hair cells that receive and transmit vestibular impulses. **m. utri′culi,** a thickening in the wall of the utricle where the epithelium contains hair cells that are stimulated by linear acceleration and deceleration and by gravity.

macule (măk′ūl) a macula.

maculocerebral (măk″ūl-o-ser′ĭ-bril) pertaining to the macula lutea and the brain.

madarosis (mad″ah-ro′sis) loss of eyelashes or eyebrows.

Madurella (mad″ūr-el′ah) a genus of imperfect fungi. *M. gris′ea* and *M. myceto′mi* are etiologic agents of maduromycosis.

maduromycosis (mah-doo″ro-mi-ko′sis) a chronic disease due to various fungi or actinomycetes, affecting the foot, hands, legs, or the internal organs; the most common form is that of the foot (*Madura foot*), marked by sinus formation, necrosis, and swelling.

mafenide (maf′in-īd) an antibacterial, $C_7H_{10}N_2$-O_2S, used topically in superficial infections.

magaldrate (mag′al-drāt) a combination of aluminum hydroxide and magnesium hydroxide used as an antacid.

magenta (mah-jen′tah) fuchsin or other salt of rosaniline.

maggot (mag′it) the soft-bodied larva of an insect, especially a form living in decaying flesh.

magma (mag′mah) 1. a suspension of finely divided material in a small amount of water. 2. a thin, pastelike substance composed of organic material. **dihydroxyaluminum aminoacetate m.,** a white viscous suspension of dihydroxyaluminum aminoacetate in water, used as a gastric antacid.

magnesia (mag-ne′zhah) magnesium oxide.

magnesium (mag-ne′ze-um) chemical element (*see table*), at. no. 12, symbol Mg; its salts are essential in nutrition, being required for the activity of many enzymes, especially those concerned with oxidative phosphorylation. **m. carbonate,** a basic hydrated magnesium carbonate containing the equivalent of 40–43.5% magnesium oxide; an antacid. **m. citrate,** a mild cathartic. **m. hydroxide,** $Mg(OH)_2$; a laxative and antacid. **m. oxide,** MgO; an antacid. **m. phosphate,** a bulky, white powder, Mg_3-$(PO_4)_2 \cdot 5H_2O$, used as an antacid. **m. salicylate,** the magnesium salt of salicylic acid, used as an antiarthritic. **m. sulfate,** Epsom salt: $MgSO_4 \cdot 7H_2O$ used as an anticonvulsant and electrolyte replenisher, and as a cathartic and local anti-inflammatory. **m. trisilicate,** a combination of magnesium oxide and silicon dioxide with varying proportions of water; an antacid.

magnet (mag′nit) an object having polarity and capable of attracting iron.

magnetropism (mag-ne″trah-pizm) a growth response in a nonmotile organism under the influence of a magnet.

magnification (mag″nĭ-fĭ-ka′shĭn) 1. apparent increase in size, as under the microscope. 2. the process of making something appear larger, as by use of lenses. 3. the ratio of apparent (image) size to real size.

mal (mal) [Fr.] illness; disease. **m. de caderas,** a trypanosomiasis of horses, mules, and dogs in South America, with weakness, especially of the hind quarters, and a staggering, swinging gait. **grand m.,** see under *epilepsy.* **m. de Meleda,** symmetrical keratosis of the palms and soles with an ichthyotic thickening of the wrists and ankles. **m. de mer,** seasickness. **petit m.,** see under *epilepsy.* **m. del pinto,** pinta.

mala (ma′lah) 1. the cheek. 2. the zygomatic bone. **ma′lar,** adj.

malabsorption (mal″ub-sorp′shin) impaired intestinal absorption of nutrients.

malacia (mah-la′she-ah) 1. morbid softening or softness of a part or tissue; also used as word termination, as in osteomalacia. 2. morbid craving for highly spiced foods.

malacoma (mal″ah-ko′mah) a morbidly soft part or spot.

malacoplakia (mal″ah-ko-pla′ke-ah) the formation of soft patches of the mucous membrane of a hollow organ. **m. vesi′cae,** a soft, yellowish, fungus-like growth on the mucosa of the bladder and ureters.

malacosis (mal″ah-ko′sis) malacia.

malacosteon (mal″ah-kos′te-on) osteomalacia.

maladjustment (mal″ah-just′ment) in psychiatry, defective adaptation to the environment, marked by anxiety.

malady (mal″ah-de) a disease or illness.

malaise (mal-āz′) a vague feeling of discomfort.

malalignment (mal″ah-līn′mint) displacement, especially of teeth from their normal relation to the line of the dental arch.

malaria (mah-lār′e-ah) an infectious febrile disease caused by protozoa of the genus *Plasmodium,* which are parasitic in red blood cells; it is transmitted by *Anopheles* mosquitoes and marked by attacks of chills, fever, and sweating occurring at intervals that depend on the time required for development of a new generation of parasites in the body. **malar′ial,** adj. **falciparum m.,** the most serious form, due to *Plasmodium falciparum,* with severe constitutional symptoms and sometimes causing death. **ovale m.,** a mild form due to *Plasmodium ovale,* with recurring tertian febrile paroxysms and a tendency to end in spontaneous recovery. **quartan m.,** that in which the febrile paroxysms occur every 72 hours, or every fourth day counting the day of occurrence as the first day of each cycle; due to *Plasmodium malariae.* **quotidian m.,** vivax malaria in which the febrile paroxysms occur daily. **tertian m.,** vivax malaria in which the febrile paroxysms occur every 42 to 47 hours, or every third day counting the day of occurrence as the first day of the cycle. **vivax m.,** that due to *Plasmodium vivax,* in which the febrile paroxysms commonly occur every other day (*tertian m.*), but may occur daily (*quotidian m.*), if there are two broods of parasites segmenting on alternate days.

Malassezia (mal″ah-se′ze-ah) *Pityrosporon.* **M. fur′fur, M. trop′ica,** *Pityrosporon orbiculare.*

malassimilation (mal″ah-sim″il-a′shin) 1. imperfect, or disordered assimilation. 2. the inability of the gastrointestinal tract to take up ingested nutrients, due to faulty digestion (maldigestion) or to impaired intestinal mucosal transport (malabsorption).

malate (ma′lāt) any salt of malic acid.

malathion (mal-ah-thi′on) an organophosphorus compound used as an insecticide.

malaxation (mal″ak-sa′shin) an act of kneading.

maldevelopment (-dĭ-vel′op-mint) abnormal growth or development.

male (māl) the sex that produces spermatozoa.

maleate (mal′e-āt) any salt or ester of maleic acid.

maleic acid (mah-le′ik) an unsaturated dibasic acid, $C_4H_4O_4$; the *cis*-isomer of fumaric acid.

maleruption (mal″e-rup′shin) eruption of a tooth out of its normal position.

malformation (-for-ma′shin) defective or abnormal formation; an anatomical aberration, especially one acquired during development.

malic acid (mal′ik) a crystalline acid, $C_4H_6O_5$, from juices of many fruits and plants, and an intermediate in the tricarboxylic acid cycle.

malignant (mah-lig′nint) becoming worse and ending in death. Having the properties of anaplasia, invasiveness, and metastasis; said of tumors.

malignin (mah-lig′nin) a protein fragment present in the serum of patients with malignant glial tumors.

malingering (-ing) willful, fraudulent feigning or exaggeration of the symptoms of illness or injury to attain a consciously desired end.

malleable (mal′e-ah-b′l) susceptible of being beaten out into a thin plate.

malleoincudal (mal″e-o-ing′kūd′l) pertaining to the malleus and incus.

malleolus (mah-le′ah-lus), pl. *malle′oli* [L.] a rounded process, such as the protuberance on either side of the ankle joint, at the lower end of the fibula, or of the tibia. **malle′olar,** adj.

malleotomy (mal″e-ot′ah-me) 1. operative division of the malleus. 2. operative separation of the malleoli.

malleus (mal′e-us) [L.] 1. see *Table of Bones.* 2. glanders.

malnutrition (mal″noo-trish′in) any disorder of nutrition.

malocclusion (-ah-kloo′zhin) improper relations of apposing teeth when the jaws are in contact.

malposition (-pah-zish′in) abnormal or anomalous placement.

malpractice (mal-prak′tis) improper or injurious practice; unskillful and faulty medical or surgical treatment.

malpresentation (mal″prez-in-ta′shin) faulty fetal presentation.

malrotation (-rah-ta′shin) abnormal or pathologic rotation, as of the vertebral column; failure of normal rotation of an organ, as of the gut, during embryological development.

maltose (mawl′tōs) a disaccharide formed when starch is hydrolyzed by amylase.

malum (ma′lum) [L.] disease. **m. articulo′rum seni′lis,** a painful degenerative state of a joint as a result of aging.

malunion (mal-ūn′yin) faulty union of the fragments of a fractured bone.

mamilla (mah-mil′ah), pl. *mamil′lae* [L.] 1. the nipple of the breast. 2. any nipple-like prominence. **mam′illary,** adj.

mamillation (mam″ĭ-la′shin) a nipple-like elevation or projection.

mamilliplasty (-plas″te) theleplasty.

mamillitis (mam″il-īt′is) thelitis.

mamm(o)- word element [L.], *breast; mammary gland.*

mamma (mam′ah), pl. *mam′mae* [L.] the breast.

mammal (mam″l) an individual of Mammalia.

mammalgia (mah-mal′je-ah) mastalgia.

Mammalia (mah-māl′e-ah) a class of warm-blooded vertebrate animals, including all that have hair and suckle their young.

mammary (mam′ah-re) pertaining to the mammary gland, or breast.

mammectomy (mah-mek′tah-me) mastectomy.

mammillitis (mam″il-īt′is) thelitis.

mammitis (mah-mīt′is) mastitis.

mammography (mah-mog′rah-fe) radiography of the mammary gland.

mammoplasia (mam″ah-pla′ze-ah) development of breast tissue.

mammoplasty (mam″ah-plas″te) plastic reconstruction of the breast, either to augment or reduce its size.

mammose (mam′ōs) 1. having large breasts. 2. mamillated.

mammotomy (mah-mot′ah-me) mastotomy.

mammotrope (mam′ah-trōp) one of the acidophils of the adenohypophysis that secrete prolactin.

mammotrophic (mam″ah-trof′ik) mammotropic.

mammotropic (-trop′ik) having a stimulating effect on the mammary gland.

mammotropin (-trōp′in) prolactin.

mandelic acid (man-del′ik) $C_8H_8O_3$, from amygdalin; used, usually as the ammonium, calcium, or sodium salt, as a urinary antiseptic.

mandible (man′dĭ-b'l) the lower jaw; see *Table of Bones*. **mandib′ular,** adj.

mandibula (man-dib′ūl-ah), pl. *mandib′ulae* [L.] mandible.

mandrel (man′dril) the shaft on which a dental tool is held in the dental handpiece, for rotation by the dental engine.

mandrin (man′drin) a metal guide for a flexible catheter.

maneuver (mah-noo′ver) a skillful or dextrous procedure. **Bracht's m.,** a method of extraction of the aftercoming head in breech presentation. **Brandt-Andrews m.,** a method of expressing the placenta from the uterus. **forward-bending m.,** a method of detecting retraction signs in neoplastic changes in the mammae; the patient bends forward from the waist with chin held up and arms extended toward the examiner. If retraction is present, an asymmetry in the breast is seen. **Heimlich m.,** a method of dislodging food or other material from the throat of a choking victim: wrap your arms around the victim, and allow his upper torso to hang forward; then make a fist with one hand and grasp it with the other, and then with both hands placed against the victim's abdomen slightly above the navel and below the rib cage, forcefully press into the abdomen with a quick upward thrust. Repeat several times if necessary. **Pajot's m.,** a method of forceps extraction

of the fetal head. **Pinard's m.,** a method of bringing down the foot in breech extraction. **Prague m.,** a method of extracting the aftercoming head in breech presentation. **Scanzoni's m.,** double application of forceps blades for delivery of a fetus in the occiput posterior position. **Toynbee m.,** pinching the nostrils and swallowing; if the auditory tube is patent, the tympanic membrane will retract medially. **Valsalva's m.,** 1. increase in intrathoracic pressure by forcible exhalation effort against the closed glottis. 2. increase in the pressure in the eustachian tube and middle ear by forcible exhalation effort against occluded nostrils and closed mouth.

manganese (man′gah-nēs) chemical element (*see table*), at. no. 25, symbol Mn; its salts occur in the body tissue in very small amounts and serve as an activator of liver arginase and other enzymes. Poisoning, usually due to inhalation of manganese dust, is manifested by symptoms including mental disorders accompanying a syndrome resembling paralysis agitans, and inflammation of the respiratory system.

mange (mānj) a skin disease of domestic animals, due to mites.

mania (ma′ne-ah) disordered mental state of extreme excitement; specifically, the manic type of manic-depressive psychosis. Also used as a word termination to denote obsessive preoccupation with something, as in tomomania. **mani′acal, ma′nic,** adj.

manic-depressive (man″ik-de-pres′iv) alternating between attacks of mania and depression; see under *psychosis*.

manikin (man′ĭ-kin) a model to illustrate anatomy or on which to practice surgical or other manipulations.

manipulation (mah-nip″ūl-a-shin) skillful or dextrous treatment by the hands.

mannitol (man′ĭ-tol) a sugar alcohol widely distributed in plants and fungi; used in diagnostic tests of kidney function and as a diuretic.

mannose (man′ōs) a monosaccharide produced by oxidation of mannitol.

mannosidosis (man″ōs-ĭ-do′sis) an inborn error of metabolism marked by a defect in α-mannosidase activity that results in lysosomal accumulation of mannose-rich substrates.

manometer (mah-nom′it-er) an instrument for measuring the pressure of liquids or gases. **manomet′ric,** adj.

Mansonella (man″son-el′ah) a genus of filarial nematodes. *M. ozzar'di* is found in the mesentery and visceral fat of man in Panama, Yucatan, Guyana, Surinam, and Argentina.

Mansonia (man-so′ne-ah) a genus of mosquitoes, several species of which transmit *Brugia malayi;* some may also transmit viruses, such as those of equine encephalomyelitis.

mantle (man′t'l) an enveloping cover or layer, such as the brain mantle, or cerebrel cortex.

manubrium (mah-noo′bre-um), pl. *manu'bria* [L.] the handle-like part of the sternum or malleus. **m. of malleus,** the longest process of the malleus; it is attached to the inner surface of the tympanic membrane and has the tensor tympani muscle attached to it. **m. of sternum,** the cranial part of the sternum, articulating with the clavicles and first two pairs of ribs.

manus (ma′nus), pl. *ma′nus* [L.] hand.

MAO monoamine oxidase.

map (map) a two-dimensional graphic representation of arrangement in space. **fate m.,** a graphic representation of a blastula or other early stage of an embryo, showing prospective significance of certain areas in normal development. **gene m.,** a graphic representation of the linear arrangement of genes on a chromosome.

marasmus (mah-raz′mis) a protein-calorie malnutrition in the first year of life, with growth retardation and wasting of subcutaneous fat and muscle. **maran′tic, maras′mic,** adj.

Marax (mār′ax) trademark for a fixed combination preparation of ephedrine sulfate, theophylline, and hydroxyzine hydrochloride.

marfanoid (mar′fan-oid) having the characteristic symptoms of Marfan's syndrome.

margarine (mar′jah-rin) a food product containing 80 per cent fat (refined cottonseed and soybeam oils, which are sources of vitamin E and essential fatty acids), and fortified to supply at least 15,000 U.S.P. units of vitamin A per pound.

margin (mar′jin) an edge or border. **mar′ginal,** adj. **dentate m.,** pectinate line. **gingival m., gum m.,** the border of the gingiva surrounding, but unattached to, the substance of the teeth.

margination (mar′jĭ-na′shin) accumulation and adhesion of leukocytes to the epithelial cells of blood vessel walls at the site of injury in the early stages of inflammation.

marginoplasty (mar′jin-o-plas″te) surgical restoration of a border, as of the eyelid.

margo (mar′go), pl. *mar′gines* [L.] margin.

marihuana, marijuana (mar″ĭ-wahn′ah) a preparation of the leaves and flowering tops of hemp plants (*Cannabis sativa*), usually smoked in cigarettes for its euphoric properties.

mark (mark) a spot, blemish, or other circumscribed area visible on a surface. **birth m.,** see *birthmark.* **port-wine m.,** nevus flammeus. **strawberry m.,** cavernous hemangioma.

marrow (mar′o) the soft organic material filling the cavities of bones (*bone marrow*). **spinal m.,** the spinal cord.

Marsupialia (mar-soo″pe-āl′e-ah) an order of mammals characterized by the possession of a marsupium, including opossums, kangaroos, wallabies, koala bears, and wombats.

marsupialization (mar-soo″pe-il-ĭ-za′shin) conversion of a closed cavity into an open pouch, by incising it and suturing the edges of its wall to the edges of the wound.

marsupium (mar-soo′pe-um), pl. *marsu′pia* [L.] 1. the scrotum. 2. an external abdominal pouch or skin fold for carrying the young and containing the mammary gland; it occurs in marsupials and spiny anteaters; also, a similar structure for carrying eggs and/or young, as in the male sea horse.

masculine (mas′kūl-in) pertaining to the male sex, or having qualities normally characteristic of the male.

masculinization (mas″kūl-in-ĭ-za′shin) the normal development of the male sex characters in the male; also, the development of male secondary sex characters in the female.

masculinovoblastoma (mas″kūl-in-o″vo-blasto′mah) lipoid cell tumor of the ovary.

maser (ma′zer) a device which produces an extremely intense, small and nearly nondivergent beam of monochromatic radiation in the microwave region, with all the waves in phase.

mask (mask) 1. to cover or conceal, as the masking of the nature of a disorder by the presence of unrelated signs, organisms, etc.; in audiometry, to obscure or diminish a sound by the presence of another sound of different frequency. 2. an appliance for shading, protecting, or medicating the face. 3. in dentistry, to camouflage metal parts of a prosthesis by covering with opaque material.

masochism (mas′ah-kizm) a perversion in which infliction of pain gives sexual gratification to the recipient. **masochis′tic,** adj.

mass (mas) 1. a lump or collection of cohering particles. 2. a cohesive mixture to be made into pills. 3. that characteristic of matter which gives it inertia. **atomic m.,** the mass of a neutral atom of a nuclide, usually expressed as atomic mass units (amu). **inner cell m.,** the cell cluster at the embryonic pole of a blastocyst from which the embryo proper develops. **lean body m.,** that part of the body including all its components except neutral storage lipid; in essence, the fat-free mass of the body.

massa (mas′ah), pl. *mas′sae* [L.] mass (1).

massage (mah-sahzh′) systematic therapeutic friction, stroking, or kneading of the body. **cardiac m.,** intermittent compression of the heart by pressure applied over the sternum (*closed cardiac m.*) or directly to the heart through an opening in the chest wall (*open cardiac m.*); done to reinstate and maintain circulation. **vibratory m.,** massage by rapidly repeated light percussion with a vibrating hammer or sound.

masseter (mas-ēt′er) see *Table of Muscles.* **masseter′ic,** adj.

masseur (mah-sur′) [Fr.] 1. a man who performs massage. 2. an instrument for performing massage.

masseuse (mah-suz′) [Fr.] a woman who performs massage.

MAST acronym for Military Anti-Shock Trousers, inflatable trousers used to induce autotransfusion of blood from the lower to the upper part of the body.

mastadenitis (mast″ad-in-īt′is) mastitis.

mastadenoma (mas″tad-ĕ-no′mah) a tumor of the breast.

mastalgia (mas-tal′je-ah) pain in the breast.

mastatrophy (mast-ă′trah-fe) atrophy of the breast.

mastectomy (mast-ek′tah-me) excision of the breast. **modified radical m.,** total mastectomy with axial node dissection, but leaving the pectoral muscles intact. **radical m.,** amputation of the breast with wide excision of the pectoral muscles and axillary lymph nodes. **subcutane-**

ous m., excision of breast tissue with preservation of overlying skin, nipple, and areola so that the breast form may be reconstructed.

mastication (mas″tĭ-ka′shin) the process of chewing food.

Mastigophora (mas″tĭ-gof′o-rah) a subphylum of Protozoa comprising those having one or more flagella throughout most of their life cycle, and a simple, centrally located nucleus; many are parasitic in both invertebrates and vertebrates, including man.

mastigote (mas′tĭ-gōt) any member of the Mastigophora.

mastitis (mas-tīt′is) inflammation of the breast. **m. neonato′rum,** any abnormal condition of the breast in the newborn. **periductal m.,** inflammation of the tissues about the ducts of the mammary gland. **plasma cell m.,** infiltration of the breast stroma with plasma cells and proliferation of the cells lining the ducts.

masto- word element [Gr.], breast; mastoid process.

mastocyte (mas′tah-sīt) a mast cell.

mastocytosis (-si-to′sis) an accumulation, local or systemic, of mast cells in the tissues; known as urticaria pigmentosa when widespread in the skin.

mastoid (mas′toid) 1. breast-shaped. 2. mastoid process. 3. pertaining to the mastoid process.

mastoidalgia (mas″toid-al′je-ah) pain in the mastoid region.

mastoideocentesis (mas-toid″e-o-sen-te′sis) paracentesis of the mastoid cells.

mastoiditis (mas″toid-īt′is) inflammation of the mastoid antrum and cells.

mastoncus (mas-tong′kus) a tumor or swelling of the breast.

mastopathy (mas-top′ah-the) any disease of the mammary gland.

mastopexy (mas′to-pek″se) surgical fixation of a pendulous breast.

mastoplasty (mas′to-plas″te) mammoplasty

mastoptosis (mas″top-to′sis) pendulous breasts.

mastoscirrhus (-skir′us) hardening of the mammary gland.

mastosquamous (-skwa′mus) pertaining to the mastoid and squama of the temporal bone.

masturbation (mas″ter-ba′shin) induction of orgasm by self-stimulation of the genitals.

matching (mach′ing) comparison to select objects having similar or identical characteristics; in transplantation immunology, a method of measuring tissue compatibility between individuals. **cross m.,** determination of the compatibility of the blood of a donor and that of a recipient before transfusion by placing the donor's cells in the recipient's serum and the recipient's cells in the donor's serum; absence of agglutination, hemolysis, and cytotoxicity indicates compatibility.

materia (mah-tēr′e-ah) [L.] material; substance. **m. al′ba,** whitish deposits on the teeth, composed of mucus and epithelial cells containing bacteria and filamentous organisms. **m. med′ica,** pharmacology.

maternity (mah-turn′it-e) 1. motherhood. 2. a lying-in hospital.

mating (māt′ing) pairing of individuals of opposite sexes, especially for reproduction. **assortative m., assorted m., assortive m.,** the mating of individuals having similar qualities or constitutions. **random m.,** the mating of individuals without regard to any similarity between them.

matrix (ma′triks), pl. ma′trices [L.] 1. the intercellular substance of a tissue, as bone matrix, or the tissue from which a structure develops, as hair or nail matrix. 2. a metal band used to provide form to a dental restoration. **bone m.,** the intercellular substance of bone consisting of collagenous fibers, ground substance, and inorganic salts. **cartilage m.,** the intercellular substance of cartilage consisting of cells and extracellular fibers embedded in an amorphous ground substance. **interterritorial m.,** a paler staining region among the darker territorial matrices. **nail m.,** m. unguis. **territorial m.,** basophilic matrix about groups of cartilage cells. **m. un′guis,** nail bed; also, the proximal part of the nail bed where growth occurs.

matter (mat′er) 1. substance; anything that occupies space. 2. pus. **gray m.,** see under substance. **white m.,** see under substance.

maturation (mă-cher-ra′shin) 1. the process of becoming mature; attainment of emotional and intellectual maturity. In biology, a process of cell division during which the number of chromosomes in the germ cells is reduced to one half the number characteristic of the species. 2. suppuration.

matutinal (mah-too′tĭ-nil) occurring in the morning.

maxilla (mak-sil′ah), pl. maxil′lae [L.] the bone of the upper jaw; see Table of Bones. **max′illary,** adj. **inferior m.,** the mandible.

maxilloethmoidectomy (mak″sil-o-eth″moid-ek′tah-me) excision of the portion of the maxilla surrounding the maxillary sinus and of the cribriform plate and anterior ethmoid cells.

maxillomandibular (-man-dib′ūl-er) pertaining to the upper and lower jaws.

maxillotomy (mak″sil-ot′ah-me) surgical sectioning of the maxilla which allows movement of all or part of the maxilla into the desired position.

maximum (mak′sĭ-mum) 1. the greatest possible or actual effect or quantity. 2. largest; utmost. **maximal,** adj. **tubular m.,** the highest rate in milligrams per minute at which the renal tubules can transfer a substance either from the tubular luminal fluid to the interstitial fluid or from the latter to the former.

maze (māz) a complicated system of intersecting paths used in intelligence tests and in demonstrating learning in experimental animals.

mazindol (ma′zin-dōl) an adrenergic, $C_{16}H_{13}Cl$-N_2O, having amphetamine-like actions; used as an anorexic.

mazopexy (ma′zo-pek″se) mastopexy.

mazoplasia (ma″zo-pla′ze-ah) degenerative epithelial hyperplasia of the mammary acini.

M.B. [L.] Medici′nae Baccalau′reus (Bachelor of Medicine).

M.C. [L.] Magis'ter Chirur'giae (*Master of Surgery*); Medical Corps.

mC millicurie.

μC microcurie.

mcg. microgram.

MCH mean corpuscular hemoglobin.

MCHC mean corpuscular hemoglobin concentration.

μChr. microcurie-hour.

MCV mean corpuscular volume.

M.D. [L.] Medici'nae Doc'tor (*Doctor of Medicine*).

Md chemical symbol, *mendelevium.*

meal (mēl) a portion of food or foods taken at some particular and usually stated or fixed time. **Boyden m.,** a test meal for the study of gallbladder evacuation, containing three or four egg yolks combined with milk and seasoned with sugar, port wine, etc. **test m.,** a meal containing material given to aid in diagnostic examination of the stomach.

mean (mēn) an average; a numerical value intermediate between two extremes. **arithmetic m.,** the sum of *n* numbers divided by *n.* **geometric m.,** the *n*th root of the product of *n* numbers.

measles (mēz″lz) rubeola; a highly contagious viral infection, usually of childhood, involving primarily the respiratory tract and reticuloendothelial tissues, marked by an eruption of discrete, red papules, which become confluent, flatten, turn brown, and desquamate. **atypical m.,** a form of natural measles infection affecting those who previously received killed measles virus vaccine. **black m.,** a severe form in which the eruption is very dark and petechial. **German m.,** rubella. **hemorrhagic m.,** black m.

measure (mezh′er) see *Tables of Weights and Measures,* accompanying *weight.*

meatorrhaphy (me″ah-tor′ah-fe) suture of the wound made in meatotomy.

meatoscopy (me″ah-tos′ko-pe) inspection of any meatus, especially the urethral meatus.

meatus (me-āt′is), pl. *mea′tus* [L.] an opening or passage. **mea′tal,** adj. **acoustic m., m. acus′ticus,** either of two passages in the ear, one leading to the tympanic membrane (*external acoustic m.*), and one through which the facial, intermediate, and vestibulocochlear nerves and the labyrinthine artery pass (*internal acoustic m.*). **auditory m.,** acoustic m. **m. na′si, m. of nose,** one of the four portions (common, inferior, middle, and superior) of the nasal cavity on either side of the septum. **m. urina′rius, urinary m.,** the opening of the urethra on the body surface through which urine is discharged.

mebendazole (mě-ben′dah-zōl) an anthelmintic, $C_{16}H_{13}N_3O_3$, used against trichuriasis, enterobiasis, ascariasis, and hookworm disease.

mecamylamine (mek″ah-mil′ah-min) a ganglionic blocking agent, $C_{11}H_{21}N$, used in the form of the hydrochloride salt as an antihypertensive.

mechanics (mě-kan′iks) the science dealing with the motions of bodies. **body m.,** the application of kinesiology to prevent and correct problems related to posture.

mechanism (mek′ah-nizm) 1. a machine or machine-like structure. 2. the manner of combination of parts, processes, etc., which subserve a common function. **defense m.,** a mental mechanism by which psychic tension is diminished, e.g., repression, rationalization, etc. **mental m.,** 1. the organization of mental operations. 2. an unconscious and indirect manner of gratifying a repressed desire.

mechanoreceptor (mek″ah-no-re-sep′ter) a receptor that is excited by mechanical pressures or distortions, as those responding to touch and muscular contractions.

mechlorethamine (mě″klor-eth′ah-mēn) one of the nitrogen mustards, $C_5H_{11}Cl_2N$; used in the form of the hydrochloride salt as an antineoplastic.

meclizine (mek′lĭ-zēn) an antinauseant, $C_{25}H_{27}ClN_2$, used as the hydrochloride salt.

meconium (mĭ-ko′ne-um) dark green mucilaginous material in the intestine of the full-term fetus.

media (me′de-ah) 1. plural of *medium.* 2. middle.

medial (me′de-il) situated toward the midline of the body or a structure.

medialis (me″de-a′lis) [L.] medial.

median (me′de-in) pertaining to or situated in the midline.

medianus (me″de-a′nus) [L.] median.

mediastinitis (me″de-as″tĭ-nīt′is) inflammation of the mediastinum.

mediastinography (me″de-as″tĭ-nog′rah-fe) radiography of the mediastinum.

mediastinopericarditis (me″de-as″tĭ-no-per″ĭ-kar-dīt′is) pericarditis with adhesions extending from the pericardium to the mediastinum.

mediastinoscopy (me″de-as″ti-nos′kah-pe) examination of the mediastinum by means of an endoscope inserted through an anterior midline incision just above the thoracic inlet.

mediastinum (me″de-ah-sti′num), pl. *mediasti′na* [L.] 1. a median septum or partition. 2. the mass of tissues and organs separating the sternum in front and the vertebral column behind, containing the heart and its large vessels, trachea, esophagus, thymus, lymph nodes, and other structures and tissues; it is divided into anterior, middle, posterior, and superior regions. **mediasti′nal,** adj. **m. tes′tis,** a partial septum of the testis formed near its posterior border by a continuation of the tunica albuginea.

mediate 1. (me′de-āt) to serve as an intermediate agent. 2. (me′de-it) indirect; accomplished by means of an intervening medium.

medicable (med′ĭ-kah-b'l) subject to treatment with reasonable expectation of cure.

medical (med′ĭ-k'l) pertaining to medicine.

medicament (mĭ-dik′ah-mint, med′ĭ-kah-mint) a medicinal agent.

Medicare (med′ĭ-kār) a program of the Social Security Administration which provides medical care to the aged.

medicated (med′ĭ-kāt″id) imbued with a medicinal substance.

medication (med″ĭ-ka′shin) 1. impregnation

with a medicine. 2. the administration of remedies. 3. a medicament. **ionic m.,** iontophoresis.

medicinal (mĭ-dis′in-il) having healing qualities; pertaining to a medicine.

medicine (med′ĭ-sin) 1. any drug or remedy. 2. the diagnosis and treatment of disease and the maintenance of health. 3. the nonsurgical treatment of disease. **aviation m.,** that dealing with the physiologic, medical, psychologic, and epidemiologic problems involved in aviation. **clinical m.,** 1. the study of disease by direct examination of the living patient. 2. the last two years of the usual curriculum in a medical college. **emergency m.,** that specialty which deals with the acutely ill or injured who require immediate medical treatment. **environmental m.,** that dealing with the effects of the environment on man, including rapid population growth, water and air pollution, travel, etc. **experimental m.,** the study of diseases based on experimentation in animals. **family m.,** see under *practice*. **forensic m.,** medical jurisprudence. **group m.,** the practice of medicine by a group of physicians, usually representing various specialties, who are associated together for the cooperative diagnosis, treatment, and prevention of disease. **internal m.,** that dealing especially with diagnosis and medical treatment of diseases and disorders of internal structures of the body. **legal m.,** medical jurisprudence. **nuclear m.,** that branch of medicine concerned with the use of radionuclides in the diagnosis and treatment of disease. **patent m.,** a drug or remedy protected by a trademark, available without a prescription. **physical m.,** physiatrics. **preclinical m.,** 1. preventive m. 2. the first two years of the usual curriculum in a medical college. **preventive m.,** science aimed at preventing disease. **proprietary m.,** a remedy whose formula is owned exclusively by the manufacturer and which is marketed usually under a name registered as a trademark. **psychosomatic m.,** the study of the relations between bodily processes and emotional life. **socialized m.,** a system of medical care controlled by the government. **space m.,** that branch of aviation medicine concerned with conditions encountered in space. **sports m.,** the field of medicine concerned with injuries sustained in athletics, including their prevention, diagnosis, and treatment. **tropical m.,** medical science applied to diseases occurring in the tropics and subtropics. **veterinary m.,** the diagnosis and treatment of diseases of animals.

medicolegal (med′ĭ-ko-le′g′l) pertaining to medical jurisprudence.

medicosocial (-so′shil) having both medical and social aspects.

mediolateral (me″de-o-lat′er-il) pertaining to the midline and one side.

medionecrosis (-nĕ-kro′sis) necrosis of the tunica media of a blood vessel.

medium (me′de-um) pl. *mediums, me′dia* [L.] 1. a means. 2. a substance that transmits impulses. 3. culture medium; see under *C.* 4. a preparation used in treating histologic specimens. **active m.,** the aggregated atoms, ions, or molecules contained in a laser's optical cavity,

in which stimulated emission will occur under the proper excitation. **clearing m.,** a substance to render histologic specimens transparent. **contrast m.,** radiopaque substance used in roentgenography to permit visualization of internal body structures. **culture m.,** see under *C.* **dioptric media,** refracting media. **disperse m., dispersion m.,** the continuous phase of a colloid system; the medium in which a colloid is dispersed, corresponding to the solvent in a true solution. **nutrient m.,** a culture medium to which nutrient materials have been added. **refracting media,** the transparent tissues and fluid in the eye through which light rays pass and by which they are refracted and focused on the retina. **transport m.,** a culture medium used for transport of clinical specimens for bacteriological examination.

medius (me′de-us) [L.] situated in the middle.

Medrol (med′rol) trademark for a preparation of methylprednisolone.

medroxyprogesterone (mĕ-drok″sĭ-pro-jes′ter-ōn) a progestational agent, $C_{24}H_{34}O_4$, used as the acetate salt.

medulla (mĕ-dul′ah), pl. *medul′lae* [L.] the innermost part; marrow; applied to the marrow of bones (*m. os′sium*), the spinal cord (*m. spina′lis*), and the central portion of such organs as the adrenal gland and the kidney (*m. re′nis*). **med′ullary,** adj. **adrenal m.,** the inner, reddish brown, soft part of the adrenal gland; it synthesizes, stores, and releases catecholamines. **m. of bone,** bone marrow. **m. ne′phrica,** m. renis. **m. oblonga′ta,** that part of the brain stem continuous with the pons above and the spinal cord below. **m. os′sium,** bone marrow. **m. re′nis,** the inner part of the kidney substance, composed chiefly of collecting elements and loops of Henle, organized grossly into pyramids. **m. spina′lis,** spinal cord. **m. of thymus,** the central portion of each lobule of the thymus; it contains many more reticular cells and far fewer lymphocytes than does the surrounding cortex.

medullated (med′il-āt″id) myelinated.

medullization (med″il-ĭ-za′shin) enlargement of marrow spaces, as in rarefying osteitis.

medulloblast (mĕ-dul′ah-blast) an undifferentiated cell of the neural tube which may develop into either a neuroblast or spongioblast.

medulloepithelioma (ep″ĭ-thēl-e-o′mah) a brain tumor composed of primitive neuroepithelial cells lining the tubular spaces.

mega- word element [Gr.], *large;* used in naming units of measurement to designate an amount 10^6 (one million) times the size of the unit to which it is joined, as megacuries (10^6 curies); symbol M.

megacalycosis (-kal″ĭ-ko′sis) nonobstructive dilatation of the renal calices due to malformation of the renal papillae.

megacaryocyte (-kar′e-o-sīt) megakaryocyte.

megacolon (-kōl′in) dilatation and hypertrophy of the colon. **acquired m.,** colonic enlargement associated with chronic constipation, but with normal ganglion cell innervation. **aganglionic m., congenital m.,** that due to congenital absence of myenteric ganglion cells in a distal segment of the large bowel, with loss of motor function in the aganglionic segment and massive hypertrophic dilatation of the normal proximal colon. **idiopathic m.,** acquired m. **toxic m.,** that associated with amebic or ulcerative colitis.

megaesophagus (meg″ah-ĕ-sof′ah-gus) see *achalasia.*

megahertz (meg′ah-hertz) one million (10^6) hertz (cycles per second). Abbreviated MHz.

megakaryoblast (meg″ah-kar′e-o-blast″) the earliest cytologically identifiable precursor in the thrombocytic series, which matures to form the promegakaryocyte.

megakaryocyte (-sīt″) the giant cell of bone marrow containing a greatly lobulated nucleus, from which mature blood platelets originate.

megakaryophthisis (-thi′sis) deficiency of megakaryocytes in bone marrow or blood.

megal(o)- word element [Gr.], *large; abnormal enlargement.*

megalgia (meg-al′je-ah) a severe pain.

megaloblast (meg′ah-lo-blast″) a large, nucleated, immature progenitor of an abnormal erythrocytic series. **megaloblas′tic,** adj.

megalocardia (meg″ah-lo-kar′de-ah) cardiomegaly.

megalocephaly (-sef′ah-le) 1. macrocephaly. 2. leontiasis ossea. **megalocephal′ic,** adj.

megalocheiria (-ki′re-ah) abnormal largeness of the hands.

megalocyte (meg′ah-lo-sīt″) an extremely large erythrocyte.

megalodactyly (meg″ah-lo-dak′tĭ-le) excessive size of the fingers or toes. **megalodac′tylous,** adj.

megaloenteron (-en′ter-on) enlargement of the intestine.

megaloesophagus (-ĕ-sof′ah-gus) see *achalasia.*

megalogastria (-gas′tre-ah) enlargement or abnormally large size of the stomach.

megalokaryoblast (-kar′e-o-blast″) megakaryoblast.

megalokaryocyte (-kar′e-o-sīt″) megakaryocyte.

megalomania (-ma′ne-ah) unreasonable conviction of one's own extreme greatness, goodness, or power.

megalopenis (-pe′nis) abnormal largeness of the penis.

megalophthalmos (meg″ah-lof-thal′mos) buphthalmos.

megalopia (meg″al-o′pe-ah) macropsia.

megalopodia (meg″ah-lo-po′de-ah) abnormal largeness of the feet.

megalopsia (meg″ah-lop′se-ah) macropsia.

megalosyndactyly (-sin-dak′tĭ-le) a condition in which the digits are very large and more or less webbed together.

megaloureter (-ūr-ēt′er) congenital ureteral dilatation without demonstrable cause.

-megaly word element [Gr.], *enlargement.*

megavitamin (-vĭt′ah-min) a dose of vitamin(s)

vastly exceeding the amount recommended for nutritional balance.

megavolt (meg′ah-volt) one million volts.

megestrol (mĕ-jes′trōl) a synthetic progestational agent, $C_{24}H_{32}O_4$.

meglumine (meg′loo-mēn) methylglucamine; a crystalline base, $C_7H_{17}NO_5$, used in preparing salts of certain acids for use as diagnostic radioopaque media (*m. diatrizoate, m. iodipamide, m. iothalamate*).

megohm (meg′ōm) one million ohms.

megophthalmos (meg″of-thal′mos) buphthalmos; hydrophthalmos.

megrim (me′grim) migraine.

meiosis (mi-o′sis) cell division occurring in maturation of sex cells, wherein, over two successive cell divisions, each daughter nucleus receives half the number of chromosomes typical of the somatic cells of the species, so that the gametes are haploid. **meiot′ic,** adj.

mel (mel) [L.] honey.

melagra (mel-ag′rah) muscular pain in the limbs.

melalgia (mel-al′je-ah) pain in the limbs.

melan(o)- word element [Gr.], *black; melanin.*

melancholia (mel″an-kōl′e-ah) a depressed and unhappy emotional state with abnormal inhibition of mental and bodily activity. **m. agita′ta, agitated m.,** a form with constant motion and signs of great emotional excitement. **m. hypochondri′aca,** extreme hypochondria. **involutional m.,** an affective disorder occurring in late middle life, with agitation, worry, anxiety, somatic preoccupations, insomnia, and sometimes paranoid reactions. **m. sim′plex,** a mild form without delusions or great excitement. **stuporous m.,** a form in which the patient lies motionless and silent, with fixed eyes and indifference to surroundings, sometimes with hallucinations.

melanin (mel′ah-nin) the dark pigment of the skin, hair, choroid coat of the eye, substantia nigra, and various tumors; it is produced by polymerization of oxidation products of tyrosine and dihydroxyphenol compounds.

melanism (mel′ah-nizm) excessive pigmentation or blackening of the integuments or other tissues, usually of genetic origin.

melanoameloblastoma (mel″ah-no-ah-mel″o-blas-to′mah) melanotic neuroectodermal tumor.

melanoblast (mel′ah-no-blast″) a cell originating from the neural crest, which develops into a melanocyte.

melanoblastoma (mel″ah-no-blas-to′mah) melanotic neuroectodermal tumor.

melanocarcinoma (-kar″sĭ-no′mah) malignant melanoma.

melanocyte (mel′ah-no-sīt, mĕ-lan′o-sīt) any of the dendritic clear cells of the epidermis that synthesize tyrosinase and, within their melanosomes, the pigment melanin; the melanosomes are then transferred from melanocytes to keratinocytes. **melanocyt′ic,** adj.

melanocytoma (mel″ah-no-si-to′mah) a neoplasm or hamartoma composed of melanocytes.

melanoderma (-der′mah) an abnormally increased amount of melanin in the skin.

melanodermatitis (-der″mah-tīt′is) dermatitis with deposit of melanin in the skin.

melanogen (mĭ-lan′ah-jen) a colorless chromogen, convertible into melanin, which may occur in the urine in certain diseases.

melanogenesis (mel″ah-no-jen′ĭ-sis) the production of melanin.

melanoglossia (-glos′e-ah) black tongue.

melanoid (mel′ah-noid) 1. resembling melanin. 2. a substance resembling melanin.

melanoleukoderma (mel″ah-no-loo″kah-der′-mah) a mottled appearance of the skin. **m. col′li,** syphilitic leukoderma about the neck.

melanoma (mel″ah-no′mah) 1. any tumor composed of melanin-pigmented cells. 2. malignant melanoma. **juvenile m.,** a benign, pink to purplish red papule, usually on the face, especially the cheeks, most commonly originating before puberty; histologically, it suggests and has been mistaken for malignant melanoma. **malignant m.,** a malignant tumor usually developing from a nevus and consisting of black masses of cells with a marked tendency to metastasis.

melanonychia (-nik′e-ah) blackening of the nails by melanin pigmentation.

melanophage (mel′ah-no-fāj″) a histiocyte laden with phagocytosed melanin.

melanophore (-fōr″) a pigment cell containing melanin, especially such a cell in fishes, amphibians, and reptiles.

melanoplakia (mel″ah-no-pla′ke-ah) the formation of melanotic patches on the oral mucosa.

melanosis (mel″ah-no′sis), pl. *melano′ses.* 1. a condition characterized by dark pigmentary deposits. 2. disorder of pigment metabolism. **m. co′li,** black or dark brown discoloration of the mucosa of the colon, due to the presence of pigment-laden (not true melanin) macrophages within the lamina propria.

melanosome (mel′ah-no-sōm″) any of the granules within the melanocytes that contain tyrosinase and synthesizes melanin; they are transferred from the melanocytes to keratinocytes.

melanotroph (mel′ah-no-trōf″) a pituitary cell that elaborates melanocyte-stimulating hormone (MSH).

melanuria (mel″an-ūr′e-ah) the excretion of darkly stained urine. **melanu′ric,** adj.

melarsoprol (mel-ar′so-prōl) an antiprotozoal effective against *Trypanosoma,* $C_{12}H_{15}AsN_6$-OS_2.

melasma (mĕ-laz′mah) dark pigmentation of the skin.

melatonin (mel″ah-to′nin) a catecholamine hormone synthesized and released by the pineal body, which influences sexual maturation.

melena (mĕ-le′nah) the passage of dark stools stained with altered blood.

melioidosis (mel″e-oid-o′sis) a glanders-like disease of rodents, transmissible to man, and caused by *Pseudomonas pseudomallei.*

melitoptyalism (mel″it-o-ti′il-izm) secretion of saliva containing glucose.

melituria (mel″ĭ-tūr′e-ah) the presence of any sugar in the urine.

Mellaril (mel′ah-ril) trademark for a preparation of thioridazine.

meloplasty (mel′ah-plas″te) plastic surgery of the cheek.

melorheostosis (mel″ah-re″os-to′sis) a form of osteosclerosis, with linear tracks extending through a long bone; see *rheostosis.*

melphalan (mel′fah-lan) a cytotoxic nitrogen mustard alkylating agent, $C_{13}H_{18}Cl_2N_2O_2$, used as an antineoplastic.

MEM macrophage electrophoretic mobility (test).

member (mem′ber) a distinct part of the body, especially a limb.

membra (mem′bra) [L.] plural of *membrum.*

membrana (mem-bra′nah), pl. *membra′nae* [L.] membrane.

membrane (mem′brān) a thin layer of tissue that covers a surface, lines a cavity, or divides a space or organ. **mem′branous,** adj. **alveolocapillary m.,** a thin tissue barrier through which gases are exchanged between the alveolar air and the blood in the pulmonary capillaries. **alveolodental m.,** periodontium. **arachnoid m.,** arachnoid (2). **atlanto-occipital m.,** either of two midline ligamentous structures, one (the *anterior)* passing from the anterior arch of the atlas to the anterior margin of the foramen magnum, the other (the *posterior)* connecting the posterior aspects of the same structures. **basement m.,** the delicate layer underlying the epithelium of mucous membranes and secreting glands. **basilar m.,** lamina basilaris. **Bichat's m.,** fenestrated m. **Bowman's m.,** a thin layer of cornea between the outer layer of stratified epithelium and the substantia propria. **Bruch's m.,** the inner layer of the choroid, separating it from the pigmentary layer of the retina. **Brunn's m.,** the epithelium of the olfactory region of the nose. **cloacal m.,** the thin temporary barrier between the embryonic hindgut and the exterior. **Corti's m.,** a gelatinous mass resting on the organ of Corti, connected with the hairs of the hair cells. **croupous m.,** the false membrane of true croup. **decidual m., deciduous m.,** decidua. **Descemet's m.,** a thin hyaline membrane between the substantia propria and endothelial layer of the cornea. **diphtheritic m.,** a false membrane characteristic of diphtheria, formed by coagulation necrosis. **drum m.,** tympanic m. **elastic m.,** one made up largely of elastic fibers. **enamel m.,** 1. dental cuticle. 2. the inner layer of cells within the enamel organ of the fetal dental germ. **extraembryonic m's,** those that protect the embryo or fetus and provide for its nutrition, respiration, and excretion; the yolk sac (umbilical vesicle), allantois, amnion, chorion, decidua, and placenta. **fenestrated m.,** one of the perforated elastic sheets of the tunica intima and tunica media of arteries. **fetal m's,** extraembryonic m's. **fibroelastic m.,** the fibroelastic layer beneath the mucous coat of the larynx. **germinal m.,** blastoderm. **glomerular m.,** the membrane covering a glomerular capillary. **hyaline m.,** 1. a membrane between the outer root sheath and inner fibrous layer of a hair follicle. 2. a layer of eosinophilic hyaline material lining alveoli, alveolar ducts, and bronchioles, found at autopsy in infants who have died of respiratory distress syndrome of the newborn. **hyaloid m.,** vitreous m. (1). **Jackson's m.,** a web of adhesions sometimes covering the cecum and causing obstruction of the bowel. **keratogenous m.,** matrix unguis. **limiting m.,** one which constitutes the border of some tissue or structure. **medullary m.,** endosteum. **mucous m.,** the membrane lining various canals and cavities of the body. **Nasmyth's m.,** dental cuticle. **nictitating m.,** a transparent fold of skin lying deep to the eyelids, which may be drawn over the front of the eyeball; found in reptiles, birds, and many mammals. **nuclear m.,** 1. either of the membranes, inner and outer, comprising the nuclear envelope. 2. nuclear envelope. **olfactory m.,** the olfactory portion of the mucous membrane lining the nasal fossa. **ovular m.,** vitelline m. **peridental m.,** periodontium. **periodontal m.,** see under *ligament.* **placental m.,** the membrane separating the fetal from the maternal blood in the placenta. **Reissner's m.,** the thin anterior wall of the cochlear duct, separating it from the scala vestibuli. **reticular m.,** a netlike membrane over the spiral organ of the ear, through which pass the free ends of the outer hair cells. **Ruysch's m., ruyschian m.,** lamina choroidocapillaris. **Scarpa's m.,** secondary tympanic m. **schneiderian m.,** the mucous membrane lining the nose. **serous m.,** tunica serosa. **Shrapnell's m.,** the thin upper part of the tympanic membrane. **striated m.,** zona pellucida. **synaptic m.,** the layer separating the neuroplasm of an axon from that of the body of the nerve cell with which it makes synapsis. **synovial m.,** the inner of the two layers of the articular capsule of a synovial joint, composed of loose connective tissue, having a free smooth surface that lines the joint cavity. **tectorial m.,** Corti's m. **tympanic m.,** the thin partition between the external acoustic meatus and the middle ear. **tympanic m., secondary,** the membrane enclosing the fenestra cochlearis. **undulating m.,** a protoplasmic membrane running like a fin along the bodies of certain protozoa. **unit m.,** the trilaminar structure of the plasma membrane and other cellular membranes (e.g., nuclear m's, mitochondrial m's) revealed by the electron microscope. **vestibular m.,** the thin anterior wall of the cochlear duct, separating it from the scala vestibuli. **vitelline m.,** the cytoplasmic, noncellular membrane surrounding the eggs of various animals. **vitreous m.,** 1. a delicate boundary layer investing the vitreous body. 2. Bruch's m. 3. Descemet's m. 4. hyaline m. (1). **yolk m.,** vitelline m. **Zinn's m.,** ciliary zonule.

membranocartilaginous (mem''brah-no-kart''-il-aj'ĭ-nus) 1. developed in both membrane and cartilage. 2. partly cartilaginous and partly membranous.

membranoid (mem'brah-noid) resembling a membrane.

membranolysis (mem''brān-ol'ĭ-sis) disruption of a cell membrane.

membrum (mem'brum), pl. *mem'bra* [L.] a limb or member of the body; an entire arm of leg. **m. mulie'bre,** clitoris. **m. viri'le,** penis.

memory (mem'o-re) that faculty by which sensations, impressions, and ideas are stored and recalled. **screen m.,** a consciously tolerable memory serving as a "screen" for another memory that may be disturbing or emotionally painful if recalled.

menacme (mĕ-nak'me) the period of a woman's life which is marked by menstrual activity.

menadiol (men''ah-di'ol) a vitamin K analogue; its sodium diphosphate salt is used as a prothrombinogenic vitamin.

menaquinone (men''ah-kwin'ōn) any of a series of compounds having vitamin K activity in which the phytyl side chain of phytonadione (vitamin K_1) is replaced by a side chain of prenyl units.

menarche (mĕ-nar'ke) establishment or beginning of the menstrual function. **menar'chial,** adj.

mendelevium (men''dĕ-le've-um) chemical element (*see table*), at. no. 101, symbol Md.

mening(o)- word element [Gr.], *meninges; membrane.*

meninges (mĕn-in'jēz) (plural of *meninx*) the three membranes covering the brain and spinal cord: dura mater, arachnoid, and pia mater. **menin'geal,** adj.

meningioma (mĕ-nin''je-o'mah) a hard, usually vascular tumor, occurring mainly along the meningeal vessels and superior longitudinal sinus, invading the dura and skull and leading to erosion and thinning of the skull.

meningism (men'in-jizm) 1. the symptoms of meningitis with acute febrile illness or dehydration without infection of the meninges. 2. hysterical simulation of meningitis.

meningismus (men''in-jiz'mus) meningism.

meningitis (men''in-jīt'is), pl. *meningi'tides* [Gr.] inflammation of the meninges. **meningit'ic,** adj. **m. of the base, basilar m.,** that affecting the meninges at the base of the brain. **cerebral m.,** inflammation of the membranes of the brain. **cerebrospinal m.,** inflammation of the meninges of the brain and spinal cord. **epidemic cerebrospinal m.,** an acute infectious, usually epidemic, disease attended by a seropurulent meningitis, due to *Neisseria meningitidis,* usually with an erythematous, herpetic, or hemorrhagic skin eruption. **meningococcal m.,** epidemic cerebrospinal m. **occlusive m.,** leptomeningitis of children, with closure of the lateral and median apertures of the fourth ventricle. **m. ossi'ficans,** ossification of the cerebral meninges. **otitic m.,** that secondary to otitis media. **septicemic m.,** that due to septic blood poisoning. **serous m.,** that with serous exudation into the ventricles and subarachnoid spaces and slight to moderate spinal fluid changes. **spinal m.,** inflammation of the membranes of the spinal cord. **tubercular m., tuberculous m.,** severe meningitis due to *Mycobacterium tuberculosis.* **viral m.,** that due to various viruses, e.g., coxsakieviruses, mumps viruses, and the virus of lymphocytic choriomeningitis, marked by malaise, fever, headache, nausea, cerebrospinal fluid pleocytosis (mainly lymphocytic), abdominal pain, stiff neck and back, and a short uncomplicated course.

meningocele (mĕ-ning′gah-sēl) hernial protrusion of the meninges through a defect in the cranium or vertebral column.

meningococcemia (-kok-sēm′e-ah) invasion of the blood by meningococci.

meningococcus (-kok′us), pl. *meningococ′ci.* An individual organism of *Neisseria meningitidis.* **meningococ′cal, meningococ′cic,** adj.

meningocyte (mĕ-ning′go-sīt) a histiocyte of the meninges.

meningoencephalitis (mĕ-ning″go-en-sef″ah-līt′is) inflammation of the brain and meninges.

meningoencephalocele (-en-sef′ah-lah-sēl″) hernial protrusion of the meninges and brain substance through a skull defect.

meningoencephalopathy (-en-sef″ah-lop′ah-the) noninflammatory disease of the cerebral meninges and brain.

meningogenic (-jen′ik) arising in the meninges.

meningomalacia (-mah-la′she-ah) softening of a membrane.

meningo-osteophlebitis (-os″te-o-flĭ-bīt′is) periostitis with inflammation of the veins of a bone.

meningopathy (men″in-gop′ah-the) any disease of the meninges.

meningoradicular (mĕ-ning″go-rah-dik′ūl-er) pertaining to the meninges and the cranial or spinal nerve roots.

meningorhachidian (-rah-kid′e-in) pertaining to spinal cord and meninges.

meningorrhagia (-ra′je-ah) hemorrhage from cerebral or spinal membranes.

meningosis (men″ing-go′sis) attachment of bones by membrane.

meninx (me′ninks), pl. *menin′ges* [Gr.] a membrane, especially one of the membranes of the brain or spinal cord—the dura mater, arachnoid, and pia mater.

meniscitis (men″ĭ-sīt′is) inflammation of a meniscus of the knee joint.

meniscocyte (mĕ-nis′kah-sīt) a sickle cell.

meniscocytosis (mĕ-nis″ko-si-to′sis) sickle cell anemia.

meniscosynovial (-sin-o′ve-il) pertaining to a meniscus and the synovial membrane.

meniscus (mĕ-nis′kus), pl. *menis′ci* [L.] something of crescent shape, as the concave or convex surface of a column of liquid in a pipet or buret, or a crescent-shaped fibrocartilage in the knee joint. **menis′cal,** adj.

meno- word element [Gr.], *menstruation.*

menolipsis (men″ah-lip′sis) temporary cessation of menstruation.

menometrorrhagia (-mĕ-trah-ra′je-ah) excessive uterine bleeding at and between menstrual periods.

menopause (men′ah-pawz) cessation of menstruation. **men′opausal,** adj.

menorrhalgia (-al′je-ah) dysmenorrhea.

menoschesis (mĕ-nos′kĕ-sis, men″o-ske′sis) retention of the menses.

menostasis (mĕ-nos′tah-sis) amenorrhea.

menostaxis (men″ah-stak′sis) a prolonged menstrual period.

menotropins (-tro′pins) a purified preparation of gonadotropins extracted from the urine of postmenopausal women containing folliclestimulating hormone (FSH) and luteinizing hormone (LH); used in the treatment of infertility.

menses (men′sēz) the monthly flow of blood from the female genital tract. **men′strual,** adj.

menstruation (men″stroo-a′shin) the cyclic, physiologic discharge through the vagina of blood and muscosal tissues from the nonpregnant uterus; it is under hormonal control and normally recurs usually at approximately four-week intervals, except during pregnancy and lactation throughout the reproductive period (puberty through menopause). **anovular m., anovulatory m.,** periodic uterine bleeding without preceding ovulation. **vicarious m.,** discharge of blood from an extragenital source at the time menstruation is normally expected.

menstruum (men′stroo-um) a solvent medium.

mensuration (men″ser-a′shin) the act or process of measuring.

mental (ment′′l) 1. pertaining to the mind. 2. pertaining to the chin.

menthol (men′thol) an alcohol from various mint oils; used locally to relieve itching and in inhalers to treat upper respiratory tract disorders.

mentoplasty (men′tah-plas″te) plastic surgery of the chin; surgical correction of deformities and defects of the chin.

mentum (men′tum) [L.] chin.

mepenzolate (me-pen′zol-āt) an anticholinergic, $C_{21}H_{26}NO_3$, used to relieve abdominal pain, gaseous distention, and diarrhea associated with colonic disease.

meperidine (mĕ-per′ĭ-dēn) a narcotic analgesic, $C_{15}H_{21}NO_2$, used as the hydrochloride salt.

mephentermine (mĕ-fen′ter-mēn) a sympathomimetic and pressor substance, $C_{11}H_{17}N$, used as the sulfate salt.

mephenytoin (mĕ-fen′ĭ-to″in) an anticonvulsant, $C_{12}H_{14}N_2O_2$.

mephitic (mĕ-fit′ik) emitting a foul odor.

mephobarbital (mef″o-bar′bĭ-tal) an anticonvulsant and sedative, $C_{13}H_{14}N_2O_3$.

mepivacaine (mĕ-piv′ah-kān) a lidocaine analogue, $C_{14}H_{21}NO_2$; its hydrochloride salt is used as a local anesthetic.

meprednisone (mĕ-pred′nĭ-sōn) an oral glucocorticoid, $C_{22}H_{28}O_5$, used as an anti-inflammatory, antiallergic, and antineoplastic steroid.

meprobamate (mĕ-pro′bah-māt, mep″ro-bam′āt) a minor tranquilizer, $C_9H_{18}N_2O_4$.

mEq. milliequivalent.

meralgia (mĕ-ral′je-ah) pain in the thigh. **m. paresthe′tica,** paresthesia, pain, and numbness in the outer surface of the thigh due to entrapment of the lateral femoral cutaneous nerve at the inguinal ligament.

merbromin (mer-bro′min) a topical antibacterial, $C_{20}H_8Br_2HgNa_2O_6$.

mercaptan (mer-kap′tan) any compound containing the —SH group bound to carbon.

mercaptomerin (mer-kap″to-mer′in) an organic mercurial diuretic; used as the disodium salt, $C_{16}H_{25}HgNNa_2O_6S$.

mercaptopurine (-pūr′ēn) an antineoplastic, $C_5H_4N_4S$.

mercurial (mer-kūr′e-il) 1. pertaining to mercury. 2. a preparation containing mercury.

mercuric (mer-kūr′ik) pertaining to mercury as a bivalent element. **m. oxide, yellow,** an anti-infective, HgO, used in ophthalmology.

Mercurochrome (mer-kūr′ah-krōm) trademark for preparations of merbromin.

mercurous (mer′kūr-us) pertaining to mercury as a monovalent element. **m. chloride,** calomel.

mercury (mer′kūr-e) chemical element (*see table*), at. no. 80, symbol Hg. Acute mercury poisoning, due to ingestion, is marked by severe abdominal pain, vomiting, bloody diarrhea with watery stools, oliguria or anuria, and corrosion and ulceration of the digestive tract; in the chronic form, due to absorption through skin and mucous membranes, inhalation, or ingestion, there is stomatitis, blue line along the gum border, sore hypertrophied gums that bleed easily, loosening of teeth, erethism, ptyalism, tremors, and incoordination. **ammoniated m.,** a topical anti-infective, HgNH₂Cl. **m. oleate,** a mixture of yellow mercuric oxide and oleic acid, used topically in various skin diseases.

merethoxylline (mer″ĕ-thok′sil-ēn) a mercurial diuretic.

meridian (mĕ-rid′e-in) an imaginary line on the surface of a globe or sphere, connecting the opposite ends of its axis. **merid′ional,** adj.

meridianus (mĕ-rid″e-a′nus), pl. *meridia′ni* [L.] meridian.

mero- word element [Gr.], *part.*

meroblastic (mer-ah-blas′tik) partially dividing; undergoing cleavage in which only part of the ovum participates.

merocrine (mer′ah-krin) discharging only the secretory product and maintaining the secretory cell intact (e.g., salivary glands, pancreas).

merogenesis (mer″o-jen′ĭ-sis) cleavage of an ovum. **merogenet′ic,** adj.

merogony (mĕ-rog′ah-ne) the development of only a portion of an ovum. **merogon′ic,** adj.

meromyosin (-mi′ah-sin) a fragment of the myosin molecule isolated by treatment with proteolytic enzyme; there are two types, heavy (H-meromyosin) and light (L-meromyosin).

meropia (mĕ-ro′pe-ah) partial blindness.

merorhachischisis (mēr″o-rah-kis′kĭ-sis) fissure of part of the spinal cord.

merotomy (mĕ-rot′ah-me) dissection into segments, especially dissection of a cell.

merozoite (mer″ah-zo′it) one of the organisms formed by multiple fission (schizogony) of a sporozoite within the body of the host.

Merthiolate (mer-thi′ol-āt) trademark for preparations of thimerosal.

merycism (mer′ĭ-sizm) rumination.

mes(o)- word element [Gr.], *middle.*

mesangiocapillary (mes-an″je-o-kap′il-er″e) pertaining to or affecting the mesangium and the associated capillaries.

mesangium (mes-an′je-um) the thin membrane supporting the capillary loops in renal glomeruli. **mesan′gial,** adj.

mesatipellic (mes-at″ĭ-pel′ik) having a transverse diameter of the pelvic inlet almost the same as that of the true conjugated diameter.

mesaxon (mes-ak′son) a pair of parallel membranes marking the line of edge-to-edge contact of Schwann cells encircling an axon.

mescaline (mes′kah-lēn) a poisonous alkaloid from the flowering heads (mescal buttons) of a Mexican cactus, *Lophophora williamsii;* it produces an intoxication with delusions of color and sound.

mesectoderm (mĕ-sek′tah-derm) embryonic migratory cells derived from the neural crest of the head that contribute to the formation of the meninges and become pigment cells.

mesencephalon (mes″-en-sef′ah-lon) the midbrain. **mesencephal′ic,** adj.

mesencephalotomy (-en-sef″ah-lot′ah-me) surgical production of lesions in the midbrain, especially for relief of intractable pain.

mesenchyma (mĕ-seng′kĭ-mah) the meshwork of embryonic connective tissue in the mesoderm from which are formed the connective tissues of the body and the blood and lymphatic vessels. **mesen′chymal,** adj.

mesenchyme (mes′eng-kīm) mesenchyma.

mesenchymoma (mes″en-ki-mo′mah) a mixed mesenchymal tumor composed of two or more cellular elements not commonly associated, exclusive of fibrous tissue.

mesenteriopexy (-en-ter′e-o-pek″se) fixation or suspension of a torn mesentery.

mesenteriplication (-en-ter″ĭ-pli-ka′shin) shortening of the mesentery by plication.

mesenterium (-en-tēr′e-um) [L.] mesentery.

mesenteron (mes-en′ter-on) the midgut.

mesentery (mes′en-tĕ″re) a membranous fold attaching various organs to the body wall; especially the peritoneal fold attaching the small intestine to the dorsal body wall. **mesenter′ic,** adj.

mesiad (me′ze-ad) toward the middle or center.

mesial (me′ze-il) nearer the center of the dental arch.

mesially (me′ze-il″e) toward the median line.

mesiobuccal (me″ze-o-buk′l) pertaining to or formed by the mesial and buccal surfaces of a tooth or of a tooth cavity.

mesioclusion (-kloo′zhin) anteroclusion; malrelation of the dental arches with the mandibular arch anterior to the maxillary arch (prognathism).

mesiodens (me′ze-o-dens), pl. *mesioden′tes.* A small supernumerary tooth, occurring singly or paired, generally palatally between the maxillary central incisors.

mesion (me′ze-on) the plane dividing the body into right and left symmetrical halves.

mesioversion (-ver′zhin) displacement of a tooth along the dental arch toward the midline of the face.

mesmerism (mes′mer-izm) hypnotism.

mesoappendix (mes″o-ah-pen′diks) the peritoneal fold connecting the appendix to the ileum.

mesobilirubinogen (-bil″ĭ-roo-bin′ah-jen) a reduced form of bilirubin, formed in the intestine, which on oxidation forms stercobilin.

mesoblast (mes′o-blast) the mesoderm, especially in the early stages.

mesoblastema (mes″o-blas-tēm′ah) the cells composing the mesoblast.

mesobronchitis (-brong-kīt′is) inflammation of middle coat of bronchi.

mesocardia (-kar′de-ah) atypical location of the heart, with the apex in the midline of the thorax.

mesocardium (-kar′de-um) that part of the embryonic mesentery connecting the heart with the body wall in front and the foregut behind.

mesocecum (-se′kum) the occasionally occurring mesentery of the cecum.

mesocephalon (-sef′ah-lon) the midbrain.

mesocolon (-kōl′on) the peritoneal process attaching the colon to the posterior abdominal wall, and called ascending, descending, etc., according to the portion of colon to which it attaches. **mesocol′ic,** adj.

mesocolopexy (-kōl′o-pek″se) suspension or fixation of the mesocolon.

mesocoloplication (-kōl″o-pli-ka′shin) plication of the mesocolon to limit its mobility.

mesocord (mes′o-kord) an umbilical cord adherent to the placenta.

mesoderm (-derm) the middle of the three primary germ layers of the embryo, lying between the ectoderm and entoderm; from it are derived the connective tissue, bone, cartilage, muscle, blood and blood vessels, lymphatics, lymphoid organs, notochord, pleura, pericardium, peritoneum, kidneys, and gonads. **mesoder′mal, mesoder′mic,** adj.

mesodiastolic (mes″o-di″ah-stol′ik) pertaining to the middle of the diastole.

mesoduodenum (-doo″o-de′num) the mesenteric fold enclosing the duodenum of the early fetus.

mesoepididymis (-ep″ĭ-did′ĭ-mis) a fold of tunica vaginalis sometimes connecting the epididymis and testis.

mesogastrium (-gas′tre-um) the portion of the primitive mesentery which encloses the stomach and from which the greater omentum develops. **mesogas′tric,** adj.

mesoglia (me-sog′le-ah) 1. microglia. 2. oligodendroglia.

mesogluteus (mes″o-glōōt′e-us) gluteus medius muscle; *see Table of Muscles.* **mesoglu′teal,** adj.

mesoileum (mes″o-il′e-um) the mesentery of the ileum.

mesojejunum (-jĕ-joo′num) the mesentery of the jejunum.

mesolymphocyte (-lim′fo-sīt) a medium-sized lymphocyte.

mesomere (mes′o-mēr) 1. a blastomere of size intermediate between a macromere and a micromere. 2. a midzone of the mesoderm between the epimere and hypomere.

mesometrium (mes″o-me′tre-um) the portion of the broad ligament below the mesovarium.

mesomorph (mez′o-morf, mes′o-morf) 1. an individual having the type of body build in which mesodermal tissues predominate: there is relative preponderance of muscle, bone, and connective tissue, usually with heavy, hard physique of rectangular outline. 2. a well-proportioned individual.

meson (me′zon, mes′on) 1. mesion. 2. a subatomic particle having a rest mass intermediate between the mass of the electron and that of the proton, carrying either a positive or a negative electric charge.

mesonephroma (mez″o-nĕ-fro′mah) a malignant tumor of the female genital tract, usually the ovary, formerly thought to arise from mesonephric rests.

mesonephros (-nef′ros), pl. *mesoneph′roi* [Gr.] the excretory organ of the embryo, arising caudad to the pronephric rudiments or the pronephros and using its ducts. **mesoneph′ric,** adj.

mesophile (-fīl) an organism which grows best at 20°–55° C. **mesophil′ic,** adj.

mesophlebitis (mes″o-fle-bīt′is) inflammation of the middle coat of a vein.

mesophryon (mes-of′re-on) the glabella, or its central point.

mesopulmonum (mes″o-pul-mōn′um) the embryonic mesentery enclosing the laterally expanding lung.

mesorchium (mes-or′ke-um) the portion of the primitive mesentery enclosing the fetal testis, represented in the adult by a fold between the testis and epididymis. **mesor′chial,** adj.

mesorectum (mes″o-rek′tum) the fold of peritoneum connecting the upper portion of the rectum with the sacrum.

mesoridazine (-rid′ah-zēn) a member of the phenothiazine group, $C_{21}H_{26}N_2OS_2$, used as a major tranquilizer.

mesosalpinx (mes″o-sal′pinks) the portion of the broad ligament above the mesovarium.

mesosigmoid (-sig′moid) the peritoneal fold attaching the sigmoid flexure to the posterior abdominal wall.

mesosigmoidopexy (-sig-moid′ah-pek″se) fixation of the mesosigmoid for prolapse of the rectum.

mesosome (mes′o-sōm) an invagination of the bacterial cell membrane, forming organelles thought to be the site of cytochrome enzymes and the enzymes of oxidative phosphorylation and the citric acid cycle.

mesosternum (mes″o-stern′um) corpus sterni.

mesotendineum (-ten-din′e-um) the connective tissue sheath attaching a tendon to its fibrous sheath.

mesothelium (-thēl′e-um) the layer of cells, derived from mesoderm, lining the body cavity of the embryo; in the adult, it forms the simple squamous epithelium that covers all true serous membranes (peritoneum, pericardium, pleura). **mesothe'lial,** adj.

mesotympanum (-tim'pah-num) the portion of the middle ear medial to the tympanic membrane.

mesovarium (-vār'e-um) the portion of the broad ligament between the mesometrium and mesosalpinx, which encloses and holds the ovary in place.

Mesozoa (-zo'ah) a small group of tiny parasites whose relationship to the Protozoa and Metazoa is uncertain.

mestranol (mes'trah-nōl) an estrogenic agent, $C_{21}H_{26}O_2$, used in combination with various progestogens as an oral contraceptive.

mesylate (mes'ĭ-lāt) USAN contraction for methanesulfonate.

meta- word element [Gr.], (1) *change; transformation; exchange;* (2) *after; next;* (3) the 1,3-position in derivatives of benzene.

metabasis (mĕ-tab'ah-sis) a change in the manifestations or course of a disease.

metabiosis (met"ah-bi-o'sis) dependence of one organism upon another for its existence; commensalism.

metabolism (mĕ-tab'o-lizm) the sum of all the physical and chemical processes by which living organized substance is produced and maintained (anabolism), and also the transformation by which energy is made available for the uses of the organism (catabolism). **metabol'ic,** adj. **basal m.,** the minimal energy expended to maintain respiration, circulation, peristalsis, muscle tonus, body temperature, glandular activity, and the other vegetative functions of the body. **inborn error of m.,** a genetically determined biochemical disorder in which a specific enzyme defect causes a metabolic block that may have pathologic consequences at birth or in later life.

metabolite (mĕ-tab'ah-līt) any substance produced by metabolism or by a metabolic process.

metacarpal (met"ah-kar'pil) 1. pertaining to the metacarpus. 2. a bone of the metacarpus.

metacarpus (-kar'pus) the part of the hand between the wrist and fingers, its skeleton being five bones (metacarpals) extending from the carpus to the phalanges.

metacentric (-sen'trik) having the centromere near the middle, so that the arms of the replicating chromosome are approximately equal in length.

metacercaria (-ser-ka're-ah), pl. *metacerca'riae.* The encysted resting or maturing stage of a trematode parasite in the tissues of an intermediate host or on vegetation.

metachromasia (-kro-ma'ze-ah) 1. failure to stain true with a given stain. 2. the different coloration of different tissues produced by the same stain. 3. change of color produced by staining. **metachromat'ic,** adj.

metachromophil (-kro'mah-fil) not staining in the usual manner with a given stain.

metachrosis (-kro'sis) change of color in animals.

metacone (met'ah-kōn) the distobuccal cusp of an upper molar tooth.

metaconid (met"ah-kōn'id) the mesiolingual cusp of a lower molar tooth.

metagenesis (-jen'ĭ-sis) alternation of generations; alternation in regular sequence of asexual with sexual reproductive methods, as in certain fungi.

Metagonimus (-gon'ĭ-mus) a genus of trematodes, including *M. yokoga'wai,* which is parasitic in the small intestine of man and mammals in Japan, China, Indonesia, the Balkans, and Israel.

metal (met'l) any element marked by luster, malleability, ductility, and conductivity of electricity and heat and which will ionize positively in solution. **metal'lic,** adj. **alkali m.,** any of a group of monovalent metals, including lithium, sodium, potassium, rubidium, and cesium.

metalloenzyme (mĕ-tal"o-en'zīm) any enzyme containing tightly bound metal atoms, e.g., the cytochromes.

metalloporphyrin (mĕ-tal"o-por'fĭ-rin) a combination of a metal with porphyrin, as in heme.

metalloprotein (-prōt'e-in, -pro'tēn) a protein molecule bound to a metal ion, e.g., hemoglobin.

metallurgy (me'al-urj-e) the science and art of using metals.

metamere (-mēr) one of a series of homologous segments of the body of an animal. In genetic theory, one of a varying number of common repeating units that make up the repressor segment of a chromosome segment.

metamorphosis (-mor'fah-sis) change of structure or shape, particularly, transition from one developmental stage to another, as from larva to adult form. **metamor'phic,** adj. **fatty m.,** any normal or pathologic transformation of fat.

metamyelocyte (-mi"il-o-sīt") a precursor in the granulocytic series, being a cell intermediate in development between a promyelocyte and the mature, segmented (polymorphonuclear) granular leukocyte, and having a U-shaped nucleus.

metanephrine (met"ah-nef'rin) a metabolite of epinephrine excreted in urine and found in certain tissues.

metanephros (-nef'ros), pl. *metaneph'roi* [Gr.] the permanent embryonic kidney, developing later than and caudad to the mesonephros. **metaneph'ric,** adj.

metaphase (met'ah-fāz) the second stage of cell division (mitosis or meiosis), in which the chromosomes, each consisting of two chromatids, are arranged in the equatorial plane of the spindle prior to separation.

metaphosphoric acid (met"ah-fos-for'ik) a polymer of phosphoric acid, $H(HPO_3)_x$ OH.

metaphysis (mĕ-taf'ĭ-sis), pl. *metaph'yses* [Gr.] the wider part at the end of the shaft of a long bone, adjacent to the epiphyseal disk. **metaphys'eal,** adj.

metaplasia (met"ah-pla'ze-ah) the change in the type of adult cells in a tissue to a form abnormal for that tissue. **metaplas'tic,** adj. **myeloid m., agnogenic,** a condition characterized by foci of extramedullary hematopoiesis and by spleno-megaly, immature blood cells in the peripheral blood, and mild to moderate anemia.

metaplasm (met'ah-plazm) deuteroplasm.

metapneumonic (met"ah-noo-mon'ik) succeeding or following pneumonia.

metaproterenol (-pro-tĕ'rĭ-nōl) a bronchodilator, $(C_{11}H_{17}NO_3)_2$, used as the sulfate salt.

metapsychology (-si-kol'ah-je) the branch of speculative psychology that deals with the significance of mental processes that are beyond empirical verification.

metaraminol (-ram'ĭ-nol) a sympathomimetic and pressor agent, $C_9H_{13}NO_2$.

metarubricyte (-roo"brĭ-sīt) orthochromatic normoblast.

metastasis (mě-tas'tah-sis) 1. transfer of disease from one organ or part of the body to another not directly connected with it, due either to transfer of pathogenic microorganisms or to transfer of cells; all malignant tumors are capable of metastasizing. 2. (pl. *metas'tases*) a growth of pathogenic microorganisms or of abnormal cells distant from the site primarily involved by the morbid process. **metastat'ic**, adj.

metatarsal (met"ah-tar'sil) 1. pertaining to the metatarsus. 2. a bone of the metatarsus.

metatarsalgia (-tar-sal'je-ah) pain and tenderness in the metarsal region.

metatarsus (-tar'sus) the part of the foot between the ankle and the toes, its skeleton being the five bones (metatarsals) extending from the tarsus to the phalanges.

metathalamus (-thal'ah-mus) the part of the diencephalon composed of the medial and lateral geniculate bodies; often considered to be part of the thalamus.

metathesis (mĭ-tath'ĭ-sis) 1. artificial transfer of a morbid process. 2. a chemical reaction in which an element or radical in one compound exchanges places with another element or radical in another compound.

metatrophic (met"ah-trof'ik) utilizing organic matter for food.

metaxalone (mĭ-taks'ah-lōn) a smooth muscle relaxant, $C_{12}H_{15}NO_3$.

Metazoa (met"ah-zo'ah) that division of the animal kingdom embracing the multicellular animals whose cells differentiate to form tissues, i.e., all animals except the Protozoa. **metazo'al, metazo'an,** adj.

metazoon (-zo'on), pl. *metazo'a* [Gr.] an individual organism of the Metazoa.

metencephalon (met"en-sef'ah-lon) [Gr.] 1. the anterior part of the hindbrain, comprising the cerebellum and pons. 2. the anterior of two brain vesicles formed by specialization of the hindbrain in embryonic development.

meteorism (mēt'e-ah-rizm") tympanites.

meteorotropism (mēt"e-o-rah'trah-pizm) response to influence by meteorologic factors noted in certain biological events. **meteorotrop'ic**, adj.

meter (mēt'er) 1. the basic unit of linear measure of the metric system, equal to 39.371 inches. 2.

an apparatus to measure the quantity of anything passing through it.

-meter word element [Gr.], *relationship to measurement; instrument for measuring.*

methacrylate (meth-ak'rĭ-lāt) an acrylic resin widely used in denture bases and as an adhesive for joint prostheses.

methacycline (meth"ah-si'klēn) a semisynthetic tetracycline derivative; its hydrochloride is used as an oral broad-spectrum antibiotic.

methadone (meth'ah-dōn) a synthetic compound, $C_{21}H_{27}NO$, with pharmacologic action similar to that of morphine and heroin, and almost equal in addiction liability; the hydrochloride is used as an antitussive and analgesic and as a substitute narcotic in the management of heroin addiction.

methamphetamine (meth"-am-fet'ah-mēn) a central nervous system stimulant and pressor substance, $C_{10}H_{15}N$, used as the hydrochloride salt. Abuse may lead to dependence.

methandrostenolone (meth-an"dro-sten'ah-lōn) an anabolic steroid with androgenic effects, $C_{20}H_{28}O_2$.

methane (meth'ān) an inflammable, explosive gas, CH_4, from decomposition of organic matter.

methanogen (meth'ah-nah-jen") an anaerobic microorganism that grows in the presence of carbon dioxide and produces methane gas. Methanogens are found in the stomach of cows, in swamp mud, and in other environments in which oxygen is not present.

methanol (meth'ah-nol) a clear, colorless, flammable liquid, CH_3OH, used as a solvent.

methantheline (mě-than'thě-lin) an anticholinergic, $C_{21}H_{26}NO$, used to depress gastric activity.

methapyrilene (meth"ah-pir"ĭ-lēn) an antihistaminic, $C_{14}H_{19}N_3S$, with sedative action; the hydrochloride salt is used in the treatment of allergic disorders and insomnia, and as a local anesthetic.

methaqualone (kwa'lōn) a hypnotic, $C_{16}H_{14}$-N_2O.

metharbital (meth-ar'bit-al) an anticonvulsant, $C_9H_{14}N_2O_3$, used in controlling myoclonic seizures and in conditions due to organic brain damage.

methdilazine (-di'lah-zēn) an antihistaminic, $C_{18}H_{20}N_2S$.

methemalbumin (met"hem-al-bu'min) a brownish pigment formed in the blood by the binding of albumin with heme; indicative of intravascular hemolysis.

methemoglobin (met-he"mah-glo'bin) a compound formed from hemoglobin by oxidation of the iron atom from the ferrous to the ferric state. A small amount of methemoglobin is present in the blood normally, but injury or toxic agents convert a larger proportion of hemoglobin into methemoglobin, which does not function as an oxygen carrier.

methenamine (meth"en-am'in) an antibacterial, $C_6H_{12}N_4$, used in urinary tract infections. **m. mandelate,** a salt of methenamine and mandelic acid, used in infections of the urinary tract.

methicillin (meth″ĭ-sil′in) a semisynthetic penicillin highly resistant to inactivation by penicillinase; its sodium salt is used parenterally.

methimazole (meth-im′ah-zōl) a thyroid inhibitor, $C_4H_6N_2S$.

methionine (mĕ-thi′ah-nēn) a naturally occurring amino acid, $C_5H_{11}NO_2S$, which is an essential component of the diet, furnishing both methyl groups and sulfur necessary for normal metabolism.

methixene (mĕ-thiks′ēn) a smooth muscle relaxant, $C_{20}H_{23}NS$, used as the hydrochloride salt.

methocarbamol (meth″ah-kar′bah-mol) a skeletal muscle relaxant, $C_{11}H_{15}NO_5$.

method (meth′id) the manner of performing any act or operation; a procedure or technique.

methodology (meth″id-ol′ah-je) the science of method; the science dealing with principles of procedure in research and study.

methohexital (-hek′sit-al) an ultrashort-acting barbiturate; its sodium salt, $C_{14}H_{17}N_2NaO_3$, is used intravenously as a general anesthetic.

methotrexate (-trek′sāt) a folic acid antagonist, $C_{20}H_{22}N_8O_5$, used as an antineoplastic agent.

methotrimeprazine (-tri-mep′rah-zēn) an analgesic, $C_{19}H_{24}N_2OS$, given intramuscularly.

methoxamine (mĕ-thok′sah-mēn) an adrenergic vasopressor, $C_{11}H_{17}NO_3$, used as the hydrochloride salt.

methoxsalen (mĕ-thok′sah-len) an acrylic acid compound, $C_{12}H_8O_4$, which induces melanin production on exposure of the skin to ultraviolet light; used in the treatment of idiopathic vitiligo and as a suntan accelerator and protectant.

methoxyflurane (mĕ-thok″se-floor′ān) a general inhalation anesthetic, $C_3H_4Cl_2F_2O$.

methoxyphenamine (-fen′ah-mēn) a sympathomimetic, $C_{11}H_{17}NO$, used as a bronchodilator and nasal decongestant in the form of the hydrochloride salt.

methscopolamine bromide (meth″skah-pol′ah-min) an anticholinergic, $C_{18}H_{24}BrNO_4$.

methsuximide (meth-suk′sĭ-mīd) an anticonvulsant, $C_{12}H_{13}NO_2$, used to treat petit mal and psychomotor epilepsy.

methyclothiazide (meth″ĭ-klo-thi′ah-zīd) a diuretic and antihypertensive, $C_9H_{11}Cl_2N_3O_4S_2$.

methyl (meth′il) the chemical group or radical CH_3—. **m. salicylate**, an oily liquid obtained from leaves of *Gaultheria procumbens* or bark of *Betula lenta*, or produced synthetically; used as a flavoring agent and as a topical analgesic in rheumatic disorders, lumbago, and sciatica.

methylamine (meth″il-am′in) a gaseous ptomaine from decaying fish and from cultures of *Vibrio cholerae*.

methylate (meth′ĭ-lāt) 1. a compound of methyl alcohol and a base. 2. to add a methyl group to a substance.

methylbenzethonium (meth″il-ben″zĕ-tho′ne-um) a local anti-infective, $C_{28}H_{44}NO_2$; used as the chloride salt.

methylcellulose (-sel′ūl-ōs) a methyl ester of cellulose; used as a bulk laxative and as a suspending agent for drugs and applied topically to the conjunctiva to protect and lubricate the cornea during certain ophthalmic procedures.

methyldopa (-do′pah) an antihypertensive, $C_{10}H_{13}NO_4$.

methyldopate (-do′pāt) the ethyl ester of methyldopa; its hydrochloride salt is given intravenously as an antihypertensive.

methylene (meth″ĭ-lēn) the divalent hydrocarbon radical CH_2.

methylergonovine (meth″il-urg″o-no′vēn) an oxytocic, $C_{20}H_{25}N_3O_2$, used as the maleate salt.

methylglucamine (-gloo′kah-mēn) meglumine.

methylphenidate (-fen′ĭ-dāt) a central stimulant, $C_{14}H_{19}NO_2$; used in the treatment of hyperkinetic children, various types of depressions, and narcolepsy.

methylprednisolone (-pred-nis′ah-lōn) a glucocorticoid, $C_{22}H_{30}O_5$, with anti-inflammatory activity slightly greater than prednisolone; also used as the 21-acetate ester and sodium succinate salt.

methyltestosterone (-tes-tos′ter-ōn) a synthetic androgenic hormone with actions and uses similar to those of testosterone.

methyltransferase (-trans′fer-ās) any enzyme that catalyzes transmethylation.

methyprylon (meth″ĭ-pri′lon) a sedative, $C_{10}H_{17}NO_2$.

methysergide (-sur′jĭd) a potent serotonin antagonist used in prophylaxis of migraine; also available as the maleate salt.

metmyoglobin (met-mi″ah-glo′bin) a compound formed from myoglobin by oxidation of the ferrous to the ferric state.

metocurine iodide (met″o-kūr′ēn) a skeletal muscle relaxant, $C_{40}H_{48}I_2N_2O_6$.

metolazone (mĕ-tōl′ah-zōn) a diuretic, saluretic, and antihypertensive, $C_{16}H_{16}ClN_3O_3S$; used in the treatment of hypertension and edema.

metopic (mĕ-top′ik) pertaining to the forehead.

metopion (mĕ-to′pe-on) glabella.

metoprolol (mĕ-to′prol-ōl) an antiadrenergic, $C_{15}H_{25}NO_3$, which is chiefly a beta₁ blocker; used in the treatment of hypertension.

metoxenous (mĕ-tok′si-nus) requiring two hosts for the life cycle; said of parasites.

metr(o)- word element [Gr.], *uterus*.

metra (me′trah) the uterus.

metratonia (me″trah-to′ne-ah) uterine atony.

metratrophia (-tro′fe-ah) atrophy of the uterus.

metrectopia (me″trek-to′pe-ah) uterine displacement.

metreurynter (me″troo-rin′ter) an inflatable bag for dilating the cervical canal.

metreurysis (me-troor′ĭ-sis) dilation of the cervix uteri by means of the metreurynter.

metric (mĕ′trik) 1. pertaining to measures or measurement. 2. having the meter as a basis.

metritis (me-trīt′is) inflammation of the uterus.

metrizamide (mĕ-triz′ah-mīd) a nonionic, water-soluble, iodinated radiographic contrast medium, $C_{18}H_{22}I_3N_3O_8$, used in myelography and cisternography.

metrocele (me′tro-sēl) hernia of the uterus.

metrocolpocele (me″tro-kol′pah-sēl) hernia of uterus with prolapse into the vagina.

metrocystosis (-sis-to′sis) formation of cysts in the uterus.

metrocyte (me′tro-sīt) a mother cell.

metrodynia (me″tro-din′e-ah) metralgia.

metroleukorrhea (-loo″kah-re′ah) leukorrhea of uterine origin.

metromalacia (-mah-la′she-ah) abnormal softening of the uterus.

metronidazole (-ni′dah-zōl) an antitrichomonal and antiamebic, $C_6H_9N_3O_3$.

metroparalysis (-pah-ral′ĭ-sis) paralysis of the uterus.

metropathia (-path′e-ah) metropathy. **m. hemorrha′gica,** essential uterine hemorrhage.

metropathy (me-trop′ah-the) any uterine disease or disorder. **metropath′ic,** adj.

metroperitonitis (me″tro-per″ĭ-ton-it′is) inflammation of the peritoneum about the uterus.

metrophlebitis (-flĕ-bīt′is) inflammation of the uterine veins.

metroptosis (me″trop-to′sis) downward displacement, or prolapse of the uterus.

metrorrhagia (-ra′je-ah) uterine bleeding, usually of normal amount, occurring at completely irregular intervals, the period of flow sometimes being prolonged.

metrorrhea (-re′ah) a free or abnormal uterine discharge.

metrosalpingography (-sal″ping-gog′rah-fe) hysterosalpingography.

metrostaxis (me″tro-stak′sis) slight but persistent uterine bleeding.

metrostenosis (-stĕ-no′sis) contraction or stenosis of the uterine cavity.

-metry word element [Gr.], *measurement.*

metyrapone (mĕ-tēr′ah-pōn) a synthetic compound, $C_{14}H_{14}N_2O$, that selectively inhibits an enzyme responsible for the biosynthesis of corticosteroids; it is used as a diagnostic aid for determination of hypothalamicopituitary-adrenocortical reserve.

MeV, Mev. megaelectron volt.

μF microfarad.

Mg chemical symbol, *magnesium.*

mg. milligram.

μg. microgram.

MHC major histocompatibility complex.

mho (mo) siemens.

MHz megahertz.

mication (mi-ka′shin) a quick motion, such as winking.

miconazole (mĭ-kon′ah-zōl) an antifungal agent, $C_{18}H_{14}Cl_4N_2O$, used against tinea pedis, tinea cruris, tinea corpora, tinea versicolor, and cutaneous and vulvovaginal candidiasis.

micr(o)- word element [Gr.], *small;* used in naming units of measurement to designate an amount 10^{-6} (one millionth) the size of the unit to which it is joined, e.g., microgram.

micracoustic (mi″krah-koos′tik) 1. rendering very faint sounds audible. 2. an instrument for rendering faint sounds audible.

micrencephaly (mi″kren-sef′ah-le) abnormal smallness and underdevelopment of the brain.

microadenoma (-ad″in-o′mah) an adenoma, as of the anterior pituitary gland, less than 10 mm. in diameter.

microaerophilic (-a″er-o-fil′ik) requiring oxygen for growth but at lower concentration than is present in the atmosphere; said of bacteria.

microaggregate (-ag′rĭ-gat) a microscopic collection of particles, as of platelets, leukocytes, and fibrin, that occurs in stored blood.

microanalysis (-ah-nal′ĭ-sis) the chemical analysis of minute quantities of material.

microanatomy (-ah-nat′ah-me) histology.

microaneurysm (-an′ūr-izm) a microscopic aneurysm, a characteristic of thrombotic purpura.

microangiopathy (-an″je-op′ah-the) disease of the small blood vessels. **microangiopath′ic,** adj. **thrombotic m.,** formation of thrombi in the arterioles and capillaries.

microbe (mi′krōb) a microorganism, especially a pathogenic bacterium. **micro′bial, micro′bic,** adj.

microbicide (mi-kro′bĭ-sīd) an agent that destroys microbes.

microbiology (-bi-ol′ah-je) the science dealing with the study of microorganisms. **microbiolog′ical,** adj.

microbiophotometer (-bi″o-fo-tom′it-er) an instrument for measuring the growth of bacterial cultures by the turbidity of the medium.

microbiota (-bi-ōt′ah) the microscopic living organisms of a region. **microbiot′ic,** adj.

microblast (mi′kro-blast) an erythroblast of 5 microns or less in diameter.

microblepharia (mi″kro-blĕ-fār′e-ah) abnormal shortness of the vertical dimensions of the eyelids.

microbody (mi′kro-bod″e) any of the membrane-bound, ovoid or spherical, granular cytoplasmic particles containing enzymes and other substances, which originate in the endoplasmic reticulum of vertebrate liver and kidney cells and other cells, and in protozoa, yeast, and many cell types of higher plants.

microburet (-būr-et′) a buret with a capacity of the order of 0.1 to 10 ml., with graduated intervals of 0.001 to 0.02 ml.

microcalix, microcalyx (-kal′iks) a very small renal calix arising by caliceal branching, usually at the side of a calix of normal size.

microcardia (-kar′de-ah) abnormal smallness of the heart.

microcheilia (-ki′le-ah) abnormal smallness of the lip.

microcheiria (-ki′re-ah) abnormal smallness of the hands.

microchemistry (-kem′is-tre) chemistry concerned with exceedingly small quantities of chemical substances.

microcinematography (-sin″ĭ-mah-tog′rah-fe) moving picture photography of microscopic objects.

microcirculation (-sur″kūl-a′shin) the flow of blood through the fine vessels (arterioles, capillaries, and venules). **microcirculato′ry,** adj.

Micrococcaceae (-kok-a′se-e) a family of gram-positive, aerobic or facultatively anaerobic bacteria of the order Eubacteriales, made up of spherical cells dividing primarily in two or three planes.

Micrococcus (-kok′us) a genus of gram-positive bacteria (family Micrococcaceae) found in soil, water, etc.

micrococcus (-kok′us), pl. *micrococ′ci.* 1. an organism of the genus *Micrococcus.* 2. a very small, spherical microorganism.

microcoria (-kor′e-ah) smallness of the pupil.

microcrystalline (-kris′tah-lin) made up of minute crystals.

microcurie (-kūr′e) one millionth (10⁻⁶) curie; abbreviated μC.

microcurie-hour (mi′kro-kūr″e-owr″) a unit of exposure equivalent to that obtained by exposure for one hour to radioactive material disintegrating at the rate of 3.7×10^4 atoms per second; abbreviated μChr.

microcyte (-sīt) an erythrocyte 5 microns or less in diameter.

microcytotoxicity (-si″to-tok-sis′it-e) the capability of lysing or damaging cells as detected in procedures (e.g., lymphocytotoxicity procedures) using extremely minute amounts of material.

microdetermination (-de-tur″mi′na-shin) chemical examination of minute quantities of substance.

microdissection (-di-sek′shin) dissection of tissue or cells under the microscope.

microdrepanocytic (-drep″ah-no-sit′ik) containing microcytic and drepanocytic elements.

microenvironment (-in-vi′rin-mint) the environment at the microscopic or cellular level.

microerythrocyte (-ĕ-rith′rah-sīt) microcyte.

microfarad (-far′ad) one millionth (10⁻⁶) farad; symbol μF.

microfauna (-faw′nah) the microscopic animal organisms of a special region.

microfilament (-fil′ah-mint) any of the submicroscopic filaments composed chiefly of actin, found in the cytoplasmic matrix of almost all cells, often with the microtubules.

microfilaria (-fi-la′re-ah), pl. *microfila′riae* [L.] the prelarval stage of Filarioidea in the blood of man and in the tissues of the vector; sometimes incorrectly used as a genus name.

microflora (-flor′ah) the microscopic vegetable organisms of a special region.

microgamete (-gam′ēt) the smaller, actively motile male gamete which fertilizes the macrogamete in anisogamy.

microgametocyte (-gah-mēt′ah-sīt) 1. a cell that produces microgametes. 2. the male gametocyte of certain Sporozoa, such as malarial plasmodia.

microglia (mi-krog′le-ah) non-neural cells forming part of the adventitial structure of the central nervous system. They are migratory and act as phagocytes to waste products. **micro-g′lial,** adj.

microgliocyte (mi-krog′le-o-sīt) a precursor of a microglial cell.

microglobulin (-glob′ūl-in) any globulin, or any fragment of a globulin, of low molecular weight.

micrognathia (-nath′e-ah) unusual smallness of the jaws, especially the lower jaw. **micrognath′ic,** adj.

microgonioscope (-go′ne-o-skōp) a gonioscope with a magnifying lens.

microgram (mi′kro-gram) one millionth (10⁻⁶) gram; abbreviated μg. or mcg.

micrograph (-graf) 1. an instrument used to record very minute movements by making a greatly magnified photograph of the minute motions of a diaphragm. 2. a photograph of a minute object or specimen as seen through a microscope.

microgyria (mi″kro-ji′re-ah) polymicrogyria.

microgyrus (-ji′rus), pl. *microgy′ri.* An abnormally small, malformed convolution of the brain.

microincineration (mi″kro-in-sin″er-a′shin) the oxidation of a small quantity of material, for identification from the ash of the elements composing it.

microinfarct (-in-farkt) a very small infarct due to obstruction of circulation in capillaries, arterioles, or small arteries.

microinjector (-in-jek′ter) an instrument for infusion of very small amounts of fluids or drugs.

microinvasion (-in-va′zhin) microscopic extension of malignant cells into adjacent tissue in carcinoma in situ. **microinva′sive,** adj.

microliter (-lēt″er) one millionth (10⁻⁶) liter; abbreviated μl.

microlithiasis (mi″kro-li-thi′ah-sis) the formation of minute concretions in an organ. **m. alveola′ris pulmo′num, pulmonary alveolar m.,** a condition due to deposition of minute calculi in the pulmonary alveoli, appearing radiographically as fine, sandlike mottling.

micromanipulator (-mah-nip′ūl-āt-er) an instrument for the moving, dissecting, etc., of minute specimens under the microscope.

micromere (mi′kro-mēr) one of the small blastomeres formed by unequal cleavage of a fertilized ovum (at the animal pole).

micrometer¹ (mi-krom′it-er) an instrument for measuring objects seen through the microscope.

micrometer² (mi′kro-mēt″er) micron; one thousandth (10⁻³) of a millimeter or one millionth (10⁻⁶) of a meter. Abbreviated μm.

micromethod (-meth″id) any technique dealing with exceedingly small quantities of material.

micromicro- word element designating 10⁻¹² (one trillionth); now supplanted by *pico-.*

micromyelia (-mi-ēl′e-ah) abnormal smallness of the spinal cord.

micromyeloblast (-mi′il-o-blast) a small, immature myelocyte. **micromyeloblas′tic,** adj.

micron (mi′kron) micrometer; one thousandth (10⁻³) of a millimeter or one millionth (10⁻⁶) of a meter; abbreviated μ.

microneedle (mi″kro-ne′d′l) a fine glass needle used in micromanipulation.

microneurosurgery (-nōōr″o-sur′jĕ-re) surgery conducted under high magnification with miniaturized instruments on microscopic vessels and structures of the nervous system.

micronucleus (-noo′kle-us) 1. in ciliate protozoa, the smaller of two types of nucleus in each cell, which functions in sexual reproduction; cf. *macronucleus*. 2. a small nucleus. 3. nucleolus.

microorganism (-or′gah-nizm) a microscopic organism; those of medical interest include bacteria, rickettsiae, viruses, fungi, and protozoa.

micropathology (-pah-thol′ah-je) 1. the sum of what is known about minute pathologic change. 2. pathology of diseases caused by microorganisms.

microperfusion (-per-fu′zhin) perfusion of a minute amount of a substance.

microphage (mi′kro-fāj) a small phagocyte; an actively motile neutrophilic leukocyte capable of phagocytosis.

microphakia (mi″kro-fa′ke-ah) abnormal smallness of the crystalline lens.

microphone (mi′krah-fōn) a device to pick up sound for amplification or transmission.

microphonic (-fon′ik) 1. serving to amplify sound. 2. cochlear m. **cochlear m.,** any of the electrical potentials generated in the hair cells of the organ of Corti in response to acoustic stimulation.

microphotograph (-fōt′ah-graf) a photograph of small size.

microphthalmos (mi″krof-thal′mus) abnormal smallness in all dimensions of one or both eyes.

micropinocytosis (mi″kro-pi″no-si-to′sis) the taking up into a cell of specific macromolecules by invagination of the plasma membrane which is then pinched off, resulting in small vesicles in the cytoplasm.

micropipet (-pi-pet′) a pipet for handling small quantities of liquids (up to 1 ml.).

microplethysmography (-pleth″is-mog′rah-fe) the recording of minute changes in the size of a part as produced by circulation of blood.

microprobe (mi′kro-prōb″) a minute probe, as one used in microsurgery.

micropsia (mi-krop′se-ah) a visual disorder in which objects appear smaller than their actual size.

micropyle (mi′kro-pīl) an opening in the investing membrane of certain ova, through which a spermatozoon enters.

microradiography (mi″kro-ra″de-og′rah-fe) radiography under conditions which permit subsequent microscopic examination or enlargement of the radiograph up to several hundred linear magnifications.

microrefractometer (-re″frak-tom′it-er) a refractometer for the discernment of variations in minute structures.

microrespirometer (-res″pi-rom′it-er) an apparatus to investigate oxygen usage in isolated tissues.

microscope (mi′krah-skōp) an instrument used to obtain an enlarged image of small objects and reveal details of structure not otherwise distinguishable. **acoustic m.,** one using very high frequency ultrasound waves, which are focused on the object; the reflected beam is con-

verted to an image by electronic processing. **binocular m.,** one with two eyepieces, permitting use of both eyes. **compound m.,** one consisting of two lens systems. **corneal m.,** one with a lens of high magnifying power, for observing minute changes in the cornea and iris. **darkfield m.,** one designed to permit diversion of light rays and illumination from the side, so that details appear light against a dark background. **electron m.,** one in which an electron beam, instead of light, forms an image for viewing on a fluorescent screen, or for photography. **fluorescence m.,** one used for the examination of specimens stained with fluorochromes or fluorochrome complexes, e.g., a fluorescein-labeled antibody, which fluoresces in ultraviolet light. **infrared m.,** one in which radiation of 800 nm. or longer wavelength is used as the image-forming energy. **light m.,** one in which the specimen is viewed under visible light. **phase m., phase-contrast m.,** one altering the phase relationships of the light passing through and that passing around the object, the contrast permitting visualization without the necessity of staining or other special preparation. **scanning m., scanning electron m.,** an electron microscope in which a beam of electrons scans over a specimen point by point and builds up an image on the fluorescent screen of a cathode ray tube. **simple m.,** one consisting of a single lens. **slit lamp m.,** a corneal microscope with a special attachment that permits examination of the endothelium on the posterior surface of the cornea. **stereoscopic m.,** a binocular microscope modified to give a three-dimensional view of the specimen. **ultraviolet m.,** one that utilizes reflecting optics or quartz and other ultraviolet-transmitting lenses. **x-ray m.,** one in which x-rays are used instead of light, the image usually being reproduced on film.

microsecond (mi′kro-sek″ind) one millionth (10^{-6}) of a second; abbreviated μs. or μsec.

microsmatic (mi″kros-mat′ik) having a feebly developed sense of smell, as in man.

microsome (mi′krah-sōm) any of the vesicular fragments of endoplasmic reticulum formed after disruption and centrifugation of cells. **microso′mal,** adj.

microspectroscope (-spek′trah-skōp) a spectroscope and microscope combined.

microspherocyte (-sfēr′ah-sīt) spherocyte.

microspherocytosis (-sfēr″o-si-to′sis) spherocytosis.

microsphygmia (-sfig′me-ah) a pulse that is difficult to perceive by the finger.

microsplenia (-sple′ne-ah) smallness of the spleen.

Microsporon (mi″kro-spor′on) *Microsporum.*

Microsporum (-spor′um) a genus of fungi which cause various diseases of skin and hair, including *M. audoui′ni, M. ca′nis, M. ful′vum,* and *M. gyp′seum.*

Microstix-3 (mi′kro-stiks) trademark for a reagent strip with a chemical test area for recognition of nitrite in urine, which turns pink on contact with nitrate, and two culture areas for semiquantification of bacterial growth after

18–24 hours of incubation; one culture area supports both gram-negative and gram-positive organisms, the other, only gram-negative organisms.

microsurgery (-sur′jĕ-re) dissection of minute structures under the microscope by means of hand-held instruments.

microsyringe (-sī-rinj′) a syringe fitted with a screw-thread micrometer for accurate measurement of minute quantities.

microtia (mi-kro′she-ah) abnormal smallness of the pinna of the ear.

microtome (mi′krah-tōm) an instrument for cutting thin sections for microscopic study.

microtubule (-too′būl) any of the slender, tubular structures composed chiefly of tubulin, found in the cytoplasmic ground substance of nearly all cells; they are involved in maintenance of cell shape and in the movements of organelles and inclusions, and form the spindle fibers of mitosis.

microvasculature (-vas′kūl-ah-cher) the finer vessels of the body, as the arterioles, capillaries, and venules. **microvas′cular,** adj.

microvillus (-vil′us), pl. *microvil′li.* A minute process from the free surface of a cell, especially cells of the proximal convolution in renal tubules and of the intestinal epithelium.

microvolt (mi′krah-volt) one millionth of a volt; symbol μV.

microwave (-wāv) a wave of electromagnetic radiation between far infrared and radio waves, regarded as extending from 300,000 to 100 megacycles (wavelength of 1 mm. to 30 cm.).

microzoon (mi″kro-zo′on) a microscopic animal organism.

micrurgy (mi-krur′je) manipulative technique in the field of a microscope. **micrur′gic,** adj.

micturate (mik′cher-āt) urinate.

midbrain (mid′brān) mesencephalon; the part of the brain developed from the middle of the three primary brain vesicles, comprising the tectum and the cerebral peduncles and traversed by the aqueduct.

midget (mij′it) a normal dwarf; a person who is undersized but perfectly formed.

midgut (mid′gut) the region of the embryonic digestive tube into which the yolk sac opens; ahead of it is the foregut and caudal to it is the hindgut.

midriff (-rif) the diaphragm; the region between the breast and waistline.

midwife (-wīf) an individual who practices midwifery; see *nurse-midwife.*

migraine (mi′grān, me′grān) a symptom complex of periodic headaches, usually temporal and unilateral, often with irritability, nausea, vomiting, constipation or diarrhea, and photophobia, preceded by constriction of the cranial arteries, usually with resultant prodromal sensory (especially ocular) symptoms, and commencing with the vasodilation that follows. **mi′grainous,** adj. **abdominal m.,** that in which abdominal symptoms are predominant.

migration (mi-gra′shin) 1. an apparently spontaneous change of place, as of symptoms. 2. diapedesis.

mikr(o)- for words beginning thus, see those beginning *micr(o)-.*

mildew (mil′doo) colloquialism for any superficial fungous growth on plants or any organic material.

miliaria (mil″e-a′re-ah) a cutaneous condition with retention of sweat, which is extravasated at different levels in the skin; when used alone, it refers to *m. rubra.* **m. ru′bra,** heat rash; prickly heat; a condition due to obstruction of the ducts of the sweat glands; the sweat escapes into the epidermis, producing pruritic red papulovesicles.

miliary (mil′e-er″e) 1. like millet seeds. 2. characterized by lesions resembling millet seeds.

milium (mil′e-um), pl. *mi′lia* [L.] a tiny, spheroidal, white epithelial cyst lying superficially within the skin usually of the face, containing lamellated keratin and often associated with vellus hair follicles.

milk (milk) 1. the fluid secretion of the mammary gland forming the natural food of young mammals. 2. any whitish milklike substance, e.g., coconut milk or plant latex. 3. a liquid (emulsion or suspension) resembling the secretion of the mammary gland. **acidophilus m.,** milk fermented with cultures of *Lactobacillus acidophilus;* used in gastrointestinal disorders to modify the bacterial flora of the intestinal tract. **certified m.,** milk whose purity is certified by a committee of physicians or a medical milk commission. **condensed m.,** milk partly evaporated and sweetened with sugar. **m. of magnesia,** a suspension containing 7–8.5 per cent of magnesium hydroxide; used as an antacid and cathartic. **modified m.,** cow's milk made to correspond to the composition of human milk. **vitamin D m.,** cow's milk fortified by addition of vitamin D. **witch's m.,** milk secreted in the breast of the newborn infant.

milking (milk′ing) the pressing out of the contents of a tubular structure by running the finger along it.

milkpox (-poks) variola minor.

milli- word element [L.], *one thousandth;* used in naming units of measurement to designate an amount 10^{-3} the size of the unit to which it is joined, e.g., milligram.

milliamperage (mil″e-am′per-ij) in radiography, the x-ray tube current during an exposure, measured in milliamperes.

milliampere (-am′pēr) one thousandth of an ampere.

milliampere-second (-sek′ind) a unit of radiographic exposure equal to the product of the milliamperage and the exposure time in seconds. Abbreviated mAs.

millicurie (mil″ĭ-kūr′e) one thousandth (10^{-3}) curie; abbreviated mC.

milliequivalent (mil″e-e-kwiv′ah-lint) one thousandth (10^{-3}) of a chemical equivalent; abbreviated mEq.

milligram (mil′ĭ-gram) one thousandth (10^{-3}) gram; abbreviated mg.

milliliter (-lēt''er) one thousandth (10^{-3}) liter; abbreviated ml.

millimeter (-mēt''er) one thousandth (10^{-3}) meter; abbreviated mm.

millimicro- word element designating 10^{-9} (one billionth) part of the unit to which it is joined; nano-.

millimole (mil′ĭ-mōl) one thousandth part of a mole; symbol mmol.

milliosmole (mil′′e-os′mōl) one thousandth of an osmole.

millisecond (mil′′ĭ-sek′ond) one thousandth (10^{-3}) of a second; abbreviated ms. or msec.

millivolt (mil′ĭ-volt) one thousandth of a volt; abbreviated mV.

milphosis (mil-fo′sis) the falling out of the eyelashes.

mimesis (mi-me′sis) stimulation of one disease or bodily process by another.

min. minim; minimum; minute.

mind (mīnd) the psyche; the faculty, or brain function, by which one is aware of his surroundings, and by which one experiences feelings, emotions, and desires, and is able to attend, reason, and make decisions.

mineral (min′er-il) any nonorganic homogeneous solid substance of the earth's crust.

mineralocorticoid (min′′er-il-o-kor′tĭ-koid) 1. any of the group of corticosteroids, principally aldosterone, predominately involved in the regulation of electrolyte and water balance through their effect on ion transport in epithelial cells of the renal tubules, resulting in retention of sodium and loss of potassium. Cf. *glucocorticoid.* 2. of, pertaining to, or resembling a mineralocorticoid.

minilaparotomy (min′′ĭ-lap′′ah-rot′ah-me) a small abdominal incision for liver biopsy, open transhepatic cholangiography, or sterilization by tubal occlusion.

minim (min′im) a unit of capacity (liquid measure), being $\frac{1}{60}$ fluid dram, or the equivalent of 0.0616 ml.

Minipress (min′ĭ-pres) trademark for a preparation of prazosin hydrochloride.

Minocin (mĭ-no′sin) trademark for preparations of minocycline hydrochloride.

minocycline (mĭ-no-si′klēn) a semisynthetic broad-spectrum antibiotic of the tetracycline group, $C_{23}H_{27}N_3O_7$.

minoxidil (mi-noks′ĭ-dil) a potent, long-acting vasodilator, $C_9H_{15}N_5O$, acting primarily on arterioles, used as an antihypertensive.

miocardia (mi′′ah-kar′de-ah) systole.

miosis (mi-o′sis) contraction of the pupil.

miotic (mi-ot′ik) 1. pertaining to, characterized by, or producing miosis. 2. an agent that causes contraction of the pupil.

miracidium (mi′′rah-sid′e-um), pl. *miraci′dia* [Gr.] the first stage larva of a trematode which undergoes further development in the body of a snail.

mire (mēr) [Fr.] one of the figures on the arm of an ophthalmometer whose images are reflected on the cornea; measurement of their variations measures the amount of corneal astigmatism.

mirror (mir′er) a polished surface that reflects sufficient light to yield images of objects in front of it. **dental m.,** mouth m. **frontal m., head m.,** a circular mirror strapped to the head of the examiner; used to reflect light into a cavity, especially in nasal, pharyngeal, and laryngeal examinations. **mouth m.,** a small mirror attached at an angle to a handle, for use in dentistry.

misanthropy (mis-an′thrah-pe) hatred of mankind.

miscarriage (mis-kar′ij) loss of the products of conception from the uterus before the fetus is viable; spontaneous abortion.

miscegenation (mis′′ĭ-jĭ-na′shin) intermarriage or interbreeding between persons of different races.

miscible (mis′ĭ-b'l) susceptible of being mixed.

misogamy (mĭ-sog′ah-me) morbid aversion to marriage.

misogyny (mĭ-soj′ĭ-ne) aversion to women.

mite (mīt) any arthropod of the order Acarina except the ticks; they are minute animals, usually transparent or semitransparent, and may be parasitic on man and domestic animals, causing various skin irritations. **harvest m.,** chigger. **itch m., mange m.,** see *Notoedres* and *Sarcoptes.*

mithramycin (mith′′rah-mi′sin) an antineoplastic antibiotic produced by *Streptomyces argillaceus* and *S. tanashiensis.*

mithridatism (mith′rĭ-dāt′′izm) acquisition of immunity to a poison by ingestion of gradually increasing amounts of it.

miticide (mīt′ĭ-sīd) an agent destructive to mites.

mitochondria (mīt′′ah-kon′dre-ah), sing. *mitochon′drion* [Gr.] small, spherical to rod-shaped cytoplasmic organelles, enclosed by two membranes separated by an intramembraneous space; the inner membrane is infolded forming a series of projections (cristae). Mitochondria are the principal sites of ATP synthesis; they contain enzymes of the citric acid cycle and for fatty oxidation, oxidative phosphorylation, and many other biochemical pathways. They contain their own DNA and ribosomes, replicate independently, and synthesize some of their own proteins. **mitochon′drial,** adj.

mitogen (mīt′′ah-jen) a substance that induces mitosis and cell tranformation, especially lymphocyte transformation. **mitogen′ic,** adj.

mitomycin (mīt′′ah-mi′sin) a group of antitumor antibiotics (mitomycin A, B, and C) produced by *Streptomyces caespitosus.*

mitosis (mi-to′sis) a method of indirect cell division in which the two daughter nuclei normally receive identical complements of the number of chromosomes characteristic of the somatic cells of the species. **mitot′ic,** adj.

mitotane (mīt′o-tān) an antineoplastic, $C_{14}H_{10}Cl_4$, used for the treatment of inoperable adrenocortical carcinoma.

mitral (mi′tril) shaped like a miter; pertaining to the mitral valve.

mitralization (mi′′tril-ĭ-za′shin) a straightening of the left border of the cardiac shadow, commonly seen radiographically in mitral stenosis.

mixture (miks'cher) a combination of different drugs or ingredients, as a fluid with other fluids or solids, or of a sclid with a liquid.

Miyagawanella (mi''yah-gah''wah-nel'ah) a genus of organisms, the species of which are now assigned to the genus *Chlamydia* as follows: *M. lymphogranulomato'sis* and *M. bronchopneumo'niae* are assigned to *C. trachomatis,* and *M. bo'vis, M. fe'lis, M. illi'nii, M. louisia'nae, M. opos'sumi, M. ornitho'sis, M. o'vis, M. pe'coris, M. pneumo'niae,* and *M. psit'taci* are assigned to *C. psittaci.*

ml milliliter.

μl microliter.

M.L.A. Medical Library Association.

M.L.D. minimum lethal dose.

mm millimeter.

Mn chemical symbol, *manganese.*

mnemonics (ne-mon'iks) improvement of memory by special methods or techniques. **mnemon'ic,** adj.

M.O. Medical Officer.

Mo chemical symbol, *molybdenum.*

mobilization (mo''bĭ-lĭ-za'shin) the rendering of a fixed part movable. **stapes m.,** surgical correction of immobility of the stapes in treatment of deafness.

modality (mo-dal'it-e) 1. in homeopathy, a condition that modifies drug action; a condition under which symptoms develop, becoming better or worse. 2. a method of application of, or the employment of, any therapeutic agent; limited usually to physical agents. 3. a specific sensory entity, such as taste.

mode (mōd) in statistics, the value or item in a variations curve showing the maximum frequency of occurrence.

modification (mod''i-fĭ-ka'shin) the process or result of changing the form or characteristics of an object or substance. **behavior m.,** see under *therapy.*

modiolus (mo-di'o-lus) the central pillar or columella of the cochlea.

modulation (moj''il-a'shin) the normal capacity of cell adaptability to its environment. **antigenic m.,** the alteration of antigenic determinants in a living cell surface membrane following interaction with antibody.

moiety (moi'it-e) any equal part; a half; also any part or portion, as a portion of a molecule.

mol (mol) mole (3).

molal (mo'lil) containing one mole of solute per kilogram of solvent. NOTE: *molal* refers to the weight of the solvent, *molar* to the volume of solvent.

molality (mo-lal'it-e) the number of moles of a solute per kilogram of pure solvent.

molar (mo'ler) 1. pertaining to a mass; not molecular. 2. adapted for grinding; see under *tooth* and see Plate XV. 3. containing one mole of solute per liter of solution. Cf. *molal.*

molarity (mo-lar'it-e) the number of moles of a solute per liter of solution.

mold (mōld) 1. any of a group of parasitic and saprophytic fungi causing a cottony growth on organic substances; also the deposit or growth produced by such fungi. 2. a form in which an object is shaped, or cast. 3. in dentistry, the shape of an artificial tooth.

molding (mold'ing) the adjusting of the shape and size of the fetal head to the birth canal during labor.

mole (mōl) 1. a fleshy mass formed in the uterus by degeneration or abortive development of an ovum. 2. a nevocytic nevus; also, any pigmented fleshy growth. 3. the amount of a substance that contains as many elementary entities (atoms, ions, molecules, or free radicals) as there are atoms in 12 grams of pure carbon-12, i.e., Avogadro's number, 6.023×10^{23}, of elementary entities; equivalent to the amount of a chemical compound having a mass in grams equal to its molecular weight. **hydatid m., hydatidiform m.,** a condition resulting from deterioration of circulation of the chorionic villi in a pathologic ovum, marked by trophoblastic proliferation and by edematous dissolution and cystic cavitation of the avascular stroma of the villi, which come to resemble grapelike cysts. **pigmented m.,** see under *nevus.*

molecule (mol'ĭ-kūl) a small mass of matter; the smallest amount of a substance which can exist alone; an aggregation of atoms, specifically a chemical combination of two or more atoms forming a specific chemical substance.

molimen (mo-li'men), pl. *molim'ina* [L.] a laborious effort made for the performance of any normal body function, especially that manifested by a variety of unpleasant symptoms preceding or accompanying menstruation.

molindone (mo-lin'dōn) a sedative and tranquilizer, $C_{16}H_{24}N_2O_2$, used for schizophrenia.

mollities (mo-lish'e-ēz) [L.] softness; abnormal softening. **m. os'sium,** osteomalacia.

molluscum (mŏ-lus'kum) 1. any of various skin diseases marked by the formation of soft rounded cutaneous tumors. 2. m. contagiosum. **mollus'cous,** adj. **m. contagio'sum,** a viral skin disease, with firm, round, translucent, crateriform papules containing caseous matter and peculiar capsulated bodies.

molt (mōlt) to shed skin, cuticle, or feathers.

Mol. wt. molecular weight.

molybdate (mo-lib'dāt) any salt of molybdic acid.

molybdenum (mo-lib'dĭ-num) chemical element (*see table*), at. no. 42, symbol Mo.

molybdoprotein (mo-lib''do-prōt'e-in, -pro'tēn) an enzyme containing molybdenum (q.v.).

monad (mo'nad) 1. a single-celled protozoon or coccus. 2. a univalent radical or element. 3. in meiosis, one member of a tetrad.

monarthritis (mon''ar-thrīt'is) inflammation of a single joint.

monarticular (-tik'u-ler) pertaining to a single joint.

monaster (mon-as'ter) the single star-shaped figure at the end of prophase in mitosis.

monathetosis (-ath''ĭ-to'sis) athetosis of one limb.

monatomic (mon''ah-tom'ik) 1. univalent. 2. monobasic. 3. containing one atom.

monecious (mon-e′shus) monoecious.

monesthetic (mon″es-thet′ik) pertaining to or affecting a single sense or sensation.

mongolism (mon′gol-izm) Down's syndrome.

monilethrix (mo-nil′ĭ-thriks) a hereditary condition in which the hairs exhibit marked multiple constrictions, giving a beading effect, and are very brittle.

Monilia (mo-nil′e-ah) *Candida*.

monilial (mo-nil′e-il) pertaining to or caused by *Monilia* (*Candida*).

moniliform (mo-nil′ĭ-form) beaded.

Moniliformis (mo-nil″ĭ-for′mis) a genus of acanthocephalan worms. *M. monilifor′mis*, a parasite of rodents, is an occasional facultative parasite of man.

Monistat (mo′nĭ-stat) trademark for a preparation of miconazole nitrate.

monitor (mon′it-er) 1. to check constantly on a given condition or phenomenon, e.g., blood pressure or heart or respiratory rate. 2. an apparatus by which such conditions can be constantly observed or recorded.

mono- word element [Gr.] *one; single; limited to one part; combined with one atom.*

monoamide (mon″o-am′id) an amide compound with only one amide group.

monoamine (-am′ēn) a molecule containing one amino group, e.g., serotonin, dopamine, and norepinephrine.

monoaminergic (-am″in-ur′jik) of or pertaining to neurons that secrete the monoamine neurotransmitters dopamine, norepinephrine, and serotonin.

monoamniotic (-am″ne-ot′ik) having or developing within a single amniotic cavity; said of monozygotic twins.

monobasic (-ba′sik) having but one atom of replaceable hydrogen.

monoblast (mon′ah-blast) the earliest precursor in the monocytic series, which matures to develop into the promocyte.

monoblepsia (mon″ah-blep′se-ah) 1. a condition in which vision is better when only one eye is used. 2. blindness to all colors but one.

monochorea (-kor-e′ah) chorea affecting only one limb.

monochorionic (-kor″e-on′ik) having or developing in a common chorionic sac; said of monozygotic twins.

monochromatic (-kro-mat′ik) 1. existing in or having only one color. 2. pertaining to or affected by monochromatism. 3. staining with only one dye at a time.

monochromatism (-kro′mah-tizm) complete color blindness; inability to discriminate hues, all colors of the spectrum appearing as neutral grays with varying shades of light and dark. **cone m.,** that in which there is some cone function. **rod m.,** that in which there is complete absence of cone function.

monochromatophil (-kro-mat′ah-fil) 1. stainable with only one kind of stain. 2. any cell or other element taking only one stain.

monoclonal (-klōn″l) derived from a single cell; pertaining to a single clone.

monocular (mon-ok′ūl-er) 1. pertaining to or having only one eye. 2. having only one eyepiece, as in a microscope.

monocyte (mon′ah-sīt) a mononuclear, phagocytic leukocyte, 13μ to 25μ in diameter, with an ovoid or kidney-shaped nucleus, and azurophilic cytoplasmic granules. Formed in the bone marrow from promonocytes, monocytes are transported to tissues, such as the lung and liver, where they develop into macrophages. **monocyt′ic,** adj.

monocytopenia (mon″o-si″to-pe′ne-ah) deficiency of monocytes in the blood.

monodermoma (-durm-o′mah) a tumor developed from one germinal layer.

monoecious (mon-e′shus) having reproductive organs typical of both sexes in a single individual.

monoethanolamine (mon″o-eth″ah-nōl′ah-mēn) a moderately viscous liquid, C_2H_7NO, used as a surfactant.

monoiodotyrosine (-i-o″do-ti′ro-sēn) an iodinated amino acid intermediate in the synthesis of thyroxine and triiodothyronine.

monokine (mon′o-kīn) a general term for soluble mediators of immune responses that are not antibodies or complement components and that are produced by mononuclear phagocytes (monocytes or macrophages).

monolocular (-lok′u-lar) having but one cavity or compartment, as a cyst.

monomania (-ma′ne-ah) psychosis on a single subject or class of subjects.

monomer (mon′ah-mer) a simple molecule of relatively low molecular weight, capable of reacting to form by repetition a dimer, trimer, or polymer.

monomeric (mon″ah-mer′ik) 1. pertaining to a single segment. 2. in genetics, determined by a gene or genes at a single locus. 3. consisting of monomers.

monomolecular (-mo-lek′ūl-er) pertaining to a single molecule or to a layer one molecule thick.

monomorphic (-mor′fik) existing in only one form; maintaining the same form throughout all developmental stages.

mononeuritis (-nōōr-īt′is) inflammation of a single nerve. **m. mul′tiplex,** simultaneous inflammation of individual peripheral nerves at sites remote from one another.

mononuclear (-noo′kle-er) having but one nucleus.

mononucleosis (-noo″kle-o′sis) excess of mononuclear leukocytes (monocytes) in the blood. **cytomegalovirus (CMV) m.,** a syndrome similar to infectious mononucleosis associated with CMV infection. **infectious m.,** an acute infectious disease associated with the Epstein-Barr virus; symptoms include fever, malaise, sore throat, lymphadenopathy, atypical lymphocytes (resembling monocytes) in the peripheral blood, and high titers of agglutinins against sheep cells.

mononucleotide (-noo′kle-ah-tīd″) nucleotide.

monophasia (mon″o-fa′ze-ah) aphasia with ability to utter only one word or phrase. **monopha′sic,** adj.

monophthalmus (mon″of-thal′mus) cyclops.

monophyletic (mon″o-fi-let′ik) descended from a common ancestor or stem cell.

monoplegia (-ple′je-ah) paralysis of a single part. **monople′gic,** adj.

monorchidism, monorchism (mon-or′kid-izm; mon′or-kizm) the condition of having only one testis or one descended testis.

monosaccharide (mon″o-sak′ah-rīd) a simple sugar; a carbohydrate that cannot be decomposed by hydrolysis.

monosomy (-so′me) existence in a cell of only one instead of the normal diploid pair of a particular chromosome. **monoso′mic,** adj.

monospasm (mon′o-spazm) spasm of a single limb or part.

monospecific (mon″o-spĕ-sif′ik) having an effect only on a particular kind of cell or tissue or reacting with a single antigen, as a monospecific antiserum.

Monosporium (-spor′e-um) a genus of fungi, including *M. apiosper′mum,* a cause of maduromycosis.

monostratal (mon″o-strāt′al) pertaining to a single layer or stratum.

monosynaptic (-sĭ-nap′tik) pertaining to or passing through a single synapse.

monothermia (-thurm′e-ah) maintenance of the same body temperature throughout the day.

monotocous (mo-not′ah-kis) giving birth to but one offspring at a time.

monotrichous (mon-ah′trĭ-kis) having a single polar flagellum.

monovalent (mon″o-vāl′int) 1. having a valency of one. 2. capable of combining with only one antigenic specificity or with only one antibody specificity.

monoxenic (-zen′ik) associated with a single known species of microorganisms; said of otherwise germ-free animals.

monoxenous (mon-ok′sin-is) requiring only one host to complete the life cycle.

monoxide (mon-ok′sīd) an oxide with one oxygen atom in the molecule.

monozygotic (mon″o-zi-got′ik) derived from a single zygote (fertilized ovum); said of twins.

mons (mons), pl. *mon′tes* [L.] a prominence. **m. pu′bis, m. ve′neris,** the rounded fleshy prominence over the symphysis pubis in the female.

monster (mon′ster) a fetus or infant with such pronounced developmental anomalies as to be grotesque and usually nonviable. **autositic m.,** one capable of independent life, the circulation of which supplies nutrition to its parasitic partner. **compound m.,** one showing some duplication of parts. **double m.,** one arising from a single ovum but with duplication or doubling of head, trunk, or limbs. **parasitic m.,** an imperfect fetus unable to exist alone and attached to an autositic partner. **triplet m.,** one with triplication of body parts. **twin m.,** double m.

monticulus (mon-tik′ūl-us), pl. *montic′uli* [L.] a small eminence. **m. cerebel′li,** the projecting or superior part of the vermis.

mood (mōōd) the emotional state of an individual.

MOPP a regimen of mechlorethamine, Oncovin (vincristine), procarbazine, and prednisone, used in cancer chemotherapy.

Moraxella (mo-rak-sel′ah) a genus of bacteria found as parasites and pathogens in warm-blooded animals. **M. lacuna′ta,** *Haemophilus duplex.*

morbid (mor′bid) 1. pertaining to, affected with, or inducing disease; diseased. 2. unhealthy or unwholesome.

morbidity (mor-bid′it-e) 1. the condition of being diseased or morbid. 2. the sick rate; the ratio of sick to well persons in a community.

morbilli (mor-bil′i) [L.] measles.

morbilliform (mor-bil′ĭ-form) measles-like; resembling the eruption of measles.

morbus (mor′bus) [L.] disease.

morcellation (mor″sil-a′shin) the division of solid tissue (as a tumor) into pieces, followed by its removal piecemeal.

mordant (mord′int) 1. a substance capable of intensifying or deepening the reaction of a specimen to a stain. 2. to subject to the action of a mordant before staining.

morgue (morg) a place where dead bodies may be kept for identification or until claimed for burial.

moria (mor′e-ah) dementia or fatuity; in psychiatry, a morbid tendency to joke.

moribund (mor′ĭ-bund) in a dying state.

moronity (mor-on′it-e) former category of mental retardation comprising persons with an I.Q. of 50–69.

-morph word element [Gr.], *shape; form.*

morphea (mor-fe′ah) a condition in which there is connective tissue replacement of the skin and sometimes the subcutaneous tissues, with formation of firm ivory white or pinkish patches, bands, or lines.

morphine (mor′fēn) the principal and most active alkaloid of opium, $C_{17}H_{19}NO_3$; its hydrochloride and sulfate salts are used as narcotic analgesics.

morphogen (mor′fah-jen) a diffusible substance in embryonic tissue postulated to form a concentration gradient that influences morphogenesis.

morphogenesis (mor″fo-jen′is-is) the evolution and development of form, as the development of the shape of a particular organ or part of the body, or the development undergone by individuals who attain the type to which the majority of the individuals of the species approximate. **morphogenet′ic,** adj.

morphology (mor-fol′ah-je) the science of the forms and structure of organisms; the form and structure of a particular organism, organ, or part. **morpholog′ic,** adj.

morphosis (mor-fo′sis) the process of formation of a part or organ. **morphot′ic,** adj.

morrhuate (mor′u-āt) the fatty acids of cod liver oil; used as a sclerosing agent, especially for the treatment of varicose veins and hemorrhoids.

mors (mōrs) [L.] death.

morsus (mor'sus) [L.] bite. **m. dia'boli,** the fimbriae at the ovarian end of an oviduct.

mortal (mort''l) 1. destined to die. 2. causing or terminating in death; fatal.

mortality (mor-tal'it-e) 1. the quality of being mortal. 2. see *death rate.* 3. the ratio of actual deaths to expected deaths.

mortar (mort'er) a bell- or urn-shaped vessel in which drugs are beaten, crushed, or ground with a pestle.

mortification (mort''i-fi-ka'shin) gangrene.

morula (mor'ūl-ah) the solid mass of cells formed by cleavage of a fertilized ovum.

mosaicism (mo-za'i-sizm) in genetics, the presence in an individual of two or more cell lines that are karyotypically or genotypically distinct and are derived from a single zygote.

mOsm milliosmole.

mosquito (mos-kēt'o) a bloodsucking and venomous insect of the family Culicidae, including the genera *Aedes, Anopheles, Culex,* and *Mansonia.*

motilin (mo-til'in) a polypeptide hormone secreted by enterochromaffin cells of the gut; it causes increased motility of several portions of the gut and stimulates pepsin secretion. Its release is stimulated by the presence of acid and fat in the duodenum.

motility (mo-til'ite) the ability to move spontaneously. **mo'tile,** adj.

motoneuron (mōt''o-nōor'on) motor neuron; a neuron having a motor function; an efferent neuron conveying motor impulses. **lower m's,** peripheral neurons whose cell bodies lie in the ventral gray columns of the spinal cord and whose terminations are in skeletal muscles. **peripheral m's,** neurons in a peripheral reflex arc that receive impulses from interneurons and transmit them to voluntary muscles. **upper m's,** neurons in the cerebral cortex that conduct impulses from the motor cortex to the motor nuclei of the cerebral nerves or to the ventral gray columns of the spinal cord.

motor (mōt'er) 1. a muscle, nerve, or center that effects or produces motion. 2. producing or subserving motion.

Motrin (mo'trin) trademark for a preparation of ibuprofen.

mottling (mot'ling) discoloration in irregular areas.

moulage (moo-lahzh') [Fr.] the making of molds or models in wax or plaster; also, a mold or model so produced.

mounding (mownd'ing) the rising in a lump of a wasting muscle when struck.

mount (mownt) to prepare specimens and slides for study.

mouse (mows) 1. a small rodent, various species of which are used in laboratory experiments. 2. a small weight or movable structure. **joint m.,** a movable fragment of cartilage or other body within a joint. **peritoneal m.,** a free body in the peritoneal cavity, probably a small detached mass of omentum, sometimes visible radiographically.

mouth (mowth) an opening, especially the ante-

rior opening of the alimentary canal, the cavity containing the tongue and teeth. **trench m.,** necrotizing ulcerative gingivitis.

mouthwash (mowth'wosh) a solution for rinsing the mouth, e.g., a preparation of potassium bicarbonate, sodium borate, thymol, eucalyptol, methyl salicylate, amaranth solution, alcohol, glycerin, and purified water.

movement (mōōv'mint) 1. an act of moving; motion. 2. an act of defecation. **ameboid m.,** movement like that of an ameba, accomplished by protrusion of cytoplasm of the cell. **associated m.,** movement of parts which act together, as the eyes. **brownian m.,** the dancing motion of minute particles suspended in a liquid, due to thermal agitation. **vermicular m's,** the wormlike movements of the intestines in peristalsis.

mover (moo'ver) that which produces motion. **prime m.,** a muscle that acts directly to bring about a desired movement.

M.P.D. maximum permissible dose.

M.P.H. Master of Public Health.

mR milliroentgen.

M.R.A. Medical Record Administrator.

M.R.C. Medical Reserve Corps.

M.R.C.P. Member of Royal College of Physicians.

M.R.C.S. Member of Royal College of Surgeons.

M.R.L. Medical Record Librarian.

mRNA messenger RNA.

MS multiple sclerosis.

M.S. Master of Science; Master of Surgery.

MSH melanocyte-stimulating hormone.

M.T. Medical Technologist.

muco- word element [L.] *mucus,* or pertaining to a mucous membrane.

muciferous (mu-sif'er-is) secreting mucus.

mucigen (mu'si-jen) the substance from which mucin is derived.

mucilage (mu'si-lij) an aqueous solution of a gummy substance, used as a vehicle or demulcent. **mucilag'inous,** adj.

mucin (mu'sin) a mucopolysaccharide or glycoprotein, the chief constituent of mucus.

mucinogen (mu-sin'ah-jen) a precursor of mucin.

mucinoid (mu'si-noid) 1. resembling mucin. 2. mucoid (2).

mucinosis (mu''si-no'sis) a state with abnormal deposits of mucins in the skin. **follicular m.,** a disease of unknown cause, characterized by plaques of folliculopapules and alopecia.

mucinous (mu'si-nis) resembling, or marked by formation of, mucin.

mucinuria (mu''sin-ūr'e-ah) the presence of mucin in the urine, suggesting vaginal contamination.

muciparous (mu-sip'ah-ris) secreting mucin.

mucocele (mu'kah-sēl) 1. dilatation of a cavity with mucous secretion. 2. a mucous polyp.

mucoenteritis (-en''tĕ-rīt'is) mucous colitis.

mucoepidermoid (-ep''i-durm'oid) composed of mucus-producing epithelial cells.

mucoid (mu'koid) 1. mucinoid. 2. any of a group

of mucus-like conjugated proteins of animal origin, differing from mucin in solubility.

mucolipidosis (mu″ko-lip″ĭ-do′sis) pl. *mucolipido′ses.* any of a group of genetic disorders in which both mucopolysaccharides and lipids accumulate in tissues but without excess of mucopolysaccharides in the urine.

mucoperichondrium (mu″ko-pĕ″re-kon′dre-um) perichondrium having a mucosal surface, as that of the nasal septum. **mucoperichon′drial,** adj.

mucoperiosteum (-os′te-um) periosteum having a mucous surface. **mucoperios′teal,** adj.

mucopolysaccharide (-sak′ah-rīd) a group of polysaccharides which contain hexosamine, which may or may not be combined with protein, and which, dispersed in water, form many of the mucins.

mucopolysaccharidosis (-sak″ah-rĭ-do′sis) any of a group of genetically determined disorders due to a defect in mucopolysaccharide metabolism, marked by skeletal changes, mental retardation, visceral involvement, corneal clouding, with widespread tissue deposits and mucopolysacchariduria.

mucoprotein (prōt′e-in, -pro′tēn) a compound present in all connective and supporting tissues, containing mucopolysaccharides as prosthetic groups; they are relatively resistant to denaturation.

mucopurulent (-pūr′ah-lint) containing both mucus and pus.

mucopus (mu′ko-pus) mucus blended with pus.

Mucor (mu′kor) a genus of fungi, some species of which cause mucormycosis.

Mucorales (mu″kor-a′lēz) an order of fungi, including bread molds and related fungi, most of which are saprophytic.

mucormycosis (-mi-ko′sis) mycosis due to fungi of the order Mucorales, including species of *Absidia, Mucor,* and *Rhizopus,* usually occurring in debilitated patients, often beginning in the upper respiratory tract or lungs, from which mycelial growths metastasize to other organs.

mucosa (mu-ko′sah), pl. *muco′sae* [L.] mucous membrane. **muco′sal,** adj.

mucous (mu′kis) pertaining to or resembling mucus; secreting mucus.

mucoviscidosis (mu″ko-vis″ĭ-do′sis) cystic fibrosis of the pancreas.

mucus (mu′kis) the free slime of the mucous membranes, composed of secretion of the glands, various salts, desquamated cells, and leukocytes.

muliebria (mu″le-eb′re-ah) the female genitalia.

multi- word element [L.], *many.*

Multiceps (mul′tĭ-seps) a genus of tapeworms, including *M. mul′ticeps,* whose adult stage is parasitic in dogs and whose larval stage (*Coenurus cerebralis*) usually develops in the central nervous system of goats and sheep and occasionally in man.

multifid (mul′tĭ-fid) cleft into many parts.

multiform (mul′tĭ-form) polymorphic.

multigravida (-grav′ĭ-dah) a woman who is pregnant and has been pregnant at least twice before.

multi-infection (mul″te-in-fek′shin) infection with several kinds of pathogens.

multipara (mul-tip′ah-rah) a woman who has had two or more pregnancies resulting in viable fetuses, whether or not the offspring were alive at birth. **multip′arous,** adj. **grand m.,** a woman who has had six or more pregnancies resulting in viable fetuses.

multiparity (mul″tĭ-par′it-e) 1. the condition of being a multipara. 2. the production of several offspring in one gestation.

multivalent (-vāl′int) 1. having the power of combining with three or more univalent atoms. 2. active against several strains of an organism.

mummification (mum″ĭ-fĭ-ka′shin) the shriveling up of a tissue, as in dry gangrene, or of a dead, retained fetus.

mumps (mumps) an acute contagious paramyxovirus disease seen mainly in childhood, involving chiefly the salivary glands, most often the parotids, but other tissues, e.g., the meninges and testes (in postpubertal males), may be affected.

mural (mūr′l) pertaining to or occurring in the wall of a body cavity.

muramidase (mu-ram′ĭ-das) lysozyme.

murexine (mu-rek′sin) a neurotoxin from the hypobranchial gland of the snail *Murex.*

murine (mūr′ēn) pertaining to mice or rats.

murmur (mur′mer) an auscultatory sound, particularly a periodic sound of short duration of cardiac or vascular origin. **anemic m.,** a cardiac murmur heard in anemia. **aortic m.,** a sound generated by blood flowing through a diseased aorta or aortic valve. **arterial m.,** a murmur over an artery, sometimes aneurysmal and sometimes constricted. **Austin Flint m.,** a presystolic murmur heard at the apex in aortic regurgitation. **blood m.,** one due to an abnormal, commonly anemic, condition of the blood. **cardiac m.,** a murmur of finite length generated by blood flow through the heart. **Carey-Coombs m.,** a rumbling mid-diastolic murmur occurring in the early stages of rheumatic fever. **continuous m.,** a humming murmur heard throughout systole and diastole. **Cruveilhier-Baumgarten m.,** one heard at the abdominal wall over veins connecting the portal and caval systems. **diastolic m.,** one heard during diastole; due to mitral obstruction, or to aortic or pulmonary regurgitation. **Duroziez's m.,** a double murmur over the femoral or other large peripheral artery; due to aortic insufficiency. **ejection m.,** systolic murmurs heard predominantly in midsystole when ejection volume and velocity of blood flow are at their maximum. **friction m.,** see *rub.* **functional m.,** a cardiac murmur generated within a structurally normal heart. **Gibson m.,** a long, rumbling sound occupying most of systole and diastole, usually localized in the second left interspace near the sternum, and usually indicative of patent ductus arteriosus. **Graham Steell's m.,** one due to pulmonary regurgitation in patients with pulmonary hypertension and mitral stenosis. **innocent m.**, functional m. **machinery m.**, Gibson m. **musical m.**, a cardiac murmur having a periodic harmonic pattern. **organic m.**, one due to structural change in the heart, a vessel, or the lung. **pansystolic m.**, one heard throughout systole. **pericardial m.**, see under *rub.* **prediastolic m.**, one occurring just before and with diastole; due to mitral obstruction, or to aortic or pulmonary regurgitation. **presystolic m.**, one shortly before the onset of ventricular ejection, usually associated with a narrowed atrial ventricular valve. **pulmonic m.**, one due to disease of the valves of the pulmonary artery. **regurgitant m.**, one due to regurgitation of blood through a diseased valvular orifice. **seagull m.**, a raucous murmur with musical qualities heard occasionally in aortic insufficiency. **Still's m.**, a functional cardiac murmur of childhood, heard in midsystole. **systolic m.**, one heard during systole; usually due to mitral or tricuspid regurgitation, or to aortic or pulmonary obstruction. **vascular m.**, one heard over a blood vessel. **vesicular m.**, the normal breath sounds heard over the lungs.

Mus (mus) a genus of mice, including *M. mus'culus*, the common house mouse; *M. decuma'nus* or *norve'gicus*, the brown rat; *M. rat'tus rat'tus*, the black rat; and *M. Alexandri'nus*, the Egyptian or roof rat.

Musca (mus'kah) a genus of flies, including the common housefly, *M. domes'tica*, which may serve as a vector of various pathogens; its larvae may cause myiasis.

musca (mus'kah), plural *mus'cae* [L.] a fly. **mus'cae volitan'tes**, specks seen as floating before the eyes.

muscarine (-rin) a deadly alkaloid from various mushrooms, e.g., *Amanita muscaria* (the fly agaric), and also from rotten fish.

muscarinic (mus''kah-rin'ik) denoting the cholinergic effects of muscarine on postganglionic parasympathetic neural impulses.

muscle (mus''l) an organ which by contraction produces movement of an animal organism; see *Table of Muscles,* and see Plates I and XIV. **agonistic m.**, one opposed in action by another muscle (the antagonist). **antagonistic m.**, one that counteracts the action of another muscle (agonist). **articular m.**, one that has one end attached to a joint capsule. **Bell's m.**, the muscular strands between the ureteric orifices and the uvula vesicae, bounding the trigone of the urinary bladder. **Brücke's m.**, the longitudinal fibers of the ciliary muscle. **cardiac m.**, the muscle of the heart, composed of striated muscle fibers. **extraocular m's**, the six voluntary muscles that move the eyeball: superior, inferior, middle, and lateral recti, and superior and inferior oblique muscles. **extrinsic m.**, one not originating in the limb or part in which it is inserted. **fixation m's, fixator m's,** accessory muscles that serve to steady a part. **hamstring m's,** the muscles of the back of the thigh: biceps femoris, semitendinous, and semimembranous muscles. **Horner's m.**, the lacrimal part of the orbicularis oculi muscle. **Houston's m.**, fibers of the bulbocavernosus muscle compressing the dorsal vein of the penis. **intrinsic m.**, one whose origin and insertion are in the same part or organ. **involuntary m.**, one that is not under the control of the will. **Landström's m.**, minute muscle fibers in the fascia around and behind the eyeball, attached in front to the anterior orbital fascia and eyelids. **Müller's m.**, the circular fibers of the ciliary muscle. **orbicular m.**, one that encircles a body opening, e.g., the eye or mouth. **Reisseisen's m's,** the smooth muscle fibers of the smallest bronchi. **Ruysch's m.**, the muscular tissue of the fundus uteri. **skeletal m's,** striated muscles attached to bones, which cross at least one joint. **smooth m.**, nonstriated, involuntary muscle. **striated m., striped m.**, any muscle whose fibers are divided by transverse bands into striations; such muscles are voluntary. **synergistic m's,** those that assist one another in action. **thenar m's,** the abductor and flexor muscles of the thumb. **voluntary m.**, any muscle that is normally under the control of the will. **yoked m's,** those that normally act simultaneously and equally, as in moving the eyes.

muscularis (mus''ku-la'ris) [L.] relating to muscle, specifically a muscular layer (lamina muscularis) or coat (tunica muscularis).

musculature (mus'kūl-ah-cher) the muscular apparatus of the body or of a part.

musculoaponeurotic (mus''kūl-o-ap''o-nōōr-ot'ik) pertaining to a muscle and its aponeurosis.

musculophrenic (-fren'ik) pertaining to or supplying the diaphragm and adjoining muscles.

musculoskeletal (-skel'it'l) pertaining to or comprising the skeleton and muscles.

musculotropic (-trop'ik) having a special affinity for or exerting its principal effect on muscular tissue.

musculus (mus'ku-lus), pl. *mus'culi* [L.] muscle; see NA terms in *Table of Muscles.*

mustard (mus'tird) 1. a plant of the genus *Brassica.* 2. the ripe seeds of *Brassica alba* and *B. nigra,* whose oils have irritant and stimulant properties. **nitrogen m.**, mechlorethamine. **nitrogen m's,** a group of toxic, blistering alkylating agents homologous to dichlorodiethyl sulfide (mustard gas), some of which have been used as antineoplastics. The group includes mechlorethamine (nitrogen m.), cyclophosphamide, thiotepa, chlorambucil, and melphalan.

mutagen (mūt'ah-jen) an agent which induces genetic mutation.

mutagenicity (-jĕ-nis'it-e) the property of being able to induce genetic mutation.

mutant (mūt''nt) 1. an organism that has undergone genetic mutation. 2. produced by mutation.

mutarotase (mūt''ah-ro'tās) an enzyme that catalyzes the conversion of α-D- to β-D-glucose.

mutarotation (-ro-ta'shin) the change in optical rotation of an optically active compound in solution.

mutase (mu'tās) a group of enzymes (transferases) that catalyze the intramolecular shifting of a chemical group from one position to another.

mutation (mu-ta'shin) a permanent transmissi-

TABLE OF MUSCLES

COMMON NAME*	NA TERM†	ORIGIN*	INSERTION*	INNERVATION	ACTION
abductor m. of great toe	m. abductor hallucis	medial tubercle of calcaneus, plantar fascia	medial surface of base of proximal phalanx of great toe	medial plantar	abducts, flexes great toe
abductor m. of little finger	m. abductor digiti minimi manus	pisiform bone, tendon of ulnar flexor m. of wrist	medial surface of base of proximal phalanx of little finger	ulnar	abducts little finger
abductor m. of little toe	m. abductor digiti minimi pedis	medial and lateral tubercle of calcaneus, plantar fascia	lateral surface of base of proximal phalanx of little toe	lateral plantar	abducts little toe
abductor m. of thumb, long	m. abductor pollicis longus	posterior surfaces of radius and ulna	lateral side of bone of first metacarpal bone	posterior interosseous	abducts, extends thumb
abductor m. of thumb, short	m. abductor pollicis brevis	tubercles of scaphoid and trapezium, transverse carpal ligament	lateral surface of base of proximal phalanx of thumb	median	abducts thumb
adductor m., great	m. adductor magnus	deep part—inferior ramus of pubis, ramus of ischium; superficial part—ischial tuberosity	deep part—linea aspera of femur; superficial part—adductor tubercle of femur	deep part—obturator; superficial part—sciatic	deep part—adducts thigh; superficial part—extends thigh
adductor m. of great toe	m. adductor hallucis	oblique head—bases of second, third, fourth metatarsals, sheath of long peroneal m.; transverse head—capsules of metatarsophalangeal joints of three lateral toes	lateral side of proximal phalanx of great toe	lateral plantar	flexes, adducts great toe
adductor m., long	m. adductor longus	crest and symphysis of pubis	linea aspera of femur	obturator	adducts, rotates, flexes thigh
adductor m., short	m. adductor brevis	inferior ramus of pubis	upper part of linea aspera of femur	obturator	adducts, rotates, flexes thigh
adductor m. of thumb	m. adductor pollicis	oblique head—sheath of radial flexor m. of wrist, anterior carpal ligament, capitate bone, bases of second and third metacarpals; transverse head—front of third metacarpal	medial surface of base of proximal phalanx of thumb	ulnar	adducts, opposes thumb
anconeus m.	m. anconeus	back of lateral epicondyle of humerus	olecranon and posterior surface of ulna	radial	extends forearm
antitragus m.	m. antitragicus	outer part of antitragus	caudate process of helix and antihelix	temporal, posterior auricular branches of facial	

arrector m's of hair	mm. arrectores pilorum	dermis	hair follicles	sympathetic	elevate hairs of skin
articular m. of elbow	m. articularis cubiti	a name applied to a few fibers of the deep surface of the triceps m. of arm that insert into the posterior ligament and synovial membrane of the elbow joint			
articular m. of knee	m. articularis genus	front of lower part of femur	upper part of capsule of knee joint	femoral	raises capsule of knee joint
aryepiglottic m.	m. aryepiglotticus	a name applied to inconstant fibers of oblique arytenoid m., from apex of arytenoid cartilage to lateral margin of epiglottis			
arytenoid m., oblique	m. arytenoideus obliquus	muscular process of arytenoid cartilage	apex of opposite arytenoid cartilage	recurrent laryngeal	closes inlet of larynx
arytenoid m., transverse	m. arytenoideus transversus	medial surface of arytenoid cartilage	medial surface of opposite arytenoid cartilage	recurrent laryngeal	approximates arytenoid cartilage
auricular m., anterior	m. auricularis anterior	superficial temporal fascia	cartilage of ear	facial	draws auricle forward
auricular m., posterior	m. auricularis posterior	mastoid process	cartilage of ear	facial	draws auricle backward
auricular m., superior	m. auricularis superior	galea aponeurotica	cartilage of ear	facial	raises auricle
biceps m. of arm	m. biceps brachii	long head—supraglenoid tubercle of scapula; short head—apex of coracoid process	tuberosity of radius, antebrachial fascia	musculocutaneous	flexes, supinates forearm
biceps m. of thigh	m. biceps femoris	long head—ischial tuberosity; short head—linea aspera of femur	head of fibula, lateral condyle of tibia	long head—tibial; short head—peroneal, popliteal	flexor, rotates leg laterally, extends thigh
brachial m.	m. brachialis	anterior surface of humerus	coronoid process of ulna	musculocutaneous, radial	flexes forearm
brachioradial m.	m. brachioradialis	lateral supracondylar ridge of humerus	lateral surface of lower end of radius	radial	flexes forearm
bronchoesophageal m.	m. bronchoesophageus	a name applied to muscle fibers arising from wall of left bronchus, reinforcing musculature of esophagus			
buccinator m.	m. buccinator	buccinator ridge of mandible, alveolar processes of maxilla, pterygomandibular ligament	orbicular m. of mouth at angle of mouth	buccal branch of facial	compresses cheek and retracts angle of mouth
bulbocavernous m.	m. bulbospongiosus	tendinous center of perineum, median raphe of bulb	fascia of penis or clitoris	pudendal	constricts urethra in male, vagina in female
canine m. See levator m. of angle of mouth					
ceratocricoid m.	m. ceratocricoideus	a name applied to muscle fibers from cricoid cartilage to inferior horn of thyroid cartilage			
chin m.	m. mentalis	incisive fossa of mandible	skin of chin	facial	wrinkles skin of chin

*m. = muscle; m's = (pl.) muscles
†m. = [L.] musculus; mm. = ([L.] pl.) musculi

TABLE OF MUSCLES—*Continued*

COMMON NAME*	NA TERM†	ORIGIN*	INSERTION*	INNERVATION	ACTION
chondroglossus m.	m. chondroglossus	lesser horn and body of hyoid bone	substance of tongue	hypoglossal	depresses, retracts tongue
ciliary m.	m. ciliaris	scleral spur	outer layers of choroid and ciliary processes	oculomotor, parasympathetic	affects shape of lens in visual accommodation
coccygeus m.	m. coccygeus	ischial spine	lateral border of lower part of sacrum, coccyx	third and fourth sacral	supports and raises coccyx
constrictor m. of pharynx, inferior	m. constrictor pharyngis inferior	undersurfaces of cricoid and thyroid cartilages	median raphe of posterior wall of pharynx	glossopharyngeal, pharyngeal plexus, external branch of superior laryngeal and recurrent laryngeal	constricts pharynx
constrictor m. of pharynx, middle	m. constrictor pharyngis medius	horns of hyoid bone, stylohyoid ligament	median raphe of posterior wall of pharynx	pharyngeal plexus of vagus, glossopharyngeal	constricts pharynx
constrictor m. of pharynx, superior	m. constrictor pharyngis superior	pterygoid plate, pterygomandibular raphe, mylohyoid ridge of mandible, mucous membrane of floor of mouth	median raphe of posterior wall of pharynx	pharyngeal plexus of vagus	constricts pharynx
coracobrachial m.	m. coracobrachialis	coracoid process of scapula	medial surface of shaft of humerus	musculocutaneous	flexes, adducts arm
corrugator m., superciliary	m. corrugator supercilii	medial end of superciliary arch	skin of eyebrow	facial	draws eyebrow downward and medially
cremaster m.	m. cremaster	inferior margin of internal oblique m. of abdomen	pubic tubercle	genital branch of genitofemoral	elevates testis
cricoarytenoid m., lateral	m. cricoarytenoideus lateralis	lateral surface of cricoid cartilage	muscular process of arytenoid cartilage	recurrent laryngeal	approximates vocal folds
cricoarytenoid m., posterior	m. cricoarytenoideus posterior	back of lamina of cricoid cartilage	muscular process of arytenoid cartilage	recurrent laryngeal	separates vocal folds
cricothyroid m.	m. cricothyroideus	front and side of cricoid cartilage	lamina of thyroid cartilage	superior laryngeal	tenses vocal folds
dartos m.	m. dartos	the nonstriated muscle fibers of the tunica dartos, the deeper layers of which form the septum of the scrotum			
deltoid m.	m. deltoideus	clavicle, acromion, spine of scapula	deltoid tuberosity of humerus	axillary	abducts, flexes, extends arm
depressor m. of angle of mouth	m. depressor anguli oris	lateral border of mandible	angle of mouth	facial	pulls down angle of mouth
depressor m. of lower lip	m. depressor labii inferioris	anterior surface of lower border of mandible	orbicular m. of mouth and skin of lower lip	facial	depresses lower lip
depressor m. of septum of nose	m. depressor septi nasi	incisive fossa of maxilla	ala and septum of nose	facial	constricts nostril and depresses ala

374

Term	Latin name	Description	Nerve	Function
depressor m., supercil- iary. See	m. depressor supercilii	a name applied to a few fibers of orbital part of orbicu- lar m. of eye that are inserted into the eyebrow, which they depress		
detrusor of bladder	m. detrusor vesicae	bundles of smooth muscle fibers forming the muscular coat of the urinary bladder, which are arranged in a longitudinal and a circular layer and on contraction serve to expel urine		
detrusor urinae. See detrusor m. of blad- der.				
diaphragm	diaphragma	back of xiphoid process, inner surfaces of lower 6 costal cartilages and lower 4 ribs, medial and lateral arcuate liga- ments, bodies of upper lumbar vertebrae	central tendon of dia- phragm	phrenic	increases volume of thorax in inspiration
digastric m.	m. digastricus	anterior belly—digastric fossa on lower border of mandible near symphy- sis; posterior belly— mastoid notch of tem- poral bone	intermediate tendon on hyoid bone	anterior belly—mylo- hyoid; posterior belly—digastric branch of facial	elevates hyoid bone, low- ers jaw
dilator m. of pupil	m. dilator pupillae	a name applied to fibers extending radially from sphincter of pupil to ciliary margin		sympathetic	dilates iris
epicranial m.	m. epicranius	a name applied to muscular covering of scalp, includ- ing occipitofrontal and temporoparietal m's and galea aponeurotica			
erector m. of spine	m. erector spinae	a name applied to fibers of the more superficial of deep muscles of back, originating from sacrum, spines of lumbar and eleventh and twelfth thoracic vertebrae, and iliac crest, which split and insert as iliocostal, longissimus, and spinal m's			
extensor m. of fingers	m. extensor digitorum	lateral epicondyle of hu- merus	common extensor tendon of each finger	posterior interosseous	extends wrist joint and phalanges
extensor m. of great toe, long	m. extensor hallucis longus	front of fibula, interos- seous membrane	base of distal phalanx of great toe	deep peroneal	extends great toe, dorsi- flexes ankle joint
extensor m. of great toe, short	m. extensor hallucis brevis	a name applied to portion of short extensor m. of toes that goes to great toe			
extensor m. of index finger	m. extensor indicis	posterior surface of ulna, interosseous membrane	common extensor tendon of index finger	posterior interosseous	extends index finger
extensor m. of little finger	m. extensor digiti min- imi	common extensor tendon	tendon of extensor m. of fingers to little finger	deep branch of radial	extends little finger
extensor m. of thumb, long	m. extensor pollicis longus	posterior surface of ulna and interosseous mem- brane	back of distal phalanx of thumb	posterior interosseous	extends, adducts thumb

COMMON NAME*	NA TERM†	ORIGIN*	INSERTION*	INNERVATION	ACTION
extensor m. of thumb, short	m. extensor pollicis brevis	posterior surface of radius	back of proximal phalanx of thumb	posterior interosseous	extends thumb
extensor m. of toes, long	m. extensor digitorum longus	anterior surface of fibula, lateral condyle of tibia, interosseous membrane	common extensor tendon of 4 lateral toes	deep peroneal	extends toes
extensor m. of toes, short	m. extensor digitorum brevis	upper surface of calcaneus	extensor tendons of first, second, third, fourth toes	deep peroneal	extends toes
extensor m. of wrist, radial, long	m. extensor carpi radialis longus	lateral supracondylar ridge of humerus	back of base of second metacarpal bone	radial	extends, abducts wrist joint
extensor m. of wrist, radial, short	m. extensor carpi radialis brevis	lateral epicondyle of humerus	base of second metacarpal bone	radial	extends, abducts wrist joint
extensor m. of wrist, ulnar	m. extensor carpi ulnaris	*humeral head*—lateral epicondyle of humerus; *ulnar head*—posterior border of ulna	base of fifth metacarpal bone	deep branch of radial	extends, abducts wrist joint
fibular m. *See* peroneal m's					
flexor m. of fingers, deep	m. flexor digitorum profundus	shaft of ulna, coronoid process	bases of distal phalanges of 4 medial fingers	anterior interosseous, ulnar	flexes distal phalanges
flexor m. of fingers, superficial	m. flexor digitorum superficialis	*humeroulnar head*—medial epicondyle of humerus, coronoid process of ulna; *radial head*—anterior border of radius	sides of middle phalanges of 4 medial fingers	median	flexes middle phalanges
flexor m. of great toe, long	m. flexor hallucis longus	posterior surface of fibula	base of distal phalanx of great toe	tibial	flexes great toe
flexor m. of great toe, short	m. flexor hallucis brevis	undersurface of cuboid, lateral cuneiform	both sides of base of proximal phalanx of great toe	medial plantar	flexes great toe
flexor m. of little finger, short	m. flexor digiti minimi brevis manus	hook of hamate bone, transverse carpal ligament	medial side of proximal phalanx of little finger	ulnar	flexes little finger
flexor m. of little toe, short	m. flexor digiti minimi brevis pedis	base of fifth metatarsal, sheath of long peroneal m.	lateral surface of base of proximal phalanx of little toe	lateral plantar	flexes little toe
flexor m. of thumb, long	m. flexor pollicis longus	anterior surface of radius, coronoid process of ulna	base of distal phalanx of thumb	anterior interosseous	flexes thumb
flexor m. of thumb, short	m. flexor pollicis brevis	tubercle of trapezium, flexor retinaculum	lateral side of base proximal phalanx of thumb	median, ulnar	flexes, adducts thumb

376

flexor m. of toes, long	m. flexor digitorum longus pedis	posterior surface of shaft of tibia	distal phalanges of 4 lateral toes	tibial	flexes toes, extends foot
flexor m. of toes, short	m. flexor digitorum brevis pedis	medial tuberosity of calcaneus, plantar fascia	middle phalanges of 4 lateral toes	medial plantar	flexes toes
flexor m. of wrist, radial	m. flexor carpi radialis	medial epicondyle of humerus	bases of second and third metacarpal bones	median	flexes, abducts wrist joint
flexor m. of wrist, ulnar	m. flexor carpi ulnaris	*humeral head*—medial epicondyle of humerus; *ulnar head*—olecranon and posterior border of ulna	pisiform bone, hook of hamate bone, base of fifth metacarpal bone	ulnar	flexes, adducts wrist joint
gastrocnemius m.	m. gastrocnemius	*medial head*—popliteal surface of femur, upper part of medial condyle, capsule of knee; *lateral head*—lateral condyle, capsule of knee	aponeurosis unites with tendon of soleus to form Achilles tendon	tibial	plantar flexes foot, flexes knee joint
gemellus m., inferior	m. gemellus inferior	tuberosity of ischium	greater trochanter of femur	nerve to quadrate m. of thigh	rotates thigh laterally
gemellus m., superior	m. gemellus superior	spine of ischium	greater trochanter of femur	nerve to internal obturator	rotates thigh laterally
genioglossus m.	m. genioglossus	superior mental spine	hyoid bone, undersurface of tongue	hypoglossal	protrudes, depresses tongue
geniohyoid m.	m. geniohyoideus	inferior mental spine	body of hyoid bone	a branch of first cervical nerve through hypoglossal	elevates, draws hyoid bone forward
glossopalatine m. *See* palatoglossus m.					
gluteus maximus m., (gluteal m., greatest)	m. gluteus maximus	lateral surface of ilium, dorsal surfaces of sacrum and coccyx, sacrotuberous ligament	iliotibial tract of fascia lata, gluteal tuberosity of femur	inferior gluteal	extends, abducts, rotates thigh laterally
gluteus medius m., (gluteal m., middle)	m. gluteus medius	lateral surface of ilium between anterior and posterior gluteal lines	greater trochanter of femur	superior gluteal	abducts, rotates thigh medially
gluteus minimus m., (gluteal m., least)	m. gluteus minimus	dorsal aspect of ilium between anterior and posterior gluteal lines	greater trochanter of femur	superior gluteal	abducts, rotates thigh medially
gracilis m.	m. gracilis	body and inferior ramus of pubis	medial surface of shaft of tibia	obturator	adducts thigh, flexes knee joint
m. of helix, greater	m. helicis major	spine of helix	anterior border of helix	auriculotemporal, posterior auricular	tenses skin of acoustic meatus
m. of helix, smaller	m. helicis minor	anterior rim of helix	concha	temporal, posterior auricular	
hyoglossus m.	m. hyoglossus	body and greater horn of hyoid bone	side of tongue	hypoglossal	depresses, retracts tongue

377

TABLE OF MUSCLES—Continued

COMMON NAME*	NA TERM†	ORIGIN*	INSERTION*	INNERVATION	ACTION
iliac m.	m. iliacus	iliac fossa, base of sacrum	greater psoas tendon, lesser trochanter of femur	femoral	flexes thigh, trunk on limb
iliococcygeus m.	m. iliococcygeus	a name applied to posterior portion of levator ani m., including fibers originating as far forward as obturator canal, and inserting on side of coccyx and on anococcygeal body			
iliocostal m.	m. iliocostalis	a name applied to lateral division of erector m. of spine			
iliocostal m. of loins	m. iliocostalis lumborum	iliac crest	angles of lower 6 or 7 ribs	thoracic and lumbar	extends lumbar spine
iliocostal m. of neck	m. iliocostalis cervicis	angles of third, fourth, fifth, and sixth ribs	transverse processes of lower fourth, fifth, and sixth cervical vertebrae	cervical	extends cervical spine
iliocostal m. of thorax	m. iliocostalis thoracis	upper borders of angles of 6 lower ribs	angles of upper ribs and transverse process of seventh cervical vertebra	thoracic	keeps thoracic spine erect
iliopsoas m.	m. iliopsoas	a name applied collectively to iliac and greater psoas m's			
incisive m's of inferior lip		incisive fossae of mandible	angle of mouth	facial	make vestibule of mouth shallow
incisive m's of superior lip		incisive fossae of maxilla	angle of mouth	facial	make vestibule of mouth shallow
m. of incisure of helix	m. incisurae helicis	a name applied to inconstant slips of fibers continuing forward from m. of tragus to bridge the notch of cartilaginous part of meatus			
infraspinous m.	m. infraspinatus	infraspinous fossa of scapula	greater tubercle of humerus	suprascapular	rotates arm laterally
intercostal m's, external	mm. intercostales externi	inferior border of rib	superior border of rib below	intercostal	act on ribs in inspiration
intercostal m's, innermost	mm. intercostales intimi	the layer of muscle fibers separated from the internal intercostal m's by the intercostal nerves			
intercostal m's, internal	mm. intercostales interni	inferior border of rib and costal cartilage	superior border of rib and costal cartilage below	intercostal	act on ribs in expiration
interosseous m's of foot, dorsal	mm. interossei dorsales pedis	adjacent sides of metatarsal bones	base of proximal phalanges of second, third, and fourth toes	lateral plantar	flex, abduct toes
interosseous m's of hand, dorsal	mm. interossei dorsales manus	each by two heads from adjacent sides of metacarpal bones	extensor tendons of second, third, and fourth fingers	ulnar	abduct, flex proximal, extend middle and distal phalanges

378

Common name	Latin name	Origin/Description	Insertion	Nerve	Action
interosseous m's, palmar	mm. interossei palmares	sides of first, second, fourth, and fifth metacarpal bones	extensor tendons of first, second, fourth, and fifth fingers	ulnar	adduct, flex proximal, extend middle and distal phalanges
interosseous m's, plantar	mm. interossei plantares	medial side of third, fourth, and fifth metatarsal bones	medial side of base of proximal phalanges of third, fourth, and fifth toes	lateral plantar	flex, abduct toes
interspinal m's	mm. interspinales	a name applied to short bands of muscle fibers extending on each side between spinous processes of contiguous vertebrae		spinal	extend vertebral column
intertransverse m's	mm. intertransversarii	a name applied to small muscles passing between transverse processes of adjacent vertebrae		spinal	bend vertebral column laterally
ischiocavernous m.	m. ischiocavernosus	ramus of ischium	crus of penis or clitoris	perineal	maintains erection of penis or clitoris
latissimus dorsi m.	m. latissimus dorsi	spines of lower thoracic vertebrae, spines of lumbar and sacral vertebrae through attachment to thoracolumbar fascia, iliac crest, lower ribs, inferior angle of scapula	floor of intertubercular groove of humerus	thoracodorsal	adducts, extends, rotates humerus medially
levator m. of angle of mouth	m. levator anguli oris	canine fossa of maxilla	orbicular m. of mouth, skin at angle of mouth	facial	raises angle of mouth
levator ani m.	m. levator ani	a name applied collectively to important muscular components of pelvic diaphragm, arising mainly from back of body of pubis and running backward toward coccyx; includes pubococcygeus (levator m. of prostate in male and pubovaginal in female), puborectal, and iliococcygeus m's		third and fourth sacral	helps support pelvic viscera and resist increases in intra-abdominal pressure
levator m. of palatine velum	m. levator veli palatini	apex of pars petrosa of temporal bone and cartilage of auditory tube	aponeurosis of soft palate	pharyngeal plexus	raises and draws back soft palate
levator m. of prostate	m. levator prostatae	a name applied to part of anterior portion of pubococcygeus m., which in male is inserted into prostate and tendinous center of perineum		sacral, pudendal	supports, compresses prostate, helps control micturition
levator m's of ribs	mm. levatores costarum	transverse processes of seventh cervical and first 11 thoracic vertebrae	medial to angle of rib below	intercostal	aid elevation of ribs in respiration
levator m. of scapula	m. levator scapulae	transverse processes of 4 upper cervical vertebrae	vertebral border of scapula	third and fourth cervical	raises scapula
levator m. of thyroid gland	m. levator glandulae thyroideae	an inconstant muscle originating on the isthmus or pyramid of the thyroid gland and inserting on the hyoid bone			
levator m. of upper eyelid	m. levator palpebrae superioris	sphenoid bone above optic foramen	skin and tarsal plate of upper eyelid	oculomotor	raises upper eyelid

TABLE OF MUSCLES—Continued

COMMON NAME*	NA TERM†	ORIGIN*	INSERTION*	INNERVATION	ACTION
levator m. of upper lip	m. levator labii superioris	lower margin of orbit	musculature of upper lip	facial	raises upper lip
levator m. of upper lip and ala of nose	m. levator labii superioris alaeque nasi	frontal process of maxilla	skin and cartilage of ala of nose, upper lip	infraorbital branch of facial	raises upper lip, dilates nostril
long m. of head	m. longus capitis	transverse processes of third to sixth cervical vertebrae	basilar portion of occipital bone	cervical	flexes head
long m. of neck	m. longus colli	superior oblique portion—transverse processes of third to fifth cervical vertebrae; inferior oblique portion—bodies of first to third thoracic vertebrae; vertical portion—bodies of 3 upper thoracic and 3 lower cervical vertebrae	superior oblique portion—tubercle of anterior arch of atlas; inferior oblique portion—transverse processes of fifth and sixth cervical vertebrae; vertical portion—bodies of second to fourth cervical vertebrae	anterior cervical	flexes, supports cervical vertebrae
longissimus m. of head	m. longissimus capitis	transverse processes of 4 or 5 upper thoracic vertebrae, articular processes of 3 or 4 lower cervical vertebrae	mastoid process of temporal bone	cervical	draws head backward, rotates head
longissimus m. of neck	m. longissimus cervicis	transverse processes of 4 or 5 upper thoracic vertebrae	transverse processes of second or third to sixth cervical vertebrae	lower cervical and upper thoracic	extends cervical vertebrae
longissimus m. of thorax	m. longissimus thoracis	transverse and articular processes of lumbar vertebrae and thoracolumbar fascia	transverse processes of all thoracic vertebrae, 9 or 10 lower ribs	lumbar and thoracic	extends thoracic vertebrae
longitudinal m. of tongue, inferior	m. longitudinalis inferior linguae	undersurface of tongue at base	tip of tongue	hypoglossal	changes shape of tongue in mastication and deglutition
longitudinal m. of tongue, superior	m. longitudinalis superior linguae	submucosa and septum of tongue	margins of tongue	hypoglossal	changes shape of tongue in mastication and deglutition
lumbrical m's of foot	mm. lumbricales pedis	tendons of long flexor m. of toes	extensor tendons of 4 lateral toes	medial and lateral plantar	flex metatarsophalangeal joints, extend distal phalanges
lumbrical m's of hand	mm. lumbricales manus	tendons of deep flexor m. of fingers	extensor tendons of 4 lateral fingers	median, ulnar	flex metacarpophalangeal joints, extend middle and distal phalanges
masseter m.	m. masseter	superficial part—zygomatic process of maxilla, lower border of zygomatic arch; deep part—lower border and medial surface of zygomatic arch	superficial part—angle and ramus of mandible; deep part—upper half of ramus and lateral surface of coronoid process of mandible	mandibular	raises mandible, closes jaws

380

multifidus m's	mm. multifidi	sacrum, sacroiliac ligament, mamillary processes of lumbar, transverse processes of thoracic, and articular processes of cervical vertebrae	spines of contiguous vertebrae above	spinal	extend, rotate vertebral column
mylohyoid m.	m. mylohyoideus	mylohyoid line of mandible	body of hyoid bone, median raphe	mylohyoid branch of inferior alveolar	elevates hyoid bone, supports floor of mouth
nasal m.	m. nasalis	maxilla	*alar part*—ala of nose; *transverse part*—by aponeurotic expansion with fellow of opposite side	facial	*alar part*—aids in widening nostril; *transverse part*—depresses cartilage of nose
oblique m. of abdomen, external	m. obliquus externus abdominus	lower 8 ribs at costal cartilages	crest of ilium, linea alba through rectus sheath	lower thoracic	flexes, rotates vertebral column, compresses abdominal viscera
oblique m. of abdomen, internal	m. obliquus internus abdominis	thoracolumbar fascia, iliac crest, inguinal ligament	lower 3 or 4 costal cartilages, linea alba, conjoined tendon to pubis	lower thoracic	flexes, rotates vertebral column, compresses abdominal viscera
oblique m. of auricle	m. obliquus auriculae	cranial surface of concha	cranial surface of auricle above concha	posterior auricular, temporal	
oblique m. of eyeball, inferior	m. obliquus inferior bulbi	orbital surface of maxilla	sclera	oculomotor	rotates eyeball upward and outward
oblique m. of eyeball, superior	m. obliquus superior bulbi	lesser wing of sphenoid above optic foramen	sclera	trochlear	rotates eyeball downward and outward
oblique m. of head, inferior	m. obliquus capitis inferior	spinous process of axis	transverse process of atlas	spinal	rotates atlas and head
oblique m. of head, superior	m. obliquus capitis superior	transverse process of atlas	occipital bone	spinal	extends and moves head laterally
obturator m., external	m. obturatorius externus	pubis, ischium, external surface of obturator membrane	trochanteric fossa of femur	obturator	rotates thigh laterally
obturator m., internal	m. obturatorius internus	pelvic surface of hip bone, margin of obturator foramen, ramus of ischium, inferior ramus of pubis, internal surface of obturator membrane	greater trochanter of femur	fifth lumbar, first and second sacral	rotates thigh laterally
occipitofrontal m.	m. occipitofrontalis	*frontal belly*—galea aponeurotica; *occipital belly*—highest nuchal line of occipital bone	*frontal belly*—skin of eyebrow, root of nose; *occipital belly*—galea aponeurotica	*frontal belly*—temporal branch of facial; *occipital belly*—posterior auricular branch of facial	*frontal belly*—raises eyebrow; *occipital belly*—draws scalp backward
omohyoid m.	m. omohyoideus	superior border of scapula	body of hyoid bone	upper cervical through ansa cervicalis	depresses hyoid bone

COMMON NAME*	NA TERM†	ORIGIN*	INSERTION*	INNERVATION	ACTION
opposing m. of little finger	m. opponens digiti minimi manus	hook of hamate bone	front of fifth metacarpal	eighth cervical through ulnar	abducts, flexes, rotates fifth metacarpal
opposing m. of thumb	m. opponens pollicis	tubercle of trapezium, flexor retinaculum	lateral side of first metacarpal	sixth and seventh metacarpal through median	flexes, opposes thumb
orbicular m. of eye	m. orbicularis oculi	*orbital part*—medial margin of orbit, including frontal process of maxilla; *palpebral part*—medial palpebral ligament; *lacrimal part*—posterior lacrimal crest	*orbital part*—near origin after encircling orbit; *palpebral part*—fibers intertwine to form lateral palpebral raphe; *lacrimal part*—lateral palpebral raphe, upper and lower tarsi	facial	closes eyelids, wrinkles forehead, compresses lacrimal sac
orbicular m. of mouth	m. orbicularis oris	a name applied to complicated sphincter muscle of mouth, comprising 2 parts; *labial part*—consisting of fibers restricted to lips; *marginal part*—consisting of fibers blending with those of adjacent muscles		facial	closes, protrudes lips
orbital m.	m. orbitalis	a thin layer of nonstriated muscle that bridges the inferior orbital fissure		sympathetic fibers	
palatoglossus m.	m. palatoglossus	undersurface of soft palate	side of tongue	pharyngeal plexus	elevates tongue, constricts fauces
palatopharyngeal m.	m. palatopharyngeus	soft palate	posterior border of thyroid cartilage, aponeurosis of pharynx	pharyngeal plexus	constricts pharynx, aids swallowing
palmar m., long	m. palmaris longus	medial epicondyle of humerus	flexor retinaculum, palmar aponeurosis	median	flexes wrist
palmar m., short	m. palmaris brevis	palmar aponeurosis	skin of medial border of hand	ulnar	assists in deepening hollow of palm
papillary m's	mm. papillares	a name applied to conical muscular projections from walls of cardiac ventricles, attached to cusps of atrioventricular valves by chordae tendineae			steady and strengthen atrioventricular valves and prevent eversion of their cusps
pectinate m's	mm. pectinati	a name applied to small ridges of muscular fibers projecting from inner walls of auricles of heart, and extending in right atrium from auricle to crista terminalis			
pectineal m.	m. pectineus	pectineal line of pubis	pectineal line of femur	femoral, obturator	flexes, adducts thigh
pectoral m., greater	m. pectoralis major	clavicle, sternum, 6 upper costal cartilages, aponeurosis of external oblique m. of abdomen	crest of intertubercular groove of humerus	lateral and medial pectoral	adducts, flexes, rotates arm medially
pectoral m., smaller	m. pectoralis minor	second, third, fourth, and fifth ribs	coracoid process of scapula	medial and lateral pectoral	draws shoulder forward and downward, raises third, fourth, and fifth ribs in forced inspiration

382

peroneal m., long	m. peroneus longus	lateral condyle of tibia, head of fibula, lateral surface of fibula	superficial peroneal	plantar flexes, everts, abducts foot
peroneal m., short	m. peroneus brevis	lateral surface of fibula	superficial peroneal	everts, abducts, plantar flexes foot
peroneal m., third	m. peroneus tertius	anterior surface of fibula, interosseous membrane	deep peroneal	everts, dorsiflexes foot
piriform m.	m. piriformis	ilium, second to fourth sacral vertebrae	first and second sacral	rotates thigh laterally
plantar m.	m. plantaris	oblique popliteal ligament, lateral supracondylar line of femur	tibial	plantar flexes foot
platysma	platysma	a name applied to a platelike muscle originating from the fascia of cervical region and inserting on mandible, and skin around mouth	cervical branch of facial	wrinkles skin of neck, depresses jaw
pleuroesophageal m.	m. pleuroesophageus	a name applied to a bundle of smooth muscle fibers, usually connecting esophagus with left mediastinal pleura		
popliteal m.	m. popliteus	lateral condyle of femur, lateral meniscus	tibial	flexes leg, rotates leg medially
procerus m.	m. procerus	fascia over nasal bone	facial	draws medial angle of eyebrows down
pronator m., quadrate	m. pronator quadratus	anterior surface and border of distal third or fourth of shaft of ulna	anterior interosseous	pronates hand
pronator m., round	m. pronator teres	*humeral head*—medial epicondyle of humerus; *ulnar head*—coronoid process of ulna	median	pronates hand, flexes elbow
psoas m., greater	m. psoas major	lesser trochanter of femur	second and third lumbar	flexes thigh or trunk
psoas m., smaller	m. psoas minor	last thoracic and first lumbar vertebrae	first lumbar	flexes trunk
pterygoid m., lateral (external)	m. pterygoideus lateralis	*upper head*—infratemporal surface of greater wing of sphenoid, infratemporal crest; *lower head*—lateral surface of lateral pterygoid plate	mandibular	protrudes mandible, opens jaws, moves mandible from side to side
pterygoid m., medial (internal)	m. pterygoideus medialis	medial surface of lateral pterygoid plate, tuber of maxilla	mandibular	closes jaws
pubococcygeus m.	m. pubococcygeus	a name applied to anterior portion of levator ani m., originating in front of obturator canal and inserting in anococcygeal ligament and side of coccyx	third and fourth sacral	helps support pelvic viscera and resist increases in intra-abdominal pressure

COMMON NAME*	NA TERM†	ORIGIN*	INSERTION*	INNERVATION	ACTION
puboprostatic m.	m. puboprostaticus	a name applied to smooth muscle fibers contained within medial puboprostatic ligament, which pass from prostate anteriorly to pubis			
puborectal m.	m. puborectalis	a name applied to portion of levator ani m., with a more lateral origin from pubic bone, and continuous posteriorly with corresponding muscle of opposite side		third and fourth sacral	helps support pelvic viscera and resist increases in intra-abdominal pressure
pubovaginal m.	m. pubovaginalis	a name applied to part of anterior portion of pubococcygeus m., which is inserted into urethra and vagina		sacral and pudendal	helps control micturition
pubovesical m.	m. pubovesicalis	a name applied to smooth muscle fibers extending from neck of urinary bladder to pubis			
pyloric sphincter m.	m. sphincter pyloricus	a thickening of the circular muscle of the stomach around its opening into the duodenum			
pyramidal m.	m. pyramidalis	body of pubis	linea alba	last thoracic	tenses abdominal wall
pyramidal m. of auricle	m. pyramidalis auriculae	a name applied to inconstant prolongation of fibers of m. of tragus to spine of helix			
quadrate m. of loins	m. quadratus lumborum	iliac crest, thoracolumbar fascia, lumbar vertebrae	twelfth rib, transverse processes of 4 upper lumbar vertebrae	first and second lumbar, twelfth thoracic	flexes trunk laterally
quadrate m. of lower lip. See depressor m. of lower lip					
quadrate m. of sole	m. quadratus plantae	calcaneus, plantar fascia	tendons of long flexor m. of toes	lateral plantar	aids in flexing toes
quadrate m. of thigh	m. quadratus femoris	tuberosity of ischium	quadrate tubercle of femur, intertrochanteric crest	fourth and fifth lumbar, first sacral	adducts, rotates thigh laterally
quadrate m. of upper lip. See levator m. of upper lip					
quadriceps m. of thigh	m. quadriceps femoris	a name applied collectively to rectus m. of thigh and intermediate, lateral and medial vastus m's, inserting by a common tendon that surrounds patella and ends on tuberosity of tibia		femoral	extends leg upon thigh
rectococcygeus m.	m. rectococcygeus	a name applied to smooth muscle fibers originating on anterior surface of second and third coccygeal vertebrae and inserting on posterior surface of rectum		autonomic	retracts, elevates rectum
rectourethral m.	m. rectourethralis	a name applied to band of smooth muscle fibers in male, extending from perineal flexure of rectum to membranous part of urethra			
rectouterine m.	m. rectouterinus	a name applied to band of fibers in female, running between cervix uteri and rectum, in rectouterine fold			
rectovesical m.	m. rectovesicalis	a name applied to band of fibers in male, connecting longitudinal musculature of rectum with external muscular coat of bladder			

384

rectus m. of abdomen	m. rectus abdominis	pubis	xiphoid process, fifth, sixth and seventh costal cartilages	lower thoracic	flexes lumbar vertebrae, supports abdomen
rectus m. of eyeball, inferior	m. rectus inferior bulbi	common tendinous ring	underside of sclera	oculomotor	adducts, rotates eyeball downward and medially
rectus m. of eyeball, lateral	m. rectus lateralis bulbi	common tendinous ring	lateral side of sclera	abducens	abducts eyeball
rectus m. of eyeball, medial	m. rectus medialis bulbi	common tendinous ring	medial side of sclera	oculomotor	adducts eyeball
rectus m. of eyeball, superior	m. rectus superior bulbi	common tendinous ring	upper side of sclera	oculomotor	adducts, rotates eyeball upward and medially
rectus m. of head, anterior	m. rectus capitis anterior	lateral mass of atlas	basilar part of occipital bone	first and second cervical	flexes, supports head
rectus m. of head, lateral	m. rectus capitis lateralis	transverse process of atlas	jugular process of occipital bone	first and second cervical	flexes, supports head
rectus m. of head, posterior, greater	m. rectus capitis posterior major	spinous process of axis	occipital bone	suboccipital, greater occipital	extends head
rectus m. of head, posterior, smaller	m. rectus capitis posterior minor	tubercle on posterior arch of atlas	occipital bone	suboccipital, greater occipital	extends head
rectus m. of thigh	m. rectus femoris	anterior inferior iliac spine, rim of acetabulum	base of patella, tuberosity of tibia	femoral	extends leg, flexes thigh
rhomboid m., greater	m. rhomboideus major	spinous processes of second, third, fourth and fifth thoracic vertebrae	vertebral margin of scapula	dorsal scapular	retracts and fixes scapula
rhomboid m., smaller	m. rhomboideus minor	spinous processes of seventh cervical and first thoracic vertebrae, lower part of nuchal ligament	vertebral margin of scapula at root of spine	dorsal scapular	retracts and fixes scapula
risorius m.	m. risorius	fascia over masseter	skin at angle of mouth	buccal branch of facial	draws angle of mouth laterally
rotator m's	mm. rotatores	a name applied to a series of small muscles deep in groove between spinous and transverse processes of vertebrae		spinal	extend and rotate vertebral column toward opposite side
sacrococcygeal m., dorsal (posterior)	m. sacrococcygeus dorsalis	a name applied to muscular slip passing from dorsal surface of sacrum to coccyx			
sacrococcygeal m., ventral (anterior)	m. sacrococcygeus ventralis	a name applied to musculotendinous slip passing from lower sacral vertebrae to coccyx			
sacrospinal m. *See* erector m. of spine					
salpingopharyngeal m.	m. salpingopharyngeus	auditory tube near its orifice	posterior part of palatopharyngeus	pharyngeal plexus	raises nasopharynx
sartorius m.	m. sartorius	anterior superior iliac spine	upper part of medial surface of tibia	femoral	flexes thigh and leg

385

COMMON NAME*	NA TERM†	ORIGIN*	INSERTION*	INNERVATION	ACTION
scalene m., anterior	m. scalenus anterior	transverse processes of third to sixth cervical vertebrae	scalene tubercle of first rib	second to seventh cervical	raises first rib, flexes cervical vertebrae forward and laterally, rotates cervical vertebrae to opposite side
scalene m., middle	m. scalenus medius	transverse processes of first to seventh cervical vertebrae	upper surface of first rib	second to seventh cervical	raises first rib, flexes cervical vertebrae laterally
scalene m. of pleura. See smallest scalene m.					
scalene m., posterior	m. scalenus posterior	transverse processes of fourth to sixth cervical vertebrae	second rib	second to seventh cervical	raises first and second ribs, flexes cervical vertebrae laterally
scalene m., smallest	m. scalenus minimus	a name applied to muscular band occasionally found between anterior and middle scalene m's			
semimembranous m.	m. semimembranosus	tuberosity of ischium	medial condyle and border of tibia, lateral condyle of femur	tibial	flexes and rotates leg medially, extends thigh
semispinal m. of head	m. semispinalis capitis	transverse processes of upper thoracic and lower cervical vertebrae	occipital bone	suboccipital, greater occipital, branches of cervical	extends head
semispinal m. of neck	m. semispinalis cervicis	transverse processes of upper thoracic vertebrae	spinous processes of second to fifth cervical vertebrae	branches of cervical	extends, rotates vertebral column
semispinal m. of thorax	m. semispinalis thoracis	transverse processes of lower thoracic vertebrae	spinous processes of lower cervical and upper thoracic vertebrae	spinal	extends, rotates vertebral column
semitendinous m.	m. semitendinosus	tuberosity of ischium	upper part of medial surface of tibia	tibial	flexes and rotates leg medially, extends thigh
serratus m., anterior	m. serratus anterior	8 or 9 upper ribs	medial border of scapula	long thoracic	draws scapula forward, rotates scapula to raise shoulder in abduction of arm
serratus m., posterior, inferior	m. serratus posterior inferior	spines of lower thoracic and upper lumbar vertebrae	4 lower ribs	ninth to twelfth thoracic	lowers ribs in expiration
serratus m., posterior, superior	m. serratus posterior superior	nuchal ligament, spinous processes of upper thoracic vertebrae	second, third, fourth and fifth ribs	first 4 thoracic	raises ribs in inspiration
soleus m.	m. soleus	fibula, popliteal fascia, tibia	calcaneus by Achilles tendon	tibial	plantar flexes foot
sphincter m. of anus, external	m. sphincter ani externus	tip of coccyx, anococcygeal ligament	tendinous center of perineum	inferior rectal, perineal branch of fourth sa-	closes anus

386

sphincter m. of anus, internal	m. sphincter ani internus	a name applied to a thickening of circular layer of muscular tunic at caudal end of rectum		
sphincter m. of bile duct	m. sphincter ductus choledochi	a name applied to annular sheath of muscle fibers investing bile duct within wall of duodenum		
sphincter m. of hepatopancreatic ampulla	m. sphincter ampullae hepatopancreaticae	a name applied to annular band of muscle fibers investing hepatopancreatic ampulla		
sphincter m. of pupil	m. sphincter pupillae	a name applied to circular fibers of iris	parasympathetic through ciliary	constricts pupil
sphincter m. of pylorus	m. sphincter pylori	a name applied to a thickening of circular muscle of stomach around its opening into duodenum		
sphincter m. of urethra	m. sphincter urethrae	median raphe behind and in front of urethra	perineal	compresses membranous urethra
sphincter m. of urinary bladder	m. sphincter vesicae urinariae	a name applied to circular layer of fibers surrounding internal urethral orifice	vesical	closes internal orifice of urethra
spinal m. of head	m. spinalis capitis	occipital bone	spinal	extends head
spinal m. of neck	m. spinalis cervicis	spinous processes of upper thoracic and lower cervical vertebrae	branches of cervical	extends vertebral column
spinal m. of thorax	m. spinalis thoracis	spinous process of seventh cervical and sometimes first and second thoracic vertebrae, nuchal ligament	branches of spinal	extends vertebral column
splenius m. of head	m. splenius capitis	spinous processes of upper lumbar and lower thoracic vertebre	cervical	extends, rotates head
splenius m. of neck	m. splenius cervicis	lower half of nuchal ligament, spinous processes of seventh cervical and upper thoracic vertebrae	cervical	extends, rotates head and neck
stapedius m.	m. stapedius	spinous process of upper thoracic vertebrae	facial	dampens movement of stapes
sternal m.	m. sternalis	interior of pyramidal eminence of tympanic cavity		
		transverse processes of upper cervical vertebrae		
		neck of stapes		
		a name applied to muscular band occasionally found parallel to sternum on sternocostal head of greater pectoral m.		
sternocleidomastoid m.	m. sternocleidomastoideus	*sternal head*—manubrium sterni; *clavicular head*—medial third of clavicle	accessory, cervical plexus	extends, rotates head and neck
sternocostal m. *See* transverse m. of thorax		mastoid process, superior nucha line of occipital bone		flexes vertebral column, rotates head to opposite side

387

COMMON NAME*	NA TERM†	ORIGIN*	INSERTION*	INNERVATION	ACTION
sternohyoid m.	m. sternohyoideus	manubrium sterni, clavicle	body of hyoid bone	ansa cervicalis	depresses hyoid bone and larynx
sternothyroid m.	m. sternothyroideus	manubrium sterni	lamina of thyroid cartilage	ansa cervicalis	depresses thyroid cartilage
styloglossus m.	m. styloglossus	styloid process	margin of tongue	hypoglossal	raises, retracts tongue
stylohyoid m.	m. stylohyoideus	styloid process	body of hyoid bone	facial	draws hyoid bone and tongue upward and backward
stylopharyngeus m.	m. stylopharyngeus	styloid process	thyroid cartilage, pharyngeal constrictors	glossopharyngeal, pharyngeal plexus	raises, dilates pharynx
subclavius m.	m. subclavius	first rib and its cartilage	lower surface of clavicle	fifth and sixth cervical	depresses lateral end of clavicle
subcostal m's	mm. subcostales	inner surface of ribs	inner surface of second or third rib below	intercostal	draw adjacent ribs together, lower ribs
subscapular m.	m. subscapularis	subscapular fossa of scapula	lesser tubercle of humerus	subscapular	rotates arm medially
supinator m.	m. supinator	lateral epicondyle of humerus, ligaments of elbow, ulna	radius	deep branch of radial	supinates hand
supraspinous m.	m. supraspinatus	supraspinous fossa of scapula	greater tubercle of humerus	suprascapular	abducts arm
suspensory m. of duodenum	m. suspensorius duodeni	a name applied to flat band of smooth muscle fibers originating from left crus of diaphragm and inserting continuous with muscular coat of duodenum at its junction with jejunum			
tarsal m., inferior	m. tarsalis inferior	inferior rectus m. of eyeball	tarsal plate of lower eyelid	sympathetic	widens palpebral fissure
tarsal m., superior	m. tarsalis superior	levator m. of upper eyelid	tarsal plate of upper eyelid	sympathetic	widens palpebral fissure
temporal m.	m. temporalis	temporal fossa and fascia	coronoid process of mandible	mandibular	closes jaws
temporoparietal m.	m. temporoparietalis	temporal fascia above ear	galea aponeurotica	temporal branches of facial	tightens scalp
tensor m. of fascia lata	m. tensor fasciae latae	iliac crest	iliotibial tract of fascia lata	superior gluteal	flexes, rotates thigh medially

388

tensor m. of palatine velum	m. tensor veli palatine	scaphoid fossa of pterygoid process, wall of auditory tube, spine of sphenoid	aponeurosis of soft palate, wall of auditory tube	mandibular	tenses soft palate, opens auditory tube
tensor m. of tympanum	m. tensor tympani	cartilaginous portion of auditory tube	handle of malleus	mandibular	tenses tympanic membrane
teres major m.	m. teres major	inferior angle of scapula	crest of intertubercular sulcus of humerus	lower subscapular	adducts, extends, and rotates arm medially
teres minor m.	m. teres minor	lateral margin of scapula	greater tubercle of humerus	axillary	rotates arm laterally
thyroarytenoid m.	m. thyroarytenoideus	lamina of thyroid cartilage	muscular process of arytenoid cartilage	recurrent laryngeal	relaxes, shortens vocal folds
thyroepiglottic m.	m thyroepigloticus	lamina of thyroid cartilage	epiglottis	recurrent laryngeal	closes inlet to larynx
thyrohyoid m.	m. thyrohyoideus	lamina of thyroid cartilage	greater horn of hyoid bone	first cervical	raises and changes form of larynx
tibial m., anterior	m. tibialis anterior	lateral condyle and lateral surface of tibia, interosseous membrane	medial cuneiform, base of first metatarsal	deep peroneal	dorsiflexes, inverts foot
tibial m., posterior	m. tibialis posterior	tibia, fibula, interosseous membrane	bases of second to fourth metatarsal and tarsal bones, except talus	tibial	plantar flexes, inverts foot
tracheal m.	m. trachealis	a name applied to transverse smooth muscle fibers filling gap at back of each cartilage of trachea		autonomic	lessens caliber of trachea
m. of tragus	m. tragicus	a name applied to a short, flattened vertical band on lateral surface of tragus, innervated by auriculotemporal and posterior auricular nerves			
transverse m. of abdomen	m. transversus abdominis	lower 6 costal cartilages, thoracolumbar fascia, iliac crest, inguinal ligament	linea alba through rectus sheath, conjoined tendon to pubis	lower thoracic	compresses abdominal viscera
transverse m. of auricle	m. transversus auriculae	cranial surface of auricle	circumference of auricle	posterior auricular branch of facial	retracts helix

TABLE OF MUSCLES—*Continued*

COMMON NAME*	NA TERM†	ORIGIN*	INSERTION*	INNERVATION	ACTION
transverse m. of chin	m. transversus menti	a name applied to superficial fibers of depressor m. of angle of mouth which turn medially and cross to opposite side			
transverse m. of nape	m. transversus nuchae	a name applied to small muscle often present, passing from occipital protuberance to posterior auricular m.; it may be either superficial or deep to trapezius			
transverse m. of perineum, deep	m. transversus perinei profundus	ramus of ischium	tendinous center of perineum	perineal	fixes tendinous center of perineum
transverse m. of perineum, superficial	m. transversus perinei superficialis	ramus of ischium	tendinous center of perineum	perineal	fixes tendinous center of perineum
transverse m. of thorax	m. transversus thoracis	posterior surface of body of sternum and of xiphoid process	second to sixth costal cartilages	intercostal	draws ribs downward
transverse m. of tongue	m. transversus linguae	median septum of tongue	dorsum and margins of tongue	hypoglossal	changes shape of tongue in mastication and deglutition
transversospinal m.	m. transversospinalis	a name applied collectively to semispinal, multifidus, and rotator m's			
trapezius m.	m. trapezius	occipital bone, nuchal ligament, spinous processes of seventh cervical and all thoracic vertebrae	clavicle, acromion, spine of scapula	accessory nerve, cervical plexus	rotates scapula to raise shoulder in abduction of arm, draws scapula backward
triangular m. *See* depressor m. of angle of mouth					

triceps m. of arm (triceps brachii m.)	m. triceps brachii	*long head*—infraglenoid tubercle of scapula; *lateral head*—posterior surface of humerus; *medial head*—posterior surface of humerus below groove for radial nerve	olecranon of ulna	radial	extends forearm; *long head* adducts, extends arm
triceps m. of calf (triceps surae m.)	m. triceps surae	a name applied collectively to gastrocnemius and soleus m's			
m. of uvula	m. uvulae	posterior nasal spine of palatine bone and aponeurosis of soft palate	uvula	pharyngeal plexus	raises uvula
vastus m., intermediate	m. vastus intermedius	anterior and lateral surfaces of femur	patella, common tendon of quadriceps m. of thigh	femoral	extends leg
vastus m., lateral	m. vastus lateralis	lateral aspects of femur	patella, common tendon of quadriceps m. of thigh	femoral	extends leg
vastus m., medial	m. vastus medialis	medial aspect of femur	patella, common tendon of quadriceps m. of thigh	femoral	extends leg
vertical m. of tongue	m. verticalis linguae	dorsal fascia of tongue	sides and base of tongue	hypoglossal	changes shape of tongue in mastication and deglutition
vocal m.	m. vocalis	angle between laminae of thyroid cartilage	vocal process of arytenoid cartilage	recurrent laryngeal	shortens and relaxes vocal folds
zygomatic m., greater	m. zygomaticus major	zygomatic bone	angle of mouth	facial	draws angle of mouth upward and backward
zygomatic m., smaller	m. zygomaticus minor	zygomatic bone	orbicular m. of mouth, levator m. of upper lip	facial	draws upper lip upward and laterally

ble change in the genetic material. Also, an individual exhibiting such change; a sport. **point m.,** a mutation resulting from a change in a single base pair in the DNA molecule. **somatic m.,** a genetic mutation occurring in a somatic cell, providing the basis for a mosaic condition. **suppressor m.,** the correction of the effect of a mutation at one locus by a mutation at another locus.

mute (mūt) 1. unable to speak. 2. a person who is unable to speak.

mutilation (mūt″ĭ-la′shin) the act of depriving an individual of a limb, member, or other important part. Also, the condition resulting therefrom.

mutism (mūt′izm) inability or refusal to speak. **akinetic m.,** a state in which the person makes no spontaneous movement or vocal sound. **elective m.,** a mental disorder of childhood characterized by continuous refusal to speak in social situations by a child who is able and willing to speak to selected persons.

muton (mu′ton) the smallest element of DNA whose alteration can give rise to a mutant organism.

mutualism (mu′choo-il-izm″) the biologic association of two individuals or populations of different species, both of which are benefited by the relationship and sometimes unable to exist without it.

M.V. [L.] *Medicus Veterinarius* (veterinary physician).

Mv chemical symbol, *mendelevium*.

mV millivolt.

μV microvolt.

my(o)- word element [Gr.], *muscle.*

myalgia (mi-al′je-ah) muscular pain. **epidemic m.,** see under *pleurodynia.*

myasthenia (mi″as-the′ne-ah) muscular debility or weakness. **myasthen′ic,** adj. **angiosclerotic m.,** intermittent claudication. **m. gas′trica,** weakness and loss of tone in the muscular coats of the stomach; atony of the stomach. **m. gra′vis, m. gra′vis pseudoparaly′tica,** a disorder of neuromuscular function, thought to be due to the presence of antibodies to acetycholine receptors at the neuromuscular junction; clinically, there is fatigue and exhaustion of the muscular system with a tendency to fluctuate in severity and without sensory disturbance or atrophy. **neonatal m.,** a transient myasthenia affecting offspring of myasthenic women.

myatonia (mi″-ah-to′ne-ah) amyotonia. **m. conge′nita,** amyotonia congenita.

myatrophy (mi-at′ro-fe) atrophy of a muscle.

myc(o)- word element [Gr.], *fungus.*

mycelium (mi-sēl′e-um), pl. *myce′lia.* The mass of threadlike processes (hyphae) constituting the fungal thallus. **myce′lial,** adj.

mycete (mi′sēt) a fungus.

mycetismus (mi″sĕ-tiz′mus) fungus poisoning, especially mushroom poisoning; see also *Amanita.*

mycetoma (mi″sĕ-to′mah) 1. maduromycosis. 2. a tumor-like tangled mass of fungal mycelia.

Mycobacteriaceae (mi″ko-bak-tēr″e-a′se-e) a family of bacteria (order Actinomycetales) found in soil and dairy products and as parasites in man and other animals.

Mycobacterium (-bak-tēr′e-um) a genus of gram-positive, acid-fast bacteria (family Mycobacteriaceae), including *M. bal′nei* (*M. mari′num*), the cause of swimming pool granuloma; *M. bo′vis,* the cause of cattle tuberculosis, transmitted to man through milk; *M. kansa′sii,* the cause of a tuberculosis-like disease in man; *M. le′prae,* the cause of leprosy; *M. paratuberculo′sis,* the cause of Johne's disease; and *M. tuberculo′sis* (the tubercle bacillus), the cause of tuberculosis, most commonly of the lungs, in man.

mycobacterium (-bak-tēr′e-um), pl. *mycobacte′ria* [L.] 1. an individual organism of the genus *Mycobacterium.* 2. a slender, acid-fast microorganism resembling *Mycobacterium tuberculosis.* **anonymous mycobacteria,** acid-fast bacteria resembling the tubercle bacilli, found in human pulmonary infections, for which species names have not been established; they are divided into the chromogens (including photochromogens [Group I] and scotochromogens [Group II]) and nonchromogens (subdivided into filamentous forms [Group III] and rapid growers [Group IV]). **Group I–IV m.,** see *anonymous m.*

mycodermatitis (-durm″ah-tīt′is) candidiasis.

Mycolog (mi′ko-log) trademark for a fixed combination preparation of nystatin, neomycin sulfate, gramicidin, and triamcinolone acetonide.

mycology (mi-kol′ah-je) the science and study of fungi.

mycomyringitis (mi″ko-mir″in-jīt′is) myringomycosis.

Mycoplasma (-plaz′mah) a genus of highly pleomorphic, gram-negative, aerobic to facultatively anerobic microorganisms that lack cell walls (family Mycoplasmataceae) including the pleuropneumonia-like organisms (PPLO), separated into 15 species, including *M. ho′minis,* found associated with nongonococcal urethritis and reported to cause mild pharyngitis in humans; *M. mycoi′des,* the type species, which causes pleuropneumonia (2); and *M. pneumo′niae,* a cause of primary atypical pneumonia.

Mycoplasmataceae (-plaz″mah-ta′se-e) a family of schizomycetes, made up of a single genus, *Mycoplasma.*

mycosis (mi-ko′sis) any disease caused by fungi. **m. fungoi′des,** a chronic, malignant, lymphoreticular neoplasm of the skin and, in late stages, lymph nodes and viscera, with development of large, painful, ulcerating tumors.

Mycostatin (mi″ko-stat′in) trademark for preparations of nystatin.

mycotic (mi-kot′ik) pertaining to a mycosis; caused by fungi.

mycotoxicosis (mi″ko-tok-sĭ-ko′sis) 1. poisoning due to a fungal or bacterial toxin. 2. poisoning due to ingestion of fungi.

mycotoxin (-tok′sin) a fungal toxin.

mydriatic (mi″dre-at′ik) 1. dilating the pupil. 2. a drug that dilates the pupil.

myectomy (mi-ek′tah-me) excision of a muscle.

myectopia (mi″ek-to′pe-ah) displacement of a muscle.

myel(o)- word element [Gr.], *marrow* (often with specific reference to the *spinal cord*).

myelapoplexy (mi″il-ap′ah-plek″se) hematomyelia.

myelatelia (-ah-tēl′e-ah) imperfect development of the spinal cord.

myelatrophy (-a′trah-fe) atrophy of the spinal cord.

myelemia (-ēm′e-ah) myelocytosis.

myelencephalon (-en-sef′ah-lon) 1. the posterior part of the hindbrain, comprising the medulla oblongata and the lower part of the fourth ventricle. 2. the posterior of two brain vesicles formed by specialization of the hindbrain in embryonic development.

myelin (mi′il-in) 1. the lipid substance surrounding the axon of myelinated nerve fibers. 2. any of a certain group of lipid substances found in various normal and pathologic tissues, differing from fats in being doubly refractive. **myelin′ic**, adj.

myelinization (mi″ĕ-lin″ĭ-za′shun) production of myelin around an axon.

myelinolysis (mi″il-in-ol′ĭ-sis) destruction of myelin; demyelination.

myelinosis (mi″il-in-o′sis) fatty degeneration, with formation of myelin.

myelinotoxic (mi″il-in-o-tok′sik) having a deleterious effect on myelin; causing demyelination.

myelitis (mi″il-īt′is) inflammation of the spinal cord or bone marrow (osteomyelitis). **myelit′ic**, adj.

myeloblast (mi′il-o-blast″) an immature cell found in the bone marrow and not normally in the peripheral blood; it is the most primitive precursor in the granulocytic series, which matures to develop into the promyelocyte and eventually the granular leukocyte.

myeloblastemia (mi″il-o-blas-tēm′ah) the presence of myeloblasts in the blood.

myeloblastoma (-blas-to′mah) a focal malignant tumor composed of myeloblasts observed in acute myelocytic leukemia.

myelocele (mi′il-o-sēl″) protrusion of the spinal cord through a defect in the vertebral column.

myelocyst (-sist″) a benign cyst developed from rudimentary medullary canals.

myelocystocele, myelocystomeningocele (mi″il-o-sis′tah-sēl; -sis″to-mī-ning′gah-sēl) myelomeningocele.

myelocyte (mi′il-o-sīt″) 1. a precursor in the granulocyte series, being a cell intermediate in development between a promyelocyte and a metamyelocyte. 2. any cell of the gray matter of the nervous system. **myelocyt′ic**, adj.

myelocytoma (-si-to′mah) myeloma.

myelodysplasia (-dis-pla′ze-ah) defective development of any part of the spinal cord.

myeloencephalitis (-en-sef″ah-līt′is) inflammation of the spinal cord and brain.

myelofibrosis (-fi-bro′sis) replacement of bone marrow by fibrous tissue.

myelogenesis (-jen′ĭ-sis) 1. development of the central nervous system. 2. the deposition of myelin around the axon.

myelogenous (mi″il-oj′ĭ-nus) produced in bone marrow.

myelogone (mi′il-o-gōn″) a white blood cell of the myeloid series having a reticulate violaceous nucleus, well-stained nucleolus, and deep blue rim of cytoplasm. **myelogon′ic**, adj.

myelography (mi″ilog′rah-fe) radiography of the spinal cord after injection of a contrast medium into the subarachnoid space.

myeloid (mi′il-oid) 1. pertaining to, derived from, or resembling bone marrow. 2. pertaining to the spinal cord. 3. having the appearance of myelocytes, but not derived from bone marrow.

myeloidosis (mi″il-oi-do′sis) formation of myeloid tissue, especially hyperplastic development of such tissue.

myelolipoma (mi″il-o-lip′o-mah) a rare benign tumor of the adrenal gland composed of adipose tissue, lymphocytes, and primitive myeloid cells.

myeloma (mi″il-o′mah) a tumor composed of cells of the type normally found in the bone marrow. **giant cell m.,** see under *tumor* (1). **multiple m.,** a malignant neoplasm of plasma cells, usually arising in bone marrow, manifested by skeletal destruction, pathologic fractures, bone pain, the presence of anomalous circulating immunoglobulins, Bence Jones proteinuria, and anemia; it is the most common form of monoclonal gammopathy; see also *plasmacytoma*. **plasma cell m.,** multiple m.

myelomalacia (mi″il-o-mah-la′she-ah) morbid softening of the spinal cord.

myelomatosis (-mah-to′sis) multiple myeloma.

myelomeningitis (-men″in-jīt′is) inflammation of the spinal cord and meninges.

myelomeningocele (-mĕ-ning′go-sēl) hernial protrusion of the spinal cord and its meninges through a defect in the vertebral column.

myelomere (-mēr″) any segment of the embryonic brain or spinal cord.

myelopathy (mi″il-op′ah-the) 1. any functional disturbance and/or pathological change in the spinal cord; often used to denote nonspecific lesions, as opposed to *myelitis.* 2. pathological bone marrow changes. **myelopath′ic**, adj. **sclerosing m.,** that marked by hardening of the spinal cord and overgrowth of the glia. **spondylotic cervical m.,** that secondary to encroachment of cervical spondylosis upon a congenitally small cervical spinal canal. **transverse m.,** that extending across the spinal cord.

myeloperoxidase (mi″il-o-per-ok′sĭ-das) a hemoprotein with peroxidase activity, occurring in the primary granules of promyelocytes, myelocytes, and neutrophils, and exhibiting bactericidal, fungicidal, and viricidal properties.

myelopetal (mi″il-op′it′l) moving toward the spinal cord.

myelophthisis (mi″il-o-thi′sis) 1. wasting of the spinal cord. 2. reduction of the cell-forming functions of bone marrow.

myeloplast (mi′il-o-plast″) any leukocyte of the bone marrow.

myelopoiesis (mi″il-o-poi-e′sis) the formation of marrow or the cells arising from it. **myelopoiet′ic,** adj.

myeloproliferative (-pro-lif′er-ah″tiv) pertaining to or characterized by medullary and extramedullary proliferation of bone marrow constituents; see under *syndrome.*

myeloradiculitis (-rah-dik″ūl-īt′is) inflammation of the spinal cord and posterior nerve roots.

myeloradiculodysplasia (-rah-dik″ūl-o-displa′ze-ah) abnormal development of the spinal cord and spinal nerve roots.

myelorrhagia (-ra′je-ah) hematomyelia.

myelosarcoma (-sar-ko′mah) a sarcomatous growth made up of myeloid tissue or bone marrow cells.

myelosclerosis (-sklĕ-ro′sis) 1. sclerosis of the spinal cord. 2. obliteration of the marrow cavity by small spicules of bone. 3. myelofibrosis.

myelosis (mi″il-o′sis) 1. proliferation of bone marrow tissue, producing the blood changes of myelocytic leukemia. 2. formation of a tumor of the spinal cord. **erythremic m.,** a malignant blood dyscrasia, one of the myeloproliferative disorders, with progressive anemia, megaloblastic erythroid hyperplasia, myeloid dysplasia, hepatosplenomegaly, and hemorrhagic phenomena.

myelospongium (mi″il-o-spun′je-um) a network developing into the neuroglia.

myelosuppressive (-sŭ-pres′iv) 1. inhibiting bone marrow activity, resulting in decreased production of blood cells and platelets. 2. an agent having such properties.

myenteron (mi-en′ter-on) the muscular coat of the intestine. **myenter′ic,** adj.

myesthesia (mi″es-the′ze-ah) muscle sensibility; sensibility to impressions coming from the muscles.

myiasis (mi-i′ah-sis) invasion of the body by the larvae of flies, characterized as cutaneous (subdermal tissue), gastrointestinal, nasopharyngeal, ocular, or urinary, depending on the region invaded.

mylohyoid (mi″lo-hi′oid) pertaining to the hyoid bone and molar teeth.

myo- word element [Gr.], *muscle.*

myoarchitectonic (mi″o-ar″kĭ-tek-ton′ik) pertaining to structural arrangement of muscle fibers.

myoatrophy (-ă′trah-fe) muscular atrophy.

myoblast (mi′ah-blast) an embryonic cell which becomes a cell of muscle fiber. **myoblas′tic,** adj.

myoblastoma (mi″o-blas-to′mah) a benign circumscribed tumor-like lesion of soft tissue; see *granular cell tumor.* **granular cell m.,** see under *tumor.*

myocardiograph (-kar′de-ah-grof″) instrument for making tracings of heart movements.

myocardiopathy (-kar′de-op′ah-the) any noninflammatory disease of the myocardium.

myocarditis (-kar-dīt′is) inflammation of the myocardium. **acute isolated m., Fiedler's m.,** a frequently fatal, idiopathic, acute myocarditis affecting chiefly the interstitial fibrous tissue.

myocardium (-kar′de-um) the middle and thickest layer of the heart wall, composed of cardiac muscle. **myocar′dial,** adj.

myocardosis (-kar-do′sis) any degenerative, noninflammatory disease of the myocardium.

myocele (mi′ah-sēl) protrusion of a muscle through its ruptured sheath.

myocerosis (mi″o-sĕ-ro′sis) waxy degeneration of muscle.

myoclonus (mi-ok′lin-is) shocklike contractions of a muscle or a group of muscles. **myoclon′ic,** adj. **palatal m.,** rapid rhythmic, up-and-down movement of one or both sides of the palate, often with ipsilateral synchronous clonic movements of the face, tongue, pharynx, and diaphragm muscles.

myocoele (mi′ah-sēl) the cavity within a myotome (2).

myocyte (-sīt) a muscle cell. **Anichkov's m.,** a myocyte found in Aschoff's bodies, having a serrated bar of chromatin in its nucleus.

myodemia (-de′me-ah) fatty degeneration of muscle.

myodystonia (-dis-to′ne-ah) disorder of muscular tone.

myodystrophy (-dis′trah-fe) 1. muscular dystrophy. 2. myotonic dystrophy.

myoedema (-ĕ-de′mah) 1. mounding. 2. edema of a muscle.

myoepithelioma (-ep″ĭ-thēl″e-o′mah) a tumor composed of outgrowths of myoepithelial cells from a sweat gland.

myoepithelium (-ep″ĭ-thēl′le-um) tissue made up of contractile epithelial cells. **myoepithe′lial,** adj.

myofascitis (-fah-sīt′is) inflammation of a muscle and its fascia.

myofibril (-fi′bril) a muscle fibril, one of the slender threads of a muscle fiber, composed of numerous myofilaments. See Plate XIV. **myofi′brillar,** adj.

myofibroblast (-fi′brah-blast) an atypical fibroblast combining the ultrastructural features of a fibroblast and a smooth muscle cell.

myofibrosis (-fi-bro′sis) replacement of muscle tissue by fibrous tissue.

myofibrositis (-fi″bro-sīt′is) perimysiitis.

myofilament (-fil′ah-mint) any of the ultramicroscopic threadlike structures composing the myofibrils of striated muscle fibers; thick ones contain myosin, thin ones actin. See Plate XIV.

myogenesis (mi″o-jen′ĭ-sis) the development of muscle tissue, especially its embryonic development. **myogenet′ic,** adj.

myogenous (mi-oj′in-is) originating in muscular tissue.

myoglobin (mi″ah-glo′bin) the oxygen-transporting pigment of muscle, a conjugated protein resembling a single subunit of hemoglobin, being composed of one globin polypeptide chain and one heme group.

myoglobulin (-glob′ūl-in) a globulin from muscle serum.

myograph (-graf) apparatus for recording effects of muscular contraction.

myography (mi-og′rah-fe) 1. the use of a myograph. 2. description of muscles. 3. radiography of muscle tissue after injection of a radiopaque medium. **myograph′ic,** adj.

myoid (mi′oid) resembling muscle.

myokinase (mi″o-ki′nās) adenylate kinase; an enzyme of muscle that catalyzes the phosphorylation of ADP to molecules of ATP and AMP.

myokinesimeter (-kin″ĕ-sim′it-er) an apparatus for measuring muscular contraction aroused by electrical stimulation.

myokinetic (-ki-net′ik) pertaining to the motion or kinetic function of muscle, as contrasted with the myotonic or tonic function.

myokymia (-ki′me-ah) a benign condition marked by brief spontaneous tetanic contractions of motor units or groups of muscle fibers, usually adjacent groups of fibers contracting alternately.

myology (mi-ol′ah-je) the scientific study or description of the muscles and accessory structures (bursae and synovial sheath).

myolysis (mi-ol′ĭ-sis) disintegration or degeneration of muscle tissue.

myoma (mi-o′mah) a tumor formed of muscular tissue. **myom′atous,** adj.

myomatosis (-mah-to′sis) the formation of multiple myomas.

myomelanosis (-mel″ah-no′sis) melanosis of muscle tissue.

myomere (mi′o-mēr) myotome (2).

myometer (mi-om′it-er) an apparatus for measuring muscle contraction.

myometritis (mi″o-me-trīt′is) inflammation of the myometrium.

myometrium (-me′tre-um) the tunica muscularis of the uterus. **myome′trial,** adj.

myoneme (mi′o-nēm) a fine contractile fiber found in the cytoplasm of certain protozoa.

myoneural (mi″ah-nōōr′l) pertaining to nerve terminations in muscles.

myopalmus (-pal′mus) muscle twitching.

myoparalysis (-pah-ral′ĭ-sis) paralysis of a muscle.

myoparesis (-pah-re′sis) slight muscle paralysis.

myopathy (mi-op′ah-the) any disease of muscle. **myopath′ic,** adj. **centronuclear m.,** myotubular m. **myotubular m.,** that marked by myofibers resembling those of early fetal muscle, i.e., myotubules. **nemaline m.,** a congenital abnormality of myofibrils in which small threadlike fibers are scattered through the muscle fibers; marked by hypotonia and proximal muscle weakness. **ocular m.,** a slowly progressive form affecting the extraocular muscles, with ptosis and progressive immobility of the eyes.

myopericarditis (mi″o-per″ĭ-kar-dīt′is) myocarditis combined with pericarditis.

myopia (mi-o′pe-ah) nearsightedness; ametropia in which parallel rays come to a focus in front of the retina, vision being better for near objects than for far. **myop′ic,** adj. **curvature m.,** myopia due to changes in curvature of the refracting surfaces of the eye. **index m.,** myopia due to abnormal refractivity of the media of the eye. **malignant m., pernicious m.,** progressive myopia with disease of the choroid, leading to

retinal detachment and blindness. **progressive m.,** myopia increasing in adult life.

myoplasm (mi′ah-plazm) the contractile part of a muscle cell, or myofibril.

myoplasty (-plas″te) plastic surgery on muscle. **myoplas′tic,** adj.

myorrhexis (mi″o-rek′sis) rupture of a muscle.

myosarcoma (-sar-ko′mah) a malignant tumor derived from myogenic cells.

myosclerosis (-sklĕ-ro′sis) hardening of muscle tissue.

myosin (mi′ah-sin) a protein of the myofibril, occurring chiefly in the A band; with actin it forms actomyosin, which is responsible for the contractile properties of muscle.

myositis (mi″o-sīt′is) inflammation of a voluntary muscle. **m. fibro′sa,** a type in which connective tissue forms within the muscle. **multiple m.,** polymyositis. **m. ossi′ficans,** myositis marked by bony deposits or by ossification of muscle. **trichinous m.,** that due to the presence of *Trichinella spiralis.*

myospasm (mi′ah-spazm) spasm of a muscle.

myotactic (mi″ah-tak′tik) pertaining to the proprioceptive sense of muscles.

myotasis (mi-ot′ah-sis) stretching of muscle. **myotat′ic,** adj.

myotenositis (mi″ah-te″nah-sīt′is) inflammation of a muscle and tendon.

myotome (mi′ah-tōm) 1. an instrument for performing myotomy. 2. the muscle plate or portion of a somite, from which voluntary muscles develop. 3. a group of muscles innervated from a single spinal segment. **myotom′ic,** adj.

myotonia (mi″ah-to′ne-ah) any disorder involving tonic spasm of muscle. **myoton′ic,** adj. **m. atro′phica,** myotonic dystrophy. **m. conge′nita,** a hereditary disease marked by tonic spasm and rigidity of certain muscles when attempts are made to move them after rest. **m. dystro′phica,** myotonic dystrophy.

myotonoid (mi-ot′n-oid) denoting muscle reactions marked by slow contraction or relaxation.

myotonus (mi-ot′n-is) tonic spasm of a muscle or a group of muscles.

myotrophic (mi′ah-tro′fik) 1. increasing the weight of muscle. 2. pertaining to myotrophy.

myotrophy (mi-ah′trah-fe) nutrition of muscle.

myotubule (mi″o-too′būl) a developing muscle fiber with a centrally located nucleus. **myotu′bular,** adj.

Myriapoda (mir″e-ap′ah-dah) a superclass of arthropods, including centipedes and millipedes.

myring(o)- word element [L.], *tympanic membrane.*

myringa (mĭ-ring′gah) the tympanic membrane.

myringectomy (mir″in-jek′tah-me) myringodectomy.

myringitis (mir″in-jīt′is) inflammation of the tympanic membrane. **m. bullo′sa, bullous m.,** a form of viral otitis media in which serous or hemorrhagic blebs appear on the tympanic membrane and often on the adjacent wall of the auditory meatus.

myringodectomy (mĭ-ring″go-dek′tah-me) excision of the tympanic membrane.

myringomycosis (-mi-ko'sis) fungal disease of the tympanic membrane.

myristic acid (mir-is'tik) a saturated fatty acid, $C_{14}H_{28}O_2$, found in spermaceti, nutmeg butter, and other fats.

Mysoline (mi'sah-lēn) trademark for preparations of primidone.

mysophilia (mi"so-fil'i-ah) paraphilia marked by lustful attitude toward excretions.

mysophobia (-fo'be-ah) morbid dread of contamination and filth.

myx(o)- word element [Gr.], *mucus; slime.*

myxadenitis (mik"sad'n-īt'is) inflammation of a mucous gland.

myxadenoma (-sad'n-o'mah) an epithelial tumor with the structure of a mucous gland.

myxasthenia (-sas-the'ne-ah) deficient secretion of mucus.

myxedema (-sĕ-de'mah) a dry, waxy type of swelling (nonpitting edema) with abnormal deposits of mucin in the skin (mucinosis) and other tissues, associated with hypothyroidism; the facial changes are distinctive, with swollen lips and thickened nose. **myxedem'atous,** adj. **congenital m.,** cretinism. **papular m.,** lichen myxedematosus. **pituitary m.,** that due to deficient secretion of the pituitary hormone thyrot-ropin. **pretibial m.,** localized edema associated with preceding hyperthyroidism and exophthalmos, occurring typically on the anterior (pretibial) surface of the legs, the mucin deposits appearing as both plaques and papules.

myxochondroma (mik"so-kon-dro'mah) chondroma with stroma resembling primitive mesenchymal tissue.

myxofibroma (mik"so-fi-bro'mah) a fibroma containing myxomatous tissue.

myxofibrosarcoma (-fi"bro-sar-ko'mah) fibrosarcoma with myxomatous areas.

myxoid (mik'soid) resembling mucus.

myxoma (mik-so'mah) a tumor composed of primitive connective tissue cells and stroma resembling mesencyhma. **myxo'matous,** adj.

myxomatosis (mik"so-mah-to'sis) 1. the development of multiple myxomas. 2. myxomatous degeneration.

myxorrhea (-re'ah) excessive flow of mucus.

myxosarcoma (-sar-ko'mah) a sarcoma with myxomatous tissue.

myxovirus (-vi'ris) any of a group of RNA viruses, including the viruses of influenza, parainfluenza, mumps, and Newcastle disease, characteristically causing agglutination of erythrocytes.

N

N 1. symbol, *newton.* 2. chemical symbol, *nitrogen.* 3. symbol, *normal* (solution); the expressions 2N (double normal), N/2 or 0.5N (half-normal), N/10 or 0.1N (tenth-normal), etc., denote the strength of a solution in comparison with the normal.

n symbol, *nano-.*

NA Nomina Anatomica.

Na chemical symbol, *sodium* (L. *natrium*).

nacreous (na'kre-us) having a pearl-like luster.

NAD nicotinamide-adenine dinucleotide.

NAD$^+$ the oxidized form of NAD.

NADH the reduced form of NAD.

nadolol (na'do-lol) a β-adrenergic blocking agent, $C_{17}H_{27}NO_4$, affecting both β_1 and β_2-receptors; used for the treatment of hypertension.

NADP nicotinamide-adenine dinucleotide phosphate.

NADP$^+$ the oxidized form of NADP.

NADPH the reduced form of NADP.

nafcillin (naf-sil'in) a semisynthetic, acid- and penicillinase-resistant penicillin that is effective against staphylococcal infections.

nail (nāl) 1. the horny cutaneous plate on the dorsal surface of the distal end of a finger or toe. 2. a rod of metal, bone, or other material for fixation of fragments of fractured bones. **ingrown n.,** aberrant growth of a toenail, with one or both lateral margins pushing deeply into adjacent soft tissue. **racket n.,** a short broad thumbnail. **spoon n.,** one with a concave surface.

Nalfon (nal'fon) trademark for a preparation of fenoprofen calcium.

nalidixic acid (nal-id-ik'sik) a synthetic antibacterial agent, $C_{12}H_{12}N_2O_3$, used in the treatment of genitourinary infections caused by gram-negative organisms.

nalorphine (nal'or-fēn) a semisynthetic congener of morphine, $C_{19}H_{21}NO_3$; used as an antagonist to morphine and related narcotics and in the diagnosis of narcotic addiction.

naloxone (nal-oks'ōn) a narcotic antagonist structurally related to oxymorphone, $C_{19}H_{21}$-NO_4; used as an antidote to narcotic overdosage and as an antagonist for pentazocine overdosage.

nandrolone (nan'dro-lōn) an androgenic, anabolic steroid, $C_{18}H_{26}O_2$; used as the decanoate and phenpropionate esters mainly as adjunctive therapy in senile and postmenopausal osteotherapy and in the treatment of severe growth retardation in children.

nanism (na'nizm) dwarfism.

nano- word element [Gr.], *dwarf; small size;* used in naming units of measurement to designate an amount 10^{-9} (one billionth) the size of the unit to which it is joined, e.g., nanocurie.

nanocephaly (na"no-sef'ah-le) microcephaly. **nanoceph'alous,** adj.

nanocormia (-kor'me-ah) abnormal smallness of the body or trunk.

nanogram (na′nah-gram) one billionth (10^{-9}) gram.

nanoid (na′noid) dwarfish.

nanomelus (na-nom′ĕ-lus) micromelus.

nanometer (na″no-mēt′er) one billionth (10^{-9}) meter.

nanophthalmia (nan″of-thal′me-ah) nanophthalmos.

nanophthalmos (nan″of-thal′mus) abnormal smallness in all dimensions of one or both eyes in the absence of other ocular defects; pure microphthalmos.

nanosecond (-sek′ind) one billionth (10^{-9}) second.

nanous (na′nus) dwarfed; stunted.

nanukayami (nah-noo-kah-yah′me) a leptospirosis marked by fever and jaundice, first reported in Japan, due to *Leptospira hebdomidis.*

nape (nāp) the back of the neck.

naphazoline (naf-az′ah-lēn) a vasoconstrictor, $C_{14}H_{14}N_2$, used as the hydrochloride salt to decongest nasal and ocular mucosae.

naphtha (naf′thah) petroleum benzin.

N.A.P.N.E.S. National Association for Practical Nurse Education and Services.

Naprosyn (nah-pro′sin) trademark for a preparation of naproxen.

napsylate (nap′sĭ-lāt) USAN contraction for 2-naphthalenesulfonate.

narcissism (nar′sĭ-sizm) dominant interest in one's self; self-love. **narcissis′tic,** adj.

narco- word element [Gr.], *stupor; stuporous state.*

narcoanalysis (nar″ko-ah-nal′ĭ-sis) psychotherapy utilizing barbiturates to release suppressed or repressed thoughts.

narcohypnosis (-hip-no′sis) hypnotic suggestions made while the patient is narcotized.

narcolepsy (nar′ko-lep″se) recurrent uncontrollable desire for sleep. **narcolep′tic,** adj.

narcosis (nar-ko′sis) reversible depression of the central nervous system produced by drugs, marked by stupor or insensibility.

narcotic (nar-kot′ic) 1. pertaining to or producing narcosis. 2. a drug that produces insensibility or stupor, especially an opioid.

narcotize (nar′kah-tīz) to put under the influence of a narcotic.

nares (na′rēs), sing. *na′ris* [L.] the nostrils; the external openings of the nasal cavity.

nasal (na′zil) pertaining to the nose.

nasalis (na-za′lis) [L.] nasal.

nascent (nas′int, na′sint) 1. being born; just coming into existence. 2. just liberated from a chemical combination, and hence more reactive because uncombined.

nasion (na′ze-on) the middle point of the frontonasal suture.

naso- word element [L.], *nose.*

nasoantral (na″zo-an′tril) pertaining to the nose and maxillary antrum.

nasoantrostomy (-an-tros′tah-me) surgical formation of a nasoantral window for drainage of an obstructed maxillary sinus.

nasociliary (-sil′e-ĕ″re) pertaining to the eyes, brow, and root of the nose.

nasofrontal (-frunt′l) pertaining to the nasal and frontal bones.

nasogastric (-gas′trik) pertaining to the nose and stomach.

nasolabial (-la′be-il) pertaining to the nose and lip.

nasolacrimal (-lak′rim′l) pertaining to the nose and lacrimal apparatus.

nasopalatine (-pal′ah-tīn) pertaining to the nose and palate.

nasopharyngitis (-far″in-jīt′is) inflammation of the nasopharynx.

nasopharyngolaryngoscope (-fah-ring″go-lah-ring′gah-skōp) a flexible fiberoptic endoscope for examining the nasopharynx and larynx.

nasopharynx (-far′inks) the part of the pharynx above the soft palate. **nasopharyn′geal,** adj.

nasosinusitis (-si″nis-īt′is) inflammation of the accessory sinuses of the nose.

nasus (na′sus) nose.

natal (nāt′l) 1. pertaining to birth. 2. pertaining to the nates (buttocks).

natality (na-tal′it-e) the birth rate.

natimortality (nāt″e-mor-tal′it-e) the proportion of stillbirths to the general birth rate.

National Formulary a book of standards for certain pharmaceuticals and preparations not included in the USP; revised every 5 years, and recognized as a book of official standards by the Pure Food and Drug Act of 1906. Abbreviated NF.

natrium (na′tre-um) [L.] sodium (symbol Na).

natriuresis (na″tre-ūr-e′sis) excretion of abnormal amounts of sodium in the urine.

natriuretic (-ūr-et′ik) 1. pertaining to or promoting natriuresis. 2. an agent that promotes natriuresis.

naturopathy (na″cher-op′ah-the) a drugless system of healing by the use of physical methods.

nausea (naw′ze-ah) an unpleasant sensation vaguely referred to the epigastrium and abdomen, with a tendency to vomit. **n. gravida′rum,** the morning sickness of pregnancy. **n. mari′na, n. nava′lis,** seasickness.

nauseant (naw′ze-int) 1. inducing nausea. 2. an agent causing nausea.

nauseate (naw′ze-āt) to affect with nausea.

nauseous (naw′shis, naw′ze-is) pertaining to or producing nausea.

navel (na′vil) the umbilicus.

navicular (nah-vik′ūl-er) boat-shaped, as the navicular bone.

NB chemical symbol, *niobium.*

NCI National Cancer Institute.

N.C.N. National Council of Nurses.

Nd chemical symbol, *neodymium.*

N.D.A. National Dental Association.

Ne chemical symbol, *neon.*

nearsightedness (nēr-sīt′id-nis) myopia.

nearthrosis (ne″ar-thro′sis) a false or artificial joint.

nebula (neb′ūl-ah) 1. a slight corneal opacity. 2. an oily preparation for use in an atomizer.

nebulization (neb″ūl-ĭ-za′shin) 1. conversion into a spray. 2. treatment by a spray.

nebulizer (neb′ūl-īz″er) an atomizer; a device for throwing a spray.

Necator (ne-kāt′er) a genus of hookworms, including *N. america′nus* (American or New World hookworm), a cause of hookworm disease.

necatoriasis (ne-kāt″or-i′ah-sis) infection with *Necator;* see *hookworm disease.*

neck (nek) a constricted portion, such as the part connecting the head and trunk, or the constricted part of an organ or other structure. **anatomic n.,** a constriction of the humerus just below its proximal articular surface. **n. of femur,** the heavy column of bone connecting the head of the femur and the shaft. **Madelung's n.,** diffuse symmetrical lipomas of the neck. **surgical n.,** the constricted part of the humerus just below the tuberosities. **n. of tooth,** the narrowed part of a tooth between the crown and the root. **uterine n., n. of uterus,** cervix uteri. **webbed n.,** pterygium colli. **wry n.,** torticollis.

necklace (nek′lis) a structure encircling the neck. **Casal's n.,** an eruption in pellagra, encircling the lower part of the neck.

necrectomy (nĕ-krek′tah-me) excision of necrotic tissue.

necro- word element [Gr.], *death.*

necrobacillosis (nek″ro-bas″ĭ-lo′sis) infection of animals with *Fusobacterium necrophorum.*

necrobiosis (-bi-o′sis) swelling, basophilia, and distortion of collagen bundles in the dermis, sometimes with obliteration of normal structure, but short of actual necrosis. **necrobiot′ic,** adj.

necrocytosis (-si-to′sis) death and decay of cells.

necrogenic (-jen′ik) productive of necrosis or death.

necrogenous (nĕ-kroj′ĭ-nis) originating or arising from dead matter.

necrology (nĕ-krol′ah-je, ne-krol′ah-je) statistics or records of death.

necrolysis (nĕ-krol′ĭ-sis) separation or exfoliation of necrotic tissue.

necrophagous (ne-krof′ah-gus) feeding upon carrion.

necrophilia (nek″ro-fil′e-ah) morbid attraction to death or to dead bodies; sexual intercourse with a dead body.

necrophilic (-fil′ik) 1. pertaining to necrophilia. 2. necrophilous.

necrophilous (nĕ-krof′ĭ-lus) showing a preference for dead tissue; said of microorganisms.

necrophobia (nek″rah-fo′be-ah) morbid dread of death or of dead bodies.

necropsy (nek′rop-se) examination of a body after death; autopsy.

necrose (ne-krōs′) to become necrotic or to undergo necrosis.

necrosis (nĕ-kro′sis), pl. *necro′ses* [Gr.] the morphological changes indicative of cell death caused by progressive enzymatic degradation; it may affect groups of cells or part of a structure or an organ. **necrot′ic,** adj. **aseptic n.,** necrosis without infection. **Balser's fatty n.,** gangrenous pancreatitis with omental bursitis and disseminated patches of necrosis of fatty tissues. **caseous n.,** that in which the tissue is soft, dry, and cheesy. **central n.,** that affecting the central portion of an affected bone, cell, or lobule of the liver. **cheesy n.,** that in which the tissue resembles cottage cheese; most often seen in tuberculosis and syphilis. **coagulation n.,** death of cells, the protoplasm of the cells becoming fixed and opaque by coagulation of the protein elements, the cellular outline persisting for a long time. **colliquative n.,** liquefactive n. **fat n.,** that in which the neutral fats in adipose tissue are split into fatty acids and glycerol, usually affecting subcutaneous fat depots as a result of trauma. **liquefactive n.,** that in which the necrotic material becomes softened and liquefied. **postpartum pituitary n.,** necrosis of the pituitary during the postpartum period, often associated with shock and excessive uterine bleeding during delivery, and leading to variable patterns of hypopituitarism. **subcutaneous fat n. of newborn,** a benign condition seen in the first few weeks of life, in which there is induration of the subcutaneous fat. **n. ustilagi′nea,** that due to ergotism. **Zenker's n.,** see under *degeneration.*

necrospermia (nek″ro-sperm′e-ah) a condition in which the spermatozoa of the semen are dead or motionless. **necrosper′mic,** adj.

necrotizing (nek′rah-tīz″ing) causing necrosis.

necrotomy (nĕ-krot′ah-me) 1. dissection of a dead body. 2. excision of a sequestrum.

needle (ne′d′l) 1. a sharp instrument for suturing or puncturing. 2. to puncture or separate with a needle. **aneurysm n.,** one with a handle, used in ligating blood vessels. **aspirating n.,** a long, hollow needle for removing fluid from a cavity. **cataract n.,** one used in removing a cataract. **discission n.,** a special form of cataract needle. **hypodermic n.,** a short, slender, hollow needle, used in injecting drugs beneath the skin. **stop n.,** one with a shoulder that prevents too deep penetration.

negativism (neg′it-iv-izm) opposition to suggestion or advice; behavior opposite to that appropriate to a specific situation.

Neisseria (ni-sēr′e-ah) a genus of gram-negative bacteria (family Neisseriaceae), including *N. gonorrhoe′ae,* the etiologic agent of gonorrhea, *N. meningi′tidis,* a prominent cause of meningitis and the specific etiologic agent of meningococcal meningitis.

Neisseriaceae (ni-sēr″e-a′se-e) a family of parasitic bacteria (order Eubacteriales).

neisserial (nīs-sēr′e-il) of, relating to, or caused by *Neisseria.*

Nemathelminthes (nem″ah-thel-min′thēz) in some classifications, a phylum including the Acanthocephala and Nematoda.

nematocide (nem′it-to-sīd″) 1. destroying nematodes. 2. an agent which destroys nematodes.

Nematoda (nem″ah-to′dah) a class of helminths (phylum Aschelminthes), the roundworms many of which are parasites; in some classifications, considered to be a phylum, and sometimes known as Nemathelminthes, or a class of that phylum.

nematode (nem′ah-tōd) a roundworm; any individual of the class Nematoda.

neo- word element [Gr.], *new; recent.*

neoantigen (ne″o-an′tĭ-jen) an intranuclear antigen, e.g., a T antigen, present in cells infected by oncogenic viruses.

neoblastic (-blas′tik) originating in or of the nature of new tissue.

neocerebellum (-sĕ″rĭ-bel′um) phylogenetically, the newer parts of the cerebellum, consisting of those parts predominately supplied by corticopontocerebellar fibers.

neocortex (-kor′teks) neopallium.

neodymium (-dim′e-um) chemical element (*see table*), at. no. 60, symbol Nd.

neoglottis (-glot′is) a glottis created by suturing the pharyngeal mucosa over the superior end of the transected trachea above the primary tracheostoma and making a permanent stoma in the mucosa; done to permit phonation after laryngectomy. **neoglot′tic,** adj.

neokinetic (-ki-net′ik) pertaining to the nervous motor mechanism regulating voluntary muscular control.

neologism (ne-ol′ah-jizm) a newly coined word; in psychiatry, a new word whose meaning may be known only to the patient using it.

neomembrane (ne″o-mem′brān) a false membrane.

neomycin (-mi′sin) a broad-spectrum antibacterial antibiotic produced by *Streptomyces fradiae,* effective against a wide range of gram-negative organisms.

neon (ne′on) chemical element (*see table*), at. no. 10, symbol Ne.

neonatal (ne″o-nāt′′l) pertaining to the first four weeks after birth.

neonate (ne′o-nāt) a newborn infant.

neonatology (-na-tol′ah-je) the diagnosis and treatment of disorders of the newborn.

neopallium (-pal′e-um) that part of the pallium (cerebral cortex) showing stratification and organization of the most highly evolved type; cf. *archipallium* and *paleopallium.*

neoplasia (-pla′ze-ah) the formation of a neoplasm.

neoplasm (ne′ah-plazm) tumor; any new and abnormal growth, specifically one in which cell multiplication is uncontrolled and progressive. Neoplasms may be benign or malignant.

neoplastic (ne″o-plas′tik) pertaining to neoplasia or to a neoplasm.

Neorickettsia (-rĭ-ket′sĭ-ah) a genus of rickettsiae (tribe Ehrlichieae), including a single species, *N. helmin′thoeca.* It is found in the salmon fluke (*Troglotrema salmincola*), a parasite of various fish, especially salmon and trout, and causes hemorrhagic enteritis in those ingesting raw infected fish.

neostigmine (-stig′min) a quaternary ammonium compound with cholinergic activity; used therapeutically as the bromide salt in the treatment of myasthenia gravis and glaucoma, and as the methylsulfate salt in the prevention and treatment of postoperative distention and urinary retention, as a screening test for pregnancy, in the treatment of delayed menstruation and myasthenia gravis, as a diagnostic test for myasthenia gravis, and as an antidote for curare principles.

neothalamus (ne″o-thal′ah-mus) the part of the thalamus connected to the neocortex.

nephelometer (nef″il-om′it-er) an instrument for measuring the concentration of substances in suspension by means of light scattering by the suspended particles.

nephr(o)- word element [Gr.], *kidney.*

nephralgia (ne-fral′je-ah) pain in a kidney.

nephrectasia (nef″rek-ta′ze-ah) distention of the kidney.

nephrectomy (ne-frek′tah-me) excision of a kidney.

nephric (nef′rik) pertaining to the kidney.

nephridium (nĕ-frid′e-um), pl. *nephri′dia* [L.] either of the paired excretory organs of certain invertebrates, having the inner end of the tubule opening into the coelomic cavity.

nephritic (nĕ-frit′ik) 1. pertaining to or affected with nephritis. 2. pertaining to the kidneys; renal. 3. an agent useful in kidney disease.

nephritis (nĕ-frīt′is), pl. *nephri′tides* [Gr.] inflammation of the kidney; a focal or diffuse proliferative or destructive disease that may involve the glomerulus, tubule, or interstitial renal tissue. **glomerular n.,** glomerulonephritis. **interstitial n.,** primary or secondary disease of the renal interstitial tissue. **lupus n.,** glomerulonephritis associated with systemic lupus erythematosus. **parenchymatous n.,** that affecting the parenchyma of kidney. **salt-losing n.,** intrinsic renal disease causing abnormal urinary sodium loss in persons ingesting normal amounts of sodium chloride, with vomiting, dehydration, and vascular collapse. **scarlatinal n.,** an acute nephritis due to scarlet fever. **transfusion n.,** nephropathy following transfusion from an incompatible donor.

nephritogenic (nĕ-frit″ah-jen′ik) causing nephritis.

nephrocalcinosis (-kal″sĭ-no′sis) precipitation of calcium phosphate in the renal tubules, with resultant renal insufficiency.

nephrocapsectomy (-kap-sek′tah-me) excision of the renal capsule.

nephrocele (nef′rah-sēl) hernia of a kidney.

nephrocolic (nef″ro-kol′ik) 1. pertaining to the kidney and colon. 2. renal colic.

nephrocoloptosis (-ko″lop-to′sis) downward displacement of the kidney and colon.

nephrocystitis (-sis-tit′is) inflammation of the kidney and bladder.

nephrogenic (-jen′ik) producing kidney tissue.

nephrogenous (nĕ-froj′ĭ-nus) arising in a kidney.

nephrography (nĕ-frog′rah-fe) roentgenography of the kidney.

nephrolith (nef′rah-lith) a calculus in a kidney.

nephrolithotomy (-lĭ-thot′ah-me) incision of the kidney for removal of calculi.

nephrology (nĕ-frol′ah-je) the branch of medical science that deals with the kidneys.

nephrolysis (nĕ-frol′ĭ-sis) 1. freeing of a kidney from adhesions. 2. destruction of kidney substance. **nephrolyt′ic,** adj.

nephroma (nĕ-fro′mah) a tumor of kidney tissue.

nephromegaly (nef″ro-meg′ah-le) enlargement of the kidney.

nephron (nef′ron) the structural and functional unit of the kidney, numbering about a million in the renal parenchyma, each being capable of forming urine; see also *renal tubules.*

nephronophthisis (nef″ron-of′thĭ-sis) wasting disease of the kidney substance. **familial juvenile n.,** a progressive hereditary kidney disease, marked by anemia, polyuria, renal loss of sodium, progressing to chronic renal failure, tubular atrophy, interstitial fibrosis, glomerular sclerosis, and medullary cysts.

nephropathy (nĕ-frop′ah-the) disease of the kidneys. **nephropath′ic,** adj. **IgA n.,** see under *glomerulonephritis.* **membranous n.,** see under *glomerulonephritis.* **reflux n.,** childhood pyelonephritis in which the renal scarring results from vesicoureteric reflux, with radiological appearance of intrarenal reflux.

nephropexy (nef″ro-pek″se) fixation or suspension of a hypermobile kidney.

nephroptosis (nef″rop-to′sis) downward displacement of a kidney.

nephropyelitis (nef″ro-pi″il-īt′is) pyelonephritis.

nephropyelography (-pi″il-og′rah-fe) radiography of the kidney and its pelvis.

nephropyosis (-pi-o′sis) suppuration of a kidney.

nephrorrhagia (-ra′je-ah) hemorrhage from the kidney.

nephrorrhaphy (nef-ror′ah-fe) suture of the kidney.

nephrosclerosis (nef″ro-sklĕ-ro′sis) hardening of the kidney; the condition of the kidney due to renovascular disease. **arteriolar n.,** that involving chiefly the arterioles, with degeneration of the renal tubules and fibrotic thickening of the glomeruli.

nephroscope (nef′rah-skōp) an instrument inserted into an incision in the renal pelvis for viewing the inside of the kidney.

nephrosis (nĕ-fro′sis), pl. *nephro′ses* [Gr.] any kidney disease, especially disease marked by purely degenerative lesions of the renal tubules. **nephrot′ic,** adj. **amyloid n.,** chronic nephrosis with amyloid degeneration of the median coat of the arteries and glomerular capillaries. **lipid n.,** nephrosis marked by edema, albuminuria, and changes in the protein and lipids of the blood and accumulation of globules of cholesterol esters in the tubular epithelium of the kidney. **lower nephron n.,** renal insufficiency leading to uremia, due to necrosis of the lower nephron cells, blocking the tubular lumens of this region; seen after severe injuries,

especially crushing injury to muscles (*crush syndrome*).

nephrosonephritis (nĕ-fro″so-nĕ-frīt′is) renal disease with nephrotic and nephritic components.

nephrostomy (nĕ-fros′tah-me) creation of a permanent fistula leading into the renal pelvis.

nephrotome (nef′rah-tōm″) one of the segmented divisions of the mesoderm connecting the somite with the lateral plates of unsegmented mesoderm; the source of much of the urogenital system.

nephrotomography (-tah-mog′rah-fe) radiologic visualization of the kidney by tomography. **nephrotomograph′ic,** adj.

nephrotomy (nĕ-frot′ah-me) incision of a kidney.

nephrotoxic (nef″ro-tok′sik) destructive to kidney cells.

nephrotoxin (-tok′sin) a toxin having a specific destructive effect on kidney cells.

nephrotropic (-trop′ik) having a special affinity for kidney tissue.

nephrotuberculosis (-too-burk″ūl-o′sis) renal disease due to *Mycobacterium tuberculosis.*

neptunium (nep-toon′e-um) chemical element (*see table*), at. no. 93, symbol Np.

nerve (nurv) a macroscopic, cordlike structure comprising a collection of nerve fibers that convey impulses between a part of the central nervous system and some other body region. See *Table of Nerves* and Plates X and XI. **accelerator n′s,** the cardiac sympathetic nerves, which, when stimulated, accelerate action of the heart. **afferent n.,** any nerve that transmits impulses from the periphery toward the central nervous system; see *sensory n.* **centrifugal n.,** efferent n. **centripetal n.,** afferent n. **depressor n.,** 1. one that lessens the activity of an organ. 2. an inhibitory nerve whose stimulation depresses a motor center. **efferent n.,** any that carries impulses from the central nervous system to the periphery, e.g., a motor nerve. **exciter n.,** one that transmits impulses resulting in an increase in functional activity. **excitoreflex n.,** a visceral nerve that produces reflex action. **furcal n.,** the fourth lumbar nerve. **fusimotor n′s,** those with nerve endings that innervate intrafusal fibers of the muscle spindle. **gangliated n.,** any nerve of the sympathetic nervous system. **inhibitory n.,** one that transmits impulses resulting in a decrease in functional activity. **Jacobson's n.,** tympanic n. **medullated n.,** myelinated n. **mixed n.,** one composed of both sensory and motor fibers. **motor n.,** an efferent nerve that stimulates muscle contraction. **myelinated n.,** one whose axons are encased in a myelin sheath. **peripheral n.,** any nerve outside the central nervous system. **pressor n.,** an afferent nerve, irritation of which stimulates a vasomotor center and increases intravascular tension. **secretory n.,** any efferent nerve whose stimulation increases glandular activity. **sensory n.,** a peripheral nerve that conducts impulses from a sense organ to the spinal cord or brain. **somatic n′s,** the motor and sensory nerves supplying skeletal

COMMON NAME* [MODALITY]	NA TERM†	ORIGIN*	BRANCHES†	DISTRIBUTION
abducent n. (6th cranial) [motor]	n. abducens	a nucleus in the pons, beneath floor of fourth ventricle		lateral rectus muscle of eyeball
accessory n. (11th cranial) [parasympathetic, motor]	n. accessorius	by cranial roots from side of medulla oblongata, and by spinal roots of spinal cord		internal branch to vagus, thereby to palate, pharynx, larynx, and thoracic viscera; external to sternocleidomastoid and trapezius muscles
acoustic n. See vestibulocochlear n.				
alveolar n., inferior [motor, general sensory]	n. alveolaris inferior	mandibular n.	mylohyoid, inferior dental, mental, and inferior gingival nerves	teeth and gums of lower jaw, skin of chin and lower lip, mylohyoid muscle and anterior belly of digastric muscle
alveolar n's, superior	nn. alveolares superiores	superior alveolar branches (anterior, middle, and posterior) that arise from infraorbital and maxillary n's, innervating teeth of upper jaw and maxillary sinus, and forming superior dental plexus		
ampullary n., anterior	n. ampullaris anterior	branch of vestibular n. that innervates ampulla of anterior semicircular duct, ending around hair cells of ampullary crest		
ampullary n., inferior. See ampullary n., posterior				
ampullary n., lateral	n. ampullaris lateralis	branch of vestibular n. that innervates ampulla of lateral semicircular duct, ending around hair cells of ampullary crest		
ampullary n., posterior	n. ampullaris posterior	branch of vestibular part of eighth cranial (vestibulocochlear) n. that innervates ampulla of posterior semicircular duct, ending around hair cells of ampullary crest		
ampullary n., superior. See ampullary n., anterior				
anal n's, inferior. See rectal n's, inferior				
anococcygeal n's [general sensory]	nn. anococcygei	coccygeal plexus		sacrococcygeal joint, coccyx, skin over coccyx
auditory n. See vestibulocochlear n.				
auricular n's, anterior [general sensory]	nn. auriculares anteriores	auriculotemporal n.		skin of anterosuperior part of external ear
auricular n., great [general sensory]	n. auricularis magnus	cervical plexus—C2–C3	anterior and posterior branches	skin over parotid gland and mastoid process, both surfaces of auricle
auricular n., posterior [motor, general sensory]	n. auricularis posterior	facial n.	occipital branch	posterior auricular and occipitofrontal muscles, skin of external acoustic meatus

401

*n. = nerve; n's = (pl.) nervus.
†n. = [L.] nervus; nn. = ([L.] pl.) nervi.

COMMON NAME* [MODALITY]	NA TERM†	ORIGIN*	BRANCHES*	DISTRIBUTION*
auriculotemporal n. [general sensory]	n. auriculotemporalis	by two roots from mandibular n.	anterior auricular n., n. of external acoustic meatus, parotid branches, branch to tympanic membrane, branches communicating with facial n.; terminal branches superficial temporal to scalp	parotid gland, scalp in temporal region, tympanic membrane. *See also* auricular n's, anterior *and* n. of external acoustic meatus
axillary n. [motor, general sensory]	n. axillaris	posterior cord of brachial plexus—C5–C6	lateral superior brachial cutaneous n., muscular branches	deltoid and teres minor muscles, skin over back of arm
buccal n. [general sensory]	n. buccalis	mandibular n.		skin and mucous membrane of cheeks, gums, and perhaps first two molars and the premolars
cardiac n., cervical, inferior [sympathetic (accelerator), visceral afferent (chiefly pain)]	n. cardiacus cervicalis inferior	cervicothoracic ganglion		heart via cardiac plexus
cardiac n., cervical, middle [sympathetic (accelerator), visceral afferent (chiefly pain)]	n. cardiacus cervicalis medius	middle cervical ganglion		heart
cardiac n., cervical, superior [sympathetic (accelerator)]	n. cardiacus cervicalis superior	superior cervical ganglion		heart
cardiac n., inferior. *See* cardiac n., cervical, inferior				
cardiac n., middle. *See* cardiac n., cervical, middle				
cardiac n., superior *See* cardiac n., cervical, superior				
cardiac n's, thoracic [sympathetic (accelerator), visceral afferent (chiefly pain)]	nn. cardiaci thoracici	ganglia T2–T4 or T5 of sympathetic trunk		heart
caroticotympanic n's [sympathetic]	nn. caroticotympanici	internal carotid plexus	help form tympanic plexus	tympanic region, parotid gland
carotid n's, external [sympathetic]	nn. carotici externi	superior cervical ganglion		cranial blood vessels and glands via external carotid plexus
carotid n., internal [sympathetic]	n. caroticus internus	superior cervical ganglion		cranial blood vessels and glands via internal carotid plexus
cavernous n's of clitoris [parasympathetic, sympathetic, visceral afferent]	nn. cavernosi clitoridis	uterovaginal plexus		erectile tissue of clitoris

402

Term	Latin	Definition	Distribution
cavernous n's of penis [sympathetic, parasympathetic, visceral afferent]	nn. cavernosi penis	prostatic plexus	
cerebral n's. See cranial n's			
cervical n's	nn. cervicales	the 8 pairs of n's that arise from cervical segments of spinal cord and, except last pair, leave vertebral column above correspondingly numbered vertebra; ventral branches of upper 4 on either side unite to form cervical plexus; those of lower 4, together with ventral branch of first thoracic n., form most of brachial plexus	
cervical n., transverse [general sensory]	n. transversus colli	cervical plexus—C2–C3; superior and inferior branches	skin on side and front of neck
ciliary n's, long [sympathetic, general sensory]	nn. ciliares longi	nasociliary n., from ophthalmic n.	dilator muscle of pupil, uvea, cornea
ciliary n's, short [parasympathetic, sympathetic, general sensory]	nn. ciliares breves	ciliary ganglion	smooth muscle and tunics of eye
clunial n's, inferior [general sensory]	nn. clunium inferiores	posterior femoral cutaneous n.	skin of lower part of buttock
clunial n's, middle [general sensory]	nn. clunium medii	plexus formed by lateral branches of dorsal branches of first 4 sacral nerves behind sacrum and coccyx	ligaments of sacrum and skin over posterior part of buttock
clunial n's, superior [general sensory]	nn. clunium superiores	lateral branches of dorsal branch of upper lumbar n's	skin of upper part of buttock
coccygeal n.	n., coccygeus	one of the pair of nerves arising from coccygeal segment of spinal cord	
cochlear n.	n. cochlearis	the part of the vestibulocochlear n. concerned with hearing, consisting of fibers that arise from the bipolar cells in the spiral ganglion and have their receptors in the spiral organ of the cochlea	
cranial n's	nn. craniales	the 12 pairs of n's connected with brain, including olfactory (I), optic (II), oculomotor (III), trochlear (IV), trigeminal (V), abducens (VI), facial (VII), vestibulocochlear (VIII), glossopharyngeal (IX), vagus (X), accessory (XI), and hypoglossal (XII) nerves	
cubital n. See ulnar n.			
cutaneous n. of arm, lateral, inferior [general sensory]	n. cutaneus brachii lateralis inferior	radial n.	skin of lateral surface of lower arm
cutaneous n. of arm, lateral, superior [general sensory]	n. cutaneus brachii lateralis superior	axillary n.	skin of back of arm
cutaneous n. of arm, medial [general sensory]	n. cutaneus brachii medialis	medial cord of brachial plexus (T1)	skin on medial and posterior aspects of arm
cutaneous n. of arm, posterior [general sensory]	n. cutaneous brachii posterior	radial n. in axilla	skin on back of arm

COMMON NAME* [MODALITY]	NA TERM†	ORIGIN*	BRANCHES*	DISTRIBUTION*
cutaneous n. of calf, lateral [general sensory]	n. cutaneus surae lateralis	common peroneal n.		skin of lateral side of back of leg, rarely may continue as sural n.
cutaneous n. of calf, medial [general sensory]	n. cutaneus surae medialis	tibial n.; usually joins fibular communicating branch of common peroneal n. to form sural n.		may continue as sural n.
cutaneous n., dorsal, intermediate [general sensory]	n. cutaneus dorsalis intermedius	superficial peroneal n.	dorsal digital n's of foot	skin of front of lower third of leg and dorsum of foot; ankle; skin and joints of adjacent sides of third and fourth, and of fourth and fifth toes
cutaneous n., dorsal, lateral [general sensory]	n. cutaneus dorsalis lateralis	continuation of sural n.		skin and joints of lateral side of foot and fifth toe
cutaneous n., dorsal, medial [general sensory]	n. cutaneus dorsalis medialis	superficial peroneal n.		skin and joints of medial side of foot and big toe; adjacent sides of second and third toes
cutaneous n. of forearm, lateral [general sensory]	n. cutaneus antebrachii lateralis	continuation of musculocutaneous n.		skin over radial skin of forearm; sometimes an area of skin of back of hand
cutaneous n. of forearm, medial [general sensory]	n. cutaneus antebrachii medialis	medial cord of brachial plexus (C8, T1)	anterior, ulnar	skin of front, medial, and posteromedial aspects of forearm
cutaneous n. of forearm, posterior [general sensory]	n. cutaneus antebrachii posterior	radial n.		skin of dorsal aspect of forearm
cutaneous n. of thigh, lateral [general sensory]	n. cutaneus femoris lateralis	lumbar plexus—L2–L3		skin of lateral aspect and front of thigh
cutaneous n. of thigh, posterior [general sensory]	n. cutaneus femoris posterior	sacral plexus—S1–S3	inferior clunial n's, perineal branches	skin of buttock, external genitalia, back of thigh and calf
digital n's, dorsal, radial. *See* digital n's of radial n., dorsal				
digital n's, dorsal, ulnar. *See* digital n's of ulnar n., dorsal				
digital n's of foot, dorsal [general sensory]	nn. digitales dorsales pedis	intermediate dorsal cutaneous n.		skin and joint of adjacent sides of third and fourth, and of fourth and fifth toes
digital n's of lateral plantar n., plantar, common [motor, general sensory]	nn. digitales plantares communes nervi plantaris lateralis	superficial branch of lateral plantar n.	medial n. gives rise to 2 proper plantar digital n's	lateral one to short flexor muscle of little toe; skin and joints of lateral side of sole and little toe; medial one to adjacent sides of fourth and fifth toes

n., plantar, proper [motor, general sensory]	proprii nervi plantaris lateralis			skin and joints of lateral side of sole and little toe, adjacent surfaces of fourth and fifth toes
digital n's of lateral surface of great toe and medial surface of second toe, dorsal [general sensory]	nn. digitales dorsales hallucis lateralis et digiti secundi medialis	medial terminal division of deep peroneal n.		skin and joints of adjacent sides of first and second toes
digital n's of medial plantar n., plantar, common [motor, general sensory]	nn. digitales plantares communes nervi plantaris medialis	medial plantar n.	muscular and proper plantar digital n's	flexor hallucis brevis muscles and first lumbrical muscles, skin and joints of medial side of foot and first toe, and adjacent sides of first and second, second and third, and third and fourth toes
digital n's of medial plantar n., plantar, proper [general sensory]	nn. digitales plantares proprii nervi plantaris medialis	common plantar digital n's		skin and joints of first toe, and adjacent sides of first and second, second and third, and third and fourth toes; the nerves extend to the dorsum to supply nail beds and tips of toes
digital n's of median n., palmar, common [motor, general sensory]	nn. digitales palmares communes nervi mediani	lateral and medial divisions of median n.		thumb, index, middle, and ring fingers, and first two lumbrical muscles
digital n's of median n., palmar, proper [motor, general sensory]	nn. digitales palmares proprii nervi mediani	common palmar digital n's	proper palmar digital n's	first two lumbrical muscles, skin and joints of both sides and palmar aspect of thumb, index, and middle fingers, radial side of ring finger, back of distal aspect of these digits
digital n's of radial n., dorsal [general sensory]	nn. digitales dorsales nervi radialis	superficial branch of radial n.		skin and joints of back of thumb, index finger, and part of middle finger, as far distally as digital phalanx
digital n's of ulnar n., dorsal [general sensory]	nn. digitales dorsales nervi ulnaris	dorsal branch of ulnar n.		skin and joints of medial side of little finger, dorsal aspects of adjacent sides of little and ring fingers and of ring and middle fingers
digital n's of ulnar n., palmar, common [general sensory]	nn. digitales palmares communes nervi ulnaris	superficial branch of ulnar n.	proper palmar digital n's	little and ring fingers
digital n's of ulnar n., palmar, proper [general sensory]	nn. digitales palmares proprii nervi ulnaris	the lateral of the two common palmar digital n's from superficial branch of ulnar n.		skin and joints of adjacent sides of fourth and fifth fingers

TABLE OF NERVES—*Continued*

COMMON NAME* [MODALITY]	NA TERM†	ORIGIN*	BRANCHES*	DISTRIBUTION*
dorsal n. of clitoris [general sensory, motor]	n. dorsalis clitoridis	pudendal n.		deep transverse muscle of perineum, sphincter muscle of urethra, corpus cavernosum of clitoris, and skin, prepuce, and glans of clitoris
dorsal n. of penis [general sensory, motor]	n. dorsalis penis	pudendal n.		deep transverse muscle of perineum, sphincter muscle of urethra, corpus cavernosum of penis, and skin, prepuce, and glans of penis
dorsal scapular n. [motor]	n. dorsalis scapulae	brachial plexus—ventral branch of C5		rhomboid muscles and occasionally the levator muscle of scapula
ethmoidal n., anterior [general sensory]	n. ethmoidalis anterior	continuation of nasociliary n., from ophthalmic n.	internal, external, lateral, and medial nasal branches	mucosa of upper and anterior nasal septum, lateral wall of nasal cavity, skin of lower bridge and tip of nose
ethmoidal n., posterior [general sensory]	n. ethmoidalis posterior	nasociliary n., from ophthalmic n.		mucosa of posterior ethmoid cells and of sphenoidal sinus
n. of external acoustic meatus [general sensory]	n. meatus acustici externi	auriculotemporal n.		skin lining external acoustic meatus, tympanic membrane
facial n. (7th cranial) [motor, parasympathetic, general sensory, special sensory]. *See also* intermediate n.	n. facialis	inferior border of pons, between olive and inferior cerebellar peduncle	stapedius, posterior auricular n.'s; parotid plexus; digastric, temporal, zygomatic, buccal, lingual, marginal mandibular, and cervical branches; communicating branch with tympanic plexus	various structures of face, head, and neck (see also individual branches in this table)
femoral n. [general sensory, motor]	n. femoralis	lumbar plexus—L2–L4; descending behind inguinal ligament to femoral triangle	saphenous n., muscular and anterior cutaneous branches	skin of thigh and leg, muscles of front of thigh, and hip and knee joints (see also individual branches in this table)
fibular n's. *See* entries under peroneal n.				
frontal n. [general sensory]	n. frontalis	ophthalmic division of trigeminal n.; enters orbit through superior orbital fissure	supraorbital and supratrochlear n's	chiefly to forehead and scalp (see individual branches listed in this table)
genitofemoral n. [general sensory, motor]	n. genitofemoralis	lumbar plexus—L1–L2	genital and femoral branches	cremaster muscle, skin of scrotum or labium majus and of adjacent area of thigh and femoral triangle

Term	Latin	Origin	Branches	Distribution
glossopharyngeal n. (9th cranial) [motor, parasympathetic, general sensory, special sensory, visceral sensory]	n., glossopharyngeus	several rootlets from lateral side of upper medulla oblongata, between olive and inferior cerebellar peduncle	tympanic n., pharyngeal, tonsillar, and lingual branches, branch to carotid sinus, communicating branch with auricular branch of vagus n.	has two enlargements (superior and inferior ganglia) and supplies tongue, pharynx, (see also individual branches in this table)
gluteal n., inferior [motor] gluteal n., superior [motor, general sensory]	n. gluteus inferior n. gluteus superior	sacral plexus—L5–S2 sacral plexus—L4–S1		gluteus maximus muscle gluteus medius and minimus muscles, tensor fasciae latae, and hip joint
hemorrhoidal n's, inferior See rectal n's, inferior				
hypogastric n.	n. hypogastricus (dexter/sinister)	a nerve trunk situated on either side (right and left), interconnecting superior and inferior hypogastric plexuses		
hypoglossal n. (12th cranial) [motor]	n. hypoglossus	several rootlets in anterolateral sulcus between olive and pyramid of medulla oblongata; passes through hypoglossal canal to tongue	lingual branches	styloglossus, hyoglossus, and genioglossus muscles, intrinsic muscles of tongue
iliohypogastric n. [motor, general sensory]	n. iliohypogastricus	lumbar plexus—L1 (sometimes T12)	lateral and anterior cutaneous branches	skin above pubis and over lateral side of buttock, and occasionally pyramidal muscle
ilioinguinal n. [general sensory]	n. ilio-inguinalis	lumbar plexus—L1 (sometimes T12); accompanies spermatic cord through inguinal canal	anterior scrotal or labial branches	skin of scrotum or labia majora, and adjacent part of thigh
infraoccipital n. See suboccipital n.				
infraorbital n. [general sensory]	n. infraorbitalis	continuation of maxillary n., entering orbit through inferior orbital fissure, occupying in succession infraorbital groove, canal, and foramen	middle and anterior superior alveolar, inferior palpebral, internal and external nasal, and superior labial branches	incisor, cuspid, and premolar teeth of upper jaw, skin and conjunctiva of lower eyelid, mobile septum and skin of side of nose, mucous membrane of mouth, skin of upper lip
infratrochlear n. [general sensory]	n. infratrochlearis	nasociliary n., from ophthalmic n.	palpebral branches	skin of root and upper bridge of nose and lower eyelid, conjunctiva, lacrimal duct
intercostobrachial n's [general sensory]	nn. intercostobrachiales	second and third intercostal n's		skin on back and medial aspect of arm
intermediate n. [parasympathetic, special sensory]	n. intermedius	smaller root of facial n., between main root and vestibulocochlear n.	greater petrosal n., chorda tympani	lacrimal, nasal, palatine, submandibular, and sublingual glands, and anterior two thirds of tongue

COMMON NAME* [MODALITY]	NA TERM†	ORIGIN*	BRANCHES*	DISTRIBUTION*
intermediofacial n. *See* facial n. and intermediate n.	n. intermediofacialis (NA alternative for facial and intermediate n's considered together)			
interosseous n. of forearm, anterior [motor, general sensory]	n. interosseus [antebrachii] anterior	median n.		long flexor muscle of thumb, deep flexor muscle of fingers, quadrate pronator muscle, wrist and intercarpal joints
interosseous n. of forearm, posterior [motor, general sensory]	n., interosseus [antebrachii] posterior	continuation of deep branch of radial n.		long abductor muscle of thumb, extensor muscles of thumb and index finger, wrist, and intercarpal joints
interosseous n. of leg [general sensory]
ischiadic n. *See* sciatic n.	interosseus cruris	tibial n.		interosseous membrane and ti-biofemoral syndesmosis
jugular n.	n. jugularis	a branch of the superior cervical ganglion which communicates with glossopharyngeal and vagus n's		
labial n's, anterior [general sensory]	nn. labiales anteriores	ilioinguinal n.		skin of anterior labial region of labia majora and adjacent part of thigh
labial n's, posterior [general sensory]	nn. labiales posteriores	pudendal n.		labium majus
lacrimal n. [general sensory]	n. lacrimalis	ophthalmic division of trigeminal n. entering orbit through superior orbital fissure		lacrimal gland, conjunctiva, lateral commissure of eye, skin of upper eyelid
laryngeal n., inferior [motor]	n. laryngeus inferior	recurrent laryngeal n., especially the terminal portion		intrinsic muscles of larynx, except cricothyroid; communicates with internal laryngeal n.
laryngeal n., recurrent [parasympathetic, visceral afferent, motor]	n. laryngeus recurrens	vagus n. (chiefly the cranial part of the accessory n.)	inferior laryngeal n., tracheal, esophageal, and inferior cardiac branches	tracheal mucosa, esophagus, cardiac plexus
laryngeal n., superior [motor, general sensory, visceral afferent, parasympathetic]	n. laryngeus superior	inferior ganglion of vagus n.	external, internal, and communicating branches	cricothyroid muscle and inferior constrictor muscle of pharynx, mucous membrane of back of tongue and larynx
lingual n. [general sensory]	n. lingualis	mandibular n., descending to tongue, first medial to mandible and then under cover of mucosa of mouth	sublingual n., lingual branch, branch to isthmus of fauces, branch communicating with hypoglossal n. and chorda tympani	anterior two thirds of tongue, adjacent areas of mouth, gums, isthmus of fauces
lumbar n's	nn. lumbales	the 5 pairs of n's that arise from lumbar segments of spinal cord, each pair leaving vertebral column below corresponding numbered vertebrae; ventral branches of these nerves		

408

Name	Latin	Origin	Branches	Distribution
mandibular n. [third division of trigeminal n.] [general sensory, motor]	n. mandibularis	trigeminal ganglion	meningeal branch, masseteric, deep temporal, lateral and medial pterygoid, buccal, auriculotemporal, lingual, and inferior alveolar n's	extensive distribution to muscles of mastication, skin of face, mucous membrane of mouth, and teeth (see also individual branches in this table)
masseteric n. [motor, general sensory]	n. massetericus	mandibular division of trigeminal n.		masseter muscle, temporomandibular joint
maxillary n. [second division of trigeminal n.] [general sensory]	n. maxillaris	trigeminal ganglion	meningeal branch, zygomatic n., posterior superior alveolar branches, infraorbital n., pterygopalatine n's, and indirectly branches of pterygopalatine ganglion	extensive distribution to skin of face and scalp, mucous membrane of maxillary sinus and nasal cavity, and teeth
median n. [general sensory]	n. medianus	lateral and medial cords of brachial plexus—C6–T1	anterior interosseous n. of forearm, common palmar digital n's, muscular and palmar branches, communicating branch with ulnar n.	ultimately, skin on front of lateral part of hand, most of flexor muscles of front of forearm, most of short muscles of thumb, elbow joint, and many joints of hand
mental n. [general sensory]	n. mentalis	inferior alveolar n.	mental and inferior labial branches	skin of chin, lower lip
musculocutaneous n. [general sensory, motor]	n. musculocutaneus	lateral cord of brachial plexus—C5–C7	lateral cutaneous n. of forearm, muscular branches	coracobrachial, biceps, brachial muscles, elbow joint, skin of radial side of forearm
mylohyoid n. [motor]	n. mylohyoideus	inferior alveolar n.		mylohyoid muscle, anterior belly of digastric muscle
nasociliary n. [general sensory]	n. nasociliaris	ophthalmic division of trigeminal nerve	long ciliary, posterior ethmoidal, anterior ethmoidal, infratrochlear n's and a communicating branch to ciliary ganglion	(see individual branches in this table)
nasopalatine n. [parasympathetic, general sensory]	n. nasopalatinus	pterygopalatine ganglion		mucosa and glands of most of nasal septum and anterior part of hard palate
obturator n. [general sensory, motor]	n. obturatorius	lumbar plexus—L3–L4	anterior, posterior, muscular branches	gracilis and adductor muscles, skin of medial part of thigh, and hip joints
obturator n., accessory [general sensory, motor]	n. obturatorius accessorius	ventral branches of L3–L4		pectineus muscle, hip joint, obturator nerve
obturator n., internal [general sensory, motor]	n. obturatorius internus	ventral branches of L5, S1–S2		posterior superior gemellus, obturator internus muscles
occipital n., greater [general sensory, motor]	n. occipitalis major	medial branch of dorsal branch of C2		semispinal muscle of head and skin of head as far forward as vertex

TABLE OF NERVES—Continued

COMMON NAME* [MODALITY]	NA TERM†	ORIGIN*	BRANCHES*	DISTRIBUTION*
occipital n., lesser [general sensory]	n. occipitalis minor	superficial cervical plexus—C2–C3		ascends behind auricle and supplies some of skin of side of head and on cranial surface of auricle
occipital n., third [general sensory]	n. occipitalis tertius	medial branch of dorsal branch of C3		skin of upper part of back of neck and head
oculomotor n. (3rd cranial) [motor, parasympathetic]	n. oculomotorius	brain stem, emerging medial to cerebral peduncles, running forward in the cavernous sinus	superior and inferior branches	entering orbit through superior orbital fissure, the branches supply levator muscle of upper lid, all extrinsic eye muscles except lateral rectus and superior oblique, and carry parasympathetic fibers from ciliary muscle to sphincter of pupil
olfactory n's (1st cranial) [special sensory]	nn. olfactorii	the n's of smell, consisting of about 20 bundles arising in olfactory epithelium and passing through cribriform plate of ethmoid bone to olfactory bulb		
ophthalmic n. (first division of trigeminal n.) [general sensory]	n. ophthalmicus	trigeminal ganglion	tentorial branches, frontal, lacrimal, nasociliary n's	eyeball and conjunctiva, lacrimal sac and gland, nasal mucosa and frontal sinus, external nose, eyelid, forehead, and scalp (see also individual branches in this table)
optic n. (2nd cranial) [special sensory]	n. opticus	the nerve of sight, consisting chiefly of axons and central processes of cells of the ganglionic layer of retina leaving the orbit through the optic canal, joining the optic chiasm (the medial ones crossing over to opposite side), and continuing as the optic tract		
palatine n., anterior. See palatine n., greater				
palatine n., greater [parasympathetic, sympathetic, general sensory]	n. palatinus major	pterygopalatine ganglion	posterior inferior [lateral] nasal branches	emerges through greater palatine foramen and supplies palate
palatine n's, lesser [parasympathetic, sympathetic, general sensory]	nn. palatini minores	pterygopalatine ganglion		emerge through lesser palatine foramen and supply soft palate and tonsil
pectoral n., lateral [motor, general sensory]	n. pectoralis lateralis	lateral cord of brachial plexus or anterior divisions of upper and middle trunks (C5–C7)		usually several n's supplying lesser pectoral muscle and acromioclavicular and shoulder joints
pectoral n., medial [motor]	n. pectoralis medialis	medial cord or lower trunk of brachial plexus (C8, T1)		usually several n's supplying greater and lesser pectoral muscles

Name [modality]	Latin	Origin	Branches	Distribution
perineal n's [motor, general sensory]	mn. perineales	pudendal n. in pudendal canal	muscular branches and posterior scrotal or labial nerves	muscular branches supply bulbospongiosus, ischiocavernosus, superficial transverse perinei muscles and bulb of penis and, in part, external sphincter muscle of anus and levator ani muscle; the scrotal (labial) n's supply the scrotum or labium majus
peroneal n., common [general sensory, motor]	n. fibularis communis	sciatic n. in lower part of thigh		supplies short head of biceps femoris muscle; gives off lateral sural cutaneous n. and communicating branch as it descends in popliteal fossa, supplies knee and superior tibiofibular joints and tibialis anterior muscle; divides into superficial and deep peroneal n's
peroneal n., deep [general sensory, motor]	n. fibularis profundus	a terminal branch of common peroneal n.		winds around neck of fibula and descends on the interosseous membrane to front of ankle; muscular branches given off to tibialis anterior, extensor digitorum longus, and third peroneal muscles, and a twig to ankle joint; a lateral terminal division supplies extensor brevis muscle and tarsal joints; medial terminal division, or digital branch, divides into dorsal digital n's for skin and joints of adjacent sides of first and second toes
peroneal n., superficial [general sensory, motor]	n. fibularis superficialis	a terminal branch of common peroneal n.		descends in front of fibula, supplies peroneus longus and brevis muscles and, in the lower part of the leg, divides into the muscular branches, medial and intermediate dorsal cutaneous n's
petrosal n., deep [sympathetic]	n. petrosus profundus	internal carotid plexus		joins greater petrosal n. to form n. of pterygoid canal and supplies lacrimal, nasal, and palatine glands via pterygopalatine ganglion and its branches
petrosal n., greater [parasympathetic, general sensory]	n. petrosus major	intermediate n. via geniculate ganglion		running forward from geniculate ganglion, joins deep petrosal n. of pterygoid canal and reaches lacrimal, nasal, and palatine glands and nasopharynx via pterygopalatine ganglion and its branches
petrosal n., lesser [parasympathetic]	n. petrosus minor	tympanic plexus		parotid gland via otic ganglion and auriculotemporal n.
phrenic n. [motor, general sensory]	n. phrenicus	cervical plexus—C4-C5	pericardial and phrenicoabdominal branches	pleura, pericardium, diaphragm, peritoneum, sympathetic plexuses
phrenic n's, accessory	mn. phrenici accessorii	inconstant contribution of fifth cervical n. to phrenic n.; when present, they run a separate course to root of neck or into thorax before joining phrenic n.		

411

COMMON NAME* [MODALITY]	NA TERM†	ORIGIN*	BRANCHES*	DISTRIBUTION*
piriform n. [general sensory, motor]	n. piriformis	dorsal branches of ventral rami of S1–S2		anterior piriform muscle
plantar n., lateral [general sensory, motor]	n. plantaris lateralis	smaller of terminal branches of tibial n.	muscular, superficial, and deep branches	lying between first and second layers of muscles of sole, supplies quadratus plantae, abductor digiti minimi, flexor digiti minimi brevis, adductor hallucis, interossei, and second, third, and fourth lumbrical muscles, and gives off cutaneous and articular twigs to lateral side of sole and fourth and fifth toes (see also individual branches in this table)
plantar n., medial [general sensory, motor]	n. plantaris medialis	larger of terminal branches of tibial n.	common plantar digital n's and muscular branches	abductor hallucis, flexor digitorum brevis, flexor hallucis brevis, and first lumbrical muscles and cutaneous and articular twigs to medial side of sole and first to fourth toes (see also individual branches in this table)
pneumogastric n. See vagus n.				
pterygoid n., lateral [motor] pterygoid n., medial [motor]	n. pterygoideus lateralis n. pterygoideus medialis	mandibular n. mandibular n.		lateral pterygoid medial pterygoid, tensor tympani, tensor veli palatini muscles
n. of pterygoid canal [parasympathetic, sympathetic]	n. canalis pterygoidei	union of deep and greater petrosal n's		pterygopalatine ganglion and branches
pterygopalatine n's [general sensory]	nn. pterygopalatini	two nerves connecting maxillary n. to pterygopalatine ganglion; they are the sensory roots of the ganglion		
pudendal n. [general sensory, motor, parasympathetic]	n. pudendus	sacral plexus—S2–S4	enters pudendal canal, gives off inferior rectal n., then divides into perineal n. and dorsal n. of penis (clitoris)	muscles, skin, and erectile tissue of perineum (see also individual branches in this table)
n. of quadrate muscle of thigh [sensory, motor]	n. musculi quadrati femoris	ventral branches of ventral rami of L4–L5		inferior gemellus, anterior quadratus femoris muscles, hip joint

radial n. [general sensory, motor]	n. radialis	posterior cord of brachial plexus—C6-C8, and sometimes C5 and T1	posterior cutaneous and inferior lateral cutaneous n's of arm, posterior cutaneous n. of forearm, muscular, deep, and superficial branches	descending in back of arm and forearm, ultimately distributed to skin on back of forearm, arm, and hand, extensor muscles on back of arm and forearm, and elbow joint and many joints of hand
rectal n's, inferior [general sensory, motor]	nn. rectales inferiores	pudendal n., or independently from sacral plexus		external sphincter muscle of anus, skin around anus, lining of anal canal up to pectinate line
recurrent n. *See* laryngeal n., recurrent				
saccular n.	n. saccularis	the branch of vestibular part of eighth cranial (vestibulocochlear) nerve that innervates macular of saccule		
sacral n's	nn. sacrales	the 5 pairs of n's that arise from sacral segments of spinal cord; the ventral branches of first 4 pairs participate in formation of sacral plexus		
saphenous n. [general sensory]	n. saphenus	termination of femoral n.	infrapatellar and medial crural cutaneous branches	knee joint, subsartorial and patellar plexuses, skin on medial side of leg and foot (see individual branches in this table)
sciatic n. [general sensory, motor]	n. ischiadicus	sacral plexus—L4–S3; leaves pelvis through greater sciatic foramen	divides into common peroneal and tibial n's, usually in lower third of thigh	
scrotal n's, anterior [general sensory]	nn. scrotales anteriores	ilioinguinal n.		skin of anterior scrotal region
scrotal n's, posterior [general sensory]	nn. scrotales posteriores	perineal n's		skin of scrotum
spinal n's	nn. spinales	the 31 pairs of n's that arise from the spinal cord and pass between the vertebrae, including 8 cervical, 12 thoracic, 5 lumbar, 5 sacral, and 1 coccygeal		
splanchnic n., greater. *See* thoracic splanchnic n., greater				
splanchnic n., lesser. *See* thoracic splanchnic n., lesser				
splanchnic n., lowest. *See* thoracic splanchnic n., lowest				
splanchnic n's, lumbar [preganglionic sympathetic, visceral afferent]	nn. splanchnici lumbales	lumbar ganglia or sympathetic trunk		upper nerves join celiac and adjacent plexuses, middle ones go to mesenteric and adjacent plexuses, lower ones descend to superior hypogastric plexus

COMMON NAME* [MODALITY]	NA TERM†	ORIGIN*	BRANCHES*	DISTRIBUTION*
splanchnic n's, pelvic [preganglionic sympathetic, visceral afferent]	nn. splanchnici pelvini	sacral plexus—S3–S4		leaving sacral plexus, enter inferior hypogastric plexus and supply pelvic organs
splanchnic n's, sacral [preganglionic sympathetic, visceral afferent]	nn. splanchnici sacrales	sacral part of sympathetic trunk		pelvic organs and blood vessels via inferior hypogastric plexus
stapedius n. [motor]	n. stapedius	facial n.		stapedius muscle
subclavian n. [motor, general sensory]	n. subclavius	upper trunk of brachial plexus—C5		subclavius muscle, sternoclavicular joint
subcostal n. [general sensory, motor]	n. subcostalis	ventral branch of T12		skin of lower abdomen and lateral side of gluteal region, parts of transverse, oblique, and rectus muscles, and usually pyramidal muscle, and adjacent peritoneum
sublingual n. [parasympathetic, general sensory]	n. sublingualis	lingual n.		sublingual gland and overlying mucous membrane
suboccipital n. [motor]	n. suboccipitalis	dorsal branch of C1		emerges above posterior arch of atlas, supplies muscles of suboccipital triangle and semispinal muscle of head
subscapular n. [motor]	n. subscapularis	posterior cord of brachial plexus—C5		usually two or more nerves, upper and lower, supplying subscapular and teres major muscles
supraclavicular n's, anterior. *See supraclavicular n's, medial*				
supraclavicular n's, intermediate [general sensory]	nn. supraclaviculares intermedii	cervical plexus—C3–C4		descend in posterior triangle, cross clavicle, supplying skin over pectoral and deltoid regions
supraclavicular n's, lateral [general sensory]	nn. supraclaviculares laterales	cervical plexus—C3–C4		descend in posterior triangle, cross clavicle, supplying skin of superior and posterior aspects of shoulder
supraclavicular n's, medial [general sensory]	nn. supraclaviculares mediales	cervical plexus—C3–C4		descend in posterior triangle, cross clavicle, supplying skin of medial infraclavicular region
supraclavicular n's, middle. *See supraclavicular n's, intermediate*				
supraclavicular n's, posterior. *See supraclavicular*				

414

			lateral and medial branches	leaves orbit through supraorbital notch or foramen, supplying skin of upper eyelid, forehead, anterior part of scalp (to vertex), mucosa of frontal sinus
supraorbital n. [general sensory]	n. supraorbitalis	continuation of frontal n.		
suprascapular n. [motor, general sensory]	n. suprascapularis	brachial plexus—C5–C6		descends through suprascapular and spinoglenoid notches, supplying acromioclavicular and shoulder joints, and supraspinous and infraspinous muscles
supratrochlear n. [general sensory]	n. supratrochlearis	frontal n.		leaves orbit at end of supraorbital margin, supplying forehead and upper eyelid
sural n. [general sensory]	n. suralis	medial sural n. and communicating branch of common peroneal n.	lateral dorsal cutaneous n. and lateral calcaneal branches	skin on back of leg, and skin and joints on lateral side of foot and heel
temporal n's, deep [motor]	nn. temporales profundi	mandibular n.		temporal muscles
n. of tensor tympani muscle [motor]	n. musculi tensoris tympani	mandibular n. via n. to medial pterygoid muscle and otic ganglion		tensor muscle of tympanum
n. of tensor veli palatini muscle [motor]	n. musculi tensoris veli palatini	mandibular n. via n. to medial pterygoid muscle and otic ganglion		tensor muscle of palatine velum
thoracic n's	nn. thoracici	the 12 pairs of spinal n's that arise from thoracic segments of spinal cord, each pair leaving vertebral column below correspondingly numbered vertebra		body wall of thorax and upper part of abdomen
thoracic n., long [motor]	n. thoracicus longus	brachial plexus—ventral branches of C5–C7		descends behind brachial plexus to anterior serratus muscle
thoracic splanchnic n., greater [preganglionic sympathetic, visceral afferent]	n. splanchnicus thoracicus major	thoracic sympathetic trunk, thoracic ganglia T5–T10		descends through diaphragm or its aortic openings and ends in celiac ganglia and plexuses with a splanchnic ganglion commonly near the diaphragm
thoracic splanchnic n., lesser [preganglionic sympathetic, visceral afferent]	n. splanchnicus thoracicus minor	thoracic ganglia T9, T10 of sympathetic trunk	renal ramus	pierces diaphragm, joins aorticorenal ganglion and celiac plexus, communicates with the renal and mesenteric plexuses
thoracic splanchnic n., lowest [sympathetic, visceral afferent]	n. splanchnicus thoracicus imus	last ganglion of sympathetic trunk or lesser splanchnic n.		aorticorenal ganglion and adjacent plexus
thoracodorsal n. [motor]	n. thoracodorsalis	posterior cord of brachial plexus—C7–C8		latissimus dorsi muscle

TABLE OF NERVES—Continued

COMMON NAME* [MODALITY]	NA TERM†	ORIGIN*	BRANCHES*	DISTRIBUTION*
tibial n. [general sensory, motor]	n. tibialis	sciatic n. in lower thigh	interosseous n. of leg, medial cutaneous n. of calf, sural and medial and lateral plantar n's, muscular and medial calcaneal branches	while still incorporated in sciatic n., supplies semimembranous and semitendinous muscles, long head of biceps, and adductor magnus muscle; supplies knee joint as it descends in popliteal fossa; continuing into leg, supplies muscles and skin of calf, sole, and toes (see also individual branches in this table)
trigeminal n. (5th cranial) [general sensory, motor]	n. trigeminus	emerges from lateral surface of pons as a motor and a sensory root, the latter expanding into trigeminal ganglion, from which the 3 divisions of nerve arise (see mandibular n., maxillary n., and ophthalmic n.)		face, teeth, mouth, nasal cavity, muscles of mastication
trochlear n. (4th cranial) [motor]	n. trochlearis	fibers of each nerve (one on either side) decussate across median plane, and emerge from back of brain stem below corresponding inferior colliculus		runs forward in lateral wall of cavernous sinus and traverses superior orbital fissure, supplying superior oblique muscle of eyeball
tympanic n. [general sensory, parasympathetic]	n. tympanicus	inferior ganglion of glossopharyngeal n.	helps form tympanic plexus	mucous membrane of tympanic cavity, mastoid air cells, auditory tube, and, via lesser petrosal n. and otic ganglion, parotid gland
ulnar n. [general sensory, motor]	n. ulnaris	medial and lateral cords of brachial plexus—C7–T1	muscular, dorsal, palmar, superficial, deep branches	ultimately to skin on front and medial part of hand, some flexor muscles on front of forearm, many short muscles of hand, elbow joint, many joints of hand
utricular n. utriculoampullary n.	n. utricularis n. utriculoampullaris	the branch of vestibular n. that innervates macula of utricle a n. that arises by peripheral division of vestibular n. and supplies utricle and ampullae of semicircular ducts		
vaginal n's [sympathetic, parasympathetic]	mn. vaginales	uterovaginal plexus		vagina

416

vagus n. (10th cranial) [parasympathetic, visceral afferent, motor, general sensory]	n. vagus	by numerous rootlets from lateral side of medulla oblongata in groove between olive and inferior cerebellar peduncle	superior and recurrent laryngeal n's, meningeal, auricular, pharyngeal, cardiac, bronchial, gastric, hepatic, celiac, and renal branches, pharyngeal, pulmonary, and esophageal plexuses, and anterior and posterior trunks	descending through jugular foramen, presents as a superior and inferior ganglion, continues through neck and thorax into abdomen, supplying sensory fibers to ear, tongue, pharynx, and larynx, motor fibers to pharynx, larynx, esophagus, and parasympathetic and parasympathetic fibers to thoracic and abdominal viscera (see also individual branches in this table)
vertebral n. [sympathetic]	n. vertebralis	cervicothoracic and vertebral ganglia		ascends with vertebral artery and gives fibers to spinal meninges, cervical n's, and posterior cranial fossa
vestibular n.	n. vestibularis	the posterior part of the vestibulocochlear n., concerned with equilibration, consisting of fibers arising from bipolar cells in vestibular ganglion; divides peripherally into rostral and caudal parts, with receptors in ampullae of semicircular canals, ventricle, and saccule		
vestibulocochlear n. (8th cranial)	n. vestibulocochlearis	emerges from brain between pons and medulla oblongata, at cerebellopontine angle and behind facial n.; divides near lateral end of internal acoustic meatus into two functionally distinct and incompletely united components, the vestibular n. and the cochlear n., and is connected with brain by corresponding roots (vestibular and cochlear roots)		
vidian n. See n. of pterygoid canal				
vidian n., deep. See petrosal n., deep				
zygomatic n. [general sensory]	n. zygomaticus	maxillary n., entering orbit through inferior orbital fissure	zygomaticofacial and zygomaticotemporal branches	communicates with lacrimal nerve, supplying skin of temple and adjacent part of face

muscle and somatic tissues. **splanchnic n's,** those of the blood vessels and viscera, especially the visceral branches of the thoracic, lumbar, and pelvic parts of the sympathetic trunks. **sympathetic n.,** 1. see under *trunk.* 2. any nerve of the sympathetic nervous system. **unmyelinated n.,** one whose axons are not encased in a myelin sheath. **vasoconstrictor n.,** one whose stimulation contracts blood vessels. **vasodilator n.,** one whose stimulation dilates blood vessels. **vasomotor n.,** one concerned in controlling the caliber of vessels, whether as a vasoconstrictor or vasodilator.

nervimotor (nurv″ĭ-mōt′er) pertaining to a motor nerve.

nervous (nurv′is) 1. pertaining to a nerve or nerves. 2. unduly excitable.

nervous breakdown (nurv′is brāk′down) a popular name for any mental disorder that interferes with the affected individual's normal activities and may include neurosis, depression, or psychosis.

nervus (nurv′is), pl. *ner'vi* [L.] nerve.

nesidiectomy (ne-sid″e-ek′tah-me) excision of the islet cells of the pancreas.

nesidioblast (ne-sid′e-o-blast″) any of the cells giving rise to islet cells of the pancreas.

neur(o)- word element [Gr.], *nerve.*

neurad (noor′ad) toward the neural axis or aspect.

neural (nōōr′'l) 1. pertaining to a nerve or to the nerves. 2. situated in the region of the spinal axis, as the neural arch.

neuralgia (nōōr-al′je-ah) paroxysmal pain extending along the course of one or more nerves. **neural′gic,** adj. **n. facia′lis ve′ra,** geniculate n. **Fothergill's n.,** trigeminal n. **geniculate n.,** Ramsay Hunt syndrome (1). **glossopharyngeal n.,** that affecting the petrosal and jugular ganglion of the glossopharyngeal nerve, marked by severe paroxysmal pain originating on the side of the throat and extending to the ear. **Hunt's n.,** Ramsay Hunt syndrome (1). **intercostal n.,** neuralgia of the intercostal nerves. **mammary n.,** neuralgic pain in the breast. **migrainous n.,** cluster headache. **Morton's n.,** see under *toe.* **postherpetic n.,** persistent burning pain and hyperesthesia along the distribution of a cutaneous nerve following an attack of herpes zoster. **red n.,** erythromelalgia. **trifacial n., trigeminal n.,** excruciating episodic pain in the area of the trigeminal nerve, often precipitated by stimulation of well-defined trigger points.

neuraminic acid (nōōr-ah-min′ik) an acid, $C_9H_{17}NO_8$, whose acyl derivatives are the sialic acids.

neuraminidase (nōōr″ah-min′ĭ-dās) an enzyme of the surface coat of myxoviruses that destroys the neuraminic acid of the cell surface during attachment, thereby preventing hemagglutination.

neuranagenesis (nōōr″an-ah-jen′ĭ-sis) regeneration of nerve tissue.

neurapophysis (nōōr″ah-pof′ĭ-sis) a structure forming either side of the neural arch; also, the part supposedly homologous with this structure in a so-called cranial vertebra.

neurapraxia (-prak′se-ah) usually temporary failure of nerve conduction in the absence of structural changes, due to blunt injury, compression, or ischemia.

neurasthenia (nōōr″as-the′ne-ah) an obsolete category of neurosis, marked by chronic weakness and easy fatigability.

neuratrophic (-trof′ik) characterized by atrophy of the nerves; also, a person so affected.

neurectasia (nōōr″ek-ta′ze-ah) neurotony.

neurectomy (nōōr-ek′tah-me) excision of a part of a nerve.

neurectopia (nōōr″ek-to′pe-ah) displacement of or abnormal situation of a nerve.

neurenteric (nōōr″en-ter′ik) pertaining to the neural tube and archenteron of the embryo.

neurergic (nōōr-ur′jik) pertaining to or dependent on nerve action.

neurilemma (nōōr″ĭ-lem′ah) the plasma membrane of a Schwann cell forming the sheath of Schwann of a myelinated or unmyelinated peripheral nerve. **neurilem′mal,** adj.

neurilemmitis (-lĕ-mīt′is) inflammation of the neurilemma.

neurilemoma (-lĕ-mo′mah) a tumor of a peripheral nerve sheath (neurilemma).

neurinoma (-no′mah) neurilemoma.

neuritis (nōōr-īt′is), pl. *neurit′ides.* Inflammation of a nerve; also used to denote noninflammatory lesions of the peripheral nervous system (see *neuropathy*). **neurit′ic,** adj. **endemic n.,** beriberi. **interstitial n.,** inflammation of the connective tissue of a nerve trunk. **multiple n.,** polyneuritis. **optic n.,** inflammation of the optic nerve, affecting part of the nerve within the eyeball (*neuropapillitis*) or the part behind the eyeball (*retrobulbar n.*). **parenchymatous n.,** that affecting chiefly the axons and myelin of the peripheral nerves. **retrobulbar n.,** see *optic n.* **toxic n.,** that due to some poison. **traumatic n.,** that following and due to an injury.

neuroanastomosis (nōōr″o-ah-nas″tah-mo′sis) surgical anastomosis of one nerve to another.

neuroanatomy (-ah-nat′ah-me) anatomy of the nervous system.

neuroarthropathy (-ar-throp′ah-the) any disease of joint structures associated with disease of the central or peripheral nervous system.

neuroastrocytoma (-as″tro-si-to′mah) a glioma composed mainly of astrocytes, found mostly in the floor of the third ventricle and the temporal lobes.

neurobehavioral (-be-hāv′ūr′l) relating to neurologic status as assessed by observation of behavior.

neurobiology (-bi-ol′ah-je) biology of the nervous system.

neuroblast (nōōr′ah-blast) an embryonic cell from which nervous tissue is formed.

neuroblastoma (nōōr′o-blas-to′mah) sarcoma of nervous system origin, composed chiefly of neuroblasts, affecting mostly infants and children up to 10 years of age, usually arising in the autonomic nervous system (sympathicoblastoma) or in the adrenal medulla.

neurocardiac (-kar'de-ak) pertaining to the nervous system and the heart.

neurocentrum (-sen'trum) one of the embryonic vertebral elements from which the spinous processes of the vertebrae develop. **neurocen'tral,** adj.

neurochemistry (kem'is-tre) that branch of neurology dealing with the chemistry of the nervous system.

neurochorioretinitis (-ko''re-o-ret''in-īt'is) inflammation of the optic nerve, choroid, and retina.

neurochoroiditis (-ko''roi-dīt'is) inflammation of the optic nerve and choroid.

neurocirculatory (surk'ūl-ah-tor''e) pertaining to the nervous and circulatory systems.

neurocladism (nōōr-ok'lah-dizm) the formation of new branches by the process of a neuron.

neuroclonic (nōōr'o-klon'ik) marked by nervous spasm.

neurocommunications (-kah-mūn''ĭ-ka'shinz) the branch of neurology dealing with the transfer and integration of information within the nervous system.

neurocranium (-kra'ne-um) the part of the cranium enclosing the brain. **neurocra'nial,** adj.

neurocrine (nōōr'ah-krīn) 1. denoting an endocrine influence on or by the nerves. 2. pertaining to neurosecretion.

neurocristopathy (nōōr''o-kris-top'ah-the) any disease arising from maldevelopment of the neural crest.

neurocutaneous (-ku-ta'ne-us) pertaining to the nerves and skin, or the cutaneous nerves.

neurocyte (nōōr'ah-sīt) a nerve cell of any kind.

neurocytolysin (nōōr''o-si-tol'ĭ-sin) a constituent of certain snake venoms which lyses nerve cells.

neurocytoma (-si-to'mah) a brain tumor consisting of undifferentiated nerve cells of nervous origin, i.e., cells resembling medullary neural epithelium.

neurodermatitis (-durm''ah-tīt'is), pl. *neurodermati'tides* [Gr.] a general term for a dermatosis presumed to be caused by itching due to emotional causes; also used to refer to n. circumscripta (*lichen simplex chronicus*) and sometimes n. disseminata (*atopic dermatitis*).

neurodynia (-din'e-ah) pain in a nerve.

neuroectoderm (-ek'tah-durm) the portion of the ectoderm of the early embryo which gives rise to the central and peripheral nervous systems, including some glial cells. **neuroectoder'mal,** adj.

neuroeffector (-ĕ-fek'ter) of or relating to the junction between a neuron and the effector organ it innervates.

neuroencephalomyelopathy (-en-sef''ah-lo-mi''il-op'ah-the) disease involving the nerves, brain, and spinal cord.

neuroendocrine (-en'do-krin) pertaining to neural and endocrine influence, and particularly to the interaction between the nervous and endocrine systems.

neuroendocrinology (-en''do-krĭ-nol'ah-je) the study of the interactions of the nervous and endocrine systems.

neuroepithelioma (-ep''ĭ-thēl''e-o'mah) neurocytoma.

neuroepithelium (-ep''ĭ-thēl'e-um) 1. epithelium made up of cells specialized to serve as sensory cells for reception of external stimuli. 2. the ectodermal epithelium, from which the central nervous system is derived.

neurofibril (-fi'bril) one of the delicate threads running in every direction through the cytoplasm of a nerve cell, extending into the axon and dendrites.

neurofibroma (-fi-bro'mah) a tumor of peripheral nerves due to abnormal proliferation of Schwann cells.

neurofibromatosis (-fi''bro-mah-to'sis) a familial condition characterized by developmental changes in the nervous system, muscles, bones, and skin, and marked by the formation of neurofibromas over the entire body associated with areas of pigmentation.

neurofilament (-fil'ah-mint) any of the slender, fibrillar elements which, along with the neurotubules, forms a neurofibril.

neurogenesis (-jen'ĭ-sis) the development of nervous tissue.

neurogenic (-jen'ik) 1. forming nervous tissue, or stimulating nervous energy. 2. originating in the nervous system.

neurogenous (nu-roj'ĭ-nus) arising in the nervous system, or from some lesion of the nervous system.

neuroglia (nōōr-og'le-ah) the supporting structure of nervous tissue, consisting, in the central nervous system, of astrocytes, oligodendrocytes, and microglia. **neurog'lial,** adj.

neurogliocyte (nōōr-og'le-o-sīt) one of the cells composing the neuroglia.

neuroglioma (nōōr''o-gli-o'mah) a tumor composed of neuroglial tissue. **n. gangliona're,** ganglioneuroma.

neurogliosis (nōōr-og''le-o'sis) a condition marked by numerous neurogliomas.

neuroglycopenia (nōōr''o-gli''ko-pe'ne-ah) chronic hypoglycemia of a degree sufficient to impair brain function, resulting in personality changes and intellectual deterioration.

neurohistology (nōōr''o-his-tol'ah-je) histology of the nervous system.

neurohormone (nōōr'o-hor''mōn) a hormone stimulating the neural mechanism.

neurohypophysis (nōōr''o-hi-pof'ĭ-sis) the posterior (or neural) lobe of the pituitary gland. **neurohypophys'eal,** adj.

neuroimmunology (nōōr''o-im''ūn-ol'ah-je) the study of the effects of the autonomic nervous activity on the immune response. **neuroimmunolog'ic,** adj.

neurokeratin (-kĕ'rit-in) a protein network seen in histological specimens of the myelin sheath.

neuroleptanalgesia (-lep''tan-al-je'ze-ah) a state of quiescence, altered awareness, and analgesia produced by a combination of a narcotic analgesic and a neuroleptic.

neuroleptic (-lep′tik) antipsychotic agent; see *antipsychotic*.

neurology (nōōr-ol′ah-je) that branch of medical science which deals with the nervous system, both normal and in disease. **neurolog′ic**, adj. **clinical n.**, that especially concerned with the diagnosis and treatment of disorders of the nervous system.

neurolysin (nōōr-ol′ĭ-sin) a cytolysin with a specific destructive action on neurons.

neurolysis (nōōr-ol′ĭ-sis) 1. release of a nerve sheath by cutting it longitudinally. 2. operative breaking up of perineural adhesions. 3. relief of tension upon a nerve obtained by stretching. 4. exhaustion of nervous energy. 5. destruction or dissolution of nerve tissue. **neurolyt′ic**, adj.

neuroma (nōōr-o′mah) a tumor or new growth largely made up of nerve cells and nerve fibers; a tumor growing from a nerve. **neurom′atous**, adj. **acoustic n.**, a benign tumor within the auditory canal arising from the eighth cranial (acoustic) nerve. **amputation n.**, traumatic neuroma occurring after amputation of an extremity or part. **n. cu′tis**, neuroma in the skin. **false n.**, one which does not contain nerve elements. **plexiform n.**, one made up of contorted nerve trunks. **n. telangiecto′des**, one containing an excess of blood vessels. **traumatic n.**, an unorganized bulbous or nodular mass of nerve fibers and Schwann cells produced by hyperplasia of nerve fibers and their supporting tissues after accidental or purposeful sectioning of the nerve.

neuromalacia (nōōr″o-mah-la′she-ah) morbid softening of the nerves.

neuromatosis (-mah-to′sis) a condition marked by the presence of many neuromas.

neuromere (nōōr′ah-mēr) 1. any of a series of transitory segmental elevations in the wall of the neural tube in the developing embryo; also, such elevations in the wall of the mature rhombencephalon. 2. a part of the spinal cord to which a pair of dorsal roots and a pair of ventral roots are attached.

neuromuscular (nōōr″o-mus′kūl-er) pertaining to nerves and muscles.

neuromyelitis (-mi″il-īt′is) inflammation of nervous and medullary substance; myelitis attended with neuritis.

neuromyopathic (-mi″ah-path′ik) pertaining to or affecting the nervous system and muscle, including the heart.

neuromyositis (-mi″ah-sīt′is) neuritis blended with myositis.

neuron (nōōr′on) nerve cell; any of the conducting cells of the nervous system, consisting of a cell body, containing the nucleus and its surrounding cytoplasm and the axon and dendrites. See Plate XI. **neuro′nal**, adj. **afferent n.**, one that conducts a nervous impulse from a receptor to a center. **efferent n.**, one that conducts a nervous impulse from a center to an organ of response. **Golgi n's**, 1. (*type I*): pyramidal cells with long axons, which leave the gray matter of the central nervous system, traverse

the white matter, and terminate in the periphery. 2. (*type II*): stellate neurons with short axons in the cerebral and cerebellar cortices and in the retina. **motor n.**, motoneuron. **postganglionic n's**, neurons whose cell bodies lie in the autonomic ganglia and whose purpose is to relay impulses beyond the ganglia. **preganglionic n's**, neurons whose cell bodies lie in the central nervous system and whose efferent fibers terminate in the autonomic ganglia. **sensory n.**, any neuron having a sensory function; an afferent neuron conveying sensory impulses.

neuronevus (nōōr″o-ne′vus) a cellular or nevocytic nevus, especially a mature one with differentiation toward neural skin structures.

neuro-ophthalmology (nōōr″o-of″thal-mol′ah-je) the specialty dealing with the portions of the nervous system related to the eye.

neuropapillitis (-pap″il-īt′is) optic neuritis.

neuroparalysis (-pah-ral′ĭ-sis) paralysis due to disease of a nerve or nerves.

neuropathogenicity (-path″ah-jin-is′it-e) the quality of producing or the ability to produce pathologic changes in nerve tissue.

neuropathology (-pah-thol′ah-je) pathology of diseases of the nervous system.

neuropathy (nōōr-op′ah-the) any functional disturbances and/or pathological changes in the peripheral nervous system; also used to denote nonspecific lesions, in contrast to inflammatory lesions (see *neuritis*). **neuropath′ic**, adj. **diabetic n.**, a chronic, symmetrical sensory polyneuropathy affecting first the nerves of the lower limbs and often affecting autonomic nerves; pathologically, there is segmental demyelination of the peripheral nerves. **entrapment n.**, any of a group of neuropathies, e.g., carpal tunnel syndrome, due to mechanical pressure on a peripheral nerve. **progressive hypertrophic interstitial n.**, a slowly progressive familial disease beginning in early life, marked by hyperplasia of interstitial connective tissue, causing thickening of peripheral nerve trunks and posterior roots, and by sclerosis of the posterior columns of the spinal cord.

neuropeptide (-pep′tĭd) any of the molecules composed of short chains of amino acids (endorphins, enkephalins, vasopressin, etc.) found in brain tissue.

neuropharmacology (-far″mah-kol′ah-je) the scientific study of the effects of drugs on the nervous system.

neurophthisis (nōōr-of′thĭ-sis) wasting of nerve tissue.

neurophysin (-fi′sin) any of a group of soluble proteins secreted in the hypothalamus that serve as binding proteins for vasopressin and oxytocin, playing a role in their transport in the neurohypophyseal tract and their storage in the posterior pituitary.

neurophysiology (-fiz″e-ol′ah-je) physiology of the nervous system.

neuropil (nōōr′ah-pil) a feltwork of interwoven dendrites and axons and of neuroglial cells in the central nervous system and in some parts of the peripheral nervous system.

neuroplasm (-plazm) the protoplasm of a nerve cell. **neuroplas′mic,** adj.

neuroplasty (-plas″te) plastic repair of a nerve.

neuropore (no͞or′ah-por) the open anterior or posterior end of the neural tube of the early embryo; they close as the embryo develops.

neuropsychiatry (-si-ki′ah-tre) the combined specialties of neurology and psychiatry.

neuroradiology (-ra″de-ol′ah-je) radiology of the nervous system.

neuroretinitis (-ret′n-it′is) inflammation of the optic nerve and retina.

neuroretinopathy (-ret′n-op′ah-the) pathologic involvement of the optic disk and retina.

neurorrhaphy (no͞or-or′ah-fe) suture of a divided nerve.

neurosarcokleisis (no͞or-o-sar″ko-kli′sis) an operation performed for neuralgia, done by relieving pressure on the affected nerve by partial resection of the bony canal through which it passes, and transplanting the nerve among soft tissues.

neurosarcoma (-sar-ko′mah) a sarcoma with neuromatous elements.

neurosclerosis (-sklĕ-ro′sis) hardening of nerve tissue.

neurosecretion (-si-kre′shun) 1. secretory activities of nerve cells. 2. the product of such activities; a neurosecretory substance. **neurosecre′tory,** adj.

neurosis (no͞or-o′sis), pl. *neuro′ses.* An emotional disorder due to unresolved conflicts, anxiety being its chief characteristic; in contrast with psychoses, neuroses do not involve gross distortions of external reality or disorganization of personality. **neurot′ic,** adj. **anxiety n.,** anxiety reaction; neurosis characterized by morbid and unjustified dread, sometimes extending to panic and often associated somatic symptoms. **character n.,** a neurosis in which certain personality traits have become exaggerated or overdeveloped. **combat n.,** a neurosis resulting from battle experiences and conditions of military life. **compensation n.,** a neurosis following injury and motivated in part by prospects of financial compensation. **compulsive n.,** an urge to perform unacceptable or senseless acts. **conversion n.,** see under *reaction.* **depersonalization n.,** one with a feeling of unreality and of estrangement from the self, one's body, or one's surroundings. **depressive n.,** one with an excessive reaction of depression, due to an internal conflict or to an identifiable event. **hypochondriacal n.,** one with persistent preoccupation with the body and fear of presumed diseases of various organs. **hysterical n.,** sudden involuntary psychogenic loss of function in response to emotional stress: the *conversion type* is manifested by disorders of the special senses or the voluntary nervous system; the *dissociative type* is manifested by alterations in the state of consciousness or in identity. **obsessional n.,** that marked by obsessions that dominate the patient's conduct. **obsessive-compulsive n.,** that marked by the persistent intrusion of repetitive thoughts or urges, compelling the performance of ritual acts. **occupational n.,**

neurosis in which the symptoms are related to the patient's occupation and interfere with its pursuit. **phobic n.,** one with intense fear, usually leading to avoidance, of an object or situation that the individual consciously recognizes as harmless. **traumatic n.,** neurosis resulting from an injury.

neurospasm (no͞or′ah-spazm) nervous twitching of a muscle.

neurosplanchnic (no͞or-o-splank′nik) pertaining to the cerebrospinal and sympathetic nervous systems.

neurospongioma (-spun″je-o′mah) glioma.

neurospongium (-spun′je-um) 1. the fibrillar component of neurons. 2. a meshwork of nerve fibers, especially the inner reticular layer of the retina.

neurosurgery (-surj′er-e) surgery of the nervous system.

neurosuture (no͞or′ah-soo-cher) neurorrhaphy.

neurosyphilis (no͞or′o-sif′il-is) syphilis of the central nervous system.

neurotendinous (-ten′di-nis) pertaining to both nerve and tendon.

neurotensin (-ten′sin) a tridecapeptide that induces vasodilation and hypotension; present in human brain tissue and postulated to be a neurotransmitter.

neurotic (no͞or-ot′ik) 1. pertaining to or affected with a neurosis. 2. pertaining to the nerves. 3. a nervous person in whom emotions predominate over reason.

neurotization (no͞or-ot″ĭ-za′shin) 1. regeneration of a nerve after its division. 2. the implantation of a nerve into a paralyzed muscle.

neurotmesis (no͞or-ot-me′sis) partial or complete severance of a nerve, with disruption of the axon and its myelin sheath and the connective tissue elements.

neurotome (no͞or′ah-tōm) 1. a needle-like knife for dissecting nerves. 2. neuromere.

neurotomography (no͞or″o-tah-mog′rah-fe) tomography of the central nervous system.

neurotomy (no͞or-ot′o-me) dissection or cutting of nerves.

neurotony (no͞or-ot′ne) stretching of a nerve.

neurotoxicity (no͞or″o-tok-sis′it-e) the quality of exerting a destructive or poisonous effect upon nerve tissue. **neurotox′ic,** adj.

neurotoxin (-tok′sin) a substance that is poisonous or destructive to nerve tissue.

neurotransducer (-tranz-doo′ser) a neuron that synthesizes and releases hormones which serve as the functional link between the nervous system and the pituitary gland.

neurotransmitter (-tranz′mit-er) a substance released from the axon terminal of a presynaptic neuron on excitation, which diffuses across the synaptic cleft to either excite or inhibit the target cell. **false n.,** an amine that can be stored in and released from presynaptic vesicles but that has little effect on postsynaptic receptors.

neurotrauma (-traw′mah) mechanical injury to a nerve.

neurotropism (no͞or-ah′trah-pizm) 1. the quality of having a special affinity for nervous tissue. 2. the alleged tendency of regenerating nerve fibers to grow toward specific portions of the periphery. **neurotrop'ic,** adj.

neurotubule (noor″o-too'būl) any of the long, straight, parallel tubules within neurons, which along with the neurofilaments, form neurofibrils.

neurovaccine (-vak'sēn) vaccine virus prepared by growing the virus in a rabbit's brain.

neurovascular (-vas'kūl-er) pertaining to both nervous and vascular elements, or to nerves controlling the caliber of blood vessels.

neurovisceral (-vis'er'l) neurosplanchnic.

neurula (noor'il-ah) the early embryonic stage following the gastrula, marked by the first appearance of the nervous system.

neurulation (noor-il-a'shin) formation in the early embryo of the neural plate, followed by its closure with development of the neural tube.

neutral (noo'tril) neither basic nor acid.

neutrocyte (noo'trah-sīt) neutrophil (2).

neutron (noo'tron) an electrically neutral or uncharged particle of matter existing along with protons in the atoms of all elements except the mass 1 isotope of hydrogen.

neutropenia (noo″tro-pe'ne-ah) diminished number of neutrophils in the blood.

neutrophil (noo'trah-fil) 1. a granular leukocyte having a nucleus with three to five lobes connected by threads of chromatin, and cytoplasm containing very fine granules; cf. *heterophil.* 2. any cell, structure, or histologic element readily stainable with neutral dyes. **stab n.,** one whose nucleus is not divided into segments.

neutrophilia (noo-trah-fil'e-ah) increase in the number of neutrophils in the blood.

neutrophilic (-fil'ik) 1. pertaining to neutrophils. 2. stainable by neutral dyes.

nevoid (ne'void) resembling a nevus.

nevus (ne'vus), pl. *ne'vi* [L.] a circumscribed stable malformation of the skin and occasionally of the oral mucosa, which is not due to external causes; the excess (or deficiency) of tissue may involve epidermal, connective tissue, adnexal, nervous, or vascular elements. **blue n.,** a dark blue nodular lesion composed of closely grouped melanocytes and melanophages situated in the mid-dermis. **blue rubber bleb n.,** a hereditary condition marked by multiple bluish cutaneous hemangiomas with soft raised centers, frequently associated with hemangiomas of the gastrointestinal tract. **n. flam'meus,** port-wine stain; a poorly defined, pink to dark bluish red area involving otherwise normal skin. **giant congenital pigmented n., giant hairy n., giant pigmented n.,** any of a group of large, darkly pigmented, hairy nevi, present at birth; they are associated with other cutaneous and subcutaneous lesions, neurofibromatosis, and leptomeningeal melanocytosis and exhibit a predisposition to the development of malignant melanoma. **halo n.,** a pigmented nevus surrounded by a ring of depigmentation. **intradermal n.,** a nevocytic nevus in which the nevus cells occur in nests in the upper part of the dermis, with no evidence of the proliferative process by which they originated. **n. of Ito,** a

mongolian spot in the distribution of the posterior supraclavicular and lateral cutaneous brachial nerves, over the shoulder. **junction n.,** a brownish, smooth, flat or slightly raised nevocytic nevus; histologically, there are nests of melanin-containing nevus cells at the dermoepidermal junction. **n. lipomato'sus,** one containing much fibrofatty tissue. **n. of Ota,** a mongolian spot, usually unilateral, involving the conjunctiva and lids, as well as adjacent facial skin, sclera, ocular muscles, and periosteum; rarely malignant melanoma may develop, usually in the iris. **sebaceous n., sebaceous n. of Jadassohn,** an epidermal nevus of the scalp or less often the face, frequently growing larger during puberty or early adult life, and rarely giving rise to a variety of new growths, including basal cell carcinoma. **n. spi'lus,** a smooth, tan to brown, macular nevus composed of melanocytes, and speckled with smaller, darker macules. **n. spongio'sus al'bus,** white sponge n. **n. uni'us la'teris,** a verrucous epidermal nevus occurring as a linear band, patch, or streak, usually along the margin between two neuromeres. **vascular n., n. vasculo'sus,** a reddish swelling or patch on the skin due to hypertrophy of the skin capillaries. **white sponge n.,** a white spongy nevus of a mucous membrane, occurring as a hereditary condition.

newborn (noo'born″) 1. recently born. 2. a recently born infant.

newton (noot'n) the SI unit of force: the force which, when applied to a body having a mass of one kilogram, accelerates it at the rate of one meter per second squared. Symbol, N.

nexus (nek'sis) 1. a bond, as between members of a series or group. 2. gap junction.

NF National Formulary.

N.F.L.P.N. National Federation for Licensed Practical Nurses.

ng. nanogram.

N.H.I. National Health Insurance; National Heart Institute.

N.H.L.I. National Heart and Lung Institute.

Ni chemical symbol, *nickel.*

niacin (ni'ah-sin) nicotinic acid; a water-soluble vitamin of the B complex, $C_6H_5NO_2$, occurring in various animal and plant tissues. It is required by the body for the formation of the coenzymes NAD and NADP important in biochemical oxidations; it also has a pellagra-curative property and a vasodilating action.

niacinamide (ni″ah-sin'im-īd) the amide of niacin, $C_6H_6N_2O$, which lacks the vasodilating action of the parent compound; used in the prophylaxis and treatment of pellagra.

NIAID National Institute of Allergy and Infectious Diseases.

NIAMD National Institute of Arthritis and Metabolic Diseases.

niche (nich) a defect in an otherwise even surface, especially a depression or recess in the wall of a hollow organ, as seen in a roentgenogram, or such a depression in an organ visible to the naked eye. **enamel n.,** either of two depressions between the dental lamina and the developing tooth germ, one pointing distally (*distal enamel n.*) and the other mesially (*mesial enamel n.*). **Haudek's n.,** see under *sign.*

NICHHD National Institute of Child Health and Human Development.

nickel (nik′′l) chemical element (*see table*), at. no. 28, symbol Ni.

nicking (nik′ing) localized constriction of the retinal blood vessels.

nicotinamide (nik′′ah-tin′ah-mīd) niacinamide. **n.-adenine dinucleotide (NAD),** the dinucleotide of nicotinamide and adenine, a coenzyme involved in numerous enzymatic reactions, in which it serves as an electron carrier by being alternately oxidized (NAD⁺) and reduced (NADH). **n.-adenine dinucleotide phosphate (NADP),** a coenzyme similar to involved nicotinamide-adenine dinucleotide except for the inclusion of 3 phosphate units; it serves as an electron carrier linking catabolic reactions (in the reduced form, NADPH) to biosynthetic (anabolic) reactions, where it gives up an electron (oxidized form, NADP⁺).

nicotine (nik′ah-tēn) a very poisonous alkaloid, $C_{10}H_{14}N_2$, obtained from tobacco or produced synthetically; used as an agricultural insecticide, and in veterinary medicine as an external parasitide.

nicotinic (nik′′ah-tin′ik) denoting the effect of nicotine and other drugs in initially stimulating and subsequently, in high doses, inhibiting neural impulses at autonomic ganglia and the neuromuscular junction.

nicotinic acid (nik′′o-tin′ik) niacin.

nicotinism (nik′ah-tēn-izm) nicotine poisoning, marked by stimulation and subsequent depression of the central and autonomic nervous systems, with death due to respiratory paralysis.

nictitation (nik′′tĭ-ta′shin) the act of winking.

nidal (nīd′′l) pertaining to a nidus.

nidation (ni-da′shun) implantation of the conceptus in the endometrium.

NIDR National Institute of Dental Research.

nidus (ni′dus), pl. *ni′di* [L.] 1. the point of origin or focus of a morbid process. 2. nucleus (2). **n. a′vis, n. hirun′dinis** [L., swallow's nest], a depression in the cerebellum between the posterior velum and uvula.

nightmare (nīt′mār′′) a terrifying dream.

nightshade (nīt′shād′′) a plant of the genus *Solanum.* **deadly n.,** belladonna leaf.

NIGMS National Institute of General Medical Sciences.

nigra (ni′grah) [L., black] substantia nigra. **ni′gral,** adj.

nigrosin (ni′grah-sin) an aniline dye, $C_{36}H_{27}N_3$, having a special affinity for ganglion cells.

nigrostriatal (ni′′gro-stri-āt′′l) projecting from the substantia nigra to the corpus striatum; said of a bundle of nerve fibers.

N.I.H. National Institutes of Health.

nikethamide (nĭ-keth′ah-mīd) a central and respiratory stimulant, $C_{10}H_{14}N_2O$.

NIMH National Institute of Mental Health.

NINDB National Institute of Neurological Diseases and Blindness.

niobium (ni-o′be-um) chemical element (*see table*), at. no. 41, symbol Nb.

nipple (nip′′l) the pigmented projection on the anterior surface of the mammary gland, surrounded by the areola; it gives outlet to milk from the breast. Also, any similarly shaped structure.

nit (nit) the egg of a louse.

nitrate (ni′trāt) any salt of nitric acid; organic nitrates are used in the treatment of angina pectoris.

nitric (ni′trik) pertaining to or containing nitrogen in one of its higher valences.

nitric acid a colorless liquid, HNO_3, which fumes in moist air and has a characteristic choking odor; used as a cauterizing agent. Its potassium salt (*potassium nitrate*) is used in potassium deficiencies and as a diuretic; its sodium salt (*sodium nitrate*) as a reagent.

nitrification (ni′′trĭ-fĭ-ka′shin) the bacterial oxidation of ammonia to nitrite and then to nitrate in the soil.

nitrite (ni′trīt) any salt of nitrous acid; organic nitrites are used in the treatment of angina pectoris.

Nitrobid (ni′tro-bid) trademark for preparations of nitroglycerin.

nitrocellulose (ni′′tro-sel′ūl-ōs) pyroxylin.

nitrofuran (-fu′ran) any of a group of antibacterials, including nitrofurantoin, nitrofurazone, etc., that are effective against a wide range of bacteria.

nitrofurantoin (-fu-ran′to-in) an antibacterial, $C_8H_6N_4O_5$, used in urinary tract infections.

nitrofurazone (-fūr′ah-zōn) an antibacterial, $C_6H_6N_4O_4$, used topically as a local anti-infective.

nitrogen (ni′trah-jin) chemical element (*see table*), at. no. 7, symbol N. It forms about 78% of the atmosphere and is a constituent of all proteins and nucleic acids. **n. mustards,** see under *mustard.* **nonprotein n.,** the nitrogenous constituents of the blood exclusive of the protein bodies, consisting of the nitrogen of urea, uric acid, creatine, creatinine, amino acids, polypeptides, and an undetermined part known as *rest nitrogen.*

nitrogenous (ni-troj′in-is) containing nitrogen.

nitroglycerin (ni′′tro-glis′er-in) a vasodilator, $C_3H_5N_3O_9$, used especially in the prophylaxis and treatment of angina pectoris.

nitromersol (-murs′ol) a local anti-infective, $C_7H_5HgNO_3$, used topically in solution or tincture.

nitrosourea (ni-tro′′so-ūr-e′ah) any of a group of lipid-soluble biological alkylating agents, including carmustine and lomustine, which cross the blood-brain barrier and are used as antineoplastic agents.

Nitrostat (ni′trah-stat) trademark for a preparation of nitroglycerin.

nitrous (ni′tris) pertaining to nitrogen in its lowest valency. **n. oxide,** a gas, N_2O, used as a general anesthetic and analgesic.

nitrous acid an unstable weak acid, HNO_2, with which free amino groups react to form hydroxyl groups and liberate gaseous nitrogen; used in the determination of urea, the N_2 being collected and measured. Its salts (*sodium nitrite* and sometimes *potassium nitrite*) are used for the relief of pain in certain conditions.

nl. nanoliter.

N.L.N. National League for Nursing.

nm. nanometer.

NMR nuclear magnetic resonance.

nn. nervi (L. pl.), *nerves*.

No chemical symbol, *nobelium*.

nobelium (no-bēl′e-im) chemical element (*see table*), at. no. 102, symbol No.

Nocardia (no-kar′de-ah) a genus of bacteria (family Actinomycetaceae), including *N. aster-oi′des*, which produces a tuberculosis-like infection in man, and *N. farci′nica* (probably identical with *N. asteroides*), which produces a tuberculosis-like infection in cattle.

nocardial (no-kar′de-il) pertaining to or caused by *Nocardia*.

nocardiosis (no-kar″de-o′sis) infection with *Nocardia*.

noci- word element [L.], *harm; injury*.

nociassociation (no″se-ah-so″se-a′shun) unconscious discharge of nervous energy under the stimulus of trauma.

nociceptor (-sep′ter) a receptor that is stimulated by injury; a receptor for pain. **nociceptive,** adj.

nociperception (-per-sep′shin) the perception of traumatic stimuli.

noctalbuminuria (nokt′al-būm″in-ūr′e-ah) excess of albumin in urine secreted at night.

nocturia (nok-tūr′e-ah) excessive urination at night.

node (nōd) a small mass of tissue in the form of a swelling, knot, or protuberance, either normal or pathological. **no′dal,** adj. **atrioventricular n.,** a collection of Purkinje fibers beneath the endocardium of the right atrium, continuous with the atrial muscle fibers and atrioventricular bundle. **Bouchard's n's,** cartilaginous and bony enlargements of the proximal interphalangeal joints of the fingers in degenerative joint disease. **Dürck's n's,** granulomatous perivascular infiltrations in the cerebral cortex in trypanosomiasis. **Flack's n.,** sinoatrial n. **Haygarth's n's,** joint swelling in arthritis deformans. **Heberden's n's,** small hard nodules, usually at the distal interphalangeal joints of the fingers, formed by calcific spurs of the articular cartilage and associated with osteoarthritis. **Hensen's n.,** primitive knot. **Keith's n., Keith-Flack n.,** sinoatrial n. **lymph n.,** any of the accumulations of lymphoid tissue organized as definite lymphoid organs along the course of lymphatic vessels, consisting of an outer cortical and an inner medullary part; they are the main source of lymphocytes of the peripheral blood and, as part of the reticuloendothelial system, serve as a defense mechanism by removing noxious agents, e.g., bacteria and toxins, and probably play a role in antibody formation. **Meynet's n's,** nodules in the capsules of joints and in tendons in rheumatic conditions, especially in children. **Osler's n's,** small, raised, swollen, tender areas, bluish or sometimes pink or red, occurring commonly in the pads of the fingers or toes, in the thenar or hypothenar eminences or the soles of the feet; they are practically pathognomonic of subacute bacterial endocarditis. **n's of Ranvier,** constrictions of myelinated nerve fibers at regular intervals at which the myelin sheath is absent and the axon is enclosed only by Schwann cell processes; see Plate XI. **Schmorl's n.,** an irregular or hemispherical bone defect in the upper or lower margin of the body of a vertebra. **sentinel n., signal n.,** an enlarged supraclavicular lymph node; often the first sign of a malignant abdominal tumor. **singer's n.,** a small, white nodule on the vocal cord in those who use their voice excessively. **sinoatrial n., sinus n.,** a collection of atypical muscle fibers (Purkinje fibers) at the junction of the superior vena cava and right atrium, in which the cardiac rhythm normally originates and which is therefore called the pacemaker of the heart. **teacher's n.,** singer's n. **Troisier's n., Virchow's n.,** sentinel n.

nodi (no′di) plural of *nodus.*

nodose (no′dōs) having nodes or projections.

nodosity (no-dos′it-e) 1. a node. 2. the quality of being nodose.

nodule (nah′jōōl) a small node or boss which is solid and can be detected by touch. **nod′ular,** adj. **Albini's n's,** gray nodules of the size of small grains, sometimes seen on the free edges of the atrioventricular valves of infants; they are remains of fetal structures. **apple jelly n's,** minute, yellowish or reddish brown, translucent nodules, seen on diascopic examination of the lesions of lupus vulgaris. **n's of Arantius,** see under *body.* **Aschoff's n's,** see under *body.* **Bianchi's n's,** bodies of Arantius. **Gamna's n's, Gandy-Gamna n's,** brown or yellow pigmented nodules sometimes seen in the enlarged spleen, e.g., in Gamna's disease and siderotic splenomegaly. **Jeanselme's n's, juxta-articular n's,** gummata of tertiary syphilis and of nonvenereal treponemal diseases, located on joint capsules, bursae, or tendon sheaths. **lymphatic n.,** 1. lymph node. 2. lymph follicle. **milker's n's,** hard circumscribed nodules on the hands of those who milk cows affected with cowpox. **Morgagni's n's,** bodies of Arantius. **pulp n.,** denticle (2). **rheumatic n's,** small round or oval, mostly subcutaneous nodules composed chiefly of a mass of Aschoff bodies; seen in rheumatic fever. **Schmorl's n.,** an irregular or hemispherical bone defect in the upper or lower margin of the body of the vertebra. **triticeous n.,** see under *cartilage.* **typhus n's,** minute nodes in the skin, formed by perivascular infiltration of mononuclear cells in typhus. **n. of vermis,** the part of the vermis of the cerebellum, on the ventral surface, where the inferior medullary velum attaches.

nodulus (nod′u-lus), pl. *no′duli* [L.] nodule.

nodus (no′dus), pl. *no′di* [L.] node.

noma (no′mah) gangrenous processes of the mouth or genitalia. In the mouth (*cancrum oris, gangrenous stomatitis*), it begins as a small gingival ulcer and results in gangrenous necrosis of surrounding facial tissues; on the genitalia (*cancrum pudendi, n. pudendi, n. vulvae*), it affects one labium majus and then the other.

nomenclature (no′men-kla″cher, no-men′klah-cher) a classified system of names, as of anatomical structures, organisms, etc. **binomial n.**, the system of designating plants and animals by two latinized words signifying the genus and species.

Nomina Anatomica (no′mǐ-nah an-ah-tom′ǐ-kah) [L.] the internationally approved official body of anatomical nomenclature; abbreviated NA.

nomogram (nom′ah-gram) a graph with several scales arranged so that a straightedge laid on the graph intersects the scales at related values of the variables; the values of any two variables can be used to find the values of the others.

non compos mentis (non kom′pos men′tis) [L.] not of sound mind.

nonconductor (non′kon-duk′ter) a substance that does not readily transmit electricity, light, or heat.

nondisjunction (-dis-junk′shin) failure (*a*) of two homologous chromosomes to pass to separate cells during the first division of meiosis, or (*b*) of the two chromatids of a chromosome to pass to separate cells during mitosis or during the second meiotic division. As a result, one daughter cell has two chromosomes or two chromatids, and the other has none.

nonelectrolyte (-e-lek′trah-līt) a substance which in solution is a nonconductor of electricity.

nonheme (non′hēm′) not bound within a porphyrin ring; said of iron so contained within a protein.

non-neuronal (non″nŏŏr-o′n′l) pertaining to or composed of nonconducting cells of the nervous system, e.g., neuroglial cells.

nonsecretor (non″sǐ-krēt′er) a person with A or B type blood whose body secretions do not contain the particular (A or B) substance.

nonself (non′self′) in immunology, pertaining to foreign antigens.

nonspecific (-spǐ-sif′ik) 1. not due to any single known cause. 2. not directed against a particular agent, but rather having a general effect.

nonunion (-ūn′yin) failure of the ends of a fractured bone to unite.

nonviable (-vi′ah-b′l) not capable of living.

N.O.P.H.N. National Organization for Public Health Nursing.

nor- chemical prefix denoting (*a*) a compound of normal structure (having an unbranched chain of carbon atoms) that is isomeric with one having a branched chain, or (*b*) a compound whose chain or ring contains one less methylene (CH_2) group than does that of its homologue.

noradrenalin (-ah-dren′ah-lin) norepinephrine.

noradrenergic (-ah-dren-urj′ik) activated by or secreting norepinephrine.

norepinephrine (-ep-ĭ-nef′rin) a catecholamine, which is the principal neurotransmitter of postganglionic adrenergic neurons, having predominately α-adrenergic activity; also secreted by the adrenal medulla in response to splanchnic

stimulation, being released predominantly in response to hypotension. It is a powerful vasopressor and is used to restore blood pressure in certain hypotensive states. Called also *levartererenol.*

norethindrone (nor-eth′in-drōn) a progestin, $C_{20}H_{26}O_2$, having some anabolic, estrogenic, and androgenic properties; used in the treatment of amenorrhea, abnormal uterine bleeding due to hormonal imbalance, and endometriosis, and in combination with an estrogen as an oral contraceptive.

norethynodrel (nor″ĕ-thi′nah-drel) a progestin, $C_{20}H_{26}O_2$, used in combination with an estrogen as an oral contraceptive, to control endometriosis, for the treatment of hypermenorrhea, to produce cyclic withdrawal bleeding, and to produce amenorrhea.

norgestrel (-jes′trel) a progestin, $C_{21}H_{28}O_2$, used in combination with an estrogen as an oral contraceptive.

norm (norm) a fixed or ideal standard.

norm(o)- word element [L.], *normal; usual; conforming to the rule.*

normal (norm′l) 1. agreeing with the regular and established type; when said of a solution, denoting one containing in each 1000 ml., 1 gram equivalent weight of the active substance; see also *N* (3). 2. in bacteriology, not immunized or otherwise bacteriologically treated.

normetanephrine (nor″met-ah-nef′rin) a metabolite of norepinephrine excreted in the urine and found in certain tissues.

normoblast (nor′mah-blast) a nucleated precursor cell in the erythrocytic series; four developmental stages are recognized: the *pronormoblast* (q.v.); the *basophilic n.*, in which the cytoplasm is basophilic, the nucleus is large with clumped chromatin, and the nucleoli have disappeared; the *polychromatic n.*, in which the nuclear chromatin shows increased clumping and the cytoplasm begins to acquire hemoglobin and takes on an acidophilic tint; and the *orthochromatic n.*, the final stage before nuclear loss, in which the nucleus is small and ultimately becomes a blue-black, homogenous structureless mass. **normoblas′tic,** adj.

normoblastosis (nor″mo-blas-to′sis) excessive production of normoblasts by the bone marrow.

normocalcemia (-kal-sēm′e-ah) a normal level of calcium in the blood. **normocalce′mic,** adj.

normochromia (-krōm′e-ah) normal color of erythrocytes.

normocyte (nor′mah-sīt) an erythrocyte that is normal in size, shape, and color.

normocytosis (nor″mo-si-to′sis) a normal state of the blood in respect to erythrocytes.

normoglycemia (-gli-sēm′e-ah) normal glucose content of the blood. **normoglyce′mic,** adj.

normokalemia (-kah-lēm′e-ah) normal level of potassium in the blood. **normokale′mic,** adj.

normospermic (-sperm′ik) producing spermatozoa normal in number and motility.

normotensive (-ten′siv) 1. characterized by normal tone, tension, or pressure, as by normal blood pressure. 2. a person with normal blood pressure.

normothermia (-therm′e-ah) a normal state of temperature. **normother′mic,** adj.

normovolemia (-vo-lēm′e-ah) normal blood volume.

nortriptyline (nor-trip′tĭ-lēn) an antidepressant, $C_{19}H_{21}N$, used as the hydrochloride salt.

nos(o)- word element [Gr.], *disease.*

nose (nōz) the specialized facial structure serving as an organ of the sense of smell and as part of the respiratory apparatus; see Plate XVI. **saddle n.,** a nose with a sunken bridge.

Nosema (no-se′mah) a genus of sporozoan parasites, including *N. a′pis,* causing disease in bees, and *N. bomby′cis,* causing disease in silkworms.

nosepiece (nōz′pēs″) the portion of a microscope nearest to the stage, which bears the objective or objectives.

nosocomial (nos″o-ko′me-il) pertaining to or originating in a hospital.

nosogeny (no-soj′ĭ-ne) pathogenesis.

nosology (no-sol′ah-je) the science of the classification of diseases. **nosolog′ic,** adj.

nosoparasite (nos″o-par′ah-sīt) an organism found in a disease which it is able to modify, but not to produce.

Nosopsyllus (-sil′us) a genus of fleas, including *N. fascia′tus,* the common rat flea of North America and Europe, a vector of murine typhus and probably of plague.

nosotaxy (nos′o-tak″se) the classification of disease.

nostril (nos′tril) either of the nares.

nostrum (nos′trum) a quack, patent, or secret remedy.

not(o)- word element [Gr.], *the back.*

notalgia (no-tal′je-ah) pain in the back.

notch (noch) an indentation on the edge of a bone or other organ. **aortic n.,** dicrotic n. **dicrotic n.,** a small downward deflection in the arterial pulse or pressure contour immediately following the closure of the semilunar valves, sometimes used as a marker for the end of systole or the ejection period. **parotid n.,** the notch between the ramus of the mandible and the mastoid process of the temporal bone.

notifiable (nōt″ĭ-fi′ah-b'l) required to be reported to the board of health.

notochord (nōt′o-kord) the rod-shaped cord of cells below the primitive groove of the embryo, defining the primitive axis of the body; the common factor of all chordates. It is the center of development of the axial skeleton.

Notoedres (nōt″o-ed′rēz) a genus of mites, including *N. ca′ti,* an itch mite causing a persistent, often fatal, mange in cats; it also infests domestic animals, and may temporarily infest man.

notum (nōt′im) the dorsal part of the body.

novobiocin (no″vo-bi′o-sin) an antibacterial, $C_{31}H_{36}N_2O_{11}$, produced by *Streptomyces niveus;* used in treatment of infections due to staphylococci and other gram-positive organisms.

Novocain (no′vah-kān) trademark for preparations of procaine.

noxious (nok′shis) hurtful; injurious; pernicious

Np chemical symbol, *neptunium.*

NPN nonprotein nitrogen.

NREM non-rapid eye movements (see under *sleep*).

ns., nsec. nanosecond.

N.S.N.A. National Student Nurse Association.

nucha (noo′kah) the nape, or back, of the neck. **nu′chal,** adj.

nuclear (noo′kle-er) pertaining to a nucleus.

nuclease (noo′kle-ās) any of a group of enzymes that split nucleic acids into nucleotides and other products.

nucleated (noo′kle-āt″id) having a nucleus or nuclei.

nuclei (nu′kle-i) plural of *nucleus.*

nucleic acids high-molecular-weight polymeric substances composed of nucleotides that constitute the acidic groups of the nucleoproteins and contain phosphoric acid, sugars, and purine and pyrimidine bases; see *deoxyribonucleic a.* and *ribonucleic a.*

nucleocapsid (noo″kle-o-kap′sid) a unit of viral structure, consisting of a capsid with the enclosed nucleic acid.

nucleofugal (noo″kle-of′u-gil) moving away from a nucleus.

nucleohistone (noo″kle-o-his′tōn) the nucleoprotein complex made up of DNA and histones, the principal constituent of chromatin.

nucleoid (noo′kle-oid) 1. resembling a nucleus. 2. a nucleus-like body sometimes seen in the center of an erythrocyte. 3. the genetic material (nucleic acid) of a virus situated in the center of the virion. 4. the nuclear region of a bacterium, which contains the chromosome but is not limited by a nuclear membrane.

nucleolonema (noo″kle-o″lon-e′mah) a network of strands formed by organization of a finely granular substance, perhaps containing RNA, in the nucleolus of a cell.

nucleolus (noo-kle′ah-lis), pl. *nucle′oli* [L.] a rounded refractile body in the nucleus of most cells, which is the site of synthesis of ribsomal RNA.

nucleopetal (noo″kle-op′it'l) moving toward a nucleus.

nucleophagocytosis (noo″kle-o-fag″o-si-to′sis) the engulfing of the nuclei of other cells by phagocytes.

nucleophile (noo″kle-ah-fīl) an electron donor in chemical reactions involving covalent catalysis in which the donated electrons bond other chemical groups (electrophiles). **nucleophil′ic,** adj.

nucleoplasm (noo′kle-ah-plazm″) the protoplasm of the nucleus of a cell.

nucleoprotein (noo″kle-o-pro′te-in) a substance composed of a simple basic protein (e.g., a histone) combined with a nucleic acid.

nucleosidase (-si′dās) an enzyme that catalyzes the splitting of nucleosides.

nucleoside (noo′kle-ah-sīd″) one of the compounds into which a nucleotide is split by the action of nucleotidase or by chemical means; it consists of a sugar (a pentose) with a purine or pyrimidine base.

nucleosome (-sōm) any of the complexes of histone and DNA in eukaryotic cells, seen under the electron microscope as beadlike bodies on a string of DNA.

nucleotidase (noo″kle-ot′ĭ-dās) an enzyme that splits nucleotides into nucleosides and phosphoric acid.

nucleotide (noo′kle-ah-tīd″) one of the compounds into which nucleic acid is split by action of nuclease; nucleotides are composed of a base (purine or pyrimidine), a sugar (ribose or deoxyribose), and a phosphate group. **cyclic n's,** those in which the phosphate group bonds to two atoms of the sugar forming a ring, as in cyclic AMP and cyclic GMP, which act as intracellular second messengers.

nucleotidyl (noo″kle-o-tīd′il) a nucleotide residue.

nucleotoxin (nu″kle-o-tok′sin) 1. a toxin from cell nuclei. 2. any toxin affecting cell nuclei.

nucleus (noo′kle-is), pl. *nu′clei* [L.] 1. cell nucleus; a spheroid body within a cell, consisting of a thin nuclear membrane, organelles, one or more nucleoli, chromatin, linin, and nucleoplasm. 2. a group of nerve cells, usually within the central nervous system, bearing a direct relationship to the fibers of a particular nerve. 3. in organic chemistry, the combination of atoms forming the central element or basic framework of the molecule of a specific compound or class of compounds. 4. see *atomic n.* **nu′clear,** adj. **ambiguous n.,** the nucleus of origin of motor fibers of the vagus, glossopharyngeal, and accessory nerves in the medulla oblongata. **arcuate nuclei, nu′clei arcua′ti,** small irregular areas of gray substance on the ventromedial aspect of the pyramid of the medulla oblongata. **atomic n.,** the central core of an atom composed of protons and neutrons, constituting most of its mass, but only a small part of its volume. **caudate n., n. cauda′tus,** an elongated, arched gray mass closely related to the lateral ventricle throughout its entire extent, which, together with the putamen, forms the neostriatum. **central n. of thalamus, n. centra′lis tha′lami,** a collection of cells close to the wall of the third ventricle, between the medial and posterior ventral nuclei of the thalamus. **cochlear nuclei, ventral and dorsal,** the nuclei of termination of sensory fibers of the cochlear part of the vestibulocochlear nerve, which partly encircle the inferior cerebellar peduncle at the junction of the medulla oblongata and pons. **cuneate n., n. cunea′tus,** a nucleus in the medulla oblongata, in which the fibers of the fasciculus cuneatus synapse. **Deiters' n.,** lateral vestibular n. **dentate n., n. denta′tus,** the largest of the deep cerebellar nuclei lying in the white matter of the cerebellum. **n. dorsa′lis, n.** thoracicus. **fastigial n., n. fasti′gii,** the most medial of the deep cerebellar nuclei, near the midline in the roof of the fourth ventricle. **n. gra′cilis,** a nucleus in the medulla oblongata, in which the fibers of the fasciculus gracilis of the spinal cord synapse. **hypoglossal n.,** the nucleus of origin of the hypoglossal nerve in the medulla oblongata. **interpeduncular n., n. interpeduncula′re,** a nucleus between the cerebral peduncles immediately dorsal to the in-

terpeduncular fossa. **lenticular n., lentiform n.,** the part of the corpus striatum just lateral to the internal capsule, comprising the putamen and globus pallidus. **motor n.,** any collection of cells in the central nervous system giving origin to a motor nerve. **olivary n., n. oliva′ris,** 1. a folded band of gray substance enclosing a white core and producing the elevation (olive) of the medulla oblongata. 2. olive (2). **n. of origin,** any collection of nerve cells giving origin to the fibers, or a part of the fibers, of a peripheral nerve. **paraventricular n., n. paraventricula′ris,** a band of cells in the wall of the third ventricle in the supraoptic part of the hypothalamus; many of its cells are neurosecretory in function (secreting oxytocin) and project to the neurohypophysis. **pontine nuclei, nu′clei pon′tis,** groups of nerve cell bodies in the part of the pyramidal tract within the ventral part of the pons upon which the fibers of the corticopontine tract synapse, and whose axons in turn cross to the opposite side and form the middle cerebellar peduncle. **n. pulpo′sus, pulpy n.,** a semifluid mass of fine white and elastic fibers forming the center of an intervertebral disk. **red n.,** a distinctive oval nucleus (pink in fresh specimens) centrally placed in the upper mesencephalic reticular formation. **n. of roof of cerebellum,** fastigial n. **n. ru′ber,** red n. **sensory n.,** the nucleus of termination of the afferent (sensory) fibers of a peripheral nerve. **subthalamic n., n. subthala′micus,** a nucleus on the medial side of the junction of the internal capsule and crus cerebri. **supraoptic n., n. supraop′ticus,** one just above the lateral part of the optic chiasm; many of its cells are neurosecretory in function (secreting antidiuretic hormone) and project to the neurohypophysis; other cells are osmoreceptors which respond to increased osmotic pressure to signal the release of antidiuretic hormone by the neurohypophysis. **tegmental nuclei,** several nuclear masses of the reticular formations of the pons and midbrain, especially of the latter, where they are in close approximation to the superior cerebellar peduncles. **terminal nuclei,** groups of nerve cells within the central nervous system on which the axons of primary afferent neurons of various cranial nerves synapse. **thoracic n., n. thorac′icus,** a column of cells in the posterior gray column of the spinal cord, extending from the 7th or 8th cervical segments to the 2nd or 3rd lumbar level. **vestibular nuclei, nu′clei vestibula′res,** the four (superior, lateral, medial, and inferior) cellular masses in the floor of the fourth ventricle in which the branches of the vestibulocochlear nerve terminate.

nuclide (noo′klīd) a species of atom characterized by the charge, mass, number, and quantum state of its nucleus, and capable of existing for a measurable lifetime (usually more than 10^{-10} sec.).

nullipara (nul-ip′ah-rah) para 0; a woman who has never borne a viable child. See *para.* **nullip′arous,** adj.

nulliparity (nul″ĭ-par′it-e) the state of being a nullipara.

number (num′ber) a symbol, as a figure or word, expressive of a certain value or a specified quantity determined by count. **atomic n.,** a number expressive of the number of protons in an atomic nucleus, or the positive charge of the nucleus expressed in terms of the electronic charge. **Avogadro's n.,** the number of particles in one mole of a substance; the value assigned to the number is 6.023×10^{23}. **mass n.,** the number expressive of the mass of a nucleus, being the total number of protons and neutrons in the nucleus of an atom or nuclide. **oxidation n.,** a number assigned to each atom in a molecule or ion that represents the number of electrons theoretically lost (negative numbers) or gained (positive numbers) in converting the atom to the elemental form (which has an oxidation number of zero). The sum of the oxidation numbers for all atoms in a neutral compound is zero; for polyatomic ions, it is equal to the ionic charge. **turnover n.,** the number of molecules of substrate acted upon by one molecule of enzyme per minute.

numbness (num′nis) a lack or diminution of sensation in a part.

nummular (num′ūl-er) 1. coin-sized and coin-shaped. 2. made up of round, flat disks. 3. arranged like a stack of coins.

nurse (nurs) 1. one who is especially prepared in the scientific basis of nursing and who meets certain prescribed standards of education and clinical competence. 2. to provide services essential to or helpful in the promotion, maintenance, and restoration of health and well-being. 3. to breast-feed an infant. **n. anesthetist,** a specially trained professional nurse who administers intravenous, spinal, and other anesthetics to render persons insensible during surgical operations, deliveries, and other medical and dental procedures. **charge n.,** one who is in charge of a patient care unit of a hospital or similar health agency. **clinical n. specialist,** a registered nurse with a high degree of knowledge, skill, and competence in a specialized area of nursing, and usually having a master's degree in nursing. **n. clinician,** a registered nurse, referred to as a *nurse clinician* or as a *nurse practitioner,* who has well-developed competencies in utilizing a broad range of cues, which are used for prescribing and implementing both direct and indirect nursing care and for articulating nursing therapies with other planned therapies. They demonstrate expertise in nursing practice and insure ongoing development of expertise through clinical experience and continuing education; generally, minimal preparation for this role is the baccalaureate degree. **community n.,** in Great Britain, a public health nurse. **community health n.,** public health n. **district n.,** community n. **general duty n.,** a registered nurse, usually one who has not undergone training beyond the basic nursing program, who sees to the general nursing care of patients in a hospital or other health agency. **graduate n.,** a graduate of a school of nursing; often used to designate one who has not been registered or licensed. **head n.,** charge n. **licensed practical n.,** a graduate of a school

of practical nursing whose qualifications have been examined by a state board of nursing and who has been legally authorized to practice as a licensed practical or vocational nurse (L.P.N. or L.V.N.), under supervision of a physician or registered nurse. **licensed vocational n.,** see *licensed practical n.* **n. practitioner,** see *n. clinician.* **private n., private duty n.,** one who attends an individual patient, usually on a fee-for-service basis, and who may specialize in a specific class of diseases. **probationer n.,** a person who has entered a school of nursing and is under observation to determine fitness for the nursing profession; applied principally to nursing students enrolled in hospital schools of nursing. **public health n.,** an especially prepared registered nurse employed in a community agency to safeguard the health of persons in the community, giving care to the sick in their homes, promoting health and well-being by teaching families how to keep well, and assisting in programs for the prevention of disease. **Queen's Nurse,** in Great Britain, a district nurse who has been trained at or in accordance with the regulations of the Queen Victoria Jubilee Institute for Nurses. **registered n.,** a graduate nurse who has been legally authorized (registered) to practice after examination by a state board of nurse examiners or similar regulatory authority, and who is legally entitled to use the designation R.N. **scrub n.,** one who directly assists the surgeon in the operating room. **n. specialist,** clinical n. specialist. **visiting n.,** public health n. **wet n.,** a woman who breast-feeds the infant of another.

nurse-midwife (-mid′wīf) an individual educated in the two disciplines of nursing and midwifery, who possesses evidence of certification according to the requirements of the American College of Nurse-Midwives. Abbreviated C.N.M. (Certified Nurse-Midwife).

nurse-midwifery (-mid′wi-fer-e) the independent management of care of essentially normal newborns and women, antepartally, intrapartally, postpartally, and/or gynecologically, occurring within a health care system which provides for medical consultation, collaborative management, or referral, and is in accord with the functions, standards, and qualifications as defined by the American College of Nurse-Midwives.

nursery (nurs′er-e) the department in a hospital where the newborn are cared for.

nursing (nurs′ing) the provision, at various levels of preparation, of services essential to or helpful in the promotion, maintenance, and restoration of health and well-being or in prevention of illness, as of infants, of sick and injured, or of others for any reason unable to provide such services for themselves.

nutation (noo-ta′shin) the act of nodding, especially involuntary nodding.

nutrient (noo′tre-int) 1. nourishing; affording nutriment. 2. a nutritious substance; or a component of food.

nutriment (noo′trĭ-mint) nourishment; nutritious material; food.

nutrition (noo-trish′in) 1. the sum of the processes involved in taking in nutriments and assimilating and utilizing them. 2. nutriment. **nutri′tional**, adj. **total parenteral n. (TPN)**, parenteral hyperalimentation.

nutritious (noo-trish′is) affording nourishment.

nutritive (noo′trit-iv) pertaining to or promoting nutrition.

nutriture (noo′trĭ-cher) the status of the body in relation to nutrition.

nyct(o)- word element [Gr.], *night; darkness.*

nyctalopia (nik″tah-lo′pe-ah) 1. night blindness. 2. in French (and incorrectly in English), day blindness.

nyctohemeral (nik″to-hem′er-il) pertaining to both day and night.

nyctophilia (-fil′e-ah) a preference for darkness or for night.

nylidrin (nil′ĭ-drin) a synthetic adrenergic, C_{19}-$H_{25}NO_2$, used as a peripheral vasodilator.

nymph (nimf) a developmental stage in certain arthropods, e.g., ticks, between the larval form and the adult, and resembling the latter in appearance.

nymph(o)- word element [Gr.], *nymphae* (labia minora).

nympha (nim′fah), pl. *nym′phae* [L.] labium minus.

nymphectomy (nim-fek′tah-me) excision of the nymphae (labia minora).

nymphitis (nim-fit′is) inflammation of the nymphae (labium minora).

nymphomania (nim″fah-ma′ne-ah) exaggerated sexual desire in a female.

nymphoncus (nim-fong′kis) swelling of the nymphae (labia minora).

nymphotomy (nim-fot′ah-me) surgical incision of the nymphae (labia minora) or clitoris.

nystagmiform (nis-tag′mĭ-form) nystagmoid.

nystagmograph (nis-tag′mah-graf) an instrument for recording the movements of the eyeball in nystagmus.

nystagmoid (nis-tag′moid) resembling nystagmus.

nystagmus (nis-tag′mis) involuntary rapid movement (horizontal, vertical, rotatory, or mixed, i.e., of two types) of the eyeball. **nystag′mic**, adj. **aural n.**, labyrinthine n. **caloric n.**, Bárány's symptom (2). **Cheyne's n.**, a peculiar rhythmical eye movement. **dissociated n.**, that in which the movements in the two eyes are dissimilar. **end-position n.**, that occurring only at extremes of gaze. **fixation n.**, that occurring only on gazing fixedly at an object. **gaze n.**, nystagmus made apparent by looking to the right or to the left. **labyrinthine n.**, vestibular nystagmus due to labyrinthine disturbance. **latent n.**, that occurring only when one eye is covered. **lateral n.**, involuntary horizontal movement of the eyes. **optokinetic n.**, the normal nystagmus occurring when looking at objects passing across the field of vision, as in viewing from a moving vehicle. **pendular n.**, that which consists of to-and-fro movements of equal velocity. **positional n.**, that which occurs, or is altered in form or intensity, on assumption of certain positions of the head. **retraction n.**, **n. retracto′rius**, a spasmodic backward movement of the eyeball occurring on attempts to move the eye; a sign of midbrain disease. **rotatory n.**, involuntary rotation of eyes about the visual axis. **spontaneous n.**, that occurring without specific stimulation of the vestibular system. **undulatory n.**, pendular n. **vertical n.**, involuntary up-and-down movement of the eyes. **vestibular n.**, that due to disturbance of the labyrinth or of the vestibular nuclei; the movements are usually jerky.

nystatin (nis′tah-tin) an antifungal antibiotic, $C_{46}H_{77}NO_{19}$, produced by growth of *Streptomyces noursei;* used in treatment of infections with *Candida albicans.*

nyxis (nik′sis) puncture, or paracentesis.

O

O chemical symbol, *oxygen.*

Ω symbol for *ohm.*

o- symbol, *ortho-.*

OB obstetrics.

ob- word element [L.], *against; in front of; toward.*

obesity (o-bēs′it-e) an increase in body weight beyond the limitation of skeletal and physical requirements, as the result of excessive accumulation of body fat. **obese′**, adj. **adult-onset o.**, that beginning in adulthood and characterized by increase in size (hypertrophy) of adipose cells with no increase in number. **lifelong o.**, that beginning in childhood and characterized by an increase both in number (hyperplasia) and in size (hypertrophy) of adipose cells. **morbid o.**, the condition of weighing two or more times the ideal weight; so called because

it is associated with many serious and life-threatening disorders.

obex (o′beks) the ependyma-lined junction of the teniae of the fourth ventricle of the brain at the inferior angle.

objective (ob-jek′tiv) 1. perceptible by the external senses. 2. a result for whose achievement an effort is made. 3. the lens or system of lenses of a microscope (or telescope) nearest the object that is being examined.

obligate (ob′lĭ-gāt) [L.] pertaining to or characterized by the ability to survive only in a particular environment or to assume only a particular role, as an obligate anaerobe.

obliquity (ob-lik′wit-e) the state of being inclined or slanting. **Litzmann's o.**, inclination of the fetal head so that the posterior parietal bone presents to the birth canal. **Nägele's o.**,

obliteration (ob-lit″er-a′shin) complete removal by disease, degeneration, surgical procedure, irradiation, etc.

oblongata (ob-long-gah′tah) medulla oblongata. **oblonga′tal**, adj.

obsession (ob-sesh′in) a persistent unwanted idea or impulse that cannot be eliminated by reasoning. **obses′sive**, adj.

obsessive-compulsive (ob-ses′iv-kom-pul′siv) marked by compulsion to repetitively perform certain acts or carry out certain rituals.

obstetrician (ob″stĭ-trish′in) one who practices obstetrics.

obstetrics (ob-stet′riks) the branch of medicine dealing with pregnancy, labor, and the puerperium. **obstet′ric, obstet′rical**, adj.

obstipation (ob″stĭ-pa′shin) intractable constipation.

obtund (ob-tund′) to render dull or blunt.

obtundent (ob-tun′dint) 1. having the power to dull sensibility or to soothe pain. 2. a soothing or partially anesthetic medicine.

obturator (ob′tu-rāt″er) a disk or plate, natural or artificial, that closes an opening.

obtusion (ob-too′shin) a deadening or blunting of sensitiveness.

occipitalization (ok-sip″it-il-iz-a′shin) synostosis of the atlas with the occiput.

occipitocervical (ok-sip″it-o-surv′ik′l) pertaining to the occiput and neck.

occipitofrontal (-front′′l) pertaining to the occiput and the face.

occipitomastoid (-mas′toid) pertaining to the occipital bone and mastoid process.

occipitomental (-ment′′l) pertaining to the occiput and chin.

occipitoparietal (-pah-ri′it′l) pertaining to the occipital and parietal bones or lobes of the brain.

occipitotemporal (-tem′per-il) pertaining to the occipital and temporal bones.

occipitothalamic (-thah-lam′ik) pertaining to the occipital lobe and thalamus.

occiput (ok′si-put) the back part of the head. **occip′ital**, adj.

occlude (ah-klōōd′) to fit close together; to close tight; to obstruct or close off.

occlusal (ah-kloo′z′l) pertaining to closure; applied to the masticating surfaces of the premolar and molar teeth.

occlusion (ah-kloo′shin) 1. the act of closure or state of being closed; an obstruction or a closing off. 2. the relation of the teeth of both jaws when in functional contact during activity of the mandible. **abnormal o.**, malocclusion. **balanced o.**, occlusion in which the teeth are in harmonious working relation. **centric o.**, occlusion of the teeth when the mandible is in centric relation to the maxilla, with full occlusal surface contact of the upper and lower teeth in habitual occlusion. **coronary o.**, complete obstruction of an artery of the heart. **eccentric o.**, occlusion of the teeth when the lower jaw has

moved from the centric position. **habitual o.**, the consistent relationship of the teeth in the maxilla to those of the mandible when the teeth in both jaws are brought into maximum contact. **lateral o.**, occlusion of the teeth when the lower jaw is moved to the right or left of centric occlusion. **lingual o.**, malocclusion in which the tooth is lingual to the line of the normal dental arch. **mesial o.**, the position of a lower tooth when it is mesial to its opposite number in the maxilla. **normal o.**, the contact of the upper and lower teeth in the centric relationship. **protrusive o.**, anteroclusion. **retrusive o.**, distoclusion.

occlusive (ah-kloo′siv) pertaining to or effecting occlusion.

occult (ah-kult′) obscure or hidden from view.

ocellus (ah-sel′us) [L.] 1. a simple eye in insects and other invertebrates. 2. one of the elements of a compound eye of insects. 3. a roundish, eyelike patch of color.

ochrometer (ah-krom′it-er) an instrument for measuring capillary blood pressure.

ochronosis (o″kron-o′sis) a peculiar discoloration of certain body tissues caused by deposit of alkapton bodies as the result of a metabolic disorder. **ochronot′ic**, adj. **ocular o.**, brown or gray discoloration of the sclera, sometimes involving also the conjunctivae and eyelids.

octa- word element [Gr., L.], *eight*.

octopamine (ok″tah-pam′ēn) a sympathomimetic amine thought to result from inability of the diseased liver to metabolize tyrosine; a false neurotransmitter, since it can be stored in presynaptic vesicles, replacing norepinephrine, but has little effect on postsynaptic receptors.

ocul(o)- word element [L.], *eye*.

ocular (ok′ūl-er) 1. pertaining to the eye. 2. eyepiece.

oculist (ok′ūl-ist) ophthalmologist.

oculocutaneous (ok″ūl-o-ku-ta′ne-us) pertaining to or affecting the eyes and the skin.

oculofacial (-fa′shil) pertaining to the eyes and the face.

oculogyration (-ji-ra′shin) movement of the eye about the anteroposterior axis. **oculogy′ric**, adj.

oculomotor (-mōt′er) pertaining to or effecting eye movements.

oculomotorius (-mo-tor′e-us) the oculomotor nerve.

oculomycosis (-mi-ko′sis) any fungal disease of the eye.

oculonasal (-na′z′l) pertaining to the eye and the nose.

oculopupillary (-pu′pil-ĕ″re) pertaining to the pupil of the eye.

oculozygomatic (-zi″go-mat′ik) pertaining to the eye and the zygoma.

oculus (ok′ūl-us), pl. *oc′uli* [L.] eye.

O.D. Doctor of Optometry; [L.] *o′culus dex′ter* (right eye); overdose.

odont(o)- word element [Gr.], *tooth*.

odontalgia (o″don-tal′je-ah) toothache.

odontectomy (o″don-tek′tah-me) excision of a tooth.

odontic (o-don′tik) pertaining to the teeth.

odontoblast (o-don′tah-blast) one of the connective tissue cells that deposit dentin and form the outer surface of the dental pulp.

odontoblastoma (o-don″to-blas-to′mah) a tumor made up of odontoblasts.

odontoclast (o-don′tah-klast) an osteoclast associated with absorption of the roots of deciduous teeth.

odontogenesis (o-don″to-jen′ĭ-sis) the origin and histogenesis of the teeth. **odontogenet′ic,** adj. **o. imperfec′ta,** dentinogenesis imperfecta.

odontogenic (-jen′ik) 1. forming teeth. 2. arising in tissues that give origin to the teeth.

odontoid (o-don′toid) like a tooth.

odontology (o″don-tol′ah-je) 1. scientific study of the teeth. 2. dentistry.

odontolysis (o″don-tol′ĭ-sis) the resorption of dental tissue.

odontoma (o″don-to′mah) any odontogenic tumor, especially a composite odontoma. **composite o.,** one consisting of both enamel and dentin in an abnormal pattern. **radicular o.,** one associated with a tooth root, or formed when the root was developing.

odontopathy (o″don-top′ah-the) any disease of the teeth. **odontopath′ic,** adj.

odontotomy (o″don-tot′ah-me) incision of a tooth.

odor (o′der) a volatile emanation perceived by the sense of smell.

odorant (o′der-int) any substance capable of stimulating the sense of smell.

-odynia word element [Gr.], *pain.*

odynometer (o″din-om′it-er) an instrument for measuring pain.

odynophagia (o-din″o-fa′je-ah) painful swallowing of food.

oe- for words beginning thus, see also those beginning *e-.*

oedipal (ed′ĭ-pil) pertaining to the Oedipus complex.

oesophagostomiasis (e-sof″ah-go-sto-mi′ah-sis) infection with *Oesophagostomum.*

Oesophagostomum (e-sof″ah-gos′tah-mum) a genus of nematode worms found in the intestines of various animals.

Oestrus (es′trus) a genus of botflies, including *O. o′vis,* a species whose larvae may infest nasal cavities and sinuses of sheep, and may cause ocular myiasis in man.

official (ŏ-fish′′l) authorized by pharmacopeias and recognized formularies.

officinal (o-fis′in-il) regularly kept for sale in druggists' shops.

ohm (ōm) the SI unit of electrical resistance, being that of a resistor in which a current of 1 ampere is produced by a potential difference of 1 volt. Symbol Ω.

ohmmeter (ōm′mēt-er) an instrument that measures electrical resistance in ohms.

-oid word element [Gr.], *resembling.*

oil (oil) 1. an unctuous, combustible substance that is liquid, or easily liquefiable, on warming, and is soluble in ether but not in water. Oils may be animal, vegetable, or mineral in origin, and volatile or nonvolatile (fixed). A number of oils are used as flavoring or perfuming agents in pharmaceutical preparations. 2. a fat that is liquid at room temperature. **castor o.,** a fixed oil obtained from the seed of *Ricinus communis;* used as a cathartic, bland emollient to the skin in certain dermatoses, and plasticizer for pharmaceuticals. **clove o.,** a volatile oil from cloves (dried flowerbuds of *Eugenia caryophyllus*); used as a topical dental analgesic, flavoring agent, germicide, and counterirritant. **cod liver o.,** partially destearinated, fixed oil from fresh livers of *Gadus morrhua* and other fish of the family Gadidae; used as a source of vitamins A and D. **cod liver o., nondestearinated,** entire fixed oil from fresh livers of *Gadus morrhua* and other fish of the family Gadidae; used as a source of vitamins A and D. **corn o.,** a refined fixed oil obtained from embryo of *Zea mays;* used as a solvent and vehicle for various medicinal agents and as a vehicle for injections. It has also been promoted as a source of polyunsaturated fatty acids in special diets. **cottonseed o.,** refined, fixed oil from seeds of cultivated plants of various species of *Gossypium;* used as a solvent and vehicle for drugs and as an emollient and laxative in veterinary medicine. **essential o., ethereal o.,** volatile o. **ethiodized o.,** an iodine addition product of the ethyl ester of fatty acids of poppyseed oil; used as a radiopaque medium in hysterosalpingography and lymphography. **eucalyptus o.,** a volatile oil from fresh leaf of species of *Eucalyptus;* used as a flavoring agent for drugs, and as an expectorant and local antiseptic with mild anesthetic effect. **expressed o., fatty o.,** fixed o. **fixed o.,** a nonvolatile oil, i.e., one that does not evaporate on warming; such oils consist of a mixture of fatty acids and their esters, and are classified as solid, semisolid, and liquid. **flaxseed o.,** linseed o. **iodized o.,** a sterile preparation of vegetable oil or oils containing 38–42% of organically combined iodine; used as a contrast medium in hysterosalpingography. **mineral o.,** a mixture of liquid hydrocarbons from petroleum; used as a levigating agent, lubricant laxative, and drug vehicle. **mineral o., light,** a mixture of hydrocarbons from petrolatum; used as a drug vehicle and laxative. **olive o.,** a fixed oil obtained from ripe fruit of *Olea europaea;* used as a setting retardant for dental cements, topical emollient, and laxative. **peanut o.,** a refined fixed oil from seed kernels of cultivated varieties of *Arachis hypogaea;* used as a solvent and vehicle for drugs, and as a laxative in veterinary medicine. **peppermint o.,** a volatile oil from fresh overground parts of flowering plant of *Mentha piperita;* used as a flavoring agent for drugs, gastric stimulant, and carminative. **persic o.,** oil expressed from kernels of varieties of *Prunus armeniaca* (apricot) or *P. persica* (peach); used as a drug vehicle. **sesame o.,** a refined, fixed oil from seeds of cultivated varieties of *Sesamum indicum;* used as a solvent for drugs. **volatile o.,** a readily evaporating substance of plant origin, containing aromatic hydrocarbons, aldehydes, alcohols, ethers, acids, terpenes, or camphors.

ointment (oint′mint) a semisolid preparation for external application to the body, usually containing a medicinal substance. **hydrophilic o.,** a water-in-oil emulsion consisting of methylparaben, propylparaben, sodium lauryl sulfate, propylene glycol, stearyl alcohol, white petrolatum, and purified water; used as an ointment base. **rose water o.,** a preparation of spermaceti, white wax, almond oil, sodium borate, stronger rose water, purified water, and rose oil; used as an emollient and ointment base. **white o.,** an oleaginous ointment base prepared from white wax and white petrolatum. **yellow o.,** a mixture of yellow wax and petrolatum; used as an ointment base.

O.L. [L.] *oc′ulus lae′vus* (left eye).

-ol word termination indicating an alcohol or a phenol.

olamine (ol′ah-mēn) USAN contraction for ethanolamine.

oleaginous (o″le-aj′ĭ-nus) oily; greasy.

oleate (o′le-āt) 1. a salt of oleic acid. 2. a solution of a substance in oleic acid.

olecranarthritis (o-lek″ran-ar-thri′tis) inflammation of the elbow joint.

olecranarthrocace (-ar-throk′ah-se) tuberculosis of the elbow joint.

olecranarthropathy (-ar-throp′ah-the) disease of the elbow joint.

olecranon (o-lek′rah-non) bony projection of the ulna at the elbow. **olec′ranal,** adj.

oleic acid (o-le′ik) an unsaturated fatty acid, $C_{17}H_{33}COOH$, found in animal and vegetable fats.

oleo- word element [L.], *oil.*

oleoresin (o″le-o-rez′in) 1. a compound of a resin and a volatile oil, such as exudes from pines, etc. 2. a compound extracted from a drug by percolation with a volatile solvent, such as acetone, alcohol, or ether, and evaporation of the solvent.

oleovitamin (-vīt′ah-min) a preparation of fish liver oil or edible vegetable oil containing one or more fat-soluble vitamins or their derivatives.

oleum (o′le-um), pl. *o′lea* [L.] oil.

olfact (ol′fakt) a unit of odor, the *minimum perceptible odor,* being the minimum concentration of a substance in solution that can be perceived by a large number of normal individuals; expressed in grams per liter.

olfaction (ol-fak′shin) 1. the act of smelling. 2. the sense of smell.

olfactology (ol″fak-tol′ah-je) the science of the sense of smell.

olfactometer (ol″fak-tom′it-er) an instrument for testing the sense of smell.

olfactory (ol-fak′ter-e) pertaining to the sense of smell.

olig(o)- word element [Gr.], *few; little; scanty.*

oligemia (ol″ĭ-gēm′e-ah) deficiency in volume of the blood. **olige′mic,** adj.

oligocardia (ol″ĭ-go-kar′de-ah) bradycardia.

oligochromemia (-kro-mēm′e-ah) deficiency of hemoglobin in the blood.

oligocystic (-sis′tik) containing few cysts.

oligocythemia (-si-thēm′e-ah) deficiency of the cellular elements of the blood. **oligocythe′mic,** adj.

oligodactyly (-dak′tĭ-le) congenital absence of one or more fingers or toes.

oligodendrocyte (-den′drah-sīt) a cell of oligodendroglia.

oligodendroglia (-den-drog′le-ah) 1. the nonneural cells of ectodermal origin forming part of the adventitial structure (neuroglia) of the central nervous system. 2. the tissue composed of such cells.

oligodendroglioma (-den″dro-gli-o′mah) a neoplasm derived from and composed of oligodendrocytes.

oligodipsia (-dip′se-ah) abnormally diminished thirst.

oligodontia (-don′she-ah) presence of fewer than the normal number of teeth.

oligogalactia (-gah-lak′she-ah) deficient secretion of milk.

oligohydramnios (-hi-dram′ne-os) deficiency in the amount of amniotic fluid.

oligohydruria (-hi-drōōr′e-ah) abnormally high concentration of urine.

oligomeganephronia (-meg″ah-nĕ-fro′ne-ah) congenital renal hypoplasia in which there is a reduction in the number of lobes and of the total number of nephrons, and hypertrophy of the nephrons. **oligomeganephron′ic,** adj.

oligomenorrhea (-men″or-e′ah) abnormally infrequent menstruation.

oligonucleotide (-noo′kle-o-tīd) a polymer made up of a few (2–10) nucleotides.

oligophosphaturia (-fos″fah-tūr′e-ah) deficiency of phosphates in the urine.

oligoplasmia (-plaz′me-ah) deficiency of blood plasma.

oligosaccharide (-sak′ah-rīd) a carbohydrate which on hydrolysis yields a small number of monosaccharides.

oligospermia (-spurm′e-ah) deficiency of spermatozoa in the semen.

oligosynaptic (-sin-ap′tik) involving a few synapses in series and therefore a sequence of only a few neurons.

oligotrophia, oligotrophy (-tro′fe-ah; ol″ĭ-gah′trah-fe) a state of poor (insufficient) nutrition.

oligozoospermia (ol″ĭ-go-zo″o-spurm′e-ah) oligospermia.

oliguria (ol″ĭ-gūr′e-ah) diminished urine secretion in relation to fluid intake. **oligu′ric,** adj.

oliva (o-li′vah), pl. *oli′vae* [L.] olive.

olivary (ol′ĭ-ver″e) shaped like an olive.

olive (ol′iv) 1. the tree *Olea europaea* and its fruit. 2. olivary body; a rounded elevation lateral to the upper part of each pyramid of the medulla oblongata.

olivifugal (ol″ĭ-vif′u-gil) moving or conducting away from the olive.

olivipetal (ol″ĭ-vip′it′l) moving or conducting toward the olive.

olivopontocerebellar (ol″ĭ-vo-pon″to-ser″ĭ-bel′er) pertaining to the olive, the middle peduncles, and the cerebellar cortex.

olophonia (ol″ah-fo′ne-ah) defective speech due to malformed vocal organs.

-oma word element [Gr.], *tumor; neoplasm.*

omasitis (o″mah-sīt′is) inflammation of the omasum.

omasum (o-ma′sum) the third division of the stomach of a ruminant animal.

omentectomy (o″men-tek′tah-me) excision of all or part of the omentum.

omentitis (o″men-tīt′is) inflammation of the omentum.

omentopexy (o-men′tah-pek″se) fixation of the omentum, especially to establish collateral circulation in portal obstruction.

omentorrhaphy (o″men-tor′ah-fe) suture or repair of the omentum.

omentum (o-men′tum), pl. *omen′ta* [L.] a fold of peritoneum extending from the stomach to adjacent abdominal organs. **omen′tal,** adj. **gastrocolic o.,** greater o. **gastrohepatic o.,** lesser o. **greater o.,** a peritoneal fold attached to the anterior surface of the transverse colon. **lesser o.,** a peritoneal fold joining the lesser curvature of the stomach and the first part of the duodenum to the porta hepatis. **o. ma′jus,** greater o. **o. mi′nor,** lesser o.

Omnipen (om′nĭ-pen) trademark for preparations of ampicillin.

omoclavicular (o″mo-klah-vik′ūl-er) pertaining to the shoulder and clavicle.

omohyoid (-hi′oid) pertaining to the shoulder and the hyoid bone.

omphal(o)- word element [Gr.], *umbilicus.*

omphalectomy (om″fah-lek′tah-me) excision of the umbilicus.

omphalelcosis (om″fil-el-ko′sis) ulceration of the umbilicus.

omphalic (om-fal′ik) pertaining to the umbilicus.

omphalitis (om″fah-līt′is) inflammation of the umbilicus.

omphalocele (om′fah-lo-sēl″) protrusion, at birth, of part of the intestine through a defect in the abdominal wall at the umbilicus.

omphalomesenteric (om″fah-lo-mes″en-ter′ik) pertaining to the umbilicus and mesentery.

omphalophlebitis (-fle-bīt′is) 1. inflammation of the umbilical veins. 2. an infectious condition characterized by markedly suppurative lesions of the umbilicus in young animals; see *navel ill.*

omphalorrhagia (-ra′je-ah) hemorrhage from the umbilicus.

omphalorrhea (-re′ah) effusion of lymph at the umbilicus.

omphalorrhexis (-rek′sis) rupture of the umbilicus.

omphalosite (om′fah-lo-sīt″) the underdeveloped member of allantoidoangiopagous twins, joined to the more developed member (autosite) by the vessels of the umbilical cord.

omphalotomy (om″fah-lot′ah-me) the cutting of the umbilical cord.

onanism (o′nah-nizm) 1. coitus interruptus. 2. masturbation.

Onchocerca (ong″ko-ser′kah) a genus of nematode parasites of the superfamily Filarioidea, including *O. vol′vulus,* which causes human infection by invading the skin, subcutaneous tissues, and other tissues, producing fibrous nodules; blindness occurs after ocular invasion.

onchocerciasis (-ser-ki′ah-sis) infection by nematodes of the genus *Onchocerca.*

onchocercoma (ong″ko-ser-ko′mah) one of the dermal or subcutaneous nodules containing *Onchocerca volvulus* in human onchocerciasis.

onco- word element [Gr.], *tumor; swelling; mass.*

oncocyte (on′ko-sīt″) a large epithelial cell with an extremely acidophilic and granular cytoplasm, containing vast numbers of mitochondria; such cells may undergo neoplastic transformation. **oncocyt′ic,** adj.

oncodnavirus (on-kod′nah-vi″rus) any DNA virus that causes cancer.

oncofetal (on″ko-fēt′l) carcinoembryonic.

oncogenesis (-jen′ĭ-sis) the production or causation of tumors. **oncogenet′ic,** adj.

oncogenic (-jen′ik) giving rise to tumors or causing tumor formation; said especially of tumor-inducing viruses.

oncogenous (ong-koj′ĭ-nus) arising in or originating from a tumor.

oncology (ong-kol′ah-je) the sum of knowledge regarding tumors; the study of tumors.

oncolysate (on-kol′ĭ-sāt) any agent that lyses or destroys tumor cells.

oncolysis (ong-kol′ĭ-sis) destruction or dissolution of a neoplasm. **oncolyt′ic,** adj.

oncornavirus (on-kor′nah-vi″rus) any RNA virus that causes cancer.

oncosis (ong-ko′sis) a morbid condition marked by the development of tumors.

oncosphere (ong′ko-sfēr) the larva of the tapeworm contained within the external embryonic envelope and armed with six hooks.

oncotherapy (ong″ko-thĕ′rah-pe) the treatment of tumors.

oncotic (ong-kot′ik) pertaining to swelling.

oncotomy (ong-kot′ah-me) the incision of a tumor or swelling.

oncotropic (ong″ko-trop′ik) having special affinity for tumor cells.

Oncovin (on′ko-vin) trademark for a preparation of vincristine sulfate.

oncovirus (on′ko-vi″rus) any virus that causes cancer.

oneir(o)- word element [Gr.], *dream.*

oneiric (o-ni′rik) pertaining to dreams.

oneirism (o-ni′rizm) a waking dream state.

onlay (on′la″) a graft applied or laid on the surface of an organ or structure.

onomatomania (on″ah-mat″ah-ma′ne-ah) mental derangement with regard to words or names.

ontogenesis (on″tah-jen′ĭ-sis) ontogeny.

ontogeny (on-toj′ĭ-ne) the complete developmental history of an individual organism. **ontogenet′ic, ontogen′ic,** adj.

onyalai, onyalia (o″ne-al′a-e; o″ne-a′le-ah) a form of thrombopenic purpura due to a nutritional disorder occurring in Africa.

onych(o)- word element [Gr.], *the nails.*

onychatrophia (o-nik″ah-tro′fe-ah) atrophy of a nail or the nails.

onychauxis (on″ĭ-kawk′sis) hypertrophy of the nails.

onychectomy (on″ĭ-kek′tah-me) excision of a nail or nail bed, or of animal claws.

onychia (o-nik′e-ah) inflammation of the nail bed, resulting in loss of the nail.

onychitis (on″ĭ-kīt′is) onychia.

onychocryptosis (on″ĭ-ko-krip-to′sis) ingrown nail.

onychodystrophy (-dis′trah-fe) malformation of a nail.

onychogenic (-jen′ik) producing nail substance.

onychograph (o-nik′o-graf) an instrument for observing and recording the nail pulse and capillary circulation.

onychogryphosis, onychogryposis (on″ĭ-ko-grĭ-fo′sis; -grĭ-po′sis) hypertrophy and curving of the nails, giving them a clawlike appearance.

onychoheterotopia (-het″er-o-to′pe-ah) abnormal location of the nails.

onycholysis (on″ĭ-kol′ĭ-sis) loosening or separation of a nail from its bed.

onychomadesis (on″ĭ-ko-mah-de′sis) complete loss of the nails.

onychomalacia (-mah-la′she-ah) softening of the fingernail.

onychomycosis (-mi-ko′sis) fungal disease of the fingernails; the nails become opaque, white, thickened, and friable.

onychopathy (on″ĭ-kop′ah-the) any disease of the nails. **onychopath′ic,** adj.

onychophagia, onychophagy (on″ĭ-ko-fa′je-ah; on″ĭ-kof′ah-je) biting of the nails.

onychorrhexis (on″ĭ-ko-rek′sis) spontaneous splitting or breaking of the nails.

onychoschizia (-skiz′e-ah) onycholysis.

onychosis (on″ĭ-ko′sis) disease or deformity of a nail or the nails.

onychotillomania (on″ĭ-ko-til″o-ma′ne-ah) neurotic picking or tearing at the nails.

onychotomy (on″ĭ-kot′ah-me) incision into a fingernail or toenail.

onyx (on′iks) 1. a variety of hypopyon. 2. a fingernail or toenail.

oo- word element [Gr.], *egg; ovum.*

ooblast (o′ah-blast) a primitive cell from which an ovum ultimately develops.

oocyst (-sist) the encysted or encapsulated ookinete in the wall of a mosquito's stomach; also, the analogous stage in the development of any sporozoon.

oocyte (-sīt) an immature ovum; it is derived from an oogonium and is called a *primary o.* prior to completion of the first maturation division, and a *secondary o.* in the period between the first and second maturation division.

oogamy (o-og′ah-me) 1. fertilization of a large nonmotile egg by a small, motile male gamete or sperm, as seen in certain algae. 2. conjugation of two dissimilar gametes; heterogamy. **oog′amous,** adj.

oogenesis (o″ah-jen′ĭ-sis) the process of formation of female gametes (ova). **oogenet′ic,** adj.

oogonium (-go′ne-um), pl. *oogo′nia* [Gr.] an ovarian egg during fetal development; near the time of birth it becomes a primary oocyte.

ookinesis (-ki-ne′sis) the mitotic movements of an ovum during maturation and fertilization.

ookinete (-kĭ-nēt′) the fertilized form of the malarial parasite in a mosquito's body, formed by fertilization of a macrogamete by a microgamete and developing into an oocyst.

oolemma (-lem′ah) zona pellucida (1).

oophor(o)- word element [Gr.], *ovary.*

oophorectomy (o″ah-fah-rek′tah-me) excision of one or both ovaries.

oophoritis (-rit′is) inflammation of an ovary.

oophorocystectomy (o-ah″fah-ro-sis-tek′tah-me) excision of an ovarian cyst.

oophorocystosis (-sis-to′sis) the formation of ovarian cysts.

oophorohysterectomy (-his″ter-ek′tah-me) excision of the ovaries and uterus.

oophoron (o-of′ah-ron) an ovary.

oophoropexy (o-of′ah-ro-pek″se) ovariopexy.

oophoroplasty (-plas″te) plastic repair of an ovary.

oophorostomy (o-of″ah-ros′tah-me) incision of an ovarian cyst for drainage purposes.

oophorotomy (o-of″ah-rot′ah-me) incision of an ovary.

ooplasm (o′ah-plazm) cytoplasm of an ovum.

oosperm (-sperm) a fertilized ovum.

ootid (-tid) the cell produced by meiotic division of a secondary oocyte, which develops into the ovum. In mammals, this second maturation division is not completed unless fertilization occurs.

opacification (o-pah″sĭ-fĭ-ka′shun) 1. the development of an opacity. 2. the rendering opaque to x-rays of a tissue or organ by introduction of a contrast medium.

opacity (o-pas′it-e) 1. the condition of being opaque. 2. an opaque area.

opalescent (o″pah-les′int) showing a milky iridescence, like an opal.

opaque (o-pāk′) impervious to light rays or, by extension, to x-rays or other electromagnetic radiation.

opening (o′pin-ing) an aperture, orifice, or open space. **aortic o.,** 1. the aperture of the ventricle into the aorta. 2. the aperture in the diaphragm for passage of the descending aorta. **cardiac o.,** the opening from the esophagus into the stomach. **pyloric o.,** the opening between the stomach and duodenum. **saphenous o.,** see under *hiatus.*

operable (op′er-ah-b'l) subject to being operated upon with a reasonable degree of safety; appropriate for surgical removal.

operant (op′ah-rint) in psychology, any response that is not elicited by specific external stimuli but that recurs at a given rate in a particular set of circumstances.

operation (op″er-a′shin) 1. any action performed with instruments or by the hands of a surgeon; a surgical procedure. 2. any effect produced by a therapeutic agent. **op′erative,** adj. **Albee's o.,** an operation for ankylosis of the hip. **Babcock's o.,** a technique for eradication of varicose veins by extirpation of the saphenous vein. **Bassini's o.,** plastic repair of inguinal hernia. **Beer's o.,** a flap method for cataract. **Belsey Mark IV o.,** an operation for gastroesophageal reflux performed through a thoracic incision; the fundus is wrapped 270 degrees around the circumference of the esophagus, leaving its posterior wall free. **Billroth's o.,** partial resection of the stomach with anastomosis to the duodenum (Billroth I) or to the jejunum (Billroth II). **Blalock-Taussig o.,** anastomosis of the subclavian artery to the pulmonary artery to shunt some of the systemic circulation into the pulmonary circulation; done in congenital pulmonary stenosis. **Bricker's o.,** surgical creation of an ileal conduit for the collection of urine. **Browne o.,** urethroplasty for hypospadias repair, in which an intact strip of epithelium is left on the ventral surface of the penis to form the roof of the urethra, and the floor of the urethra is formed by epithelialization from the lateral wound margins. **Brunschwig's o.,** pancreatoduodenectomy performed in two stages. **Caldwell-Luc o.,** radical maxillary sinusotomy. **Cotte's o.,** removal of the presacral nerve. **Daviel's o.,** extraction of a cataract through a corneal incision without cutting the iris. **Dührssen's o.,** vaginal fixation of the uterus. **Dupuy-Dutemps o.,** blepharoplasty of the lower lid with tissue from the upper lid. **Elliot's o.,** sclerectomy by trephine. **equilibrating o.,** tenotomy of the direct antagonist of a paralyzed eye muscle. **exploratory o.,** incision into a body area to determine the cause of unexplained symptoms. **flap o.,** any operation involving the raising of a flap of tissue. **Fothergill o.,** an operation for uterine prolapse by fixation of the cardinal ligaments. **Frazier-Spiller o.,** division of the sensory root of the gasserian ganglion for relief of trigeminal neuralgia. **Fredet-Ramstedt o.,** pyloromyotomy. **Freyer's o.,** suprapubic enucleation of the hypertrophied prostate. **Frost-Lang o.,** insertion of a gold ball in place of an enucleated eyeball. **Gonin's o.,** thermocautery of the fissure in the retina, for retinal detachment. **Hartmann's o.,** resection of a diseased portion of the colon, with the proximal end of the colon brought out as a colostomy and the distal stump or rectum being closed by suture. **Kelly's o., King's o.,** arytenoidopexy. **Kraske's o.,** removal of the coccyx and part of the sacrum for access to a rectal carcinoma. **Lagrange's o.,** sclerectoiridectomy. **Le Forte's o.,** partial colpectomy. **Lorenz's o.,** an operation for congenital dislocation of the hip. **McBurney's o.,** radical surgery for the cure of inguinal hernia. **Macewen's o.,** supracondylar section of the femur for genu valgum. **McGill's o.,** suprapubic transvesical prostatectomy. **Madlener o.,** sterilization by crushing and ligating the middle portion of the fallopian tube. **Manchester o.,** Fothergill o. **Motais o.,** transplantation of a portion of the tendon of the superior rectus muscle of the eyeball into the upper lid, for ptosis. **Partsch o.,** a technique for marsupialization of a dental cyst. **Pomeroy's o.,** sterilization by ligation of a loop of fallopian tube and resection of the tied loop. **radical o.,** one involving extensive resection of tissue for complete extirpation of disease. **Ramstedt o.,** pyloromyotomy. **Saemisch's o.,** transfixion of the cornea and of the base of the ulcer for cure of hypopyon. **Torkildsen's o.,** ventriculocisternostomy. **Wertheim's o.,** radical hysterectomy. **Ziegler's o.,** V-shaped iridectomy for forming an artificial pupil.

operculum (o-per′kūl-um), pl. *oper′cula* [L.] a lid or covering; the folds of pallium from the frontal, parietal, and temporal lobes of the cerebrum overlying the insula. **oper′cular,** adj. **dental o.,** the hood of gingival tissue overlying the crown of an erupting tooth. **trophoblastic o.,** the plug of trophoblast that helps close the gap in the endometrium made by the implanting blastocyst.

operon (op′er-on) a segment of a chromosome comprising an operator gene and closely linked structural genes having related functions.

ophiasis (o-fi′ah-sis) a form of alopecia areata involving the temporal and occipital margins of the scalp in a continuous band.

ophidism (o′fī-dizm) poisoning by snake venom.

ophryon (o′fre-on) the middle point of the transverse supraorbital line.

ophryosis (of″re-o′sis) spasm of the eyebrow.

ophthalm(o)- word element [Gr.], *eye.*

ophthalmagra (of″thal-mag′rah) sudden pain in the eye.

ophthalmalgia (of″thal-mal′je-ah) pain in the eye.

ophthalmectomy (of″thal-mek′tah-me) excision of an eye; enucleation of the eyeball.

ophthalmencephalon (of″thal-men-sef′ah-lon) the retina, optic nerve, and visual apparatus of the brain.

ophthalmia (of-thal′me-ah) severe inflammation of the eye. **Egyptian o.,** trachoma. **gonorrheal o.,** acute and severe purulent ophthalmia due to gonorrheal infection. **o. neonato′rum,** any hyperacute purulent conjunctivitis occurring during the first 10 days of life, usually contracted during birth from infected vaginal discharge of the mother. **periodic o.,** a form of uveitis affecting horses. **phlyctenular o.,** see under *keratoconjunctivitis.* **purulent o.,** a form with a purulent discharge, commonly due to gonorrheal infection. **sympathetic o.,** granulomatous inflammation of the uveal tract of the uninjured eye following a wound involving the uveal tract of the other eye, resulting in bilateral granulomatous inflammation of the entire uveal tract.

ophthalmic (of-thal′mik) pertaining to the eye.

ophthalmitis (of″thal-mīt′is) inflammation of the eyeball. **ophthalmit′ic,** adj.

ophthalmoblennorrhea (of-thal″mo-blen″ah-re′ah) gonorrheal ophthalmia.

ophthalmocele (of-thal′mah-sēl) exophthalmos.

ophthalmodynamometry (-di″nah-mom′ĭ-tre) determination of the blood pressure in the retinal artery.

ophthalmodynia (-din′e-ah) pain in the eye.

ophthalmoeikonometer (-i-ko-nom′it-er) an

instrument for determining both the refraction of the eye and the relative size and shape of the ocular images.

ophthalmography (of″thal-mog′rah-fe) description of the eye and its diseases.

ophthalmogyric (of-thal″mah-ji′rik) oculogyric.

ophthalmolith (of-thal′mo-lith) a lacrimal calculus.

ophthalmologist (of″thal-mol′ah-jist) a physician who specializes in ophthalmology.

ophthalmology (of″thal-mol′ah-je) that branch of medicine dealing with the eye, its anatomy, physiology, pathology, etc. **ophthalmolog′ic,** adj.

ophthalmomalacia (of-thal″mo-mah-la′she-ah) abnormal softness of the eyeball.

ophthalmometry (of″thal-mom′ĭ-tre) determination of the refractive powers and defects of the eye.

ophthalmomycosis (of-thal″mo-mi-ko′sis) any disease of the eye caused by a fungus.

ophthalmomyotomy (-mi-ot′ah-me) surgical division of the muscles of the eyes.

ophthalmoneuritis (-nōōr-īt′is) inflammation of the ophthalmic nerve.

ophthalmopathy (of″thal-mop′ah-the) any disease of the eye.

ophthalmoplasty (of-thal′mo-plas″te) plastic surgery of the eye or its appendages.

ophthalmoplegia (of-thal″mo-ple′je-ah) paralysis of the eye muscles. **ophthalmople′gic,** adj. **o. exter′na,** paralysis of extraocular muscles. **o. inter′na,** paralysis of the iris and ciliary apparatus. **nuclear o.,** that due to a lesion of nuclei of motor nerves of eye. **Parinaud's o.,** paralysis of conjugate upward movement of the eyes without paralysis of convergence, associated with midbrain lesions. **partial o.,** that affecting some of the eye muscles. **progressive o.,** gradual paralysis of all the eye muscles. **total o.,** paralysis of all the eye muscles, both intraocular and extraocular.

ophthalmorrhagia (-ra′je-ah) hemorrhage from the eye.

ophthalmorrhea (-re′ah) oozing of blood from the eye.

ophthalmorrhexis (-rek′sis) rupture of an eyeball.

ophthalmoscope (of-thal′mah-skōp) an instrument containing a perforated mirror and lenses used to examine the interior of the eye. **direct o.,** one that produces an upright, or unreversed, image of approximately 15 times magnification. **indirect o.,** one that produces an inverted, or reversed, direct image of two to five times magnification.

ophthalmoscopy (of″thal-mos′kah-pe) examination of the eye by means of the ophthalmoscope. **medical o.,** that performed for diagnostic purposes. **metric o.,** that performed for measurement of refraction.

ophthalmostasis (of″thal-mos′tah-sis) fixation of the eye with the ophthalmostat.

ophthalmostat (of-thal′mah-stat) an instrument for holding the eye steady during operation.

ophthalmotomy (of″thal-mot′ah-me) incision of the eye.

ophthalmotrope (of-thal′mah-trōp) a mechanical eye that moves like a real eye.

opiate (o′pe-it) 1. any drug derived from opium. 2. any sleep-inducing drug.

opioid (o′pe-oid) 1. any synthetic narcotic that has opiate-like activities but is not derived from opium. 2. denoting naturally occurring peptides, e.g., enkephalins, that exert opiate-like effects by interacting with opiate receptors of cell membranes.

opisthion (o-pis′the-on) the midpoint of the lower border of the foramen magnum.

opisthorchiasis (o″pis-thor-ki′ah-sis) infection of the biliary tract by *Opisthorchis.*

Opisthorchis (o″pis-thor′kis) a genus of flukes parasitic in the liver and biliary tract of various birds and mammals; *O. felineus* and *O. viverrini* cause opisthorchiasis in humans.

opisthotonos (o″pis-thot′ah-nos) a form of spasm in which the head and heels are bent backward and the body bowed forward. **opisthoton′ic,** adj.

opium (o′pe-um) air-dried milky exudation from incised unripe capsules of *Papaver somniferum* or its variety *album,* containing some 25 alkaloids, the more important being morphine, narcotine, codeine, papaverine, thebaine, and narceine; the alkaloids are used for their narcotic and analgesic effect. Because it is highly addictive, opium production and cultivation of the plants from which it is obtained is prohibited by most nations under an international agreement.

opportunistic (op″er-tōōn-is′tik) 1. denoting a microorganism which does not ordinarily cause disease but becomes pathogenic under certain circumstances. 2. denoting a disease or infection caused by such an organism.

opsin (op′sin) a protein of the retinal rods (scotopsin) and cones (photopsin) that combines with 11-*cis*-retinal to form visual pigments.

opsinogen (op-sin′ah-jen) a substance (antigen) capable of inducing the formation of opsonins. **opsinog′enous,** adj.

opsiuria (op″se-u′re-ah) excretion of urine more rapidly during fasting than after a meal.

opsoclonia, opsoclonus (op″sah-clo′ne-ah; -clo′nus) involuntary, nonrhythmic horizontal and vertical oscillations of the eyes.

opsonin (op′son-in) an antibody which renders bacteria and other cells susceptible to phagocytosis. **opson′ic,** adj. **immune o.,** an antibody which sensitizes a particulate antigen to phagocytosis, after combination with the homologous antigen *in vivo* or *in vitro.*

opsonization (op″son-i-za′shin) the rendering of bacteria and other cells subject to phagocytosis.

opsonocytophagic (op″son-o-sīt″o-faj′ik) denoting the phagocytic activity of blood in the presence of serum opsonins and homologous leukocytes.

opsonometry (op″son-om′ĭ-tre) measurement of the opsonic index.

optesthesia (op″tes-the′ze-ah) visual sensibility; ability to perceive visual stimuli.

optic (op′tik) of or pertaining to the eye.

optical (op′tik′l) pertaining to vision.

optician (op-tish′in) a specialist in opticianry.

opticianry (op-tish′in-re) the translation, filling, and adapting of ophthalmic prescriptions, products, and accessories.

opticochiasmatic (op″tĭ-ko-ki″az-mat′ik) pertaining to the optic nerves and chiasma.

opticociliary (op″tĭ-ko-sil′e-ĕ″re) pertaining to the optic and ciliary nerves.

opticopupillary (-pu′pil-ĕ″re) pertaining to the optic nerve and pupil.

optics (op′tiks) the science of light and vision.

opto- word element [Gr.], *visible; vision; sight.*

optogram (op′tah-gram) the retinal image formed by the bleaching of visual purple under the influence of light.

optokinetic (op″to-ki-net′ik) pertaining to movement of the eyes, as in nystagmus.

optometer (op-tom′it-er) a device for measuring the power and range of vision.

optometrist (op-tom′ĭ-trist) a specialist in optometry.

optometry (op-tom′ĭ-tre) the professional practice of primary eye and vision care for the diagnosis, treatment, and prevention of associated disorders and for the improvement of vision by the prescription of spectacles and by use of other functional, optical, and pharmaceutical means regulated by state law.

optomyometer (op″to-mi-om′it-er) a device for measuring the power of ocular muscles.

OPV poliovirus vaccine live oral.

O.R. operating room.

ora[1] (o′rah), pl. *o′rae* [L.] an edge or margin. **o. serra′ta re′tinae,** the zigzag margin of the retina of the eye.

ora[2] (o′rah) [L.] plural of *os,* mouth.

orad (o′rad) toward the mouth.

oral (o′ril) pertaining to the mouth, taken through or applied in the mouth, as an oral medication or an oral thermometer. 2. denoting that aspect of the teeth which faces the oral cavity or tongue.

orality (o-ral′it-e) a term embracing all of the aspects and components (sucking, mouthing, etc.) of the oral stage of psychosexual development.

orange (or′inj) 1. the tree, *Citrus aurantium,* and its edible yellow fruit; the peel of two varieties is used in making various pharmaceuticals. 2. a color between yellow and red. **Agent O.,** see under *agent.*

orbicular (or-bik′ūl-er) circular; rounded.

orbiculare (or-bik″u-la′re) a small oval knob on the long limb of the incus, articulating with or ossified to the head of the stapes.

orbiculus (or-bik′ūl-us), pl. *orbic′uli* [L.] a small disk.

orbit (or′bit) the bony cavity containing the eyeball and its associated muscles, vessels, and nerves. **or′bital,** adj.

orbita (or′bit-ah), pl. *or′bitae* [L.] orbit.

orbitale (or″bĭ-ta′le) the lowest point on the inferior edge of the orbit.

orbitalis (or″bĭ-ta′lis) [L.] pertaining to the orbit.

orbitonasal (or″bit-o-na′zil) pertaining to the orbit and nose.

orbitonometer (-nom′it-er) an instrument for measuring backward displacement of the eyeball produced by a given pressure on its anterior aspect.

orbitotomy (or″bĭ-tot′ah-me) incision into the orbit.

orbivirus (or′bĭ-vi″rus) a group of RNA viruses, a subgroup of the diplornavirus.

orcein (or-se′in) a brownish-red coloring substance obtained from orcinol; used as a stain for elastic tissue.

orchi(o)- word element [Gr.], *testis.*

orchialgia (or″ke-al′je-ah) pain in a testis.

orchidectomy (or″kĭ-dek′tah-me) orchiectomy.

orchidic (or-kid′ik) pertaining to a testis.

orchidorrhaphy (or″kĭ-dor′ah-fe) orchiopexy.

orchiectomy (or″ke-ek′tah-me) excision of one or both testes.

orchiepididymitis (-ep″ĭ-did″ĭ-mi′tis) inflammation of the testis and epididymis.

orchiocele (or′ke-o-sēl) 1. hernial protrusion of a testis. 2. scrotal hernia. 3. tumor of a testis.

orchiomyeloma (or″ke-o-mi″ĕ-lo′mah) plasmacytoma of the testis.

orchiopathy (or″ke-op′ah-the) any disease of the testis.

orchiopexy (or′ke-o-pek″se) fixation of an undescended testis in the scrotum.

orchioplasty (-plas″te) plastic surgery of a testis.

orchioscheocele (or″ke-os′ke-o-sēl″) scrotal tumor with scrotal hernia.

orchiotomy (or″kĭ-ot′ah-me) incision and drainage of a testis.

orchitis (or-kit′is) inflammation of a testis. **orchit′ic,** adj.

order (or′der) a taxonomic category subordinate to a class and superior to a family (or suborder).

orderly (or′der-le) a male hospital attendant who does general work, attending especially to needs of male patients.

ordinate (or′d′n-it) the vertical line in a graph along which is plotted one of two sets of factors considered in the study.

orexigenic (or-ek″sĭ-jen′ik) increasing or stimulating the appetite.

orf (orf) 1. a contagious pustular viral dermatitis of sheep, communicable to man. 2. sheep-pox.

organ (or′gin) a somewhat independent body part that performs a special function. **o. of Corti,** the organ lying against the basilar membrane in the cochlear duct, containing special sensory receptors for hearing, and consisting of neuroepithelial hair cells and several types of supporting cells. **effector o.,** a muscle or gland that contracts or secretes, respectively, in direct response to nerve impulses. **end o.,** end-organ. **enamel o.,** a process of epithelium forming a cap over a dental papilla and developing into the enamel. **genital o's,** reproductive o's. **Golgi**

tendon o., any of the mechanoreceptors arranged in series with muscle in the tendons of mammalian muscles, being the receptor for stimuli responsible for the lengthening reaction. **Jacobson's o.,** vomeronasal o. **sense o's, sensory o's,** organs that receive stimuli that give rise to sensations, i.e., organs that translate certain forms of energy into nerve impulses which are perceived as special sensations. **spiral o.,** o. of Corti. **vestigial o.,** an undeveloped organ that, in the embryo or in some ancestor, was well developed and functional. **vomeronasal o.,** a small sac just above the vomeronasal cartilage; rudimentary in adult man but well developed in many lower animals. **Weber's o.,** prostatic utriculus. **o's of Zuckerkandl,** paraaortic bodies.

organelle (or″gah-nel′) a specialized structure of a cell, such as a mitochondrion, Golgi complex, lysosome, endoplasmic reticulum, ribosome, centriole, chloroplast, cilium, or flagellum.

organic (or-gan′ik) 1. pertaining to an organ or organs. 2. having an organized structure. 3. arising from an organism. 4. pertaining to substances derived from living organisms. 5. denoting chemical substances containing carbon. 6. pertaining to or cultivated by use of animal or vegetable fertilizers, rather than synthetic chemicals.

organism (or′gin-izm) an individual living thing, whether animal or plant.

organization (or″gin-ĭ-za′shin) the replacement of blood clots by fibrous tissue. **health maintenance o.,** see under *H.*

organize (or′gin-īz) to provide with an organic structure; to form into organs.

organizer (or′gin-īz″er) a special region of the embryo which is capable of determining the differentiation of other regions. **primary o.,** the dorsal lip region of the blastopore.

organo- word element [Gr.], *organ.*

organogenesis, organogeny (or″gin-o-jen′ĭ-sis; or″gin-oj′ĭ-ne) the origin or development of organs.

organoid (or′gin-oid) 1. resembling an organ. 2. a structure that resembles an organ.

organomegaly (or″gin-o-meg′il-e) enlargement of the viscera; visceromegaly.

organomercurial (-mer-kūr′e-il) any mercury-containing organic compound.

organometallic (-mĭ-tal′ik) consisting of a metal combined with an organic radical.

organon (or′gah-non) pl. *or′gana* [Gr.] organ.

organophosphate (or″gin-o-fos′fāt) an organic ester of phosphoric or thiophosphoric acid; such compounds are powerful acetylcholinesterase inhibitors and are used as insecticides and nerve gases. **organophos′phorous,** adj.

organotrophic (-trof′ik) 1. relating to the nutrition of organs of the body. 2. deriving energy from the oxidation of organic compounds; said of bacteria.

organotropism (or-gin-ah′trah-pizm) the special affinity of chemical compounds or pathogenic agents for particular tissues or organs of the body. **organotrop′ic,** adj.

organ-specific (or′gin-spah-sif′ik) restricted to, or having an effect only on, a particular organ, as an organ-specific antigen.

organum (or′gah-num), pl. *or′gana* [L.] organ.

orgasm (or′gazm) the apex and culmination of sexual excitement.

orientation (or″e-en-ta′shin) the recognition of one's position in relation to time and space.

orifice (or′ĭ-fis) 1. the entrance or outlet of any body cavity. 2. any foramen, meatus, or opening. **orific′ial,** adj. **cardiac o.,** see under *opening.*

orificium (or″i-fish′e-um), pl. *orifi′cia* [L.] orifice.

origin (or′ĭ-jin) [L.] the source or beginning of anything, especially the more fixed end or attachment of a muscle (as distinguished from its insertion), or the site of emergence of a peripheral nerve from the central nervous system.

Orinase (or′ĭ-nās) trademark for a preparation of tolbutamide.

ornithine (or′nĭ-thēn) an amino acid obtained from arginine by splitting of urea; it is an intermediate in urea biosynthesis.

Ornithodoros (or″nĭ-thod′ah-ris) a genus of soft-bodied ticks, many species of which are reservoirs and vectors of the spirochetes (*Borrelia*) of relapsing fevers.

ornithosis (or″nĭ-tho′sis) a disease of birds and domestic fowl, transmissible to man, caused by a strain of *Chlamydia psittaci;* in man and psittacine birds, it is known as *psittacosis.*

orolingual (o″ro-ling′gwil) pertaining to the mouth and tongue.

oronasal (-na′zil) pertaining to the mouth and nose.

oropharynx (-phar′inks) the part of the pharynx between the soft palate and the upper edge of the epiglottis.

orphenadrine (or-fen′ah-drēn) a drug, $C_{18}H_{23}$-NO, having antihistaminic, antitremor, and antispasmodic activities; its citrate and hydrochloride salts are used as skeletal muscle relaxants.

orth(o)- word element [Gr.], *straight; normal; correct.* In chemistry, *ortho-* indicates an isomer; also, a cyclic derivative having two substitutes in adjacent positions.

orthochorea (or″tho-ko-re′ah) choreic movements in the erect posture.

orthochromatic (-kro-mat′ik) staining normally.

orthodeoxia (-de-ok′se-ah) accentuation of arterial hypoxemia in the erect position.

orthodontics (-don′tiks) that branch of dentistry concerned with irregularities of teeth and malocclusion, and associated facial abnormalities. **orthodon′tic,** adj.

orthodontist (-don′tist) a dentist who specializes in orthodontics.

orthodromic (-drom′ik) conducting impulses in the normal direction; said of nerve fibers.

orthograde (or′tho-grād) walking with the body upright.

orthometer (or-thom′it-er) instrument for determining relative protrusion of the eyeballs.

orthomolecular (or″tho-mol-ek′ūl-er) pertaining to the theory that certain diseases are associated with biochemical abnormalities resulting in increased needs for certain nutrients, e.g., vitamins, and can be treated by administration of large doses of these substances.

orthomyxovirus (-mik″so-vi′rus) a subgroup of myxoviruses that includes the viruses of human and animal influenza.

orthopedic (-pe′dik) pertaining to the correction of deformities of the musculoskeletal system; pertaining to orthopedics.

orthopedics (-pe′diks) that branch of surgery dealing with the preservation and restoration of the function of the skeletal system, its articulations, and associated structures.

orthopedist (-pe′dist) an orthopedic surgeon.

orthopercussion (-per-kush′in) percussion with the distal phalanx of the finger held perpendicularly to the body wall.

orthophoria (-for′e-ah) normal equilibrium of the eye muscles, or muscular balance. **orthophor′ic**, adj.

orthophosphoric acid (or″thah-fos-for′ik) phosphoric acid.

orthopnea (or″thop-ne′ah) difficult breathing except in the upright position. **orthopne′ic**, adj.

orthopraxis, orthopraxy (or″thah-prak′sis; -prak′se) mechanical correction of deformities.

orthoptic (or-thop′tik) correcting obliquity of one or both visual axes.

orthoptics (or-thop′tiks) treatment of strabismus by exercise of the ocular muscles.

orthoscope (or′thah-skōp) an apparatus which neutralizes corneal refraction by means of a layer of water.

orthoscopic (or″thah-skop′ik) 1. affording a correct and undistorted view. 2. pertaining to orthoscopy.

orthosis (or-tho′sis), pl. **ortho′ses**. An orthopedic appliance or apparatus used to support, align, prevent, or correct deformities or to improve function of movable parts of the body.

orthostatic (or-thah-stat′ik) pertaining to or caused by standing erect.

orthostatism (or-thah-stat′izm) an erect standing position of the body.

orthotic (or-thot′ik) serving to protect or to restore or improve function; pertaining to the use or application of an orthosis.

orthotics (or-thot′iks) the field of knowledge relating to orthoses and their use.

orthotist (or′thot-ist) a person skilled in orthotics, and practicing its application in individual cases.

orthotonos, orthotonus (or-thot′ah-nus) tetanic spasm which fixes the head, body, and limbs in a rigid straight line.

orthotopic (or″thah-top′ik) occurring at the normal place.

O.S. [L.] *o'culus sinis'ter* (left eye).

Os chemical symbol, *osmium.*

os[1] (os), pl. *o'ra* [L.] 1. any body orifice. 2. the mouth.

os[2] (os), pl. *os'sa* [L.] bone; see *Table of Bones.*

osche(o)- word element [Gr.], *scrotum.*

oscheitis (os″ke-īt′is) inflammation of the scrotum.

oscheoma (os″ke-o′mah) tumor of the scrotum.

oscheoplasty (os′ke-o-plas″te) plastic surgery of the scrotum.

oscillation (os″ĭ-la′shin) a backward and forward motion, like that of a pendulum; also vibration, fluctuation, or variation.

oscillo- word element [L.], *oscillation.*

oscillometer (os″ĭ-lom′it-er) an instrument for measuring oscillations.

oscillopsia (os″ĭ-lop′se-ah) a visual sensation that stationary objects are swaying back and forth.

oscilloscope (ŏ-sil′ah-skōp) an instrument that displays a visual representation of electrical variations on the fluorescent screen of a cathode-ray tube.

osculum (os′kūl-um) [L.] a small aperture or minute opening.

-ose a suffix indicating that the substance is a carbohydrate.

-osis word element [Gr.], *disease; morbid state; abnormal increase.*

osm(o)- word element [Gr.], (1) *odor; smell* (2) *impulse; osmosis.*

osmate (oz′māt) a salt of osmic acid.

osmatic (oz-mat′ik) pertaining to the sense of smell.

osmic acid (oz′mik) osmium tetroxide.

osmics (oz′miks) the science dealing with the sense of smell.

osmium (oz′me-um) chemical element (*see table*), at. no. 76, symbol Os. **o. tetroxide**, a fixative used in preparing histologic specimens, OsO_4.

osmolality (oz″mo-lal′it-e) the concentration of a solution in terms of osmoles of solutes per kilogram of solvent.

osmolar (oz-mōl′er) pertaining to the concentration of osmotically active particles in solution.

osmolarity (oz″mo-lar′it-e) the concentration of a solution in terms of osmoles of solutes per liter of solution.

osmole (oz′mol) a unit of osmotic pressure equivalent to the amount of solute substances that dissociates in solution to form one mole (Avogadro's number) of particles (molecules and ions). Abbreviated Osm.

osmometer (oz-mom′it-er) 1. a device for testing the sense of smell. 2. an instrument for measuring osmotic pressure.

osmophilic (oz″mah-fil′ik) having an affinity for solutions of high osmotic pressure.

osmophore (oz″mah-fōr) the group of atoms responsible for the odor of a compound.

osmoreceptor (oz″mo-re-sep′ter) 1. any of a group of specialized neurons in the supraoptic nuclei of the hypothalamus that are stimulated by increased osmolality (chiefly, increased sodium concentration) of the extracellular fluid; their excitation promotes the release of antidiuretic hormone by the posterior pituitary. 2. a specialized sensory nerve ending sensitive to stimulation giving rise to the sensation of odors.

osmoregulation (-reg″ūl-a′shin) adjustment of

internal osmotic pressure of a simple organism or body cell in relation to that of the surrounding medium. **osmoreg′ulatory,** adj.

osmosis (oz-mo′sis, os-mo′sis) [Gr.] the passage of pure solvent from a solution of lesser to one of greater solute concentration when the two solutions are separated by a membrane which selectively prevents the passage of solute molecules, but is permeable to the solvent. **osmot′ic,** adj.

osmostat (oz′mo-stat″) the regulatory centers that control the osmolality of the extracellular fluid.

osphresiology (os-fre″ze-ol′ah-je) the science of odors and the sense of smell.

osphresiometer (os-fre″ze-om′it-er) an instrument for measuring acuteness of the sense of smell.

osphresis (os-fre′sis) the sense of smell. **osphret′ic,** adj.

ossein (os′e-in) the collagen of bone.

osseocartilaginous (os″e-o-kart″il-aj′ĭ-nus) composed of bone and cartilage.

osseofibrous (-fi′brus) made up of fibrous tissue and bone.

osseomucin (-mu′sin) the ground substance that binds together the collagen and elastic fibrils of bone.

osseous (os′e-us) of the nature or quality of bone; bony.

ossicle (os′ĭ-k'l) a small bone, especially one of those in the middle ear. **ossic′ular,** adj. **Andernach's o's,** sutural bones. **auditory o's,** the small bones of the middle ear: incus, malleus, and stapes. See Plate XII.

ossiculectomy (os″ĭ-kūl-ek′tah-me) excision of one or more ossicles of the middle ear.

ossiculotomy (os″ĭ-kūl-ot′ah-me) incision of the auditory ossicles.

ossiculum (ŏ-sik′ūl-um), pl. *ossic′ula* [L.] ossicle.

ossiferous (ŏ-sif′er-us) producing bone.

ossific (ŏ-sif′ik) forming or becoming bone.

ossification (os″ĭ-fĭ-ka′shin) formation of or conversion into bone or a bony substance. **ectopic o.,** a pathological condition in which bone arises in tissues not in the osseous system and in connective tissues usually not manifesting osteogenic properties. **endochondral o.,** ossification which occurs in and replaces cartilage. **intramembranous o.,** ossification that occurs in and replaces connective tissue.

ossify (os′ĭ-fi) to change or develop into bone.

oste(o)- word element [Gr.], *bone.*

ostealgia (os″te-al′je-ah) pain in the bones.

ostearthrotomy (-ar-throt′ah-me) excision of an articular end of a bone.

ostectomy (os-tek′tah-me) excision of a bone or part of a bone.

osteectopia (os″te-ek-to′pe-ah) displacement of a bone.

osteitis (os″te-īt′is) inflammation of bone. **condensing o.,** osteitis with hard deposits of earthy salts in affected bone. **o. defor′mans,** rarefying osteitis resulting in weakened deformed bones of increased mass, which may lead to bowing of long bones and deformation of flat bones; when the bones of the skull are affected, deafness may result. **o. fibro′sa cys′tica, o. fibro′sa cys′tica generalisa′ta, o. fibro′sa osteoplas′tica,** rarefying osteitis with fibrous degeneration and formation of cysts and with the presence of fibrous nodules on the affected bones, due to marked osteoclastic activity secondary to hyperparathyroidism. **o. frag′ilitans,** osteogenesis imperfecta. **o. fungo′sa,** chronic osteitis in which the haversian canals are dilated and filled with granulation tissue. **parathyroid o.,** o. fibrosa cystica. **sclerosing o.,** 1. sclerosing nonsuppurative osteomyelitis. 2. condensing o.

ostempyesis (ost″em-pi-e′sis) suppuration within a bone.

osteoanagenesis (os″te-o-an′ah-jen″ĭ-sis) regeneration of bone.

osteoarthritis (-ar-thrīt′is) noninflammatory degenerative joint disease marked by degeneration of the articular cartilage, hypertrophy of bone at the margins, and changes in the synovial membrane, accompanied by pain and stiffness.

osteoarthropathy (-ar-throp′ah-the) any disease of the joints and bones. **hypertrophic pulmonary o., secondary hypertrophic o.,** symmetrical osteitis of the four limbs, chiefly localized to the phalanges and terminal epiphyses of the long bones of the forearm and leg; it is often secondary to chronic lung and heart conditions.

osteoarthrosis (-ar-thro′sis) chronic noninflammatory bone disease.

osteoarthrotomy (-ar-throt′ah-me) ostearthrotomy.

osteoblast (os′te-o-blast″) a cell arising from a fibroblast, which, as it matures, is associated with bone production.

osteoblastoma (os″te-o-blas-to′mah) a benign, painful, rather vascular tumor of bone marked by formation of osteoid tissue and primitive bone.

osteocampsia (-kamp′se-ah) curvature of a bone.

osteochondral (-kon′dril) pertaining to bone and cartilage.

osteochondritis (-kon-drīt′is) inflammation of bone and cartilage. **o. defor′mans juveni′lis,** osteochondrosis of the capitular epiphysis of the femur. **o. defor′mans juveni′lis dor′si,** osteochondrosis of vertebrae. **o. dis′secans,** that resulting in splitting of pieces of cartilage into the affected joint.

osteochondrodysplasia (-kon″dro-dis-pla′ze-ah) any disorder of cartilage and bone growth.

osteochondrodystrophy (-kon″dro-dis′trah-fe) Morquio's syndrome.

osteochondrolysis (-kon-drol′ĭ-sis) osteochondritis dissecans.

osteochondroma (-kon-dro′mah) a benign bone tumor consisting of projecting adult bone capped by cartilage.

osteochondromatosis (-kon″dro-mah-to′sis) occurrence of multiple osteochondromas.

osteochondrosis (-kon-dro′sis) a disease of the growth ossification centers in children, beginning as a degeneration or necrosis followed by regeneration or recalcification; known by various names, depending on the bone involved.

osteoclasis (os″te-ok′lah-sis) surgical fracture or refracture of bones.

osteoclast (os′te-ah-klast″) 1. a large multinuclear cell associated with absorption and removal of bone. 2. an instrument used for osteoclasis. **osteoclas′tic,** adj.

osteoclastoma (os″te-o-klas-to′mah) giant cell tumor of bone.

osteocope (os′te-ah-kōp″) severe pain in a bone. **osteocop′ic,** adj.

osteocranium (os″te-o-kra′ne-um) the fetal skull during the period of ossification.

osteocystoma (-sis-to′mah) a bone cyst.

osteocyte (os′te-ah-sīt″) an osteoblast that has become embedded within the bone matrix, occupying a bone lacuna and sending, through the canaliculi, slender cytoplasmic processes that make contact with processes of other osteocytes.

osteodiastasis (-di-as′tah-sis) the separation of two adjacent bones.

osteodynia (-din′e-ah) ostealgia.

osteodystrophy (-dis′trah-fe) abnormal development of bone. **renal o.,** a condition due to chronic kidney disease, marked by impaired kidney function, elevated serum phosphorus levels, and low or normal serum calcium levels, and by stimulation of parathyroid function, resulting in a variable admixture of bone disease.

osteoepiphysis (-e-pif′ĭ-sis) any bony epiphysis.

osteofibroma (-fi-bro′mah) osteoma blended with fibroma.

osteogen (os′te-ah-jen″) the substance composing the inner layer of the periosteum, from which bone is formed.

osteogenesis (os″te-ah-jen′ĭ-sis) the formation of bone; the development of the bones. **o. imperfec′ta,** several types of collagen disorder, of variable inheritance, due to defective biosynthesis of type I collagen and characterized by brittle, osteoporotic, easily fractured bones; other defects are blue sclerae, wormian bones, and dentinogenesis imperfecta.

osteogenic (-jen′ik) derived from or composed of any tissue concerned in bone growth or repair.

osteohalisteresis (os″te-o-hah-lis″ter-e′sis) deficiency in mineral elements of bone.

osteoid (os′te-oid) 1. resembling bone. 2. the organic matrix of bone; young bone that has not undergone calcification.

osteolipochondroma (os″te-o-lip″o-kon-dro′mah) osteochondroma with fatty elements.

osteology (os″te-ol′ah-je) scientific study of the bones.

osteolysis (os″te-ol′ĭ-sis) dissolution of bone; applied especially to the removal or loss of the calcium of bone. **osteolyt′ic,** adj.

osteoma (os″te-o′mah) a tumor composed of bony tissue; a hard tumor of bonelike structure developing on a bone (*homoplastic o.*) and sometimes on other structures (*heteroplastic o.*). **o. cu′tis,** a condition in which bone-containing nodules form in the skin. **o. du′rum, o. ebur′-neum,** one containing hard bony tissue. **o.**

medulla′re, one containing marrow spaces. **osteoid o.,** a small, benign but painful, circumscribed tumor of spongy bone, occurring especially in the bones of the extremities and vertebrae, most often in young persons. **o. spongi-o′sum,** one containing cancelled bone.

osteomalacia (os″te-o-mah-la′she-ah) softening of the bones (due to impaired mineralization, with excess accumulation of osteoid), resulting from vitamin D deficiency. **osteomala′cic,** adj. **hepatic o.,** osteomalacia as a complication of cholestatic liver disease, which may lead to severe bone pain and multiple fractures. **infantile o., juvenile o.,** late rickets.

osteomere (os′te-o-mēr″) one of a series of similar bony structures, such as the vertebrae.

osteometry (os″te-om′ĭ-tre) measurement of the bones.

osteomyelitis (os″te-o-mi″il-īt′is) inflammation of bone, localized or generalized, due to pyogenic infection. **osteomyelit′ic,** adj. **Garré's o., sclerosing nonsuppurative o.,** a chronic form involving the long bones, especially the tibia and femur, marked by a diffuse inflammatory reaction, increased density and spindle-shaped sclerotic thickening of the cortex, and an absence of suppuration.

osteomyelodysplasia (-mi″il-o-dis-pla′ze-ah) a condition characterized by thinning of the osseous tissue of bones and increase in size of the marrow cavities, attended with leukopenia and fever.

osteomyxochondroma (-mik″so-kon-dro′mah) osteochondromyxoma.

osteon (os′te-on) the basic unit of structure of compact bone, comprising a haversian canal and its concentrically arranged lamellae.

osteonecrosis (os″te-o-nĕ-kro′sis) necrosis of a bone.

osteoneuralgia (-nōōr-al′je-ah) neuralgia of a bone.

osteopath (os′te-ah-path″) a practitioner of osteopathy.

osteopathia (os″te-ah-path′e-ah) osteopathy (1). **o. conden′sans dissemina′ta,** osteopoikilosis. **o. stria′ta,** an asymptomatic condition characterized radiographically by multiple condensations of cancellous bone tissue, giving a striated appearance.

osteopathy (os″te-op′ah-the) 1. any disease of a bone. 2. a system of therapy based on the theory that the body is capable of making its own remedies against disease and other toxic conditions when it is in normal structural relationship and has favorable environmental conditions and adequate nutrition; it utilizes generally accepted physical methods of diagnosis and therapy, while emphasizing the importance of normal body mechanics and manipulative methods of detecting and correcting faulty structure. **osteopath′ic,** adj.

osteopenia (os″te-o-pe′ne-ah) 1. reduced bone mass due to a decrease in the rate of osteoid synthesis to a level insufficient to compensate normal bone lysis. 2. any decrease in bone mass below the normal. **osteopen′ic,** adj.

osteoperiosteal (-per″e-os′te-il) pertaining to bone and its periosteum.

osteoperiostitis (-per″e-os-tīt′is) inflammation of a bone and its periosteum.

osteopetrosis (-pĭ-tro′sis) a hereditary disease marked by abnormally dense bone, and by the common occurrence of fractures of affected bone.

osteophlebitis (os″te-o-fleb-īt′is) inflammation of the veins of a bone.

osteophyma, osteophyte (os″te-ah-fi′mah; os′te-ah-fit″) a bony excrescence or outgrowth.

osteoplasty (os′te-ah-plas″te) plastic surgery of the bones.

osteopoikilosis (os″te-o-poi″kĭ-lo′sis) a mottled condition of bones, apparent radiographically, due to the presence of multiple sclerotic foci and scattered stippling. **osteopoikilot′ic,** adj.

osteoporosis (-por-o′sis) abnormal rarefaction of bone; it may be idiopathic or occur secondary to other diseases. **osteoporot′ic,** adj.

osteoradionecrosis (-ra″de-o-nĕ-kro′sis) necrosis of bone as a result of exposure to radiation.

osteorrhagia (-ra″je-ah) hemorrhage from bone.

osteorrhaphy (os″te-or′ah-fe) fixation of fragments of bone with sutures or wires.

osteosarcoma (os″te-o-sar-ko′mah) osteogenic sarcoma. **osteosarco′matous,** adj.

osteosclerosis (-sklĭ-ro′sis) the hardening or abnormal density of bone. **osteosclerot′ic,** adj. **o. conge′nita,** achondroplasia. **o. fra′gilis,** osteopetrosis. **o. fra′gilis generalisa′ta,** osteopetrosis.

osteosis (os″te-o′sis) the formation of bony tissue. **o. cu′tis,** osteoma cutis.

osteosuture (os″te-o-soo′cher) osteorrhaphy.

osteosynovitis (-sin″ah-vīt′is) synovitis with osteitis of neighboring bones.

osteosynthesis (-sin″this-is) surgical fastening of the ends of a fractured bone.

osteotabes (-ta′bēz) a disease, chiefly of infants, in which bone marrow cells are destroyed and the marrow disappears.

osteothrombosis (-throm-bo′sis) thrombosis of the veins of a bone.

osteotome (os′te-ah-tōm″) a chisel-like knife for cutting bone.

osteotomy (os″te-ot′ah-me) incision or transection of a bone. **cuneiform o.,** removal of a wedge of bone. **displacement o.,** surgical division of a bone and shifting of the divided ends to change the alignment of the bone or to alter weight-bearing stresses. **linear o.,** the sawing or linear cutting of a bone.

ostitis (os-tīt′is) osteitis.

ostium (os′te-um), pl. **os′tia** [L.] a mouth or orifice. **os′tial,** adj. **o. abdomina′le,** the fimbriated end of an oviduct. **coronary o.,** either of the two openings in the aortic sinus which mark the origin of the (left and right) coronary arteries. **o. inter′num,** o. uterinum tubae. **o. pharyn′geum,** the pharyngeal opening of the auditory tube. **o. pri′mum,** an opening in the lower portion of the membrane dividing the embryonic heart into right and left sides. **o. secun′dum,** an opening high in the septum of the embryonic heart, approximately where the foramen ovale will later appear. **tympanic o., o. tympan′icum,** the opening of the auditory tube on the carotid wall of the tympanic cavity. **o. u′teri,** the external opening of the uterine cervix into the vagina. **o. uteri′num tu′bae,** the point where the cavity of the uterine tube becomes continuous with that of the uterus. **o. vagi′nae,** external orifice of the vagina.

ostomate (os′tah-māt) one who has undergone enterostomy or ureterostomy.

ostomy (os′tah-me) general term for an operation in which an artificial opening is formed, as in colostomy, ureterostomy, etc.

OT *old term* in anatomy; old tuberculin.

ot(o)- word element [Gr.], *ear.*

otalgia (o-tal′je-ah) pain in the ear; earache.

OTC over the counter; said of drugs not required by law to be sold on prescription only.

otic (ōt′ik) pertaining to the ear; aural.

otitis (o-tīt′is) inflammation of the ear. **otit′ic,** adj. **aviation o.,** barotitis media. **o. exter′na,** inflammation of the external ear. **furuncular o.,** formation of furuncles in the external meatus. **o. inter′na, o. labyrin′thica,** labyrinthitis. **o. mastoi′dea,** inflammation of the mastoid spaces. **o me′dia,** inflammation of the middle ear. **o. me′dia, secretory,** a painless accumulation of mucoid or serous fluid in the middle ear, due to obstruction of the eustachian tube and causing conduction deafness. **o. myco′tica,** that due to parasitic fungi. **o. parasi′tica,** otoacariasis. **o. sclero′tica,** otitis marked by hardening of the ear structures.

otoacariasis (ōt″o-ak″ah-ri′ah-sis) infection of the ears of cats, dogs, and domestic rabbits with mites of the genus *Otodectes.*

otoantritis (-an-trīt′is) inflammation of the attic of the tympanum and the mastoid antrum.

Otobius (o-to′be-us) a genus of soft-bodied ticks parasitic in the ears of various animals and known also to infest man.

otocephaly (-sef′ah-le) a congenital malformation characterized by lack of a lower jaw and by ears that are united below the face.

otocranium (-kra′ne-um) 1. the chamber in the petrous bone lodging the internal ear. 2. the auditory portion of the cranium. **otocra′nial,** adj.

otocyst (ōt′ah-sist) 1. the auditory vesicle of the embryo. 2. the auditory sac of some lower animals.

Otodectes (ōt″ah-dek′tēz) a genus of mites; see also *otoacariasis.*

otoencephalitis (-en-sef″ah-lit′is) inflammation of the brain due to extension from an inflamed middle ear.

otoganglion (-gang′gle-on) the otic ganglion.

otogenic, otogenous (ōt″ah-jen′ik; o-toj′i-nus) originating within the ear.

otolaryngology (ōt″o-lar″in-gol′ah-je) that branch of medicine dealing with disease of the ear, nose, and throat.

otolith (ōt′ah-lith) 1. see *statoconia.* 2. a calcareous mass in the inner ear of vertebrates or in the otocyst of invertebrates.

otology (o-tol′ah-je) the branch of medicine dealing with the ear, its anatomy, physiology, and pathology. **otolog′ic,** adj.

otomucormycosis (ōt″o-mu″kor-mi-ko′sis) mucormycosis of the ear.

otomycosis (-mi-ko′sis) fungal infection of the external auditory meatus and ear canal.

otoneurology (-nōōr-ol′ah-je) that branch of otology dealing especially with those portions of the nervous system related to the ear. **otoneurolog′ic,** adj.

otopathy (o-top′ah-the) any disease of the ear.

otopharyngeal (ōt″o-fah-rin′je-il) pertaining to the ear and pharynx.

otoplasty (ōt′ah-plas″te) plastic surgery of the ear.

otopolypus (ōt″o-pol′ĭ-pus) polyp in the ear.

otopyorrhea (-pi″or-e′ah) a copious purulent discharge from the ear.

otopyosis (-pi-o′sis) suppurative disease of the ear.

otorhinolaryngology (-ri″no-lar″in-gol′ah-je) the branch of medicine dealing with the ear, nose, and throat.

otorhinology (-ri-nol′ah-je) the branch of medicine dealing with the ear and nose.

otorrhagia (-ra′je-ah) hemorrhage from the ear.

otorrhea (-re′ah) a discharge from the ear.

otosalpinx (ōt″o-sal′pinks) the auditory tube.

otosclerosis (-sklĭ-ro′sis) a condition in which otospongiosis may cause bony ankylosis of the stapes, resulting in conductive hearing loss. **otosclerot′ic,** adj.

otoscope (ōt′ah-skōp) an instrument for inspecting or auscultating the ear.

otospongiosis (ōt″o-spon″je-o′sis) the formation of spongy bone in the bony labyrinth of the ear.

otosteal (o-tos′te-il) pertaining to the ossicles of the ear.

ototoxic (ōt″o-tok′sik) having a deleterious effect upon the eighth nerve or on the organs of hearing and balance.

O.U. [L.] *oculus uterque* (each eye).

ouabain (wah-ba′in) a cardiac glycoside, $C_{29}H_{44}O_{12}$, from *Strophanthus gratus*, which has the same actions as digitalis but produces digitalization more rapidly.

ounce (owns) a measure of weight in both the avoirdupois ($\frac{1}{16}$ lb., 437.5 gr., 28.3495 gm.) and apothecaries ($\frac{1}{12}$ lb., 480 gr., 31.103 gm.) system; abbreviated oz. **fluid o.,** a unit of liquid measure of the apothecaries' system, being 8 fluid-drams, or the equivalent of 29.57 ml.

outbreeding (owt′brēd″ing) the mating of unrelated individuals, which often produces more vigorous offspring than the parents are in terms of growth, survival, and fertility.

outlet (owt′let) a means or route of exit or egress. **pelvic o.,** the inferior opening of the pelvis.

outpatient (owt′pa″shint) a patient who comes to the hospital, clinic, or dispensary for diagnosis and/or treatment but does not occupy a bed.

outpocketing (-pok″it-ing) evagination.

outpouching (owt′powch″ing) obtrusion of a layer or part to form a pouch; evagination.

output (-put) the yield or total of anything produced by any functional system of the body. **cardiac o.,** the effective volume of blood expelled by either ventricle of the heart per unit of time (usually volume per minute). **stroke o.,** the amount of blood ejected by each ventricle at each beat of the heart. **urinary o.,** the amount of urine excreted by the kidneys.

ova (o′vah) plural of *ovum*.

ovari(o)- word element [Gr.], *ovary*.

ovariectomy (o-vār″e-ek′tah-me) oophorectomy.

ovariocele (o-vār′e-o-sēl″) hernia of an ovary.

ovariocentesis (o-vār″e-o-sen-te′sis) surgical puncture of an ovary.

ovariopexy (-pek′se) the operation of elevating and fixing an ovary to the abdominal wall.

ovariorrhexis (-rek′sis) rupture of an ovary.

ovariosalpingectomy (-sal″pin-jek′tah-me) excision of an ovary and oviduct.

ovariostomy (o-vār″e-os′tah-me) oophorostomy.

ovariotomy (-ot′ah-me) surgical removal of an ovary, or removal of an ovarian tumor.

ovariotubal (o-vār″e-o-too′b'l) pertaining to an ovary and oviduct.

ovaritis (o″vah-rīt′is) oophoritis.

ovarium (o-vār′e-um), pl. *ova′ria* [L.] ovary.

ovary (o′vah-re) the female gonad: either of the paired female sexual glands in which ova are formed. **ova′rian,** adj. **polycystic o.,** one containing multiple, small follicular cysts filled with yellow or bloodstained, thin serous fluid; it may lead to Stein-Leventhal syndrome.

overbite (o′ver-bīt″) the extension of the upper incisor teeth over the lower ones vertically when the opposing posterior teeth are in contact.

overcompensation (o″ver-kom″pin-sa′shin) exaggerated correction of a real or imagined physical or psychologic defect.

overdenture (-den′cher) a complete denture supported both by mucosa and by a few remaining natural teeth that have been altered to permit the denture to fit over them.

overdetermination (-de-ter″min-a′shin) the unconscious mechanism through which every emotional reaction or symptom is the result of multiple factors.

overdose (o′ver-dōs″) 1. to administer an excessive dose. 2. an excessive dose.

overdosage (o″ver-do′sij) 1. the administration of an excessive dose. 2. the condition resulting from an excessive dose.

overhydration (-hi-dra′shin) a state of excess fluids in the body.

overjet (o′ver-jet) extension of the incisal or buccal cusp ridges of the upper teeth labially or buccally to the incisal margins and ridges of the lower teeth when the jaws are closed normally.

overlay (-la) a later component superimposed on a preexisting state or condition. **psychogenic o.,** an emotionally determined increment to a preexisting symptom or disability of organic or physically traumatic origin.

overventilation (o″ver-vent″il-a′shin) hyperventilation.

ovi-, ovo- word element [L.], *egg; ovum.*

ovicide (o′vĭ-sīd) an agent destructive to the ova of certain organisms.

oviduct (-dukt) a passage through which ova leave the maternal body or pass to an organ communicating with exterior of the body; see *uterine tube.* **ovidu′cal, oviduct′al,** adj.

oviferous (o-vif′er-is) producing ova.

oviform (o′vĭ-form) egg-shaped.

ovigenesis (o″vĭ-jen′is-is) oogenesis.

oviparous (o-vip′ah-rus) producing eggs in which the embryo develops outside the maternal body, as in birds.

ovipositor (-pos′it-er) a specialized organ by which many female insects deposit their eggs.

ovoplasm (o′vah-plazm) the cytoplasm of an unfertilized ovum.

ovotestis (o″vo-tes′tis) a gonad containing both testicular and ovarian tissue.

ovoviviparous (-vi-vip′ah-rus) bearing living young that hatch from eggs inside the maternal body, the embryo being nourished by food stored in the egg; said of lizards, etc.

ovular (o′vūl-er) pertaining to an ovule or an ovum.

ovulation (o″vūl-a′shin) the discharge of the ovum from the graafian follicle. **ov′ulatory,** adj.

ovule (o′vūl) 1. the ovum within a graafian follicle. 2. any small, egglike structure.

ovum (o′vum), pl. *o′va* [L.] an egg; the female reproductive or germ cell which, after fertilization, is capable of developing into a new member of the same species.

oxacillin (ok″sah-sil′in) a semisynthetic penicillin used as the sodium salt in infections due to penicillin-resistant, gram-positive organisms.

oxalate (ok′sil-āt) any salt of oxalic acid. **calcium o.,** a salt of oxalic acid which may be deposited in urinary calculi.

oxalemia (ok″sil-ēm′e-ah) excess of oxalates in the blood.

oxalic acid (ok-sal′ik) a dibasic acid, HOOC-COOH, occurring in various fruits and vegetables and as a metabolic product of ascorbic acid.

oxalism (ok′sil-izm) poisoning by oxalic acid or by an oxalate.

oxaloacetate (ok″sil-o-as′ĭ-tāt) a salt or ester of oxaloacetic acid.

oxaloacetic acid (ok″sah-lo-ah-sēt′ik) a metabolic intermediate in the tricarboxylic acid cycle, HOOCCOCH₂COOH, which is also a substrate of aspartate aminotransferase.

oxalosis (ok″sil-o′sis) generalized deposition of calcium oxalate, in renal and extrarenal tissues, as may occur in primary hyperoxaluria.

oxaluria (ok″sil-ūr′e-ah) hyperoxaluria.

oxandrolone (ok-san′drah-lōn) an androgenic steroidal lactone, $C_{19}H_{30}O_3$, used to accelerate anabolism and/or to arrest excessive catabolism.

oxazepam (oks-az′ah-pam) a benzodiazepine tranquilizer $C_{15}H_{11}ClN_2O_2$; used as an antianxiety agent and as an adjunct for acute withdrawal symptoms in chronic alcoholics.

oxethazaine (ok-seth′ah-zān) a topical anes-

thetic, $C_{28}H_{41}N_3O_3$, used orally to relieve gastric distress.

oxidant (ok′sĭ-dint) the electron acceptor in an oxidation-reduction (redox) reaction.

oxidase (ok′sĭ-dās) any of a class of enzymes that catalyze the reduction of molecular oxygen independently of hydrogen peroxide.

oxidation (ok″sĭ-da′shin) the act of oxidizing or state of being oxidized.

oxidation-reduction (-re-duk′shin) the chemical reaction whereby electrons are removed (oxidation) from atoms of the substance being oxidized and transferred to those being reduced (reduction).

oxide (ok′sīd) a compound of oxygen with an element or radical.

oxidize (ok′sĭ-dīz) to cause to combine with oxygen or to remove hydrogen.

oxidoreductase (ok″sĭ-do-re-duk′tās) a class of enzymes that catalyze the reversible transfer of electrons from one substance to another (oxidation-reduction, or redox reaction).

oxim, oxime (ok′sim) any of a series of compounds formed by action of hydroxylamine on an aldehyde or ketone.

oxolinic acid (ok″sah-lin′ik) a synthetic antibacterial, $C_{13}H_{11}NO_5$, used in the treatment of urinary tract infections due to susceptible gram-negative organisms.

5-oxoproline (ok″sah-pro′lēn) an acidic lactam of glutamic acid occurring at the N-terminus of several peptides and proteins.

5-oxoprolinuria (-pro″lin-ūr′e-ah) an inborn error of metabolism marked by abnormally increased levels of 5-oxoproline in the urine, metabolic acidosis, and an increase in the rate of hemolysis.

oxtriphylline (oks-trif′ĭ-lēn) a compound of choline and theophylline, $C_{12}H_{21}N_5O_3$; used chiefly as a bronchodilator.

oxy- word element [Gr.], *sharp; quick; sour; presence of oxygen in a compound.*

oxybenzone (ok″se-ben′zōn) a topical sunscreening agent, $C_{14}H_{12}O_3$.

oxybutynin (ok″se-būt′′nin) an anticholinergic, $C_{22}H_{31}NO_3$, having direct antispasmodic effect on smooth muscle; used in the treatment of uninhibited neurogenic bladder and reflex neurogenic bladder.

oxycephaly (-sef′ah-le) a condition in which the top of the skull is pointed or conical owing to premature closure of the coronal and lambdoid sutures. **oxycephal′ic,** adj.

oxychlorosene (ok″se-klor′ah-sēn) a stabilized organic complex of hypochlorous acid used as a topical antiseptic in the treatment of localized infections.

oxycodone (-ko′dōn) a semisynthetic narcotic analgesic, $C_{18}H_{21}NO$, derived from morphine.

oxygen (ok′sĭ-jin) chemical element (*see table*), at. no. 8, symbol O. It constitutes about 20% of atmospheric air; is the essential agent in the respiration of plants and animals; and, although noninflammable, is necessary to support combustion. **o. debt,** deficiency of oxygen occurring in violent exercise. **hyperbaric o.,**

oxygen under greater than atmospheric pressure.

oxygenase (-jĭ-nās″) any oxidoreductase that catalyzes the incorporation of both atoms of molecular oxygen into the substrate.

oxygenate (-jĭ-nāt) to saturate with oxygen.

oxyhematoporphyrin (-hem″ah-to-por′fĭ-rin) a pigment sometimes found in the urine, closely allied to hematoporphyrin.

oxyhemoglobin (-he″mah-glo′bin) hemoglobin that contains bound O_2, a compound formed from hemoglobin on exposure to alveolar gas in the lungs.

oxylalia (-lāl′e-ah) rapidity of speech.

oxymetazoline (-mĭ-taz′ah-lēn) a vasoconstrictor, $C_{16}H_{24}N_2O$, used topically as the hydrochloride salt in nasal congestion.

oxymetholone (-meth′ah-lōn) an anabolic-androgenic steroid, $C_{21}H_{32}O_3$, which promotes retention of nitrogen, phosphorus, and calcium.

oxymorphone (-mor′fōn) a narcotic analgesic, $C_{17}H_{19}NO_4$; used as the hydrochloride salt.

oxymyoglobin (-mi″ah-glo′bin) myoglobin charged with oxygen.

oxyntic (ok-sint′ik) secreting acid, as the parietal (oxyntic) cells.

oxyphenbutazone (-fen-būt′ah-zōn) a phenylbutazone derivative, $C_{19}H_{20}N_2O_3$, having similar anti-inflammatory, analgesic, and antipyretic actions; used in the treatment of arthritis, gout, and similar conditions.

oxyphencyclimine (-si′klĭ-mēn) an anticholinergic, $C_{20}H_{28}N_2O_3$, with antisecretory, antimotility, and antispasmodic actions; the hydrochloride salt is used in the treatment of peptic ulcer and other gastrointestinal disorders.

oxyphenisatin (-fĕ-ni′sah-tin) a cathartic, $C_{20}H_{15}NO_3$; administered as an enema to cleanse the bowel before surgery or colon examination.

oxyphenonium (-fĕ-no′ne-um) an anticholinergic, $C_{21}H_{34}NO_3$, used as the bromide ester in the treatment of peptic ulcer and gastrointestinal hypermotility or spasm.

oxyphil (ok′sĭ-fil) 1. Hürthle cell. 2. oxyphilic.

oxyphilic, oxyphilous (ok″sĭ-fil′ik; ok-sif′ĭ-lus) stainable with an acid dye.

oxytetracycline (ok″se-tĕ-trah-si′klēn) a broad-spectrum antibiotic of the tetracycline group, produced by *Streptomyces rimosus*, $C_{22}H_{24}N_2O_9$, used chiefly as an antibacterial.

oxytocia (-to′se-ah) rapid labor.

oxytocic (-to′sik) 1. pertaining to, marked by, or promoting oxytocia. 2. an agent that promotes rapid labor by stimulating contractions of the myometrium.

oxytocin (-to′sin) an octapeptide hypothalamic hormone stored in the posterior pituitary, which has uterine-contracting and milk-releasing actions; it may also be prepared synthetically or obtained from the posterior pituitary of domestic animals; used to induce active labor, increase the force of contractions in labor, contract uterine muscle after delivery of the placenta, control postpartum hemorrhage, and stimulate milk ejection.

oxyuriasis (-ūr-i′ah-sis) infection with *Enterobius vermicularis* (in humans) or with other oxyurids; enterobiasis.

oxyuricide (-ūr′ĭ-sīd) an agent that destroys oxyurids.

oxyurid (-ūr′id) a pinworm, seatworm, or threadworm; any individual of the superfamily Oxyuroidea.

Oxyuris (-ūr′is) a genus of intestinal nematode worms (superfamily Oxyuroidea). **O. equi**, a species found in horses. **O. vermicula′ris**, *Enterobius vermicularis*.

Oxyuroidea (-ūr″oi-de′ah) a superfamily of small nematodes—the pinworms, seatworms, or threadworms—parasitic in the cecum and colon of vertebrates and sometimes infecting invertebrates.

oz. ounce.

ozena (o-ze′nah) an atrophic rhinitis marked by a thick mucopurulent discharge, mucosal crusting, and fetor.

ozone (o′zōn) a bluish explosive gas or blue liquid, being an allotropic form of oxygen, O_3; it is antiseptic and disinfectant, and irritating and toxic to the pulmonary system.

P

P chemical symbol, *phosphorus*.

P₁ parental generation.

P₂ pulmonic second sound.

p symbol for (1) the short arm of a chromosome or (2) the frequency of the more common allele of a pair.

p- symbol, *para-*.

P.A. physician assistant.

Pa 1. chemical symbol, *protactinium*. 2. symbol for *pascal*.

PAB, PABA para-aminobenzoic acid.

pabulum (pab′ŭl-um) food or aliment.

pacemaker (pās′māk″er) that which sets the pace at which a phenomenon occurs; often used alone to indicate the natural cardiac pacemaker or an artificial cardiac pacemaker. **cardiac p., artificial,** a device designed to stimulate, by electrical impulses, contraction of the heart muscle at a certain rate; worn by or implanted in the body of the patient. **demand p.,** an implanted cardiac pacemaker in which the generator stimulus is inhibited by a signal derived from the heart's electrical activation (depolarization), thus minimizing the risk of pacemaker-induced fibrillation. **fixed-rate p.,** an implanted cardiac pacemaker in which the generator stimulates the heart at a predetermined rate, regardless of cardiac rhythm. **wandering p.,** a condition in which the site of origin of the impulses controlling the heart rate shifts from the head of the sinoatrial node to a lower part of the node or to another part of the atrium.

pachy- word element [Gr.], *thick*.

pachyacria (pak″e-a′kre-ah) enlargement of the soft parts of the extremities.

pachyblepharon (pak″e-blef′ah-ron) thickening of the eyelids.

pachycephaly (-sef′ah-le) abnormal thickness of the bones of the skull. **pachycephal′ic,** adj.

pachycheilia (-ki′le-ah) thickening of the lips.

pachychromatic (-kro-mat′ik) having the chromatin in thick strands.

pachydactyly (-dak′tĭ-le) enlargement of the fingers and toes.

pachyderma (-der′mah) abnormal thickening of the skin. **pachyder′matous,** adj.

pachydermatocele (-der-mat′ah-sēl) plexiform neuroma attaining large size, producing an elephantiasis-like condition.

pachydermoperiostosis (-durm″o-pĕ″re-os-to′-sis) pachyderma affecting the face and scalp, thickening of the bones of the distal extremities, and acropachy.

pachyglossia (-glos′e-ah) abnormal thickness of the tongue.

pachygyria (-ji′re-ah) macrogyria.

pachyleptomeningitis (-lep″to-men″in-jīt′is) inflammation of dura mater and pia mater.

pachymeningitis (-men″in-jīt′is) inflammation of the dura mater.

pachymeningopathy (-men″ing-gop′ah-the) noninflammatory disease of the dura mater.

pachymeninx (-me′ninks) the dura mater.

pachynsis (pah-kin′sis) an abnormal thickening. **pachyn′tic,** adj.

pachyonychia (pak″e-o-nik′e-ah) abnormal thickening of the nails. **p. conge′nita,** a rare, congenital, dominantly inherited disorder marked by great thickening of the nails, hyperkeratosis of palms and soles, and leukoplakia.

pachyperiostitis (pak″ĭ-pĕ″re-os-tītis) periostitis of the long bones resulting in abnormal thickness of affected bones.

pachyperitonitis (-pĕ″rit′n-īt-is) inflammation and thickening of the peritoneum.

pachypleuritis (-plōōr-īt′is) fibrothorax.

pachysalpingitis (-sal″pin-jīt′is) chronic salpingitis with thickening.

pachysalpingo-ovaritis (-sal-ping″go-o″vah-rīt′is) chronic inflammation of the ovary and uterine tube, with thickening.

pachysomia (-so′me-ah) abnormal thickening of parts of the body.

pachytene (pak′ĭ-tēn) in the prophase of meiosis, the stage following zygotene during which the chromosomes shorten, thicken, and separate into two sister chromatids joined at their centromeres. Paired homologous chromosomes, which were joined by synapsis, now form a tetrad of four chromatids. Where crossing over has occurred between nonsister chromatids, they are joined by X-shaped chiasmata.

pachyvaginalitis (pak″ĭ-vaj″in-il-it′is) inflammation and thickening of the tunica vaginalis.

pachyvaginitis (-vaj″in-īt′is) chronic vaginitis with thickening of the vaginal walls.

pack (pak) 1. treatment by wrapping a patient in blankets or sheets or a limb in towels, either wet or dry and hot or cold; also, the blankets or towels used for this purpose. 2. a tampon.

packer (pak′er) an instrument for introducing a dressing into a cavity or a wound.

packing (pak′ing) the filling of a wound or cavity with gauze, sponges, pads, or other material; also, the material used for this purpose.

pad (pad) a cushion-like mass of soft material. **abdominal p.,** a pad for the absorption of discharges from abdominal wounds, or for packing off abdominal viscera to improve exposure during surgery. **dinner p.,** a pad placed over the stomach before a plaster jacket is applied; the pad is then removed, leaving space under the jacket to accommodate expansion of the stomach after eating. **fat p.,** a large pad of fat lying behind and below the patella. **knuckle p's,** nodular thickenings of the skin on the dorsal surface of the interphalangeal joints. **retromolar p.,** a cushion-like mass of tissue situated at the distal termination of the mandibular residual ridge. **sucking p., suctorial p.,** a lobulated mass of fat which occupies the space between the masseter and the external surface of the buccinator; it is well developed in infants.

pae- for words beginning thus, see those beginning with *pe-*.

PAF platelet activating factor.

-pagus word element [Gr.], *conjoined twins.*

PAH, PAHA para-aminohippuric acid.

pain (pān) a feeling of distress, suffering, or agony, caused by stimulation of specialized nerve endings. **bearing-down p.,** pain accompanying uterine contractions during the second stage of labor. **false p's,** ineffective pains resembling labor pains, not accompanied by cervical dilatation. **growing p's,** recurrent quasirheumatic limb pains peculiar to early youth. **hunger p.,** pain coming on at the time for feeling hunger for a meal; a symptom of gastric disorder. **intermenstrual p.,** pain accompanying ovulation, occurring during the period between the menses, usually about midway. **labor p's,** the rhythmic pains of increasing severity and frequency due to contraction of the uterus at childbirth. **phantom limb p.,** pain felt as though arising in an absent (amputated) limb. **psychogenic p.,** symptoms of physical pain having psychological origin. **referred p.,** pain felt in a part other than that in which the cause that produced it is situated. **rest p.,** a continuous burning pain due to ischemia of the lower leg, which begins or is aggravated after reclining and is relieved by sitting or standing.

paint (pānt) 1. a liquid designed for application to a surface, as of the body or a tooth. 2. to apply a liquid to a specific area as a remedial or protective measure.

palae(o)- word element [Gr.], *old.*

palaeocerebellum (pāl″e-o-ser″ah-bel′im) those parts of the cerebellum whose afferent inflow is predominantly supplied by spinocerebellar fibers. **palaeocerebel′lar,** adj.

palaeocortex (pāl″e-o-kor′teks) that portion of the cortex cerebri that, with the archaeocortex, develops in association with the olfactory system and is phylogenetically older and less stratified than the neocortex. **palaeocor′tical,** adj.

palat(o)- word element [L.], *palate.*

palate (pal′it) roof of the mouth; the partition separating the nasal and oral cavities. **pal′atal, pal′atine,** adj. **cleft p.,** congenital fissure of median line of palate. **hard p.,** the anterior portion of the palate, separating the oral and nasal cavities, consisting of the bony framework and covering membranes. **soft p.,** the fleshy part of the palate, extending from the posterior edge of the hard palate; the uvula projects from its free inferior border.

palatitis (pal″ah-tīt′is) inflammation of the palate.

palatognathous (pal″ah-tog′nah-this) having a congenitally cleft palate.

platoplasty (pal′it-o-plas″te) plastic reconstruction of the palate.

palatoplegia (pal″it-o-ple′je-ah) paralysis of the palate.

palatorrhaphy (pal″ah-tor′ah-fe) surgical correction of a cleft palate.

palatoschisis (pal″ah-tos′kĭ-sis) cleft palate.

palatum (pah-lah′tum) [L.] palate.

pale(o)- see *palae(o).*

paleencephalon (pa″le-en-sef′ah-lon) the (phylogenetically) old brain; all of the brain except the cerebral cortex and its dependencies.

paleokinetic (-ki-net′ik) old kinetic; applied to the nervous motor mechanism concerned in automatic associated movements.

paleopathology (-pah-thol′ah-je) study of disease in bodies which have been preserved from ancient times.

paleostriatum (-stri-āt′um) the phylogenetically older portion of the corpus striatum, represented by the globus pallidus. **paleostria′tal,** adj.

paleothalamus (-thal′ah-mus) the phylogenetically older part of the thalamus, i.e., the medial portion which lacks reciprocal connections with the neopallium.

pali(n)- word element [Gr.], *again; pathologic repetition.*

palindromia (pal″in-dro′me-ah) a recurrence of relapse. **palindrom′ic,** adj.

palinopsia (pal″in-op′se-ah) visual perseveration; the continuance of a visual sensation after the stimulus is gone.

palladium (pah-la′de-um) chemical element (*see table*), at. no. 46, symbol Pd.

pallanesthesia (pal″an-es-the′ze-ah) loss or absence of pallesthesia.

pallesthesia (pal″es-the′ze-ah) sensibility to vibrations; the peculiar vibrating sensation felt when a vibrating tuning-fork is placed against a subcutaneous bony prominence of the body. **pallinesthet′ic,** adj.

palliative (pal′e-ah-tiv, -āt″iv) affording relief; also, a drug that so acts.

pallidectomy (pal″ĭ-dek′tah-me) extirpation of the globus pallidus.

pallidoansotomy (-an-sot′ah-me) production of lesions in the globus pallidus and ansa lenticularis.

pallidotomy (-dot′ah-me) a stereotaxic surgical techique for the production of lesions in the globus pallidus for treatment of extrapyramidal disorders.

pallidum (pal′ĭ-dum) the globus pallidus. **pal′lidal,** adj.

pallium (pal′e-um) the cerebral cortex viewed in its entirety, i.e., the mantle of gray matter covering both cerebral hemispheres. Also, the cerebral cortex during its development.

pallor (pal′er) paleness, as of the skin.

palm (pahm) the hollow or flexor surface of the hand. **pal′mar,** adj.

palma (pahl′mah), pl. *pal′mae* [L.] palm.

palmaris (pahl-ma′ris) palmar.

palmitic acid (pal-mit′ik) a saturated fatty acid, $C_{15}H_{31}COOH$, from animal and vegetable fats; see also *stearic acid.*

palmitoleic acid (pal-mit-o-le′ik) an unsaturated fatty acid, $C_{15}H_{29}COOH$, found in various oils and a common constituent of glycerides in human adipose tissue.

palmus (pahl′mus) 1. palpitation. 2. clonic

spasm of leg muscles, producing jumping motion.

palpation (pal-pa′shin) the act of feeling with the hand; the application of the fingers with light pressure to the surface of the body for the purpose of determining the condition of the parts beneath in physical diagnosis.

palpebra (pal′pah-brah), pl. *pal′pebrae* [L.] eyelid. **pal′pebral,** adj.

palpebralis (pal″pah-brāl′is) [L.] palpebral.

palpebritis (pal″pah-brīt′is) blepharitis.

palpitation (pal″pĭ-ta′shun) a subjective sensation of an unduly rapid or irregular heart beat.

palsy (pawl′ze) paralysis. **Bell's p.,** unilateral facial paralysis of sudden onset due to lesion of the facial nerve, resulting in characteristic facial distortion. **cerebral p.,** persisting qualitative motor disorder appearing before age three, due to nonprogressive damage to the brain. **Erb's p.,** Erb-Duchenne paralysis. **facial p.,** Bell's p. **shaking p.,** paralysis agitans. **wasting p.,** spinal muscular atrophy.

pamoate (pam′ah-wāt) USAN contraction for 4,4′-methylenebis[3-hydroxy-2-naphthoate].

pampiniform (pam-pin′ĭ-form) shaped like a tendril.

pan- word element [Gr.], *all.*

panagglutinin (pan″ah-glōōt′n-in) an agglutinin which agglutinates the erythrocytes of all human blood groups.

pananxiety (pan″ang-zi′ĭt-e) diffuse, all-pervading anxiety.

panatrophy (pan-ă′trah-fe) atrophy of several parts; diffuse atrophy.

panautonomic (-awt″ah-nom-ik) pertaining to or affecting the entire autonomic (sympathetic and parasympathetic) nervous system.

pancarditis (pan″kar-dīt′is) diffuse inflammation of the heart.

pancolectomy (-ko-lek′tah-me) excision of the entire colon, with creation of an outlet from the ileum on the body surface.

pancreas (pan′kre-is), pl. *pancre′ata* [Gr.] a large, elongated, racemose gland situated transversely behind the stomach, between the spleen and duodenum. Its external secretion contains digestive enzymes. An internal secretion, insulin, is produced by the beta cells, and glucagon is produced by the alpha cells. The alpha, beta, and delta cells form aggregates, called islands of Langerhans. See Plate IV. **pancreat′ic,** adj.

pancreatectomy (-tek′tah-me) excision of the pancreas.

pancreatico- word element [Gr.], *pancreatic duct.*

pancreaticoduodenal (pan″kre-at″ĭ-ko-doo″ah-dēn′l; -doo-ad″′n-il) pertaining to the pancreas and duodenum.

pancreaticoduodenostomy (-dod′n-os′tah-me) anastomosis of the pancreatic duct to a different site on the duodenum.

pancreaticoenterostomy (-en″ter-os′tah-me) anastomosis of the pancreatic duct to the intestine.

pancreaticogastrostomy (-gas-tros′tah-me) anastomosis of the pancreatic duct to the stomach.

pancreaticojejunostomy (-je″joo-nos′tah-me) anastomosis of the pancreatic duct to the jejunum.

pancreatin (pan′kre-it-in) a substance from the pancreas of the hog or ox containing enzymes, principally amylase, protease, and lipase; used as a digestive aid.

pancreatitis (pan″kre-ah-tīt′is) inflammation of the pancreas. **acute hemorrhagic p.,** a condition due to autolysis of pancreatic tissue caused by escape of enzymes into the substance, resulting in hemorrhage into the parenchyma and surrounding tissues.

pancreato- word element [Gr.], *pancreas.*

pancreatoduodenectomy (pan″kre-it-o-doo″od′n-ek′tah-me) excision of the head of the pancreas along with the encircling loop of the duodenum.

pancreatogenous (pan″kre-ah-toj′ĭ-nus) arising in the pancreas.

pancreatography (pan″kre-ah-tog′rah-fe) roentgenography of the pancreas.

pancreatolithectomy (pan″kre-it-o-lĭ-thek′tah-me) excision of a calculus from the pancreas.

pancreatolithiasis (-lĭ-thi′ah-sis) presence of calculi in the ductal system or parenchyma of the pancreas.

pancreatolithotomy (-lĭ-thot′ah-me) incision of the pancreas for the removal of calculi.

pancreatolysis (pan″kre-ah-tol′ĭ-sis) destruction of pancreatic tissue. **pancreatolyt′ic,** adj.

pancreatotomy (-tot′ah-me) incision of the pancreas.

pancreatotropic (pan″kre-it-o-trop′ik) having an affinity for the pancreas.

pancrelipase (pan″kre-li′pās) a preparation of hog pancreas containing enzymes, principally lipase with amylase and protease, having the same actions as pancreatic juice; used as a digestive aid.

pancreoprivic (pan″kre-o-priv′ik) lacking a pancreas.

pancreozymin (-zi′min) a hormone of the duodenal mucosa that stimulates the external secretory activity of the pancreas, especially its production of amylase; identical with cholecystokinin.

pancuronium (pan″kūr-o′ne-um) a skeletal muscle relaxant used as the bromide salt, C_{35}-$H_{60}Br_2N_2O_4$.

pancystitis (pan″sis-tīt′is) cystitis involving the entire thickness of the wall of the urinary bladder, as occurs in interstitial cystitis.

pancytopenia (pan″sīt-ah-pe′ne-ah) abnormal depression of all the cellular elements of the blood.

pandemic (pan-dem′ik) a widespread epidemic disease; widely epidemic.

panencephalitis (pan″en-sef″ah-līt′is) encephalitis, probably of viral origin, which produces intranuclear or intracytoplasmic inclusion bodies that result in parenchymatous lesions of both the gray and white matter of the brain.

papilla

panendoscope (pan-en′dah-skōp) a cystoscope that permits wide-angle viewing of the urinary bladder.

panhypopituitarism (pan-hi″po-pĭ-tu′it-er) generalized hypopituitarism due to absence or damage of the pituitary gland, which, in its complete form, leads to absence of gonadal function and insufficiency of thyroid and adrenal function. When cachexia is a prominent feature, it is called *Simmonds' disease* or *pituitary cachexia.*

panhysterosalpingectomy (-his-ter-o-sal″pin-jek′tah-me) excision of the body of the uterus, cervix, and uterine tubes.

panhysterosalpingo-oophorectomy (-salping″go-o″of-ah-rek′tah-me) excision of the uterus, cervix, uterine tubes, and ovaries.

panic (pan′ik) extreme and unreasoning fear and anxiety. **acute homosexual p., homosexual p.,** an acute reaction due to unconscious conflicts involving homosexuality, marked by severe anxiety, excitement, and great activity, often accompanied by assaultiveness and auditory hallucinations accusing the patient of homosexual inclinations.

panleukopenia (-loo-ko-pe′ne-ah) a viral disease of cats, marked by leukopenia and by inactivity, refusal of food, diarrhea, and vomiting.

panmyelophthisis (-mi-il-of′thĭ-sis) aplastic anemia.

panneurosis (pan″nŏŏr-o′sis) the simultaneous occurrence of all neurotic symptoms (anxiety, conversion symptoms, obsessions, and phobias).

panniculectomy (pah-nik″ŭl-ek′tah-me) surgical excision of the abdominal apron of superficial fat in the obese.

panniculitis (-lĭt′is) inflammation of the panniculus adiposus, especially of the abdomen. **nodular nonsuppurative p., relapsing febrile nonsuppurative p.,** a disease marked by fever and the formation of crops of tender nodules in subcutaneous fatty tissues.

panniculus (pah-nik′ŭl-is), pl. *panni′culi* [L.] a layer of membrane. **p. adipo′sus,** the subcutaneous fat: a layer of fat underlying the corium. **p. carno′sus,** a muscular layer in the superficial fascia of certain lower animals; represented in man mainly by the platysma.

pannus (pan′is) 1. superficial vascularization of the cornea with infiltration of granulation tissue. 2. an inflammatory exudate overlying the synovial cells on the inside of a joint. 3. panniculus adiposus. **p. trachomato′sus,** pannus of the cornea secondary to trachoma.

panophthalmitis (pan″of-thal-mīt′is) inflammation of all the eye structures or tissues.

panotitis (-o-tīt′is) inflammation of all the parts or structures of the ear.

panphobia (-fo′be-ah) fear of everything; vague and persistent dread of an unknown evil.

Panstrongylus (pan-stron′jĭ-lis) a genus of hemipterous insects, species of which transmit trypanosomes.

pant(o)- word element [Gr.], *all; the whole.*

pantetheine (pan″tĭ-the′in) an amide of pantothenic acid, an intermediate in the biosynthesis of CoA, a growth factor for *Lactobacillus bul-*

garicus, and a cofactor in certain enzyme complexes.

pantothenate (pan″tah-then′āt) any salt of pantothenic acid.

pantothenic acid (pan″tah-then′ik) $C_9H_{17}NO_5$, a component of coenzyme A and a member of the vitamin-B complex; necessary for nutrition in some animal species, but of uncertain importance for humans.

papain (pah-pa′in, pah-pi′in) a proteolytic enzyme from the latex of papaw, *Carica papaya,* which catalyzes the hydrolysis of proteins and polypeptides to amino acids; used as a protein digestant and as a topical application for enzymatic débridement.

papaverine (pah-pav′er-in) an alkaloid, $C_{20}H_{21}$-NO_4, obtained from opium or prepared synthetically; the hydrochloride salt is used as a smooth muscle relaxant.

paper (pa′per) a material manufactured in thin sheets from fibrous substances which have first been reduced to a pulp. **litmus p.,** moisture-absorbing paper impregnated with a solution of litmus: if slightly acid, it is red, and alkalis turn it blue; if slightly alkaline, it is blue and acid turns it red. **test p.,** paper stained with a compound which changes visibly on occurrence of a chemical reaction.

papilla (pah-pil′ah), pl. *papil′lae* [L.] a small nipple-shaped projection or elevation. **pap′illary,** adj. **circumvallate p.,** vallate p. **conical p.,** one of the sparsely scattered elevations on the tongue, often considered to be modified filiform papillae. **papillae of corium,** conical extensions of the fibers, capillary blood vessels, and sometimes nerves of the corium into corresponding spaces among downward- or inward-projecting rete ridges on the undersurface of the epidermis. **dental p., dentinal p.,** the small mass of condensed mesenchyme capped by each of the enamel organs. **duodenal p.,** either of the small elevations (major and minor) on the mucosa of the duodenum, the *major* at the entrance of the conjoined pancreatic and common bile ducts, the *minor* at the entrance of the accessory pancreatic duct. **filiform p.,** one of the threadlike elevations covering most of the tongue surface. **foliate p.,** one of the parallel mucosal folds on the tongue margin at the junction of its body and root. **fungiform p.,** one of the knoblike projections of the tongue scattered among the filiform papillae. **hair p.,** the fibrovascular mesodermal papilla enclosed within the hair bulb. **incisive p.,** an elevation at the anterior end of the raphe of the palate. **interdental p.,** gingival p. **lacrimal p.,** an elevation on the margin of either eyelid, near the medial angle of the eye. **lingual p.,** see *conical, filiform, foliate, fungiform,* and *vallate p.* **mammary p.,** the nipple of the breast. **optic p.,** optic disk. **palatine p.,** incisive p. **p. pi′li,** hair p. **renal p.,** the blunted apex of a renal pyramid. **tactile papillae,** see under *corpuscle.* **urethral p.,** a slight elevation in the vestibule of the vagina at the external orifice of the urethra. **vallate p.,** one of the 8 to 12 large papillae arranged in a V near the base of the tongue.

papilledema (pap″il-ĭ-de′mah) edema of the optic disk.

papillitis (pap″il-īt′is) inflammation of the optic disk.

papilloadenocystoma (pap″il-o-ad″ĭ-no-sis-to′mah) papillary cystadenoma.

papilloma (pap″il-o′mah) a benign tumor derived from epithelium. **papillo′matous,** adj.

papillomatosis (pap″il-o″mah-to′sis) development of multiple papillomas.

papilloretinitis (pap″il-o-ret″in-īt′is) inflammation of the optic disk and retina.

papillotomy (pap″il-ot′ah-me) incision of a papilla, as of a duodenal papilla.

papovavirus (pap″o-vah-vi′ris) a group of relatively small, ether-resistant DNA viruses, many of which are oncogenic or potentially oncogenic.

papulation (pap″ūl-a′shin) the formation of papules.

papule (pap′ūl) a small circumscribed, solid, elevated lesion of the skin. **pap′ular,** adj.

papulosis (pap″ūl-o′sis) the presence of multiple papules.

papyraceous (pap″ĭ-ra′shis) like paper.

para (par′ah) a woman who has produced one or more viable offspring. **p. I,** primipara. **p. II,** secundipara, etc.

para- word element [Gr.], *beside; beyond; accessory to; apart from; against, etc.* In chemistry, indicating the substitution in a derivative of the benzene ring of two atoms linked to opposite carbon atoms in the ring.

para-aminobenzoic acid (PAB, PABA) (par″.ah-ah-me″no-ben-zo′ik) $NH_2C_6H_4COOH$, a precursor of folic acid and a growth factor for certain microorganisms; used in medicine as a sunscreen.

para-anesthesia (par″ah-an″es-the′ze-ah) anesthesia of the lower part of the body.

parabiosis (-bi-o′sis) 1. the union of two individuals, as conjoined twins, or of experimental animals by surgical operation. 2. temporary suppression of conductivity and excitability. **parabiot′ic,** adj.

paracasein (-ka′se-in) the chemical product of the action of rennin on casein.

paracentesis (-sen-te′sis) surgical puncture of a cavity for the aspiration of fluid. **paracentet′ic,** adj.

parachlorophenol (-klor″ah-fe′nol) a local anti-infective, C_6H_5ClO, used in dentistry.

paracholera (-kol′er-ah) a disease resembling Asiatic cholera but not caused by *Vibrio cholerae.*

paraclinical (-klin′ik′l) pertaining to abnormalities (e.g., morphological or biochemical) underlying clinical manifestations (e.g., chest pain or fever).

Paracoccidioides (-kok-sid″ĭ-oi′dēz) a genus of fungi that proliferate by multiple budding yeast cells in the tissues; it includes *P. brasilien′sis,* the etiologic agent of paracoccidioidomycosis.

paracoccidioidomycosis (-kok-sid″e-oi″do-mi-ko′sis) an often fatal, chronic granulomatous disease caused by *Paracoccidioides brasiliensis,* primarily involving the lungs, but spreading to the skin, mucous membranes, lymph nodes, and internal organs.

paracolitis (-kol-īt′s) inflammation of the outer coat of the colon.

paracrine (par′ah-krin) 1. denoting a type of hormone function in which hormone synthesized in and released from endocrine cells binds to its receptor in nearby cells and affects their function. 2. denoting the secretion of a hormone by an organ other than an endocrine gland.

paracusis (-ku′sis) any perversion of hearing.

paradidymis (-did″ĭ-mis) a small, vestigial structure found occasionally in the adult in the anterior spermatic cord.

paradox (par′ah-doks) a seemingly contradictory occurrence. **paradox′ic, paradox′ical,** adj. **Weber's p.,** elongation of a muscle which has been so stretched that it cannot contract.

paraffin (-fin) 1. a purified hydrocarbon wax used for embedding histological specimens. 2. formerly, an *alkane.* **light liquid p.,** light mineral oil. **liquid p.,** mineral oil.

paraffinoma (par″ah-fĭ-no′mah) a chronic granuloma produced by prolonged exposure to paraffin.

paraganglioma (-gang″gle-o′mah) a tumor of the tissue composing the paraganglia. **nonchromaffin p.,** chemodectoma.

paraganglion (-gang′gle-in), pl. *paragan′glia.* A collection of chromaffin cells derived from neural ectoderm, occurring outside the adrenal medulla, usually near the sympathetic ganglia and in relation to the aorta and its branches.

paragonimiasis (-gon″ĭ-mi′ah-sis) infection with flukes of the genus *Paragonimus.*

Paragonimus (-gon-ĭ-mis) a genus of trematode parasites, having two invertebrate hosts, the first a snail, the second a crab or crayfish; it includes *P. westerma′ni,* the lung fluke, occurring especially in Asia, found in cysts in the lungs and sometimes the pleura, liver, abdominal cavity, and elsewhere in man and lower animals who ingest infected freshwater crayfish and crabs.

paragranuloma (-gran″ūl-o′mah) the most benign form of Hodgkin's disease, largely confined to the lymph nodes.

parahemophilia (-hēm″o-fil′e-ah) a hereditary hemorrhagic tendency due to deficiency of coagulation Factor V.

parahormone (-hor′mōn) a substance, not a true hormone, which has a hormone-like action in controlling the functioning of some distant organ.

parakeratosis (-ker″ah-to′sis) persistence of the nuclei of keratinocytes as they rise into the horny layer of the skin. It is normal in the epithelium of the true mucous membrane of the mouth and vagina.

parakinesia (-ki-ne′se-ah) perversion of motor function; in ophthalmology, irregular action of an individual ocular muscle.

paralalia (-lāl′e-ah) a disorder of speech, especially the production of a vocal sound different from the one desired, or the substitution in speech of one letter for another.

paralbumin (par″al-bu′min) an albumin or protein substance found in ovarian cysts.

paraldehyde (pah-ral′dĕ-hīd) a polymerization product of acetaldehyde, $C_6H_{12}O$, having rapid-acting sedative and hypnotic properties; used to control insomnia, excitement, agitation, delirium, and convulsions.

parallagma (par″ah-lag′mah) displacement of a bone or of the fragments of a broken bone.

parallergy (par-al′er-je) a condition in which an allergic state, produced by specific sensitization, predisposes the body to react to other allergens with clinical manifestations that differ from the original reaction. **paraller′gic**, adj.

paralysis (pah-ral′ĭ-sis) loss or impairment of motor function in a part due to lesion of the neural or muscular mechanism; also, by analogy, impairment of sensory function (*sensory p.*). **p. a′gitans**, a slowly progressive form of parkinsonism, usually seen late in life, marked by masklike facies, tremor of resting muscles, slowing of voluntary movements, festinating gait, peculiar posture, muscular weakness, and sometimes excessive sweating and feelings of heat. **ascending p.**, spinal paralysis which progresses cephalad. **bulbar p.**, that due to changes in motor centers of the medulla oblongata; the chronic form is marked by progressive paralysis and atrophy of the lips, tongue, pharynx, and larynx, and is due to degeneration of the nerve nuclei of the floor of the fourth ventricle. **central p.**, that due to a lesion of the brain or spinal cord. **compression p.**, that caused by pressure on a nerve. **conjugate p.**, loss of ability to perform some parallel ocular movements. **crossed p.**, that affecting one side of face and the other side of the body. **decubitus p.**, that due to pressure on a nerve from lying for a long time in one position. **divers' p.**, that resulting from too rapid reduction of pressure on deep-sea divers. **Duchenne's p.**, 1. Erb-Duchenne p. 2. progressive bulbar p. **Erb-Duchenne p.**, paralysis of the upper roots of the brachial plexus due to destruction of the fifth and sixth cervical roots, without involvement of the small muscles of the hand. **facial p.**, weakening or paralysis of the facial nerve, as in Bell's palsy. **familial periodic p.**, a rare dominantly inherited disorder with recurring attacks of rapidly progressive flaccid paralysis, associated with a fall in (hypokalemic type), a rise in (hyperkalemic type), or normal (normokalemic type) serum potassium levels. **hyperkalemic periodic p.**, see *familial periodic p.* **hypokalemic periodic p.**, see *familial periodic p.* **immune p., immunological p.**, the absence of immune response to a specific antigen, usually induced with very large doses of antigen. **Klumpke's p., Klumpke-Dejerine p.**, atrophic paralysis of the lower arm and hand, due to lesion of the eighth cervical and first dorsal nerves. **Landry's p.**, acute febrile polyneuritis. **mixed p.**, combined motor and sensory paralysis. **motor p.**, paralysis of voluntary muscles. **musculospiral p.**, paralysis of the extensor muscles of the wrist and fingers. **normokalemic periodic p.**, see *familial periodic p.* **periodic p.**, a recurrent paralysis; see

also *familial periodic p.* **progressive bulbar p.**, see *bulbar p.* **pseudobulbar p.**, spastic weakness of the muscles innervated by the cranial nerves, i.e., the facial muscles, the pharynx, and tongue, due to bilateral lesions of the corticospinal tract, often accompanied by uncontrolled weeping or laughing. **pseudohypertrophic muscular p.**, see under *dystrophy.* **sensory p.**, loss of sensation due to a morbid process. **spastic spinal p.**, lateral sclerosis. **Todd's p.**, transient hemiplegia or monoplegia occurring after an epileptic seizure. **vasomotor p.**, cessation of vasomotor control.

paralyzant (par′ah-līz″int) 1. causing paralysis. 2. a drug that causes paralysis.

paramania (par″ah-ma′ne-ah) parathymia in which one manifests joy by complaining.

paramastigote (-mas′tĭ-gōt) having an accessory flagellum by the side of a larger one.

paramastitis (-mas-tīt′is) inflammation of tissues around the mammary gland.

Paramecium (-me′she-um) a genus of ciliate protozoa.

paramecium (-me′she-um), pl. *parame′cia.* An organism of the genus *Paramecium.*

paramenia (-me′ne-ah) disordered or difficult menstruation.

parameter (pah-ram′it-er) 1. in mathematics and statistics, an arbitrary constant, such as a population mean or standard deviation. 2. a property of a system that can be measured numerically.

paramethadione (par″ah-meth″ah-di′ōn) an anticonvulsant, $C_7H_{11}NO_3$, used in petit mal epilepsy.

paramethasone (-meth′ah-sōn) a glucocorticoid, $C_{22}H_{29}FO_5$, used as the 21-acetate ester for its anti-inflammatory and antiallergic effects.

parametric 1. (-me′trik) situated near the uterus; parametrial. 2. (-mĕ′trik) pertaining to or defined in terms of a parameter.

parametritis (-me-trīt′is) inflammation of parametrium.

parametrium (-me′tre-um) the extension of the subserous coat of the supracervical portion of the uterus laterally between the layers of the broad ligament. **parame′trial**, adj.

paramnesia (par″am-ne′ze-ah) an unconsciously false memory.

paramucin (par″ah-mu′sin) a colloid substance from ovarian cysts, differing from mucin and pseudomucin in that it reduces Fehling's solution before boiling with acid.

paramyloidosis (par-am″ĭ-loi-do′sis) accumulation of an atypical form of amyloid in tissues.

paramyoclonus (par″ah-mi-ok′lo-nus) a condition characterized by myoclonic contractions of various muscles. **p. mul′tiplex**, a condition characterized by sudden shocklike muscular contractions.

paramyotonia (-mi″ah-to′ne-ah) a disease marked by tonic spasms due to disorder of muscular tonicity, especially a hereditary and congenital affection. **p. congen′ita**, see under *myotonia.*

paramyxovirus (-mik″sah-vi′ris) any of a subgroup of myxoviruses, including the viruses of human and animal parainfluenza, mumps, and Newcastle disease.

paraneoplastic (par″ah-ne″o-plas′tik) pertaining to changes produced in tissue remote from a tumor or its metastases.

paranephric (-nef′rik) 1. near the kidney. 2. pertaining to the adrenal gland.

paranephritis (-nĕ-frīt′is) 1. inflammation of the adrenal gland. 2. inflammation of the connective tissue around the kidney.

paranephros (-nef′ros) an adrenal gland.

paranesthesia (par″an-es-the′ze-ah) para-anesthesia.

paranoia (-noi′ah) a psychotic disorder marked by well-systematized, logically consistent delusions of grandeur, persecution, or jealousy, with no other psychotic feature. There are five types: persecutory, jealous, erotomanic, somatic, and grandiose. **parano′ic,** adj.

paranomia (par″ah-no′me-ah) aphasia marked by inability to name objects felt (*myotactic p.*) or seen (*visual p.*).

paranucleus (-noo′kle-is) a body sometimes seen in cell protoplasm near the nucleus. **paranu′clear,** adj.

paraparesis (-pah-re′sis, par′ĭ-sis) partial paralysis of the lower extremities.

parapertussis (par″ah-per-tus′is) an acute respiratory disease clinically indistinguishable from mild or moderate pertussis, caused by *Bordetella parapertussis.*

paraphasia (-fa′ze-ah) partial aphasia in which the patient employs wrong words, or uses words in wrong and senseless combinations (*choreic p.*).

paraphemia (-fēm′e-ah) aphasia marked by the employment of the wrong words.

paraphia (par-a′fe-ah) perversion of the sense of touch.

paraphilia (par″ah-fil′e-ah) a psychosexual disorder marked by sexual urges and fantasies involving objects, the suffering or humiliation of oneself or one's partner, children, or other nonconsenting partners. **paraphil′iac,** adj.

paraphrasia (-fra′ze-ah) disorderly arrangement of spoken words.

paraplasm (par′ah-plazm) 1. any abnormal growth. 2. hyaloplasm (1). **paraplas′tic,** adj.

paraplectic (par″ah-plek′tik) paraplegic.

paraplegia (-ple′je-ah) paralysis of the lower part of the body including the legs. **paraple′gic,** adj.

parapraxia (par″ah-prak′se-ah) 1. irrational behavior. 2. inability to perform purposive movements properly.

parapraxis (-prak′sis) a lapse of memory or mental error, such as a slip of the tongue or misplacement of an object, which, in psychoanalytic theory, is due to unconscious associations and motives.

paraprotein (-pro′tēn, prōt′e-in) immunoglobulin produced by a clone of neoplastic plasma cells proliferating abnormally, e.g., myeloma proteins and cryoglobulins.

paraproteinemia (-pro″tēn-ēm′e-ah) presence in the blood of paraproteins.

parapsis (par-ap′sis) paraphia.

parapsoriasis (par″ah-sor-i′ah-sis) a group of slowly developing, persistent, maculopapular scaly erythrodermas, devoid of subjective symptoms and resistant to treatment.

paraquat (par′ah-qwat) a poisonous dipyridilium compound whose dichloride and dimethylsulfate salts are used as a contact herbicide. Contact with concentrated solutions causes irritation of the skin, cracking and shedding of the nails, and delayed healing of cuts and wounds. After ingestion of large doses, renal and hepatic failure may develop, followed by pulmonary insufficiency.

pararosaniline (-ro-zan′ĭ-lin) a basic dye; a triphenylmethane derivative, $HOC(C_6H_4NH_2)_3$, one of the components of basic fuchsin.

pararrhythmia (-rith′me-ah) parasystole.

parasexual (-sek′shoo-il) accomplished by other than sexual means, as by genetic study of *in vitro* somatic cell hybrids.

parasite (par′ah-sīt) 1. a plant or animal that lives upon or within another living organism at whose expense it obtains some advantage; see *symbiosis.* 2. the smaller, less complete member of asymmetrical conjoined twins, attached to and dependent upon the autosite. **parasit′ic,** adj. **malarial p.,** *Plasmodium.* **obligate p., obligatory p.,** one that is entirely dependent upon a host for its survival.

parasitemia (par″ah-si-te′me-ah) the presence of parasites, especially malarial forms, in the blood.

parasitism (par′ah-sīt″izm, -sit-izm) 1. symbiosis in which one population (or individual) adversely affects another, but cannot live without it. 2. infection or infestation with parasites.

parasitogenic (par″ah-sīt″ah-jen′ik) due to parasites.

parasitology (-si-tol′ah-je) the scientific study of parasites and parasitism.

parasitotropic (-sīt″ah-trop′ik) having an affinity for parasites.

paraspadias (-spa′de-as) a congenital condition in which the urethra opens on one side of the penis.

parasuicide (-soo′ĭ-sīd) an apparent attempt at suicide, as by self-poisoning or self-mutilation, in which death is not the desired outcome.

parasympathetic (-sim″pah-thet′ik) see under *system.*

parasympatholytic (-sim″pah-tho-lit′ik) anticholinergic: producing effects resembling those of interruption of the parasympathetic nerve supply of a part; having a destructive effect on the parasympathetic nerve fibers or blocking the transmission of impulses by them. Also, an agent that produces such effects.

parasympathomimetic (-mi-met′ik) producing effects resembling those of stimulation of the parasympathetic nerve supply of a part. Also, an agent that produces such effects.

parasynapsis (par″ah-sĭ-nap′sis) the union of chromosomes side by side during meiosis.

parasystole (-sis'tah-le) a cardiac irregularity attributed to the interaction of two foci independently initiating cardiac impulses at different rates.

paratenon (-ten'on) the fatty areolar tissue filling the interstices of the fascial compartment in which a tendon is situated.

parathion (-thi'on) an agricultural insecticide, $C_{10}H_{14}NO_5PS$, highly toxic to humans and animals.

parathormone (-thor'mōn) parathyroid hormone.

parathymia (-thi'me-ah) a perverted, contrary, or inappropriate mood.

parathyroid (-thi'roid) 1. see under *gland*. 2. a preparation containing parathyroid hormone from the parathyroid glands of animals; used for treatment and diagnosis of hypoparathyroidism.

parathyrotropic (-thi''ro-trop'ik) having an affinity for the parathyroid glands.

paratope (par'ah-tōp) the site on the antibody molecule that attaches to an antigen.

paratrophy (par-ă'trah-fe) dystrophy.

paratuberculosis (par''ah-too-burk''ūl-o'sis) 1. a tuberculosis-like disease not due to *Mycobacterium tuberculosis*. 2. Johne's disease.

paratyphoid (-ti'foid) infection due to *Salmonella* of all groups except *S. typhosa*.

paravaginitis (-vaj''in-īt'is) inflammation of the tissues alongside the vagina.

parazone (par'ah-zōn) one of the white bands alternating with dark bands (diazones) seen in cross section of a tooth.

paregoric (par''ĭ-gor'ik) a mixture of powdered opium, anise oil, benzoic acid, camphor, diluted alcohol, and glycerin; used as an antiperistaltic, especially in the treatment of diarrhea.

parenchyma (pah-reng'kĭ-mah) the essential or functional elements of an organ, as distinguished from its stroma or framework. **paren'chymal**, adj.

parenteral (pah-ren'ter-il) not through the alimentary canal, but rather by injection through some other route, as subcutaneous, intramuscular, etc.

parepididymis (par''ep-ĭ-did'ĭ-mis) paradidymis.

paresis (pah-re'sis, par'ĭ-sis) 1. slight or incomplete paralysis. 2. dementia paralytica. **paret'ic**, adj. **general p.**, dementia paralytica.

paresthesia (par''es-the'ze-ah) morbid or perverted sensation; an abnormal sensation, as burning, prickling, formication, etc.

pargyline (par'gĭ-lēn) an antihypertensive, $C_{11}H_{13}N$, used as the hydrochloride salt.

paries (pār'e-ez), pl. *pari'etes* [L.] a wall, as of an organ or cavity.

parietal (pah-ri'it'l) 1. of or pertaining to the walls of a cavity. 2. pertaining to or located near the parietal bone.

parietofrontal (pah-ri''it-o-front''l) pertaining to the parietal and frontal bones, gyri, or fissures.

parity (par'it-e) 1. para; the condition of a women with respect to having borne viable offspring. 2. equality; close correspondence or similarity.

parkinsonism (par'kin-sin-izm'') a group of neurological disorders marked by hypokinesia, tremor, and muscular rigidity; see *parkinsonian syndrome*, under *syndrome*, and see *paralysis agitans*. **parkinson'ian**, adj.

paroccipital (par''ok-sip'it'l) beside the occipital bone.

paromomycin (par'ah-mo-mi'sin) a broad-spectrum antibiotic derived from *Streptomyces rimosus* var. *paromomycinus*; the sulfate salt is used as an antiamebic.

paronychia (par''-ah-nik'e-ah) inflammation involving the folds of tissue around the fingernail.

paronychial (-ah-nik'e-il) pertaining to paronychia or to the nail folds.

paroophoron (-o-of'ah-ron) an inconstantly present, small group of coiled tubules between the layers of the mesosalpinx, being a remnant of the excretory part of the mesonephros.

parophthalmia (-of-thal'me-ah) inflammation of the connective tissue around the eye.

parorchidium (par''or-kid'e-im) displacement of a testis or testes.

parostosis (par''os-to'sis) ossification of tissues outside the periosteum.

parotid (pah-rot'id) near the ear.

parotiditis (pah-rot''ĭ-dīt'is) parotitis.

parotitis (par''o-tīt'is) inflammation of the parotid gland. **epidemic p.,** mumps.

parovarian (par''o-vār'e-in) 1. beside the ovary. 2. pertaining to the epoophoron.

paroxysm (par'ok-sizm) 1. a sudden recurrence or intensification of symptoms. 2. a spasm or seizure. **paroxys'mal**, adj.

pars (pars), pl. *par'tes* [L.] a division or part. **p. mastoi'dea,** the mastoid portion of the temporal bone, being the irregular, posterior part. **p. petro'sa,** the petrous portion of the temporal bone, containing the inner ear and located at the base of the cranium. **p. pla'na,** the thin part of the ciliary body; the ciliary disk. **p. squamo'sa,** the flat scalelike, anterior and superior portion of the temporal bone. **p. tympa'nica,** the part of the temporal bone forming the anterior and inferior walls and part of the posterior wall of the external acoustic meatus.

pars planitis (pars pla-ni'tis) granulomatous uveitis of the pars plana of the ciliary body.

particle (part'ik'l) a tiny mass of material. **Dane p.,** an intact hepatitis B viral particle. **elementary p's of mitochondria,** numerous minute, club-shaped granules with spherical heads attached to the inner membrane of a mitochondrion. **viral p.,** virion.

partitioning (par-tish'un-ing) dividing into parts. **gastric p.,** a form of gastroplasty in which a small stomach pouch is formed whose filling signals satiety; used in the treatment of morbid obesity.

parturient (par-tūr'e-int) giving birth or pertaining to birth; by extension, a woman in labor.

parturiometer (par-tūr″e-om′it-er) device used in measuring expulsive power of the uterus.

parturition (part″ah-rish′in) the act or process of giving birth to a child; see *labor.*

parulis (pah-roo′lis) a subperiosteal abscess of the gum.

parvicellular (par″vĭ-sel′ūl-er) composed of small cells.

parvovirus (par″vo-vi′ris) a group of extremely small, morphologically similar, ether-resistant DNA viruses, including the adeno-associated viruses.

PAS, PASA para-aminosalicylic acid.

pascal (pas-kal′, pas′kal) the SI unit of pressure, which corresponds to a force of one newton per square meter; symbol, Pa.

pastern (pas′tern) the part of a horse's foot occupied by the first and second phalanges.

Pasteurella (pas″ter-el′ah) a genus of gram-negative bacteria (family Pasteurellaceae), including *P. multo′cida,* the etiologic agent of the hemorrhagic septicemias.

pasteurellosis (pas″ter-il-o′sis) infection with organisms of the genus *Pasteurella.*

pasteurization (pas″cher-ĭ-za′shin) heating of milk and other liquids to moderate temperature for a definite time, often 60° C. for 30 min., which kills most pathogenic bacteria and considerably delays other bacterial development.

patch (pach) a small area differing from the rest of a surface. **Peyer's p's,** oval elevated patches of closely packed lymph follicles on the mucosa of the small intestines.

patella (pah-tel′ah), pl. *patel′lae* [L.] see *Table of Bones.* **patel′lar,** adj.

patellectomy (pat″il-ek′tah-me) excision of the patella.

patent (pāt′nt) 1. open, unobstructed, or not closed. 2. apparent, evident.

path(o)- word element [Gr.], *disease.*

pathergy (path′er-je) 1. a condition in which the application of a stimulus leaves the organism unduly susceptible to subsequent stimuli of a different kind. 2. a condition of being allergic to numerous antigens. **pather′gic,** adj.

pathfinder (path′fīnd″er) 1. an instrument for locating urethral strictures. 2. a dental instrument for tracing the course of root canals.

pathoanatomical (path″o-an″ah-tom′ik′l) pertaining to the anatomy of diseased tissues.

pathobiology (-bi-ol′ah-je) pathology.

pathoclisis (-klis′is) a specific sensitivity to specific toxins, or a specific affinity of certain toxins for certain systems or organs.

pathogen (path′ah-jen) any disease-producing agent or microorganism. **pathogen′ic,** adj.

pathogenesis (path″ah-jen′ĭ-sis) the development of morbid conditions or of disease; more specifically the cellular events and reactions and other pathologic mechanisms occurring in the development of disease. **pathogenet′ic,** adj.

pathognomonic (path″ug-no-mon′ik) specifically distinctive or characteristic of a disease or pathologic condition; denoting a sign or symptom on which a diagnosis can be made.

pathologic (path″ah-loj′ik) 1. indicative of or caused by some morbid condition. 2. pertaining to pathology.

pathology (pah-thol′ah-je) 1. that branch of medicine treating of the essential nature of disease, especially of the changes in body tissues and organs which cause or are caused by disease. 2. the structural and functional manifestations of disease. **cellular p.,** that which regards the cells as starting points of the phenomena of disease and which recognizes that every cell descends from some preexisting cell. **clinical p.,** pathology applied to the solution of clinical problems, especially the use of laboratory methods in clinical diagnosis. **comparative p.,** that which considers human disease processes in comparison with those of the lower animals. **oral p.,** that treating of conditions causing or resulting from morbid anatomic or functional changes in the structures of the mouth. **speech p.,** a field of the health sciences dealing with the evaluation of speech, language, and voice disorders and the rehabilitation of patients with such disorders not amenable to medical or surgical treatment. **surgical p.,** the pathology of disease processes that are surgically accessible for diagnosis or treatment.

pathomimesis (path″o-mi-me′sis) malingering.

pathomorphism (-mor′fizm) perverted or abnormal morphology.

pathophysiology (-fiz″e-ol′ah-je) the physiology of disordered function.

pathopsychology (-si-kol′ah-je) the psychology of mental disease.

pathosis (pah-tho′sis) a diseased condition.

pathway (path′wa) a course usually followed. In neurology, the nerve structures through which a sensory impression is conducted to the cerebral cortex (*afferent p.*) or through which an impulse passes from the brain to the skeletal musculature (*efferent p.*). Also used alone to indicate a sequence of reactions that convert one biological material to another (*metabolic p.*). **amphibolic p.,** a group of metabolic reactions providing small metabolites for further metabolism to end products or for use as precursors in synthetic, anabolic reactions. **Embden-Meyerhof p.** (of glucose metabolism), the series of enzymatic reactions in the anaerobic conversion of glucose to lactic acid, resulting in energy in the form of adenosine triphosphate (ATP). **properidin p.,** alternative complement p.

-pathy word element [Gr.], *morbid condition* or *disease;* generally used to designate a noninflammatory condition.

patrilineal (pat″rĭ-lin′e-il) descended through the male line.

patulous (pach′il-is) spread widely apart; open; distended.

pauci- word element [L.], *few.* Cf. *olig(o).*

paucisynaptic (paw″se-sin-ap′tik) oligosynaptic.

pause (pawz) an interruption, or rest. **compensatory p.,** the pause after a premature ventricular systole, related to blockage of one beat of the basic pacemaker.

pavor (pa′vor) [L.] terror. **p. noctur′nus,** a

nightmare of children causing them to cry out in fright and awake in panic.

Pb chemical symbol, *lead* (L. *plumbum*).

PBI protein-bound iodine.

p.c. [L.] *post ci'bum* (after meals).

PCO₂ carbon dioxide partial pressure or tension; also written P_{CO_2}, pCO_2, or pCO_2.

PCV packed-cell volume.

Pd chemical symbol, *palladium.*

pearl (purl) 1. a small medicated granule, or a glass globule with a single dose of volatile medicine, such as amyl nitrite. 2. a rounded mass of tough sputum as seen in the early stages of an attack of bronchial asthma. **epidermic p's, epithelial p's,** rounded concentric masses of epithelial cells found in certain papillomas and epitheliomas. **Laennec's p's,** soft casts of the smaller bronchial tubes expectorated in bronchial asthma.

pecten (pek'tin), pl. *pec'tines* [L.] 1. a comb; in anatomy, applied to certain comblike structures. 2. a narrow zone in the anal canal, bounded above by the pectinate line. **p. os'sis pu'bis,** pectineal line.

pectenosis (pek″tin-o'sis) stenosis of the anal canal due to an inelastic ring of tissue between the anal groove and anal crypts.

pectin (pek'tin) a homosaccharidic polymer of sugar acids of fruit that forms gels with sugar at the proper pH; a purified form obtained from the acid extract of the rind of citrus fruits or from apple pomace is used as a protectant and in cooking. **pec'tic,** adj.

pectinate (pek'tĭ-nāt) comb-shaped.

pectineal (pek-tin'e-il) pertaining to the os pubis.

pectiniform (pek-tin'ĭ-form) comb-shaped.

pectoral (pek'ter-il) 1. of or pertaining to the breast or chest. 2. relieving disorders of the respiratory tract, as an expectorant.

pectoralis (pek″tah-ra'lis) [L.] pertaining to the chest or breast.

pectus (pek'tis) the breast, chest, or thorax. **p. carina'tum,** pigeon breast. **p. excava'tum,** funnel chest.

ped(o)- word element, (1) [Gr.], *child*; (2) [L.], *foot.*

pedal (ped'l) pertaining to the foot or feet.

pederasty (ped″er-as'te) homosexual anal intercourse between men and boys with the latter as passive partners.

pediatrics (pe″de-at'riks) that branch of medicine dealing with the child and its development and care and with the diseases of children and their treatment. **pediat'ric,** adj.

pedicel (ped'ĭsil) a footlike part, especially any of the secondary processes of a podocyte.

pedicellation (ped″ĭ-sil-a'shin) the development of a pedicle.

pedicle (ped'ik'l) a footlike, stemlike, or narrow basal part or structure.

pedicular (pĭ-dik'ūl-er) pertaining to or caused by lice.

pediculation (pĭ-dik″ūl-a'shin) 1. the process of forming a pedicle. 2. infestation with lice.

pediculicide (pĭ-dik'ūl-ĭ-sīd) 1. destroying lice. 2. an agent that destroys lice.

pediculosis (pĭ-dik″ūl-o'sis) infestation with lice of the family Pediculidae, especially infestation with *Pediculus humanus.*

pediculous (pĭ-dik'ūl-is) infested with lice.

Pediculus (pĭ-dik'ūl-is) a genus of lice. *P. huma'-nus,* a species feeding on human blood, is a major vector of typhus, trench fever, and relapsing fever; two subspecies are recognized: *P. huma'-nus* var. *capitis* (head louse) found on the scalp hair, and *P. huma'nus* var. *corporis* (body, or clothes, louse) found on the body.

pediculus (pĭ-dik'ūl-is), pl. *pedi'culi* [L.] pedicle.

pedigree (ped'ĭ-gre') a table, chart, diagram, or list of an individual's ancestors, used in genetics in the analysis of mendelian inheritance.

peditis (pĭ-dit'is) pedal osteitis.

pedodontics (-don'tiks) that branch of dentistry dealing with the teeth and mouth conditions of children.

pedophilia (-fil'e-ah) 1. abnormal fondness for children; sexual activity of adults with children. 2. a sexual perversion in which there are intense, recurrent urges or phantasies of engaging in sex with a prepubertal child. *pedophilic,* adj.

pedorthics (pi-dor'thiks) the design, manufacture, fitting, and modification of shoes and related foot appliances as prescribed for the amelioration of painful or disabling conditions of the foot and leg. **pedor'thic,** adj.

peduncle (pe-dunk″l) a stemlike connecting part, especially, (*a*) a collection of nerve fibers coursing between different areas in the central nervous system, or (*b*) the stalk by which a nonsessile tumor is attached to normal tissue. **pedun'cular,** adj. **cerebellar p's,** three sets of paired bundles of the hindbrain (*superior, middle,* and *inferior*) connecting the cerebellum to the midbrain, pons, and medulla oblongata, respectively. **cerebral p.,** the ventral half of the midbrain, divisible into a dorsal part (*tegmentum*) and a ventral part (*crus cerebri*), which are separated by the substantia nigra. **pineal p.,** habenula (2).

pedunculotomy (pĭ-dunk″ūl-ot'ah-me) incision of a cerebral peduncle.

pedunculus (pĭ-dunk'ūl-is) [L.] peduncle.

peg (peg) a projecting structure. **rete p's,** inward projections of the epidermis into the dermis, as seen histologically in verticle sections.

pelage (pel'ij, pĕ-lahzh') [Fr.] the hairy coat of mammals; hairs of the body, limbs, and head collectively.

peliosis (pe″le-o'sis) purpura. **p. he'patis,** mottled blue liver, due to blood-filled lacunae in the parenchyma.

pellagra (pah-la'grah, pah-lag'rah) a syndrome due to niacin deficiency or failure to convert tryptophan to niacin), marked by dermatitis on parts of the body exposed to light or trauma, inflammation of the mucous membranes, diarrhea, and psychic disturbances. **pellag'rous,** adj.

pellagroid (pah-lag'roid) resembling pellagra.

pellicle (pel′ik′l) a thin scum forming on the surface of liquids.

pellucid (pel-oo′sid) translucent.

pelvicaliceal, pelvicalyceal (pel″ve-kal″ĭ-se-il) pertaining to the renal pelves and calices.

pelvicephalometry (-sef″ah-lom″ĭ-tre) measurement of the fetal head in relation to the maternal pelvis.

pelvifixation (-fik-sa′shin) surgical fixation of a displaced pelvic organ.

pelvimetry (pel-vim′ĭ-tre) measurement of the capacity and diameter of the pelvis.

pelviotomy (pel″ve-ot′ah-me) 1. incision or transection of a pelvic bone. 2. pyelotomy.

pelvis (pel′vis), pl. *pel′ves*. The lower (caudal) portion of the trunk of the body, bounded anteriorly and laterally by the hip bones and posteriorly by the sacrum and coccyx. Also applied to any basin-like structure, e.g., the renal pelvis. **pel′vic**, adj. **android p.**, one with a wedge-shaped inlet and narrow anterior segment, typically found in the male. **anthropoid p.**, one in which the anteroposterior diameter of the inlet equals or exceeds the transverse diameter. **assimilation p.**, one in which the ilia articulate with the vertebral column higher (*high assimilation p.*) or lower (*low assimilation p.*) than normal, the number of lumbar vertebrae being correspondingly decreased or increased. **beaked p.**, one with the pelvic bones laterally compressed and their anterior junction pushed forward. **brachypellic p.**, one in which the transverse diameter exceeds the anteroposterior diameter by 1 to 3 cm. **contracted p.**, one showing a decrease of 1.5 to 2 cm. in any important diameter; when all dimensions are proportionately diminished it is a *generally contracted p.* **dolichopellic p.**, an elongated pelvis, the anteroposterior diameter being greater than the transverse diameter. **false p.**, the part of the pelvis superior to a plane passing through the ileopectineal lines. **flat p.**, one in which the anteroposterior dimension is abnormally reduced. **funnel p.**, one with a normal inlet but a greatly narrowed outlet. **gynecoid p.**, the normal female pelvis: a rounded oval pelvis with well-rounded anterior and posterior segments. **p. jus′to ma′jor**, an unusually large gynecoid pelvis, with all dimensions increased. **p. jus′to mi′nor**, a small gynecoid pelvis, with all dimensions symmetrically reduced. **juvenile p.**, infantile p. **p. ma′jor**, false p. **mesatipellic p.**, one in which the transverse diameter is equal to the anteroposterior diameter or exceeds it by no more than 1 cm. **p. mi′nor**, true p. **Nägele's p.**, one contracted in an oblique diameter, with complete ankylosis of the sacroiliac synchondrosis of one side and imperfect development of the sacrum and coxa on the same side. **platy-pellic p., platypelloid p.**, one shortened in the anteroposterior aspect, with a flattened transverse, oval shape. **rachitic p.**, one distorted as a result of rickets. **renal p.**, the funnel-shaped expansion of the upper end of the ureter into which the renal calices open; it is usually within the renal sinus, but under certain conditions, a large part of it may be outside the kidney (*extrarenal p.*). **Robert's p.**, a transversely

contracted pelvis caused by osteoarthritis affecting both sacroiliac joints, the inlet becoming a narrow wedge. **scoliotic p.**, one deformed as a result of scoliosis. **split p.**, one with a congenital separation at the symphysis pubis. **spondylolisthetic p.**, one in which the last, or rarely the fourth or third, lumbar vertebra is dislocated in front of the sacrum, more or less occluding the pelvic brim. **true p.**, the part of the pelvis inferior to a plane passing through the ileopectineal lines.

pelvospondylitis (pel″vo-spon″dĭ-līt′is) inflammation of the pelvic portion of the spine. **p. ossi′ficans**, rheumatoid spondylitis.

pemoline (pem′ah-lēn) a central nervous system stimulant, $C_9H_8N_2O_2$.

pemphigoid (pem′fĭ-goid) 1. resembling pemphigus. 2. a group of dermatological syndromes similar to but clearly distinguishable from the pemphigus group.

pemphigus (pem′fĭ-gus) 1. a distinctive group of diseases marked by successive crops of bullae. 2. p. vulgaris. **benign familial p.**, a hereditary, recurrent vesiculobullous dermatitis, usually involving the axillae, groin, and neck, with crops of lesions that regress over several weeks or months. **p. erythemato′sus**, a chronic form in which the lesions, limited to the face and chest, resemble those of disseminated lupus erythematosus. **p. folia′ceus**, a chronic, generalized, vesicular and scaling eruption somewhat resembling dermatitis herpetiformis or, later in its course, exfoliative dermatitis. **p. ve′getans**, a variant of pemphigus vulgaris in which the bullae are replaced by verrucoid hypertrophic vegetative masses. **p. vulga′ris**, a rare relapsing disease with suprabasal, intraepidermal bullae of the skin and mucous membranes; invariably fatal if untreated.

pendelluft (pen′del-looft) the movement of air back and forth between the lungs, resulting in increased dead space ventilation.

pendulous (pen′jil-is, pen′dūl-is) hanging loosely; dependent.

penetrance (pen′ĭ-trins) the frequency with which a heritable trait is manifested by individuals carrying the principal gene or genes conditioning it.

penetrometer (pen″ĭ-trom′it-er) an instrument for measuring the penetrating power of x-rays.

-penia word element [Gr.], *deficiency.*

penicillamine (pen″ĭ-sil-am′in) a product of penicillin, $C_5H_{11}NO_2S$, which chelates copper and other metals; used mainly to remove excess copper from the body in hepatolenticular degeneration.

penicillic acid (pen-ĭ-sil′ik) an antibiotic substance, $C_8H_{10}O_4$, isolated from cultures of various species of *Penicillium* and *Aspergillus*.

penicillin (pen″ĭ-sil′in) any of a large group of natural or semisynthetic antibacterial antibiotics derived directly or indirectly from strains of fungi of the genus *Penicillium* and other soil-inhabiting fungi, which exert a bacteriocidal as well as a bacteriostatic effect on susceptible bacteria by interfering with the final stages of the synthesis of peptidoglycan, a substance in the bacterial cell wall. The penicillins, despite their relatively low toxicity for the host, are active against many bacteria, especially gram-positive pathogens (streptococci, staphylococci, pneumococci); clostridia; some gram-negative forms (gonococci, meningococci); some spirochetes (*Treponema pallidum* and *T. pertenue*); and some fungi. Certain strains of some target species, e.g., staphylococci, secrete the enzyme penicillinase, which inactivates penicillin and confers resistance to the antibiotic.

penicillinase (pen″ĭ-sil′ĭ-nās) an enzyme produced by certain bacteria which inactivates penicillin, thus increasing resistance to the antibiotic; a purified form from *Bacillus cereus* is used in the treatment reactions to penicillin.

Penicillium (-sil′e-im) a genus of fungi.

penicilloyl-polylysine (pen″ĭ-sil′oil-pol″ĭ-li′-sēn) an agent prepared from polylysine and a penicillenic acid; intradermal reaction elicits a wheal and erythema response in those sensitive to penicillin.

penicillus (pen″ĭ-sil′is), pl. *penicil′li* [L.] any of the brushlike groups of arterial branches in the lobules of the spleen.

penile (pe′nīl) of or pertaining to the penis.

penis (pe′nis) the male organ of urination and copulation.

penitis (pe-nīt′is) inflammation of the penis.

penniform (pen′ĭ-form) shaped like a feather.

pent(a)- word element [Gr.], *five.*

pentaerythritol (pen″tah-ĭ-rith′rĭ-tol″) an alcohol, $(CH_2OH)_4C$, used in the form of the tetranitrate ester as a vasodilator in the treatment of angina pectoris.

pentagastrin (-gas′trin) a synthetic pentapeptide consisting of β-alanine and the C-terminal tetrapeptide of gastrin; used as a test of gastric secretory function.

pentazocine (pen-taz′ah-sēn) a synthetic narcotic, $C_{27}H_{27}NO$, used as an analgesic.

pentetic acid (pen-tēt′ik) diethylenetriaminepentaacetic acid.

pentobarbital (pen″tah-bar′bĭ-tal) a short- to intermediate-acting barbiturate, $C_{11}H_{17}N_2O_3$; the sodium salt is used as a hypnotic and sedative.

pentose (pen′tōs) a monosaccharide containing five carbon atoms in a molecule.

pentosuria (pen″tōs-ūr′e-ah) a benign inborn error of metabolism due to a defect in the activity of the enzyme L-xylulose dehydrogenase, resulting in high levels of L-xylulose in the urine.

pentylenetetrazol (pen″tĭ-lēn-tē′trah-zol) a convulsant analeptic, $C_6H_{10}N_4$.

peotillomania (pe″o-til″o-ma′ne-ah) constant but nonmasturbatory, pulling at the penis.

peplomer (pep′lo-mer) a subunit of a peplos.

peplos (pep′lohs) the lipoprotein envelope of some types of virions, assembled in some cases from subunits (peplomers).

pepsin (pep′sin) the proteolytic enzyme of gastric juice which catalyzes the hydrolysis of native or denatured proteins to form a mixture of polypeptides; it is formed from pepsinogen in

the presence of acid or, autocatalytically, in the presence of pepsin.

pepsinogen (pep-sin′ah-jin) a zymogen secreted by the chief cells of the gastric glands and converted into pepsin in the presence of gastric acid or of pepsin itself.

peptic (pep′tik) pertaining to pepsin or to digestion or to the action of gastric juices.

peptidase (pep′tĭ-dās) any of a subclass of proteolytic enzymes that catalyze the hydrolysis of peptide linkages.

peptide (pep′tīd, pep′tid) any of a class of compounds of low molecular weight which yield two or more amino acids on hydrolysis; known as di-, tri-, tetra-, (etc.) peptides, depending on the number of amino acids in the molecule. Peptides form the constituent parts of proteins.

peptidergic (pep″tĭ-der′jik) of or pertaining to neurons that secrete peptide hormones.

peptidoglycan (-gli′kan) a glycan (polysaccharide) attached to short cross-linked peptides; found in bacterial cell walls.

peptogenic (pep″tah-jen′ik) 1. producing pepsin or peptones. 2. promoting digestion.

peptolysis (pep-tol′ĭ-sis) the splitting up of peptones. **peptolyt′ic,** adj.

peptone (pep′tōn) a derived protein, or a mixture of cleavage products produced by partial hydrolysis of native protein. **pepton′ic,** adj.

peptotoxin (pep″to-tok′sin) any toxin or poisonous base developed from a peptone; also, a poisonous alkaloid or ptomaine occurring in certain peptones and putrefying proteins.

per- word element [L.], (1) *throughout; completely; extremely;* (2) in chemistry, *a large amount; combination of an element in its highest valence.*

peracid (per-as′id) an acid containing more than the usual quantity of oxygen.

peracute (per″ah-kūt′) very acute.

per anum (per a′num) [L.] through the anus.

percept (per′sept″) the object perceived; the mental image of an object in space perceived by the senses.

perception (per-sep′shin) the conscious mental registration of a sensory stimulus. **percep′tive,** adj.

perceptivity (per″sep-tiv′it-e) ability to receive sense impressions.

perchloric acid (per-klor′ik) a colorless volatile liquid, $HClO_4$, which can cause powerful explosions in the presence of organic matter or anything reducible.

percolate (per′kah-lāt) 1. to strain; to submit to percolation. 2. to trickle slowly through a substance. 3. a liquid that has been submitted to percolation.

percolation (per″kah-la′shin) the extraction of soluble parts of a drug by passing a solvent liquid through it.

percussion (per-kush′in) the act of striking a part with short, sharp blows as an aid in diagnosing the condition of the underlying parts by the sound obtained. **auscultatory p.,** auscultation of the sound produced by percussion. **immediate p.,** that in which the blow is struck directly against the body surface. **mediate p.,** that in which a pleximeter is used. **palpatory p.,** a combination of palpation and percussion, affording tactile rather than auditory impressions.

percussor (per-kus′or) an instrument for performing percussion.

percutaneous (per″ku-ta′ne-us) performed through the skin.

perencephaly (per″en-sef′ah-le) porencephaly.

perforans (per′fo-rans) [L.] penetrating; applied to various muscles and nerves.

perfusate (per-fu′zāt) a liquid that has been subjected to perfusion.

perfusion (per-fu′zhin) 1. the act of pouring over or through, especially the passage of a fluid through the vessels of a specific organ. 2. a liquid poured over or through an organ or tissue.

peri- word element [Gr.], *around; near.* See also words beginning *para-*.

periacinal, periacinous (per″e-as′ĭ-nil; -as′ĭ-nis) around an acinus.

periadenitis (-ad″′n-īt′is) inflammation of tissues around a gland. **p. muco′sa necro′tica recur′rens,** the more severe form of aphthous stomatitis, marked by recurrent attacks of aphtha-like lesions that begin as small, firm nodules, which enlarge, ulcerate, and heal by scar formation, leaving numerous atrophied scars on the oral mucosa.

periampullary (-am′pūl-ĕ-re) situated around an ampulla.

periapical (-a′pĭ-kil) surrounding the apex of the root of a tooth.

periappendicitis (-ah-pen″dĭ-sīt′is) inflammation of the tissues around the vermiform appendix.

periarteritis (-ar″ter-īt′is) inflammation of the outer coat of an artery and of the tissues around it.

periarthritis (-ar-thrīt′is) inflammation of tissues around a joint.

periarticular (-ar-tik′ūl-er) around a joint.

periblast (per′ĭ-blast) the portion of the blastoderm of telolecithal eggs, the cells of which lack complete cell membranes.

peribronchiolitis (-bronk″e-o-līt′is) inflammation of tissues around the bronchioles.

peribronchitis (-bronk-īt′is) a form of bronchitis consisting of inflammation and thickening of the tissues around the bronchi.

pericaliceal, pericalyceal (-kal″′ĭ-se′il) situated near to or around a renal calix.

pericallosal (-kah-lo′sil) situated around the corpus callosum.

pericardiectomy (-kar″de-ek′tah-me) excision of a portion of the pericardium.

pericardiocentesis (-kar″de-o-sen-te′sis) surgical puncture of the pericardial cavity for the aspiration of fluid.

pericardiolysis (-kar″de-ol′ĭ-sis) the operative freeing of adhesions between the visceral and parietal pericardium.

pericardiophrenic (-kar″de-o-fren′ik) pertaining to the pericardium and diaphragm.

pericardiorrhaphy (per″ĭ-kar″de-or′ah-fe) suture of the pericardium.

pericardiostomy (-kar″de-os′tah-me) creation of an opening into the pericardium, usually for the drainage of effusions.

pericardiotomy (-kar″de-ot′ah-me) incision of the pericardium.

pericarditis (-kar-dīt′is) inflammation of the pericardium. **pericardit′ic,** adj. **adhesive p.,** a condition due to the presence of dense fibrous tissue between the parietal and visceral layers of the pericardium. **constrictive p.,** pericarditis leading to thickening and sometimes calcification, with impaired diastolic filling, inflow stasis, or constrictive effect. **fibrinous p., fibrous p.,** chronic pericarditis with formation of fibrous tissue and probably adhesions. **p. obli′terans, obliterating p.,** adhesive pericarditis that leads to obliteration of the pericardial cavity.

pericardium (-kar′de-im) the fibroserous sac enclosing the heart and the roots of the great vessels. **pericar′dial,** adj. **adherent p.,** one abnormally connected with the heart by dense fibrous tissue.

pericecitis (-se-sīt′is) inflammation of the tissues around the cecum.

pericementitis (-se″men-tīt′is) periodontitis.

pericholangitis (-ko″lan-jīt′is) inflammation of the tissues around the bile ducts.

pericholecystitis (-ko″le-sis-tīt′is) inflammation of tissues around the gallbladder.

perichondrium (-kon′dre-im) the layer of fibrous connective tissue investing all cartilage except the articular cartilage of synovial joints. **perichon′dral,** adj.

perichordal (-kord′l) surrounding the notochord.

perichoroidal (-ko-roid′l) surrounding the choroid coat.

pericolitis, pericolonitis (-kol-i′tis; -kol″on-īt′is) inflammation around the colon, especially of its peritoneal coat.

pericolpitis (-kol-pīt′is) inflammation of tissues around the vagina.

pericoronal (-kŏ-ro′nil) around the crown of a tooth.

pericranitis (-kra-nīt′is) inflammation of the pericranium.

pericranium (-kra′ne-im) the periosteum of the skull. **pericra′nial,** adj.

pericyte (per′ĭ-sīt) one of the peculiar elongated, contractile cells found wrapped about precapillary arterioles outside the basement membrane.

pericytial (per″ĭ-si′shil) around a cell.

periderm (per′ĭ-durm) the outer layer of the bilaminar fetal epidermis, generally disappearing before birth. **periderm′al,** adj.

peridesmium (-dez′me-im) the areolar membrane that covers the ligaments.

perididymis (-did′ĭ-mis) tunica vaginalis.

perididymitis (-did″ĭ-mīt′is) inflammation of the tunica vaginalis.

peridiverticulitis (-di″ver-tik″ūl-īt′is) inflammation around an intestinal diverticulum.

periduodenitis (-du″od′n-īt′is) inflammation around the duodenum.

periencephalitis (per″e-en-sef′ah-līt′is) inflammation of the surface of the brain.

perienteritis (-en″ter-īt′is) inflammation of the peritoneal coat of the intestines.

periesophagitis (-e-sof″ah-jīt′is) inflammation of tissues around the esophagus.

perifolliculitis (-fah-lik″ūl-īt′is) inflammation around the hair follicles.

perigangliitis (-gang″gle-īt′is) inflammation of tissues around a ganglion.

perigastritis (-gas-trīt′is) inflammation of the peritoneal coat of stomach.

perihepatitis (-hep″ah-tīt′is) inflammation of the peritoneal capsule of the liver and the surrounding tissue.

peri-islet (per″e-i′lit) situated around the islets of Langerhans.

perijejunitis (per″ĭ-je″joo-nīt′is) inflammation around the jejunum.

perikaryon (-kar′e-on) the cell body of a neuron.

perilabyrinthitis (-lab″ĭ-rin-thīt′is) inflammation of tissues around the labyrinth.

perilaryngitis (-lar″in-jīt′is) inflammation of tissues around the larynx.

perilymph, perilympha (per′ĭ-limf; per″ĭ-lim′fah) the fluid within the space separating the membranous and osseous labyrinth of the ear.

perilymphangitis (per″ĭ-lim″fan-jīt′is) inflammation around a lymphatic vessel.

perimeningitis (-men″in-jīt′is) pachymeningitis.

perimetrium (pe″rĭ-me′tre-im) the serous membrane enveloping the uterus.

perimyelitis (pe″rĭ-mi″il-īt′is) inflammation of (a) the pia of the spinal cord, or (b) the endosteum.

perimyositis (-mi″ah-sīt′is) inflammation of connective tissue around a muscle.

perimysiitis (-mis″e-īt′is) inflammation of the perimysium; myofibrositis.

perimysium (-mis′e-um) the connective tissue demarcating a fascicle of skeletal muscle fibers. See Plate XIV. **perimys′ial,** adj.

perinatal (-nāt′l) relating to the period shortly before and after birth; from the twentieth to twenty-ninth week of gestation to one to four weeks after birth.

perinatology (-na-tol′ah-je) the branch of medicine (obstetrics and pediatrics) dealing with the fetus and infant during the perinatal period.

perineal (-ne′il) pertaining to the perineum.

perineocele (-ne′ah-sēl) a hernia between the rectum and the prostate or between the rectum and the vagina.

perineoplasty (-ne′ah-plas″te) plastic repair of the perineum.

perineorrhaphy (-ne-or′ah-fe) suture of the perineum.

perineotomy (-ne-ot′ah-me) incision of the perineum.

perineovaginal (-ne″ah-vaj′ĭ-nil) pertaining to or communicating with the perineum and vagina.

perinephritis (-ně-frīt′is) inflammation of the perinephrium.

perinephrium (-nef′re-im) the peritoneal envelope and other tissues around the kidney. **perineph′rial,** adj.

perineum (-ne′im) 1. the pelvic floor and associated structures occupying the pelvic outlet, bounded anteriorly by the pubic symphysis, laterally by the ischial tuberosities, and posteriorly by the coccyx. 2. the region between the thighs, bounded in the male by the scrotum and anus and in the female by the vulva and anus.

perineuritis (-nōōr-īt′is) inflammation of the perineurium.

perineurium (-nōōr′e-im) the sheath surrounding each bundle of fibers in a peripheral nerve. See Plate XI. **perineu′rial,** adj.

period (pēr′e-id) an interval or division of time. **latency p.,** 1. latent p. 2. in psychoanalytic theory, the period, usually between 5 years of age and adolescence, of relative quiescence in psychosexual development, with a cessation of interest in persons of the opposite sex and a tendency to associate mainly with persons of one's own sex. **latent p.,** a seemingly inactive period, as that between exposure of tissue to an injurious agent and the manifestations of response, or that between the instant of stimulation and the beginning of response. **postsphygmic p.,** the short period (0.08 second) of ventricular diastole, after the sphygmic period, and lasting until the atrioventricular valves open. **presphygmic p.,** the first phase of ventricular systole, being the period (0.04–0.06 sec.) immediately after closure of the atrioventricular valves and lasting until the semilunar valves open. **refractory p.,** the period of depolarization and repolarization of the cell membrane after excitation; during the first portion (*absolute refractory p.*), the nerve or muscle fiber cannot respond to a second stimulus, whereas during the *relative refractory period,* it can respond only to a strong stimulus. **sphygmic p.,** the second phase of ventricular systole (0.21–0.30 sec.), between the opening and closing of the semilunar valves, while the blood is discharged into the aorta and pulmonary artery. **Wenckebach p.,** a usually repetitive sequence seen in partial heart block, marked by progressive lengthening of the P-R interval until ventricular response occurs.

periodicity (pēr″e-ah-dis′it-e) recurrence at regular intervals of time.

periodontics (-don′tiks) the branch of dentistry dealing with the study and treatment of diseases of the periodontium.

periodontitis (-don-tīt′is) inflammation of the periodontium.

periodontium (-don′she-im), pl. *periodon′tia.* the tissues investing and supporting the teeth, including the cementum, periodontal ligament, alveolar bone, and gingiva. In NA, restricted to the periodontal ligament.

periodontosis (-don-to′sis) a degenerative disorder of the periodontal structures, marked by tissue destruction.

perionychium (-o-nik'e-um) the epidermis bordering a nail.

perioophoritis (-o''of-or-īt'is) inflammation of tissues around the ovary.

perioophorosalpingitis (-o-of''or-o-sal''pin-jīt'is) inflammation of tissues around an ovary and uterine tube.

perioperative (-op'er-it-iv) pertaining to the period extending from the time of hospitalization for surgery to the time of discharge.

periophthalmic (-of-thal'mik) around the eye.

periople (pĕ're-o''p'l) the smooth, shiny layer on the outer surface of the hoofs of ungulates.

perioptometry (per''e-op-tom'ĭ-tre) measurement of acuity of peripheral vision or of limits of the visual field.

periorbita (-or'bit-ah) periosteum of the bones of the orbit, or eye socket. **perior'bital,** adj.

periorbitis (-or-bīt'is) inflammation of the periorbita.

periorchitis (-or-kīt'is) vaginalitis.

periosteitis (-os''te-it'is) periostitis.

periosteoma (-os-te-o'mah) a morbid bony growth surrounding a bone.

periosteomyelitis (-os''te-o-mi''il-īt'is) inflammation of the entire bone, including periosteum and marrow.

periosteophyte (-os'te-ah-fīt'') a bony growth on the periosteum.

periosteotomy (-os''te-ot'ah-me) incision of the periosteum.

periosteum (-os'te-im) a specialized connective tissue covering all bones and having bone-forming potentialities. **perios'teal,** adj.

periostitis (-os-tīt'is) inflammation of the periosteum.

periostosis (-os-to'sis) abnormal deposition of periosteal bone; the condition manifested by development of periosteomas.

periotic (-ōt'ik) 1. situated about the ear, especially the internal ear. 2. the petrous and mastoid portions of the temporal bone, at one stage a distinct bone.

peripachymeningitis (per''ĭ-pak''ĭ-men''in-jīt'is) inflammation of tissue between the dura mater and its bony covering.

peripapillary (-pap'ĭ-lĕ''re) around the optic papilla.

peripartum (-part'im) occurring during the last month of gestation or the first few months after delivery, with reference to the mother.

periphacitis (-fah-sīt'is) inflammation of the capsule of the eye lens.

peripherad (per-if'er-ad) toward the periphery.

periphery (per-if'er-e) an outward surface or structure; the portion of a system outside the central region. **periph'eral,** adj.

periphlebitis (pĕ''rĭ-flĭ-bīt'is) inflammation of tissues around a vein, or of the external coat of a vein.

periplasmic (-plas'mik) around the plasma membrane; between the plasma membrane and the cell wall of a bacterium.

periproctitis (-prok-tīt'is) inflammation of tissues around the rectum and anus.

periprostatitis (-pros''tah-tīt is) inflammation of tissues around the prostate.

peripylephlebitis (-pi''le-flĕ-bīt'is) inflammation of tissues around the portal vein.

perirectitis (-rek-tīt'is) periproctitis.

perisalpingitis (-sal''pin-jīt'is) inflammation of tissues around the uterine tube.

perisigmoiditis (-sig''moid-īt'is) inflammation of the peritoneum of the sigmoid flexure.

perisinusitis (-si''nis-īt'is) inflammation of tissues about a sinus.

perispermatitis (-spurm''ah-tīt'is) inflammation of tissues about the spermatic cord.

perisplanchnitis (-splank-nīt'is) inflammation of tissues around the viscera.

perisplenitis (-splin-īt'is) inflammation of the peritoneal surface of the spleen.

perispondylitis (-spon''dĭ-līt'is) inflammation of tissues around a vertebra.

peristalsis (per''ĭ-stal'sis) the wormlike movement by which the alimentary canal or other tubular organs having both longitudinal and circular muscle fibers propel their contents, consisting of a wave of contraction passing along the tube for variable distances. **peristal'tic,** adj.

peristaphyline (-staf'ĭ-lin) around the uvula.

peritectomy (-tek'tah-me) excision of a ring of conjunctiva around the cornea in treatment of pannus.

peritendineum (-ten-din'e-im) connective tissue investing larger tendons and extending between the fibers composing them.

peritendinitis, peritenonitis (-ten''dĭ-nīt'is, -ten''in-nīt'is) tenosynovitis.

perithelioma (-thēl''e-o'mah) hemangiopericytoma.

perithelium (-thēl'e-im) the connective tissue layer surrounding the capillaries and smaller vessels.

perithyroiditis (-thi''roid-īt'is) inflammation of the capsule of the thyroid gland.

peritomy (per-it'ah-me) 1. incision of the conjunctiva and subconjunctival tissue about the entire circumference of the cornea. 2. circumcision.

peritoneal (per''it-ah-ne'il) pertaining to the peritoneum.

peritonealgia (per''it-ah-ne-al'je-ah) pain in the peritoneum.

peritoneocentesis (per''it-ah-ne'-o-sen-te'sis) paracentesis of the abdominal cavity.

peritoneoclysis (per''it-ah-ne-ok'lĭ-sis) injection of fluid into the peritoneal cavity.

peritoneoscopy (per''it-ah-ne-os'kah-pe) visual examination of the organs of the abdominal (peritoneal) cavity with an endoscope.

peritoneotomy (per''it-ah-ne-ot'ah-me) incision into the peritoneum.

peritoneovenous (per''it-ah-ne''o-ve'nis) communicating with the peritoneal cavity and the venous system.

peritoneum (per''it-ah-ne'im) the serous membrane lining the walls of the abdominal and pelvic cavities (*parietal p.*) and investing the contained viscera (*visceral p.*), the two layers enclosing a potential space, the peritoneal cavity. **peritone′al**, adj.

peritonitis (-itah-nīt′is) inflammation of the peritoneum, which may be due to chemical irritation or bacterial invasion.

peritonsillar (-ton′sĭ-ler) around a tonsil.

peritonsillitis (-ton″sĭ-lit′is) inflammation of peritonsillar tissues.

peritrichous (pĭ-rĭ′trĭ-kis) 1. having flagella around the entire surface; said of bacteria. 2. having flagella around the cytostome only; said of Ciliophora.

periumbilical (pĕ″re-um-bil′ik′l) around the umbilicus.

periureteritis (-ūr-ēt″er-īt′is) inflammation of tissues around the ureter.

perivaginitis (-vaj″ĭ-nīt′is) pericolpitis.

perivasculitis (-vas″kūl-īt′is) inflammation of a perivascular sheath and surrounding tissue.

perivesical (-ves′ĭ-k′l) around the bladder.

perivesiculitis (-vĭ-sik″ūl-īt′is) inflammation of tissues around the seminal vesicles.

perlèche (per-lesh′) inflammation with exudation, maceration, and fissuring at the labial commissures.

permanganate (per-man′gah-nāt) a salt containing the MnO_4^- ion.

permeable (per′me-ah-b′l) not impassable; pervious; permitting passage of a substance.

permease (pur′me-ās) a general term for carrier proteins involved in the transport of substances across cell membranes.

permeate (pur′me-āt″) 1. to penetrate or pass through, as through a filter. 2. the constituents of a solution or suspension that pass through a filter.

pernicious (per-nish′is) tending to a fatal issue.

pernio (pur′ne-o) chilblain.

pero- word element [Gr.], *deformity; maimed.*

peromelia (-mēl′e-ah) congenital deformity of the limbs.

peroneal (per″o-ne′al) pertaining to the fibula or to the outer side of the leg; fibular.

peroral (per-or′il) performed or administered through the mouth.

per os (per os) [L.] by mouth.

peroxidase (per-ok′sĭ-dās) any of a group of iron-porphyrin enzymes that catalyze the oxidation of some organic substrates in the presence of hydrogen peroxide.

peroxide (per-ok′sīd) that oxide of any element containing more oxygen than any other; more correctly applied to compounds having such linkage as —O—O—.

peroxisome (per-oks′ĭ-sōm) any of the microbodies present in vertebrate animal cells, especially liver and kidney cells, which are rich in the enzymes perioxidase, catalase, D-amino acid oxidase, and, to a lesser extent, urate oxidase.

perphenazine (per-fen′ah-zēn) a major tranquilizer and antiemetic, $C_{21}H_{26}ClN_3OS$.

per primam (intentionem) (per pri′mam in-ten″she-o′nem) [L.] by first intention.

per rectum (per rek′tim) [L.] by way of the rectum.

Persantine (per-san′tēn) trademark for preparations of dipyridamole.

per secundam (intentionem) (per se-kun′dam in-ten″she-o′nem) [L.] by second intention.

perseveration (per-sev″er-a′shin) persistent repetition of the same verbal or motor response to varied stimuli; continuance of activity after cessation of the causative stimulus.

persona (per-so′nah) Jung's term for the personality "mask" or façade presented by a person to the outside world, as opposed to the anima.

personality (pers″in-al′it-e) the characteristic way a person thinks, feels, and behaves, including conscious attitudes, values, and styles, and also unconscious conflicts and defense mechanisms. **alternating p.**, see *multiple p.* **antisocial p. disorder**, a personality disorder characterized by continuous and chronic antisocial behavior in which the rights of others are violated; associated personality traits include impulsiveness, egocentricity, inability to tolerate boredom or frustration, irritability and aggressiveness, recklessness, disregard for truth, and inability to maintain consistent, responsible functioning at work, at school, or as a parent. The concept of a personality disorder that predisposes an individual toward criminality has a long history; those exhibiting this personality have been called psychopaths and sociopaths. **avoidant p. disorder**, a personality disorder characterized by social discomfort, hypersensitivity to criticism, and an aversion to activities that involve significant interpersonal contact; there is a proclivity to anxiety, an exaggeration of difficulties, a general timidity, and a desire for affection and acceptance that is restrained for fear of rejection. **borderline p. (disorder)**, a personality disorder marked by a pervasive instability of mood, self-image, and interpersonal relationships; impulsive and self-damaging acts are common, as are uncontrolled anger, fears of abandonment, chronic feelings of boredom or emptiness, and recurrent self-mutilating behavior and suicide threats. **cyclothymic p. disorder**, cyclothymia. **dependent p. (disorder)**, a personality disorder marked by feelings of helplessness when alone or when close relationships end, as well as a general preoccupation with fears of being abandoned; other features include difficulty in decision-making without substantial advice and reassurance, low self-esteem, and hypersensitivity to criticism or disapproval. **double p., dual p.,** see *multiple p.* **explosive p.,** intermittent explosive disorder. **histrionic p. (disorder),** a personality disorder marked by excessive emotionality and attention-seeking behavior; there is overconcern with physical attractiveness, sexual seductiveness, intolerance of delayed gratification, and rapid shifting and shallow expression of emotions. **hysterical p.,** histrionic p. **inadequate p.,** a diagnostic category referring to persons who are generally ineffectual or inept, socially, intellectually, and physically; it does not correspond to any particular pattern of personality traits. **multiple p.,** a functional mental disorder characterized by the existence in an individual of two or more distinct personalities, each having unique memories, charactersitic behavior, and social relationships that determine the individual's actions when that personality is dominant. Transitions from one personality to another are abrupt; the original personality usually is totally unaware of the other personalities (subpersonalities), experiencing only gaps of time when the others are in control. Subpersonalities may or may not have awareness of the others. **narcissistic p. disorder,** a personality disorder characterized by grandiosity (in fantasy or behavior), a lack of social empathy combined with a hypersensitivity to the judgment of others, interpersonal exploitiveness, a sense of entitlement, and a need for constant signs of admiration. **obsessive p., obsessive-compulsive p. disorder,** a personality disorder characterized by an emotionally constricted manner that is unduly conventional, serious, formal, and stingy, by preoccupation with trivial details, rules, order, organization, schedules, and lists, by stubborn insistance on having things one's own way without regard for the effects on others, by excessive devotion to work and productivity to the detriment of interpersonal relationships, and by indecisiveness due to fear of making mistakes. **paranoid p. (disorder),** a personality disorder marked by a view of other people as hostile, devious, and untrustworthy and a combative response to disappointments or to events experienced as rebuffs or humiliations. Notable are a questioning of the loyalty of friends, the bearing of grudges, and a tendency to read threatening meanings into benign remarks. It differs from paranoia or paranoid schizophrenia, in which there is delusional or hallucinatory persecution, in that the paranoid personality is overreacting to or misinterpreting real, if minor, slights or setbacks. **passive aggressive p. (disorder),** a personality disorder characterized by an indirect resistance to demands for adequate social and occupational performance; anger and opposition to authority and the expectations of others that is expressed covertly by obstructionism, procrastination, stubbornness, dawdling, forgetfulness, and intentional inefficiency. **psychopathic p.,** antisocial p. **sadistic p. (disorder),** a personality disorder marked by a pervasive pattern of cruel, demeaning, and aggressive behavior; satisfaction is gained in intimidating, coercing, and humiliating others; an excitable temper flares readily to argument, belligerence, and the infliction of pain; there is a fascination with violence, social intolerance, and a broad-ranging authoritarianism. **schizoid p., (disorder),** a personality disorder marked by indifference to social relationships and restricted range of emotional experience and expression. Those affected lack the capacity for social relationships, are cold and aloof, and are indifferent to praise, criticism, or the feelings of others. In previous classifications schizoid personality included some persons who are now classed as schizotypal or avoidant personalities. **schizotypal p. (disorder),** a personality disorder characterized by marked deficits in interpersonal competence and eccentricities in ideation, appearance, and behavior; ideas of reference are common, as are odd beliefs or magical thinking, a lack of close friends, excessive social anxiety, suspiciousness, and occasional paranoid ideation. In previous official classifications these persons would have been diagnosed as having simple or latent schizophrenia or schizoid personality disorder. Other terms that have been used are borderline, prepsychotic, prodromal, pseudoneurotic, and ambulatory schizophrenia. **self-defeating p. (disorder),** a personality disorder marked by feelings of martyrdom, inclination to be drawn to problematic situations or relationships, and failure to accomplish tasks crucial to life objectives; a tendency to engage in excessive self-sacrifice and an inability to enjoy the rewards of success also are notable. **sociopathic p.,** antisocial p. **split p.,** originally, a colloquial equivalent for *schizophrenia,* now more commonly used as an equivalent for *multiple personality.*

perspiration (per″spĭ-ra′shun) 1. sweating; the functional secretion of sweat. 2. sweat.

persulfate (per-sul′fāt) a salt of persulfuric acid.

per tubam (per tu′bam) [L.] through a tube.

pertussis (per-tus′is) an infectious disease caused by *Bordetella pertussis,* marked by catarrh of the respiratory tract and peculiar paroxysms of cough, ending in a prolonged crowing or whooping respiration.

pertussoid (per-tus′oid) 1. resembling whooping cough. 2. an influenzal cough resembling that of whooping cough.

per vaginam (per vah-ji′nam) [L.] through the vagina.

perversion (per-ver′zhin) deviation from the normal course. **sexual p.,** paraphilia.

pes (pes), pl. *pe′des,* gen. *pe′dis* [L.] foot; the terminal organ of the leg, or lower limb; any footlike part.

pessary (pes′ah-re) 1. an instrument placed in the vagina to support the uterus or rectum or as a contraceptive device. 2. a medicated vaginal suppository.

pestilence (pes′tĭ-lins) a virulent contagious epidemic or infectious epidemic disease. **pestilen′tial,** adj.

pestle (pes′′l, pest′′l) an implement for pounding drugs in a mortar.

peta- (pet′ah) a word element used in naming units of measurement to designate a quantity 10^{15} (a quadrillion, or thousand million million) times the unit to which it is joined.

-petal word element [L.], *directed* or *moving toward.*

petechia (pah-te′ke-ah), pl. *pete′chiae* [L.] a minute red spot due to escape of a small amount of blood. **pete′chial,** adj.

petiole (pet′e-ōl) a stalk or pedicle. **epiglottic p.,** the pointed lower end of the epiglottic cartilage, attached to the thyroid cartilage.

petiolus (pah-ti′ah-ol-is) petiole.

petit mal (pĕ-te′ mahl′) [Fr.] see under *epilepsy.*

pétrissage (pe′-trĭ-sahzh′) [Fr.] foulage.

petrolatum (pĕ″trah-la′tum) a purified mixture of semisolid hydrocarbons obtained from petroleum; used as an ointment base, protective dressing, and soothing application to the skin.

petromastoid (pĕ″trah-mas′toid) 1. pertaining to the petrous portion of the temporal bone and its mastoid process. 2. otocranium (2).

petro-occipital (-ok-sip′it′l) pertaining to the petrous portion of the temporal bone and to the occipital bone.

petrosal (pĕ-tro′sil) pertaining to the petrous portion of the temporal bone.

petrositis (pĕ″trah-sīt′is) inflammation of the petrous portion of the temporal bone.

petrosphenoid (-sfe′noid) pertaining to the petrous portion of the temporal bone and to the sphenoid bone.

petrosquamous (-skwa′mis) pertaining to the petrous and squamous portions of the temporal bone.

pexis (pek′sis) 1. the fixation of matter by a tissue. 2. surgical fixation. **pex′ic,** adj.

-pexy word element [Gr.], *surgical fixation.* **-pec′tic,** adj.

peyote (pa-ōt′e) a stimulant drug from mescal buttons, whose active principle is mescaline; used by North American Indians in certain ceremonies to produce an intoxication marked by feelings of ecstasy.

pH the symbol relating the hydrogen ion (H⁺) concentration or activity of a solution to that of a given standard solution. Numerically the pH is approximately equal to the negative logarithm of H⁺ concentration expressed in molarity. pH 7 is neutral; above it alkalinity increases and below it acidity increases.

phac(o)- word element [Gr.], *lens.* See also words beginning *phako-.*

phacoanaphylaxis (fak″o-an″ah-fi-lak′sis) hypersensitivity to the protein of the crystalline lens of the eye, induced by escape of material from the lens capsule.

phacocele (fak′ah-sēl) hernia of the eye lens.

phacocystectomy (fak″o-sis-tek′tah-me) excision of part of lens capsule for cataract.

phacocystitis (-sis-tīt′is) inflammation of capsule of eye lens.

phacoemulsification (-ĭ-mul″sĭ-fĭ-ka′shin) a method of cataract extraction in which the lens is fragmented by ultrasonic vibrations and simultaneously irrigated and aspirated.

phacoerysis (-ĕ′rĭ-sis) removal of the eye lens in cataract by suction.

phacoid (fak′oid) shaped like a lens.

phacoiditis (fak″oid-īt′is) phakitis.

phacoidoscope (fah-koid-ah-skōp) phacoscope.

phacolysis (fah-kol′ĭ-sis) dissolution or discission of the eye lens. **phacolyt′ic,** adj.

phacomalacia (fak″o-mah-la′she-ah) softening of the lens; a soft cataract.

phacometachoresis (-met″ah-kor-e′sis) displacement of the eye lens.

phacosclerosis (-sklĕ-ro′sis) hardening of the eye lens; a hard cataract.

phacoscope (fak′ah-skōp″) instrument for viewing accommodative changes of the eye lens.

phacotoxic (fak′o-tok′sik) exerting a deleterious effect upon the crystalline lens.

phaeohyphomycosis (fe″o-hi″fo-mi-ko′sis) any opportunistic infection caused by dematiacious fungi.

phag(o)- word element [Gr.], *eating; ingestion.*

phage (fāj) bacteriophage.

-phagia, -phagy word element [Gr.], *eating; swallowing.*

phagocyte (fag′ah-sīt) any cell that ingests microorganisms or other cells and foreign particles. **phagocyt′ic,** adj.

phagocytin (fag″ah-sīt′′n) a bactericidal substance from neutrophilic leukocytes.

phagocytoblast (fag″ah-sīt′ah-blast) a cell giving rise to phagocytes.

phagocytolysis (-si-tol′ĭ-sis) destruction of phagocytes. **phagocytolyt′ic,** adj.

phagocytosis (-si-to′sis) the engulfing of microorganisms or other cells and foreign particles by phagocytes. **phagocytot′ic,** adj.

phagosome (fag′ah-sōm) a membrane-bound vesicle in a phagocyte containing the phagocytized material.

phagotype (-tīp) phage type; see under *type.*

phak(o)- see *phac(o)-.*

phakitis (fa-kīt′is) inflammation of the crystalline lens.

phakoma (fah-ko′mah) 1. an occasional small, grayish white tumor seen microscopically in the retina in tuberous sclerosis. 2. a patch of myelinated nerve fibers seen very infrequently in the retina in neurofibromatosis.

phakomatosis (fak″o-mah-to′sis) any of four hereditary syndromes (neurofibromatosis, tuberous sclerosis, Sturge-Weber syndrome, and von Hippel-Lindau disease) marked by disseminated hamartomas of the eye, skin, and brain.

phalang(o)- word element [Gr.], *phalanx* or *phalanges.*

phalangeal (fah-lan′je-il) pertaining to a phalanx.

phalangectomy (fal″an-jek′tah-me) excision of a phalanx.

phalangitis (fal″an-jīt′is) inflammation of one or more phalanges.

phalanx (fa′lanks), pl. *phalan′ges* [Gr.] any bone of a finger or toe; see *phalanges* in *Table of Bones.* **phalan′geal,** adj.

phallectomy (fal-ek′tah-me) amputation of the penis.

phallitis (fal-īt′is) penitis.

phalloidin, phalloidine (fah-loid′in) a hexapeptide poison from the mushroom *Amanita phalloides,* which causes asthenia, vomiting, diarrhea, convulsions, and death.

phallus (fal′is) the penis. **phal′lic,** adj.

phanerosis (fan″er-o′sis) the process of becoming visible.

phantasm (fan′tazm) phantom (1).

phantom (fant′im) 1. an image or impression not evoked by actual stimuli. 2. a model of the body or of a specific part thereof. 3. a device for simulating the *in vivo* effect of radiation on tissues.

phar., pharm. *pharmacy; pharmaceutical; pharmacopeia.*

pharmac(o)- word element [Gr.], *drug; medicine.*

pharmaceutical 464

pharmaceutical (fahr″mah-sōōt′ĭ-kil) 1. pertaining to pharmacy or drugs. 2. a medicinal drug.

pharmacist (fahr′mah-sist) one who is licensed to prepare and sell or dispense drugs and compounds, and to make up prescriptions.

pharmacodynamics (-di-nam′iks) the study of the biochemical and physiological effects of drugs and the mechanisms of their actions, including the correlation of actions and effects of drugs with their chemical structure. **pharmacodynam′ic,** adj.

pharmacogenetics (-jĭ-net′iks) the study of the relationship between genetic factors and the nature of responses to drugs.

pharmacognosy (fahr″mah-kog′nah-se) the branch of pharmacology dealing with natural drugs and their constituents.

pharmacokinetics (fahr″mah-ko-ki-net′iks) the action of drugs in the body over a period of time, including the processes of absorption, distribution, localization in tissues, biotransformation, and excretion. **pharmacokinet′ic,** adj.

pharmacology (fahr″mah-kol′ah-je) the science that deals with the origin, nature, chemistry, effects, and uses of drugs; it includes pharmacognosy, pharmocokinetics, pharmacodynamics, pharmacotherapeutics, and toxicology. **pharmacolog′ic,** adj.

pharmacopeia (-pe′ah) an authoritative treatise on drugs and their preparations. See also *U.S.P.* **pharmacopei′al,** adj.

pharmacopsychosis (-si-ko′sis) any of a group of mental diseases due to alcohol, drugs, or poisons.

pharmacotherapy (-ther′ah-pe) treatment of disease with medicines.

pharmacy (fahr′mah-se) 1. the branch of the health sciences dealing with the preparation, dispensing, and proper utilization of drugs. 2. a place where drugs are compounded or dispensed.

Pharm.D. Doctor of Pharmacy.

pharyng(o)- word element [Gr.], *pharynx.*

pharyngalgia (far″ing-gal′je-ah) pain in the pharynx.

pharyngeal (fah-rin′je-il) pertaining to the pharynx.

pharyngectomy (far″in-jek′tah-me) excision of part of the pharynx.

pharyngemphraxis (far″in-jem-frak′sis) obstruction of the pharynx.

pharyngismus (far″in-jiz′mis) muscular spasm of the pharynx.

pharyngitis (far″in-jīt′is) inflammation of the pharynx. **pharyngit′ic,** adj.

pharyngocele (fah-ring′gah-sēl″) herniation or cystic deformity of the pharynx.

pharyngomycosis (-mi-ko′sis) any fungal infection of the pharynx.

pharyngoperistole (-pĕ-ris′tah-le) pharyngostenosis.

pharyngoplegia (fah-ring″go-ple′je-ah) pharyngoparalysis.

pharyngorhinitis (-ri-nīt′is) inflammation of the nasopharynx.

pharyngorrhea (-re′ah) mucous discharge from the pharynx.

pharyngoscopy (far″ing-gos′kah-pe) direct visual examination of the pharynx.

pharyngostenosis (fah-ring″go-sten-o′sis) narrowing of the pharynx.

pharyngotomy (far″ing-got′ah-me) incision of the pharynx.

pharynx (far′inks) the throat; the musculomembranous cavity behind the nasal cavities, mouth, and larynx, communicating with them and with the esophagus.

phase (fāz) 1. one of the aspects or stages through which a varying entity may pass. 2. in physical chemistry, any physically or chemically distinct, homogeneous, and mechanically separable part of a system, e.g., the ice and steam phases of water.

phasmid (faz′mid) 1. either of the two caudal chemoreceptors occurring in certain nematodes (Phasmidia). 2. any nematode containing phasmids.

phenacetin (fĭ-nas′it-in) an analgesic, $C_{10}H_{13}$-NO_2.

phenanthrene (fĭ-nan′thrēn) a colorless, crystalline hydrocarbon, $(C_6H_4 \cdot CH)_2$.

phenazopyridine (fen″ah-zo-pēr′ĭ-dēn) a urinary analgesic, $C_{11}H_{11}N_5$, used as the hydrochloride salt.

phencyclidine (fen-si′klĭ-dēn) a potent analgesic and anesthetic, $C_{17}H_{25}N$, used in veterinary medicine. Abuse of this drug may lead to serious psychological disturbances. Abbreviated PCP.

phenelzine (fen′il-zēn) a monoamine oxidase inhibitor, $C_8H_{12}N_2$, used as an antidepressant.

Phenergan (-er-gan) trademark for a preparation of promethazine.

phenethicillin (fĭ-neth″ĭ-sil′in) a semisynthetic acid-resistant penicillin, $C_{17}H_{20}N_2O_5S$, which is a methyl analogue of penicillin V.

phenindamine (fĭnin′dah-min) an antihistaminic, $C_{19}H_{19}N$, used as the tartrate salt.

phenindione (fen-in′di-ōn) an anticoagulant, $C_{15}H_{10}O_2$.

pheniramine (fe-nir′ah-min) an antihistaminic, $C_{16}H_{20}N_2$, used as the maleate salt.

phenmetrazine (fen-met′rah-zēn) a central nervous stimulant, $C_{11}H_{15}NO$, used as an anorexic in the form of the hydrochloride salt.

phenobarbital (fe″no-bar′bĭ-tal) an anticonvulsant, sedative, and hypnotic, $C_{12}H_{12}N_2O_3$; also used as the sodium salt.

phenocopy (fe′nah-kop″e) an environmentally induced phenotype mimicking one usually produced by a specific genotype.

phenodeviant (fe″no-de′ve-ant) an individual whose phenotype differs significantly from that of the typical phenotype in the population.

phenol (fe′nol) 1. an extremely poisonous compound, $C_6H_5 \cdot OH$, obtained by distillation of coal tar; used as an antimicrobial. Ingestion or absorption of phenol through the skin causes colic, weakness, collapse, and local irritation and corrosion. 2. any organic compound containing one or more hydroxyl groups attached to an aromatic or carbon ring.

phenolate (fe'nil-āt) 1. to treat with phenol for purposes of sterilization. 2. a salt formed by union of a base with phenol, in which a monovalent metal, such as sodium or potassium, replaces the hydrogen of the hydroxyl group.

phenolphthalein (fe''nol-tha'lēn) a cathartic, $C_{20}H_{14}O_4$.

phenolsulfonphthalein (-sul''fōn-tha'lēn) a red powder, $C_{19}H_{14}O_5S$, used as a test of renal function.

phenomenon (fe-nom'ĕ-non) any sign or objective symptom; any observable occurrence or fact. **dawn p.**, the early-morning increase in plasma glucose concentration and thus insulin requirement in a patient with insulin-dependent diabetes mellitus. **Somogyi p.**, a rebound phenomenon occurring in diabetes: overtreatment with insulin induces hypoglycemia, thus initiating hormone release; this stimulates lipolysis, gluconeogenesis, and glycogenolysis, which in turn cause rebound hyperglycemia and ketosis.

phenothiazine (fe''no-thi'ah-zēn) a veterinary anthelmintic; also used to denote a group of major tranquilizers resembling phenothiazine in molecular structure.

phenotype (fe'nah-tīp) the entire physical, biochemical, and physiological makeup of an individual as determined both genetically and environmentally. Also, any one or any group of such traits. **phenotyp'ic,** adj.

phenoxybenzamine (fĭ-nok''se-ben'zah-mēn) an adrenergic blocking agent, $C_{18}H_{22}ClNO$; the hydrochloride salt is used as a vasodilator and sometimes as an antihypertensive.

phenprocoumon (fen-pro'koo-mon) an anticoagulant of the coumarin type, $C_{18}H_{16}O_3$.

phenpropionate (-pro'pe-ah-nāt'') USAN contraction for 3-phenylpropionate.

phensuximide (-suk'sĭ-mīd) an anticonvulsant, $C_{11}H_{11}NO_2$.

phentermine (fen'ter-mēn) an anorexic, $C_{10}H_{15}N$.

phentolamine (fen-tol'ah-mēn) a potent alpha-adrenergic blocking agent; it blocks the hypertensive action of epinephrine and norepinephrine and most responses of smooth muscles that involve alpha-adrenergic cell receptors. Its hydrochloride and mesylate salts are used in the diagnosis of hypertension due to pheochromocytoma.

phenyl (fen'il, fe'nil) the monovalent radical, C_6H_5. **phenyl'ic,** adj.

phenylactic acid (fen''il-ah-sēt'ik) $C_6H_5CH_2$-COOH, a product of defective phenylalanine catabolism present in the urine in phenylketonuria.

phenylalanine (fen''il-al'ah-nīn) a naturally occurring amino acid essential for optimal growth in infants and for nitrogen equilibrium in human adults.

phenylbutazone (-būt'ah-zōn) a congener of aminopyrine, $C_{19}H_{20}N_2O_2$, having analgesic, antipyretic, anti-inflammatory, and mild uricosuric properties; used in the treatment of gout,

rheumatoid arthritis, ankylosing spondylitis, and other rheumatoid conditions.

phenylephrine (-ef'rin) an adrenergic, C_9H_{13}-NO_2, used as the hydrochloride salt for its potent vasoconstrictor properties.

phenylic acid (fen-il'ik) phenol.

phenylketonuria (-ke''tōn-ūr'e-ah) an inborn error of metabolism marked by an inability to convert phenylalanine into tyrosine, permitting accumulation of phenylalanine and its metabolic products in body fluids; it results in mental retardation, neurologic manifestations, light pigmentation, eczema, and mousy odor, unless treated by a diet low in phenylalanine. **phenylketonu'ric,** adj.

phenylmercuric (-mer-kūr'ik) denoting a compound containing the radical C_6H_5Hg—, forming various antiseptic, antibacterial, and fungicidal salts; compounds of the acetate and nitrate salts are used as bacteriostatics, and the former is used as a herbicide.

phenylpropanolamine (-pro''pah-nol'am-in) an adrenergic, $C_9H_{13}NO$, used chiefly as a nasal and sinus decongestant in the form of the hydrochloride salt.

phenylpyruvic acid (fen''il-pi-roo'vik) C_6H_5-$CH_2COCOOH$, an intermediary product in the metabolism of phenylalanine, present in the urine in phenlketonuria.

phenylthiourea (-thi''o-ūr-e'ah) a compound used in genetics research; the ability to taste it is inherited as a dominant trait. It is intensely bitter to about 70% of the population, and nearly tasteless to the rest.

phenyltoloxamine (-tol-ok'sah-mēn) an antihistaminic, $C_{17}H_{21}NO$.

phenytoin (fen'ĭ-to-in) an anticonvulsant and cardiac depressant, $C_{15}H_{12}N_2O_2$, used in the treatment of all forms of epilepsy except petit mal and as an antiarrhythmic.

pheochrome (fe'ah-krōm) chromaffin.

pheochromoblast (fe''o-kro'mah-blast) any of the embryonic structures that develop into chromaffin (pheochrome) cells.

pheochromocyte (-kro'mah-sīt) a chromaffin cell.

pheochromocytoma (-kro''mah-si-to'mah) a tumor of chromaffin tissue of the adrenal medulla or sympathetic paraganglia; symptoms, notably hypertension, reflect the increased secretion of epinephrine and norepinephrine.

pheresis (fĕ-re'sis) apheresis.

pheromone (fer'ah-mōn) a substance secreted to the outside of the body and perceived (as by smell) by other individuals of the same species, releasing specific behavior in the percipient.

Ph.G. Graduate in Pharmacy.

Phialophora (fi''ah-lof'ah-rah) a genus of imperfect fungi. *P. verrucosa* is a cause of chromomycosis; *P. jeanselmi* is a cause of maduromycosis.

-philia word element [Gr.], *affinity for; morbid fondness of.* **-phil'ic,** adj.

philtrum (fil'trum) the vertical groove in the median portion of the upper lip.

phimosis (fi-mo'sis) constriction of the orifice of

the prepuce so that it cannot be drawn back over the glans. **phimot'ic,** adj.

phleb(o)- word element [Gr.], *vein.*

phlebangioma (fleb″an-je-o′mah) a venous aneurysm.

phlebarteriectasia (-ar-tēr″e-ek-ta′ze-ah) general dilatation of veins and arteries.

phlebectasia (-ek-ta′ze-ah) dilatation of a vein; a varicosity.

phlebectomy (flĕ-bek′tah-me) excision of a vein, or a segment of a vein.

phlebemphraxis (fleb″em-frak′sis) stoppage of a vein by a plug or clot.

phlebismus (flĕ-biz′mus) obstruction and consequent turgescence of veins.

phlebitis (flĭ-bīt′is) inflammation of a vein. **phlebit′ic,** adj. **sinus p.,** inflammation of a cerebral sinus.

phleboclysis (flĕ-bok′lĭ-sis) injection of fluid into a vein.

phlebography (flĕ-bog′rah-fe) 1. radiography of a vein filled with contrast medium. 2. the graphic recording of the venous pulse. 3. a description of the veins.

phlebolithiasis (fleb″o-lĭ-thi′ah-sis) the development of venous calculi or concretions.

phlebomanometer (-mah-nom′ĕ-ter) an instrument for the direct measurement of venous blood pressure.

phleborrhaphy (flĕ-bor′ah-fe) suture of a vein.

phlebosclerosis (-sklĕ-ro′sis) fibrous thickening of the walls of veins.

phlebostasis (flĭ-bos′tah-sis) 1. retardation of blood flow in veins. 2. temporary sequestration of a portion of blood from the general circulation by compressing the veins of an extremity.

phlebothrombosis (fleb″o-throm-bo′sis) the development of venous thrombi in the absence of associated inflammation.

Phlebotomus (flĭ-bot′ah-mus) a genus of biting sandflies, the females of which suck blood. They are vectors of various diseases, including kala-azar (*P. argen'tipes, P. chinen'sis, P. marti'ni, P. orienta'lis, P. pernicio'sus*), Carrión's disease (*P. nogu'chi, P. verruca'rum*), cutaneous leishmaniasis (*P. sergen'ti*), and phlebotomus fever (*P. papatas'ii*).

phlebotomy (flĭ-bot′-ah-me) incision of a vein.

phlegm (flem) viscid mucus excreted in abnormally large quantities from the respiratory tract.

phlegmasia (fleg-ma′ze-ah) [Gr.] inflammation. **p. al′ba do′lens,** phlebitis of the femoral vein, with swelling of the leg, usually without redness (milk leg), occasionally following parturition or an acute febrile illness. **p. ceru′lea do′lens,** an acute fulminating form of deep venous thrombosis, with pronounced edema and severe cyanosis of the extremity.

phlegmatic (fleg-mat′ik) of dull and sluggish temperament.

phlegmon (fleg′mon) diffuse inflammation of the soft or connective tissue due to infection. **phleg′monous,** adj.

phlog(o)- word element [Gr.], *inflammation.*

phlogogenic (flog″ah-jen′ik) producing inflammation.

phlyctena (flik-te′nah) 1. a small blister made by a burn. 2. a small vesicle containing lymph seen on the conjunctiva in certain conditions. **phlyc′tenar,** adj.

phlyctenular (flik-ten′u-lar) associated with the formation of phlyctenules, or of vesicle-like prominences.

phlyctenule (flik′tin-ūl) a minute vesicle; an ulcerated nodule of cornea or conjunctiva.

phobia (fo′be-ah) any persistent abnormal dread or fear; also, a word termination denoting abnormal fear or aversion. **pho′bic,** adj. **simple p.,** any phobia of objects, but not of situations (agoraphobia) or of functions (social phobia), e.g., fear of dogs, cats, mice, spiders, blood and injuries, claustrophobia, acrophobia, and air travel. **social p.,** any phobia of function, and not of situations (agoraphobia) or of objects (simple phobia), in which the person fears embarrassment or humiliation, e.g., public speaking or eating or using a lavatory.

phocomelia (fo″kah-me′le-ah) congenital absence of the proximal portion of a limb or limbs, the hands or feet being attached to the trunk by a small, irregularly shaped bone. **phocome′lic,** adj.

phocomelus (fo-kom′il-is) an individual exhibiting phocomelia.

phon(o)- word element [Gr.], *sound; voice; speech.*

phonasthenia (fo″nas-the′ne-ah) weakness of the voice; difficult phonation from fatigue.

phonendoscope (fo-nen′dah-skōp) a stethoscopic device that intensifies auscultatory sounds.

phoniatrics (fo″ne-ă′triks) the treatment of speech defects.

phonocardiography (-kar″de-og′rah-fe) the graphic representation of heart sounds and murmurs; by extension, the term also includes pulse tracings (carotid, apex, and jugular pulse). **phonocardiograph′ic,** adj.

phonocatheter (-kath′it-er) a device similar to a conventional catheter, with a microphone at the tip.

phonometer (fon-om′it-er) a device for measuring intensity of sounds.

phonomyoclonus (fo″nah-mi-ok′lah-nis) myoclonus in which a sound is heard on auscultation of an affected muscle, indicating fibrillar contractions.

phonomyography (-mi-og′rah-fe) the recording of sounds produced by muscle contraction.

phonopathy (fon-op′ah-the) any disease or disorder of the organs of speech.

phonoreceptor (fo″no-re-sep′ter) a receptor for sound stimuli.

phonorenogram (-re′no-gram) a record of sounds produced by pulsation of the renal artery obtained by a phonocatheter passed through a ureter into the kidney pelvis.

phonostethograph (-steth′o-graf) an instrument by which chest sounds are amplified, filtered, and recorded.

-phore word element [Gr.], *a carrier.*

-phoresis word element [Gr.], *transmission.*

phoria (fo're-ah) heterophoria.

phosgene (fos'jēn) a suffocating and highly poisonous war gas, carbonyl chloride, COCl₂.

phosphagen (fos'fah-jen) a group of compounds, including phosphocreatine and phosphoarginine, present in tissue which yield high-energy phosphate on cleavage.

phosphatase (fos'fah-tās) any of a group of enzymes capable of catalyzing the hydrolysis of esterified phosphoric acid, with liberation of inorganic phosphate.

phosphate (fos'fāt) any salt or ester of phosphoric acid. **phosphat'ic,** adj.

phosphatemia (fos″fah-tēm′e-ah) an excess of phosphates in the blood.

phosphatidic acid (fos″fah-tid′ik) any compound formed by esterification of three hydroxyl groups of glycerol with two fatty acid groups and one phosphoric acid group; found widely in animals and plants.

phosphaturia (fos″fah-tūr′e-ah) an excess of phosphates in the urine.

phosphene (fos'fēn) a sensation of light due to a stimulus other than light rays, e.g., a mechanical stimulus.

phosphoarginine (fos″fo-ar′jĭ-nin) an arginine–phosphoric acid compound homologous with phosphocreatine but found in invertebrate muscles.

phosphocreatine (-kre′ah-tin) a creatine–phosphoric acid compound occurring in muscle, being the most important storage form of high-energy phosphate, the energy source in muscle contraction.

phosphofructokinase (-fruk″to-ki′nās) an enzyme of spermatozoa, which enables them to utilize fructose as an energy source.

phosphoglyceride (-glis′er-īd) a class of phospholipids, including lecithin and cephalin, consisting of a glycerol backbone, two fatty acids, and a phosphorylated alcohol, e.g., choline, ethanolamine, serine, and inositol. They are a major component of cell membranes.

phospholipase (-lip′ās) any of four enzymes (phospholipase A to D), which catalyze the hydrolysis of a phospholipid.

phospholipid (-lip′id) any lipid that contains phosphorus, including those with a glycerol backbone (phosphoglycerides and plasmalogens) or a backbone of sphingosine or a related substance (sphingomyelins). They are the major lipids in cell membranes.

phosphonecrosis (-nĕ-kro′sis) necrosis of the jaw bone due to exposure to phosphorus.

phosphoprotein (-prōt′e-in) a conjugated protein in which phosphoric acid is esterified with a hydroxy amino acid.

phosphoric acid (fos-for′ik) a crystalline acid, H₃PO₄, formed by the oxidation of phosphorus; its salts are the phosphates.

phosphorism (fos'fer-izm) chronic phosphorus poisoning; see *phosphorus.*

phosphorolysis (fos″fer-ol′ĭ-sis) cleavage of a chemical bond with simultaneous addition of

the elements of phosphoric acid to the residues.

phosphorous acid (fos'fer-is) H₃PO₃; its salts are the phosphites.

phosphoruria (fos″fer-ūr′e-ah) free phosphorus in the urine.

phosphorus (fos'fer-is) chemical element (*see table*), at. no. 15, symbol P. Ingestion or inhalation produces toothache, phosphonecrosis (phossy jaw), anorexia, weakness, and anemia. Phosphorus is an essential element in the diet; in the form of phosphates, it is a major component of the mineral phase of bone and occurs in all tissues, being involved in almost all metabolic processes. **phos'phorous,** adj.

phosphorylase (fos-fōr′ĭ-lās) an enzyme which, in the presence of inorganic phosphate, catalyzes reversibly the conversion of glycogen into glucose-1-phosphate.

phosphorylation (fos″fōr-ĭ-la′shin) the metabolic process of introducing a phosphate group into an organic molecule. **oxidative p.,** the formation of high-energy phosphate bonds by phosphorylation of ADP to ATP; it occurs in the mitochondria.

phosphotransferase (fos″fo-trans′fer-ās) any of a subclass of enzymes that catalyze the transfer of a phosphate group.

phot(o)- word element [Gr.], *light.*

photalgia (fo-tal′je-ah) pain, as in the eye, caused by light.

photoablation (fo″to-ab-la′shun) volatilization of tissue by ultraviolet radiation emitted by a laser.

photoactive (fōt″o-ak′tiv) reacting chemically to sunlight or ultraviolet radiation.

photobiology (-bi-ol′ah-je) the branch of biology dealing with the effect of light on organisms. **photobiolog'ic, photobiolog'ical,** adj.

photobiotic (-bi-ot′ik) living only in the light.

photocatalysis (-kah-tal′ĭ-sis) promotion or stimulation of a chemical reaction by light. **photocatalyt'ic,** adj.

photocatalyst (-kat′ah-list) a substance, e.g., chlorophyll, that brings about a chemical reaction to light.

photochemistry (-kem′is-tre) the branch of chemistry dealing with the chemical properties or effects of light rays or other radiation. **photochem'ical,** adj.

photochemotherapy (-ke″mo-thĕ′rah-pe) treatment by means of drugs (e.g., methoxsalen) that react to ultraviolet radiation or sunlight.

photochromogen (-kro′mah-jen) a microorganism whose pigmentation develops as a result of exposure to light. **photochromogen'ic,** adj.

photocoagulation (-ko-ag″ūl-a′shin) condensation of protein material by the controlled use of an intense beam of light (e.g., argon laser) used especially in the treatment of retinal detachment and destruction of abnormal retinal vessels or intraocular tumor masses.

photodermatitis (-der″mah-tīt′is) an abnormal state of the skin in which light is an important causative factor.

photofluorography (-floor″og′rah-fe) the photographic recording of fluoroscopic images on small films, using a fast lens.

photogenic (-jen′ik) 1. produced by light. 2. producing or emitting light.

photoluminescence (fōt″o-loo″min-es′ins) the quality of being luminescent after exposure to light.

photolysis (fo-tol′ĭ-sis) chemical decomposition by light. **photolyt′ic,** adj.

photometry (fo-tom′ĭ-tre) measurement of the intensity of light.

photomicrograph (fōt″o-mi′kro-graf) a photograph of an object as seen through an ordinary light microscope.

photon (fo′ton) a particle (quantum) of radiant energy.

photoparoxysmal (-par″oks-iz′mil) photoconvulsive; denoting an abnormal electroencephalographic response to photic stimulation (brief flashes of light), marked by diffuse paroxysmal discharge recorded as spike-wave complexes; the response may be accompanied by minor seizures.

photoperiod (-pēr′e-id) the period of time per day that an organism is exposed to daylight (or to artificial light). **photoperiod′ic,** adj.

photoperiodism (-pēr″e-ah-dizm) the physiologic and behavioral reactions brought about in organisms by changes in the duration of daylight and darkness.

photophilic (-fil′ik) thriving in light.

photophobia (-fo′be-ah) abnormal visual intolerance to light. **photopho′bic,** adj.

photophthalmia (fōt″of-thal′me-ah) ophthalmia due to exposure to intense light, as in snow blindness.

photopia (fo-to′pe-ah) day vision. **photop′ic,** adj.

photopsia (fo-top′se-ah) appearance as of sparks or flashes, in retinal irritation.

photopsin (fo-top′sin) the protein moiety of the cones of the retina that combines with retinal to form photochemical pigments.

phototarmosis (fōt″op-tar-mo′sis) sneezing caused by the influence of light.

photoptometer (fōt″op-tom′iter) an instrument for measuring visual acuity by determining the smallest amount of light that will render an object just visible.

photoreactivation (fōt″o-re-ak″tĭ-va′shin) reversal of the biological effects of ultraviolet radiation on cells by subsequent exposure to visible light.

photoreceptor (-re-sep′ter) a nerve end-organ or receptor sensitive to light.

photoretinitis (-ret″in-īt′is) retinitis due to exposure to intense light.

photoscan (fōt′o-skan) a two-dimensional representation of gamma rays emitted by a radioactive isotope in body tissue, produced by a printout mechanism utilizing a light source to expose a photographic film.

photosensitive (fōt″o-sen′sit-iv) exhibiting abnormally heightened sensitivity to sunlight.

photosensitization (-sen″sit-iz-a′shin) the development of abnormally heightened reactivity of the skin to sunlight.

photostable (fōt′o-sta″b′l) unchanged by the influence of light.

photosynthesis (fōt″o-sin′thĭ-sis) a chemical combination caused by the action of light; specifically, the formation of carbohydrates from carbon dioxoide and water in the chlorophyll tissue of plants under the influence of light. **photosynthet′ic,** adj.

phototaxis (-tak′sis) the movement of cells and microorganisms under the influence of light. **phototac′tic,** adj.

phototherapy (-thĕ′rah-pe) treatment of disease by exposure to light.

phototoxic (-tok′sik) having a toxic effect triggered by exposure to light.

phototrophic (-trof′ik) capable of deriving energy from light.

phototropism (fo-tah′trah-pizm) 1. the tendency of an organism to turn or move toward or away from light. 2. color change produced in a substance by the action of light. **phototrop′ic,** adj.

phren(o)- word element [Gr.], (1) *diaphragm;* (2) *mind;* (3) *phrenic nerve.*

phrenemphraxis (fren″em-frak′sis) phrenicotripsy.

phrenetic (frĕ-net′ik) maniacal.

phrenic (fren′ik) pertaining to the diaphragm or to the mind.

phrenicectomy (fren″ĭ-sek′tah-me) resection of the phrenic nerve.

phrenicoexeresis (fren″ĭ-ko-ek-ser′ĕ-sis) avulsion of the phrenic nerve.

phrenicotomy (-kot′o-me) surgical division of the phrenic nerve.

phrenicotripsy (fren″ĭ-ko-trip′se) surgical crushing of the phrenic nerve.

phrenocolic (fren″o-kol′ik) pertaining to the diaphragm and colon.

phrenogastric (-gas′trik) pertaining to the diaphragm and stomach.

phrenohepatic (-hĕ-pat′ik) pertaining to the diaphragm and liver.

phrenoplegia (fren″o-ple′je-ah) paralysis of the diaphragm.

phrenosin (fren′ah-sin) a cerebroside containing cerebronic acid attached to the sphingosine.

phrenotropic (fren″o-trop′ik) exerting its principal effect upon the mind.

phrynoderma (frin″o-der′mah) a follicular hyperkeratosis probably due to deficiency of vitamin A or of essential fatty acids.

phthalein (thal′e-in) any one of a series of coloring matters formed by the condensation of phthalic anhydride with the phenols.

phthalylsulfathiazole (thal″il-sul″fah-thi′ah-zōl) an intestinal antibacterial, $C_{17}H_{13}N_3O_5S_2$.

phthiriasis (thi-ri′ah-sis) infestation with *Phthirus pubis.*

Phthirus (thir′is) a genus of lice, including *P. pu′bis* (the pubic, or crab, louse), which infests the hair of the pubic region, and sometimes the eyebrows and eyelashes.

phthisis (thi′sis) 1. a wasting of the body. 2. tuberculosis.

phyco- word element [Gr.], *seaweed; algae.*

phycology (fi-kol′ah-je) the scientific study of algae.

Phycomycetes (fi″ko-mi-sēt′ēz) a group of fungi comprising the common water, leaf, and bread molds.

phycomycosis (-mi-ko′sis) any of a group of acute fungal diseases caused by members of Phycomycetes.

phylogeny (fi-loj′ĭ-ne) the complete developmental history of a race or group of organisms. **phylogen′ic,** adj.

phylum (fi′lim), pl. *phy′la.* A primary division of the plant or animal kingdom, grouping organisms which are assumed to have a common ancestry.

phyma (fi′mah) [Gr.] a skin tumor or tubercle.

physiatrics (fiz″e-ă′triks) that branch of medicine using physical therapy; physical agents, such as light, heat, water, and electricity; and mechanical apparatus in the diagnosis, prevention, and treatment of bodily disorders.

physiatrist (ă′trist) a physician who specializes in physiatrics.

physic (fiz′ik) 1. the art of medicine and of therapeutics. 2. a medicine, especially a cathartic.

physical (fiz′ik-il) pertaining to the body, to material things, or to physics.

physician (fĭ-zish′in) 1. an authorized practitioner of medicine, one graduated from a college of medicine or osteopathy and licensed by the appropriate board; see also *doctor.* 2. one who practices medicine as distinct from surgery. **p. assistant,** one who has been trained in an accredited program and certified by an appropriate board to perform certain of a physician's duties, including history taking, physical examination, diagnostic tests, treatment, and certain minor surgical procedures, all under the responsible supervision of a licensed physician. Abbreviated P.A. **attending p.,** one who attends a hospital at stated times to visit the patients and give directions as to their treatment. **emergency p.,** a specialist in emergency medicine. **family p.,** a medical specialist who plans and provides the comprehensive primary health care of all members of a family, regardless of age or sex, on a continuous basis. **resident p.,** a graduate and licensed physician resident in a hospital.

physicochemical (fiz″ĭ-ko-kem′ik-il) pertaining to both physics and chemistry.

physics (fiz′iks) the study of the laws and phenomena of nature, especially of forces and general properties of matter and energy.

physio- word element [Gr.], *nature; physiology; physical.*

physiochemical (fiz″e-o-kem′ik-il) pertaining to both physiology and chemistry.

physiognomy (fiz″e-og′nah-me) 1. determination of mental or moral character and qualities by the face. 2. the countenance, or face. 3. the facial expression and appearance as a means of diagnosis.

physiologic, physiological (fiz″e-o-loj′ik; loj′-ik-il) pertaining to physiology; normal; not pathologic.

physiologist (fiz″e-ol′ah-jist) a specialist in physiology.

physiology (fiz″e-ol′ah-je) 1. the science which treats of the functions of the living organism and its parts, and of the physical and chemical factors and processes involved. 2. the basic processes underlying the functioning of a species or class of organism, or any of its parts or processes. **morbid p., pathologic p.,** the study of disordered function or of function in diseased tissues.

physiopathologic (fiz″e-o-path″ah-loj′ik) pertaining to pathologic physiology.

physiotherapist (-thĕ′rah-pist) physical therapist.

physiotherapy (-thĕ′rah-pe) physical therapy.

physique (fĭ-zēk′) the body organization, development, and structure.

physo- word element [Gr.], *air; gas.*

physohematometra (fi″so-hem″ah-to-me′trah) gas and blood in the uterine cavity.

physohydrometra (-hi″dro-me′trah) gas and serum in the uterine cavity.

physometra (-me′trah) gas in the uterine cavity.

physopyosalpinx (-pi″o-sal′pinks) gas and pus in the uterine tube.

physostigmine (-stig′min) an alkaloid usually obtained from dried ripe seed of *Physostigma venenosum;* used as a topical miotic in the form of the base and of the salicylate and sulfate salts.

phyt(o)- word element [Gr.], *plant; an organism of the vegetable kingdom.*

phytic acid (fīt′ik) the hexaphosphoric acid ester of inositol, found in many plants and microorganisms and in animal tissues.

phytoagglutinin (fīt″o-ah-glŏŏt′in-in) an agglutinin of plant origin.

phytobezoar (-be′zōr) a bezoar composed of vegetable fibers.

phytohemagglutinin (fīt″o-hem″ah-glŏŏt′in-in) a hemagglutinin of plant origin.

phytohormone (-hor′mōn) plant hormone; any of the hormones produced in plants which are active in controlling growth and other functions at a site remote from their place of production.

phytol (fi′tol) an unsaturated aliphatic alcohol present in chlorophyll as an ester; used in the preparation of vitamins E and K.

phytonadione (fīt″o-nah-di′ōn) vitamin K$_1$: a vitamin found in green plants or prepared synthetically, used as a prothrombinogenic agent.

phytoparasite (-par″ah-sīt) any parasitic vegetable organism or species.

phytopathogenic (-path″ah-jen′ik) producing disease in plants.

phytopathology (-pah-thol′ah-je) the pathology of plants.

phytophotodermatitis (-fōt″o-der″mah-tīt′is) phototoxic dermatitis induced by exposure to certain plants and then to sunlight.

phytoprecipitin (-pre-sip′it-in) a precipitin formed in response to vegetable antigen.

phytosis (fi-to′sis) any disease caused by a phytoparasite.

phytotoxic (fīt″ah-tok′sik) 1. pertaining to phytotoxin. 2. poisonous to plants.

phytotoxin (-tok′sin) an exotoxin produced by certain species of higher plants; any toxin of plant origin.

pia-arachnitis (pi″ah-ar″ak-nīt′is) leptomeningitis.

pia-arachnoid (-ah-rak′noid) the pia mater and arachnoid considered together as one functional unit; the leptomeninges.

pial (pi′il) pertaining to the pia mater.

pia mater (pi′ah māt′er) [L.] the innermost of the three meninges covering the brain and spinal cord.

piarachnoid (pi″ar-ak′noid) pia-arachnoid.

pica (pi′kah) craving for unnatural articles as food; a depraved appetite.

pico- word element designating 10^{-12} (one trillionth) part of the unit to which it is joined.

picogram (pi′ko-gram) one trillionth (10^{-12}) gram. Abbreviated pg.

picometer (pi″ko-mēt′er) a unit of length, 10^{-12} meter. Abbreviated pm.

picornavirus (pi-kor″nah-vi′rus) an extremely small, ether-resistant RNA virus, one of the group comprising the enteroviruses and the rhinoviruses.

picrate (pik′rāt) any salt of picric acid.

picric acid (pik′rik) trinitrophenol.

picrocarmine (pik″ro-kar′min) a histological stain consisting of a mixture of carmine, ammonia, distilled water, and aqueous solution of picric acid.

picrotoxin (-tok′sin) an active principle, $C_{30}H_{34}O_{13}$, from the seed of *Anamirta cocculus*, used as a central and respiratory stimulant in barbiturate poisoning.

piebaldism (pi-bawld′izm) a condition in which the skin is partly brown and partly white, as in partial albinism and vitiligo.

piedra (pe-a′drah) a fungal disease of the hair in which white or black nodules of fungi form on the shafts.

piesesthesia (pi-e″zes-the′ze-ah) the sense by which pressure stimuli are felt.

piesimeter (pi″ī-sim′it-er) instrument for testing the sensitiveness of the skin to pressure.

-piesis word element [Gr.], *pressure.* **-pies′ic,** adj.

PIF proliferation inhibiting factor.

pigment (pig′mint) 1. any coloring matter of the body. 2. a stain or dyestuff. 3. a paintlike medicinal preparation to be applied to the skin. **pig′mentary,** adj. **bile p.,** any of the coloring matters of the bile, including bilirubin, biliverdin, etc. **blood p.,** any of the pigments derived from hemoglobin. **respiratory p's,** substances, e.g., hemoglobin, myoglobin, or cytochromes, which take part in the oxidative processes of the animal body.

pigmentation (pig″min-ta′shin) the deposition of coloring matter; the coloration or discoloration of a part by a pigment. **hematogenous p.,** pigmentation produced by accumulation of hemoglobin derivatives, such as hematoidin or hemosiderin.

pigmented (pig-ment′id) colored by deposit of pigment.

pigmentolysin (pig″men-tol′ĭ-sin) a lysin which destroys pigment.

pigmentophage (pig-men′tah-fāj) any pigment-destroying cell, especially such a cell of the hair.

pilar, pilary (pīl′er; pil′ah-re) pertaining to the hair.

pile (pīl) 1. hemorrhoid. 2. in nucleonics, a chain-reacting fission device for producing slow neutrons and radioactive isotopes. **sentinel p.,** a hemorrhoid-like thickening of the mucous membrane at the lower end of an anal fissure.

piles (pīlz) hemorrhoids.

pileus (pil′e-is) caul.

pili (pi′li) plural of *pilus.*

pill (pil) a small globular or oval medicated mass to be swallowed; a tablet. **enteric-coated p.,** one enclosed in a substance that dissolves only when it has reached the intestines.

pillar (pil′er) a supporting column, usually occurring in pairs. **p's of the fauces,** folds of mucous membrane at sides of fauces.

pilo- word element [L.], *hair; composed of hair.*

pilocarpine (pi″lo-kar′pin) a cholinergic alkaloid, $C_{11}H_{16}N_2O_2$, from leftlets of *Pilocarpus jaborandi* and *P. microphyllus;* used as an ophthalmic miotic in the form of the hydrochloride and nitrate salts.

pilocystic (-sis′tik) hollow or cystlike, and containing hair; said of dermoid tumors.

piloerection (-ī-rek′shin) erection of the hair.

pilojection (-jek′shin) introduction of one or more hairs into an aneurysmal sac, to promote formation of a blood clot.

pilomatrixoma (-ma-trik′so-mah) a benign, circumscribed, calcifying epithelial neoplasm derived from hair matrix cells, manifested as a small firm intracutaneous spheroid mass, usually on the face, neck, or arms.

pilomotor (-mōt′er) pertaining to the arrector muscles, the contraction of which produces cutis anserina (goose flesh) and piloerection.

pilonidal (-nīd′′l) having a nidus of hairs.

pilose (pi′lōs) hairy; covered with hair.

pilosebaceous (pi″lo-sĭ-ba′shis) pertaining to the hair follicles and the sebaceous glands.

pilus (pi′lis), pl. *pi′li* [L.] 1. a hair. **pi′leal,** adj. 2. one of the minute filamentous appendages of certain bacteria associated with antigenic properties of the cell surface. **pi′leate,** adj. **p. cunicula′tus** (pl. *pi′li cunicula′ti*), burrowing hair. **p. incarna′tus** (pl. *pi′li incarna′ti*), ingrown hair. **p. tor′tus** (pl. *pi′li tor′ti*), twisted hair.

pimelic acid (pim-el′ik) HOOC(CH₂)₅COOH, an intermediate in oleic acid oxidation and a precursor of biotin.

pimelitis (pim″il-īt′is) inflammation of the adipose tissue.

pimelopterygium (pim″il-o-ter-ij′e-im) a fatty outgrowth on the conjunctiva.

pimelosis (pim″il-o′sis) 1. conversion into fat. 2. fatness, or obesity.

pimple (pim′p'l) a papule or pustule.

pin (pin) a slender, elongated piece of metal used for securing fixation of parts. **Steinmann p.,** a metal rod for the internal fixation of fractures.

pincement (pans-maw′) [Fr.] pinching of the flesh in massage.

pineal (pin′e-il) 1. pertaining to the pineal body. 2. shaped like a pine cone.

pinealectomy (pin″e-ah-lek′to-me) excision of the pineal body.

pinealism (pin′e-ah-lizm) the condition due to deranged secretion of the pineal body.

pinealoblastoma (pin″e-ah-lo-blas-to′mah) pinealoma in which the pineal cells are not well differentiated.

pinealocyte (pin′e-ah-lo-sīt″) an epithelioid cell of the pineal body.

pinealoma (pin″e-ah-lo′mah) a tumor of the pineal body composed of neoplastic nests of large epithelial cells; it may cause hydrocephalus, precocious puberty, and gait disturbances.

pinguecula (ping-gwek′ūl-ah) a benign yellowish spot on the bulbar conjunctiva.

piniform (pin′ĭ-form) conical or cone shaped.

pinkeye (pink′i″) acute contagious conjunctivitis.

pinna (pin′ah) auricle; the part of the ear outside the head. **pin′nal,** adj.

pinocyte (pin′ah-sīt) a cell that exhibits pinocytosis. **pinocyt′ic,** adj.

pinocytosis (pi″nah-si-to′sis) a mechanism by which cells ingest extracellular fluid and its contents; it involves the formation of invaginations by the cell membrane, which close and break off to form fluid-filled vacuoles in the cytoplasm. **pinocytot′ic,** adj.

pinosome (pi′no-sōm) the intracellular vacuole formed by pinocytosis.

pint (pīnt) a unit of liquid measure in the apothecaries' system, 16 fluid ounces or equivalent to 473.17 milliliters.

pinworm (pin′wurm) any oxyurid, especially *Enterobius vermicularis.*

piperacetazine (pi″per-ah-set′ah-zēn) a tranquilizer, $C_{24}H_{30}N_2O_2S$.

piperazine (pi-per′ah-zēn) a compound, C_4H_{10}-N_2, various salts of which are used as anthelmintics.

piperocaine (pi′per-o-kān″) a local anesthetic, $C_{16}H_{23}NO_2$, used as the hydrochloride salt.

pipet (pi-pet′) pipette.

pipette (pi-pet′) [Fr.] 1. a glass or transparent plastic tube used in measuring or transferring small quantities of liquid or gas. 2. to dispense by means of a pipette.

pipobroman (pi″po-bro′man) an antineoplastic, $C_{10}H_{16}Br_2N_2O_2$.

piriform (pir′ĭ-form) pear-shaped.

Piroplasma (pi″ro-plaz′mah) *Babesia.*

piroplasmosis (-plaz-mo′sis) babesiasis.

pisiform (pi′sĭ-form) resembling a pea in shape and size.

pit (pit) 1. a hollow fovea or indentation. 2. a pockmark. 3. to indent, or to become and remain for a few minutes indented, by pressure.

pitch (pich) 1. a dark, more or less viscous residue from distillation of tar and other substances. 2. natural asphalt of various kinds. 3. the quality of sound dependent on the frequency of vibration of the waves producing it.

pithecoid (pith′ĭ-koid) apelike.

pitting (pit′ing) 1. the formation, usually by scarring, of a small depression. 2. the removal from erythrocytes, by the spleen, of such structures as iron granules, without destruction of the cells. 3. remaining indented for a few minutes after removal of firm finger-pressure, distinguishing fluid edema from myxedema.

pituicyte (pĭ-tu′ĭ-sīt) the distinctive fusiform cell composing most of the neurohypophysis.

pituitarism (pĭ-tu′ĭ-ter-izm″) disorder of pituitary function; see *hyper-* and *hypopituitarism.*

pituitary (pĭ-tu′ĭ-tĕ″re) see under *gland.* **posterior p.,** 1. the posterior lobe of the pituitary gland; the neurohypophysis. 2. a preparation of animal posterior pituitary having the pharmacological actions of its hormones, oxytocin and vasopressin; used mainly as an antidiuretic in the treatment of diabetes insipidus and as a vasoconstrictor.

pityriasis (pit″ĭ-ri′ah-sis) originally, a group of skin diseases marked by the formation of fine, branny scales, but now used only with a modifier. **p. al′ba,** a chronic condition with patchy scaling and hypopigmentation of the skin of the face. **p. ro′sea,** a dermatosis marked by scaling pink oval macules arranged with the long axes parallel to the cleavage lines of the skin. **p. ru′bra pila′ris,** a chronic inflammatory skin disease marked by pink scaling macules and fine acuminate, horny, follicular papules, beginning usually with severe seborrhea of the scalp and seborrheic dermatitis of the face, and associated with keratoderma of the palms and soles. **p. versic′olor,** tinea versicolor.

pityroid (pit′ĭ-roid) furfuraceous; branny.

Pityrosporum (pit″ĭ-ros′per-im) a genus of yeastlike fungi, including *P. orbic′ulare,* a species customarily found on normal skin but capable of causing tinea versicolor in susceptible hosts.

pivalate (piv′ah-lāt) USAN contraction for trimethylacetate.

pK the negative logarithm of the ionization constant (K) of an acid, the pH of a solution in which half of the acid molecules are ionized.

PKU phenylketonuria.

placebo (plah-se′bo) [L.] an inactive substance or preparation given to satisfy the patient's symbolic need for drug therapy, and used in controlled studies to determine the efficacy of medicinal substances. Also, a procedure with no intrinsic therapeutic value, performed for such purposes.

placenta (plah-sen′tah), pl. *placentas* or *placen′-tae.* An organ characteristic of true mammals during pregnancy, joining mother and offspring, providing endocrine secretion and selective exchange of soluble bloodborne substances through apposition of uterine and trophoblastic vascularized parts. **placen'tal,** adj. **p. accre'ta,** one abnormally adherent to the myometrium, with partial or complete absence of the decidua basalis. **fetal p.,** the part of the placenta derived from the chorionic sac that encloses the embryo, consisting of a chorionic plate and villi. **p. incre'ta,** placenta accreta with penetration of the myometrium. **maternal p.,** the maternally contributed part of the placenta, derived from the decidua basalis. **p. membrana'cea,** one that is abnormally thin and spread out over an unusually large area of the uterine wall. **p. percre'ta,** placenta accreta with invasion of the myometrium to its peritoneal covering, sometimes causing rupture of the uterus. **p. pre'via,** one located in the lower uterine segment, so that it partially or entirely covers or adjoins the internal os. **p. reflex'a,** one in which the margin is thickened, appearing to turn back on itself. **p. spu'ria,** an accessory portion having no blood vessel attachment to the main placenta. **p. succenturia'ta,** an accessory portion attached to the main placenta by an artery and vein.

placentation (plas″in-ta′shin) the series of events following implantation of the embryo and leading to development of the placenta.

placentitis (-tīt′is) inflammation of the placenta.

placentography (-tog′rah-fe) radiological visualization of the placenta after injection of a contrast medium.

placentoid (plah-sen′toid) resembling the placenta.

placode (plak′ōd) a platelike structure, especially a thickened plate of ectoderm in the early embryo, from which a sense organ develops, e.g., *auditory p.* (ear), *lens p.* (eye), and *olfactory p.* (nose).

plagiocephaly (pla″je-o-sef′ah-le) an unsymmetrical and twisted condition of the head, due to irregular closure of the cranial sutures. **plagiocephal'ic,** adj.

plague (plāg) an acute febrile, infectious, fatal disease due to *Yersinia pestis,* beginning with chills and fever, quickly followed by prostration, and frequently attended by delirium, headache, vomiting, and diarrhea; primarily a disease of rats and other rodents, it is transmitted to man by flea bites, or communicated from patient to patient. **bubonic p.,** plague marked by swelling of the lymph nodes, forming buboes in the femoral, inguinal, axillary, and cervical regions; in the severe form (black death), septicemia occurs, producing petechial hemorrhages. **pulmonic p.,** a rapidly progressive, highly contagious pneumonia with extensive involvement of the lungs and productive cough with mucoid, bloody, foamy, plague bacilli-laden sputum. **sylvatic p.,** plague in wild rodents, such as the ground squirrel, which serve as a reservoir from which man may be infected.

plane (plān) 1. a flat surface determined by the position of three points in space. 2. a specified level, as the plane of anesthesia. 3. to rub away or abrade; see *planing.* 4. a superficial incision in the wall of a cavity or between tissue layers, especially in plastic surgery, made so that the precise point of entry into the cavity or between the layers can be determined. **axial p.,** one parallel with the long axis of a structure. **base p.,** an imaginary plane upon which is estimated the retention of an artificial denture. **coronal p.,** frontal p. **Frankfort horizontal p.,** a horizontal plane represented in profile by a line between the lowest point on the margin of the orbit and the highest point on the margin of the auditory meatus. **frontal p.,** one passing longitudinally through the body from side to side, at right angles to the median plane, dividing the body into front and back parts. **horizontal p.,** 1. one passing through the body, at right angles to both the frontal and median planes, dividing the body into upper and lower parts. 2. one passing through a tooth at right angles to its long axis. **median p.,** one passing longitudinally through the middle of the body from front to back, dividing it into right and left halves. **nuchal p.,** the outer surface of the occipital bone between the foramen magnum and the superior nuchal line. **occipital p.,** the outer surface of the occipital bone above the superior nuchal line. **orbital p.,** 1. the orbital surface of the maxilla. 2. visual p. **sagittal p.,** a vertical plane passing through the body parallel to the median plane (or to the sagittal suture), dividing the body into left and right portions. **temporal p.,** the depressed area on the side of the skull below the inferior temporal line. **transverse p.,** one passing horizontally through the body, at right angles to the sagittal and frontal planes, and dividing the body into upper and lower portions. **vertical p.,** one perpendicular to a horizontal plane, dividing the body into left and right, or front and back portions. **visual p.,** one passing through the visual axes of the two eyes.

planigraphy (plah-nig′rah-fe) see *body-section roentgenography.* **planigraph'ic,** adj.

planing (pla′ning) abrasion of disfigured skin to promote reepithelization with minimal scarring; done by mechanical means (dermabrasion) or by application of a caustic (chemabrasion).

planocellular (pla″no-sel′ūl-er) composed of flat cells.

planoconcave (-kon′kāv) flat on one side and concave on the other.

planoconvex (-kon′veks) flat on one side and convex on the other.

planography (plah-nog′rah-fe) planigraphy.

planta pedis (plan′tah pe′dis) the sole of the foot.

Plantago (plan-ta′go) a genus of herbs, including *P. in'dica, P. psyl'lium* (Spanish psyllium), and *P. ova'ta* (blond psyllium); see plantago seed.

plantalgia (plan-tal′je-ah) pain in the sole of the foot.

plantar (plan′tar″, plant′er) pertaining to the sole of the foot.

plantaris (plan-ta′ris) [L.] plantar.

plantigrade (plan′tĭ-grād) walking on the full sole of the foot.

planula (plan′ūl-ah) a larval coelenterate.

planum (pla′num), pl. *pla′na* [L.] plane.

plaque (plak) any patch or flat area. **attachment p's,** small regions of increased density along the sarcolemma of skeletal muscles to which myofilaments seem to attach. **bacterial p., dental p.,** a mass adhering to the enamel surface of a tooth, composed of a mixed colony of bacteria in an intercellular matrix of bacterial and salivary polymers and remnants of epithelial cells and leukocytes. It may cause caries, dental calculi and periodontal disease. **fibrous p.,** the lesion of atherosclerosis, a pearly white area within an artery that causes the intimal surface to bulge into the lumen; it is composed of lipid, cell debris, smooth muscle cells, collagen, and, in older persons, calcium. **Hollenhorst p's,** atheromatous emboli containing cholesterol crystals in the retinal arterioles, a sign of impending serious cardiovascular disease.

-plasia word element [Gr.], *development; formation.*

plasm (plazm) 1. plasma. 2. formative substance (cytoplasm, hyaloplasm, etc.).

plasma (plaz′mah) the fluid portion of the blood or lymph. **plasmat′ic,** adj. **antihemophilic human p.,** human plasma which has been processed promptly to preserve the antihemophilic properties of the original blood; used for temporary correction of bleeding tendency in hemophilia. **blood p.,** see under B. **seminal p.,** the fluid portion of the semen, in which the spermatozoa are suspended.

plasmablast (plaz′mah-blast) the immature precursor of a plasma cell.

plasmacyte (-sīt) plasma cell. **plasmacyt′ic,** adj.

plasmacytoma (plaz″mah-si-to′mah) any focal neoplasm of plasma cells, including those of multiple myeloma. Isolated plasmacytomas may occur outside the bone marrow (*extramedullary p's*), affecting such tissues as the nasal, oral, and pharyngeal mucosa and the viscera.

plasmacytosis (-si-to′sis) an excess of plasma cells in the blood.

plasmalemma (plaz″mah-lem′ah) plasma membrane.

plasmalogen (plaz-mal′ah-jen) a term applied to members of a group of phospholipids present in platelets which liberate higher fatty aldehydes on hydrolysis. Plasmalogens are also found in cell membranes of muscle and of the myelin sheath of nerve fibers.

plasmapheresis (plaz″mah-fĕ-re′sis) the removal of plasma from withdrawn blood, with retransfusion of the formed elements into the donor; generally, type-specific fresh frozen plasma or albumin is used to replace the withdrawn plasma. The procedure may be done for purposes of collecting plasma components or for therapeutic purposes.

plasmid (plaz′mid) any extrachromosomal self-replicating genetic element of a cell. In bacteria, plasmids are circular DNA molecules that reproduce themselves and are thus conserved, apart from the chromosome, through successive cell divisions; they include the F factor and R factor. Plasmids that may also be-

come integrated into the chromosome are sometimes called episomes.

plasmin (plaz′min) a proteolytic enzyme with a high specificity for fibrin and the particular ability to dissolve formed fibrin clots.

plasminogen (plaz-min′ah-jen) the inactive precursor of plasmin, occurring in plasma and converted to plasmin by the action of urokinase.

plasmocyte (plaz′mo-sīt) plasma cell.

plasmodesma (-dez′mah), pl. *plasmodes′mata.* A bridge of cytoplasm connecting adjacent cells.

plasmodicidal (plaz-mōd″ĭ-sīd′'l) destructive to plasmodia; malariacidal.

Plasmodium (plaz-mo′de-um) a genus of sporozoa (family Plasmodiidae) parasitic in the red blood cells of animals and man. Four species, *P. falci′parum, P. mala′riae, P. ova′le,* and *P. vi′vax,* cause the four specific types of malaria in man.

plasmodium (plaz-mōd′e-im), pl. *plasmo′dia* [Gr.] 1. a parasite of the genus *Plasmodium.* 2. a multinucleate continuous mass of protoplasm. **plasmo′dial,** adj.

plasmolysis (plaz-mol′ĭ-sis) contraction of cell protoplasm due to loss of water by osmosis. **plasmolyt′ic,** adj.

plasmon (plaz′mon) the hereditary factors of the egg cytoplasm.

plasmorrhexis (plaz″mo-rek′sis) erythrocytorrhexis.

plasmoschisis (plaz-mos′kĭ-sis) the splitting up of cell protoplasm.

plasmotropism (plaz-mah′trah-pizm) destruction of erythrocytes in the liver, spleen, or marrow, as contrasted with their destruction in the circulation. **plasmotrop′ic,** adj.

plaster (plas′ter) 1. plaster of Paris. 2. a pastelike mixture which can be spread over the skin and which is adhesive at body temperature; may be protectant, counterirritant, etc. **p. of Paris,** calcined calcium sulfate; on addition of water it forms a porous mass that is used in making casts and bandages to support or immobilize body parts, and in dentistry for taking dental impressions.

plastic (plas′tik) 1. tending to build up tissues to restore a lost part. 2. capable of being molded. 3. a substance produced by chemical condensation or by polymerization. 4. material that can be molded.

plastid (plas′tid) 1. any elementary constructive unit, as a cell. 2. any specialized organ of the cell other than the nucleus and centrosome, such as chloroplast or amyloplast.

-plasty word element [Gr.], *formation* or *plastic repair of.*

plate (plāt) 1. a flat structure or layer, as a thin layer of bone. 2. dental p. 3. to apply a culture medium to a Petri dish. 4. to inoculate such a plate with bacteria. **axial p.,** primitive streak. **bite p.,** biteplate. **cribriform p.,** fascia cribrosa. **dental p.,** a plate of acrylic resin, metal, or other material which is fitted to the shape of the mouth, and serves to support artificial teeth. **dorsal p.,** roof p. **epiphyseal p.,** the thin plate of cartilage between the epiphysis and the metaphysis of a growing long bone. **equatorial**

p., the collection of chromosomes at the equator of the spindle in mitosis. **floor p.,** the unpaired ventral longitudinal zone of the neural tube. **foot p.,** see *footplate.* **medullary p.,** neural p. **motor p.,** end-plate. **muscle p.,** myotome (2). **neural p.,** the thickened plate of ectoderm in the embryo which develops into the neural tube. **roof p.,** the unpaired dorsal longitudinal zone of the neural tube. **sole p.,** a mass of protoplasm in which a motor nerve ending is embedded. **tarsal p.,** one of the plates of connective tissue forming the framework of either (upper or lower) eyelid. **tympanic p.,** the bony plate forming the floor and sides of the meatus auditorius. **ventral p.,** floor p.

platelet (plāt'lit) a disk-shaped structure, 2 to 4 μm, in diameter, found in the blood of all mammals and chiefly known for its role in blood coagulation; platelets, which are formed by detachment of part of the cytoplasm of a megakaryocyte, lack a nucleus and DNA but contain active enzymes and mitochondria. Called also *thrombocyte.*

plateletpheresis (plāt'lit-fĭ-re'sis) thrombocytapheresis.

platinum (plat'nim) chemical element (*see table*), at. no. 78, symbol Pt.

platy- word element [Gr.], *flat.*

platybasia (plat''ĭ-ba'ze-ah) basilar impression.

platycelous (-sēl'is) having one surface flat and the other concave.

platycoria (-kor'e-ah) a dilated condition of the pupil of the eye.

platyhelminth (-hel'minth) one of the Platyhelminthes; a flatworm.

Platyhelminthes (-hel-min'thēz) a phylum of acoelomate, dorsoventrally flattened, bilaterally symmetrical animals, commonly known as flatworms; it includes the classes Cestoidea (tapeworms) and Trematoda (flukes).

platyhieric (-hi-er'ik) having a sacral index above 100.

platypellic, platypelloid (-pel'ik; -pel'oid) having a flat pelvis; see under *pelvis.*

platypodia (-po'de-ah) flatfoot.

platysma (plah-tiz'mah) see *Table of Muscles.*

pledge (plej) a solemn statement of intention. **Nightingale p.,** a statement of principles for the nursing profession, formulated by a committee in 1893 and subscribed to by student nurses at the time of the capping ceremonies.

pledget (plej'it) a small compress or tuft.

-plegia word element [Gr.], *paralysis; a stroke.*

pleiotropism, pleiotropy (pli-ah'trah-pizm; -trah-pe) the production by a single gene of multiple phenotypic effects. **pleiotrop'ic,** adj.

pleo- word element [Gr.], *more.*

pleocytosis (-si-to'sis) presence of a greater than normal number of cells in cerebrospinal fluid.

pleomorphism (-mor'fizm) the occurrence of various distinct forms by a single organism or within a species. **pleomor'phic, pleomor'phous,** adj.

pleonectic (ple''ah-nek'tik) characterized by having a higher than normal O₂ content at a given Po₂; said of blood.

pleonosteosis (ple''on-os''te-o'sis) abnormally increased ossification. **Léri's p.,** a hereditary syndrome of premature and excessive ossification, with short stature, limitation of movement, broadening and deformity of digits, and mongolian facies.

plessesthesia (ples''es-the'ze-ah) palpatory percussion.

plethora (pleth'ah-rah) an excess of blood. **plethor'ic,** adj.

plethysmograph (plĕ-thiz'mo-grah) an instrument for recording variations in volume of an organ, part, or limb.

plethysmography (pleth''iz-mog'rah-fe) the determination of changes in volume by means of a plethysmograph.

pleur(o)- word element [Gr.], *pleura; rib; side.*

pleura (ploor'ah), pl. *pleu'rae* [Gr.] serous membrane investing the lungs (*pulmonary p.*) and lining the walls of the thoracic cavity (*parietal p.*), the two layers enclosing a potential space, the pleural cavity. **pleu'ral,** adj.

pleuracotomy (ploor''ah-kot'ah-me) incision into the pleural cavity.

pleuralgia (ploor-al'je-ah) pain in the pleura or in the side. **pleural'gic,** adj.

pleurapophysis (ploor''ah-pof'ĭ-sis) a rib, or a vertebral process corresponding to a rib.

pleurectomy (ploor-ek'tah-me) excision of a portion of the pleura.

pleurisy (ploor'ĭ-se) inflammation of the pleura. **pleurit'ic,** adj. **adhesive p.,** that in which exudate forms dense adhesions which partially or totally obliterate the pleural space. **diaphragmatic p.,** that limited to parts near the diaphragm. **dry p.,** a variety with dry fibrinous exudate. **fibrinous p.,** that marked by deposition of large amounts of fibrin in the pleural cavity. **interlobular p.,** a form enclosed between the lobes of the lung. **plastic p.,** that characterized by deposition of a soft, semisolid exudate. **purulent p.,** thoracic empyema. **serous p.,** that marked by free exudation of fluid. **wet p., p. with effusion,** that marked by serous exudation.

pleuritis (ploor-it'is) pleurisy.

pleurocele (ploor'ah-sēl) hernia of lung tissue or of pleura.

pleurocentesis (ploor''ah-sen-te'sis) thoracentesis.

pleurocentrum (-sen'trim) the lateral element of the vertebral column.

pleurodynia (ploor''ah-din'e-ah) paroxysmal pain in the intercostal muscles. **epidemic p.,** an epidemic disease due to coxsackievirus B, marked by a sudden attack of violent pain in the chest, fever, and a tendency to recrudescence on the third day.

pleurogenic, pleurogenous (-jen'ik; ploor-oj'ĭ-nis) originating in the pleura.

pleurography (ploor-og'rah-fe) radiography of the pleural cavity.

pleurohepatitis (ploor''o-hep''ah-tīt'is) hepatitis with inflammation of a portion of the pleura near the liver.

pleurolysis (ploo-rol′ĭ-sis) surgical separation of the pleura from its attachments.

pleuroparietopexy (ploor″o-pah-ri′it-o-pek″se) fixation of the lung to the chest wall by adhesion of the visceral and parietal pleura.

pleuropericarditis (-per″ĭ-kar-dīt′is) inflammation involving the pleura and the pericardium.

pleuroperitoneal (-per″it-ah-ne′il) pertaining to the pleura and peritoneum.

pleuropneumonia (-noo-mo′ne-ah) 1. pleurisy complicated by pneumonia. 2. an infectious disease of cattle, combining pneumonia and pleurisy, due to *Mycoplasma mycoides*.

pleuropneumonia-like (-noo-mo′ne-ah-lik″) a term applied to a group of filterable microorganisms similar to *Mycoplasma mycoides*, the cause of pleuropneumonia; such organisms have been isolated from sheep and goats, dogs, rats, mice, and man. See also *Mycoplasma*.

pleurothotonos (-thot″n-is) tetanic bending of the body to one side.

pleurotomy (ploor-ot′ah-me) incision of the pleura.

plexectomy (plek-sek′tah-me) surgical excision of a plexus.

pleximeter (plek-sim′it-er) 1. a plate to be struck in mediate percussion. 2. diascope.

plexitis (plek-sīt′is) inflammation of a nerve plexus.

plexogenic (plek′sah-jen″ik) giving rise to a plexus or plexiform structure.

plexopathy (pleks-op′ah-the) any disorder of a plexus, especially of nerves. **lumbar p.,** neuropathy of the lumbar plexus.

plexor (plek′ser) a hammer used in diagnostic percussion.

plexus (plek′sis), pl. *plex′us, plex′uses* [L.] a network or tangle, chiefly of vessels or nerves. **plex′al,** adj. **brachial p.,** a nerve plexus originating from the ventral branches of the last four cervical and the first thoracic spinal nerves, giving off many of the principal nerves of the shoulder, chest, and arms. **cardiac p.,** the plexus around the base of the heart, chiefly in the epicardium, formed by cardiac branches from the vagus nerves and the sympathetic trunks and ganglia. **carotid p's,** nerve plexuses surrounding the common, external, and internal carotid arteries. **celiac p.,** a network of ganglia and nerves lying in front of the aorta behind the stomach, supplying the abdominal viscera. **cervical p.,** a nerve plexus formed by the ventral branches of the first four cervical nerves, supplying structures in the neck region. **choroid p.,** infoldings of blood vessels of the pia mater covered by a thin coat of ependymal cells that form tufted projections into the third, fourth, and lateral ventricles of the brain; they secrete the cerebrospinal fluid. **coccygeal p.,** a nerve plexus formed by the ventral branches of the coccygeal and fifth sacral nerve and by a communication from the fourth sacral nerve, giving off the anococcygeal nerves. **cystic p.,** a nerve plexus near the gallbladder. **dental p.,** either of two plexuses (inferior and superior) of nerve fibers, one from the inferior alveolar nerve, situated around the roots of the lower teeth, and the other from the superior alveolar nerve, situated around the roots of the upper teeth. **Exner's p.,** superficial tangential fibers in the molecular layer of the cerebral cortex. **Heller's p.,** an arterial network in the submucosa of the intestine. **lumbar p.,** one formed by the ventral branches of the second to fifth lumbar nerves in the psoas major muscle (the branches of the first lumbar nerve often are included). **lumbosacral p.,** the lumbar and sacral plexuses considered together, because of their continuous nature. **Meissner's p.,** a network of nerve fibers beneath the intestinal mucosa. **myenteric p.,** a nerve plexus within the muscular layers of the intestines. **pampiniform p.,** 1. a plexus of veins from the testicle and epididymis, constituting part of the spermatic cord. 2. a plexus of ovarian veins in the broad ligament. **phrenic p.,** a nerve plexus accompanying the inferior phrenic artery to the diaphragm and adrenal glands. **sacral p.,** one arising from the ventral branches of the last two lumbar and the first four sacral nerves. **solar p.,** celiac p. **tympanic p.,** a network of nerve fibers supplying the mucous lining of the tympanum, mastoid air cells, and pharyngotympanic tube.

-plexy word element [Gr.], *stroke; seizure.* **-plectic,** adj.

plica (pli′kah), pl. *pli′cae* [L.] a fold.

plicate (pli′kāt) plaited or folded.

plication (pli-ka′shin) the operation of taking tucks in a structure to shorten it.

plicotomy (pli-kot′ah-me) surgical division of the posterior fold of the tympanic membrane.

plombage (plom-bahzh′) [Fr.] the filling of a space or cavity in the body with inert material.

PLT *p*sittacosis-*l*ymphogranuloma venereum-*t*rachoma (group); see *Chlamydia*.

plug (plug) an obstructing mass. **Dittrich's p's,** masses of fat globules, fatty acid crystals, and bacteria occurring in the bronchi in putrid bronchitis or bronchiectasis. **epithelial p.,** a mass of ectodermal cells that temporarily closes the external naris of the fetus. **mucous p.,** a plug formed by secretions of the mucous glands of the cervix uteri and closing the cervical canal during pregnancy. **vaginal p.,** one consisting of a mass of coagulated sperm and mucus which forms in the vagina of animals after coitus.

plugger (plug′er) an instrument for compacting filling material in a tooth cavity.

plumbic (plum′bik) pertaining to lead.

plumbism (plum′bizm) chronic lead poisoning; see *lead*[1].

plumbum (plum′bum) [L.] lead (symbol Pb).

pluri- word element [L.], *more.*

pluripotentiality (-po-ten″she-al′it-e) ability to develop in any one of several different ways, or to affect more than one organ or tissue. **pluripo′tent, pluripoten′tial,** adj.

plutonium (ploo-to′ne-um) chemical element (*see table*), at. no. 94, symbol Pu.

Pm chemical symbol, *promethium.*

P.M.I. point of maximal impulse (of the heart).

-pnea word element [Gr.], *respiration; breathing.* **-pneic,** adj.

pneo- word element [Gr.], *breath; breathing.*

pneogram (ne′ah-gram) spirogram.

pneometer (ne-om′it-er) spirometer.

pneum(o)- word element [Gr.], *air* or *gas; lung.*

pneumarthrography (noo″mar-throg′rah-fe) radiography of a joint after injection of air or gas as a contrast medium.

pneumarthrosis (-thro′sis) gas or air in a joint.

pneumat(o)- word element [Gr.], *air* or *gas; lung.*

pneumatic (noo-mat′ik) pertaining to air or respiration.

pneumatization (noo″mut-iz-a′shin) the formation of pneumatic cells or cavities in tissue, especially such formation in the temporal bone.

pneumatocele (noo-mat′o-sēl) 1. hernia of lung tissue. 2. a usually benign, thin-walled air-containing cyst of the lung. 3. a tumor or sac containing gas, especially a gaseous swelling of the scrotum.

pneumatograph (-graf) spirograph.

pneumatometer (noo″mah-tom′it-er) pneometer.

pneumatometry (-tom′ĭ-tre) measurement of the air inspired and expired.

pneumatorrhachis (-tor″ah-kis) presence of gas in the vertebral canal.

pneumatosis (-to′sis) air or gas in an abnormal location in the body. **p. cystoi′des intestina′lis,** a condition characterized by the presence of thin-walled, gas-containing cysts in the wall of the intestine.

pneumaturia (noo″mah-tōōr′e-ah) gas or air in the urine.

pneumoangiogram (noo″mo-an′je-ah-gram″) a composite of radiographs obtained by pneumoencephalography and cerebral angiography.

pneumoarthrography (-ar-throg′rah-fe) pneumarthrography.

pneumocephalus (-sef′ah-lis) air in the intracranial cavity.

pneumococcemia (-kok-sēm′e-ah) pneumococci in the blood.

pneumococcidal (-kok-sīd′′l) destroying pneumococci.

pneumococcosis (-kok-o′sis) infection with pneumococci.

pneumococcosuria (-kok″ōs-ūr′e-ah) pneumococci in the urine.

pneumococcus (-kok′is), pl. *pneumococ′ci.* An individual organism of the species *Streptococcus pneumoniae.* **pneumococ′cal,** adj.

pneumoconiosis (-ko″ne-o′sis) any lung disease, e.g., anthracosis, silicosis, etc., due to permanent deposition of substantial amounts of particulate matter in the lungs.

pneumocranium (-kra′ne-im) pneumocephalus.

Pneumocystis (-sis′tis) a genus of organisms of uncertain status, but considered to be protozoa. *P. cari′nii* is the causative agent of interstitial plasma cell pneumonia.

pneumocystography (-sis-tog′rah-fe) radiography of the urinary bladder after injection of air or gas.

pneumoderma (-der′mah) subcutaneous emphysema.

pneumoencephalography (-en-sef″il-og′rah-fe) radiographic visualization of the fluid-containing structures of the brain after cerebrospinal fluid is intermittently withdrawn by lumbar puncture and replaced by air, oxygen, or helium.

pneumoenteritis (-en″ter-īt′is) inflammation of the lungs and intestine.

pneumography (noo-mog′rah-fe) 1. an anatomical description of the lungs. 2. graphic recording of the respiratory movements. 3. radiography of a part after injection of a gas.

pneumohemopericardium (noo″mo-he″mo-pĕ″re-kar′de-im) air or gas and blood in the pericardium.

pneumohemothorax (-thor′aks) gas or air and blood in the pleural cavity.

pneumohydrometra (noo″mo-hi″dro-me′trah) gas and fluid in the uterus.

pneumohydropericardium (-pĕ″re-kar′de-um) air or gas and fluid in the pericardium.

pneumohydrothorax (-thor′aks) air or gas with effused fluid in the thoracic cavity.

pneumolithiasis (noo″mo-lĭ-thi′ah-sis) the presence of concretions in the lungs.

pneumomediastinum (-me″de-as-ti′nim) presence of air or gas in tissues of the mediastinum, occurring pathologically or introduced intentionally.

pneumometer (noo-mom′it-er) pneograph.

pneumomycosis (noo″mo-mi-ko′sis) any fungal disease of the lungs.

pneumomyelography (-mi″il-og′rah-fe) radiography of the spinal canal after withdrawal of cerebrospinal fluid and injection of air or gas.

pneumonectomy (-nek′tah-me) excision of lung tissue; it may be total, partial, or of a single lobe (*lobectomy*).

pneumonia (noo-mo′ne-ah) inflammation of the lungs with exudation and consolidation. **p. al′ba,** a fatal desquamative pneumonia of the newborn due to congenital syphilis, with fatty degeneration of the lungs, which appear pale and virtually airless. **aspiration p.,** that due to aspiration of foreign material into the lungs. **atypical p.,** primary atypical p. **bacterial p.,** that due to bacteria, chief among which are *Streptococcus pneumoniae, Streptococcus hemolytica, Staphylococcus aureus,* and *Klebsiella pneumoniae.* **bronchial p.,** bronchopneumonia. **desquamative p.,** chronic pneumonia with hardening of the fibrous exudate and proliferation of the interstitial tissue and epithelium. **desquamative interstitial p.,** chronic pneumonia with desquamation of large alveolar cells and thickening of the walls of distal air passages; marked by dyspnea and nonproductive cough. **double p.,** that affecting both lungs. **Friedländer's p., Friedländer's bacillus p.,** a form characterized by massive mucoid inflammatory exudates in a lobe of the lung, due to *Klebsiella pneumoniae.* **hypostatic p.,** that due to dorsal decubitus in weak or aged persons. **influenza virus p., influenzal p.,** an acute, severe, usually fatal disease due to influenza virus, with high fever, prostration, sore throat, aching pains, profound dyspnea and anxiety, and massive edema and consolidation. The term is also applied to influenza complicated by bacterial pneumonia. **inhalation p.,** 1. aspiration p. 2. bronchopneumonia due to inhalation of irritating vapors. **interstitial p.,** a chronic form with increase of the interstitial tissue and decrease of the proper lung tissue, with induration. **interstitial plasma cell p.,** a form affecting infants and debilitated persons, including those receiving certain drugs, in which cellular detritus containing plasma cells appears in lung tissue; it is caused by *Pneumocystis carinii*. **lipid p., lipoid p.,** a pneumonia-like reaction of lung tissue to the aspiration of oil. **lobar p.,** an acute infectious disease due to the pneumococcus and marked by inflammation of one or more lobes of the lungs followed by consolidation. **lobular p.,** bronchopneumonia. **mycoplasmal p.,** primary atypical pneumonia caused by *Mycoplasma pneumoniae*. **parenchymatous p.,** desquamative p. **Pittsburgh p.,** pneumonia resembling legionnaires' disease, caused by *Legionella micdadei* and occurring as a nosocomial infection in immunosuppressed patients. **Pneumocystis p.,** interstitial plasma cell p. **primary atypical p.,** a general term applied to acute infectious pulmonary disease caused by *Mycoplasma pneumoniae*, species of *Rickettsia* and *Chlamydia*, or various viruses, including adenoviruses and the parainfluenza virus, with extensive but tenuous pulmonary infiltration, fever, malaise, myalgia, sore throat, and a cough that becomes productive and paroxysmal. **rheumatic p.,** a rare, usually fatal complication of acute rheumatic fever, characterized by extensive pulmonary consolidation and rapidly progressive functional deterioration and by alveolar exudate, interstitial infiltrates, and necrotizing arteritis. **varicella p.,** that developing after the skin eruption in varicella (chickenpox) and apparently due to the same virus; symptoms may be severe, with violent cough, hemoptysis, and severe chest pain. **viral p.,** that due to a virus, e.g., adenovirus, or influenza, parinfluenza, or varicella virus; see *primary atypical p.* **white p.,** p. alba.

pneumonic (noo-mon′ik) pertaining to the lung or to pneumonia.

pneumonitis (noo″mah-ni′tis) inflammation of lung tissue.

pneumono- word element [Gr.], *lung.*

pneumonocentesis (noo-mo″no-sen-te′sis) surgical puncture of a lung for aspiration.

pneumonocyte (noo-mon′ah-sīt) collective term for the alveolar epithelial cells (great alveolar cells and squamous alveolar cells) and alveolar phagocytes of the lungs.

pneumonolysis (noo″mah-nol′ĭ-sis) division of tissues attaching the lung to the wall of the chest cavity, to permit collapse of the lung.

pneumonopathy (noo″mah-nop′ah-the) any lung disease.

pneumonopexy (noo-mo′nah-pek″se) surgical fixation of the lung to the thoracic wall.

pneumonorrhaphy (noo″mon-or′ah-fe) suture of the lung.

pneumonosis (noo″mah-no′sis) any lung disease.

pneumonotomy (noo″mah-not′ah-me) incision of the lung.

pneumopericardium (-pĕ″re-kar′de-im) air or gas in the pericardial cavity.

pneumoperitoneum (-pĕ″rit′n-e′im) air or gas in the peritoneal cavity.

pneumoperitonitis (-pe″rit′n-īt′is) peritonitis with accumulation of air or gas in the peritoneal cavity.

pneumopleuritis (noo″mo-ploor-īt′is) inflammation of the lungs and pleura.

pneumopyelography (-pi″il-og′rah-fe) radiography after injection of oxygen or air into the renal pelvis.

pneumopyopericardium (-pi″o-pĕ″re-kar′de-um) air or gas and pus in the pericardium.

pneumopyothorax (-pi″o-thor′aks) air or gas and pus in the pleural cavity.

pneumoradiography (-ra″de-og′rah-fe) radiography after injection of air or oxygen.

pneumoretroperitoneum (-rĕ″tro-pĕ″rit′n-e′im) air in the retroperitoneal space.

pneumorrhagia (-ra′je-ah) hemorrhage from the lungs; severe hemoptysis.

pneumotachograph (-tak′ah-graf) an instrument for recording the velocity of respired air.

pneumotachometer (-tah-kom′it-er) a transducer for measuring expired air flow.

pneumotaxic (-tak′sik) regulating the respiratory rate.

pneumotherapy (-thĕ′rah-pe) treatment of disease of lungs.

pneumothorax (-thor′aks) air or gas in the pleural space, which may occur spontaneously (*spontaneous p.*), as a result of trauma or pathological process, or be introduced deliberately (*artificial p.*).

pneumotomy (noo-mot′ah-me) pneumonotomy.

pneumoventriculography (noo″mo-ventrik″ŭl-og′rah-fe) radiography of the cerebral ventricles after injection of air or gas.

P.O. [L.] *per os* (by mouth; orally).

Po chemical symbol, *polonium.*

Po₂ oxygen partial pressure (tension); also written P_{O_2}, pO_2, and pO_2.

pock (pok) a pustule, especially of smallpox.

pockmark (pok′mark″) a depressed scar left by a pustule.

pod(o)- word element [Gr.], *foot.*

podagra (pah-dag′rah) gouty pain in the great toe.

podalgia (pah-dal′je-ah) pain in the feet.

podalic (pah-dal′ik) accomplished by means of the feet; see under *version.*

podarthritis (pod″ar-thrīt′is) inflammation of the joints of the foot.

podiatry (pah-di′ah-tre) chiropody; the specialized field dealing with the study and care of the foot, including its anatomy, pathology, medicinal and surgical treatment, etc. **podiat′ric,** adj.

podium (po′de-im), pl. *po′dia* [L.] a footlike process; a sucker foot.

podocyte (pod′ah-sīt) an epithelial cell of the

visceral layer of a renal glomerulus, having a number of footlike radiating processes (pedicels).

pododynamometer (pod"o-di"nah-mom'it-er) a device for determining the strength of leg muscles.

pododynia (-din'e-ah) neuralgic pain of the heel and sole; burning pain without redness in the sole of the foot.

podology (pah-dol'ah-je) podiatry.

podophyllin (pod"ah-fil'in) podophyllum resin.

podophyllum (-fil'im) the dried rhizome and roots of *Podophyllum peltatum;* see under *resin.*

poe- for words beginning thus, see those beginning *pe-.*

pogoniasis (po"gin-i'ah-sis) excessive growth of the beard, or growth of a beard on a woman.

pogonion (pah-go'ne-in) the anterior midpoint of the chin.

-poiesis word element [Gr.], *formation.* **-poiet'ic,** adj.

poietin (poi-e'tin) any of the hormones involved in regulation of the numbers of the various cell types in the peripheral blood.

poikilo- word element [Gr.], *varied; irregular.*

poikiloblast (poi'ki-lah-blast") an abnormally shaped erythroblast.

poikilocyte (-sīt) an abnormally shaped erythrocyte.

poikiloderma (-der'mah) a condition characterized by pigmentary and atrophic changes in the skin, giving it a mottled appearance.

poikilotherm (poi'ki-lah-therm") an animal that exhibits poikilothermy; a cold-blooded animal.

poikilothermy (poi"ki-lah-ther'me) the state of having a body temperature which varies with that of the environment. **poikilother'mal, poikilother'mic,** adj.

point (point) 1. a small area or spot; the sharp end of an object. 2. to approach the surface, like the pus of an abscess, at a definite spot or place. **p. A,** a roentgenographic, cephalometric landmark, determined on the lateral head film; it is the most retruded part of the curved bony outline from the anterior nasal spine to the crest of the maxillary alveolar process. **auricular p.,** the center of the opening of the external auditory meatus. **p. B,** a roentgenographic cephalometric landmark, determined on the lateral head film; it is the most posterior midline point in the concavity between the infradentale and pogonion. **boiling p.,** the temperature at which a liquid will boil; at sea level, water boils at 100° C., or 212° F. **cardinal p's,** 1. the points on the different refracting media of the eye which determine the direction of the entering or emerging light rays. 2. four points within the pelvic inlet—the two sacroiliac articulations and the two iliopectineal eminences. **craniometric p's,** the established points of reference for measurement of the skull. **dew p.,** the atmospheric temperature at which moisture begins to be deposited as dew. **far p.,** the remotest point at which an object is clearly seen when the eye is at rest. **fixation p.,** the point on which the vision is fixed. **freezing p.,** the tem-

perature at which a liquid begins to freeze; for water, 0° C., or 32° F. **isobestic p.,** the wavelength at which two substances have the same absorptivity. **isoelectric p. (pI),** the pH of a solution in which molecules of a specific substance, such as a protein, have equal numbers of positively and negatively charged groups and therefore do not migrate in an electric field. **jugal p.,** the point at the angle formed by the masseteric and maxillary edges of the zygomatic bone. **lacrimal p.,** the opening on the lacrimal papilla of an eyelid, near the medial angle of the eye, into which tears from the lacrimal lake drain to enter the lacrimal canaliculi. **McBurney's p.,** a point of special tenderness in appendicitis, about ½-2 inches from the right anterior iliac spine on a line between this spine and the navel. **p. of maximal impulse,** the point on the chest where the impulse of the left ventricle is felt most strongly, normally in the fifth costal interspace inside the mamillary line. **melting p.,** the minimum temperature at which a solid begins to liquefy. **near p.,** the nearest point of clear vision, the *absolute near p.* being that for either eye alone with accommodation relaxed, and the *relative near p.* that for both eyes with the employment of accommodation. **nodal p's,** two points on the axis of an optical system situated so that a ray falling on one will produce a parallel ray emerging through the other. **pressure p.,** 1. a point of extreme sensibility to pressure. 2. one of various locations on the body at which digital pressure may be applied for the control of hemorrhage. **subnasal p.,** the central point at the base of the nasal spine. **trigger p.,** a spot on the body at which pressure or other stimulus gives rise to specific sensations or symptoms. **triple p.,** the temperature and pressure at which the solid, liquid, and gas phases of a substance are in equilibrium. **Valleix's p's,** tender points along the course of certain nerves in neuralgia.

pointer (point'er) contusion at a bony eminence. **hip p.,** a contusion of the bone of the iliac crest, or avulsion of muscle attachments at the iliac crest.

pointillage (pwahn-tēl-yahzh') [Fr.] massage with the points of the fingers.

poise (poiz) the unit of viscosity, being that of a fluid which would require a shearing force of one dyne to move a square centimeter area of a layer of fluid 1 cm. per second relative to a parallel layer of fluid 1 cm. distant.

poison (poiz'n) a substance which, on ingestion, inhalation, absorption, application, injection, or development within the body, in relatively small amounts, may cause structural damage or functional disturbance.

poisoning (poiz'ning) the morbid condition produced by a poison. **blood p.,** septicemia. **food p.,** a group of acute illnesses due to ingestion of contaminated food. It may result from allergy; toxemia from foods, such as those inherently poisonous or those contaminated by poisons; foods containing poisons formed by bacteria; or foodborne infections. **forage p.,** a disease produced in animals, especially horses, as a result of eating moldy or fermented food. **heavy**

metal p., poisoning with any of the heavy metals, particularly arsenic, antimony, lead, mercury, cadmium, or thallium. **mushroom p.,** that due to ingestion of poisonous mushrooms; see *Amanita.* **salmon p.,** see *Neorickettsia.* **sausage p.,** allantiasis. **scombroid p.,** see *Scombroidea.*

poison ivy (poiz'n i've) *Rhus radicans.*

poison oak (ōk) *Rhus diversiloba* or *R. toxicodendron.*

poison sumac (soo'mak) *Rhus vernix.*

Polaramine (pah-lar'ah-mēn) trademark for preparations of dexchlorpheniramine.

polarimetry (po''lah-rim'ĭ-tre) measurement of the rotation of plane polarized light.

polarity (pah-lar'it-e) the condition of having poles or of exhibiting opposite effects at the two extremities.

polarization (po''ler-iz-a'shin) the production of that condition in light in which its vibrations are parallel to each other in one plane, or in circles and ellipses.

polarography (po''ler-og'rah-fe) an electrochemical technique for identifying and estimating the concentration of reducible elements in an electrochemical cell by means of the dual measurement of the current flowing through the cell and the electrical potential at which each element is reduced. **polarograph'ic,** adj.

pole (pōl) 1. either extremity of any axis, as of the fetal ellipse or a body organ. 2. either one of two points which have opposite physical qualities. **po'lar,** adj. **animal p.,** that pole of an ovum to which the nucleus is approximated, and from which the polar bodies pinch off. **cephalic p.,** the end of the fetal ellipse at which the head of the fetus is situated. **frontal p.,** the most prominent part of the anterior end of each hemisphere of the brain. **germinal p.,** animal p. **negative p.,** cathode. **occipital p.,** the posterior end of the occipital lobe of the brain. **pelvic p.,** the end of the fetal ellipse at which the breech of the fetus is situated. **positive p.,** anode. **temporal p.,** the prominent anterior end of the temporal lobe of the brain. **vegetal p., vegetative p., vitelline p.,** that pole of an ovum at which the greater amount of food yolk is deposited.

poli(o)- word element [Gr.], *gray matter.*

policeman (pah-lēs'min) a glass rod with a piece of rubber tubing on one end, used as a stirring rod and transfer tool in chemical analysis.

policlinic (pol''ĭ-klin'ik) a city hospital, infirmary, or clinic; cf. *polyclinic.*

polio (pōl'e-o) poliomyelitis.

polioclastic (po''le-o-klas'tik) destroying the gray matter of the nervous system.

poliodystrophia (-dis-tro'fe-ah) poliodystrophy. **p. ce'rebri,** a rare disease of young children, marked by neuron degeneration of the cerebral cortex and elsewhere, with progressive mental deterioration, motor disturbances, sometimes cortical deafness and blindness, and early death.

poliodystrophy (-dis'trah-fe) atrophy of the cerebral gray matter.

polioencephalitis (-en-sef''il-īt'is) inflammatory disease of the gray matter of the brain. **inferior p.,** bulbar paralysis.

polioencephalomeningomyelitis (-en-sef''il-o-mĕ-ning''go-mi''il-īt'is) inflammation of the gray matter of the brain and spinal cord and of the meninges.

polioencephalomyelitis (-mi''il-īt'is) inflammation of the gray matter of the brain and spinal cord.

polioencephalopathy (-en-sef''ah-lop'ah-the) disease of the gray matter of the brain.

poliomyelitis (-mi''il-īt'is) an acute viral disease marked clinically by fever, sore throat, headache, vomiting, and often stiffness of the neck and back; these may be the only symptoms of the minor illness. In the major illness (*acute anterior p.*), which may or may not be preceded by the minor illness, there is central nervous system involvement, stiff neck, pleocytosis in spinal fluid, and perhaps paralysis; there may be subsequent atrophy of muscle groups, ending in contraction and permanent deformity. **acute anterior p.,** see *poliomyelitis.* **ascending p.,** poliomyelitis with a cephalad progression. **bulbar p.,** a severe form affecting the medulla oblongata, which may result in dysfunction of the swallowing mechanism, respiratory embarrassment, and circulatory distress. **spinal paralytic p.,** the classic form of acute anterior poliomyelitis, in which the appearance of flaccid paralysis, usually of one or more limbs, makes the diagnosis definite.

poliomyelopathy (-mi''il-op'ah-the) any disease of the gray matter of the spinal cord.

poliosis (pōl-e-o'sis) premature grayness of the hair.

poliovirus (pōl-e-o-vi'ris) the causative agent of poliomyelitis, separable, on the basis of specificity of neutralizing antibody, into three serotypes designated types 1, 2, and 3.

pollen (pol'in) the male fertilizing element of flowering plants.

pollex (pol'eks) [L.] the thumb. **p. val'gus,** deviation of the thumb toward the ulnar side. **p. va'rus,** deviation of the thumb toward the radial side.

pollicization (pol''ĭ-siz-a'shin) surgical construction of a thumb from a finger.

pollinosis (pol''ĭ-no'sis) an allergic reaction to pollen; hay fever.

polocyte (pōl'ah-sīt) see *polar bodies.*

polonium (pah-lo'ne-im) chemical element (*see table*), at. no. 84, symbol Po.

poloxamer (pol-oks'ah-mer) any of a series of nonionic surfactants of the polyoxypropylene-polyoxyethylene copolymer type, used as surfactants, emulsifiers, stabilizers, and food additives.

polus (pōl'is), pl. *po'li* [L.] pole.

poly- word element [Gr.], *many; much.*

polyacrylamide (pol''e-ah-kril'ah-mīd) a polymer of acrylamide.

polyadenitis (-ad''in-īt'is) inflammation of several glands.

polyadenosis (-ad''in-o'sis) disorder of several glands, particularly endocrine glands.

polyamine (-ah-mēn′) any compound, e.g., spermine and spermidine, containing two or more amino groups.

polyangiitis (-an″je-īt′is) inflammation involving multiple blood or lymph vessels.

polyarteritis (-ar″ter-īt′is) a condition marked by multiple sites of inflammatory and destructive lesions in the arterial system; see *periarteritis nodosa.*

polyarthric (-ar′thrik) polyarticular.

polyarthritis (-ar-thrīt′is) inflammation of several joints. **chronic villous p.,** chronic inflammation of the synovial membrane of several joints. **p. rheumat′ica,** rheumatic fever.

polyarticular (-ar-tik′ūl-er) affecting many joints.

polyatomic (-ah-tom′ik) made up of several atoms.

polybasic (-ba′sik) having several replaceable hydrogen atoms.

polyblast (pol′e-blast) free macrophage.

polycarbophil (pol″e-kar′bah-fil) polyacrylic acid cross-linked with divinyl glycol; used as a gastrointestinal absorbent.

polycholia (-kōl′e-ah) excessive flow or secretion of bile.

polychondritis (-kon-drīt′is) inflammation of many cartilages of the body. **chronic atrophic p., p. chro′nica atro′phicans, relapsing p.** an acquired, idiopathic chronic disease with a tendency to recurrence, marked by inflammatory and degenerative lesions of various cartilaginous structures.

polychromasia (-krōm-a′ze-ah) 1. variation in the hemoglobin content of erythrocytes. 2. polychromatophilia.

polychromatic (-krom-at′ik) many-colored.

polychromatocyte (-krom-at′ah-sīt) a cell stainable with various kinds of stain.

polychromatophil (-krom-at′ah-fil) a structure stainable with many kinds of stain.

polychromatophilia (-krom-at″ah-fil′e-ah) 1. the property of being stainable with various stains; affinity for all sorts of stains. 2. a condition in which the erythrocytes, on staining, show various shades of blue combined with tinges of pink. **polychromatophil′ic,** adj.

polychromemia (-krom-ēm′e-ah) increase in the coloring matter of the blood.

polyclinic (-klin′ik) a hospital and school where diseases and injuries of all kinds are studied and treated.

polyclonal (-klōn″l) derived from different cells; pertaining to several clones.

polyclonia (-klo′ne-ah) a disease marked by many clonic spasms.

polycoria (-kor′e-ah) more than one pupil in an eye.

polycrotism (pah-lik′rah-tizm) the quality of having several secondary waves to each beat of the pulse. **polycrot′ic,** adj.

polycyesis (pol″e-si-e′sis) multiple pregnancy.

polycystic (-sis′tik) containing many cysts.

polycythemia (-si-thēm′e-ah) an increase in the total cell mass of the blood. **absolute p.,** an increase in red cell mass caused by increased

erythropoiesis, which may occur as a compensatory physiologic response to tissue hypoxia or as the principal manifestation of polycythemia vera. **p. hyperto′nica,** a syndrome of increased red cell mass (without splenomegaly, leukocytosis, or thrombocytosis), hypertrophy of the heart, and labile hypertension. **relative p.,** a decrease in plasma volume without change in red blood cell mass so that the erythrocytes become more concentrated (elevated hematocrit), which may be an acute transient or a chronic condition. **p. ru′bra,** p. vera. **secondary p.,** any absolute increase in the total red cell mass other than polycythemia vera. **stress p.,** chronic relative polycythemia usually affecting white, middle-aged, mildly obese males who are active, anxiety-prone, and hypertensive. **p. ve′ra,** a myeloproliferative disorder of unknown etiology, characterized by abnormal proliferation of all hematopoietic bone marrow elements and an absolute increase in red cell mass and total blood volume, associated frequently with splenomegaly, leukocytosis, and thrombocythemia.

polydactylism, polydactyly (-dak′til-izm; -dak′tĭ-le) the presence of supernumerary digits on the hands or feet.

polydipsia (-dip′se-ah) excessive thirst.

polydysplasia (-dis-pla′ze-ah) faulty development of several tissues, organs, or systems.

polyesthesia (-es-the′ze-ah) a sensation as if several points were touched on application of a stimulus to a single point.

polyestradiol phosphate (pol″e-es″trah-di′ol) a polymer of estradiol phosphate having estrogenic activity similar to that of estradiol; used in the palliative therapy of prostatic carcinoma.

polyethylene (-eth′ĭ-lēn) polymerized ethylene, $(CH_2—CH_2)_n$, a synthetic plastic material, forms of which have been used in reparative surgery. **p. glycol,** a polymer of ethylene oxide and water, available in liquid form (polyethylene glycol 300 or 400) or as waxy solids (polyethylene glycol 1540 or 4000), used in various pharmaceutical preparations.

polygalactia (-gah-lak′she-ah) excessive secretion of milk.

polygene (pol′ĭ-jēn) a group of nonallelic genes that interact to influence the same character with additive effect.

polygenic (pol″ĭ-jēn′ik) pertaining to or determined by several different genes.

polyglactin (-glak′tin) an absorbable surgical suture material, $(C_2H_2O_2)_m(C_3H_4O_2)_n$.

polyglandular (-glan′dūl-er) pertaining to or affecting several glands.

polygraph (pol′ĭ-graf) an apparatus for simultaneously recording blood pressure, pulse, and respiration, and variations in electrical resistance of the skin; popularly known as a lie-detector.

polygyria (pol″ĭ-ji′re-ah) excess of convolutions in the brain.

polyhedral (-he′dril) having many sides or surfaces.

polyhidrosis (-hi-dro′sis) hyperhidrosis.

polyhydramnios (-hi-dram′ne-is) hydramnios.

polyhydric (-hi′drik) containing more than two hydroxyl groups.

polyinfection (-in-fek′shin) infection with more than one organism.

polyionic (-i-on′ik) containing several different ions (e.g., potassium, sodium, etc.), as a polyionic solution.

polyleptic (-lep′tik) having many remissions and exacerbations.

polymastia (-mas′te-ah) the presence of supernumerary mammary glands.

polymastigote (-mas′tĭ-gōt) 1. having several flagella. 2. a mastigote having several flagella.

polymelus (pah-lim′il-is) an individual with supernumerary limbs.

polymenorrhea (pol″ĭ-men″ah-re′ah) abnormally frequent menstruation.

polymer (pol′ĭ-mer) a compound, usually of high molecular weight, formed by the linear combination of simpler molecules (monomeres); it may be formed without formation of any other product (*addition p.*) or with simultaneous elimination of water or other simple compound (*condensation p.*).

polymerase (pol-im′er-ās) an enzyme that catalyzes polymerization.

polymeric (pol″ĭ-mer′ik) exhibiting the characteristics of a polymer.

polymerization (po-lim″er-iz-a′shin, -mer″iz-a′shin) the combining of several simpler compounds to form a polymer.

polymicrobial, polymicrobic (pol″ĭ-mi-kro′be-il; -mi-kro′bik) marked by the presence of several species of microorganisms.

polymicrogyria (-mi″kro-ji′re-ah) a brain malformation marked by development of numerous microgyri.

polymorph (pol′ĭ-morf) colloquial term for polymorphonuclear leukocyte.

polymorphic (pol″ĭ-mor′fik) occurring in several or many forms; appearing in different forms in different developmental stages.

polymorphism (-mor′fizm) the quality of existing in several different forms. **balanced p.,** an equilibrium mixture of homozygotes and heterozygotes maintained by natural selection against both homozygotes.

polymorphocellular (-mor″fah-sel′ūl-er) having cells of many forms.

polymorphonuclear (-noo″kle-er) 1. having a nucleus so deeply lobed or so divided as to appear to be multiple. 2. a polymorphonuclear leukocyte; see *neutrophil* (1).

polymorphous (-mor′fis) polymorphic.

polymyalgia (pol″ĭ-mi-al′je-ah) pain involving many muscles.

polymyoclonus (-mi-ok′lin-is) 1. a fine or minute muscular tremor. 2. polyclonia.

polymyopathy (-mi-op′ah-the) disease affecting several muscles simultaneously.

polymyositis (-mi″ah-sīt′is) inflammation of several or many muscles at once, along with degenerative and regenerative changes marked by muscle weakness out of proportion to the loss of muscle bulk.

polymyxin (-mik′sin) generic term for antibiotics derived from *Bacillus polymyxa;* they are differentiated by affixing different letters of the alphabet. **p. B,** the least toxic of the polymyxins; its sulfate is used in the treatment of various gram-negative infections.

polynesic (-ne′sik) occurring in many foci.

polyneural (-noor′il) pertaining to or supplied by many nerves.

polyneuralgia (-nōōr-al′je-ah) neuralgia of several nerves.

polyneuritis (-nōōr-īt′is) inflammation of many nerves simultaneously. **acute febrile p., acute infectious p.,** an acute, rapidly progressive, ascending paralysis, beginning in the feet and ascending to the other muscles, often occurring after an enteric or respiratory infection.

polyneuromyositis (-nōōr″o-mi-ah-sīt′is) inflammation of the muscles and peripheral nerves, with loss of reflexes, sensory loss, and paresthesias.

polyneuropathy (-nōōr-op′ah-the) a disease involving several nerves. **erythredema p.,** acrodynia.

polyneuroradiculitis (-nōōr-o-rah-dik″ūl-īt′is) inflammation of spinal ganglia, nerve roots, and peripheral nerves.

polynuclear (-noo″kle-er) 1. polynucleate. 2. polymorphonuclear.

polynucleate (-noo″kle-āt) polynuclear.

polynucleotide (-noo′kle-ah-tīd) any polymer of mononucleotides.

polyopia (-o′pe-ah) visual perception of several images of a single object.

polyorchidism (-or′kid-izm) the presence of more than two testes.

polyorchis (-or′kis) a person exhibiting polyorchidism.

polyostotic (-os-tot′ik) affecting several bones.

polyovular (-o′vūl-er) pertaining to or produced from more than one ovum, as polyovular twins.

polyovulatory (-ov′ūl-ah-tor″e) discharging several ova in one ovarian cycle.

polyoxyl stearate (-oks′il) a group of surfactants consisting of a mixture of mono- and diesters of stearate and polyoxyethylene diols; they are numbered according to the average polymer length of oxyethylene units, e.g., polyoxyl 40 stearate.

polyp (pol′ip) any growth or mass protruding from a mucous membrane. **adenomatous p.,** a benign polypoid adenoma. **fibrinous p.,** intrauterine polyp made up of fibrin from retained blood. **juvenile p's,** small, benign hemispheric hamartomas of the large intestine occurring sporadically in children. **retention p's,** juvenile p's.

polyparesis (pol″e-pah-re′sis) dementia paralytica.

polypectomy (-pek′tah-me) excision of a polyp.

polypeptide (-pep′tīd) a peptide containing more than two amino acids linked by peptide bonds.

polypeptidemia (-pep″tĭ-dēm′e-ah) the presence of polypeptides in the blood.

polyphagia (-fa′je-ah) excessive ingestion of food.

polyphalangia, polyphalangism (-fah-lan'je-ah; -fah-lan'jizm) excess of phalanges in a finger or toe.

polypharmacy (-far'mah-se) 1. administration of many drugs together. 2. administration of excessive medication.

polyplastic (-plas'tik) 1. containing many structural or constituent elements. 2. undergoing many changes of form.

polyplegia (-ple'je-ah) paralysis of several muscles.

polyploidy (-ploi"de) possession of more than two sets of homologous chromosomes.

polypnea (pol"ip-ne'ah) hyperpnea.

polypoid (pol'ĭ-poid) resembling a polyp.

polyporous (pol-ip'er-is) having many pores.

polyposis (-po'sis) the formation of numerous polyps. **familial p.,** a hereditary condition marked by multiple adenomatous polyps with high malignant potential, lining the intestinal mucosa, especially that of the colon, beginning at about puberty. Multiple intestinal polyps occur in *Gardner's, Peutz-Jeghers, Canada-Cronkhite,* and *Turcot's syndromes.*

polypous (pol'ĭ-pis) polyp-like.

polyptychial (pol"e-ti'ke-al) arranged in several layers.

polypus (pol'ĭ-pus), pl. *po'lypi* [L.] polyp.

polyradiculitis (pol"e-rah-dik"ŭl-īt'is) inflammation of the nerve roots.

polyradiculoneuritis (-rah-dik"ŭl-o-nōōr-īt'is) acute febrile polyneuritis which involves the peripheral nerves, the spinal nerve roots, and the spinal cord.

polyribosome (-ri'bah-sōm) a cluster of ribosomes connected with messenger RNA; they play a role in peptide synthesis.

polysaccharide (-sak'ah-rīd) a carbohydrate which on hydrolysis yields many monosaccharides.

polyserositis (-sēr"ah-sīt'is) general inflammation of serous membranes, with effusion.

polysome (pol'e-sōm) polyribosome.

polysomy (-so'me) an excess of a particular chromosome.

polysorbate 80 (-sor'bāt) an oleate ester of sorbitol and its anhydride (sorbitan) condensed with polymers of ethylene oxide, consisting of approximately 20 oxyethylene units; it is a surfactant used as an emulsifying, dispersing, and solubilizing agent.

polyspermy (-sper'me) fertilization of an ovum by more than one spermatozoon; occurring normally in certain species (*physiologic p.*) and sometimes abnormally in others (*pathologic p.*).

polystyrene (-sti'rēn) the resin produced by polymerization of styrol, a clear resin of the thermoplastic type, used in the construction of denture bases.

polysynaptic (-sĭ-nap'tik) pertaining to or relayed through two or more synapses.

polysyndactyly (-sin-dak'tĭ-le) hereditary association of polydactyly and syndactyly.

polytef (pol'ĭ-tef) a polymer of tetrafluoroethylene, used as a surgical implant material for many prostheses, such as artificial vessels and orbital floor implants and for many applications in skeletal augmentation and skeletal fixation.

polytene (pol'ĭ-tēn) composed of or containing many strands of chromatin (chromonemata).

polytenosynovitis (pol"ĭ-ten"o-sin"o-vīt'is) inflammation of several or many tendon sheaths at the same time.

polythelia (-thēl'e-ah) the presence of supernumerary nipples.

polythiazide (-thi'ah-zīd) a diuretic and antihypertensive, $C_{11}H_{13}ClF_3N_3O_4S_3$.

polytomogram (pol"ĭ-tom'ah-gram) the record produced by polytomography.

polytomography (-to-mog'rah-fe) tomography of tissue at several predetermined planes.

polytrichia (-trik'e-ah) hypertrichiasis.

polyunsaturated (-un-sach'er-āt-id) denoting a fatty acid, e.g., linoleic acid, having more than one double bond in its hydrocarbon chain.

polyunsaturated fatty acids fatty acids having two or more double bonds. A diet high in polyunsaturated fatty acids tends to lower plasma cholesterol levels.

polyuria (-ūr'e-ah) excessive secretion of urine.

polyvalent (-vāl'int) multivalent.

polyvinylpyrrolidine (-vi"nil-pi-rol'ĭ-dēn) povidone.

pompholyx (pom'fah-liks) an intensely pruritic skin eruption on the sides of the digits or on the palms and soles, consisting of small, discrete, round vesicles, typically occurring in repeated self-limited attacks.

pomum (po'mum), pl. *po'ma* [L.] apple. **p. ada'mi,** the prominence on the throat caused by thyroid cartilage.

pons (ponz) 1. any slip of tissue connecting two parts of an organ. 2. that part of the metencephalon lying between the medulla oblongata and the midbrain, ventral to the cerebellum; see *brain stem.* **p. he'patis,** an occasional projection partially bridging the longitudinal fissure of the liver.

pontic (pon'tik) the portion of a dental bridge which substitutes for an absent tooth.

ponticulus (pon-tik'ŭl-is), pl. *pontic'uli* [L.] delicate plates of white matter passing across the anterior end of the pyramid and just below the pons. **pontic'ular,** adj.

pontine (pon'tīn) pertaining to the pons.

pontobulbar (pon"to-bul'ber) pertaining to the pons and the region of the medulla oblongata dorsad to it.

pontocerebellar (pon"to-ser"ĭ-bel'er) pertaining to the pons and cerebellum.

pontomesencephalic (-mes"en-sef'al-ik) pertaining to or involving the pons and the mesencephalon.

popliteal (pop"lĭt'e-il) pertaining to the area behind the knee.

POR problem oriented record.

poradenitis (por"ad-in-īt'is) inflammation of lymph nodes with formation of small abscesses.

porcine (por'sīn) pertaining to swine.

pore (por) a small opening or empty space. **alveolar p's,** openings between adjacent pulmonary alveoli that permit passage of air from one to another. **nuclear p's,** small octagonal openings in the nuclear envelope at sites where the two nuclear membranes are in contact, which together with the annuli form the pore complex. **slit p's,** small slitlike spaces between the pedicels of the podocytes of the renal glomerulus.

porencephalitis (por″en-sef″il-īt′is) porencephaly associated with an inflammatory process.

porencephaly (por″en-sef′ah-le) development or presence of abnormal cysts or cavities in the brain tissue, usually communicating with a lateral ventricle. **porencephal′ic, porenceph′alous,** adj.

porokeratosis (por″o-ker″ah-to′sis) a hereditary dermatosis marked by a centrifugally spreading hypertrophy of the stratum corneum around the sweat pores followed by atrophy. Also known as *p. of Mibelli.* **porokeratot′ic,** adj.

poroma (po-ro′mah) a tumor arising in a pore. **eccrine p.,** a benign tumor arising from the intradermal portion of an eccrine sweat duct, usually on the sole.

porosis (por-o′sis) 1. the formation of the callus in repair of a fractured bone. 2. cavity formation.

porosity (por-os′it-e) the condition of being porous; a pore.

porotomy (por-ot′ah-me) meatotomy.

porous (por′is) penetrated by pores and open spaces.

porphin (por′fin) the fundamental ring structure of four linked pyrrole nuclei around which porphyrins, hemin, cytochromes, and chlorophyll are built.

porphobilinogen (por″fo-bi-lin′ah-jin) an intermediary product in the biosynthesis of heme.

porphyria (por-fēr′e-ah, por-fi′re-ah) a disturbance of porphyrin metabolism characterized by increase in formation and excretion of porphyrins or their precursors. **acute intermittent p.,** hereditary hepatic porphyria due to a defect of pyrrole metabolism, with recurrent attacks of abdominal pain, gastrointestinal and neurologic disturbances, and excessive amounts of aminolevulinic acid and porphobilinogen in the urine. **congenital erythropoietic p.,** hereditary erythropoietic porphyria, with cutaneous photosensitivity leading to mutilating lesions, hemolytic anemia, splenomegaly, excessive urinary excretion of uroporphyrin, and, invariably, erythrodontia and hypertrichosis. **p. cuta′nea tar′da heredita′ria,** hepatic porphyria resembling the variegate form except that abdominal and neurologic symptoms are absent or mild. **p. cuta′nea tar′da symptoma′tica,** a sporadic form, usually associated with chronic alcoholism, marked by chronic skin lesions ranging from slight fragility to severe scarring, and by hepatomegaly and excessive excretion of uro- and coproporphyrin. **erythropoietic p.,** that in which excessive formation of porphyrin or its precursors occurs in bone marrow normoblasts; it includes congenital erythropoietic porphyria and erythropoietic

protoporphyria. **hepatic p.,** that in which the excess formation of porphyrin or its precursors occurs in the liver. **variegate p.,** hereditary hepatic porphyria, with chronic skin manifestations, chiefly extreme mechanical fragility of the skin, mainly of areas exposed to sunlight, episodes of abdominal pain, neuropathy, and, typically, an excess of coproporhyrin and protoporphyrin in bile and feces.

porphyrin (por′fī-rin) any of a group of iron- or magnesium-free cyclic tetrapyrrole derivatives, occurring universally in protoplasm, and forming the basis of the respiratory pigments of animals and plants.

porphyrinuria (por″fī-rin-ūr′e-ah) an excess of porphyrin in the urine.

porta (port′ah), pl. *por′tae* [L.] an entrance or portal; especially the site of entrance to an organ of the blood vessels and other structures supplying or draining it. **p. he′patis,** the transverse fissure on the visceral surface of the liver where the portal vein and hepatic artery enter and the hepatic ducts leave.

portacaval (port″ah-ka′vil) pertaining to the portal vein and inferior vena cava.

portal (port′'l) 1. an avenue of entrance; porta. 2. pertaining to a porta, especially the porta hepatis.

portio (por′she-o), pl. *portio′nes* [L.] a part or division. **p. du′ra,** the facial nerve. **p. interme′dia,** intermediate nerve. **p. mol′lis,** vestibulocochlear nerve. **p. supravagina′lis,** the part of the cervix uteri that does not protrude into the vagina. **p. vagina′lis,** the portion of the uterus projecting into the vagina.

portoenterostomy (port″o-en″ter-os′tah-me) surgical anastomosis of the jejunum to a decapsulated area of liver in the porta hepatis region and to the duodenum; done to establish a conduit from the intrahepatic bile ducts to the intestine in biliary atresia.

portography (por-tog′rah-fe) radiography of the portal vein after injection of opaque material into the superior mesenteric vein or one of its branches during operation (*portal p.*), or percutaneously into the spleen (*splenic p.*).

portosystemic (por″to-sis-tem′ik) connecting the portal and systemic venous circulation.

porus (po′rus), pl. *po′ri* [L.] an opening or pore. **p. acus′ticus exter′nus,** the outer end of the external acoustic meatus. **p. acus′ticus inter′nus,** the opening of the internal acoustic meatus. **p. op′ticus,** the opening in the sclera for passage of the optic nerve.

-posia word element [Gr.], *intake of fluids.*

position (pah-zish′in) 1. a bodily posture or attitude. 2. the relationship of a given point on the presenting part of the fetus to a designated point of the maternal pelvis; see accompanying table. Cf. *presentation.* **anatomic p.,** that of the human body, standing erect, with palms turned forward, used as the position of reference in designating the site or direction of structures of the body. **Bonner's p.,** flexion, abduction, and outward rotation of the thigh in coxitis. **Bozeman's p.,** the knee-elbow position with straps used for support. **Brickner p.,** the wrist is tied to the head of the bed to obtain abduction and external rotation for shoulder disability. **decubitus p.,** that of the body lying on a horizontal surface, designated according to the aspect of the body touching the surface, *dorsal decubitus* (on the back), *left lateral decubitus* (on the left side), *right lateral decubitus* (on the right side), or *ventral decubitus* (on the abdomen). **Fowler's p.,** that in which the head of the patient's bed is raised 18–20 inches above the level, with the knees also elevated. **knee-chest p.,** the patient resting on his knees and upper chest. **knee-elbow p.,** the patient resting on his knees and elbows with the chest elevated. **lithotomy p.,** the patient on his back with hips and knees flexed and thighs abducted and externally rotated. **Mayer p.,** a roentgenographic position that gives a unilateral superoinferior view of the temporomandibular joint, external auditory canal, and mastoid and petrous processes. **Rose's p.,** a supine position with the head over the table edge in full extension. **Sims' p.,** the patient on his left side and chest, the right knee and thigh drawn up, the left arm along the back. **Trendelenburg's p.,** the patient is supine on a surface inclined 45 degrees, his head at the lower end and his legs flexed over the upper end. **verticosubmental p.,** a roentgenographic position that gives an axial projection of the mandible, including the coronoid and condyloid processes of the rami, the base of the skull and its foramina, the petrous pyramids, the sphenoidal, posterior ethmoid, and maxillary sinuses, and the nasal septum. **Waters p.,** a roentgenographic position that gives a posteroanterior view of the maxillary sinus, maxilla, orbits, and zygomatic arches.

positive (poz′it-iv) having a value greater than zero; indicating existence or presence, as chromatin-positive; characterized by affirmation or cooperation.

positron (poz′ĭ-tron) a positively charged electron.

posology (pah-sol′ah-je) the science or system of dosage. **posolog′ic,** adj.

post- word element [L.], *after; behind.*

postauricular (pōst″aw-rik′ūl-er) located or performed behind the auricle of the ear.

postaxial (pōst-ak′se-il) behind an axis; in anatomy, referring to the medial (ulnar) aspect of the upper arm, and the lateral (fibular) aspect of the lower leg.

postbrachial (-bra′ke-il) on the posterior part of the upper arm.

postcava (-ka′vah) the inferior vena cava. **postca′val,** adj.

postcibal (-si′bil) after eating; postprandial.

postcornu (-kor′noo) the posterior horn of the lateral ventricle.

postdiastolic (-di″as-tol′ik) after diastole.

postdicrotic (pōst″di-krot′ik) after the dicrotic elevation of the sphygmogram.

posterior (pos-tēr′e-er) directed toward or situated at the back; opposite of anterior.

postero- word element [L.], *the back; posterior to.*

posteroanterior (pos″ter-o-an-tēr′e-er) directed from the back toward the front.

POSITIONS OF THE FETUS IN VARIOUS PRESENTATIONS

CEPHALIC PRESENTATION

Vertex—occiput the point of direction
  Left occipitoanterior (L.O.A.)
  Left occipitotransverse (L.O.T.)
  Right occipitoposterior (R.O.P.)
  Right occipitotransverse (R.O.T.)
  Right occipitoanterior (R.O.A.)
  Left occipitoposterior (L.O.P.)
Face—chin the point of direction
  Right mentoposterior (R.M.P.)
  Left mentoanterior (L.M.A.)
  Right mentotransverse (R.M.T.)
  Right mentoanterior (R.M.A.)
  Left mentotransverse (L.M.T.)
  Left mentoposterior (L.M.P.)
Brow—the point of direction
  Right frontoposterior (R.F.P.)
  Left frontoanterior (L.F.A.)
  Right frontotransverse (R.F.T.)
  Right frontoanterior (R.F.A.)
  Left frontotransverse (L.F.T.)
  Left frontoposterior (L.F.P.)

BREECH OR PELVIC PRESENTATION

Complete breech—sacrum, the point of direction (feet crossed and thighs flexed on abdomen)
  Left sacroanterior (L.S.A.)
  Left sacrotransverse (L.S.T.)
  Right sacroposterior (R.S.P.)
  Right sacroanterior (R.S.A.)
  Right sacrotransverse (R.S.T.)
  Left sacroposterior (L.S.P.)
Incomplete breech—sacrum, the point of direction. Same designations as above, adding the qualifications footling, knee, etc.

TRANSVERSE LIE OR SHOULDER PRESENTATION

Shoulder—scapula the point of direction

Left scapuloanterior (L.Sc.A.)	Back anterior positions
Right scapuloanterior (R.Sc.A.)	
Right scapuloposterior (R.Sc.P.)	Back posterior positions
Left scapuloposterior (L.Sc.P.)	

posteroclusion (-kloo′zhin) distoclusion.

posteroexternal (-ek-ster′nil) situated on the outside of a posterior aspect.

posteroinferior (-in-fēr′e-er) behind and below.

posterolateral (-lat′er-il) situated on the side and toward the posterior aspect.

posteromedian (-me′de-in) situated on the middle of a posterior aspect.

posterosuperior (-soo-pēr′e-er) situated behind and above.

postganglionic (pōst″gang-gle-on′ik) distal to a ganglion.

posthepatitic (-hep-ah-tit′ik) occurring after or as a consequence of hepatitis.

posthioplasty (pos′the-o-plas″te) plastic repair of the prepuce.

posthitis (pos-thīt′is) inflammation of the prepuce.

posthypnotic (pōst″hip-not′ik) following the hypnotic state.

postictal (pōst-ik′til) following a seizure.

postmaturity (pōst″mah-chōōr′it-e) the condition of an infant after a prolonged gestation period. **postmature′,** adj.

post mortem (pōst mort′im) [L.] after death.

postmortem (pōst-mort′im) performed or occurring after death.

postnatal (-nāt′′l) occurring after birth, with reference to the newborn.

postoral (-or′il) in the back part of the mouth.

post partum (pōst part′im) [L.] after parturition.

postpartum (pōst-part′im) occurring after childbirth, with reference to the mother.

postprandial (-pran′de-il) after a meal; postcibal.

postpuberal, postpubertal (-pu′ber-il; -til) after puberty.

postpubescent (pōst″pu-bes′int) after puberty.

postsphygmic (pōst-sfig′mik) after the pulse wave.

poststenotic (post″stĭ-not′ik) located or occurring distal to or beyond a stenosed segment.

postsynaptic (-sĭ-nap′tik) distal to or occurring beyond a synapse.

postulate (pos′choo-lāt) anything assumed or taken for granted.

postvaccinal (pōst-vak′sĭ-nil) occurring after vaccination for smallpox.

potable (po′tah-b′l) fit to drink.

potash (pot′ash) impure potassium carbonate. **caustic p.,** potassium hydroxide. **sulfurated p.,** a mixture of potassium polysulfides and potassium thiosulfate; a source of sulfide in pharmaceuticals.

potassemia (pot″ah-se′me-ah) hyperkalemia.

potassium (pah-tas′e-um) chemical element (*see table*), at. no. 19, symbol K. Potassium is the chief cation of intracellular fluid. For potassium salts not listed here, see under the active ingredient. **p. acetate,** a systemic and urinary alkalizer, $CH_3 \cdot COOK$. **p. bicarbonate,** a transparent, crystalline salt used as an electrolyte replenisher, antacid, and urinary alkalizer. **p. chloride,** an electrolyte replenisher, KCL, for oral or intravenous administration. **p. citrate,** $C_6H_5K_3O_7 \cdot H_2O$, used in potassium deficiency and as a systemic alkalizer, diuretic, and expectorant. **p. gluconate,** $C_6H_{11}KO_7$, used as an electrolyte replenisher in the prophylaxis and treatment of hypokalemia. **p. hydroxide,** a powerful alkaline and caustic compound, KOH, used as an alkalinizing agent and occasionally as an escharotic in bites of rabid animals. **p. iodide,** KI, used as an expectorant and as an antithyroid agent. **p. metaphosphate,** KPO_3, a buffering agent in pharmaceutical preparations. **p. permanganate,** $KMnO_4$, used as a topical anti-infective, oxidizing agent, and antidote for many poisons.

potency (pōt′′n-se) power, especially (1) the ability of the male to perform coitus; (2) the power of a drug to produce the desired effects; (3) the ability of an embryonic part to develop and complete its destiny. **po′tent,** adj.

potential (pah-ten′shil) 1. existing and ready for action, but not active. 2. electric tension or pressure. **action p.,** the electrical activity developed in a muscle or nerve cell during activity. **after-p.,** the period following termination of the spike potential. **membrane p.,** the electric potential existing on the two sides of a membrane or across the cell wall. **resting p.,** the potential difference across the membrane of a normal cell at rest. **spike p.,** the initial, very large change in potential of an excitable cell membrane during excitation.

potentiation (po-ten″she-a′shin) enhancement of one agent by another so that the combined effect is greater than the sum of the effects of each one alone.

pouch (powch) a pocket-like space or sac, as of the peritoneum. **abdominovesical p.,** one formed by reflection of the peritoneum from the abdominal wall to the anterior surface of the bladder. **p. of Douglas,** rectouterine p. **Prussak's p.,** a recess in the tympanic membrane between the flaccid part of the membrane and the neck of the malleus. **Rathke's p.,** a diverticulum from the embryonic buccal cavity from which the anterior pituitary is developed. **rectouterine p.,** the space between the bladder and uterus in the peritoneal cavity. **Seessel's p.,** an outpouching of the embryonic pharynx rostrad of the pharyngeal membrane and caudal to Rathke's pouch.

poudrage (poo-drahzh′) [Fr.] application of powder to a surface, as between the visceral and parietal pleura, to promote their fusion.

poultice (pōl′tis) a soft, moist, mass about the consistency of cooked cereal, spread between layers of muslin, linen, gauze, or towels and applied hot to a given area in order to create moist local heat or counterirritation.

pound (pownd) a unit of weight in the avoirdupois (453.6 grams, or 16 ounces) or apothecaries′ (373.2 grams, or 12 ounces) system.

povidone (po′vĭ-don) polyvinylpyrrolidine, a synthetic polymer used as a dispersing and suspending agent; it has also been used as a plasma volume expander.

povidone-iodine (-i′ah-dīn) a complex produced by reacting iodine with povidone; used as a topical anti-infective.

power (pow′er) 1. capability; potency; the ability to act. 2. a measure of magnification, as of a microscope. **defining p.,** the ability of a lens to make an object clearly visible. **resolving p.,** the ability of the eye or of a lens to make small objects that are close together separately visible, thus revealing the structure of an object.

pox (poks) any eruptive or pustular disease, especially one caused by a virus, e.g., chickenpox, cowpox, etc.

poxvirus (poks-vi′ris) any of a group of morphologically similar and immunologically related DNA viruses, including the virus of vaccinia (cowpox), smallpox, and those producing pox diseases in lower animals.

P.P.D. purified protein derivative; see under *tuberculin*.

PPLO pleuropneumonia-like organisms; see *pleuropneumonia-like.*

p.p.m. parts per million.

Pr chemical symbol, *praseodymium.*

practice (prak′tis) the utilization of one's knowledge in a particular profession, the practice of medicine being the exercise of one's knowledge in the practical recognition and treatment of disease.

practitioner (prak-tish′in-er) one who has complied with the requirements and who is engaged in the practice of medicine. **nurse p.,** see *nurse clinician.*

prae- for words beginning thus, see those beginning *pre-.*

pragmatagnosia (prag″mat-ag-no′ze-ah) inability to recognize formerly known objects.

pragmatamnesia (-am-ne′ze-ah) loss of the power of remembering the appearance of objects.

pralidoxime (pral″ĭ-doks′ēm) a cholinesterase reactivator, $C_7H_9N_2O$, whose salts are used in treatment of organophosphate poisoning; it also has limited value in counteracting carbamate-type cholinesterase inhibitors.

prandial (pran′de-il) pertaining to a meal.

praseodymium (pra″ze-o-dim′e-im) chemical element (*see table*), at. no. 59, symbol Pr.

praxiology (prak″se-ol′ah-je) the science or study of conduct.

prazosin (prah′zo-sin) a quinazoline derivative with vasodilator properties, $C_{19}H_{21}N_5O_4$, used as an oral antihypertensive.

pre- word element [L.], *before* (in time or space).

preagonal (pre-ag′in′l) immediately before the death agony.

preanesthesia (pre″an-es-the″ze-ah) preliminary anesthesia; light anesthesia or narcosis induced by medication as a preliminary to administration of a general anesthetic.

preanesthetic (-an-es-thet′ik) 1. pertaining to preanesthesia. 2. an agent that induces preanesthesia. 3. occurring before administration of an anesthetic.

preantiseptic (-an-tĭ-sep′tik) pertaining to the time before the discovery of antisepsis.

preauricular (-aw-rik′ūl-er) in front of the auricle of the ear.

preaxial (pre-ak′se-il) situated before an axis; in anatomy, referring to the lateral (radial) aspect of the upper arm, and the medial (tibial) aspect of the lower leg.

prebetalipoprotein (-bāt″ah-lip″o-prōt′e-in) very low-density lipoprotein.

prebetalipoproteinemia (-bāt″ah-lip″o-prōt′e-in-ēm′e-ah) hyperprebetalipoproteinemia.

precapillary (-kap′ĭ-lĕ-re) a vessel lacking complete coats, intermediate between an arteriole and a true capillary, and containing scattered smooth muscle cells in its wall, usually having sphincter areas, which control blood flow into capillaries.

precava (-ka′vah) the superior vena cava. **preca′val,** adj.

prechordal (-kord′′l) in front of the notochord.

precipitant (-sip′it-int) a substance that causes precipitation.

precipitate (-sip′ĭ-tāt) 1. to cause settling in solid particles of substance in solution. 2. a deposit of solid particles settled out of a solution. 3. occurring with undue rapidity.

precipitin (-sip′it-in) an antibody to soluble antigen that specifically aggregates the macromolecular antigen *in vivo* or *in vitro* to give a visible precipitate.

precipitinogen (-sip″ĭ-tin′ah-jen) a soluble antigen which stimulates the formation of and reacts with a precipitin.

preclinical (-klin′ĭ-kil) before a disease becomes clinically recognizable.

precocity (-kos′it-e) unusually early development of mental or physical traits. **preco′cious,** adj.

precognition (pre″kog-nish′in) extrasensory perception of a future event.

precoma (pre-ko′mah) the neuropsychiatric state preceding coma, as in hepatic encephalopathy. **precom′atose,** adj.

preconscious (-kon′shis) not present in consciousness, but readily recalled into it.

precordia (pre-kor′de-ah) precordium.

precordium (-kor′de-um) the region over the heart and lower thorax. **precor′dial,** adj.

precornu (-kor′noo) the anterior cornu of the lateral ventricle.

precostal (-kos′til) in front of the ribs.

precuneus (-ku′ne-is), pl. *precu′nei* [L.] a small convolution on the medial surface of the parietal lobe of the cerebrum.

precursor (pre″kur-ser) something that precedes. In biological processes, a substance from which another, usually more active or mature substance is formed. In clinical medicine, a sign or symptom that heralds another.

prediabetes (-di″ah-bēt′ēz) a state of latent impairment of carbohydrate metabolism in which the criteria for diabetes mellitus are not all satisfied.

prediastole (pre″di-as′tah-le) the interval immediately preceding diastole. **prediastol′ic,** adj.

predicrotic (-di-krot′ik) occurring before the dicrotic wave of the sphygmogram.

predigestion (-di-jes′chin) partial artificial digestion of food before its ingestion.

predisposition (pre-dis″po-zish′in) a latent susceptibility to disease which may be activated under certain conditions.

prediverticular (-di″ver-tik′ūl-er) denoting a condition of thickening of the muscular wall of the colon and increased intraluminal pressure without evidence of diverticulosis.

prednisolone (pred-nis′ah-lōn) a glucocorticoid, $C_{21}H_{28}O_5$, used as an anti-inflammatory and antiallergic agent.

prednisone (pred′nĭ-sōn) a glucocorticoid, $C_{21}H_{26}O_5$, used like prednisolone.

preeclampsia (pre″e-klamp′se-ah) a toxemia of late pregnancy, characterized by hypertension, proteinuria, and edema.

preexcitation (pre-ek″si-ta′shin) premature excitation of a portion of the ventricle, occurring in Wolff-Parkinson-White syndrome and characterized by a short P-R interval and a wide QRS interval.

prefrontal (pre-front′l) 1. situated in the anterior part of the frontal lobe or region. 2. the central part of the ethmoid bone.

preganglionic (pre″gang-gle-on′ik) proximal to a ganglion.

pregenital (pre-jen′it′l) antedating the emergence of genital interests.

pregnancy (preg′nan-se) the condition of having a developing embryo or fetus in the body, after union of an ovum and spermatozoon. **abdominal p.,** ectopic pregnancy within the peritoneal cavity. **ampullar p.,** ectopic pregnancy in the ampulla of the uterine tube. **cervical p.,** ectopic pregnancy within the cervical canal. **combined p.,** simultaneous intrauterine and extrauterine pregnancies. **cornual p.,** pregnancy in a horn of the uterus. **ectopic p., extrauterine p.,** development of the fertilized ovum outside the cavity of the uterus. **false p.,** development of all the signs of pregnancy without the presence of an embryo. **interstitial p.,** pregnancy in the portion of the oviduct within the uterine wall. **intraligamentary p., intraligamentous p.,** ectopic pregnancy within the broad ligament. **multiple p.,** presence of more than one fetus in the uterus at the same time. **mural p.,** interstitial p. **ovarian p.,** pregnancy occurring in an ovary. **phantom p.,** false pregnancy due to psychogenic factors. **tubal p.,** ectopic pregnancy within a uterine tube. **tuboabdominal p.,** ectopic pregnancy occurring partly in the fimbriated end of the oviduct and partly in the abdominal cavity. **tubo-ovarian p.,** pregnancy at the fimbria of the uterine tube.

pregnane (preg′nān) a crystalline saturated steroid hydrocarbon, $C_{21}H_{36}$; β-*pregnane* is the form from which several hormones, including progesterone, are derived; α-*pregnane* is the form excreted in the urine.

pregnanediol (preg″nān′di-ol) a crystalline, biologically inactive dihydroxy derivative of pregnane, formed by reduction of progesterone and found especially in urine of pregnant women.

pregnanetriol (preg″nān-tri′ol) a metabolite of 17-hydroxyprogesterone; its excretion in the urine is greatly increased in certain disorders of the adrenal cortex.

prehallux (pre-hal′uks) a supernumerary bone of the foot growing from the medial border of the scaphoid.

prehemiplegic (pre″hem-ĭ-ple′jik) preceding hemiplegia.

prehensile (pre-hen′sil) adapted for grasping or seizing.

prehension (-hen′shin) the act of grasping.

prehormone (-hor′mōn) prohormone.

prehyoid (-hi′oid) in front of the hyoid bone.

prehypophysis (pre″hi-pof′ĭ-sis) the anterior lobe of the pituitary gland.

preictal (pre-ik′til) occurring before a stroke, seizure, or attack.

preinvasive (pre″in-va′siv) not yet invading tissues outside the site of origin.

preleukemia (-loo-kēm′e-ah) a stage of bone marrow dysfunction preceding the development of acute myelogenous leukemia. **preleuke′mic,** adj.

prelimbic (pre-lim′bik) in front of a limbus.

premalignant (pre″mah-lig′nint) precancerous.

Premarin (prem′ah-rin) trademark for preparations of conjugated estrogens.

premaxilla (pre″mak-sil′ah) incisive bone.

premaxillary (pre-mak′sĭ-le-re) 1. in front of the maxilla. 2. pertaining to the premaxilla (incisive bone).

premedication (pre″med-ĭ-ka′shin) preliminary medication, particularly internal medication to produce narcosis prior to general anesthesia.

premenarchal (-mĕ-nark″l) occurring before establishment of menstruation.

premenstrual (pre-men′stroo-il) preceding menstruation.

premenstruum (-men′stroo-um) the period immediately before menstruation.

premolar (-mōl′er) in front of the molar teeth; see under *tooth*.

premonocyte (-mon′ah-sīt) promonocyte.

premorbid (-mor′bid) occurring before development of disease.

premunition (pre″mu-nish′in) resistance to infection by the same or closely related pathogen established after an acute infection has become chronic, and lasting as long as the infecting organisms are in the body. **premu′nitive,** adj.

premyeloblast (pre-mi′ĕ-lo-blast″) precursor of a myeloblast.

premyelocyte (-sīt″) promyelocyte.

prenatal (pre-na′tal) preceding birth.

preoptic (-op′tik) in front of the optic chiasm.

preproinsulin (-pro-in′sūl-in) the precursor of proinsulin, containing an additional polypeptide sequence at the N-terminal.

preproprotein (-pro-prōt′e-in) any precursor of a proprotein.

preprosthetic (-pros-thet′ik) performed or occurring before insertion of a prosthesis.

prepuberal, prepubertal (pre-pu′ber-il; -pu′ber-til) before puberty; pertaining to the period of accelerated growth preceding gonadal maturity.

prepubescent (pre″pu-bes′int) prepubertal.

prepuce (pre′pūs) the foreskin: a cutaneous fold over the glans penis. **prepu′tial,** adj. **p. of clitoris,** a fold capping the clitoris formed by union of the labia minora and the clitoris.

preputiotomy (pre-pu″she-ot′ah-me) incision of the prepuce to relieve phimosis.

preputium (-pu′she-im) prepuce.

prepyloric (pre″pi-lor′ik) just proximal to the pylorus.

presby- word element [Gr.], *old age.*

presbycardia (prez″bĭ-kar′de-ah) impaired cardiac function attributed to aging, with senescent changes in the body and no evidence of other cause of heart disease.

presbycusis (-ku′sis) progressive, bilaterally

symmetrical perceptive hearing loss occurring with age.

presbyophrenia (prez″be-o-fre′ne-ah) loss of memory, disorientation, and confabulation, occurring in old age.

presbyopia (-o′pe-ah) diminution of accommodation of the lens of the eye occurring normally with aging. **presbyop′ic**, adj.

prescription (prĭ-skrip′shin) a written directive for the preparation and administration of a remedy; see also *inscription, signature, subscription,* and *superscription.*

presenile (-se′nīl) pertaining to a condition resembling senility, but occurring in early or middle life.

presentation (prez″in-ta′shin) lie; the relationship of the long axis of the fetus to that of the mother. Cf. *position.* **antigen p.,** the hypothesis that macrophages not only ingest and process antigen, refining and complexing it with SRNA, but also present it in concentrated form at their surfaces to lymphocytes, thus inducing an immune response by the lymphocytes. **breech p.,** presentation of the fetal buttocks or feet in labor; the feet may be alongside the buttocks (*complete breech p.*); the legs may be extended against the trunk and the feet lying against the face (*frank breech p.*); or one or both feet or knees may be prolapsed into the maternal vagina (*incomplete breech p.*). **brow p.,** presentation of the fetal brow in labor. **cephalic p.,** presentation of any part of the fetal head in labor, whether the vertex, face, or brow. **compound p.,** prolapse of an extremity of the fetus alongside the head in cephalic presentation or of one or both arms alongside a presenting breech at the beginning of labor. **footling p.,** presentation of the fetus with one (single footling) or both (double footling) feet prolapsed into the maternal vagina. **funic p.,** presentation of the umbilical cord in labor. **longitudinal p.,** that in which the long axis of the fetus lies parallel to that of the mother, with either the head or breech the presenting part. **oblique p.,** that in which the long axis of the fetal body lies obliquely to that of the mother; the shoulder presents first. **placental p.,** placenta previa. **shoulder p.,** see *oblique p.* and *transverse lie.* **transverse p.,** see under *lie.* **vertex p.,** that in which the vertex of the fetal head is the presenting part.

presomite (-so′mīt) referring to embryos before the appearance of somites.

presphenoid (-sfe′noid) the anterior portion of the body of the sphenoid bone.

presphygmic (-sfig′mik) preceding the pulse wave.

pressor (pres′or) tending to increase blood pressure.

pressoreceptive (pres″o-re-sep′tiv) sensitive to stimuli due to vasomotor activity.

pressoreceptor (-re-sep′ter) a receptor or nerve ending sensitive to stimuli of vasomotor activity.

pressosensitive (-sen′sit-iv) pressoreceptive.

pressure (presh′er) stress or strain, by compression, expansion, pull, thrust, or shear. **blood p.,** the pressure of the blood on the walls of the arteries, dependent on the energy of the heart action, elasticity of the arterial walls, and volume and viscosity of the blood; the *maximum* or *systolic* pressure occurs near the end of the stroke output of the left ventricle, and the *minimum* or *diastolic* late in ventricular diastole. **central venous p. (CVP),** the venous pressure as measured at the right atrium, done by means of a catheter introduced through the median cubital vein to the superior vena cava. **cerebrospinal p.,** the pressure or tension of the cerebrospinal fluid, normally 100–150 mm. as measured by the manometer. **intracranial p.,** pressure of the subarachnoidal fluid. **intraocular p.,** the pressure exerted against the outer coats by the contents of the eyeball. **mean circulatory filling p.,** a measure of the average (arterial and venous) pressure necessary to cause filling of the circulation with blood; it varies with blood volume and is directly proportional to the rate of venous return and thus to cardiac output. **negative p.,** pressure less than that of the atmosphere. **oncotic p.,** the osmotic pressure due to the presence of colloids in solution. **osmotic p.,** the potential pressure of a solution directly related to its solute osmolar concentration; it is the maximum pressure developed by osmosis in a solution separated from another by a semipermeable membrane, i.e., the pressure that will just prevent osmosis between two such solutions. **partial p.,** pressure exerted by each of the constituents of a mixture of gases. **positive p.,** pressure greater than that of the atmosphere. **positive end-expiratory p. (PEEP),** a method of mechanical ventilation in which pressure is maintained to increase the volume of gas remaining in the lungs at the end of expiration, thus reducing the shunting of blood through the lungs and improving gas exchange. **pulse p.,** the difference between systolic and diastolic pressures. **venous p.,** blood pressure in the veins.

presternum (pre-ster′nim) the manubrium of the sternum.

presubiculum (pre″sub-ik′ūl-im) a modified six-layered cortex between the subiculum and the main part of the parahippocampal gyrus.

presynaptic (-sĭ-nap′tik) situated or occurring proximal to a synapse.

presystole (pre-sis′tah-le) the interval just before systole.

presystolic (pre″sis-tol′ik) just before systole.

pretectal (pre-tek′til) located anterior to the tectum mesencephali.

prevalence (prev′ah-lins) the total number of cases of a specific disease in existence in a given population at a certain time.

preventive (pre-vent′iv) prophylactic.

prevesical (-ves′ĭ-kal) anterior to the bladder.

prezygotic (pre″zi-got′ik) occurring before completion of fertilization.

priapism (pri′ah-pizm) persistent abnormal erection of penis, accompanied by pain and tenderness.

prilocaine (pril′o-kān) a local anesthetic, $C_{13}H_{20}N_2O$, used as the hydrochloride salt.

primaquine (pri'mah-kwin) a compound used as an antimalarial, $C_{15}H_{21}N_3O$, being gametocidal to all forms of malaria; used as the phosphate salt.

Primates (pri-ma'tēz) the highest order of mammals, including man, apes, monkeys, and lemurs.

primidone (pri'mĭ-dōn) an anticonvulsant, $C_{12}H_{14}N_2O_2$.

primigravida (pri″mĭ-grav'ĭ-dah) a woman pregnant for the first time; gravida I.

primipara (pri-mip'ah-rah) para 1; a woman who has had one pregnancy that resulted in a viable young. See *para*. **primip'arous**, adj.

primitive (prim'ĭ-tiv) first in point of time; existing in a simple or early form; showing little evolution.

primordial (pri-mor'de-al) primitive.

primordium (pri-mor'de-um) the earliest indication during embryonic development of an organ or part.

princeps (prin'seps) [L.] principal; chief.

principle (prin'sip'l) 1. a chemical component. 2. a substance on which certain of the properties of a drug depend. 3. a law of conduct.

prion (pri'on) a slow infectious particle that lacks nucleic acids; prions are the cause of Creutzfeld-Jakob disease and scrapie.

prism (prizm) a solid with a triangular or polygonal cross section.

prismosphere (priz'mo-sfēr) a prism combined with a spherical lens.

p.r.n. [L.] *pro re na'ta* (according to circumstances).

Pro proline.

pro- word element [L., Gr.], *before; in front of; favoring.*

proaccelerin (pro″ak-sel'er-in) coagulation Factor V.

proactivator (pro-akt'ĭ-vāt-er) a precursor of an activator; a factor which reacts with an enzyme to form an activator.

proatlas (-at'lis) a rudimentary vertebra which in some animals lies in front of the atlas; sometimes seen in man as an anomaly.

proband (pro'band) propositus.

probang (-bang) a flexible rod with a ball, tuft, or sponge at one end; used to apply medications to or remove matter from the esophagus or larynx.

probe (prōb) a long, slender instrument for exploring wounds or body cavities or passages.

probenecid (pro-ben'ĕ-sid) a drug, $C_{13}H_{19}NO_4S$, used as a uricosuric agent in the treatment of gout; also used to increase serum concentration of certain antibiotics and other drugs.

procainamide (-kān'ah-mīd) a cardiac depressant, $C_{13}H_{21}N_3O$, used as the hydrochloride salt in the treatment of arrhythmias.

procaine (pro'kān) a local anesthetic, $C_{12}H_{20}N_2O_2$; the hydrochloride salt is used in solution for infiltration, nerve block, and spinal anesthesia.

procarbazine (pro-kar'bah-zēn) an antineoplastic, $C_{12}H_{19}N_3O$, used in the treatment of Hodgkin's disease.

procarboxypeptidase (pro″kar-bok″se-pep'tĭ-

dās) the inactive precursor of carboxypeptidase, which is converted to the active enzyme by the action of trypsin.

procarcinogen (-kar-sin″ah-jen) a chemical substance that becomes carcinogenic only after it is altered by metabolic processes.

Procaryotae (pro-kar″e-ōt'e) a kingdom comprising all prokaryotic organisms.

procedure (pro-se'jer) a series of steps by which a desired result is accomplished.

procelous (pro-se'lis) having the anterior surface concave; said of vertebrae.

procentriole (-sen'tre-ōl) the immediate precursor of centrioles and ciliary basal bodies.

procephalic (pro″sĕ-fal'ik) pertaining to the anterior part of the head.

procercoid (pro-ser'koid) a larval stage of fish tapeworms.

process (pros'es) 1. a prominence or projection, as from a bone. 2. a series of operations, events, or steps leading to achievement of a specific result; also, to subject to such a series to produce desired changes. **acromial p.**, acromion. **alveolar p.**, the part of the bone in either the maxilla or mandible surrounding and supporting the teeth. **basilar p.**, a quadrilateral plate of the occipital bone projecting superiorly and anteriorly from the foramen magnum. **caudate p.**, the right of the two processes on the caudate lobe of the liver. **ciliary p's**, meridionally arranged ridges or folds projecting from the crown of the ciliary body. **clinoid p.**, any of the three (anterior, medial, and posterior) processes of the sphenoid bone. **coracoid p.**, a curved process arising from the upper neck of the scapula and overhanging the shoulder joint. **coronoid p.**, 1. the anterior part of the upper end of the ramus of the mandible. 2. a projection at the proximal end of the ulna. **ensiform p.**, xiphoid p. **ethmoid p.**, a bony projection above and behind the maxillary process of the inferior nasal concha. **falciform p.**, 1. the lateral margin of the saphenous hiatus. 2. falx cerebri. **frontonasal p.**, an expansive facial process in the embryo which develops into the forehead and bridge of the nose. **funicular p.**, the portion of the tunica vaginalis surrounding the spermatic cord. **lacrimal p.**, a process of the inferior nasal concha that articulates with the lacrimal bone. **malar p.**, zygomatic p. of maxilla. **mamillary p.**, a tubercle on each superior articular process of a lumbar vertebra. **mandibular p.**, the ventral process formed by bifurcation of the first branchial arch (mandibular arch) in the embryo, which unites ventrally with its fellow to form the lower jaw. **mastoid p.**, the conical projection at the base of the mastoid portion of the temporal bone. **maxillary p.**, 1. the dorsal process formed by bifurcation of the first branchial arch (mandibular arch) in the embryo, which joins with the ipsilateral median nasal process in the formation of the upper jaw. 2. a bony process descending from the ethmoid process of the inferior nasal concha. **odontoid p.**, a toothlike projection of the axis which articulates with the atlas. **pterygoid p.**, one of the wing-shaped processes of the sphenoid. **spinous p. of vertebrae**, a part of the vertebrae projecting backward from the arch, giving attachment to the back muscles. **styloid p.,** a long pointed projection, especially a long spine projecting downward from the inferior surface of the temporal bone. **uncinate p.,** any hooklike process, as of vertebrae, the lacrimal bone, or the pancreas. **xiphoid p.,** the pointed process of cartilage, supported by a core of bone, connected with the lower end of the sternum. **zygomatic p.,** a projection from the frontal or temporal bone, or from the maxilla, by which they articulate with the zygomatic bone.

processus (pro-ses′us), pl. *proces′sus* [L.] process; used in official names of various anatomic structures.

prochlorperazine (pro-per′ah-zēn) a phenothiazine derivative, $C_{20}H_{24}ClN_3S$, used as a tranquilizer and antiemetic.

prochondral (-kon′dril) occurring before the formation of cartilage.

procidentia (pro″sĭ-den′she-ah) a state of prolapse, especially of the uterus.

procoagulant (-ko-ag′ūl-int) 1. tending to promote coagulation. 2. a precursor of a natural substance necessary to coagulation of the blood.

procollagen (-kol′ah-jen) the precursor molecule of collagen, synthesized in the fibroblast, osteoblast, etc., and cleaved to form collagen extracellularly.

proconvertin (-kon-vert′in) coagulation Factor VII.

procreation (-kre-a′shin) the act of begetting or generating.

proct(o)- word element [Gr.], *rectum;* see also words beginning *rect(o)-*.

proctalgia (prok-tal′je-ah) pain in the rectum.

proctatresia (prokt″ah-tre′ze-ah) imperforate anus.

proctectasia (prokt″ek-ta′ze-ah) dilatation of the rectum or anus.

proctectomy (prok-tek′tah-me) excision of the rectum.

procteurynter (prokt″ūr-in′ter) a baglike device used to dilate the rectum.

proctitis (prok-tīt′is) inflammation of the rectum.

proctocele (prokt′ah-sēl) rectocele.

proctoclysis (prok-tok′lĭ-sis) slow introduction of large quantities of liquid into the rectum.

proctocolpoplasty (-kol′po-plas″te) repair of a rectovaginal fistula.

proctocystoplasty (-sis′to-plas″te) repair of a rectovesical fistula.

proctocystotomy (-sis-tot′ah-me) removal of a vesical stone through the rectum.

proctodeum (-de′im) the ectodermal depression of the caudal end of the embryo, where later the anus is formed.

proctology (prok-tol′ah-je) the branch of medicine concerned with disorders of the rectum and anus. **proctolog′ic,** adj.

proctoparalysis (prok″to-pah-ral′ĭ-sis) paralysis of the anal and rectal muscles.

proctopexy (prok′to-pek″se) surgical fixation of the rectum.

proctoplasty (-plas″te) plastic repair of the rectum.

proctoplegia (prok″to-ple′je-ah) proctoparalysis.

proctoptosis (prok″top-to′sis) prolapse of the rectum.

proctorrhaphy (prok-tor′ah-fe) surgical repair of the rectum.

proctorrhea (prok″to-re′ah) a mucous discharge from the anus.

proctoscope (prok′to-skōp) a speculum or tubular instrument with illumination for inspecting the rectum.

proctosigmoiditis (-sig″moi-di′tis) inflammation of the rectum and sigmoid colon.

proctosigmoidoscopy (-sig″moi-dos′ko-pe) examination of the rectum and sigmoid colon with the sigmoidoscope.

proctostenosis (prok″to-stĭ-no′sis) stricture of the rectum.

proctostomy (prok-tos′tah-me) creation of a permanent artificial opening from the body surface into the rectum.

proctotomy (prok-tot′ah-me) incision of the rectum.

procumbent (pro-kum′bint) prone; lying on the face.

procursive (-ker′siv) tending to run forward.

procyclidine (-si′klĭ-dēn) a synthetic drug, $C_{19}H_{29}NO$, used as the hydrochloride salt in treatment of parkinsonism.

prodrome (pro′drōm) a premonitory symptom; a symptom indicating the onset of a disease. **pro-dro′mal, prodro′mic,** adj.

pro-drug (-drug) a compound that, on administration, must undergo chemical conversion by metabolic processes before becoming an active pharmacological agent; a precursor of a drug.

product (prod′ukt) something produced. **cleavage p.,** a substance formed by splitting of a compound molecule into a simpler one. **fibrin degradation p's, fibrinolytic split p's,** fragments of fibrinogen or fibrin degraded by plasmin. **fission p.,** an isotope, usually radioactive, of an element in the middle of the periodic table, produced by fission of a heavy element under bombardment with high-energy particles. **spallation p's,** the isotopes of many different chemical elements produced in small amounts in nuclear fission. **substitution p.,** a substance formed by substitution of one atom or radical in a molecule by another atom or radical.

productive (pro-duk′tiv) producing or forming; said especially of an inflammation that produces new tissue or of a cough that brings forth sputum or mucus.

proenzyme (pro-en′zīm) zymogen; an inactive precursor of an enzyme.

proestrogen (pro-es′trah-jen) a substance without estrogenic activity but which is metabolized in the body to active estrogen.

proestrus (-es′tris) the period of heightened follicular activity preceding estrus.

-profen a suffix indicating an anti-inflammatory agent of the ibuprofen type (propionic acid derivatives).

professional (prah-fesh'in'l) 1. pertaining to one's profession or occupation. 2. one who is a specialist in a particular field or occupation. **allied health p.,** a person with special training and licensed when necessary, who works under the supervision of a health professional with responsibilities bearing on patient care.

Professional Standards Review Organization see *PSRO.*

profile (pro'fil) a simple outline as of the side view of the head or face; by extension, a graph representing quantitatively a set of characteristics determined by tests.

proflavine (pro-fla'vin) a constituent of acriflavine, $C_{13}H_{11}N_3$, used as a topical and urinary antiseptic in the form of the hemisulfate salt.

profundaplasty, profundoplasty (-fun''dah-plas''te) reconstruction of an occluded or stenosed deep femoral artery.

profundus (-fun'dus) [L.] deep.

progastrin (-gas'trin) an inactive precursor of gastrin.

progeria (pro-jēr'e-ah) premature old age, a condition occurring in childhood marked by small stature, absence of facial and pubic hair, wrinkled skin, gray hair, and eventual development of atherosclerosis.

progestational (pro''jes-ta'shin'l) 1. referring to that phase of the menstrual cycle just before menstruation, when the corpus luteum is active and the endometrium is secreting. 2. denoting a class of pharmaceutical preparations having effects similar to those of progesterone.

progesterone (pro-jes'tĭ-rōn) the principal progestational hormone, $C_{21}H_{30}O_2$, liberated by the corpus luteum, adrenal cortex, and placenta, whose function is to prepare the uterus for the reception and development of the fertilized ovum by inducing transformation of the endometrium from the proliferative to the secretory stage; used as a progestin in the treatment of functional uterine bleeding, abnormalities of the menstrual cycle, and threatened abortion.

progestin (-jes'tin) originally, the crude hormone of the corpus luteum; it has since been isolated in pure form and is now known as *progesterone.* Certain synthetic and natural progestational agents are called progestins.

progestogen (-jes'tah-jen) any substance having progestational activity.

proglossis (-glos'is) the tip of the tongue.

proglottid (-glot'id) one of the segments making up the body of a tapeworm; see *strobila.*

proglottis (-glot'is) proglottid.

prognathism (prog'nah-thizm) abnormal protrusion of one or both jaws, especially the lower jaw, the gnathic index being above 103. **prognath'ic, prog'nathous,** adj.

prognosis (prog-no'sis) a forecast of the probable course and outcome of a disorder. **prognos'tic,** adj.

prograyid (-grav'id) denoting the phase of the endometrium in which it is prepared for pregnancy.

prohormone (-hor'mōn) a precursor of a hormone, such as a polypeptide that is cleaved to form a shorter polypeptide hormone or a steroid that is converted to an active hormone by peripheral metabolism.

proinsulin (-in'sūl-in) a precursor of insulin, having low biologic activity.

projection (-jek'shin) 1. a throwing forward, especially the reference of impressions made on the sense organs to their proper source, so as to locate correctly the objects producing them. 2. a connection between the cerebral cortex and other parts of the nervous system or organs of special sense. 3. the act of extending or jutting out, or a part that juts out. 4. a mental mechanism by which a repressed complex is regarded as belonging to the external world or to someone else.

prokaryon (-kar'e-on) 1. nuclear material scattered in the cytoplasm of the cell, rather than bounded by a nuclear membrane; found in some unicellular organisms, such as bacteria. 2. prokaryote.

prokaryote (-kar'e-ōt) a unicellular organism lacking a true nucleus and nuclear membrane, having genetic material composed of a single loop of naked double-stranded DNA. Prokaryotes with the exception of mycoplasmas have a rigid cell wall. **prokaryot'ic,** adj.

prolabium (-la'be-im) the prominent central part of the upper lip.

prolactin (-lak'tin) a hormone of the anterior pituitary which stimulates and sustains lactation in postpartum mammals, and shows luteotropic activity in certain mammals.

prolactinoma (-lak''tĭ-no'mah) a pituitary tumor that secretes prolactin.

prolapse (pro'laps) 1. the falling down, or downward displacement, of a part or viscus. 2. to undergo such displacement. **p. of cord,** protrusion of the umbilical cord ahead of the presenting part of the fetus in labor. **p. of the iris,** protrusion of the iris through a wound in the cornea. **Morgagni's p.,** chronic inflammatory hyperplasia of the mucosa and submucosa of the sacculus laryngis. **rectal p., p. of rectum,** protrusion of the rectal mucous membrane through the anus. **p. of uterus,** downward displacement of the uterus so that the cervix is within the vaginal orifice (*first-degree p.*), the cervix is outside the orifice (*second-degree p.*), or the entire uterus is outside the orifice (*third-degree p.*).

prolapsus (pro-lap'sis) [L.] prolapse.

prolepsis (-lep'sis) recurrence of a paroxysm before the expected time. **prolep'tic,** adj.

prolidase (pro'lĭ-dās) an enzyme which catalyzes the hydrolysis of the imide bond between an α-carboxyl group and proline or hydroxyproline.

proliferation (-lif''er-a'shin) the reproduction or multiplication of similar forms, especially of cells. **prolif'erative, prolif'erous,** adj.

proligerous (pro-lij'er-is) producing offspring.

prolinase (pro'lĭ-nās) an enzyme that catalyzes the hydrolysis of dipeptides containing proline or hydroxyproline as N-terminal groups.

proline (pro'lēn) a cyclic amino acid occurring in proteins; it is a major constituent of collagen.

prolymphocyte (pro-lim′fah-sīt) a cell of the lymphocytic series intermediate between the lymphoblast and lymphocyte.

promastigote (-mas′tĭ-gōt) the morphologic stage in the development of certain protozoa, characterized by a free anterior flagellum and resembling the typical adult form of *Leptomonas*.

promazine (pro′mah-zēn) a phenothiazine derivative, $C_{17}H_{20}N_2S$, used as a major tranquilizer in the form of the hydrochloride salt.

promegakaryocyte (pro″meg-ah-kar′e-o-sīt″) a precursor in the thrombocytic series, being a cell intermediate between the megakaryoblast and the megakaryocyte.

promegaloblast (pro-meg′ah-lo-blast″) the earliest form in the abnormal erythrocyte maturation sequence occurring in vitamin B_{12} and folic acid deficiencies; it corresponds to the pronormoblast, and develops into a megaloblast.

promethazine (-meth′ah-zēn) a phenothiazine derivative, $C_{17}H_{20}N_2S$; the hydrochloride salt is used as an antihistaminic, antiemetic, and tranquilizer.

promethestrol (-meth′es-trol) a synthetic estrogenic agent, $C_{20}H_{26}O_2$, used as the dipropionate ester.

promethium (-me′the-im) chemical element (*see table*), at. no. 61, symbol Pm.

prominence (prom′ĭ-nins) a protrusion or projection.

promonocyte (pro-mon′ah-sīt) a cell of the monocytic series intermediate between the monoblast and monocyte, with coarse chromatin structure and one or two nucleoli.

promontory (prom′in-tor″e) a projecting process or eminence.

promyelocyte (-mi′il-o-sīt″) a precursor in the granulocytic series, intermediate between myeloblast and myelocyte, containing a few, as yet undifferentiated, cytoplasmic granules.

pronation (pro-na′shin) the act of assuming the prone position, or the state of being prone. Applied to the hand, the act of turning the palm backward (posteriorly) or downward, performed by medial rotation of the forearm. Applied to the foot, a combination of eversion and abduction movements taking place in the tarsal and metatarsal joints and resulting in lowering of the medial margin of the foot, hence of the longitudinal arch.

prone (prōn) lying face downward.

pronephros (pro-nef′ros), pl. *prone′phroi* [Gr.] the primordial kidney; an excretory structure or its rudiments developing in the embryo before the mesonephros; its duct is later used by the mesonephros, which arises caudal to it.

pronograde (pro′nah-grād) walking with the body approximately horizontal; applied to quadrupeds.

pronormoblast (pro-nor′mah-blast) the earliest erythrocyte precursor, having a relatively large nucleus containing several nucleoli, surrounded by a small amount of cytoplasm; see also *normoblast*.

pronucleus (-noo′kle-is) the haploid nucleus of a sex cell.

prootic (-o′tik) in front of the ear.

propagation (prop″ah-ga′shin) reproduction. **prop′agative**, adj.

propantheline (-pan′thĭ-lēn) an anticholinergic, $C_{23}H_{30}NO_3$, used as the bromide salt, especially in the treatment of peptic ulcer.

proparacaine (-par′ah-kān) a topical anesthetic, $C_{16}H_{26}N_2O_3$, used as the hydrochloride salt.

properdin (pro′per-din) a relatively heat-labile, normal serum protein (a euglobulin) that, in the presence of complement component C3 and magnesium ions, acts nonspecifically against gram-negative bacteria and viruses and plays a role in lysis of erythrocytes. It migrates as a β-globulin, and although not an antibody, may act in conjunction with complement-fixing antibody.

prophage (-fāj) the latent stage of a phage in a lysogenic bacterium, in which the viral genome becomes inserted into a specific portion of the host chromosome and is duplicated in each cell generation.

prophase (-fāz) the first stage in cell reduplication in either meiosis or mitosis.

prophylactic (-fi-lak′tik) 1. tending to ward off disease; pertaining to prophylaxis. 2. an agent that tends to ward off disease.

prophylaxis (-fi-lak′sis) prevention of disease; preventive treatment.

propiolactone (pro″pe-o-lak′tōn) a disinfectant, $C_3H_4O_2$.

propionate (-ah-nāt) any salt of propionic acid.

Propionibacterium (-bak-tēr′e-im) a genus of gram-positive bacteria found as saprophytes in dairy products.

propionic acid (pro-pe-on′ik) CH_3CH_2COOH, found in chyme and sweat, and one of the products of bacterial fermentation of wood pulp waste; its salts (calcium and sodium propionate) are used as local antifungals, and to inhibit mold growth in bakery and dairy products.

propositus (pro-poz′it-is), pl. *propo′siti* [L.] the original person presenting a mental or physical disorder who serves as the basis for a hereditary or genetic study.

propoxyphene (-pok′se-fēn) an analgesic, $C_{22}H_{29}NO_2$, used as the hydrochloride and napsylate salts.

propranolol (-pran′ol-ōl) a β-adrenergic blocking agent, $C_{16}H_{21}NO_2$, used in the treatment of cardiac arrhythmias and hypertrophic subaortic stenosis and in the prophylaxis of migraine.

proprietary (-pri′ĭ-ter″e) 1. denoting a medicine protected against free competition as to name, composition, or manufacturing process by patent, trademark, copyright, or secrecy. 2. a medicine so protected.

proprioception (pro″pre-o-sep′shin) perception mediated by proprioceptors or proprioceptive tissues.

proprioceptor (pro″pre-o-sep′ter) any of the sensory nerve endings that give information concerning movements and position of the body; they occur chiefly in muscles, tendons, and the labyrinth. **propriocep′tive**, adj.

proprotein (pro-prōt'e-in) a protein that is cleaved to form a smaller protein, e.g., proinsulin, the precursor of insulin.

proptometer (-tom'it-er) an instrument for measuring the degree of exophthalmos.

proptosis (prop-to'sis) forward displacement or bulging, especially of the eye.

propulsion (pro-pul'shin) 1. a tendency to fall forward in walking. 2. festination.

propyl (pro'pil) the univalent radical CH_3CH_2-CH_2— from propane.

propylene (-pĭ-lēn) a gaseous hydrocarbon, $CH_3 \cdot CH \cdot CH_2$, having anesthetic properties.
p. glycol, a colorless, viscous liquid used as a humectant and solvent.

propylhexedrine (pro''pil-hek'sĭ-drēn) an adrenergic, $C_{10}H_{21}N$, given by inhalation to decongest the nasal mucosa.

propyliodone (-i'ah-dōn) a radiopaque medium, $C_{10}H_{11}I_2NO_3$, used in bronchography.

propylthiouracil (-thi''ah-ūr'ah-sil) a thyroid inhibitor, $C_7H_{10}N_2OS$.

pro re nata (pro ra nah'tah) [L.] according to circumstances. Abbreviated p.r.n.

prorennin (pro-ren'in) the zymogen (proenzyme) in the gastric glands that is converted to rennin.

prorubricyte (-roo'brĭ-sīt) basophilic normoblast.

pros(o)- word element [Gr.], *forward; anterior.*

prosecretin (-se-krēt'in) the precursor of secretin.

prosection (pro-sek'shin) carefully programmed dissection for demonstration of anatomic structure.

prosencephalon (pros''en-sef'ah-lon) forebrain.

prosodemic (pros''ah-dem'ik) passing directly from one person to another; said of disease.

prosop(o)- word element [Gr.], *face.*

prosopagnosia (-pag-no'se-ah) inability to recognize faces due to damage to the underside of both occipital lobes.

prosopalgia (-pal'je-ah) trigeminal neuralgia. **prosopal'gic**, adj.

prosopectasia (-pek-ta'ze-ah) oversize of the face.

prosoplasia (-pla'se-ah) 1. abnormal differentiation of tissue. 2. development into a higher level of organization or function.

prosopodiplegia (pros''ah-po-di-ple'je-ah) paralysis of the face and one lower extremity.

prosoponeuralgia (-nōōr-al'je-ah) facial neuralgia.

prosopoplegia (-ple'je-ah) facial paralysis. **prosopople'gic,** adj.

prosoposchisis (pros''o-pos'kĭ-sis) congenital fissure of the face.

prostacyclin (pros''tah-si'klin) an intermediate in the metabolic pathway of arachnidonic acid, formed from prostaglandin endoperoxides in the walls of arteries and veins; it is a potent vasodilator and a potent inhibitor of platelet aggregation.

prostaglandin (-glan'din) any of a group of naturally occurring, chemically related hydroxy fatty acids that stimulate contractility of the uterine and other smooth muscle and have the ability to lower blood pressure, regulate acid secretion of the stomach, regulate body temperature and platelet aggregation, and to control inflammation and vascular permeability; they also affect the action of certain hormones. Nine primary types are labeled A through I, the degree of saturation of the side chain of each being designated by subscripts 1, 2, and 3. The types of prostaglandin are abbreviated PGE_2, PGF_{2a}, and so on.

prostate (pros'tāt) a gland surrounding the neck of the bladder and urethra in the male; it contributes a secretion to the semen. **prostat'ic**, adj.

prostatectomy (pros''tah-tek'tah-me) excision of all or part of the prostate.

prostatism (pros'tah-tizm) a symptom complex resulting from compression or obstruction of the urethra, due most commonly to hyperplasia of the prostate.

prostatitis (pros''tah-tīt'is) inflammation of the prostate. **prostatit'ic,** adj. **allergic p., eosinophilic p.,** a condition seen in certain allergies, characterized by diffuse infiltration of the prostate by eosinophils, with small foci of fibrinoid necrosis. **nonspecific granulomatous p.,** prostatitis characterized by focal or diffuse tissue infiltration by peculiar, large, pale macrophages.

prostatocystitis (pros''tah-to-sis-tīt'is) inflammation of the neck of the bladder (prostatic urethra) and the bladder cavity.

prostatocystotomy (-sis-tot'ah-me) incision of the bladder and prostate.

prostatolithotomy (pros''tah-to-lĭ-thot'ah-me) incision of the prostate for removal of a calculus.

prostatomegaly (-meg'ah-le) hypertrophy of the prostate.

prostatorrhea (-re'ah) catarrhal discharge from the prostate.

prostatotomy (pros''tah-tot'ah-me) surgical incision of the prostate.

prostatovesiculectomy (pros''tah-to-vĕ-sik''ūl-ek'tah-me) excision of the prostate and seminal vesicles.

prostatovesiculitis (-vĕ-sik''ūl-īt'is) inflammation of the prostate and seminal vesicles.

prosthesis (pros-the'sis), pl. *prosthe'ses* [Gr.] an artificial substitute for a missing body part, such as an arm or leg, eye, or tooth, used for functional or cosmetic reasons, or both.

prosthion (pros'the-on) the point on the maxillary alveolar process that projects most anteriorly in the midline.

prosthodontics (pros''thah-don'tiks) that branch of dentistry concerned with the construction of artificial appliances designed to restore and maintain oral function by replacing missing teeth and sometimes other oral structures or parts of the face.

prostholith (pros'thah-lith) a preputial concretion or calculus.

prostration (pros-tra'shin) extreme exhaustion

or lack of energy or power. **heat p.,** see under *exhaustion.* **nervous p.,** neurasthenia.

protactinium (pro″tak-tin′e-im) chemical element (*see table*), at. no. 91, symbol Pa.

protamine (prōt′ah-min) one of a class of basic proteins occurring in the sperm of certain fish, having the property of neutralizing heparin; the sulfate salt is used as an antidote to heparin overdosage.

protanopia (prōt″ah-no′pe-ah) red blindness; imperfect perception of red, with confusion of reds and greens. **protanop′ic,** adj.

protease (e-ās) any proteolytic enzyme; see *peptidase.*

protectant, protective (pro-tek′tint; pro-tek′-tiv) 1. affording defense or immunity. 2. an agent affording defense against harmful influence.

protector (pro-tek′ter) a substance in a catalyst which prolongs the rate of activity in the latter.

proteid (prōt′e-id) protein.

protein (prōt′e-in) any of a group of complex organic compounds containing carbon, hydrogen, oxygen, nitrogen, and sulfur. Proteins, the principal constituents of the protoplasm of all cells, are of high molecular weight and consist of α-amino acids joined by peptide linkages. Twenty different amino acids are commonly found in proteins, each protein having a unique, genetically defined amino-acid sequence which determines its specific shape and function. They serve as enzymes, structural elements, hormones, immunoglobulins, etc., and are involved in oxygen transport, muscle contraction, electron transport, and other activities **Bence Jones p.,** a low-molecular weight, heat-sensitive urinary protein found in multiple myeloma, which coagulates when heated to 45°–55° C. and redissolves partially or wholly on boiling. **complete p.,** one containing the essential amino acids in the proportion required in the human diet. **conjugated p's,** those in which the protein is combined with nonprotein molecules or prosthetic groups, e.g., nucleoproteins, glycoproteins, lipoproteins, and metalloproteins. **C-reactive p.,** a globulin that forms a precipitate with the C-polysaccharide of the pneumonococcus; its demonstration in the serum is an indicator of inflammation of infectious or noninfectious origin. **myeloma p.,** a homogeneous monoclonal immunoglobulin produced by a plasmacytoma, or partial immunoglobulin molecules, such as Bence Jones protein, produced by plasma cells that have undergone neoplastic transformation. **partial p.,** one having a ratio of essential amino acids different from that of the average body protein. **plasma p's,** all the proteins present in the blood plasma, including the immunoglobulins. **serum p's,** proteins in the blood serum, including immunoglobulins, albumin, complement, coagulation factors, and enzymes.

proteinaceous (prōt″e-in-a′shis) pertaining to or of the nature of protein.

proteinase (prōt′e-in-ās″) any enzyme that catalyzes the splitting of interior peptide bonds in a protein; an endopeptidase.

proteinemia (prōt″e-in-ēm′e-ah) excess of protein in the blood.

proteinosis (prōt″e-in-o′sis) the accumulation of excess protein in the tissues. **lipid p.,** a hereditary defect of lipid metabolism marked by yellowish deposits of hyaline lipid-carbohydrate mixture on the inner surface of the lips, under the tongue, on the oropharynx and larynx, and by skin lesions. **pulmonary alveolar p.,** a chronic lung disease in which the distal alveoli become filled with a bland, eosinophilic, probably endogenous proteinaceous material that prevents ventilation of affected areas.

proteinuria (-ūr′e-ah) an excess of serum proteins in the urine. **proteinu′ric,** adj.

proteoglycan (prōt″e-o-gli′kan) any of a group of glycoproteins present in connective tissue and formed of subunits of disaccharides linked together and joined to a protein core; the proteoglycans, which include the mucopolysaccharides with their protein moiety, serve as a binding or cementing material.

proteolipid (-lip′id) a combination of a peptide or protein with a lipid, having the solubility characteristic of lipids.

proteolysis (ol′ĭ-sis) the splitting of proteins by hydrolysis of the peptide bonds with formation of smaller polypeptides. **proteolyt′ic,** adj.

proteometabolism (-mě-tab′ah-lizm) the metabolism of protein.

proteopeptic (-pep′tik) digesting protein.

Proteus (prōt′e-is) a genus of gram-negative, motile bacteria usually found in fecal and other putrefying matter, including *P. morga′nii,* found in the intestines and associated with summer diarrhea of infants, and *P. vulga′ris,* often found as a secondary invader in various localized suppurative pathologic processes; it is a cause of cystitis.

prothrombin (-throm′bin) coagulation Factor II.

prothrombinase (-throm′bin-ās) thromboplastin.

prothrombinogenic (pro-throm″bĭ-no-jen′ik) promoting the production of prothrombin.

protirelin (pro-ti′rah-lin) thyrotropin releasing hormone.

protist (prōt′ist) any member of the Protista.

Protista (pro-tis′tah) a kingdom comprising bacteria, algae, slime molds, fungi, and protozoa; it includes all single-celled organisms.

protium (prōt′e-um) see *hydrogen.*

proto- word element [Gr.], *first.*

protoblast (prōt′ah-blast) a blastomere from which a particular organ or part develops. **protoblas′tic,** adj.

protocol (-kol) the original notes made on a necropsy, an experiment, or on a case of disease.

protodiastolic (prōt″o-di″ah-stol′ik) pertaining to early diastole, i.e., immediately following the second heart sound.

protoduodenum (-doo″o-de′nim) the first or proximal portion of the duodenum, extending from the pylorus to the duodenal papilla.

protogaster (-gas′ter) archenteron.

protomerite (tom'er-īt) the anterior portion of certain gregarine protozoa.

proton (pro'ton) an elementary particle that is the core or nucleus of an ordinary hydrogen atom of mass 1; the unit of positive electricity, being equivalent to the electron in charge and approximately to the hydrogen ion in mass.

protoneuron (prōt''o-noor'on) the first neuron in a peripheral reflex arc.

proto-oncogene (pro''to-ongk'o-jēn) a normal gene that with slight alteration by mutation or other mechanism becomes an oncogene.

protoplasm (prōt'ah-plazm) the viscid, translucent colloid material, the essential constituent of the living cell, including cytoplasm and nucleoplasm. **protoplas'mic,** adj.

protoplast (-plast) a bacterial or plant cell deprived of its rigid wall but with its plasma membrane intact; the cell is dependent for its integrity on an isotonic or hypertonic medium.

protoporphyria (prōt''o-por-fēr'e-ah) erythropoietic p.: porphyria marked by excessive protoporphyrin in erythrocytes, plasma, and feces, and by intense itching, erythema, and edema on short exposure to sunlight; skin lesions usually fade without scarring or pigmentation but a chronic weatherbeaten appearance is characteristic.

protoporphyrin (-por'fĭ-rin) the porphyrin, $C_{34}H_{34}N_4O_4$, whose iron complex united with protein occurs in hemoglobin and other respiratory pigments.

protoporphyrinuria (-por''fĭ-rin-ūr'e-ah) protoporphyrin in the urine.

protospasm (prōt'ah-spazm) a spasm which begins in a limited area and extends to other parts.

Prototheca (pro''to-the'kah) a genus of ubiquitous yeastlike organisms generally considered to be algae; *P. wickerhamii* and *P. zop'fii* are pathogenic.

protothecosis (pro''to-the-ko'sis) infection caused by organisms of the genus *Prototheca*, varying from cutaneous lesions to systemic invasion, occurring as an opportunistic infection or as a result of traumatic implantation of organisms into the tissues.

prototroph (-trōf) an organism with the same growth factor requirements as the ancestral strain; said of microbial mutants. **prototroph'ic,** adj.

protovertebra (pro''to-vert'ah-brah) 1. somite. 2. the caudal half of a somite forming most of the vertebra.

Protozoa (-zo'ah) a phylum comprising the simplest organisms of the animal kingdom, consisting of unicellular organisms ranging in size from submicroscopic to macroscopic. It includes the Sarcodina, Mastigophora, Ciliophora, and Sporozoa.

protozoacide (-zo'ah-sīd) destructive to protozoa; an agent destructive to protozoa.

protozoiasis (-zo-i'ah-sis) any disease caused by protozoa.

protozoology (-zo-ol'ah-je) the study of protozoa.

protozoon (-zo'on), pl. *protozo'a* [Gr.] any member of the Protozoa.

protozoophage (-zo'ah-fāj) a cell having a phagocytic action on protozoa.

protraction (pro-trak'shun) a forward projection of a facial structure; in *mandibular p.*, the gnathion is anterior to the orbital plane; in *maxillary p.*, the subnasion is anterior to the orbital plane.

protractor (-trak'ter) an instrument for extracting foreign bodies from wounds.

protransglutaminase (pro-tranz''gloo-tam'in-ās) the inactive precursor of transglutaminase.

protriptyline (-trip'tĭ-lēn) a tricyclic antidepressant, $C_{19}H_{21}N$.

protrusion (-troo'zhin) extension beyond the usual limits, or above a plane surface.

protuberance (-too'ber-ins) a projecting part, or prominence.

protuberantia (-too''ber-an'she-ah), pl. *protuberan'tiae* [L.] protuberance.

provertebra (-vert'ĭ-brah) protovertebra.

provirus (-vi'ris) the genome of an animal virus integrated (by crossing over) into the chromosome of the host cell, and thus replicated in all of its daughter cells.

provitamin (-vīt'ah-min) a substance, e.g., ergosterol, from which the animal organism can form vitamin.

proximad (prok'sĭ-mad) in a proximal direction.

proximal (prok'sĭ-mil) nearest to a point of reference, as to a center or median line or to the point of attachment or origin.

proximalis (prok''sĭ-ma'lis) [L.] proximal.

proximobuccal (-buk''l) pertaining to the proximal and buccal surfaces of a posterior tooth.

prozone (pro'zōn) the phenomenon exhibited by some sera, in which agglutination or precipitation occurs at higher dilution ranges, but is not visible at lower dilutions or when undiluted.

prurigo (proo-ri'go) [L.] any of several itchy skin eruptions in which the characteristic lesion is dome-shaped with a small transient vesicle on top, followed by crusting or lichenification. **prurig'inous,** adj. **p. mi'tis,** prurigo of a mild type. **p. nodula'ris,** a form of neurodermatitis, usually occurring on the extremities in middle-aged women, marked by discrete, firm, rough-surfaced, dark brownish-gray, intensely itchy nodules. **p. sim'plex,** papular urticaria.

pruritogenic (proor''it-o-jen'ik) causing pruritus, or itching.

pruritus (proor-ī'tis) itching. **prurit'ic,** adj. **p. a'ni,** intense chronic itching in the anal region. **p. hiema'lis,** winter itch. **p. seni'lis,** itching in the aged, due to degeneration of the skin. **symptomatic p.,** that occurring secondarily to another condition. **uremic p.,** generalized itching associated with chronic renal failure and not attributable to other internal or skin disease. **p. vul'vae,** intense itching of the female external genitals.

prussic acid (prus'ik) hydrogen cyanide; see under *hydrogen*.

psalterium (sal-tēr'e-im) 1. omasum. 2. commissure of the fornix.

psammoma (sah-mo′mah) a tumor, especially a meningioma, containing psammoma bodies.

psammosarcoma (sam″o-sar-ko′mah) a sarcoma containing granular material.

pseud(o)- word element [Gr.], *false*.

pseudarthrosis (soo″dar-thro′sis) a pathologic condition in which failure of callus formation following pathologic fracture through an area of deossification in a weight-bearing long bone results in formation of a false joint.

pseudesthesia (soo″des-the′ze-ah) a subjective sensation occurring in the absence of the appropriate stimuli.

pseudoacanthosis (soo″do-ak″an-tho′sis) a condition clinically resembling acanthosis. **p. ni′gricans**, a benign form of acanthosis nigricans associated with obesity; the obesity is sometimes associated with endocrine disturbance.

pseudoagraphia (-ah-graf′e-ah) a condition in which the patient can copy writing, but cannot write independently except in a meaningless and illegible manner.

pseudoallele (-ah-lēl′) one of two or more genes which are seemingly allelic, but which can be shown to have distinctive but closely linked loci. **pseudoallel′ic**, adj.

pseudoanemia (-ah-nēm′e-ah) marked pallor with no evidence of anemia.

pseudoaneurysm (-an′ūr-izm) dilatation and tortuosity of a vessel, giving the appearance of an aneurysm.

pseudoangina (-an-ji′nah) a nervous disorder resembling angina.

pseudoapoplexy (-ap′ah-plek″se) a condition resembling apoplexy, but without hemorrhage.

pseudocast (soo′dah-kast) an accidental formation of urinary sediment resembling a true cast.

pseudocele (-sēl) the fifth ventricle.

pseudocholesteatoma (-ko″les-te″ah-to′mah) a horny mass of epithelial cells resembling cholesteatoma in the tympanic cavity in chronic middle ear inflammation.

pseudochorea (-kor-e′ah) a state of general incoordination resembling chorea.

pseudochromhidrosis (-krōm″hi-dro′sis) discoloration of sweat by surface contaminants.

pseudocirrhosis (-si-ro′sis) a condition suggestive of, but not due to, cirrhosis; often due to pericarditis (*pericardial p.*); see *Pick's disease* (2).

pseudoclaudication (-claw″di-ka′shin) intermittent claudication due to compression of the cauda equina.

pseudocoarctation (-ko″ark-ta′shin) a condition radiographically resembling coarctation but without compromise of the lumen, as occurs in a congenital anomaly of the aortic arch.

pseudocolloid (soo″do-kol′oid) a mucoid substance sometimes found in ovarian cysts.

pseudocoxalgia (-kok-sal′je-ah) osteochondrosis of the capitular epiphysis of the femur.

pseudocrisis (-kri′sis) sudden but temporary abatement of febrile symptoms.

pseudocroup (soo′dah-krōōp) 1. laryngismus stridulus. 2. thymic asthma.

pseudocyesis (soo″do-si-e′sis) false pregnancy.

pseudocylindroid (-si-lin′droid) a shred of mucin in the urine resembling a cylindroid.

pseudocyst (soo′dah-sist) an abnormal or dilated space resembling a cyst but not lined with epithelium.

pseudodementia (soo″do-de-men′she-ah) a state of general apathy resembling dementia, but without defect of intelligence.

pseudodiphtheria (-dif-the′re-ah) the presence of a false membrane not due to *Corynebacterium diphtheriae*.

pseudodominant (-dom′ĭ-nint) giving the appearance of being dominant; said of a recessive genetic trait appearing in the offspring of a homozygous and a heterozygous parent.

pseudoemphysema (-em″fĭ-ze′mah) a condition resembling emphysema, but due to temporary obstruction of the bronchi.

pseudoephedrine (-ĕ-fed′rin) one of the optical isomers of ephedrine; the hydrochloride salt is used as a nasal decongestant.

pseudoexstrophy (-ek′strah-fe) a developmental anomaly marked by the characteristic musculoskeletal defects of exstrophy of the bladder but with no major defect of the urinary tract.

pseudofolliculitis (-fah-lik″ūl-īt′is) a chronic disorder occurring chiefly in Negroes, most often in the submandibular region of the neck, the characteristic lesions of which are erythematous papules containing buried hairs.

pseudofracture (-frak′cher) a condition seen in the roentgenogram of a bone as a thickening of the periosteum and formation of new bone over what looks like an incomplete fracture.

pseudoglioma (-gli-o′mah) any condition mimicking retinoblastoma, e.g., retrolental fibroplasia or exudative retinopathy.

pseudoglottis (-glot′is) 1. the aperture between the false vocal cords. 2. neoglottis. **pseudoglot′tic**, adj.

pseudogout (soo′dah-gowt) an apparently hereditary, arthritic condition marked by attacks of goutlike symptoms, usually affecting a single joint (particularly the knee), and associated with chondrocalcinosis.

pseudohematuria (-hēm″ah-tōōr′e-a) the presence in the urine of pigments that impart a pink or red color, but with no detectable hemoglobin or blood cells.

pseudohemophilia (soo″do-hēm″o-fil′e-ah) von Willebrand's disease.

pseudohermaphroditism (-her-maf′rah-dit-izm″) a state in which the gonads are of one sex, but one or more contradictions exist in the morphologic criteria of sex.

pseudohernia (-her′ne-ah) an inflamed sac or gland simulating strangulated hernia.

pseudohypertrophy (-hi-per′trah-fe) increase in size without true hypertrophy. **pseudohypertroph′ic**, adj.

pseudohypoaldosteronism (-hi″po-al-dos′ter-ōn-izm) a hereditary disorder of infancy, characterized by severe salt loss by the kidneys; it is thought to be due to unresponsiveness of the distal renal tubule to aldosterone.

pseudohypoparathyroidism (-hi″po-par″ah-thi′roi-dizm) a hereditary condition resembling hypoparathyroidism, but caused by failure of response to parathyroid hormone, marked by hypocalcemia and hyperphosphatemia.

pseudoisochromatic (-i″so-krom-at′ik) seemingly of the same color throughout; applied to solution for testing color blindness, containing two pigments that can be distinguished by the normal eye.

pseudojaundice (-jawn′dis) skin discoloration due to blood changes and not to liver disease.

pseudomania (-ma′ne-ah) 1. false or pretended mental disorder. 2. pathologic lying.

pseudomelanosis (-mel″ah-no′sis) discoloration of tissue after death by blood pigments.

Pseudomonas (-mo′nas) a genus of gram-negative, strictly anaerobic bacteria, some species of which are pathogenic for plants and vertebrates. *P. aerugino′sa*, the only species pathogenic for man, produces the blue-green pigment, pyocyanin, which gives the color to "blue pus," and causes various human diseases; *P. mal′lei* causes glanders; *P. pseudomal′lei* causes melioidosis.

pseudomucin (-mu′sin) a mucin-like substance found in ovarian cysts. **pseudomu′cinous,** adj.

pseudomyxoma (-mik-so′mah) a mass of epithelial mucus resembling a myxoma. **p. peritone′i,** the presence in the peritoneal cavity of mucoid matter from a ruptured ovarian cyst or a ruptured mucocele of the appendix.

pseudoneuritis (-nōōr-īt′is) a congenital hyperemic condition of the optic papilla.

pseudopapilledema (-pap″ĭ-lĕ-de′mah) anomalous elevation of the optic disk.

pseudoparalysis (-pah-ral′ĭ-sis) apparent loss of muscular power without real paralysis. **arthritic general p.,** a condition resembling dementia paralytica, dependent on intracranial atheroma in arthritic patients. **Parrot's p., syphilitic p.,** pseudoparalysis of one or more extremities in infants, due to syphilitic osteochondritis of an epiphysis.

pseudoparaplegia (-par″ah-ple′je-ah) spurious paralysis of the lower limbs, as in hysteria or malingering.

pseudoparesis (-pah-re′sis) a hysterical or non-organic condition simulating paresis.

pseudopelade (-pe′lād) patchy alopecia roughly simulating alopecia areata; it may be due to various disease of the hair follicles, some of which are associated with scarring.

pseudoplegia (-ple′je-ah) hysterical paralysis.

pseudopodium (-po′de-um) a temporary protrusion of the cytoplasm of an ameba, serving for purposes of locomotion or to engulf food.

pseudopolyp (-pol′ip) a hypertrophied tab of mucous membrane resembling a polyp.

pseudopolyposis (-pol″ĭ-po′sis) numerous pseudopolyps in the colon and rectum, due to long-standing inflammation.

pseudopseudohypoparathyroidism (-soo″do-hi″po-par″ah-thi′roi-dizm) an incomplete form of pseudohypoparathyroidism marked by the same constitutional features but by normal levels of calcium and phosphorus in the blood serum.

pseudopsia (soo-dop′se-ah) false or perverted vision.

pseudopsychosis (soo-do-si-ko′sis) Ganser's syndrome.

pseudopterygium (soo″do-ter-ij′e-im) an adhesion of the conjunctiva to the cornea following a burn or other injury.

pseudoptosis (-to′sis) decrease in the size of the palpebral aperture.

pseudorabies (-ra′bēz) a highly contagious disease of the central nervous system of dogs, cats, rats, cattle, and swine, due to a herpesvirus and marked by sudden onset, late paralysis, convulsions, and death within three days; in swine, it usually runs a milder course.

pseudoreaction (-re-ak′shin) a false or deceptive reaction; a skin reaction in intradermal tests which is not due to the specific test substance but to protein in the medium employed in producing the toxin.

pseudorickets (-rik′its) renal osteodystrophy.

pseudoscarlatina (-skar″lah-te′nah) a septic condition with fever and eruption resembling scarlet fever.

pseudosclerosis (-sklĕ-ro′sis) a condition with the symptoms but without the lesions of multiple sclerosis. **Strümpell-Westphal p., Westphal-Strümpell p.,** hepatolenticular degeneration.

pseudostoma (soo-dos′tah-mah) an apparent communication between epithelial cells or opening in a membrane which is in actuality a staining artifact.

pseudotetanus (soo″do-tet′ah-nus) persistent muscular contractions resembling tetanus but unassociated with *Clostridium tetani*.

pseudotruncus arteriosus (-trunk′is ar-tēr″e-o′sis) the most severe form of tetralogy of Fallot.

pseudotuberculosis (-too-berk″ūl-o′sis) a fatal disease of rodents due to *Yersinia pseudotuberculosis*, with caseous swellings and nodules in various organs. Rarely, *Corynebacterium pseudotuberculosis* causes the disease in domestic animals.

pseudotumor (-tōōm′er) phantom tumor. **p. ce′rebri,** cerebral edema and raised intracranial pressure without neurological signs except occasional sixth-nerve palsy.

pseudoxanthoma elasticum (-zan-tho′mah e-las′tĭ-kim) a dermatosis marked by small yellowish macules and papules, and histologically by swollen, calcified elastic fibers with degeneration of the collagen fibers in the lower and middle dermis and in the gastrointestinal tract and heart.

p.s.i. pounds per square inch.

psilocin (si′lah-sin) a hallucinogenic substance closely related to psilocybin.

psilocybin (si″lah-si′bin) a hallucinogen, C_{13}-$H_{18(20)}O_9N_2P_2$, having indole characteristics, isolated from the mushroom *Psilocybe mexicana*.

psittacosis (sit″ah-ko′sis) a disease due to a strain of *Chlamydia psittaci*, first seen in parrots and later in other birds and domestic fowl; it is transmissible to man, usually taking the form of a pneumonia accompanied by fever, cough, and often splenomegaly. See also *ornithosis.*

psoralen (sor'ah-len) any of the constituents of certain plants (e.g., *Psoralea corylifolia*) that have the ability to produce phototoxic dermatitis when an individual is first exposed to a psoralen and then to sunlight; certain perfumes and drugs (e.g., methoxsalen) contain psoralens.

psoriasis (sor-i'ah-sis) a chronic, hereditary, recurrent dermatosis marked by discrete vivid red macules, papules, or plaques covered with silvery lamellated scales. **psoriat'ic,** adj.

PSRO Professional Standards Review Organization: a regional organization of physicians and in some cases allied health professionals established to monitor health care services paid for by Medicare, Medicaid, and Maternal and Child Health programs to assure that services provided are medically necessary, meet professional standards, and are provided in the most economic medically appropriate health care agency or institution.

psych(o)- word element [Gr.], *mind.*

psychalgia (si-kal'je-ah) pain of mental or hysterical origin; pain attending or due to mental effort. **psychal'gic,** adj.

psychataxia (si"kah-tak'se-ah) disordered mental state with confusion, agitation, and inability to fix the attention.

psyche (si'ke) the mind; the human faculty for thought, judgment, and emotion; the mental life, including both conscious and unconscious processes. **psy'chic,** adj.

psychedelic (si"ki-del'ik) pertaining to or causing hallucinations, distortions of perception, and, sometimes, psychotic-like behavior; also, a drug producing such effects.

psychiatry (si-ki'ah-tre) that branch of medicine dealing with the study, treatment, and prevention of mental illness. **psychiat'ric,** adj. **biological p.,** that which emphasizes physical, chemical, and neurological causes and treatment approaches. **descriptive p.,** that based on observation and study of external factors that can be seen, heard, or felt. **dynamic p.,** the study of emotional processes, their origins and the mental mechanisms underlying them. **forensic p.,** that dealing with the legal aspects of mental disorders. **organic p.,** 1. that dealing with the psychological aspects of organic brain disease. 2. biological p. **preventive p.,** a broad term referring to the amelioration, control, and limitation of psychiatric disability. **social p.,** that concerned with the cultural and social factors that engender, precipitate, intensify, or prolong maladaptive patterns of behavior and complicate treatment.

psychic (si'kik) pertaining to the mind.

psychoactive (si"ko-ak'tiv) affecting the mind or behavior, as psychoactive drugs.

psychoanaleptic (-an"ah-lep'tik) exerting a stimulating effect upon the mind.

psychoanalysis (-ah-nal'ĭ-sis) a method of diagnosing and treating mental and emotional disorders through ascertaining and analyzing the facts of the patient's mental life. **psychoanalyt'ic,** adj.

psychobiology (-bi-ol'ah-je) study of the interrelations of body and mind in the formation and functioning of personality. **psychobiolog'ical,** adj.

psychodrama (-drah'mah) group psychotherapy in which patients dramatize their individual conflicting situations of daily life.

psychodynamics (-di-nam'iks) the science of human behavior and motivation.

psychogenesis (-jen'ĭ-sis) 1. mental development. 2. production of a symptom or illness by psychic, as opposed to organic, factors.

psychogenic (-jen'ik) having an emotional or psychologic origin.

psychograph (-graf) 1. a chart for recording graphically a person's personality traits. 2. a written description of a person's mental functioning.

psycholepsy (-lep'se) a condition marked by sudden mood changes.

psychology (si-kol'ah-je) the science dealing with the mind and mental processes, especially in relation to human and animal behavior. **psycholog'ic, psycholog'ical,** adj. **analytic p.,** psychology by introspective methods. **child p.,** the study of the development of the mind of the child. **clinical p.,** the use of psychologic knowledge and techniques in the treatment of persons with emotional difficulties. **community p.,** a broad term referring to the organization of community resources for the prevention of mental disorders. **criminal p.,** the study of the mentality, motivation, and social behavior of criminals. **depth p.,** psychoanalysis. **developmental p.,** the study of behavioral change through the life span. **dynamic p.,** that stressing the element of energy in mental processes. **environmental p.,** the study of the effects of the physical and social environment on behavior. **experimental p.,** the study of the mind and mental operations by the use of experimental methods. **gestalt p.,** gestaltism. **physiologic p., physiological p.,** the branch of psychology that studies the relationship between physiologic processes and behavior. **social p.,** that treating of the social aspects of mental life.

psychometry (si-kom'ĭ-tre) the testing and measuring of mental and psychologic ability, efficiency, potentials, and functioning. **psychomet'ric,** adj.

psychomotor (si"ko-mōt'er) pertaining to motor effects of cerebral or psychic activity.

psychoneural (-nōōr'il) relating to the totality of neural events initiated by a sensory input and leading to storage, to discrimination, or an output of any kind.

psychoneurosis (-nōōr-o'sis) neurosis. **psychoneurot'ic,** adj.

psychopath (si'kah-path) a person who has an antisocial personality.

psychopathology (-pah-thol'ah-je) the branch of medicine dealing with the causes and processes of mental disorders.

psychopathy (si-kop'ah-the) any disease of the mind.

psychopharmacology (si″ko-fahr″mah-kol′-ah-je) 1. the study of the action of drugs on psychological functions and mental states. 2. the use of drugs to modify psychological functions and mental states. **psychopharmacolog′ic,** adj.

psychophysical (-fiz′ĭ-kil) pertaining to the mind and its relation to physical manifestations.

psychophysics (-fiz′iks) scientific study of quantitative relations between characteristics or patterns of physical stimuli and the sensations induced by them.

psychophysiology (-fiz″e-ol′ah-je) scientific study of the interaction and interrelations of psychic and physiologic factors. **psychophysiolog′ic,** adj.

psychoplegic (-ple′jik) an agent lessening cerebral activity or excitability.

psychosensory (-sen′ser-e) perceiving and interpreting sensory stimuli.

psychosexual (-sek′shoo-il) pertaining to the psychic or emotional aspects of sex.

psychosis (si-ko′sis), pl. *psycho′ses.* Any major mental disorder of organic or emotional origin marked by derangement of personality and loss of contact with reality, often with delusions, hallucinations, or illusions. Cf. *neurosis.* **affective p.,** mood disorder. **alcoholic p.,** mental disorder caused by excessive use of alcohol. **bipolar p.** bipolar disorder. **brief reactive p.,** an episode of psychotic symptoms that are a reaction to a recognizable, distressing life event, of sudden onset and less than one month's duration. **involutional p.,** see under *melancholia.* **Korsakoff's p.,** Korsakoff's syndrome. **manic-depressive p.,** bipolar disorder. **organic p.,** organic mental disorder. **senile p.,** mental deterioration in old age, with organic brain changes, the symptoms including impaired memory for recent events, confabulation, irritability, etc. **symbiotic p., symbiotic infantile p.,** a condition seen in two- to four-year-old children having an abnormal relationship to the mothering figure, characterized by intense separation anxiety, severe regression, giving up of useful speech, and autism. **toxic p.,** one due to ingestion of toxic agents into the body, or to the presence of toxins within the body.

psychosocial (-so′shil) pertaining to or involving both psychic and social aspects.

psychosomatic (-sah-mat′ik) pertaining to the mind-body relationship; having bodily symptoms of psychic, emotional, or mental origin.

psychostimulant (-stim′ūl-int) 1. producing a transient increase in psychomotor activity. 2. a drug that produces such effects.

psychosurgery (-ser′jer-e) brain surgery done to relieve mental and psychic symptoms.

psychotherapy (-thĕ′rah-pe) treatment designed to produce a response by mental rather than by physical effects.

psychotic (si-kot′ik) 1. pertaining to, characterized by, or caused by psychosis. 2. a person exhibiting psychosis.

psychotogenic (si-kot″ah-jen′ik) producing a psychosis.

psychotomimetic (-mi-met′ik) pertaining to, characterized by, or producing symptoms similar to those of a psychosis.

psychotropic (si″ko-trop′ik) exerting an effect on the mind; said especially of drugs.

psychr(o)- word element [Gr.], *cold.*

psychralgia (si-kral′je-ah) a painful sensation of cold.

psychrophilic (si″kro-fil′ik) fond of cold; said of bacteria growing best in the cold (15°–20° C.).

psychrophore (si′krah-fōr) a double catheter for applying cold.

psyllium (sil′ĭ-im) a plant of the genus *Plantago.*

Pt chemical symbol, *platinum.*

pt. pint.

PTA plasma thromboplastin antecedent (coagulation Factor XI).

ptarmic (tar′mik) causing sneezing.

ptarmus (tar′mis) spasmodic sneezing.

PTC plasma thromboplastin component; phenylthiocarbamide.

pterion (tēr′e-on) a point of junction of frontal, parietal, temporal, and sphenoid bones.

pteroylglutamic acid (ter″o-il-gloo-tam′ik) folic acid.

pterygium (tĕ-rij′e-im) a winglike structure, especially an abnormal triangular fold of membrane in the interpalpebral fissure, extending from the conjunctiva to the cornea. **p. col′li,** webbed neck; a thick skin fold on the side of the neck, from the mastoid region to the acromion.

pterygoid (tĕ′rĭ-goid) shaped like a wing.

pterygomandibular (tĕ″rĭ-go-man-dib′ūl-er) pertaining to the pterygoid process and the mandible.

pterygomaxillary (-mak′sĭ-lĕ″re) pertaining to the pterygoid process and the maxilla.

pterygopalatine (pal′ah-tīn) pertaining to the pterygoid process and the palate bone.

ptilosis (ti-lo′sis) falling out of the eyelashes.

ptomaine (to′mān, to-mān′) any of an indefinite class of toxic bases, usually considered to be formed by the action of bacterial metabolism or proteins.

ptosed (tōst) affected with ptosis.

ptosis (to′sis) 1. prolapse of an organ or part. 2. paralytic drooping of the upper eyelid. **ptot′ic,** adj.

-ptosis word element [Gr.], *downward displacement.* **-ptot′ic,** adj.

ptyal(o)- word element [Gr.], *saliva.* See also *sial(o).*

ptyalagogue (ti-al′ah-gog) sialagogue.

ptyalectasis (ti″ah-lek′tah-sis) 1. a state of dilatation of a salivary duct. 2. surgical dilation of a salivary duct.

ptyalin (ti′ah-lin) α-amylase occurring in saliva.

ptyalism (ti′il-izm) excessive secretion of saliva.

ptyalocele (ti-al′ah-sēl) a cystic tumor containing saliva.

ptyalogenic (ti″ah-lo-jen′ik) formed from or by the action of saliva.

ptyaloreaction (-re-ak′shin) a reaction occurring in or performed on the saliva.

ptyalorrhea (-re′ah) ptyalism.

Pu chemical symbol, *plutonium.*

pubarche (pu-bar′ke) the first appearance of pubic hair.

pubertas (pu-ber′tas) puberty. **p. prae′cox,** precocious puberty.

puberty (pu′bert-e) the period during which the secondary sex characteristics begin to develop and the capability of sexual reproduction is attained. **pu′beral, pu′bertal,** adj.

pubes (pu′bez), sing. *pu′bis* [L.] 1. the hairs growing over the pubic region. 2. the pubic region. **pu′bic,** adj.

pubescent (pu-bes′int) 1. arriving at the age of puberty. 2. covered with down or lanugo.

pubiotomy (pu″be-ot′ah-me) surgical separation of the pubic bone lateral to the symphysis.

pubis (pu′bis) pubic bone; see *Table of Bones.*

pubovesical (-ves′ĭ-kil) pertaining to the pubis and bladder.

pudendum (pu-den′dim), pl. *puden′da* [L.] vulva; the external genitalia of humans, especially of the female. **puden′dal, pu′dic,** adj. **p. femini′num, p. mulie′bre,** the female pudendum.

puerile (pu′er-il) pertaining to childhood or to children; childish.

puerpera (pu-er′per-ah) a woman who has just given birth to a child.

puerperal (-per-il) pertaining to a puerpera or to the puerperium.

puerperalism (-per-al-izm) morbid condition incident to childbirth.

puerperium (pu″er-pēr′e-im) the period or state of confinement after childbirth.

Pulex (pu′leks) a genus of fleas, including *P. ir′ritans,* the common, or human flea, which attacks man and domestic animals, and may act as an intermediate host of certain helminths.

pulicicide (pu-lis′ĭ-sīd) an agent destructive to fleas.

pullulation (pul″ul-a′shin) development by sprouting or budding.

pulmo (pul′mo), pl. *pulmo′nes* [L.] lung.

pulmoaortic (pul″mo-a-or′tik) pertaining to the lungs and aorta.

pulmonary (pul′mo-nĕ″re) pertaining to the lungs or the pulmonary artery.

pulmonic (pul-mon′ik) pulmonary.

pulmonitis (pul″mah-nīt′is) pneumonitis.

pulmotor (pul′mōt′er) an apparatus for forcing oxygen into the lungs and inducing artificial respiration.

pulp (pulp) any soft, juicy animal or vegetable tissue. **pul′pal,** adj. **coronal p.,** the part of the dental pulp contained in the crown portion of the pulp cavity. **dental p.,** richly vascularized and innervated connective tissue inside the pulp cavity of a tooth. **digital p.,** a cushion of soft tissue on the palmar or plantar surface of the distal phalanx of a finger or toe. **red p., splenic p.,** the dark reddish brown substance filling the interspaces of the splenic sinuses.

white p., sheaths of lymphatic tissue surrounding the arteries of the spleen.

pulpa (pul′pah), pl. *pul′pae* [L.] pulp.

pulpectomy (pul-pek′tah-me) removal of dental pulp.

pulpitis (pul-pīt′is), pl. *pulpi′tides* [L.] inflammation of dental pulp.

pulpotomy (pul-pot′ah-me) excision of the coronal pulp.

pulsatile (pul′sah-tīl) characterized by a rhythmic pulsation.

pulsation (pul-sa′shun) a throb, or rhythmic beat, as of the heart.

pulse (puls) the rhythmic expansion of an artery which may be felt with the finger. **alternating p.,** one with regular alternation of weak and strong beats without changes in cycle length. **anacrotic p.,** one in which the ascending limb of the tracing shows a transient drop in amplitude. **bigeminal p.,** one in which two beats occur in rapid succession, the groups of two being separated by a longer interval. **cannon ball p.,** Corrigan's p. **capillary p.,** Quincke's p. **catadicrotic p.,** one in which the descending limb of the tracing shows two small notches. **Corrigan's p.,** jerky pulse with full expansion and sudden collapse. **dicrotic p.,** a pulse characterized by two peaks, the second peak occurring in diastole and being an exaggeration of the dicrotic wave. **entoptic p.,** a phose occurring with each pulse beat. **hard p.,** one characterized by high tension. **jerky p.,** one in which the artery is suddenly and markedly distended. **paradoxical p.,** one that markedly decreases in size during inspiration, as often occurs in constrictive pericarditis. **pistol-shot p.,** one in which the arteries are subject to sudden distention and collapse. **plateau p.,** one that is slowly rising and sustained. **quadrigeminal p.,** one with a pause after every fourth beat. **Quincke's p.,** alternate blanching and flushing of the nail bed due to pulsation of subpapillary arteriolar and venous plexuses, as seen in aortic insufficiency. **Riegel's p.,** one which is smaller during respiration. **thready p.,** one that is very fine and scarcely perceptible. **tricrotic p.,** one in which the tracing shows three marked expansions in one beat of the artery. **trigeminal p.,** one with a pause after every third beat. **vagus p.,** a slow pulse. **venous p.,** the pulsation over a vein, especially over the right jugular vein. **waterhammer p.,** Corrigan's p. **wiry p.,** a small, tense pulse.

pulsion (pul′shin) a pushing outward.

pulsus (pul′sis) [L.] pulse. **p. bisferiens,** a pulse characterized by two strong systolic peaks separated by a midsystolic dip, most commonly occurring in pure aortic regurgitation and in aortic regurgitation with stenosis. **p. dif′ferens,** inequality of the pulse observable at corresponding sites on either side of the body.

pultaceous (pul-ta′shis) like a poultice; pulpy.

pulverulent (pul-ver′ūl-int) powdery; dustlike.

pulvinar (pul-vi′nar) the prominent medial part of the posterior end of the thalamus.

pumice (pum′is) a substance consisting of silicates of aluminum, potassium, and sodium; used in dentistry as an abrasive.

pump (pump) 1. an apparatus for drawing or forcing liquids or gases. 2. to draw or force liquids or gases. **breast p.**, a manual or electric pump for abstracting breast milk. **calcium p.**, the mechanism of active transport of calcium (Ca⁺⁺) across a membrane, as of the sarcoplasmic reticulum of muscle cells, against a concentration gradient; the mechanism is driven by hydrolysis of ATP. **sodium p., sodium-potassium p.**, the mechanism of active transport, driven by hydrolysis of ATP, by which sodium (Na⁺) is extruded from a cell and potassium (K⁺) is brought in, so as to maintain the low concentration of Na⁺ and the high concentration of K⁺ within the cell with respect to the surrounding medium.

pump-oxygenator (pump′ok″sĭ-jin-āt″er) an apparatus consisting of a blood pump and oxygenator, plus filters and traps, for saturating the blood with oxygen during heart surgery.

punchdrunk (punch′drunk″) a traumatic encephalopathy of prizefighters resulting from cumulative cerebral concussions, with general slowing of mental functions, bouts of confusion, and scattered memory loss.

punctate (punk′tāt) spotted; marked with points or punctures.

punctiform (-tĭ-form) like a point.

punctum (-tum), pl. *punc′ta* [L.] a point or small spot. **p. cae′cum**, blind spot. **p. lacrima′le** lacrimal point. **p. prox′imum**, near point. **p. remo′tum**, far point.

puncture (-cher) the act of piercing or penetrating with a pointed object or instrument; a wound so made. **cisternal p.**, puncture of the cisterna cerebellomedullaris through the posterior atlanto-occipital membrane to obtain cerebrospinal fluid. **lumbar p., spinal p.**, the tapping of the subarachnoid space in the lumbar region, usually between the third and fourth lumbar vertebrae. **sternal p.**, removal of bone marrow from the manubrium of the sternum through an appropriate needle.

pupa (pu′pah), pl. *pu′pae* [L.] the second stage in the development of an insect, between the larva and the imago. **pu′pal**, adj.

pupil (pu′pil) the opening in the center of the iris through which light enters the eye. See Plate XIII. **pu′pillary**, adj. **Adie's p.**, tonic p. **Argyll Robertson p.**, one which is miotic and responds to accommodative effort, but not to light. **fixed p.**, one that does not react either to light or on convergence, or in accommodation. **Hutchinson's p.**, one which is dilated while the other is not. **tonic p.**, a usually unilateral condition of the eye in which the affected pupil is larger than the other; responds to accommodation and convergence in a slow, delayed fashion; and reacts to light only after prolonged exposure to dark or light.

pupilla (pu-pil′ah) [L.] pupil.

pupillometry (-lom′ĭ-tre) measurement of the diameter or width of the pupil of the eye.

pupilloplegia (pu″pĭ-lo-ple′je-ah) tonic pupil.

pupilloscopy (pu″pĭ-los′kah-pe) retinoscopy.

pupillostatometer (pu″pĭ-lo-stah-tom′ĭt-er) an instrument for measuring the distance between the pupils.

purgation (pur-ga′shin) catharsis; purging effected by a cathartic medicine.

purgative (purg′it-iv) 1. cathartic (1); causing bowel evacuation. 2. a cathartic, particularly one stimulating peristaltic action.

purge (purj) 1. a purgative medicine or dose. 2. to cause free evacuation of feces.

purine (pūr′ēn) a compound, C₅H₄N₄, not found in nature, but variously substituted to produce a group of compounds, *purines* or *purine bases,* which include adenine and guanine found in nucleic acids and xanthine and hypoxanthine.

purple (pur′p'l) 1. a color between blue and red. 2. a substance of this color used as a dye or indicator. **visual p.**, rhodopsin.

purpura (purp′ūr-ah) a group of disorders characterized by purplish or brownish red discoloration, easily visible through the epidermis, caused by hemorrhage into the tissues. **purpu′ric**, adj. **allergic p., anaphylactoid p.,** Schönlein-Henoch p. **p. annula′ris telangiecto′des,** a rare form in which punctate erythematous lesions coalesce to form an annular or serpiginous pattern. **fibrinolytic p.,** purpura associated with increased fibrinolytic activity of the blood. **p. ful′minans,** nonthrombocytopenic purpura seen mainly in children, usually after an infectious disease, marked by fever, shock, anemia, and sudden, rapidly spreading symmetrical skin hemorrhages of the lower limbs, often associated with extensive intravascular thromboses and gangrene. **p. hemorrha′gica,** idiopathic thrombocytopenic p. **Henoch's p.,** Schönlein-Henoch purpura in which abdominal symptoms predominate. **malignant p.,** epidemic cerebrospinal meningitis. **nonthrombocytopenic p.,** purpura without any decrease in the platelet count of the blood. **Schönlein's p.,** Schönlein-Henoch purpura in which articular symptoms predominate. **Schönlein-Henoch p.,** nonthrombocytopenic purpura of unknown cause, most often seen in children, associated with various clinical symptoms, such as urticaria and erythema, arthropathy and arthritis, gastrointestinal symptoms, and renal involvement. **p. seni′lis,** dark purplish red ecchymoses occurring on the forearms and backs of the hands in the elderly. **thrombocytopenic p.,** any form in which the platelet count is decreased, occurring as a primary disease (*idiopathic thrombocytopenic p.*) or as a consequence of a primary hematologic disorder (*secondary thrombocytopenic p.*). **thrombotic thrombocytopenic p.,** a disease marked by thrombocytopenia, hemolytic anemia, neurological manifestations, azotemia, fever, and thromboses in terminal arterioles and capillaries.

purpurinuria (pur″pūr-in-ūr′e-ah) purpurin (uroerythrin) in the urine.

purulence (pūr-ah-lins) the formation or presence of pus. **pur′ulent**, adj.

puruloid (pūr′ah-loid) resembling pus.

pus (pus) a protein-rich liquid inflammation

product made up of cells (leukocytes), a thin fluid (liquor puris), and cellular debris.

pustula (pus'tu-lah), pl. *pus'tulae* [L.] pustule.

pustule (pus'tūl) a small, elevated, circumscribed, pus-containing lesion of the skin. **pus'tular,** adj.

pustulosis (pus''tūl-o'sis) a condition marked by an eruption of pustules.

putamen (pu-ta'men) the larger and more lateral part of the lentiform nucleus.

putrefaction (pu''trĭ-fak'shin) enzymatic decomposition, especially of proteins, with the production of foul-smelling compounds, such as hydrogen sulfide, ammonia, and mercaptans. **putrefac'tive,** adj.

putrescence (pu-tres'ens) the condition of undergoing putrefaction. **putres'cent,** adj.

putrescine (pu-tres'in) a polyamine, $H_2N(CH_2)_4$-NH_2, first found in decaying meat.

putrid (pu'trid) rotten; putrefied.

PVP polyvinylpyrrolodine (see *povidone*).

PVP-I povidone-iodine.

pyarthrosis (pi''ar-thro'sis) suppuration within a joint cavity; acute suppurative arthritis.

pycno- see words beginning *pykn(o)*-.

pyel(o)- word element [Gr.], *renal pelvis.*

pyelectasis (pi''il-ek'tah-sis) dilatation of the renal pelvis.

pyelitis (pi''il-īt'is) inflammation of the renal pelvis. **pyelit'ic,** adj.

pyelocaliectasis (pi''il-o-kal''e-ek'tah-sis) dilatation of the renal pelvis and calices.

pyelocystitis (-sis-tīt-is) inflammation of the renal pelvis and bladder.

pyelography (pi''il-og'rah-fe) radiography of the renal pelvis and ureter after injection of contrast material. **antegrade p.,** that in which the contrast medium is introduced by percutaneous needle puncture into the renal pelvis. **retrograde p.,** pyelography after introduction of contrast material through the ureter.

pyelointerstitial (pi''il-o-in''ter-stish'il) pertaining to the interstitial tissue of the renal pelvis.

pyelolithotomy (-lĭ-thot'ah-me) incision of the renal pelvis for removal of calculi.

pyelonephritis (-nĕ-frīt'is) inflammation of the kidney and its pelvis due to bacterial infection.

pyelonephrosis (-nĕ-fro'sis) any disease of the kidney and its pelvis.

pyelopathy (pi''il-op'ah-the) any disease of the renal pelvis.

pyeloplasty (pi''il-o-plas''te) plastic repair of the renal pelvis.

pyelostomy (pi''il-los'tah-me) surgical formation of an opening into the renal pelvis.

pyelotomy (pi''il-ot'ah-me) incision of the renal pelvis.

pyelovenous (pi''il-o-ve'nis) pertaining to the renal pelvis and renal veins.

pyemesis (pi-em'ĭ-sis) the vomiting of pus.

pyemia (pi-ēm'e-ah) septicemia in which secondary foci of suppuration occur and multiple abscesses are formed. **pye'mic,** adj. **arterial p.,** that due to dissemination of septic emboli from the heart. **cryptogenic p.,** that in which the

source of infection is in an unidentified tissue.

Pyemotes (pi''ĭ-mōt'ēz) a genus of parasitic mites. *P. ventrico'sus* attacks certain insect larvae found on straw, grain, and other plants, and causes grain itch in man.

pyencephalus (pi''en-sef'ah-lis) abscess of the brain.

pyesis (pi-e'sis) suppuration.

pygal (pi'gil) pertaining to the buttocks.

pygalgia (pi-gal'je-ah) pain in the buttocks.

pykn(o)- word element [Gr.], *thick; compact; frequent.*

pyknic (pik'nik) having a short, thick, stocky build.

pyknocyte (pik'nah-sīt) a distorted and contracted, occasionally spiculed erythrocyte.

pyknodysostosis (-dis''os-to'sis) a hereditary syndrome of dwarfism, osteopetrosis, and skeletal anomalies of the cranium, digits, and mandible.

pyknometer (pik-nom'it-er) an instrument for determining the specific gravity of fluids.

pyknomorphous (pik''nah-mor'fis) having the stained portions of the cell body compactly arranged.

pyknosis (pik-no'sis) a thickening, especially degeneration of a cell in which the nucleus shrinks in size and the chromatin condenses to a solid, structureless mass or masses. **pyknot'ic,** adj.

pyle- word element [Gr.], *portal vein.*

pylephlebectasis (pi''lĭ-flĕ-bek'tah-sis) dilatation of the portal vein.

pylephlebitis (-flĕ-bīt'is) inflammation of the portal vein.

pylor(o)- word element [Gr.], *pylorus.*

pyloralgia (pi''lor-al'je-ah) pain in the region of the pylorus.

pylorectomy (pi''lor-ek'tah-me) excision of the pylorus.

pyloristenosis (pi-lor''e-stĕ-no'sis) pyloric stenosis.

pylorodiosis (pi-lor''o-di-o'sis) dilation of a pyloric stricture with the finger during operation.

pyloroduodenitis (-doo''o-de-nīt'is) inflammation of the pyloric and duodenal mucosa.

pylorogastrectomy (-gas-trek'tah-me) excision of the pylorus and adjacent portion of the stomach.

pyloromyotomy (-mi-ot'ah-me) incision of the longitudinal and circular muscles of the pylorus.

pyloroplasty (pi-lor'ah-plas''te) plastic surgery of the pylorus. **double p.,** posterior pyloromyotomy combined with the Heineke-Mikulicz pyloroplasty. **Finney p.,** enlargement of the pyloric canal by establishment of an inverted U-shaped anastomosis between the stomach and duodenum after longitudinal incision. **Heineke-Mikulicz p.,** enlargement of a pyloric stricture by incising the pylorus longitudinally and suturing the incision transversely.

pyloroscopy (pi''lor-os'kah-pe) endoscopic inspection of the pylorus.

pylorostomy (pi''lor-os'tah-me) surgical formation of an opening through the abdominal wall into the stomach near the pylorus.

pylorotomy (-ot'ah-me) incision of the pylorus.

pylorus (pi-lor'is) the distal aperture of the stomach, opening into the duodenum; variously used to mean pyloric part of the stomach, and pyloric antrum, canal, opening, or sphincter. **pylor'ic,** adj.

pyo- word element [Gr.], *pus.*

pyccele (pi'ah-sēl) a collection of pus, as in the scrotum.

pyocephalus (pi"ah-sef'ah-lis) purulent fluid in the cerebral ventricles.

pyochezia (-ke'ze-ah) pus in the feces.

pyococcus (-kok'is) any pus-forming coccus.

pyocolpocele (-kol'pah-sēl) a vaginal tumor containing pus.

pyocyanase (-si'ah-nās) an antibacterial material from cultures of *Pseudomonas aeruginosa* (*pyocyanea*); bactericidal for many bacteria and lytic for some (*Vibrio cholerae*).

pyocyst (pi'ah-sist) a cyst containing pus.

pyoderma (pi"ah-der'mah) any purulent skin disease. **p. gangreno'sum,** a rapidly evolving cutaneous ulcer or ulcers, with marked undermining of the border.

pyogenesis (-jen'ĭ-sis) the formation of pus.

pyogenic (-jen'ik) producing pus.

pyohemothorax (-he"mo-thor'aks) pus and blood in the pleural space.

pyohydronephrosis (-hi"dro-nĕ-fro'sis) the accumulation of pus and urine in the kidney.

pyoid (pi'oid) resembling or like pus.

pyolabyrinthitis (pi"o-lab"ĭ-rin-thīt'is) inflammation of the labyrinth of the ear, with suppuration.

pyometritis (-me-trīt'is) purulent inflammation of the uterus.

pyomyositis (-mi"ah-sīt'is) purulent myositis.

pyonephritis (-nĕ-frīt'is) purulent inflammation of the kidney.

pyonephrolithiasis (-nef"ro-lĭ-thi'ah-sis) pus and stones in the kidney.

pyonephrosis (-nĕ-fro'sis) suppurative destruction of the renal parenchyma, with total or almost complete loss of kidney function.

pyo-ovarium (-o-vār'e-im) an abscess of the ovary.

pyopericardium (-per"ĭ-kar'de-im) pus in the pericardium.

pyoperitoneum (-per"it-ah-ne'um) pus in the peritoneal cavity.

pyophthalmitis (pi"of-thal-mīt'is) purulent inflammation of the eye.

pyophysometra (pi"o-fi"so-me'trah) pus and gas in the uterus.

pyopneumocholecystitis (pi"o-nōōm"o-ko"lĭ-sis-tīt'is) distention of the gallbladder, with presence of pus and gas.

pyopneumohepatitis (-hep"ah-tīt'is) abscess of the liver with pus and gas in the abscess cavity.

pyopneumopericardium (-per"ĭ-kar'de-im) pus and gas in the pericardium.

pyopneumoperitonitis (-per"it'n-īt'is) peritonitis with presence of pus and gas.

pyopneumothorax (-thor'aks) pus and air or gas in the pleural cavity.

pyopoiesis (pi"o-poi-e'sis) pyogenesis.

pyoptysis (pi-op'tĭ-sis) expectoration of purulent matter.

pyopyelectasis (pi"o-pi"il-ek'tah-sis) dilatation of the renal pelvis with pus.

pyorrhea (-re'ah) a copious discharge of pus. **pyorrhe'al,** adj. **p. alveola'ris,** compound periodontitis.

pyosalpingitis (-sal"pin-jīt'is) purulent salpingitis.

pyosalpingo-oophoritis (-sal-ping"go-o"of-ah-rīt'is) purulent inflammation of the uterine tube and ovary.

pyosalpinx (-sal'pinks) accumulation of pus in a uterine tube.

pyostatic (-stat'ik) arresting suppuration; an agent that arrests suppuration.

pyothorax (-thor'aks) an accumulation of pus in the thorax; empyema.

pyourachus (-ūr'ah-kis) pus in the urachus.

pyoureter (-ūr-ēt'er) pus in the ureter.

pyramid (pir'ah-mid) a pointed or cone-shaped structure or part; often used to indicate the pyramid of the medulla oblongata. **p. of cerebellum,** p. of vermis. **p. of Ferrein,** any of the intracortical prolongations of the renal pyramids. **Lalouette's p.,** p. of thyroid. **p. of light,** a triangular reflection seen upon the tympanic membrane. **malpighian p's,** renal p's. **p. of medulla oblongata,** either of two rounded masses, one on either side of the median fissure of the medulla oblongata. **renal p's,** the conical masses composing the medullary substance of the kidney. **p. of thyroid,** an occasional third lobe of the thyroid gland, extending upward from the isthmus. **p. of tympanum,** the hollow elevation in the inner wall of the middle ear containing the stapedius muscle. **p. of vermis,** the part of the vermis cerebelli between the tuber vermis and the uvula.

pyramis (pir'ah-mis), pl. *pyram'ides* [Gr.] pyramid.

pyrantel (pĭ-ran'tel) an anthelmintic, $C_{11}H_{14}$-N_2S, used as the pamoate and tartrate salts.

pyrectic (pi-rek'tik) 1. pertaining to fever; feverish. 2. a fever-inducing agent.

pyretic (pi-ret'ik) pertaining to fever.

pyretogenesis (pi-rēt"o-jen'ĕ-sis) the origin and causation of fever.

pyretogenous (pi"rĭ-toj'in-is) 1. caused by high body temperature. 2. pyrogenic.

pyrexia (pi-rek'se-ah) a fever, or febrile condition. **pyrex'ial,** adj.

pyridine (pir'ĭ-din) 1. a coal tar derivative, C_5-H_5N, derived also from tobacco and various organic matter. 2. any of a group of substances homologous with normal pyridine.

pyridostigmine (pir"ĭ-do-stig'mēn) a cholinesterase inhibitor, $C_9H_{13}N_2O_2$; the bromide salt is used in treatment of myasthenia gravis and as an antidote to nondepolarizing muscle relaxants, such as curariform drugs.

pyridoxal (pir"ĭ-dok'sil) a form of vitamin B6.

p. phosphate, a major coenzyme involved in amino acid metabolism.

pyridoxamine (pir″ĭ-doks′ah-mēn) one of the three active forms of vitamin B₆. **p. phosphate,** a coenzyme involved in amino acid metabolism.

pyridoxine (pir″ĭ-dok′sēn) one of the forms of vitamin B₆, $C_8H_{11}NO_3$, chiefly used, as the hydrochloride salt, in the prophylaxis and treatment of vitamin B₆ deficiency. It is also used in counteracting the neurotoxic effects of isoniazid, and sometimes in the treatment of myasthenia gravis.

pyrilamine (pi-ril′ah-mēn) an antihistaminic, $C_{17}H_{23}N_3O$, used as the maleate salt.

pyrimethamine (pi″rĭ-meth′ah-mēn) a folic acid antagonist, $C_{12}H_{13}ClN_4$, used as an antimalarial, especially for suppressive prophylaxis, and also used concomitantly with a sulfonamide in the treatment of toxoplasmosis.

pyrimidine (pi-rim′ĭ-dēn) an organic compound, $C_4H_4N_2$, the fundamental form of the pyrimidine bases, including uracil, cytosine, and thymine.

pyro- word element [Gr.], *fire; heat;* (in chemistry) *produced by heating.*

pyrogen (pi′rah-jen) a fever-producing substance. **pyrogen′ic,** adj.

pyroglobulinemia (pi″ro-glob″ūl-in-ēm′e-ah) presence in the blood of an abnormal globulin constituent which is precipitated by heat.

pyromania (-ma′ne-ah) obsessive preoccupation with fires; compulsion to set fires.

pyronin (pi′rah-nin) a red aniline histologic stain.

pyrophosphatase (-fos′fah-tās) any enzyme that catalyzes the hydrolysis of central pyrophosphate linkages.

pyrophosphate (-fos′fāt) a salt of pyrophosphoric acid.

pyrophosphoric acid (pi″ro-fos-for′ik) a dimer of phosphoric acid, $H_4P_2O_7$; its esters are important in energy metabolism and biosynthesis, e.g., ATP.

pyrosis (pi-ro′sis) heartburn.

pyrotic (pi-rot′ik) caustic; burning.

pyroxylin (pi-rok′sĭ-lin) a product of the action of a mixture of nitric and sulfuric acids on cotton, consisting chiefly of cellulose tetranitrate; a necessary ingredient of collodion.

pyrrobutamine (pir″o-būt′ah-min) an antihistaminic, $C_{20}H_{22}ClN$.

pyrrole (pir′ōl) a basic, cyclic substance, $(CH)_4$-NH, obtained by destructive distillation of various animal substances.

pyrrolidine (pĭ-rol′ĭ-din) a simple base, $(CH_2)_4$-NH, obtained from tobacco or prepared from pyrrole.

pyruvate (pi′roo-vāt) a salt, ester, or anion of pyruvic acid. Pyruvate is the end product of glycolysis and may be metabolized to lactate or to acetyl CoA.

pyruvic acid (pi-roo′vik) $CH_3CO\ COOH$, an intermediate in carbohydrate and protein metabolism; it accumulates in blood and tissue in thiamine deficiency.

pyrvinium (pir-vin′e-im) an anthelmintic used for intestinal pinworms in the form of the pamoate salt, $C_{75}H_{70}N_6O_6$.

pyuria (pi-ūr′e-ah) pus in the urine.

PZI protamine zinc insulin.

Q

q symbol for the long arm of a chromosome.

q.d. [L.] *qua′que di′e* (every day).

q.h. *qua′que ho′ra* (every hour).

q.i.d. [L.] *qua′ter in di′e* (four times a day).

q.s. [L.] *quan′tum sa′tis* (a sufficient amount).

q-sort (ku′sort) a technique of personality assessment in which the subject (or an observer) indicates the degree to which a standardized set of descriptive statements applies to the subject.

Quaalude (kwa′lōōd) trademark for a preparation of methaqualone.

quack (kwak) one who misrepresents his ability and experience in diagnosis and treatment of disease or effects to be achieved by his treatment.

quackery (kwak′er-e) the practice or methods of a quack.

quadr(i)- word element [L.], *four.*

quadrant (kwod′rint) 1. one fourth of the circumference of a circle. 2. one of four corresponding parts, or quarters, as of the surface of the abdomen or of the field of vision.

quadrantanopia (kwod″ran-tah-no′pe-ah) defective vision or blindness in one fourth of the visual field.

quadrate (kwod′rāt) square or squared.

quadriceps (kwod′rĭ-seps) having four heads.

quadrigeminal (-jem′ĭ-n'l) fourfold; in four parts; forming a group of four.

quadripara (kwod-rip′ah-rah) a woman who has had four pregnancies which resulted in viable offspring; para IV.

quadriplegia (kwod″rĭ-ple′je-ah) paralysis of all four limbs.

quadritubercular (-tu-ber′ku-ler) having four tubercles or cusps.

quadruped (kwod′roo-ped) 1. four-footed. 2. an animal having four feet.

quadruplet (kwod′rĭ-plet, kwod-roo′plet) one of four offspring produced at one birth.

quantum (kwon′tum), pl. *quan′ta* [L.] a unit of measure under the quantum theory (q.v.).

quarantine (kwor′in-tēn) 1. restriction of freedom of movement of apparently well individuals who have been exposed to infectious disease, which is imposed for the maximal incubation period of the disease. 2. a period of detention for vessels, vehicles, or travelers coming from infected or suspected ports or places. 3. the place where persons are detained for inspection. 4. to detain or isolate on account of suspected contagion.

quart (kwort) one fourth of a gallon (946 ml.).

quartan (kwor′tin) recurring in four-day cycles.

quarter (kwor′ter) the part of a horse's hoof between the heel and the toe. **false q.,** a cleft in a horse's hoof from the top to the bottom.

quartz (kworts) a crystalline form of silica (silicon dioxide).

quater in die (kwah′ter in de′a) [L.] four times a day.

quaternary (kwah′ter-nār″e, kwah-ter′nah-re) 1. fourth in order. 2. containing four elements or groups.

quenching (kwench′ing) any type of interference, such as absorption of fluorescent emission by the surrounding medium, that reduces the intensity of fluorescence.

Quibron (kwĭ′bron) trademark for a fixed combination preparation of theophylline and guanefesin. Quibron Plus also contains butabarbital.

quickening (kwik′en-ing) the first perceptible movement of the fetus in the uterus.

quinacrine (kwin′ah-krin) an antimalarial, antiprotozoal, and anthelmintic, $C_{23}H_{30}ClN_3$, used especially for suppressive therapy of malaria and in the treatment of giardiasis and tapeworm infestations.

quinestrol (kwin-es′trol) a long-acting estrogen, $C_{25}H_{32}O_2$.

quinethazone (-eth′ah-zōn) a diuretic, $C_{10}H_{12}$-ClN_3O_3S, used in the treatment of edema and hypertension.

quinidine (kwin′ĭ-din) the dextrorotatory isomer of quinine, $C_{20}H_{24}N_2O_2$, used in treatment of cardiac arrhythmias.

quinine (kwi′nīn, kwin-ēn′, kwin′in) an alkaloid of cinchona, $C_{20}H_{24}N_2O_2$, which suppresses the asexual erythrocytic forms of malarial parasites and has a slight effect on the gametocytes of *Plasmodium vivax* and *P. malariae*. Quinine also has analgesic, antipyretic, mild oxytocic, cardiac depressant, and sclerosing properties, and it decreases the excitability of the motor endplate.

quininism (kwin′ĭ-nizm) cinchonism.

quinone (kwi-nōn′, kwin′ōn) any benzene derivative in which two hydrogen atoms are replaced by two oxygen atoms.

quinsy (kwin′ze) peritonsillar abscess.

quint- word element [L.], *five.*

quintan (kwin′tan) recurring every fifth day, as a fever.

quintipara (kwin-tip′ah-rah) a woman who has had five pregnancies which resulted in viable offspring; para V.

quintuplet (kwin′tŭ-plet, kwin-tup′let) one of five offspring produced at one birth.

quittor (kwit′er) a fistulous sore on the quarters or the coronet of a horse's foot.

quotidian (kwo-tid′e-an) recurring every day; see *malaria.*

quotient (kwo′shint) a number obtained by division. **achievement q.,** the achievement age divided by the mental age, indicating progress in learning. **caloric q.,** the heat evolved (in calories) divided by the oxygen consumed (in milligrams) in a metabolic process. **intelligence q.,** a measure of intelligence obtained by dividing the mental age by the chronological age and multiplying the result by 100. **respiratory q.,** the ratio of the volume of carbon dioxide given off by the body tissues to the volume of oxygen absorbed by them; usually equal to the corresponding volumes given off and taken up by the lungs. Abbreviated R.Q.

R

R symbol for *roentgen;* chemical symbol for an *organic radical.*

℞ symbol, L. *rec′ipe* (take); prescription; treatment.

r symbol for ring chromosome.

Ra chemical symbol, *radium.*

rabid (rab′id) affected with rabies; pertaining to rabies.

rabies (ra′bēz, ra′be-ēz) an acute, usually fatal, infectious viral disease of the central nervous system of mammals, human infection resulting from the bite of a rabid animal (bats, dogs, etc.). In the later stages, it is marked by paralysis of the muscles of deglutition and glottal spasm provoked by the drinking or the sight of liquids, and by manical behavior, convulsions, tetany, and respiratory paralysis. **rab′ic,** adj.

racemase (ra′sĭ-mās) an enzyme that catalyzes the racemization of an optically active substance.

racemate (ra′sĭ-māt) a racemic compound.

racemethionine (rās″ĕ-mĕ-thi′o-nēn) a compound, $C_5H_{11}NO_2S$, used as a dietary supplement with lipotropic action.

racemic (ra-se′mik) optically inactive, being composed of equal amounts of dextrorotatory and levorotatory isomers.

racemization (ras″ĭ-mĭ-za′shun) the transformation of one half of the molecules of an optically active compound into molecules having exactly the opposite configuration, with complete loss of rotatory power.

racemose (ras′ĭ-mōs) shaped like a bunch of grapes.

rachi(o)- word element [Gr.], *spine.*

rachialgia (ra″ke-al′je-ah) pain in the spine.

rachicentesis (ra″kĭ-sen-te′sis) lumbar puncture.

rachidial, rachidian (rah-kid′e-al; rah-kid′e-an) pertaining to the spine.

rachigraph (ra′kĭ-graf) an instrument for recording the outlines of the spine and back.

rachilysis (rah-kil′ĭ-sis) correction of lateral curvature of the spine by combined traction and pressure.

rachiometer (ra″ke-om′ĕ-ter) an apparatus for measuring spinal curvature.

rachiotomy (-ot′ah-me) incision of a vertebra or the vertebral column.

rachis (ra′kis) the vertebral column.

rachischisis (rah-kis′kĭ-sis) congenital fissure of the vertebral column. **r. poste′rior,** spina bifida.

rachitic (rah-kit′ik) pertaining to rickets.

rachitis (rah-ki′tis) rickets.

rachitogenic (rah-kit″o-jen′ik) causing rickets.

rad (rad) *r*adiation *a*bsorbed *d*ose: a unit of measurement of the absorbed dose of ionizing radiation, corresponding to an energy transfer of 100 ergs per gram of any absorbing material.

rad. [L.] *ra′dix* (root).

radectomy (rah-dek′tah-me) excision of the root of a tooth.

radiad (ra′de-ad) toward the radius or radial side.

radial (ra′de-al) 1. pertaining to the radius of the arm or to the radial (lateral) aspect of the arm as opposed to the ulnar (medial) aspect; pertaining to a radius. 2. radiating; spreading outward from a common center.

radialis (ra″de-a′lis) [L.] radial.

radiatio (ra″de-a′she-o), pl. *radiatio′nes* [L.] a radiation or radiating structure.

radiation (ra″de-a′shun) 1. divergence from a common center. 2. a structure made up of divergent elements, as one of the fiber tracts in the brain. 3. energy transmitted by waves through space or through some medium; usually referring to electromagnetic radiation when used without a modifier. By extension, a stream of particles, such as electrons or alpha particles. **acoustic r.,** a fiber tract arising in the medial geniculate nucleus and passing laterally to terminate in the transverse temporal gyri of the temporal lobe. **r. of corpus callosum,** the fibers of the corpus callosum radiating to all parts of the neopallium. **corpuscular r.,** particles emitted in nuclear disintegration, including alpha and beta particles, protons, neutrons, positrons, and deuterons. **electromagnetic r.,** see under *wave.* **ionizing r.,** corpuscular or electromagnetic radiation capable of producing ionization, directly or indirectly, in its passage through matter. **optic r.,** a fiber tract starting at the lateral geniculate body, passing through the pars retrolentiformis of the internal capsule, and terminating in the striate area on the medial surface of the occipital lobe, on either side of the calcarine sulcus. **pyramidal r.,** fibers extending from the pyramidal tract to the cortex. **tegmental r.,** fibers radiating laterally from the red nucleus. **thalamic r.,** fibers which reciprocally connect the thalamus and cerebral cortex by way of the internal capsule, usually grouped into four subradiations (peduncles): an-

terior or frontal, superior or centroparietal, posterior or occipital, and inferior or temporal.

radical (rad′ĭ-k'l) 1. directed to the root or cause; designed to eliminate all possible extensions of a morbid process. 2. a group of atoms which enters and goes out of chemical combination without change.

radicle (rad′ĭ-k'l) one of the smallest branches of a vessel or nerve.

radicotomy (rad″ĭ-kot′ah-me) rhizotomy.

radiculalgia (rah-dik″u-lal′je-ah) pain due to disorder of the spinal nerve roots.

radicular (rah-dik′u-ler) pertaining to a root or radicle.

radiculitis (rah-dik″u-li′tis) inflammation of the spinal nerve roots.

radiculoganglionitis (rah-dik″u-lo-gang″gle-o-ni′tis) inflammation of the posterior spinal nerve roots and their ganglia.

radiculomeningomyelitis (-mĕ-ning″go-mi″ĕ-li′tis) inflammation of the nerve roots, meninges, and spinal cord.

radiculomyelopathy (-mi″ĕ-lop′ah-the) disease of the nerve roots and spinal cord.

radiculoneuritis (-noo-ri′tis) acute febrile polyneuritis.

radiculoneuropathy (-noo-rop′ah-the) disease of the nerve roots and spinal nerves.

radiculopathy (rah-dik″u-lop′ah-the) disease of the nerve roots. **spondylotic caudal r.,** compression of the cauda equina due to encroachment upon a congenitally small spinal canal by spondylosis, resulting in neural disorders of the lower limbs.

radio- word element [L.], *ray; radiation; emission of radiant energy; radium; radius* (bone of the forearm); affixed to the name of a chemical element to designate a radioactive isotope of that element.

radioactivity (-ak-tiv′ĭ-te) emission of corpuscular or electromagnetic radiations consequent to nuclear disintegration, a natural property of all chemical elements of atomic number above 83 and possible of induction in all other known elements. **radioac′tive,** adj. **artificial r., induced r.,** that produced by bombarding an element with high-velocity particles.

radioallergosorbent (-al″er-go-sor′bent) denoting a radioimmunoassay technique for the measurement of specific IgE antibody to a variety of allergens.

radioautograph (-aw′to-graf) autoradiograph.

radiobicipital (-bi-sip′ĭ-tal) pertaining to the radius and the biceps muscle.

radiobiology (-bi-ol′ah-je) the branch of science concerned with effects of light and of ultraviolet and ionizing radiations on living tissue or organisms. **radiobiolog′ical,** adj.

radiocardiography (-kar″de-og′rah-fe) graphic recording of variation with time of the concentration, in a selected chamber of the heart, of a radioactive isotope, usually injected intravenously.

radiocarpal (-kar′p'l) pertaining to the radius and carpus.

radiochemistry (-kem′is-tre) the branch of chemistry dealing with radioactive materials.

radiocinematograph (-sin″ĕ-mat′o-graf) a moving picture camera combined with an x-ray machine, making possible moving pictures of internal organs.

radiocystitis (-sis-ti′tis) inflammatory tissue changes in the urinary bladder caused by irradiation.

radiodensity (ra″de-o-den′sĭ-te) radiopacity.

radiodermatitis (-der″mah-ti′tis) a cutaneous inflammatory reaction to exposure to biologically effective levels of ionizing radiation.

radiodiagnosis (-di″ag-no′sis) diagnosis by means of x-rays and radiographs.

radiodontics (-don′tiks) dental radiology.

radiodontist (-don′tist) a dentist who specializes in dental radiology.

radiogold (ra′de-o-gold″) gold-198.

radiogram (-gram″) radiograph.

radiograph (-graf″) the film produced by radiography.

radiography (ra″de-og′rah-fe) the making of film records (radiographs) of internal structures of the body by passing x-rays or gamma rays through the body to act on specially sensitized film. **radiograph′ic**, adj. **body-section r.**, a special technique to show in detail images and structures lying in a predetermined plane of tissue, while blurring or eliminating detail in images in other planes; various mechanisms and methods for such radiography have been given various names, e.g., laminagraphy, tomography. **digital r.**, a technique in which x-ray absorption is quantified by assignment of a number to the amount of x-rays reaching the detector; the information is manipulated by a computer to produce an optimal image. **electron r.**, a technique in which a latent electron image is produced on clear plastic by passing x-ray photons through a gas with a high atomic number; this image is then developed into a black-and-white picture. **mucosal relief r.**, radiography after injection and evacuation of a barium enema and inflation of the intestine with air under light pressure, to reveal fine detail of the intestinal mucosa. **neutron r.**, that in which a narrow beam of neutrons from a nuclear reactor is passed through tissues, especially useful in visualizing bony tissues. **serial r.**, the making of several exposures of a particular area at arbitrary intervals. **spot-film r.**, the making of localized instantaneous radiographic exposures during fluoroscopy.

radiohumeral (ra″de-o-hu′mer-al) pertaining to the radius and humerus.

radioimmunity (-ĭ-mu′nĭ-te) diminished sensitivity to radiation.

radioimmunoassay (-im″u-no-as′a) a highly sensitive and specific assay method that uses the competition between radiolabeled and unlabeled substances in an antigen-antibody reaction to determine the concentration of the unlabeled substance, which may be an antibody or a substance against which specific antibodies can be produced.

radioimmunodiffusion (-im″u-no-dĭ-fu′zhun) immunodiffusion conducted with radioisotope-labeled antibodies or antigens.

radioimmunosorbent (-im″u-no-sor′bent) denoting a radioimmunoassay technique for measuring IgE in samples of serum.

radioiodine (-i′o-dīn) any radioactive isotope of iodine; used in diagnosis and treatment of thyroid disease and in scintiscanning.

radioisotope (-i′so-tōp) a radioactive isotope, i.e., one whose atoms undergo radioactive decay emitting alpha, beta, or gamma radiation. Radioisotopes are produced by the decay of other radioisotopes or by the irradiation of stable isotopes in a cyclotron or nuclear reactor.

radioligand (-li′gand) a radioisotope-labeled substance, e.g., an antigen, used in the quantitative measurement of an unlabeled substance by its binding reaction to a specific antibody or other receptor site.

radiologist (ra″de-ol′o-jist) a physician specializing in radiology.

radiology (ra″de-ol′ah-je) that branch of the health sciences dealing with radioactive substances and radiant energy and with the diagnosis and treatment of disease by means of both ionizing (e.g., x-rays) and nonionizing (e.g., ultrasound) radiations. **radiolog′ic radiolog′ical**, adj.

radiolucent (ra″de-o-loo′sent) permitting the passage of radiant energy, such as x-rays, with little attenuation, the representative areas appearing dark on the exposed film.

radiometer (ra″de-om′ĕ-ter) an instrument for detecting and measuring radiant energy.

radionecrosis (-nĕ-kro′sis) tissue destruction due to radiant energy.

radioneuritis (-noo-ri′tis) neuritis from exposure to radiant energy.

radionuclide (-noo′klīd) a radioactive nuclide.

radiopacity (-pas′ĭ-te) the quality or property of obstructing the passage of radiant energy, such as x-rays, the representative areas appearing light or white on the exposed film. **radiopaque′**, adj.

radiopathology (-pah-thol′ah-je) the pathology of the effects of radiation on tissues.

radiopelvimetry (-pel-vim′ĕ-tre) measurement of the pelvis by radiography.

radiopharmaceutical (-fahr″mah-soo′tĭ-k'l) a radioactive pharmaceutical used for diagnostic or therapeutic purposes.

radioreceptor (-re-sep′ter) a receptor which is stimulated by radiant energy, e.g., light.

radioresistance (-re-zis′tins) resistance, as of tissue or cells to irradiation. **radioresist′ant**, adj.

radioscopy (ra″de-os′kah-pe) fluoroscopy.

radiosensitivity (ra″de-o-sen″sĭ-tiv′ĭ-te) sensitivity, as of the skin, tumor tissue, etc., to radiant energy, such as x-rays or other radiations. **radiosen′sitive**, adj.

radiotherapy (-ther′ah-pe) treatment of disease by means of ionizing radiation; tissue may be exposed to a beam of radiation, or a radioactive element may be contained in devices (e.g., needles or wire) and inserted directly into the tissues (*interstitial r.*), or it may be introduced into a natural body cavity (*intracavitary r.*).

radiothermy (-ther′me) short-wave diathermy.

radiotoxemia (-tok-se′me-ah) toxemia produced by radiant energy.

radiotracer (-tra′ser) a radioactive tracer.

radiotransparent (-trans-pār′ent) radiolucent.

radiotropic (-trop′ik) influenced by radiation.

radioulnar (-ul′ner) pertaining to the radius and ulna.

radium (ra′de-um) a radioactive element (*see table*), at. no. 88, symbol Ra; it has a half-life of 1622 years, emitting alpha, beta, and gamma radiation. It decays to radon.

radius (ra′de-us), pl. *ra′dii* [L.] 1. a line from the center of a circle to a point on its circumference. 2. see *Table of Bones*. **r. fix′us,** straight line from the hormion to inion.

radix (ra′diks), pl. *rad′ices* [L.] root.

radon (ra′don) a gaseous radioactive element (*see table*), at. no. 86, symbol Rn, resulting from decay of radium.

rage (rāj) a state of violent anger. **sham r.,** a state resembling rage occurring in decorticated animals or in certain pathologic conditions in man.

ragocyte (rag′o-sīt) a polymorphonuclear phagocyte, found in the joints in rheumatoid arthritis, with cytoplasmic inclusions of aggregated IgG, rheumatoid factor, fibrin, and complement.

rale (rahl) an abnormal respiratory sound heard on auscultation, indicating some pathologic condition. **amphoric r.,** a coarse, musical, and tinkling rale due to the splashing of fluid in a cavity connected with a bronchus. **clicking r.,** a small sticky sound heard on inspiration, due to the passage of air through secretions in the smaller bronchi. **crackling r.,** subcrepitant r. **crepitant r.,** a fine dry, crackling sound like that made by rubbing hairs between the fingers; heard at the end of inspiration. **dry r.,** a whistling, musical, or squeaky sound, heard in asthma and bronchitis. **moist r.,** a sound produced by fluid in the bronchial tubes. **sibilant r.,** a high-pitched hissing sound due to viscid secretions in the bronchial tubes or by thickening of the tube walls; heard in asthma and bronchitis. **subcrepitant r.,** a fine moist rale heard in conditions associated with liquid in the smaller tubes.

ramal (ra′m′l) pertaining to a ramus.

ramification (ram″ĭ-fĭ-ka′shun) 1. distribution in branches. 2. a branching.

ramify (ram′ĭ-fi) 1. to branch; to diverge in different directions. 2. to traverse in branches.

ramisection (ram″ĭ-sek′shun) section of the appropriate rami communicantes of the sympathetic nervous system.

ramitis (ram-i′tis) inflammation of a ramus.

ramose (ra′mos) branching; having many branches.

ramulus (ram′u-lus), pl. *ram′uli* [L.] a small branch or terminal division.

ramus (ra′mus), pl. *ra′mi* [L.] a branch, as of a nerve, vein, or artery. **r. commu′nicans** (pl.

ra′mi communican′tes), a branch connecting two nerves or two arteries.

range (rānj) 1. the difference between the upper and lower limits of a variable or of a series of values. 2. the geographical region in which a given species is found. **r. of motion,** the range, measured in degrees of a circle, through which a joint can be extended and flexed.

ranine (ra′nīn) pertaining to (*a*) a frog; (*b*) a ranula, or to the lower surface of the tongue; (*c*) the sublingual vein.

ranula (ran′u-lah) a cystic tumor beneath the tongue. **ran′ular,** adj. **pancreatic r.,** a retention cyst of the pancreatic duct.

raphe (ra′fe) a seam; the line of union of the halves of various symmetrical parts.

rapport (rah-por′) a relation of harmony and accord, as between patient and physician.

rarefaction (rar″ĭ-fak′shun) condition of being or becoming less dense.

rash (rash) a temporary eruption on the skin. **butterfly r.,** a skin eruption across the nose and adjacent areas of the cheeks in the pattern of a butterfly, as in lupus erythematosus and seborrheic dermatitis. **diaper r.,** dermatitis occurring in infants on the areas covered by the diaper. **drug r.,** see under *eruption*. **heat r.,** miliaria rubra.

raspatory (ras′pah-tor-e) a file or rasp for surgical use.

RAST radioallergosorbent test.

rate (rāt) the speed or frequency with which an event or circumstance occurs per unit of time, population, or other standard of comparison. **basal metabolic r.,** an expression of the rate at which oxygen is utilized by the body cells, or the calculated equivalent heat production by the body, in a fasting subject at complete rest. Abbreviated B.M.R. **birth r.,** the number of births during one year for the total population (*crude birth r.*), for the female population (*refined birth r.*), or for the female population of childbearing age (*true birth r.*). Either a midyear or an average figure may be used for the population. **case fatality r.,** the ratio of the number of deaths caused by a specified disease to the number of diagnosed cases of that disease. **death r.,** an expression of the number of deaths in a population at risk during one year. The *crude death r.* is the ratio of the number of deaths to the total population of a geographic area; the *age-specific death r.* is the ratio of the number of deaths in a specific age group to the number of persons in that age group; the *cause-specific death r.* is the ratio of the number of deaths due to a specified cause to the total population. Either a midyear or an average figure may be used for the population at risk. **dose r.,** the amount of any therapeutic agent administered per unit of time. **erythrocyte sedimentation r.,** the rate at which erythrocytes sediment from a well-mixed specimen of venous blood, as measured by the distance that the top of a column of erythrocytes falls in a specified time interval under specified conditions. **fatality r.,** case fatality r. **five-year survival r.,** an expression of the number of survivors with no trace of disease five years after each has been diagnosed or treated for the same disease. **glomerular filtration r.,** an expression of the quantity of glomerular filtrate formed each minute in the nephrons of both kidneys, calculated by measuring the clearance of specific substances, e.g., inulin or creatinine. **growth r.,** an expression of the increase in size of an organic object per unit of time. **heart r.,** the number of contractions of the cardiac ventricles per unit of time. **incidence r.,** the ratio of the number of new cases of a disease in a population to the population at risk during a specified time period. **morbidity r.,** the number of cases of a given disease occurring in a specified period per unit of population. **mortality r.,** death r. **pulse r.,** the number of pulsations noted in a peripheral artery per unit of time. **respiration r.,** the number of movements of the chest wall per unit of time, indicative of inspiration and expiration. **sedimentation r.,** the rate at which a sediment is deposited in a given volume of solution, especially when subjected to the action of a centrifuge.

ratio (ra′she-o) [L.] an expression of the quantity of one substance or entity in relation to that of another; the relationship between two quantities expressed as the quotient of one divided by the other. **A-G r., albumin-globulin r.,** the ratio of albumin to globulin in blood serum, plasma, or the urine in various renal diseases. **cardiothoracic r.,** the ratio of the transverse diameter of the heart to the internal diameter of the chest at its widest point just above the dome of the diaphragm. **lecithin-sphingomyelin r. (L/S r.),** the ratio of lecithin to sphingomyelin concentration in the amniotic fluid, used to predict the degree of pulmonary maturity of the fetus and thus the risk of respiratory distress syndrome (RDS) if the fetus is delivered prematurely. **sex r.,** the number of males in a population per number of females, usually stated as the number of males per 100 females.

rationalization (rash″un-al-ĭ-za′shun) an unconscious defense mechanism by which one justifies attitudes and behavior that would otherwise be intolerable.

Rauwolfia (rou-wool′fe-ah) a genus of tropical trees and shrubs, including over 100 species, that provide numerous alkaloids, notably reserpine, of medical interest.

rauwolfia (rou-wool′fe-ah) any member of the genus *Rauwolfia;* the dried root, or extract of the dried root, of *Rauwolfia.* **r. serpenti′na,** the dried root of *Rauwolfia serpentina,* sometimes with fragments of rhizome and other parts, used as an antihypertensive and sedative.

ray (ra) a line emanating from a center, as a more or less distinct portion of radiant energy (light or heat), proceeding in a specific direction. **alpha r's, α-r's,** high-speed helium nuclei ejected from radioactive substances; they have less penetrating power than beta rays. **beta r's, β-r's,** electrons ejected from radioactive substances with velocities as high as 0.98 of the velocity of light; they have more penetrating power than alpha rays, but less than gamma rays. **cosmic r's,** very penetrating radiations

apparently moving through interplanetary space in every direction. **gamma r's, γ-r's,** electromagnetic radiation of short wavelengths emitted by an atomic nucleus during a nuclear reaction, consisting of high energy photons, having no mass and no electric charge, and traveling with the speed of light and with great penetrating power. **grenz r's,** roentgen rays having wavelengths about 2 A.U., lying between roentgen rays and ultraviolet rays. **medullary r.,** any cortical extension of a bundle of tubules from a renal pyramid. **roentgen r's,** x-rays; electromagnetic radiations of wavelengths below 5 A.U., commonly generated by passing high voltage current (about 10,000 volts) through a Coolidge tube; they are able to penetrate most substances to some extent and to affect a photographic plate. **x-r's,** roentgen r's.

Rb chemical symbol, *rubidium.*

RBC red blood cells; red blood (cell) count.

R.B.E. relative biological effectiveness.

Re chemical symbol, *rhenium.*

re- word element [L.], *back; again; contrary,* etc.

reabsorption (-sorp′shun) 1. the act or process of absorbing again, as the absorption by the kidneys of substances (glucose, proteins, sodium, etc.) already secreted into the renal tubules. 2. resorption.

reactant (re-ak′tant) a substance entering into a chemical reaction.

reaction (re-ak′shun) 1. opposite action, or counterreaction; the response to stimuli. 2. a phenomenon caused by the action of chemical agents; a chemical process in which one substance is transformed into another substance or other substances. 3. the mental and/or emotional state that develops in any particular situation. **acrosome r.,** structural changes that occur in spermatozoa in the vicinity of an ovum that facilitate entry of the spermatozoon by release of acrosomal enzymes. **alarm r.,** the physiologic effects (increase in blood pressure, cardiac output, blood flow to skeletal muscles, rate of glycolysis, and blood glucose concentration; decrease in blood flow to viscera) mediated by sympathetic nervous system discharge and release of adrenal medullary hormones in response to stress, fright, or rage. **allergic r.,** a local or general reaction characterized by altered reactivity of the animal body to an antigenic substance. **antigen-antibody r.,** the reversible binding of antigen to homologous antibody by the formation of weak bonds between antigenic determinants on antigen molecules and antigen binding sites on immunoglobulin molecules. **anxiety r.,** see under *neurosis.* **Arias-Stella r.,** nuclear and cellular hypertrophy of the endometrial epithelium, associated with ectopic pregnancy. **chain r.,** one which is self-propagating, each step initiating the succeeding step. **conversion r.,** see under *disorder.* **cross r.,** interaction between an antibody and an antigen that is closely related to the one which specifically stimulated synthesis of the antibody. **defense r.,** see under *mechanism.* **r. of degeneration,** the reaction to electrical stimulation of muscles whose nerves have degenerated, consisting of loss of response to a faradic stimulation in a muscle, and to galvanic and faradic stimulation in the nerve. **dissociative r.,** see under *disorder*. **foreign body r.,** a granulomatous inflammatory reaction evoked by the presence of exogenous material in the tissues, characterized by the formation of foreign body giant cells. **gross stress r.,** post-traumatic stress disorder. **hemiopic pupillary r.,** in certain cases of hemianopia, light thrown upon one side of the retina causes the iris to contract, while light thrown upon the other side arouses no response. **Herxheimer's r.,** Jarisch-Herxheimer r. **id r.,** a secondary skin eruption occurring in sensitized patients as a result of circulation of allergenic products from a primary site of infection. **immune r.,** see under *response.* **Jarisch-Herxheimer r.,** a transient, short-term immunologic reaction commonly seen following antibiotic treatment of early and later stages of syphilis and, less often, of certain other diseases, marked by fever, chills, headache, myalgia, and exacerbation of cutaneous lesions. **Jones-Mote r.,** a mild skin reaction of the delayed hypersensitivity type occurring after challenge with protein antigens. **lengthening r.,** reflex elongation of the extensor muscles which permits flexion of a limb. **leukemic r.,** **leukemoid r.,** a peripheral blood picture resembling that of leukemia or indistinguishable from it on the basis of morphologic appearance alone. **Neufeld's r.,** swelling of the capsules of pneumococci, seen under the microscope, on mixture with specific immune serum, owing to the binding of antibody with the capsular polysaccharide. **Pirquet's r.,** appearance of a papule with a red areola 24–48 hours after introduction of two small drops of Old tuberculin by slight scarification of the skin; a positive test indicates previous infection. **precipitin r.,** the formation of an insoluble precipitate by reaction of antigen and antibody. **Schultz-Charlton r.,** disappearance of scarlet fever rash around the site of an injection of scarlet fever antitoxin. **serum r.,** seroreaction. **startle r.,** the various psychophysiological phenomena, including involuntary motor and autonomic reactions, evidenced by an individual in reaction to a sudden, unexpected stimulus, as a loud noise. **stress r.,** 1. alarm r. 2. post-traumatic stress disorder. **Weil-Felix r.,** agglutination by blood serum of typhus patients of a bacillus of the proteus group from the urine and feces. **Wernicke's r.,** hemiopic pupillary r. **wheal-flare r.,** a cutaneous sensitivity reaction to skin injury or administration of antigen, due to histamine production and marked by edematous elevation and erythematous flare.

reaction-formation (re-ak′shun-for-ma′shun) an unconscious defense mechanism in which a person assumes an attitude that is the reverse of the wish or impulse actually harbored.

reading (rēd′ing) understanding of written or printed symbols representing words. **lip r., speech r.,** understanding of speech through observation of the speaker's lip movements.

reagent (re-a′jent) a substance used to produce a chemical reaction so as to detect, measure, produce, etc., other substances.

reagin (re′ah-jin) the antibody that mediates immediate hypersensitivity reactions; in humans, IgE. **reagin′ic,** adj.

reamer (re′mer) an instrument used in dentistry for enlarging root canals.

receptaculum (re″sep-tak′u-lum), pl. *receptac′-ula* [L.] a vessel or receptacle. **r. chy′li,** cisterna chyli.

receptor (re-sep′ter) 1. a molecule on the surface or within a cell that recognizes and binds with specific molecules, producing a specific effect in the cell; e.g., the cell-surface receptors for antigens or cytoplasmic receptors for steroid hormones. 2. a sensory nerve ending that responds to various stimuli. **adrenergic r's,** receptors for epinephrine or norepinephrine, such as those on effector organs innervated by postganglionic adrenergic fibers of the sympathetic nervous system. Classified as *α-adrenergic r's,* which are stimulated by norepinephrine and blocked by agents such as phenoxybenzamine, and *β-adrenergic r's,* which are stimulated by epinephrine and blocked by agents such as propranolol; the latter has two subtypes, $β_1$-r's (produce lipolysis and cardiostimulation) and $β_2$-r's (produce bronchodilation and vasodilation). **cholinergic r.,** receptor sites on effector organs innervated by cholinergic nerve fibers and which respond to the acetylcholine secreted by these fibers. **complement r.,** a cell-surface receptor structure capable of binding activated complement components. For example, component C3b is bound to neutrophils, B-lymphocytes, and macrophages. **histamine r's,** receptors for histamine, classified as H_1-r's, which produce bronchoconstriction and contraction of the gut and are blocked by antihistamines, such as pyrilamine or chlorpheniramine, and H_2-r's, which produce gastric acid secretion and are blocked by H_2-blockers, such as cimetidine. **muscarinic r's,** cholinergic receptors that are stimulated by the alkaloid muscarine and blocked by atropine; they are found on automatic effector cells and on central neurons in the thalamus and cerebral cortex. **nicotinic r's,** cholinergic receptors that are stimulated initially and blocked at high doses by the alkaloid nicotine and blocked by tubocurarine; they are found on automatic ganglion cells, on striated muscle cells, and on spinal central neurons.

recessive (re-ses′iv) 1. tending to recede; in genetics, incapable of expression unless the responsible allele is carried by both members of a pair of homologous chromosomes. 2. a recessive allele or trait.

recessus (re-ses′us), pl. *reces′sus* [L.] a recess.

recidivation, recidivism (re-sid″ĭ-va′shun; -sid′ĭ-vizm) 1. the repetition of an offense or crime. 2. the relapse or recurrence of a disease.

recipe (res′ĭ-pe) [L.] take; used at the head of a prescription, indicated by the symbol ℞. 2. a formula for the preparation of a specific combination of ingredients.

recipient (re-sip′e-ent) one who receives, as a blood transfusion, or a tissue or organ graft. **universal r.,** a person thought to be able to receive blood of any "type" without agglutination of the donor cells.

recognin (re-kog′nin) any of a group of protein fragments produced from cancer cells that are capable of recognizing specific cells; they include astrocytin and malignin.

recognition (rek″og-nish′un) in immunology, the interaction of immunologically competent cells with antigen, involving antigen binding to a specific receptor on the cell surface and resulting in an immune response.

recombinant (re-kom′bĭ-nant) 1. the new cell or individual that results from genetic recombination. 2. pertaining or relating to such cells or individuals. See also under *DNA.*

recombination (re″kom-bĭ-na′shun) the reunion, in the same or different arrangement, of formerly united elements that have been separated; in genetics, the formation of new gene combinations due to crossing over by homologous chromosomes.

recompression (re″kom-presh′un) return to normal environmental pressure after exposure to greatly diminished pressure.

reconstruction (re″kon-struk′shun) to reassemble or re-form from constituent parts, such as the mathematical process by which an image is assembled from a series of projections in computed tomography.

record (rek′erd) a permanent or long-lasting account of something (as on film, in writing, etc.); in dentistry, a registration. **problem-oriented r. (POR),** a method of patient care record keeping that focuses on specific health problems and a cooperative health care plan designed to cope with the identified problems. The components of the POR are: *data base,* which contains information required for each patient regardless of diagnosis or presenting problems; *problem list,* which contains the major problems currently needing attention; *plan,* which specifies what is to be done with regard to each problem; *progress notes,* which document the observations, assessments, nursing care plans, physician's orders, etc., of all health care personnel directly involved in the care of the patient. See also *SOAP.*

recrement (rek′rĭ-ment) saliva, or other secretion, which is reabsorbed into the blood. **recrementi′tious,** adj.

recrudescence (re″kroo-des′ens) recurrence of symptoms after temporary abatement. **recrudes′cent,** adj.

recruitment (re-kroot′ment) 1. the gradual increase to a maximum in a reflex when a stimulus of unaltered intensity is prolonged. 2. in audiology, an abnormally rapid increase in the loudness of a sound caused by a slight increase in its intensity.

rect(o)- word element [L.], *rectum.* See also words beginning *proct*(o)-.

rectalgia (rek-tal′je-ah) proctalgia.

rectectomy (rek-tek′tah-me) proctectomy.

rectification (rek″tĭ-fĭ-ka′shun) 1. the act of making straight, pure, or correct. 2. redistillation of a liquid to purify it.

rectitis (rek-ti′tis) proctitis.

rectoabdominal (rek″to-ab-dom′ĭ-n′l) pertaining to the rectum and abdomen.

rectocele (rek′to-sēl) hernial protrusion of part of the rectum into the vagina.

rectocolitis (rek″to-co-li′tis) coloproctitis.

rectocutaneous (-ku-ta′ne-us) pertaining to the rectum and the skin.

rectolabial (-la′be-al) relating to the rectum and a labium majus.

rectopexy (rek′to-pek″se) proctopexy.

rectoplasty (-plas″te) proctoplasty.

rectoscope (-skōp) proctoscope.

rectosigmoid (rek″to-sig′moid) the terminal portion of the sigmoid colon and the proximal portion of the rectum.

rectosigmoidectomy (-sig″moi-dek′tah-me) excision of the rectosigmoid.

rectostomy (rek-tos′tah-me) proctostomy.

rectourethral (rek″to-u-re′thral) pertaining to or communicating with the rectum and urethra.

rectouterine (-u′ter-in) pertaining to the rectum and uterus.

rectovaginal (-vaj′ĭ-n′l) pertaining to or communicating with the rectum and vagina.

rectovesical (-ves′ĭ-k′l) pertaining to or communicating with the rectum and bladder.

rectum (rek′tum) the distal portion of the large intestine. **rec′tal,** adj.

rectus (rek′tus) [L.] straight.

recumbent (re-kum′bent) lying down.

recuperation (re-koo″per-a′shun) recovery of health and strength.

recurrence (re-ker′ens) the return of symptoms after a remission. **recur′rent,** adj.

recurvation (re″kur-va′shun) a backward bending or curvature.

red (red) 1. one of the primary colors, produced by the longest waves of the visible spectrum. 2. a red dye or stain. **Congo r.,** a dark red or brownish powder used as a diagnostic aid in amyloidosis. **phenol r.,** phenolsulfonphthalein. **scarlet r.,** an azo dye having some power to stimulate cell proliferation; it has been used to enhance wound healing. **vital r.,** a dye injected into the circulation to estimate blood volume by determining the concentration of the dye in the plasma.

redia (re′de-ah), pl. *re′diae* [L.] a larval stage of certain trematode parasites, which develops in the body of a snail host and gives rise to daughter rediae, or to the cercariae.

redintegration (red″in-tĕ-gra′shun) 1. the restoration or repair of a lost or damaged part. 2. a psychic process in which part of a complex stimulus provokes the complete reaction that was previously made only to the complex stimulus as a whole.

redox (red′oks) oxidation-reduction.

reduce (re-dūs′, -dōōs′) 1. to restore to the normal place or relation of parts, as to reduce a fracture. 2. to undergo reduction. 3. to decrease in weight or size.

reductant (re-duk′tint) the electron donor in an oxidation-reduction (redox) reaction.

reductase (re-duk′tās) any enzyme that has a reducing action on chemicals. **5α-r.,** an enzyme that catalyzes the irreversible reduction of testosterone to dihydrotestosterone.

reduction (re-duk′shun) 1. the correction of a fracture, luxation, or hernia. 2. the addition of hydrogen to a substance, or more generally, the gain of electrons. **closed r.,** the manipulative reduction of a fracture without incision. **open r.,** reduction of a fracture after incision into the fracture site.

reduplication (re″du-pli-ka′shun) 1. a doubling back. 2. the recurrence of paroxysms of a double type. 3. a doubling of parts, connected at some point, the extra part being usually a mirror image of the other.

reentry (re-en′tre) in cardiology, a postulated mechanism by which a premature beat can be coupled to the normal beat.

reflex (re′fleks) a reflected action or movement; the sum total of any particular automatic response mediated by the nervous system. **abdominal r's,** contractions of the abdominal muscles on stimulating the abdominal skin. **accommodation r.,** the coordinated changes that occur when the eye adapts itself to near vision; constriction of the pupil, convergence of the eyes, and increased convexity of the lens. **Achilles tendon r.,** triceps surae jerk. **acoustic r.,** contraction of the stapedius muscle in response to intense sound. **anal r.,** contraction of the anal sphincter on irritation of the anal skin. **ankle r.,** triceps surae jerk. **auditory r.,** any reflex caused by stimulation of the auditory nerve, especially momentary closure of both eyes produced by a sudden sound. **Babinski's r.,** dorsiflexion of the big toe on stimulation of the sole, occurring in lesions of the pyramidal tract. **Babkin r.,** pressure by the examiner's thumbs on the palms of both hands of the infant results in opening of the infant's mouth. **biceps r.,** contraction of the biceps muscle when its tendon is tapped. **Brain's r.,** quadrupedal extensor r. **carotid sinus r.,** slowing of the heart beat on pressure on the carotid artery at the level of the cricoid cartilage. **Chaddock's r.,** in lesions of the pyramidal tract, stimulation below the external malleolus causes extension of the great toe. **chain r.,** a series of reflexes, each serving as a stimulus to the next one, representing a complete activity. **ciliary r.,** the movement of the pupil in accommodation. **ciliospinal r.,** dilation of the ipsilateral pupil on painful stimulation of the skin at the side of the neck. **conditioned r.,** see under *response.* **conjunctival r.,** closure of the eyelid when the conjunctiva is touched. **corneal r.,** closure of the lids on irritation of the cornea. **cough r.,** the sequence of events initiated by the sensitivity of the lining of the passageways of the lung and mediated by the medulla as a consequence of impulses transmitted by the vagus nerve, resulting in coughing, i.e., the clearing of the passageways of foreign matter. **cremasteric r.,** stimulation of the skin on the front and inner thigh retracts the testis on the same side. **deep r.,** one elicited by a sharp tap on the appropriate tendon or muscle to induce brief

stretch of the muscle, followed by contraction. **digital r.,** Hoffmann's sign (2). **diving r.,** a reflex involving cardiovascular and metabolic adaptations to conserve oxygen occurring in animals during diving into water; observed in reptiles, birds, and mammals, including man. **embrace r.,** Moro r. **gag r.,** pharyngeal r. **gastrocolic r.,** increase in intestinal peristalsis after food enters the empty stomach. **gastroileal r.,** increase in ileal motility and opening of the ileocecal valve when food enters the empty stomach. **grasp r.,** flexion or clenching of the fingers or toes on stimulation of the palm or sole. **Hoffmann's r.,** see under *sign* (2). **jaw r.,** jaw-jerk r., closure of the mouth caused by a downward blow on the passively hanging chin; rarely seen in health but very noticeable in corticospinal tract lesions. **knee r.,** see under *jerk.* **light r.,** 1. a luminous image reflected from the membrana tympani. 2. contraction of the pupil when light falls on the eye. **Magnus and de Kleijn neck r's,** extension of both ipsilateral limbs, or one, or part of a limb, and increase of tonus on the side to which the chin is turned when the head is rotated to the side, and flexion with loss of tonus on the side to which occiput points. Essentially a sign of *decerebrate rigidity.* **Mayer's r.,** opposition and adduction of the thumb combined with flexion at the metacarpophalangeal joint and extension at the interphalangeal joint, on downward pressure of the index finger. **Mendel-Bechterew r.,** dorsal flexion of the second to fifth toes on percussion of the dorsum of the foot; in certain organic nervous disorders, plantar flexion occurs. **Moro r.,** flexion of an infant's thighs and knees, fanning and then clenching of fingers, with arms first thrown outward and then brought together as though embracing something; produced by a sudden stimulus and seen normally in the newborn. **myotatic r.,** stretch r. **neck righting r.,** rotation of the trunk in the direction in which the head of the supine infant is turned; this reflex is absent or decreased in infants with spasticity. **nociceptive r.,** any reflex initiated by painful stimuli. **Oppenheim's r.,** see under *sign.* **orbicula′ris r., orbicular oculi r.,** normal contraction of the orbicularis oculi muscle, with resultant closing of the eye, on percussion at the outer aspect of the supraorbital ridge, over the glabella, or around the margin of the orbit. **palatal r.,** stimulation of the palate causes swallowing. **patellar r.,** knee jerk. **pharyngeal r.,** contraction of the pharyngeal constrictor muscle elicited by touching the back of the pharynx. **pilomotor r.,** the production of goose flesh on stroking the skin. **placing r.,** flexion followed by extension of the leg when the infant is held erect and the dorsum of the foot is drawn along the under edge of a table top; it is obtainable in the normal infant up to the age of six weeks. **plantar r.,** irritation of the sole contracts the toes. **proprioceptive r.,** one initiated by stimuli arising from some function of the reflex mechanism itself. **pupillary r.,** 1. contraction of the pupil on exposure of the retina to light. 2. any reflex involving the iris, resulting in change in the size of the pupil, occurring in response to various stimuli, e.g., change in illumination or point of fixation, sudden loud noise, or emotional stimulation. **quadriceps r.**, knee jerk. **quadrupedal extensor r.**, extension of a hemiplegic flexed arm on assumption of the quadrupedal position. **red r.**, a luminous red appearance seen upon the retina in retinoscopy. **righting r.**, the ability to assume an optimal position when there has been a departure from it. **Rossolimo's r.**, in pyramidal tract lesions, plantar flexion of the toes on tapping their plantar surface. **spinal r.**, any reflex action mediated through a center of the spinal cord. **startle r.**, Moro r. **stepping r.**, movements of progression elicited when the infant is held upright and inclined forward with the soles of the feet touching a flat surface. **stretch r.**, reflex contraction of a muscle in response to passive longitudinal stretching. **sucking r.**, sucking movements of the lips of an infant elicited by touching the lips or the skin near the mouth. **superficial r.**, any withdrawal reflex elicited by noxious or tactile stimulation of the skin, cornea, or mucous membrane, including the corneal reflex, pharyngeal reflex, cremasteric reflex, etc. **swallowing r.**, palatal r. **tendon r.**, contraction of a muscle caused by percussion of its tendon. **tonic neck r.**, extensions of the arm and sometimes of the leg on the side to which the head is forcibly turned, with flexion of the contralateral limbs; seen normally in the newborn. **triceps r.**, contraction of the belly of the triceps muscle and slight extension of the arm when the tendon of the muscle is tapped directly, with the arm flexed and fully supported and relaxed. **triceps surae r.**, see under *jerk*. **vestibular r's**, the reflexes for maintaining the position of the eyes and body in relation to changes in orientation of the head. **vestibulo-ocular r.**, nystagmus or deviation of the eyes in response to stimulation of the vestibular system by angular acceleration or deceleration or by irrigation of the ears with warm or cool water or air (caloric test).

reflexogenic, reflexogenous (re-flek″so-jen′ik, re″fleks-oj′ĕ-nus) producing or increasing reflex action.

reflexograph (re-flek′so-graf) an instrument for recording a reflex.

reflexometer (re″flek-som′ĕ-ter) an instrument for measuring the force required to produce myotatic contraction.

reflux (re′fluks) a backward or return flow. **esophageal r.**, **gastroesophageal r.**, reflux of the stomach contents into the esophagus. **hepatojugular r.**, distention of the jugular vein induced by applying manual pressure over the liver; it suggests insufficiency of the right heart. **intrarenal r.**, reflux of urine into the renal parenchymal tissue. **vesicoureteral r.**, **vesicoureteric r.**, backward flow of urine from the bladder into a ureter.

refract (re-frakt′) 1. to cause to deviate. 2. to ascertain errors of ocular refraction.

refraction (re-frak′shun) 1. the act or process of refracting; specifically, the determination of the refractive errors of the eye and their correction with glasses. 2. the deviation of light in passing obliquely from one medium to another

of different density. **refrac′tive**, adj. **double r.**, refraction in which incident rays are divided into two refracted rays, so as to produce a double image. **dynamic r.**, the normal accommodation of the eye which is continually exerted without conscious effort.

refractionist (-ist) one skilled in determining the refracting power of the eyes and correcting refracting defects.

refractometer (re″frak-tom′ĕ-ter) 1. an instrument for measuring the refractive power of the eye. 2. an instrument for determining the indexes of refraction of various substances, particularly for determining the strength of lenses for spectacles.

refractory (re-frak′tor-e) not readily yielding to treatment.

refrangible (re-fran′jĭ-b'l) susceptible to being refracted.

refresh (re-fresh′) to denude an epithelial wound to enhance tissue repair.

refrigeration (re-frij″er-a′shun) therapeutic application of low temperature.

refusion (re-fu′zhun) the return of blood to the circulation after temporary removal or stoppage of flow.

regeneration (re-jen″ĕ-ra′shun) the natural renewal of a structure, as of a lost tissue or part.

regimen (rej′ĭ-men) a strictly regulated scheme of diet, exercise, or other activity designed to achieve certain ends.

regio (re′je-o), pl. *regio′nes* [L.] region.

region (re′jun) a plane area with more or less definite boundaries. **re′gional**, adj. **abdominal r's**, the areas into which the anterior surface of the abdomen is divided, including the *epigastric*, *hypochondriac* (right and left), *inguinal* (right and left), *lateral* (right and left), *pubic*, and *umbilical*. **facial r's**, the areas into which the face is divided, including the *buccal* (side of oral cavity), *infraorbital* (below the eye), *mental* (chin), *nasal* (nose), *oral* (lips), *orbital* (eye), *parotideomasseter* (angle of the jaw), and *zygomatic* (cheek bone). **pectoral r's**, the areas into which the anterior surface of the chest is divided, including the *axillary*, *infraclavicular*, and *mammary*. **perineal r.**, the region overlying the pelvic outlet, including the *anal* and *urogenital*. **precordial r.**, the part of the anterior surface of the body covering the heart and the pit of the stomach.

registrant (rej′is-trint) a nurse listed on the books of a registry as available for duty.

registrar (rej′is-trar) 1. an official keeper of records. 2. in British hospitals, a resident specialist who acts as assistant to the chief or attending specialist.

registration (rej″is-tra′shun) the act of recording; in dentistry, the making of a record of the jaw relations present or desired, in order to transfer them to an articulator to facilitate proper construction of a dental prosthesis.

registry (rej′is-tre) 1. an office where a nurse's name may be listed as being available for duty. 2. a central agency for the collection of pathologic material and related data in a specified field of pathology.

regression (re-gresh'un) 1. return to a former or earlier state. 2. subsidence of symptoms or of a disease process. 3. in biology, the tendency in successive generations toward the mean. 4. defensive retreat to an earlier, often infantile, pattern of behavior or thought. **regres'sive**, adj.

Regroton (reg'ro-ton) trademark for a fixed combination preparation of chlorthalidone and reserpine.

regulation (reg″u-la'shun) 1. the act of adjusting or state of being adjusted to a certain standard. 2. in biology, the adaptation of form or behavior of an organism to changed conditions. 3. the power of a pregastrula stage to form a whole embryo from a part. **menstrual r.**, removal of the uterine contents, without dilatation, by application of a vacuum through a cannula introduced into the uterus.

regurgitant (re-ger'jĭ-tint) flowing backward.

regurgitation (re-ger″jĭ-ta'shun) a backward flowing, as the casting up of undigested food, or the backflow of blood through a defective heart valve. **valvular r.**, backflow of blood through the orifices of the heart valves owing to imperfect closing of the valves; named, according to the valve affected, *aortic, mitral, pulmonic,* or *tricuspid r.*

rehabilitation (re″hah-bil″ĭ-ta'shun) restoration to useful activity of persons with physical or other disability.

rehydration (re″hi-dra'shun) the restoration of water or fluid content to a body or to a substance which has become dehydrated.

reimplantation (re″im-plan-ta'shun) replacement of tissue or a structure in the site from which it was previously lost or removed.

reinfection (re″in-fek'shun) a second infection by the same agent or a second infection of an organ with a different agent.

reinforcement (re″in-fors'ment) the increasing of force or strength; in behavioral science, the presentation of a stimulus so as to modify a response; the stimulus may be a reward or a punishment.

reinfusate (re'in-fu″sāt) fluid for reinfusion into the body, usually after being subjected to a treatment process.

reinfusion (re″in-fu'zhun) infusion of body fluid that has previously been withdrawn from the same individual, e.g., reinfusion of ascitic fluid after ultrafiltration.

reinnervation (re″in-er-va'shun) restoration of nerve supply to a part from which it has been lost; it may occur spontaneously or by nerve grafting.

reintegration (re″in-tĕ-gra'shun) 1. biological integration after a state of disruption. 2. restoration of harmonious mental function after disintegration of the personality in mental illness.

rejection (re-jek'shun) an immune reaction against grafted tissue that results in failure of the graft to survive.

relapse (re-laps') the return of a disease after its apparent cessation.

relation (re-la'shun) the condition or state of one object or entity when considered in connection with another. **object r.,** the emotional bond formed between one person and another, as contrasted with interest in and love for oneself.

relaxant (re-lak'sint) 1. causing relaxation. 2. an agent which causes relaxation. **muscle r.,** an agent that specifically aids in reducing muscle tension.

relaxin (re-lak'sin) a protein-like principle secreted by the corpus luteum during pregnancy, producing relaxation of the pubic symphysis and dilation of the uterine cervix in certain animal species.

reline (re-lin') to resurface the tissue side of a denture with new base material in order to achieve a more accurate fit.

REM rapid eye movements (see under *sleep*).

rem (rem) *r*oentgen-equivalent–*m*an: the amount of any ionizing radiation which has the same biological effectiveness of 1 rad of x-rays; 1 rem = 1 rad × RBE (relative biological effectiveness).

remedy (rem'ah-de) anything that cures or palliates disease. **reme'dial,** adj.

remineralization (re-min″er-al-ĭ-za'shun) restoration of mineral elements, as of calcium salts to bone.

remission (re-mish'un) diminution or abatement of the symptoms of a disease; the period during which such diminution occurs.

remittent (re-mit'ent) having periods of abatement and of exacerbation.

remotivation (re-mo″tĭ-va'shun) in psychiatry, a group therapy technique administered by the nursing staff in a mental hospital, which is used to stimulate the communication skills and an interest in the environment of long-term, withdrawn patients.

ren (ren), pl. *re'nes* [L.] kidney. **r. mo'bilis,** hypermobile kidney.

renal (re'n'l) pertaining to the kidney.

reniform (ren'ĭ-form) kidney-shaped.

renin (re'nin) a proteolytic enzyme synthesized, stored, and secreted by the juxtaglomerular cells of the kidney; it plays a role in regulation of blood pressure by catalyzing the conversion of angiotensinogen to angiotensin 1.

reninism (-izm) a condition marked by overproduction of renin. **primary r.,** a syndrome of hypertension, hypokalemia, hyperaldosteronism, and elevated plasma renin activity, due to proliferation of juxtaglomerular cells.

renipelvic (ren″ĭ-pel'vik) pertaining to the pelvis of the kidney.

reniportal (-por'tal) pertaining to the portal system of the kidney.

rennin (ren'in) the milk-curdling enzyme found in the gastric juice of human infants (before pepsin formation) and abundantly in that of the calf and other ruminants; a preparation from the stomach of the calf is used to coagulate milk protein to facilitate its digestion.

renogastric (re″no-gas'trik) pertaining to the kidney and stomach.

renography (re-nog'rah-fe) radiography of the kidney.

renointestinal (re″no-in-tes′tĭ-n′l) pertaining to the kidney and intestine.

renopathy (re-nop′ah-the) nephropathy.

renoprival (re″no-pri′val) pertaining to or caused by lack of kidney function.

renule (ren′ūl) an area of kidney supplied by a branch of the renal artery, usually consisting of three or four medullary pyramids and their corresponding cortical substance.

reovirus (re″o-vi′rus) any of a group of ether-resistant RNA viruses isolated from healthy children, children with febrile and afebrile upper respiratory disease, children with diarrhea, and many animals.

reoxygenation (re-ok″sĭ-jen-a′shun) in radiobiology, the phenomenon in which hypoxic (and thus radioresistant) tumor cells become more exposed to oxygen (and thus more radiosensitive) by coming into closer proximity to capillaries after death and loss of other tumor cells due to previous irradiation.

repair (re-pār′) the physical or mechanical restoration of damaged or diseased tissues by the growth of healthy new cells or by surgical apposition.

repercussion (re″per-kush′un) 1. the driving in of an eruption, or scattering of a swelling. 2. ballottement.

replantation (re″plan-ta′shun) reimplantation.

replication (rep″lĭ-ka′shun) 1. a turning back of a part so as to form a duplication. 2. repetition of an experiment to ensure accuracy. 3. the process of duplicating or reproducing, as replication of an exact copy of a polynucleotide strand of DNA or RNA.

repolarization (re-po″ler-ĭ-za′shun) the reestablishment of polarity, especially the return of cell membrane potential to resting potential after depolarization.

repositor (-poz′ĭ-ter) an instrument used in returning displaced organs to the normal position.

repression (re-presh′un) 1. the act of restraining, inhibiting, or suppressing. 2. in psychiatry, an unconscious defense mechanism in which unacceptable ideas and impulses are thrust out or kept out of consciousness. 3. in genetic theory, inhibition of gene transcription by a repressor. **enzyme r.,** interference, usually by the endproduct of a pathway, with synthesis of the enzymes of that pathway.

repressor (re-pres′er) that which restrains or inhibits; a substance produced by a regulator gene that acts to prevent initiation by the operator gene of protein synthesis by the operon.

reproduction (re″pro-duk′shun) 1. the production of offspring by organized bodies. 2. the creation of a similar object or situation; duplication; replication. **reproduc′tive,** adj. **asexual r.,** reproduction without the fusion of sexual cells. **cytogenic r.,** production of a new individual from a single germ cell or zygote. **sexual r.,** reproduction by the fusion of a female sexual cell with a male sexual cell or by the development of an unfertilized egg. **somatic r.,** production of a new individual from a multicellular fragment by fission or budding.

reptilase (rep′til-ās) an enzyme from Russell's viper venom used in determining blood clotting time.

repulsion (re-pul′shun) 1. the act of driving apart or away; a force that tends to drive two bodies apart. 2. in genetics, the occurrence on opposite chromosomes in a double heterozygote of the two mutant alleles of interest.

RES reticuloendothelial system.

rescinnamine (re-sin′ah-min) an alkaloid, C_{35}-$H_{42}N_2O_9$, from various species of *Rauwolfia;* used as an antihypertensive and tranquilizer.

resect (re-sekt′) to excise part or all of an organ or other structure.

resection (re-sek′shun) excision of a portion or all of an organ or other structure. **root r.,** apicoectomy. **transurethral r.,** resection of the prostate by means of an instrument passed through the urethra. **wedge r.,** removal of a triangular mass of tissue.

resectoscope (re-sek′to-skōp) an instrument with a wide-angle telescope and an electrically activated wire loop for transurethral removal or biopsy of lesions of the bladder, prostate, or urethra.

reserpine (res′er-pēn) an alkaloid, $C_{33}H_{40}N_2O_9$, from various species of *Rauwolfia;* used as an antihypertensive and tranquilizer.

reserve (re-zerv′) 1. to hold back for future use. 2. a supply, beyond that ordinarily used, which may be utilized in emergency. **alkali r., alkaline r.,** the amount of conjugate base components of the blood buffers, the most important being bicarbonate. **cardiac r.,** potential ability of the heart to perform work beyond that necessary under basal conditions.

reservoir (rez′er-vwar) 1. a storage place or cavity. 2. an alternate host or passive carrier of a pathogenic organism. **r. of Pecquet,** cisterna chyli.

resident (rez′ĭ-dent) a graduate and licensed physician receiving training in a specialty in a hospital.

residue (rez′ĭ-du) a remainder; that remaining after removal of other substances. In biochemistry, a portion of a molecule that is incorporated in another molecule, e.g., an amino acid residue in a polypeptide.

residuum (re-zid′u-um), pl. *resid′ua* [L.] a residue or remainder.

resin (rez′in) any of a number of semisolid or amorphous solid organic substances exuded by various trees and shrubs or produced synthetically; most are soft and sticky but harden on exposure to cold. **res′inous,** adj. **acrylic r's,** products of the polymerization of acrylic or methacrylic acid or their derivatives, used in fabrication of medical prostheses and dental restorations and appliances. **anion-exchange r.,** see *ion-exchange r.* **cation-exchange r.,** see *ion-exchange r.* **cholestyramine r.,** a synthetic, strongly basic anion-exchange resin in the chloride form which chelates bile salts in the intestine, thus preventing their reabsorption; used in the symptomatic relief of pruritus associated with bile stasis. **ion-exchange r.,** a high molecular weight insoluble polymer of simple organic compounds capable of exchanging its attached ions for other ions in the surrounding medium; classified as (a) cation- or anion-exchange r's, depending on which ions the resin exchanges (the former are used to restrict intestinal sodium absorption in edematous states, and the latter as antacids in ulcer treatment); and (b) carboxylic, sulfonic, etc., depending on the nature of the active groups. **podophyllum r.,** a mixture of resins from podophyllum, used as a topical caustic in the treatment of certain papillomas.

resistance (re-zis′tans) 1. opposition, or counteracting force, as opposition of a conductor to passage of electricity or other energy or substance. 2. the natural ability of a normal organism to remain unaffected by noxious agents in its environment; see also *immunity.* 3. in studies of respiration, an expression of the opposition to flow of air produced by the tissues of the air passages, in terms of pressure per amount of air per unit of time. 4. in psychoanalysis, opposition to the coming into consciousness of repressed material. **drug r.,** the ability of a microorganism to withstand the effects of a drug that are lethal to most members of its species.

resolution (rez″o-loo′shun) 1. subsidence of a pathologic state. 2. perception as separate of two adjacent points; in microscopy, the smallest distance at which two adjacent objects can be distinguished as separate.

resolvent (re-zol′vent) 1. promoting resolution or the dissipation of a pathologic growth. 2. an agent that promotes resolution.

resonance (rez′o-nins) 1. the prolongation and intensification of sound produced by transmission of its vibrations to a cavity, especially such a sound elicited by percussion. Decrease of resonance is called *dullness;* its increase, *flatness.* 2. a vocal sound heard on auscultation. 3. mesomerism. **amphoric r.,** a sound resembling that produced by blowing over the mouth of an empty bottle. **nuclear magnetic r.,** a measure, by means of applying an external magnetic field to a solution in a constant radiofrequency field, of the magnetic moment of atomic nuclei to determine the structure of organic compounds. An application of this technique, magnetic resonance imaging, permits imaging of the soft tissues of the body by distinguishing between hydrogen atoms in different environments. **skodaic r.,** increased percussion resonance at the upper part of the chest, with flatness below it. **tympanitic r.,** peculiar sound elicited by percussing a tympanitic abdomen. **vesicular r.,** normal pulmonary resonance. **vocal r.,** the sound of ordinary speech as heard through the chest wall.

resonator (rez′o-na″ter) 1. an instrument used to intensify sounds. 2. an electric circuit in which oscillations of a certain frequency are set up by oscillations of the same frequency in another circuit.

resorb (re-sorb′) to take up or absorb again.

resorcinol (rĕ-zor′sĭ-nol) a bactericidal, fungicidal, keratolytic, exfoliative, and antipruritic agent, $C_6H_6O_2$, used especially as a topical kera-

tolytic in the treatment of acne and other dermatoses.

resorption (re-sorp′shun) 1. the lysis and assimilation of a substance, as of bone. 2. reabsorption.

respirable (rĕ-spīr′ah-b′l) suitable for respiration.

respiration (res″pĭ-ra′shun) 1. the exchange of oxygen and carbon dioxide between the atmosphere and the body cells, including inspiration and expiration, diffusion of oxygen from alveoli to the blood and of carbon dioxide from the blood to the alveoli, and the transport of oxygen to and carbon dioxide from the body cells. 2. cellular respiration; the exergonic metabolic processes in living cells by which molecular oxygen is taken in, organic substances are oxidized, free energy is released, and carbon dioxide, water, and other oxidized products are given off by the cell. **abdominal r.,** the inspiration and expiration accomplished mainly by the abdominal muscles and diaphragm. **aerobic r.,** the oxidative transformation of certain substrates into secretory products, the released energy being used in the process of assimilation. **anaerobic r.,** respiration in which energy is released from chemical reactions in which free oxygen takes no part. **artificial r.,** that which is maintained by force applied to the body, by stimulation of the phrenic nerve by application of electric current, or by *mouth-to-mouth method* (resuscitation of an apneic victim by direct application of the mouth to his, regularly taking a deep breath and blowing into the victim's lungs). **Biot's r.,** rapid, short breathing, with pauses of several seconds. **Cheyne-Stokes r.,** breathing characterized by rhythmic waxing and waning of respiration depth, with regularly recurring apneic periods. **cogwheel r.,** breathing with jerky inspiration. **electrophrenic r.,** induction of respiration by electric stimulation of the phrenic nerve. **external r.,** the exchange of gases between the lungs and the blood. **internal r.,** the exchange of gases between the body cells and the blood. **Kussmaul's r.,** air hunger. **paradoxical r.,** that in which a lung, or a portion of a lung, is deflated during inspiration and inflated during expiration. **tissue r.,** internal r.

respirator (res′per-a″ter) an apparatus to qualify the air breathed through it, or a device for giving artificial respiration or to assist in pulmonary ventilation. **cuirass r.,** a respirator applied only to the chest, either completely surrounding the trunk or applied only to the front of the chest and abdomen. **Drinker r.,** popularly, "iron lung": an apparatus for producing artificial respiration over long periods of time, consisting of a metal tank, enclosing the patient's body, with his head outside, and within which artificial respiration is maintained by alternating negative and positive pressure.

respiratory (rĕ-spi′rah-tor-e) pertaining to respiration.

respirometer (res″pĭ-rom′ĕ-ter) an instrument for determining the nature of respiration.

response (re-spons′) any action or change of condition evoked by a stimulus. **anamnestic r.,** the larger, more rapid immune response that occurs on the second exposure to an antigen. **autoimmune r.,** the immune response against an autoantigen. **conditioned r.,** a response evoked by a conditioned stimulus; a response to a stimulus that was incapable of evoking it before conditioning. **galvanic skin r.,** the alteration in the electrical resistance of the skin associated with sympathetic nerve discharge. **immune r.,** any response of the immune system to an antigenic stimulus, including antibody production, cell-mediated immunity, and immunological tolerance. **triple r. (of Lewis),** a physiologic reaction of the skin to stroking with a blunt instrument: first a red line develops at the site of stroking, owing to the release of histamine or a histamine-like substance, then a flare develops around the red line, and lastly a wheal is formed as a result of local edema. **unconditioned r.,** an unlearned response, i.e., one that occurs naturally.

rest (rest) 1. repose after exertion. 2. a fragment of embryonic tissue retained within the adult organism. 3. an extension which helps support a removable partial denture. **adrenal r.,** accessory adrenal tissue. **incisal r., lingual r., occlusal r.,** a metallic extension from a removable partial denture to aid in supporting the prosthesis. **suprarenal r.,** adrenal r **Walthard cell r's,** see under *islet.*

restenosis (re″stĕ-no′sis) recurrent stenosis, especially of a cardiac valve after surgical correction of the primary condition.

restiform (res′tĭ-form) shaped like a rope.

restitution (res″tĭ-too′shun) the spontaneous realignment of the fetal head with the fetal body, after delivery of the head.

restoration (res″to-ra′shun) 1. induction of a return to a previous state, as a return to health or replacement of a part to normal position. 2. partial or complete reconstruction of a body part, or the device used in its place.

restraint (re-strānt′) forcible control, as by means of a straitjacket.

resuscitation (re-sus″ĭ-ta′shun) restoration to life of one apparently dead. **cardiopulmonary r. (CPR),** the reestablishing of heart and lung action after cardiac arrest or apparent sudden death resulting from electric shock, drowning, respiratory arrest, and other causes. The two major components of CPR are artificial ventilation and closed chest cardiac massage.

resuscitator (re-sus′ĭ-ta″tor) an apparatus for initiating respiration in persons whose breathing has stopped.

retainer (re-tān′er) an appliance or device that keeps a tooth or partial denture in proper position.

retardate (re-tar′dāt) a mentally retarded person.

retardation (re″tar-da′shun) delay; hindrance; delayed development. **mental r.,** a mental disorder characterized by significantly subaverage general intellectual functioning associated with impairment in adaptive behavior and manifested in the developmental period; classified according to IQ as *mild* (50–70), *moderate*

(35–50), *severe* (20–35), and *profound* (less than 20).

retching (rech′ing) strong involuntary effort to vomit.

rete (re′te), pl. *re'tia* [L.] a network or meshwork, especially of blood vessels. **arterial r., r. arteri-o′sum,** an anastomotic network of minute arteries, just before they become capillaries. **articular r.,** a network of anastomosing blood vessels in or around a joint. **r. malpig′hii,** malpighian layer. **r. mirab′ile,** a vascular network formed by division of an artery or vein into many smaller vessels that reunite into a single vessel. **r. ova′rii,** a homologue of the rete testis, developed in the early female fetus, but vestigial in the adult. **r. subpapilla′re,** the network of arteries at the boundary between the papillary and reticular layers of the corium. **r. test′is,** a network formed in the mediastinum testis by the seminiferous tubules. **r. veno′-sum,** an anastomotic network of small veins.

retention (re-ten′shun) the process of holding back or keeping in position, as persistence in the body of material normally excreted, or maintenance of a dental prosthesis in proper position in the mouth.

reticula (rĕ-tik′u-lah) [L.] plural of *reticulum.*

reticular, reticulated (rĕ-tik′u-ler; rĕ-tik′u-lāt″ed) resembling a net.

reticulation (rĕ-tik″u-la′shun) the formation or presence of a network.

reticulin (rĕ-tik′u-lin) a scleroprotein from the connective fibers of reticular tissue.

reticulitis (rĕ-tik″u-li′tis) inflammation of the reticulum of a ruminant animal.

reticulocyte (rĕ-tik′u-lo-sīt) a young erythrocyte showing a basophilic reticulum under vital staining.

reticulocytopenia (rĕ-tik″u-lo-si″to-pe′ne-ah) deficiency of reticulocytes in the blood.

reticulocytosis (-si-to′sis) an excess of reticulocytes in the peripheral blood.

reticuloendothelial (-en″do-the′le-al) pertaining to the reticuloendothelium or to the reticuloendothelial system.

reticuloendothelioma (-en″do-the″le-o′mah) malignant lymphoma.

reticuloendotheliosis (-en″do-the″le-o′sis) hyperplasia of reticuloendothelial tissue. **leukemic r.,** leukemia marked by splenomegaly and by an abundance of large, mononuclear abnormal cells with numerous, irregular cytoplasmic projections that give them a flagellated or hairy appearance in the bone marrow, spleen, liver, and peripheral blood.

reticuloendothelium (-en″do-the′le-um) the tissue of the reticuloendothelial system.

reticulohistiocytoma (-his″te-o-si-to′mah) a granulomatous aggregation of lipid-laden histiocytes and multinucleated giant cells.

reticulopenia (-pe′ne-ah) reticulocytopenia.

reticulopodium (-po′de-um) a threadlike, branching pseudopod.

reticulosis (rĕ-tik″u-lo′sis) an abnormal increase in cells derived from or related to the reticuloendothelial cells. **familial histiocytic**

r., histiocytic medullary r., a fatal hereditary disorder marked by anemia, granulocytopenia, thrombocytopenia, phagocytosis of blood cells, diffuse proliferation of histiocytes, and enlargement of the liver, spleen, and lymph nodes.

reticulum (rĕ-tik′u-lum), pl. *retic′ula* [L.] 1. a small network, especially a protoplasmic network in cells. 2. reticular tissue. 3. the second stomach of a ruminant animal. **endoplasmic r.,** an ultramicroscopic organelle of nearly all higher plant and animal cells, consisting of a system of membrane-bound cavities in the cytoplasm; occurring in two types, rough-surfaced (*granular r.*), bearing large numbers of ribosomes on its outer surface, and smooth-surfaced (*agranular r.*). **sarcoplasmic r.,** a form of agranular reticulum in the sarcoplasm of striated muscle, comprising a system of smooth-surfaced tubules surrounding each myofibril. **stellate r.,** the soft, middle part of the enamel organ of a developing tooth.

retiform (re′tĭ-form, ret′ĭ-form) reticular.

retina (ret′ĭ-nah) the innermost tunic of the eyeball, containing the neural elements for reception and transmission of visual stimuli.

retinaculum (ret′′ĭ-nak′u-lum), pl. *retinac′ula* [L.] 1. a structure that retains an organ or tissue in place. 2. an instrument for retracting tissues during surgery. **r. flexo′rum ma′nus,** a fibrous band forming the carpal canal through which pass the tendons of the flexor muscles of the hand and fingers. **r. musculo′rum peroneo′-rum infe′rius,** a fibrous band across the peroneal tendons that holds them in place on the lateral calcaneus. **r. musculo′rum peroneo′-rum supe′rius,** a fibrous band across the peroneal tendons that helps hold them in place below and behind the lateral malleolus. **r. ten′dinum,** a tendinous restraining structure, such as an annular ligament.

retinal (ret′ĭ-n'l) 1. pertaining to the retina. 2. the aldehyde of retinol, having vitamin A activity. In the retina, retinal combines with opsins to form visual pigments.

retinene (ret′ĭ-nēn) the aldehyde of vitamin A, occurring in two forms: r_1 is retinal (2), and r_2 is dehydroretinal.

retinitis (ret′′ĭ-ni′tis) inflammation of the retina. **r. circina′ta, circinate r.,** circinate retinopathy. **exudative r.,** Coats' disease. **r. pigmento′sa,** a group of diseases, often hereditary, marked by progressive loss of retinal response, retinal atrophy, attenuation of retinal vessels, clumping of pigment, and contraction of the visual field. **r. prolif′erans,** a condition sometimes due to intraocular hemorrhage, with neovascularization and the formation of fibrous tissue extending into the vitreous from the retinal surface; retinal detachment may be a sequel. **suppurative r.,** that due to pyemic infection.

retinochoroiditis (-ko′′roi-di′tis) inflammation of the retina and choroid. **r. juxtapapilla′ris,** a small area of inflammation on the fundus near the papilla; seen in young healthy individuals.

retinoid (ret′ĭ-noid) 1. resembling the retina. 2. any derivative of retinal.

retinol (ret′ĭ-nol) vitamin A₁; the form, $C_{20}H_{30}O$,

of vitamin A found in mammals, which is reversibly dehydrogenated by enzymatic action into its aldehyde, retinal (2).

retinomalacia (ret′′ĭ-no-mah-la′she-ah) softening of the retina.

retinopapillitis (-pap′′ĭ-li′tis) inflammation of the retina and optic papilla.

retinopathy (ret′′ĭ-nop′ah-the) any noninflammatory disease of the retina. **circinate r.,** a condition in which a circle of white spots encloses the macula, leading to complete foveal blindness. **diabetic r.,** retinopathy associated with diabetes mellitus, which may be of the background type, progressively characterized by microaneurysms, intraretinal punctate hemorrhages, yellow, waxy exudates, cotton-wool patches, and macular edema, or of the proliferative type, characterized by neovascularization of the retina and optic disk, which may project into the vitreous, proliferation of fibrous tissue, vitreous hemorrhage, and retinal detachment. **exudative r.,** Coats' disease. **hypertensive r.,** that associated with essential or malignant hypertension; changes may include irregular narrowing of the retinal arterioles, hemorrhages in the nerve fiber layers and the outer plexiform layer, exudates and cotton-wool patches, arteriosclerotic changes, and, in malignant hypertension, papilledema. **r. of prematurity,** retrolental fibroplasia. **proliferative r.,** the proliferative type of diabetic retinopathy. **renal r.,** a retinopathy associated with renal and hypertensive disorders and presenting the same symptoms as hypertensive retinopathy. **stellate r.,** a retinopathy not associated with hypertensive, renal, or arteriosclerotic disorders, but presenting the same symptoms as hypertensive retinopathy.

retinoschisis (ret′′ĭ-nos′kĭ-sis) splitting of the retina, occurring in the nerve fiber layer (*juvenile form*), or in the external plexiform layer (*adult form*).

retinoscope (ret′ĭ-no-skōp′′) an instrument for performing retinoscopy.

retinoscopy (ret′′ĭ-nos′kah-pe) observation of the pupil under a beam of light projected into the eye, as a means of determining refractive errors.

retinosis (ret′′ĭ-no′sis) any degenerative, noninflammatory condition of the retina.

retinotopic (ret′′ĭ-no-top′ik) relating to the organization of the visual pathways and visual area of the brain.

retothelium (re′′to-the′le-um) reticuloendothelium.

retractile (re-trak′til) susceptible of being drawn back.

retraction (re-trak′shun) the act of drawing back, or condition of being drawn back. **clot r.,** the drawing away of a blood clot from a vessel wall, a function of blood platelets.

retractor (re-trak′ter) 1. an instrument for holding open the lips of a wound. 2. a muscle that retracts.

retrieval (re-tre′v'l) in psychology, the process of obtaining memory information from wherever it has been stored.

retro- word element [L.], *behind; backward.*

retroaction (ret″ro-ak′shun) action in a reversed direction; reaction.

retrobulbar (-bul′ber) 1. behind the pons. 2. behind the eyeball.

retrocervical (-ser′vĭ-k'l) behind the cervix uteri.

retrocession (-sesh′un) a going backward; backward displacement.

retrocochlear (-kok′le-ar) 1. behind the cochlea. 2. denoting the eighth cranial nerve and cerebellopontine angle as opposed to the cochlea.

retrocollic (-kol′ik) pertaining to the back of the neck; nuchal.

retrocollis (-kol′is) spasmodic wryneck in which the head is drawn back.

retrocursive (-ker′siv) marked by stepping backward.

retrodeviation (-de″ve-a′shun) a general term including retroversion, retroflexion, retroposition, etc.

retrodisplacement (-dis-plās′ment) backward or posterior displacement.

retroflexion (-flek′shun) the bending of an organ so that its top is thrust backward.

retrogasserian (-gas-ēr′e-an) pertaining to the sensory (posterior) root of the trigeminal (gasserian) ganglion.

retrognathia (-nath′e-ah) underdevelopment of the maxilla or mandible. **retrognath′ic,** adj.

retrograde (ret″ro-grād) going backward; retracing a former course; catabolic.

retrogression (ret″ro-gresh′un) degeneration; deterioration; regression; return to an earlier, less complex condition.

retromorphosis (-mor-fo′sis) retrograde metamorphosis.

retroperitoneal (-per″ĭ-to-ne′al) behind the peritoneum.

retroperitoneum (-per″ĭ-to-ne′um) the retroperitoneal space.

retroperitonitis (-per″ĭ-to-ni′tis) inflammation of the retroperitoneal space.

retropharyngitis (-far″in-ji′tis) inflammation of the posterior part of the pharynx.

retroplasia (-pla′ze-ah) retrograde metaplasia; degeneration of a tissue or cell into a more primitive type.

retroposed (-pōzd′) displaced backward.

retroposition (pah-zĭ′shun) backward displacement.

retropulsion (-pul′shun) 1. a driving back, as of the fetal head in labor. 2. tendency to walk backward, as in some cases of tabes dorsalis. 3. an abnormal gait in which the body is bent backward.

retrouterine (-u′ter-in) behind the uterus.

retroversion (-ver′zhun) the tipping backward of an entire organ.

retrovesical (-ves′ĭ-k'l) behind the urinary bladder.

retrovirus (-vi′rus) a large group of RNA viruses that includes the leukoviruses and lentiviruses; so called because they carry reverse transcriptase.

revascularization (re-vas″ku-lar-i-za′shun) 1. restoration of blood supply, as after a wound. 2. the restoration of an adequate blood supply to a part by means of a blood vessel graft, as in aortocoronary bypass.

reversion (re-ver′zhun) 1. a returning to a previous condition; regression. 2. in genetics, inheritance from some remote ancestor of a character which has not been manifest for several generations.

revulsant (re-vul′sant) revulsive.

revulsion (re-vul′shun) the act of drawing blood from one part to another, as in counterirritation.

revulsive (re-vul′siv) 1. causing revulsion. 2. an agent causing revulsion; a counterirritant.

Rf chemical symbol, *rutherfordium.*

R.F.A. right fronto-anterior (position of the fetus).

R.F.P. right frontoposterior (position of the fetus).

R.F.T. right frontotransverse (position of the fetus).

Rh 1. chemical symbol, *rhodium.* 2. symbol for *Rhesus factor.*

Rh_{null} symbol for a rare blood type in which all Rh factors are lacking.

rhabd(o)- word element [Gr.], *rod; rod-shaped.*

Rhabditis (rab-di′tis) a genus of minute nematodes found mostly in damp earth, and as an accidental parasite in man.

rhabdocyte (rab′do-sīt) metamyelocyte.

rhabdoid (rab′doid) resembling a rod; rodshaped.

rhabdomyoblastoma (rab″do-mi″o-blas-to′mah) rhabdomyosarcoma.

rhabdomyolysis (-mi-ol′ĭ-sis) disintegration of striated muscle fibers with excretion of myoglobin in the urine.

rhabdomyoma (-mi-o′mah) a tumor containing striated muscle fibers.

rhabdomyosarcoma (-mi″o-sar-ko′mah) a highly malignant tumor of striated muscle derived from primitive mesenchymal cells. The *pleomorphic* form affects predominantly the extremities of adults; the *alveolar* form occurs mainly in adolescents and young adults, and the *embryonal* form occurs predominantly in infants and children.

rhabdosarcoma (-sar-ko′mah) rhabdomyosarcoma.

rhabdovirus (-vi′rus) any of a group of morphologically similar bullet-shaped or bacilliform RNA viruses.

rhachi- for words beginning thus, see those beginning *rachi-.*

rhagades (rag′ah-dēz) fissures, cracks, or fine linear scars in the skin, especially such lesions around the mouth or other regions subjected to frequent movement.

rhaphe (ra′fe) raphe.

rhegma (reg′mah) a rupture, rent, or fracture.

rhegmatogenous (reg″mah-toj′ĕ-nus) arising from a rhegma, as rhegmatogenous detachment of the retina.

rhenium (re'ne-um) chemical element (*see table*), at. no. 75, symbol Re.

rheo- word element [Gr.], *electric current; flow* (as of fluids).

rheology (re-ol'ah-je) the science of the deformation and flow of matter, such as the flow of blood through the heart and blood vessels.

rheostosis (re''e-to'sis) a condition of hyperostosis marked by the presence of streaks in the bones; see also *melorheostosis*.

rheotaxis (re''o-tak'sis) the orientation of an organism in a stream of liquid, with its long axis parallel with the direction of flow, designated *negative* (moving in the same direction) or *positive* (moving in the opposite direction).

rheum (room) any watery or catarrhal discharge.

rheumarthritis (roo''mar-thri'tis) rheumatoid arthritis.

rheumatalgia (roo''mah-tal'je-ah) chronic rheumatic pain.

rheumatid (roo'mah-tid) any skin lesion etiologically associated with rheumatism.

rheumatism (roo'mah-tizm) any of a variety of disorders marked by inflammation, degeneration, or metabolic derangement of the connective tissue structures, especially the joints and related structures, and attended by pain, stiffness, or limitation of motion. **rheumat'ic,** adj. **acute articular r., inflammatory r.,** rheumatic fever. **muscular r.,** fibrositis. **palindromic r.,** repeated attacks of arthritis and periarthritis without fever and without causing irreversible joint changes.

rheumatoid (roo'mah-toid) resembling rheumatism.

rheumatologist (roo''mah-tol'ah-jist) a specialist in rheumatology.

rheumatology (-tol'ah-je) the branch of medicine dealing with rheumatic disorders, their causes, pathology, diagnosis, treatment, etc.

rhexis (rek'sis) the rupture of a blood vessel or of an organ.

rhigosis (rĭ-go'sis) the perception of cold.

rhin(o)- word element [Gr.], *nose; nose-like structure.*

rhinal (ri'n'l) pertaining to the nose.

rhinalgia (ri-nal'je-ah) pain in the nose.

rhinencephalon (ri''nen-sef'ah-lon) 1. the part of the brain once thought to be concerned entirely with olfactory mechanisms, including olfactory nerves, bulbs, tracts, and subsequent connections (all olfactory in function) and the limbic system (not primarily olfactory in function); homologous with olfactory portions of the brain in lower animals. 2. the area of the brain comprising the anterior perforated substance, band of Broca, subcallosal area, and paraterminal gyrus. 3. one of the parts of the embryonic telencephalon.

rhinesthesia (ri''nes-the'ze-ah) the sense of smell.

rhineurynter (ri''nu-rin'ter) a dilatable rubber bag for distending a nostril.

rhinion (rin'e-on) the lower end of the suture between the nasal bones.

rhinitis (ri-ni'tis) inflammation of the nasal mucous membrane. **allergic r., anaphylactic r.,** any allergic reaction of the nasal mucosa, occurring perennially (*nonseasonal allergic r.*) or seasonally (*hay fever*). **atrophic r.,** chronic rhinitis with wasting of the mucous membrane and glands. **r. caseo'sa,** that with a caseous, gelatinous, and fetid discharge. **fibrinous r.,** rhinitis with development of a false membrane. **hypertrophic r.,** that with thickening and swelling of the mucous membrane. **membranous r.,** chronic rhinitis with a membranous exudate. **nonseasonal allergic r.,** allergic rhinitis occurring continuously or intermittently all year round, due to exposure to a more or less ever-present allergen, marked by sudden attacks of sneezing, swelling of the nasal mucosa with profuse watery discharge, itching of the eyes, and lacrimation. **purulent r.,** chronic rhinitis with formation of pus. **vasomotor r.,** 1. nonallergic rhinitis in which transient changes in vascular tone and permeability (with the same symptoms of allergic rhinitis) are brought on by such stimuli as mild chilling, fatigue, anger, and anxiety. 2. any condition of allergic or nonallergic rhinitis, as opposed to infectious rhinitis.

rhinoantritis (ri''no-an-tri'tis) inflammation of the nasal cavity and maxillary sinus.

rhinocanthectomy (-kan-thek'tah-me) rhinommectomy.

rhinocele (ri'no-sēl) rhinocoele.

rhinocephaly (rhi''no-sef'ah-le) a developmental anomaly characterized by the presence of a proboscis-like nose above eyes partially or completely fused into one.

rhinocheiloplasty (-ki'lo-plas''te) plastic surgery of the lip and nose.

rhinocleisis (-kli'sis) obstruction of the nasal passages.

rhinocoele (ri'no-sēl) the ventricle of the olfactory lobe of the brain.

rhinodacryolith (ri''no-dak're-o-lith'') a lacrimal concretion in the nasal duct.

rhinodynia (-din'e-ah) pain in the nose.

rhinogenous (ri-noj'ĕ-nus) arising in the nose.

rhinokyphosis (ri''no-ki-fo'sis) an abnormal hump on the ridge of the nose.

rhinolalia (-la'le-ah) a nasal quality of the voice from some disease or defect of the nasal passages, such as undue patency (*r. aper'ta*) or undue closure (*r. clau'sa*) of the posterior nares.

rhinolaryngitis (-lār''in-ji'tis) inflammation of the mucosa of the nose and larynx.

rhinolith (ri'no-lith) a nasal calculus.

rhinolithiasis (ri''no-lĭ-thi'ah-sis) a condition associated with formation of rhinoliths.

rhinologist (ri-nol'ah-jist) a specialist in rhinology.

rhinology (ri-nol'ah-je) the sum of knowledge about the nose and its diseases.

rhinomanometry (-mah-nom'ĕ-tre) measurement of the airflow and pressure within the nose during respiration; nasal resistance or obstruction can be calculated from the figures obtained.

rhinommectomy (ri″nom-ek′tah-me) excision of the inner canthus of the eye.

rhinomycosis (ri″no-mi-ko′sis) fungal infection of the nasal mucosa.

rhinonecrosis (-ně-kro′sis) necrosis of the nasal bones.

rhinopathy (ri-nop′ah-the) any disease of the nose.

rhinopharyngitis (ri″no-făr″in-ji′tis) inflammation of the nasopharynx.

rhinophonia (-fo′ne-ah) a nasal twang or quality of voice.

rhinophycomycosis (ri″no-fi″ko-mi-ko′sis) a fungal disease caused by *Entomophora coronata*, marked by formation of large polyps in the subcutaneous tissues of the nose and paranasal sinuses; orbital involvement and unilateral blindness may follow. Cerebral involvement is common.

rhinophyma (-fi′mah) a form of rosacea marked by redness, sebaceous hyperplasia, and nodular swelling and congestion of the skin of the nose.

rhinoplasty (ri′no-plas″te) plastic surgery of the nose.

rhinorrhagia (-ra′je-ah) nosebleed; epistaxis.

rhinorrhea (-re′ah) the free discharge of a thin nasal mucus. **cerebrospinal r.,** discharge of cerebrospinal fluid through the nose.

rhinosalpingitis (-sal″pin-ji′tis) inflammation of the mucosa of the nose and eustachian tube.

rhinoscleroma (-sklě-ro′mah) a granulomatous disease, ascribed to *Klebsiella rhinoscleromatis*, involving the nose and nasopharynx; the growth forms hard patches or nodules, which tend to enlarge and are painful to the touch.

rhinoscope (ri′no-skōp) a speculum for use in nasal examination.

rhinoscopy (ri-nos′ko-pe) examination of the nose with a speculum, either through the anterior nares (*anterior r.*) or the nasopharynx (*posterior r.*).

rhinosporidiosis (ri″no-spo-rid″e-o′sis) a fungal disease caused by *Rhinosporidium seeberi*, marked by large polyps on the mucosa of the nose, eyes, ears, and sometimes the penis and vagina.

rhinotomy (ri-not′o-me) incision into the nose.

rhinovirus (ri″no-vi′rus) any of a large subgroup of the picornaviruses that cause the common cold and other upper respiratory ailments.

Rhipicephalus (ri″pĭ-sef′ah-lus) a genus of cattle ticks, many species of which transmit disease-producing organisms, such as *Babesia ovis*, *B. canis*, *Theileria parva*, *Borrelia theileri*, *Rickettsia rickettsii*, and *R. conorii*.

rhiz(o)- word element [Gr.], *root*.

rhizoid (ri′zoid) resembling a root.

rhizolysis (ri-zol′ĭ-sis) interruption of spinal nerve roots by coagulation with radiofrequency waves.

rhizomelic (ri″zo-mel′ik) pertaining to the hips and shoulders (the roots of the limbs).

rhizomeningomyelitis (-mě-ning″go-mi″ě-li′tis) radiculomeningomyelitis.

rhizoneure (ri′zo-nūr) a nerve cell forming a nerve root.

Rhizopoda (ri-zop′ah-dah) a superclass of protozoa of the subphylum Sarcodina, comprising the amebae.

Rhizopus (ri-zo′pus) a genus of fungi (order Mucorales), some species of which cause mucormycosis.

rhizotomy (ri-zot′ah-me) division or transection of a nerve root.

rhod(o)- word element [Gr.], *red*.

rhodamine (ro′dah-mēn, ro-dam′in) a red fluorescent dye.

rhodium (ro′de-um) chemical element (*see table*), at. no. 45, symbol Rh.

Rhodnius prolixus (rod′ne-us pro-lik′sus) a winged hemipterous insect of South America capable of transmitting *Trypanosoma cruzi*, the cause of Chagas' disease.

rhodogenesis (ro″do-jen′ě-sis) regeneration of rhodopsin after its bleaching by light.

rhodophylaxis (-fi-lak′sis) the ability of the retinal epithelium to regenerate rhodopsin. **rhodophylac′tic,** adj.

rhodopsin (ro-dop′sin) visual purple; a photosensitive purple-red chromoprotein in the retinal rods that is bleached to visual yellow (all-*trans* retinal) by light, thereby stimulating retinal sensory endings.

rhombencephalon (romb″en-sef′ah-lon) hindbrain.

rhombocoele (rom′bo-sēl) the terminal expansion of the canal of the spinal cord.

rhonchus (rong′kus), pl. *rhon′chi.* a rattling in the throat; also a dry, coarse rale in the bronchial tubes, due to a partial obstruction. See *rale.* **rhon′chal, rhon′chial,** adj.

Rhus (rus) a genus of trees and shrubs; contact with certain species produces a severe dermatitis in sensitive persons. The most important toxic species are: *R. diversilo′ba* and *R. toxicoden′dron*, or poison oak; *R. ra′dicans*, or poison ivy; and *R. ver′nix*, or poison sumac.

rhythm (rithm) a measured movement; the recurrence of an action or function at regular intervals. **rhyth′mic, rhyth′mical,** adj. **alpha r.,** electroencephalographic waves having a frequency of 8 to 13 per second, typical of a normal person awake in a quiet resting state. **beta r.,** electroencephalographic waves having a frequency of 18 to 30 per second, typical during periods of intense activity of the nervous system. **cantering r.,** gallop r. **circadian r.,** the regular recurrence in cycles of approximately 24 hours from one stated point to another, e.g., certain biological activities that occur at that interval regardless of constant darkness or other conditions of illumination. **coupled r.,** heart beats occurring in pairs, the second beat usually being a ventricular premature beat; see also *bigeminal pulse.* **delta r.,** 1. electroencephalographic waves having a frequency below 3½ per second, typical in deep sleep, in infancy, and in serious brain disorders. 2. delta waves (1). **escape r.,** a heart rhythm initiated by lower centers when the sinoatrial node fails to initiate impulses, when its rhythmicity is depressed, or when its impulses are completely blocked. **gallop r.,** an auscultatory finding of three (*triple r.*) or four heart sounds, the extra sound(s) by convention being in diastole and related either to atrial contraction (*fourth sound, presystolic gallop*), to early rapid filling of a ventricle with an altered ventricular compliance (*protodiastolic gallop*), or to concurrence of atrial contraction and ventricular early rapid filling (*summation gallop*). **infradian r.,** the regular recurrence in cycles of more than 24 hours, as certain biological activities which occur at such intervals, regardless of conditions of illumination. **nodal r.,** heart rhythm initiated in the specialized junctional tissue, i.e., the atrioventricular node and the main (His) bundle. **sinus r.,** the normal heart rhythm originating in the sinoatrial node. **theta r.,** electroencephalographic waves having a frequency of 4 to 7 per second, occurring mainly in children but also in adults under emotional stress. **triple r.,** the cadence produced when three heart sounds recur in successive cardiac cycles; see also *gallop r.* **ultradian r.,** the regular recurrence in cycles of less than 24 hours, as certain biological activities which occur at such intervals, regardless of conditions of illumination. **ventricular r.,** the ventricular contractions occurring in complete heart block.

rhythmicity (rith-mis′ĭ-te) in cardiology, the ability to beat, or the state of beating, rhythmically without external stimuli.

rhytidectomy (rit″ĭ-dek′tah-me) excision of skin for elimination of wrinkles.

rhytidoplasty (rit″ĭ-do-plas″te) plastic sugery for the elimination of skin wrinkles.

rhytidosis (rit″ĭ-do′sis) a wrinkling, as of the cornea.

rib (rib) any one of the paired bones, 12 on either side, extending from the thoracic vertebrae toward the median line on the ventral aspect of the trunk, forming the major part of the thoracic skeleton; see also *Table of Bones.* **abdominal r′s, asternal r′s,** false r′s. **cervical r.,** a supernumerary rib arising from a cervical vertebra. **false r′s,** the five lower ribs on either side, not attached directly to the sternum. **floating r′s,** the two lower false ribs on either side, usually without ventral attachment. **slipping r.,** one whose attaching cartilage is repeatedly dislocated. **true r′s,** the seven upper ribs on either side, connected to the sternum by their costal cartilages.

riboflavin (ri′bo-fla″vin) vitamin B₂; the heat-stable factor of the vitamin B complex, found in milk, muscle, liver, kidney, eggs, grass, malt, and various algae; it is an essential nutrient for man and is a component of FAD and FMN, which as coenzymes or prosthetic groups functioning as hydrogen carriers in oxidation-reduction reactions catalyzed by flavoproteins. Deficiency of the vitamin is known as *ariboflavinosis.* **r. kinase,** an enzyme (a phosphotransferase) that catalyzes the conversion of free riboflavin and ATP to flavin mononucleotide (FMN) and ADP.

ribonuclease (-noo′kle-ās) an enzyme which catalyzes the depolymerization of ribonucleic acid.

ribonucleic acid (RNA), (ri″bo-noo-kle′ik) a nu-

cleic acid found in all living cells, which on hydrolysis yields adenine, guanine, cytosine, uracil, ribose, and phosphoric acid; messenger RNA is an RNA fraction which transfers information from DNA to the protein-forming system of the cell; ribosomal RNA comprises about half the substance of ribosomes; transfer RNA (soluble RNA) is an RNA fraction which combines with one amino acid species transferring it from activating enzyme to ribosome.

ribonucleoprotein (-noo″kle-o-pro′tēn) a substance composed of both protein and ribonucleic acid.

ribonucleoside (-noo′kle-o-sīd) a nucleoside in which the purine or pyrimidine base is combined with ribose.

ribonucleotide (-noo′kle-o-tīd) a nucleotide in which the purine or pyrimidine base is combined with ribose.

ribose (ri′bōs) an aldopentose present in ribonucleic acid (RNA).

ribosome (ri′bo-sōm) any of the intracellular ribonucleoprotein particles concerned with protein synthesis; they consist of reversibly dissociable units and are found either bound to cell membranes or free in the cytoplasm. They may occur singly or occur in clusters (polyribosomes).

ribosyl (-sil) a glycosyl radical formed from ribose.

ricin (ri′sin) a phytotoxin in the seeds of the castor oil plant (*Ricinus communis*), inhalation or ingestion of which causes intoxication producing superficial inflammation of the respiratory mucosa with hemorrhages into the lungs, or edema of the gastrointestinal tract with hemorrhages.

Ricinus (ris′ĭ-nus) a genus of euphorbiaceous plants, including *R. commu′nis,* or castor oil plant, the seeds of which afford castor oil. See also *ricin.*

rickets (rik′its) a condition due to vitamin D deficiency, especially in infancy and childhood, with disturbance of normal ossification, marked by bending and distortion of the bones, nodular enlargements on the ends and sides of the bones, delayed closure of the fontanels, muscle pain, and sweating of the head. **adult r.,** osteomalacia. **fetal r.,** achondroplasia. **late r.,** that occurring in older children. **renal r.,** renal osteodystrophy. **tardy r.,** late r. **vitamin D–resistant r.,** a condition almost indistinguishable from ordinary rickets clinically but resistant to unusually large doses of vitamin D; it is often familial but may occur sporadically.

Rickettsia (rĭ-ket′se-ah) a genus of the tribe Rickettsieae, transmitted by lice, fleas, ticks, and mites to man and other animals, causing various diseases. **R. ak′ari,** the etiologic agent of rickettsialpox, transmitted by the mite *Allodermanyssus sanguineus* from the reservoir of infection in house mice. **R. austra′lis,** the etiologic agent of North Queensland tick typhus, possibly transmitted by *Ixodes* ticks. **R. cono′rii,** the etiologic agent of boutonneuse fever (Marseilles fever, Mediterranean fever) and possibly of Indian tick typhus, Kenya typhus,

and South American tick-bite fever; transmitted by *Rhipicephalus* and *Haemaphysalis* ticks.
R. prowaze′kii, the etiologic agent of epidemic typhus and the latent infection Brill's disease, which are transmitted from man to man via *Pediculus humanus.* **R. rickett′sii,** the etiologic agent of Rocky Mountain spotted fever, transmitted by *Dermacentor, Rhipicephalus, Haemaphysalis, Amblyomma,* and *Ixodes* ticks. **R. tsutsugamu′shi,** the etiologic agent of scrub typhus, transmitted by larval mites of the genus *Trombicula,* including *T. akamushi* and *T. deliensis,* from rodent reservoirs of infection.

rickettsia (rĭ-ket′se-ah), pl. *rickett′siae.* An individual organism of the Rickettsiaceae.

Rickettsiaceae (rĭ-ket″se-a′se-e) a family of the order Rickettsiales.

rickettsial (rĭ-ket′se-al) pertaining to or caused by rickettsiae.

Rickettsiales (rĭ-ket″se-a′lēz) an order of gram-negative bacteria occurring as elementary bodies that typically multiply only inside cells of the host. Parasitic for vertebrates and invertebrates, which serve as vectors, they may be pathogenic for man and other animals.

rickettsialpox (rik-et′se-al-poks″) a febrile disease with a vesiculopapular eruption, resembling chickenpox clinically, caused by *Rickettsia akari.*

rickettsicidal (rik-et″sĭ-si′d′l) destructive to rickettsiae.

Rickettsieae (rik″et-si′e-e) a tribe of the family Rickettsiaceae.

rickettsiosis (rik-et″se-o′sis) infection with rickettsiae.

ridge (rij) a linear projection or projecting structure; a crest. **dental r.,** any linear elevation on the crown of a tooth. **dermal r′s,** cristae cutis. **genital r.,** the more medial part of the urogenital ridge, giving rise to the gonad. **healing r.,** an indurated ridge that normally forms deep to the skin along the length of a healing wound. **interureteric r.,** a fold on mucous membrane extending across the bladder between the ureteric orifices. **mammary r.,** milk line. **mesonephric r.,** the more lateral portion of the urogenital ridge, giving rise to the mesonephros. **synaptic r.,** a wedge-shaped projection of a cone pedicle or of a rod spherule, on either side of which lie the horizontal cells whose dendrites are inserted into the ridge. **urogenital r.,** a longitudinal ridge in the embryo, lateral to the mesentery.

ridgling (rij′ling) an animal, especially a horse, with one or both testes undescended.

rifampicin (rif′am-pĭ-sin) rifampin.

rifampin (rif′am-pin) a semisynthetic antibacterial derived from rifamycin SV, used in treatment of pulmonary tuberculosis and carriers of *Neisseria meningitidis.*

rigidity (rĭ-jid′ĭ-te) inflexibility or stiffness. **clasp-knife r.,** increased tension in the extensors of a joint when it is passively flexed, giving way suddenly on exertion of further pressure. **cogwheel r.,** tension in a muscle which gives way in little jerks when the muscle is passively stretched. **decerebrate r.,** rigid extension of an animal's legs as a result of decerebration; occurring in man as a result of lesions in the upper brain stem.

rigor (rig′er) [L.] a chill; rigidity. **r. mor′tis,** the stiffening of a dead body accompanying depletion of adenosine triphosphate in the muscle fibers.

rim (rim) a border or edge. **bite r., occlusion r., record r.,** a border constructed on temporary or permanent denture bases in order to record the maxillomandibular relation and for positioning of the teeth.

rima (ri′mah), pl. *ri′mae* [L.] a cleft or crack. **r. glot′tidis,** the elongated opening between the true vocal cords and between the arytenoid cartilages. **r. o′ris,** the opening of the mouth. **r. palpebra′rum,** palpebral fissure. **r. puden′di,** the cleft between the labia majora.

rimula (rim′u-lah), pl. *rim′ulae* [L.] a minute fissure, as of the spinal cord or brain.

rinderpest (rin′der-pest) cattle plague.

ring (ring) 1. any annular or circular organ or area. 2. in chemistry, a collection of atoms united in a continuous or closed chain. **abdominal r., external,** superficial inguinal r. **abdominal r., internal,** deep inguinal r. **Albl's r.,** a ring-shaped shadow in radiographs of the skull, caused by aneurysm of a cerebral artery. **Bandl's r.,** pathologic retraction r.; see *retraction r.* **benzene r.,** the closed hexagon of carbon atoms in benzene, from which different benzene compounds are derived by replacement of hydrogen atoms. **Cannon's r.,** a focal contraction seen radiographically at the mid-third of the transverse colon, marking an area of overlap between the superior and inferior nerve plexuses. **conjunctival r.,** a ring at the junction of the conjunctiva and cornea. **constriction r.,** a contracted area of the uterus, where the resistance of the uterine contents is slight, as over a depression in the contour of the fetus, or below the presenting part. **deep inguinal r.,** an aperture in the transverse fascia for the spermatic cord or the round ligament. **Kayser-Fleischer r.,** a gray-green to red-gold pigmented ring at the outer margin of the cornea, seen in progressive lenticular degeneration and pseudosclerosis. **retraction r.,** a ringlike thickening and indentation occurring in normal labor at the junction of the isthmus and corpus uteri, delineating the upper contracting portion and the lower dilating portion (*physiologic retraction r.*), or a persistent retraction ring in abnormal or prolonged labor that obstructs expulsion of the fetus (*pathologic retraction r.*). **Schwalbe's r.,** a circular ridge composed of collagenous fibers surrounding the outer margin of Descemet's membrane. **superficial inguinal r.,** an opening in the aponeurosis of the external oblique muscle for the spermatic cord or the round ligament. **tympanic r.,** the bony ring forming part of the temporal bone at birth and developing into the tympanic plate. **umbilical r.,** the aperture in the fetal abdominal wall through which the umbilical cord communicates with the fetus. **vascular r.,** a developmental anomaly of the aortic arch wherein the trachea and esophagus are encircled by vascular structures, many variations being possible.

ring-bone (ring'bōn) exostosis involving the first or second phalanx of the horse, resulting in lameness if the articular surfaces are affected.

ringworm (-werm) tinea.

RIST radioimmunosorbent test.

risus (ri'sus) [L.] laughter. **r. sardon'icus,** a grinning expression produced by spasm of facial muscles.

rivalry (ri'vul-re) a state of competition or antagonism. **sibling r.,** competition between siblings for the love, affection, and attention of one or both parents or for other recognition or gain.

riziform (riz'ĭ-form) resembling grains of rice.

R.L.L. right lower lobe (of lungs).

R.M.A. right mentoanterior (position of the fetus).

R.M.P. right mentoposterior (position of the fetus).

R.M.T. right mentotransverse (position of the fetus).

R.N. Registered Nurse.

Rn chemical symbol, *radon*.

RNA ribonucleic acid.

RNase ribonuclease.

R.O.A. right occipitoanterior (position of the fetus).

roaring (ror'ing) a condition in the horse marked by a rough sound on inspiration and sometimes on expiration.

Robaxin (ro-bak'sin) trademark for preparations of methocarbamol.

Rochalimaea (ro''kah-li-me'ah) a genus of the family Rickettsiaceae resembling the genus *Rickettsia,* but usually found extracellularly in the arthropod host, including *R. quinta'na,* the etiologic agent of trench fever, transmitted by the body louse *Pediculus humanus.*

rod (rod) a straight, slim mass of substance, specifically one of the rodlike bodies of the retina. See *retinal r's.* **Corti's r's,** pillar cells. **enamel r's,** the approximately parallel rods or prisms forming the enamel of the teeth. **olfactory r.,** the slender apical portion of an olfactory bipolar neuron, a modified dendrite extending to the surface of the epithelium. **retinal r's,** highly specialized cylindrical segments of the visual cells containing rhodopsin; they serve night vision and detection of motion, and together with the retinal cones, they form the light-sensitive elements of the retina.

rodenticide (ro-den'tĭ-sīd) 1. destructive to rodents. 2. an agent destructive to rodents.

roentgen (rent'gen) the international unit of x- or γ-radiation; it is the quantity of x- or γ-radiation such that the associated corpuscular emission per 0.001293 gm. of air produces, in air, ions carrying 1 electrostatic unit of electrical charge of either sign. Abbreviated R.

roentgenkymogram (rent''gen-ki'mo-gram) the film obtained by roentgenkymography.

roentgenkymography (-ki-mog'rah-fe) a technique of graphically recording the movements of an organ on a single x-ray film.

roentgenogram (rent'gen-o-gram'') a film produced by roentgenography.

roentgenography (rent''gen-og'rah-fe) radiography. **roentgenograph'ic,** adj.

roentgenologist (rent''gen-ol'ah-jist) a specialist in roentgenology; radiologist.

roentgenology (rent''gen-ol'-ah-je) that branch of radiology dealing with the diagnostic and therapeutic use of roentgen rays (x-rays).

roentgenometry (rent''gen-om'ě-tre) 1. measurement of the intensity of x-rays. 2. the direct measurement of structures shown in the roentgenogram with or without the necessity of correcting for magnification.

roentgenoscope (rent'gen-o-skōp'') fluoroscope.

roentgenoscopy (rent''gě-nos'kah-pe) examination by means of roentgen rays (x-rays); fluoroscopy.

roentgenotherapy (rent''gen-o-ther'ah-pe) radiotherapy.

role (rōl) the behavior pattern that an individual presents to others. **gender r.,** the image projected by a person that identifies his or her sex. It is the public expression of gender identity.

rombergism (rom'berg-izm) Romberg's sign.

rongeur (raw-zhur') [Fr.] an instrument for cutting tough tissue, particularly bone.

room (rōōm) a place in a building, enclosed and set apart for occupancy or for performance of certain procedures. **operating r.,** one especially equipped for the performance of surgical operations. **recovery r.,** a hospital unit adjoining operating or delivery rooms, with special equipment and personnel for the care of patients immediately after operation or childbirth.

rooming-in (rōōm'ing-in'') the practice of keeping a newborn infant in a crib near the mother's bed instead of in a nursery during the hospital stay.

root (rōōt) that portion of an organ, such as a tooth, hair, or nail, that is buried in the tissues, or by which it arises from another structure. **anterior r.,** ventral r. **dorsal r.,** the posterior, or sensory, division of each spinal nerve, attached centrally to the spinal cord and joining peripherally with the ventral root to form the nerve before it emerges from the intervertebral foramen. **motor r.,** ventral r. **nerve r's,** the series of paired bundles of nerve fibers which emerge at each side of the spinal cord, termed dorsal (or posterior) or ventral (or anterior) according to their position. There are 31 pairs (8 cervical, 12 thoracic, 5 lumbar, 5 sacral, and 1 coccygeal), each corresponding dorsal and ventral root joining to form a spinal nerve. Certain cranial nerves, e.g., the trigeminal, also have nerve roots. **posterior r.,** dorsal r. **sensory r.,** dorsal r. **ventral r.,** the anterior, or motor, division of each spinal nerve, attached centrally to the spinal cord and joining peripherally with the dorsal root to form the nerve before it emerges from the intervertebral foramen.

R.O.P. right occipitoposterior (position of the fetus).

rosacea (ro-za'she-ah) a chronic disease of the skin of the nose, forehead, and cheeks, marked by flushing, followed by red coloration due to dilatation of the capillaries, with the appearance of papules and acne-like pustules.

rosaniline (ro-zan′ĭ-lin) a triphenylmethane derivative, $C_{20}H_{21}N_3O$, the basis of various dyes and a component of basic fuchsin.

rosary (ro′zah-re) a structure resembling a string of beads. **rachitic r.,** a succession of bead-like prominences along the costal cartilages, in rickets.

roseola (ro-ze′o-lah, ro″ze-o′lah) [L.] 1. any rose-colored rash. 2. exanthema subitum. **r. infan′tum,** exanthema subitum. **syphilitic r.,** eruption of rose-colored spots in early secondary syphilis.

rosette (ro-zet′) [Fr.] any structure or formation resembling a rose, such as (a) the clusters of polymorphonuclear leukocytes around a globule of lipid nuclear material, as observed in the test for disseminated lupus erythematosus, or (b) a figure formed by the chromosomes in an early stage of mitosis.

rosin (roz′in) solid resin obtained from species of *Pinus;* used in preparation of ointments and plasters.

rostellum (ros-tel′um) a small protruberance or beak, especially the fleshy protuberance of the scolex of a tapeworm, which may or may not bear hooks.

rostrad (ros′trad) 1. toward a rostrum; nearer the rostrum in relation to a specific point of reference. 2. cephalad.

rostral (ros′tral) 1. pertaining to or resembling a rostrum; having a rostrum or beak. 2. situated toward a rostrum or toward the beak (oral and nasal region), which may mean superior (in relationships of areas of the spinal cord) or anterior or ventral (in relationships of brain areas).

rostrate (ros′trāt) beaked.

rostrum (ros′trum), pl. *ros′tra* [L.] a beak-shaped process.

rot (rot) 1. decay. 2. a disease of sheep, and sometimes of man, due to *Fasciola hepatica.*

rotation (ro-ta′shun) the process of turning around an axis. In obstetrics, the turning of the fetal head (or presenting part) for proper orientation to the pelvic axis. **optical r.,** the quality of certain optically active substances whereby the plane of polarized light is changed, so that it is rotated in an arc the length of which is characteristic of the substance. **van Ness r.,** fusion of the knee joint and rotation of the ankle to function as the knee; done to correct a congenitally missing femur.

rotavirus (ro′tah-vi″rus) any of a group of double-stranded RNA viruses having a wheel-like appearance and responsible for acute infantile gastroenteritis and for diarrhea in mice, calves, and pigs.

rotenone (ro′tah-nōn) a poisonous compound from derris root and other roots; used as an insecticide and as a scabicide.

roughage (ruf′ij) indigestible material such as fibers or cellulose in the diet.

rouleau (roo-lo′), pl. *rouleaux′* [Fr.] a roll of red blood cells resembling a pile of coins.

roundworm (rownd′werm) any worm of the class Nematoda; a nematode.

R.P.F. renal plasma flow.

R.Ph. Registered Pharmacist.

rpm revolutions per minute.

R.Q. respiratory quotient.

-rrhage, -rrhagia word element [Gr.], *excessive flow.* **-rrhagic,** adj.

-rrhea word element [Gr.], *profuse flow.* **-rrheic,** adj.

rRNA ribosomal RNA (ribonucleic acid).

R.S.A. right sacroanterior (position of the fetus).

R.Sc.A. right scapuloanterior (position of the fetus).

R.Sc.P. right scapuloposterior (position of the fetus).

R.S.P. right sacroposterior (position of the fetus).

R.S.T. right sacrotransverse (position of the fetus).

Ru chemical symbol, *ruthenium.*

rub (rub) friction rub; an auscultatory sound caused by the rubbing together of two serous surfaces. **friction r.,** see *rub.* **pericardial r.,** a scraping or grating noise heard with the heart beat, usually a two-and-fro sound, associated with an inflamed pericardium. **pleural r., pleuritic r.,** a rub produced by friction between the visceral and costal pleurae.

rubber-dam (rub′er-dam″) a sheet of thin latex rubber used by dentists to isolate teeth from the fluids of the mouth during dental treatment.

rubefacient (roo″bĕ-fa′shint) 1. reddening the skin. 2. an agent that reddens the skin by producing hyperemia.

rubella (roo-bel′ah) German measles: a mild viral infection marked by a pink macular rash, fever, and lymph node enlargement most often affecting children and nonimmune young adults; transplacental infection of the fetus in the first trimester may produce death of the conceptus or severe developmental anomalies. See also *congenital rubella syndrome,* under *syndrome.*

rubeola (roo-be′o-lah, ru″be-o′lah) a synonym of measles in English and of German measles in French and Spanish.

rubeosis (roo″be-o′sis) redness. **r. i′ridis,** a condition characterized by a new formation of vessels and connective tissue on the surface of the iris, frequently seen in diabetics.

ruber (roo′ber) [L.] red.

rubescent (roo-bes′int) growing red; reddish.

rubidium (roo-bid′e-um) chemical element (see *table*), at. no. 37, symbol Rb.

rubor (roo′bor) [L.] redness, one of the cardinal signs of inflammation.

rubriblast (roo′brĭ-blast) pronormoblast.

rubric (roo′brik) red; specifically, pertaining to the red nucleus.

rubricyte (roo′brĭ-sīt) polychromatic normoblast.

rubrospinal (roo″bro-spi′n′l) pertaining to the red nucleus and the spinal cord.

rubrothalamic (-thah-lam′ik) pertaining to the red nucleus and the thalamus.

rubrum (roo′brum) [L.] red.

rudiment (roo'dĭ-ment) 1. a vestigial organ. 2. primordium.

rudimentary (roo''dĭ-men'ter-e) 1. imperfectly developed. 2. vestigial.

rudimentum (roo''dĭ-men'tum) rudiment; in NA, the first indication of a structure in the course of its embryonic development.

ruga (roo'gah), pl. *ru'gae* [L.] a ridge or fold. **ru'-gose,** adj.

rugosity (roo-gos'ĭ-te) 1. a condition of being rugose. 2. a fold, wrinkle, or ruga.

R.U.L. right upper lobe (of lung).

rule (rōol) a statement of conditions commonly observed in a given situation, or of a prescribed procedure to obtain a given result. **Clark's r.,** the dose of a drug for a child is obtained by multiplying the adult dose by the child's weight in pounds and dividing the result by 150. **Durham r.,** a definition of criminal responsibility from a federal appeals court case, Durham vs. United States, holding that "an accused is not criminally responsible if his unlawful act was the product of mental disease or mental defect." In 1972 the same court reversed itself and adopted the American Law Institute Formulation (see under *formulation*). **Fried's r.,** the dose of a drug for an infant less than two years old is obtained by multiplying the child's age in months by the adult dose and dividing the result by 150. **M'Naghten r.,** a definition of criminal responsibility formulated in 1843 by English judges questioned by the House of Lords as a result of the acquittal of Daniel M'Naghten on grounds of insanity. It holds that "to establish a defense on the ground of insanity, it must be clearly proved that at the time of committing the act the party accused was laboring under such a defect of reason from disease of the mind as not to know the nature and quality of the act he was doing; or, if he did know it, that he did not know that what he was doing was wrong." **Nägele's r.,** (for predicting day of labor) subtract three months from the first day of the last menstruation and add seven days. **van't Hoff's r.,** the velocity of chemical reactions is increased twofold or more for each rise of 10° C. in temperature. **Young's r.,** the dose of a drug for a child is obtained by multiplying the adult dose by the child's age in years and dividing the result by the sum of the child's age plus 12.

rumen (roo'men) the first stomach of a ruminant.

rumenitis (roo''mĕ-ni'tis) inflammation of the rumen.

ruminant (roo'mĭ-nant) 1. chewing the cud. 2. one of the order of animals, including cattle, sheep, goats, deer, and antelopes, which have a stomach with four complete cavities (rumen, reticulum, omasum, abomasum), through which the food passes in digestion.

rumination (roo''mĭ-na'shun) 1. the casting up of the food to be chewed thoroughly a second time, as in cattle. 2. meditation.

rump (rump) the buttock or gluteal region.

rupia (roo'pe-ah) thick, dark, raised, lamellated, adherent crusts on the skin, somewhat resembling oyster shells, as in late recurrent secondary syphilis. **ru'pial,** adj.

rupture (rup'chur) 1. tearing or disruption of tissue. 2. hernia.

rush (rush) peristaltic rush; a powerful wave of contractile activity that travels very long distances down the small intestine, caused by intense irritation or unusual distention.

rut (rut) the period or season of heightened sexual activity in some male mammals, coinciding with estrus in females.

ruthenium (roo-the'ne-um) chemical element (*see table*), at. no. 44, symbol Ru.

rutherford (ruth'er-ford) a unit of radioactive disintegration, representing one million disintegrations per second.

rutherfordium (ruth''er-for'de-um) chemical element (*see table*), at. no. 104, symbol Rf.

RV residual volume.

Ŗ, Rx symbol, [L.] *rec'ipe* (take); prescription; treatment.

S

S chemical symbol, *sulfur;* symbol for *siemens* and *Svedberg unit.*

s symbol for *second.*

sabulous (sab'u-lus) gritty or sandy.

saburra (sah-bur'ah) foulness of the mouth or stomach. **sabur'ral,** adj.

sac (sak) a pouch; a baglike organ or structure. **air s's,** alveolar s's. **allantoic s.,** the dilated portion of the allantois, becoming a part of the placenta in many mammals. **alveolar s's,** the spaces into which the alveolar ducts open distally, and with which the alveoli communicate. **amniotic s.,** amnion. **conjunctival s.,** the potential space, lined by conjunctiva, between the eyelids and eyeball. **dental s.,** the dense fibrous layer of mesenchyme surrounding the enamel organ and dental papilla. **endolymphatic s.,** the blind, flattened cerebral end of the endolymphatic duct. **heart s.,** the pericardium. **hernial s.,** the peritoneal pouch enclosing a hernia. **Hilton's s.,** laryngeal saccule. **lacrimal s.,** the dilated upper end of the nasolacrimal duct. **yolk s.,** the extraembryonic membrane that connects with the midgut; at the end of the fourth week of development it expands into a pear-shaped vesicle (*umbilical vesicle*) connected to the body of the embryo by a long narrow tube (*yolk stalk*). In mammals, it produces a complete vitelline circulation in the early embryo and then undergoes regression.

saccade (sah-kād') the series of involuntary,

abrupt, rapid, small movements or jerks of both eyes simultaneously in changing the point of fixation. **saccad'ic,** adj.

saccate (sak'āt) 1. shaped like a sac. 2. contained in a sac.

sacchar(o)- word element [L.], *sugar.*

saccharide (sak'ah-rīd) one of a series of carbohydrates, including the sugars.

sacchariferous (sak"ah-rif'er-us) containing or yielding sugar.

saccharin (sak'ah-rin) a white, crystalline compound several hundred times sweeter than sucrose; used as a flavor and non-nutritive sweetener.

saccharogalactorrhea (sak"ah-ro-gah-lak"to-re'ah) secretion of milk containing an excess of sugar.

saccharolytic (-lit'ik) capable of splitting up sugar.

saccharometabolism (-mě-tab'o-lizm) metabolism of sugar. **saccharometabol'ic,** adj.

Saccharomyces (sak"ah-ro-mi'sēz) a genus of yeasts, including *S. cerevis'iae,* or brewers' yeast. **saccharomycet'ic,** adj.

sacciform (sak'sĭ-form) shaped like a bag or sac.

saccular (sak'u-ler) pertaining to or resembling a sac.

sacculated (sak'u-lāt"ed) containing saccules.

sacculation (sak"u-la'shun) 1. a saccule, or pouch. 2. the quality of being sacculated.

saccule (sak'ūl) a little bag or sac; applied specifically to the smaller of the two divisions of the membranous labyrinth of the ear. **laryngeal s.,** a diverticulum extending upward from the front of the laryngeal ventricle.

sacculocochlear (sak"u-lo-kok'le-er) pertaining to the saccule and cochlea.

sacculus (sak'u-lus), pl. *sac'culi* [L.] a saccule.

saccus (sak'us), pl. *sac'ci* [L.] a sac.

sacr(o)- word element [L.], *sacrum.*

sacrad (sa'krad) toward the sacrum.

sacral (sa'kral) pertaining to the sacrum.

sacralgia (sa-kral'je-ah) pain in the sacrum.

sacralization (sa"kral-ĭ-za'shun) anomalous fusion of the fifth lumbar vertebra with the first segment of the sacrum.

sacrectomy (sa-krek'tah-me) excision or resection of the sacrum.

sacrococcygeal (sa"kro-kok-sij'e-al) pertaining to the sacrum and coccyx.

sacrodynia (-din'e-ah) sacralgia.

sacroiliac (-il'e-ak) pertaining to the sacrum and ilium, or to their articulation.

sacrolumbar (-lum'bar) pertaining to the sacrum and loins.

sacrosciatic (-si-at'ik) pertaining to the sacrum and ischium.

sacrospinal (-spi'n'l) pertaining to the sacrum and the spinal column.

sacrovertebral (-ver'tě-bral) pertaining to the sacrum and vertebrae.

sacrum (sa'krum) [L.] see *Table of Bones.*

sadism (sa'dizm, sad'izm) the derivation of sexual gratification through the infliction of pain or humiliation on others. **sadis'tic,** adj.

sadomasochism (sa"do-, sad"o-mas'o-kizm) a state characterized by both sadistic and masochistic tendencies. **sadomasochis'tic,** adj.

sagittal (saj'ĭ-t'l) 1. shaped like an arrow. 2. situated in the direction of the sagittal suture; said of an anteroposterior plane or section parallel to the median plane of the body.

sagittalis (saj"ĭ-ta'lis) [L.] sagittal.

sal (sal) [L.] salt.

salicylamide (sal"ĭ-sil-am'ĭd) an amide of salicylic acid, $C_7H_7NO_2$, used as an analgesic and antipyretic.

salicylate (sal'ĭ-sil"āt, sah-lis'ĭ-lāt) a salt of salicylic acid; a number of salicylates are used as drugs.

salicylic (sal"ĭ-sil'ik) containing the radical salicyl.

salicylic acid (sal"ĭ-sil'ik) a crystalline acid, HOC_6H_4COOH, used as a topical keratolytic and keratoplastic; its salts, e.g., sodium salicylate, are used as analgesics.

salicylism (sal"ĭ-sil'izm) toxic effects of overdosage with salicylic acid or its salts, usually marked by tinnitus, nausea, and vomiting.

salicyluric acid (sal"ĭ-sil-ūr'ik) a compound of glycol and salicylic acid, found in urine after administration of salicylic acid.

salifiable (sal"ĭ-fi'ah-b'l) capable of combining with an acid to form a salt.

saline (sa'lēn, sa'līn) salty; of the nature of a salt. **physiological s.,** an isotonic aqueous solution of NaCl for temporarily maintaining living cells.

saliva (sah-li'vah) the enzyme-containing secretion of the salivary glands. **sal'ivary,** adj.

salivant (sal'ĭ-vant) provoking a flow of saliva.

salivation (sal"ĭ-va'shun) 1. the secretion of saliva. 2. ptyalism.

Salmonella (sal"mo-nel'ah) a genus of gram-negative bacteria. The genus *Salmonella* is very complex and has been described by several different systems of nomenclature. Clinical laboratories frequently report salmonellae as one of three species, differentiated on the basis of serologic and biochemical reactions: *S. ty'phi, S. cho'leraesu'is,* and *S. enteri'tidis;* the last contains all serotypes except the first two. In this system many strains familiarly named as species are designated as serotypes of *S. enteritidis.* Salmonellae may also be grouped into five subgenera (I–V) on the basis of biochemical reactions and further into species on the basis of antigenic reactions; subgenus I contains most of the species. Pathogenic species include *S. arizo'-nae* (salmonellosis), *S. choleraesuis* (a strain pathogenic for pigs that may infect humans), *S. enteritidis* (gastroenteritis), *S. enteritidis* serotype *paratyphi A* (paratyphoid fever), *S. ty'phi* (typhoid fever), and *S. enteritidis* serotype *typhimurium* (food poisoning and paratyphoid fever).

salmonella (-nel'ah), pl. *salmonel'lae.* Any organism of the genus *Salmonella.* **salmonel'lal,** adj.

salmonellosis (-nel-o'sis) infection with *Salmonella.*

salping(o)- word element [Gr.], *tube (eustachian tube* or *uterine tube).*

salpingectomy (sal″pin-jek′tah-me) excision of a uterine tube.

salpingemphraxis (-jem-frak′sis) obstruction of an auditory tube.

salpingian (sal-pin′je-an) pertaining to the auditory or the uterine tube.

salpingitis (sal″pin-ji′tis) inflammation of the auditory or the uterine tube. **salpingit′ic**, adj.

salpingocele (sal-ping′go-sēl) hernial protrusion of a uterine tube.

salpingography (sal″ping-gog′rah-fe) radiography of the uterine tubes after injection of a radiopaque medium.

salpingolithiasis (sal-ping″go-lǐ-thi′ah-sis) the presence of calcareous deposits in the wall of the uterine tubes.

salpingolysis (sal″ping-gol′ǐ-sis) surgical separation of adhesions involving the uterine tubes.

salpingo-oophorectomy (sal-ping″go-o″ah-fah-rek′tah-me) excision of a uterine tube and ovary.

salpingo-oophoritis (-o″ah-fah-ri′tis) inflammation of a uterine tube and ovary.

salpingo-oophorocele (-o-of′o-ro-sēl″) hernia of a uterine tube and ovary.

salpingopexy (-pek′se) fixation of a uterine tube.

salpingopharyngeal (-fah-rin′je-al) pertaining to the auditory tube and the pharynx.

salpingoplasty (sal-ping′go-plas″te) plastic repair of a uterine tube.

salpingostomy (sal″ping-gos′tah-me) 1. formation of an opening or fistula into a uterine tube for the purpose of drainage. 2. surgical restoration of the patency of a uterine tube.

salpingotomy (sal″ping-got′ah-me) surgical incision of a uterine tube.

salpinx (sal′pinks) [Gr.] a tube; specifically, the auditory tube or the uterine tube.

salsalate (sal′sah-lāt) an analgesic and anti-inflammatory, $C_{14}H_{10}O_5$.

salt (sawlt) 1. sodium chloride, or common salt. 2. any compound of a base and an acid; any compound of an acid some of whose replaceable atoms have been substituted. 3. [pl.] a saline purgative. **bile s's,** glycine or taurine conjugates of bile acids, which are formed in the liver and secreted in the bile. They are powerful detergents which break down fat globules enabling them to be digested. **Epsom s.,** magnesium sulfate. **Glauber's s.,** sodium sulfate. **Rochelle s.,** potassium sodium tartrate. **smelling s's,** aromatized ammonium carbonate; stimulant and restorative.

saltation (sal-ta′shun) the action of leaping, especially (1) chorea, or the dancing which sometimes accompanies it; (2) conduction along myelinated nerves; (3) in genetics, an abrupt variation in species; a mutation. **sal′tatory,** adj.

salting out (sawl′ting owt) the precipitation of proteins by raising the salt concentration.

salubrious (sah-loo′bre-us) conducive to health; wholesome.

saluresis (sal″u-re′sis) urinary excretion of sodium and chloride ions. **saluret′ic,** adj.

Salutensin (sal″u-ten′sin) trademark for a fixed combination preparation of hydroflumethiazide and reserpine.

salve (sav) a thick ointment or cerate.

samarium (sah-mar′e-um) chemical element (*see table*), at. no. 62, symbol Sm.

sanative (san′ah-tiv) curative; healing.

sanatorium (san″ah-tor′e-um) an institution for treatment of sick persons, especially a private hospital for convalescents or patients with chronic diseases or mental disorders.

sanatory (san′ah-tor″e) conducive to health.

sand (sand) material occurring in small, gritty particles. **brain s.,** acervulus cerebri.

sandfly (sand′fli) any of various two-winged flies, especially of the genus *Phlebotomus.*

sane (sān) sound in mind.

sangui- word element [L.], *blood.*

sanguifacient (sang″gwǐ-fa′shent) hematopoietic.

sanguine (sang′gwin) 1. abounding in blood. 2. ardent; hopeful.

sanguineous (sang-gwin′e-us) abounding in blood; pertaining to the blood.

sanguinolent (sang-gwin′ah-lent) of a bloody tinge.

sanguinopurulent (sang″gwǐ-no-pu′ru-lent) containing both blood and pus.

sanguis (sang′gwis) [L.] blood.

sanies (sa′ne-ēz) a fetid ichorous discharge containing serum, pus, and blood. **sa′nious,** adj.

saniopurulent (sa″ne-o-pūr′oo-lent) partly sanious and partly purulent.

sanioserous (-sēr′us) partly sanious and partly serous.

sanitarian (san″ǐ-tār′e-an) one skilled in sanitation and public health science.

sanitarium (san″ǐ-tār′e-um) an institution for the promotion of health.

sanitary (san′ǐ-tār″e) promoting or pertaining to health.

sanitation (san″ǐ-ta′shun) the establishment of conditions favorable to health.

sanitization (san″ǐ-tǐ-za′shun) the process of making or the quality of being made sanitary.

sanity (san″ǐ-te) soundness of mind.

saphena (sah-fe′nah) [L.] the small saphenous or the great saphenous vein; see *Table of Veins.*

saphenous (sah-fe′nus) pertaining to or associated with a saphena; applied to certain arteries, nerves, veins, etc.

sapo (sa′po) [L.] soap.

saponaceous (sa″pah-na′shus) soapy; of soaplike feel or quality.

saponification (sah-pon″ǐ-fǐ-ka′shun) conversion of an oil or fat into a soap by combination with an alkali.

saponin (sap′ah-nin) a group of glycosides widely distributed in plants, which form a durable foam when their watery solutions are shaken, and which dissolve erythrocytes even in high dilutions.

sapr(o)- word element [Gr.], decay; decayed matter.

saprophyte (sap′rah-fīt) any organism living upon dead or decaying organic matter. **saprophyt′ic,** adj.

saprozoic (sap″rah-zo′ik) living on decayed organic matter; said of animals, especially protozoa.

saralasin (sar-al′ah-sin) an angiotensin II antagonist, $C_{42}H_{65}N_{13}O_{10}$, used as an antihypertensive in the treatment of severe hypertension and in the diagnosis of renin-dependent hypertension.

sarc(o)- word element [Gr.], *flesh.*

Sarcina (sar′sĭ-nah) a genus of bacteria (family Micrococcaceae) found in soil and water as saprophytes.

sarcoblast (sar′ko-blast) a primitive cell which develops into a muscle cell.

sarcocele (-sēl) any fleshy swelling or tumor of the testis.

sarcocyst (-sist) any member of, or any cyst formed by, *Sarcocystis.*

Sarcocystis (sar″ko-sis′tis) a genus of parasitic protozoa that occur as sporocysts in the muscle tissue of mammals, birds, and reptiles.

sarcocystosis (sar″ko-sis-to′sis) infection with protozoa of the genus *Sarcocystis,* which in humans is usually asymptomatic or manifested by muscle cysts associated with myositis or myocarditis or by intestinal infection. It is usually transmitted by eating undercooked beef or pork containing sporocysts or by ingestion of sporocysts from the feces of an infected animal.

Sarcodina (-di′nah) a subphylum of protozoa consisting of organisms that alter their body shape and that move about and acquire food either by means of pseudopodia or by protoplasmic flow without producing discrete pseudopodia.

sarcoid (sar′koid) 1. sarcoidosis. 2. a sarcoma-like tumor. 3. fleshlike.

sarcoidosis (sar″koi-do′sis) a chronic, progressive, generalized granulomatous reticulosis involving almost any organ or tissue, characterized histologically by the presence in all affected tissues of noncaseating epithelioid cell tubercles.

sarcolemma (sar″ko-lem′ah) the membrane covering a striated muscle fiber. **sarcolem′mic, sarcolem′mous,** adj.

sarcoma (sar-ko′mah) a malignant tumor made up of a substance like the embryonic connective tissue. **Abernethy's s.,** a malignant fatty tumor occurring mainly on the trunk. **alveolar soft part s.,** one with a reticulated fibrous stroma enclosing groups of sarcoma cells enclosed in alveoli walled with connective tissue. **ameloblastic s.,** the malignant counterpart of ameloblastic fibroma. **botryoid s., s. botryoi′des,** an embryonal rhabdomyosarcoma arising in submucosal tissue, usually in the upper vagina, cervix uteri, or neck of urinary bladder in young children and infants, presenting grossly as a polypoid grapelike structure. **endometrial stromal s.,** a pale, polypoid, fleshy, malignant tumor of the endometrial stroma.

giant cell s., malignant giant cell tumor of bone. **immunoblastic s. of B cells,** an aggressive B-cell lymphoma, in many cases associated with a preexisting immunologic disorder. **immunoblastic s. of T cells,** a group of T-cell lymphomas derived from T lymphocytes in the paracortical area arising from a mixture of small lymphocytes and many large transformed cells. **Kaposi's s.,** a multicentric, malignant neoplastic vascular proliferation, characterized by the development of bluish-red nodules on the skin, sometimes with widespread visceral involvement; a particularly virulent, disseminated form occurs in immunocompromised patients. **osteogenic s.,** a malignant primary tumor of bone composed of a malignant connective tissue stroma with evidence of osteoid, bone and/or cartilage formation; depending upon the dominant component, classified as osteoblastic, fibroblastic, and chondroblastic. **pseudo–Kaposi s.,** unilateral subacute to chronic dermatitis occurring in association with an underlying arteriovenous fistula and closely resembling Kaposi's sarcoma clinically and histologically. **reticulocytic s., reticuloendothelial s., reticulum cell s.,** histiocytic lymphoma. **Rous s.,** a virus-induced sarcoma of chickens.

sarcomatoid (-toid) resembling a sarcoma.

sarcomatosis (sar-ko″mah-to′sis) condition characterized by development of many sarcomas at various sites.

sarcomatous (sar-ko′mah-tus) pertaining to or of the nature of a sarcoma.

sarcomere (sar′ko-mēr) the contractile unit of a myofibril; sarcomeres are repeating units, delimited by the Z bands, along the length of the myofibril.

sarcomphalocele (sar″kom-fal′o-sēl) fleshy tumor of the umbilicus.

sarcoplasm (sar′ko-plazm) the interfibrillary matter of striated muscle. **sarcoplas′mic,** adj.

sarcoplast (-plast) an interstitial cell of muscle, itself capable of being transformed into muscle.

sarcopoietic (sar″ko-poi-et′ik) producing flesh or muscle.

Sarcoptes (sar-kop′tēz) a genus of mites, including *S. scabie′i,* the cause of scabies in man; other varieties cause mange in domestic animals.

sarcosis (sar-ko′sis) abnormal increase of flesh.

sarcosporidiosis (sar″ko-spo-rid″e-o′sis) sarcocystosis.

sarcostosis (sar″kos-to′sis) ossification of fleshy tissue.

sarcotubules (sar″ko-tu′būlz) the membrane-limited structures of the sarcoplasm, forming a canalicular network around each myofibril.

sarcous (sar′kus) pertaining to flesh or muscle tissue.

satellite (sat′el-īt″) 1. a vein that closely accompanies an artery, such as the brachial. 2. a minor, or attendant, lesion situated near a larger one. 3. a globoid mass of chromatin attached at the secondary constriction to the ends of the short arms of acrocentric autosomes. 4. exhibiting satellitism.

satellitism (sat′el-i-tizm) the phenomenon in

which certain bacterial species grow more vigorously in the immediate vicinity of colonies of other unrelated species, owing to the production of an essential metabolite by the latter species.

satellitosis (sat″el-i-to′sis) accumulation of neuroglial cells about neurons; seen whenever neurons are damaged.

saturated (sach′er-āt″ed) 1. denoting an organic compound that has only single bonds between carbon atoms. 2. unable to hold in solution any more of a given substance.

saturation (sach″er-a′shun) the state of being saturated, or the act of saturating. **oxygen s.,** the amount of oxygen bound to hemoglobin in the blood expressed as a percentage of the maximal binding capacity.

satyriasis (sat″ĭ-ri′ah-sis) pathologic or exaggerated sexual desire in the male.

saucerization (saw″ser-ĭ-za′shun) 1. the excavation of tissue to form a shallow shelving depression, usually performed to facilitate drainage from infected areas of bone. 2. the shallow saucer-like depression on the upper surface of a vertebra which has suffered a compression fracture.

saw (saw) a cutting instrument with a serrated edge. **Gigli's wire s.,** a flexible wire with saw teeth.

saxitoxin (sak″sĭ-tok′sin) a powerful neurotoxin synthesized and secreted by certain dinoflagellates, which accumulates in the tissues of shellfish feeding on the dinoflagellates and may cause a severe toxic reaction in persons consuming contaminated shellfish.

Sb chemical symbol, *antimony* (L. *stibium*).

Sc chemical symbol, *scandium*.

scab (skab) 1. the crust of a superficial sore. 2. to become covered with a crust or scab.

scabicide (ska′bĭ-sīd) 1. lethal to *Sarcoptes scabiei.* 2. an agent lethal to *Sarcoptes scabiei.*

scabies (ska′bēz) a contagious skin disease due to the itch mite, *Sarcoptes scabiei;* the female bores into the stratum corneum, forming burrows (cuniculi), attended by intense itching and eczema caused by scratching. **scabiet′ic,** adj. **Norwegian s.,** a rare, severe form associated with an immense number of mites with marked scales and crusts, usually accompanied by lymphadenopathy and eosinophilia.

scala (ska′lah), pl. *sca′lae* [L.] a ladder-like structure. **s. me′dia,** cochlear duct. **s. tym′pani,** the part of the cochlea below the lamina spiralis. **s. vestib′uli,** the part of the cochlea above the lamina spiralis.

scald (skawld) to burn with hot liquid or steam; a burn so produced.

scale (skāl) 1. a thin flake or compacted platelike structure, as of cornified epithelial cells on the body surface. 2. a thin fragment of tartar or other concretion on the surface of the teeth. 3. to remove material from a body surface, as incrustations from a tooth surface. 4. a scheme or device by which some property may be measured (as hardness, weight, linear dimension). **absolute s.,** a temperature scale with zero at the absolute zero of temperature. **Brazelton**

behavioral s., a method for assessing infant behavior by responses to environmental stimuli. **Celsius s.,** a temperature scale with the ice point at zero and the normal boiling point of water at 100 degrees (100° C.); see table accompanying *temperature.* **centigrade s.,** one with 100 gradations or steps between two fixed points, as the Celsius scale; see table accompanying *temperature.* **Fahrenheit s.,** a temperature scale with the ice point at 32 and the normal boiling point of water at 212 degrees (212° F.); see table accompanying *temperature.* **French s.,** a scale used for denoting the size of catheters, sounds, etc., each unit being roughly equivalent to 0.33 mm. in diameter. **gray s.,** a representation of intensities in shades of gray, as in gray scale ultrasonography. **Kelvin s.,** an absolute centigrade scale on which the unit of measurement corresponds with that of the Celsius scale, but the ice point is at 273.15 degrees (273.15° K.). **temperature s.,** one for expressing degree of heat, based on absolute zero as a reference point, or with a certain value arbitrarily assigned to such temperatures as the ice point and boiling point of water. See table accompanying *temperature.*

scalenectomy (ska″lĕ-nek″tah-me) resection of the scalenus muscle.

scalenotomy (-not′ah-me) division of the scalenus muscle.

scaler (skāl′er) a dental instrument for removal of calculus from teeth.

scalp (skalp) the skin covering the cranium.

scalpel (skal′p′l) a small surgical knife usually having a convex edge.

scan (skan) an image produced using a moving detector or a sweeping beam of radiation, as in scintiscanning, B-mode ultrasonography, scanography, or computed tomography.

scandium (skan′de-um) chemical element (*see table*), at. no. 21, symbol Sc.

scanning (skan′ning) 1. production of a scintiscan. 2. a manner of utterance characterized by somewhat regularly recurring pauses.

scapha (ska′fah), pl. *sca′phae* [L.] the curved depression separating the helix and antihelix.

scaphocephaly (skaf″o-sef′ah-le) abnormal length and narrowness of the skull as a result of premature closure of the sagittal suture. **scaphocephal′ic, scaphoceph′alous,** adj.

scaphoid (skaf′oid) boat-shaped; see *Table of Bones.*

scaphoiditis (skaf″oi-di′tis) inflammation of the scaphoid bone.

scapula (skap′u-lah), pl. *scap′ulae* [L.] see *Table of Bones.* **scap′ular,** adj.

scapulalgia (skap″u-lal′je-ah) pain in the scapular region.

scapulectomy (skap″u-lek′tah-me) excision or resection of the scapula.

scapuloclavicular (skap″u-lo-klah-vik′u-ler) pertaining to the scapula and clavicle.

scapulohumeral (-hu′mer-al) pertaining to the scapula and humerus.

scapulopexy (skap′u-lo-pek″se) surgical fixation of the scapula.

scapus (ska′pus), pl. *sca′pi* [L.] shaft.

scar (skahr) cicatrix; a mark remaining after the healing of a wound or other morbid process. By extension applied to other visible manifestations of an earlier event.

scarification (skar″ĭ-fĭ-ka′shun) production in the skin of many small superficial scratches or punctures, as for introduction of vaccine.

scarificator (skar′ĭ-fĭ-ka″ter) scarifier.

scarifier (skar′ĭ-fi″er) an instrument with many sharp points, used in scarification.

scarlatina (skahr″lah-te′nah) scarlet fever. **scarlat′inal,** adj. **s. angino′sa,** a form with severe throat symptoms.

scarlatinella (skahr-lat″ĭ-nel′ah) Duke's disease.

scarlatiniform (skahr″lah-tin′ĭ-form) resembling scarlet fever.

scat(o)- word element [Gr.], *dung; fecal matter.*

scatemia (skah-te′me-ah) alimentary toxemia in which chemical poisons are absorbed through the intestine.

scatology (skah-tol′ah-je) 1. study and analysis of feces. 2. a preoccupation with feces and filth. **scatolog′ical,** adj.

scatoscopy (skah-tos′ko-pe) examination of the feces.

Sc.D. Doctor of Science.

schindylesis (skin″dĭ-le′sis) an articulation in which one bone is received into a cleft in another.

schist(o)- word element [Gr.], *cleft; split.*

schistocephalus (shis″-, skis″to-sef′ah-lus) a fetus with a cleft head.

schistocoelia (-se′le-ah) congenital fissure of the abdomen.

schistocormus (-kor′mus) a fetus with a cleft trunk.

schistocyte (shis′-, skis′to-sīt) a fragment of a red blood corpuscle, commonly observed in the blood in hemolytic anemia.

schistocytosis (shis″-, skis″to-si-to′sis) an accumulation of schistocytes in the blood.

schistomelus (shis-, skis-tom′ĕ-lus) a fetus with a cleft limb.

schistoprosopus (shis″-, skis″to-pros′o-pus) a fetus with a cleft face.

Schistosoma (-so′mah) a genus of blood flukes, including *S. haemato′bium* of Africa, *S. japon′icum* of the Far East, *S. manso′ni* of Africa, South America, and the West Indies, and *S. intercala′tum* of West Central Africa, which cause infection in man by penetrating the skin of persons coming in contact with infected waters; the invertebrate hosts are certain snails. See specific diseases under *schistosomiasis.* **schistoso′mal,** adj.

schistosome (shis′-, skis′to-sōm) an individual of the genus *Schistosoma.*

schistosomiasis (shis″-, skis″to-so-mi′ah-sis) infection with *Schistosoma.* **s. haemato′bia,** urinary s. **s. intercala′tum,** an endemic intestinal disease of West Central Africa due to infection with *Schistosoma intercalatum,* with abdominal pain, diarrhea, and other intestinal symptoms. **s. japon′ica,** infection with *Schistosoma japonica.* The acute form is marked by fever, allergic symptoms, and diarrhea; chronic effects, which may be severe, are due to fibrosis around eggs deposited in the liver, lungs, and central nervous system. **s. manso′ni,** infection with *Schistosoma mansoni,* living chiefly in the mesenteric veins but migrating to deposit eggs in venules, primarily of the large intestine; eggs lodging in the liver may lead to peripheral fibrosis, hepatosplenomegaly, and ascites. **urinary s.,** infection with *Schistosoma haematobium* involving the urinary tract and causing cystitis and hematuria.

schistosomicide (-so′mĭ-sīd) an agent lethal to schistosomes.

schistosomus (-so′mus) a fetus with a fissure of the abdomen and with rudimentary or absent lower limbs.

schistothorax (-thor′aks) congenital fissure of the chest or sternum.

schiz(o)- word element [Gr.], *divided; division.*

schizamnion (skiz-am′ne-on) an amnion formed by cavitation over or in the inner cell mass, as in human development.

schizogenesis (skiz″o-jen′ĕ-sis) reproduction by fission. **schizog′enous,** adj.

schizogony (skĭ-zog′o-ne) the asexual reproduction of a sporozoan parasite (sporozoite) by multiple fission of the nucleus of the parasite followed by segmentation of the cytoplasm, giving rise to merozoites. **schizogon′ic,** adj.

schizogyria (skiz″o-ji′re-ah) a condition in which there are wedge-shaped cracks in the cerebral convolutions.

schizoid (skiz′oid, skit′soid) 1. denoting the traits that characterize the schizoid personality. 2. denoting schizophrenia-like traits that are held by some to indicate a predisposition to schizophrenia.

schizont (skiz′ont) the multinucleate stage in the development of some members of the Sarcodina and some sporozoans during schizogony.

schizonychia (skiz″o-nik′e-ah) splitting of the nails.

schizophasia (-fa′ze-ah) incomprehensible, disordered speech.

schizophrenia (skit″so-, skiz″o-fre′ne-ah) a mental disorder or group of disorders characterized by disturbances in the form and content of thought (e.g., delusions, hallucinations), in mood (e.g., inappropriate affect), in sense of self and relationship to the external world (e.g., loss of ego boundaries, withdrawal), and in behavior (e.g., bizarre or apparently purposeless behavior). **schizophren′ic,** adj. **catatonic s.,** a form characterized by psychomotor disturbance, which may be manifested by a marked decrease in reactivity to the environment and spontaneous activity or by excited, uncontrollable, and apparently purposeless motor activity. **childhood s.,** schizophrenia with onset before puberty, marked by autistic, withdrawn behavior, failure to develop an identity separate from the mother's, and gross developmental immaturity. **disorganized s., hebephrenic s.,** a form marked by frequent incoherence, loosening of associations, shallow and inappropriate affect, giggling, silly behavior and mannerisms, regression, and hypochondriasis. **paranoid s.,** a form characterized by delusions of grandeur or persecution, often with hallucinations. **process s.,** severe progressive schizophrenia assumed to have an endogenous origin and a poor prognosis; cf. *reactive s.* **reactive s.,** a form attributed chiefly to environmental conditions, with an acute onset and a favorable prognosis. **residual s.,** a condition manifested by individuals with symptoms of schizophrenia who, after a psychotic schizophrenic episode, are no longer psychotic. **undifferentiated s.,** a condition manifested by schizophrenic symptoms that are of mixed or indefinite type which cannot be classified under other forms of schizophrenia.

schizotrichia (skiz″o-trik′e-ah) splitting of the hairs at the ends.

schwannoma (shwahn-o′mah) a neoplasm originating from Schwann cells (of the myelin sheath) of neurons; schwannomas include neurofibromas and neurilemomas. **granular cell s.,** see under *tumor.*

sciage (se-ahzh′) [Fr.] a sawing movement in massage.

sciatic (si-at′ik) pertaining to the ischium; see also *Table of Nerves.*

sciatica (si-at′ĭ-kah) neuralgia along the course of the sciatic nerve, most often with pain radiating into the buttock and lower limb, most commonly due to herniation of a lumbar disk.

SCID severe combined immunodeficiency disease.

science (si′ens) 1. the systematic observation of natural phenomena for the purpose of discovering laws governing those phenomena. 2. the body of knowledge accumulated by such means. **scientif′ic,** adj.

scieropia (si″er-o′pe-ah) defect of vision in which objects appear in a shadow.

scintigram (sin′tĭ-gram) scintiscan.

scintigraphy (sin-tig′rah-fe) the production of two-dimensional images of the distribution of radioactivity in tissues after the internal administration of a radiopharmaceutical imaging agent, the images being obtained by a scintillation camera. **scintigraph′ic,** adj.

scintillation (sin″tĭ-la′shun) 1. an emission of sparks. 2. a subjective visual sensation, as of seeing sparks. 3. a particle emitted in disintegration of a radioactive element; see also under *counter.*

scintiscan (sin′tĭ-skan) a two-dimensional representation of the gamma rays emitted by a radioactive isotope, revealing its concentration in a specific organ or tissue.

scirrhoid (skir′oid) resembling scirrhous carcinoma.

scirrhous (skir′us) hard or indurated; see under *carcinoma.*

scissura (sĭ-su′rah), pl. *scissu′rae* [L.] an incisure; a splitting.

scler(o)- word element [Gr.], *hard; sclera.*

sclera (skler′ah), pl. *scler′ae.* the tough white outer coat of the eyeball, covering approximately the posterior five-sixths of its surface, continuous anteriorly with the cornea and posteriorly with the external sheath of the optic nerve. **scler′al,** adj.

scleradenitis (skler″ad-ĕ-ni′tis) inflammation and hardening of a gland.

sclerectasia (-ek-ta′ze-ah) a bulging state of the sclera.

sclerectoiridectomy (sklĕ-rek″to-ir″ĭ-dek′tah-me) excision of part of the sclera and of the iris.

sclerectoiridodialysis (-ir″ĭ-do-di-al′ĭ-sis) sclerectomy and iridodialysis.

sclerectomy (sklĕ-rek′tah-me) excision of part of the sclera.

scleredema (skler″ĕ-de′mah) diffuse, symmetrical, woodlike, nonpitting induration of the skin of unknown etiology, typically beginning on the head, face, or neck and spreading to involve the shoulders, arms, and thorax and sometimes extracutaneous sites. **s. neonato′rum,** sclerema.

sclerema (sklĕ-re′mah) a severe, sometimes fatal disorder of adipose tissue occurring chiefly in preterm, sick, debilitated infants, manifested by induration of the involved tissue, causing the skin to become cold, yellowish white, mottled, boardlike, and inflexible.

scleriritomy (skler″ĭ-rit′-o-me) incision of the sclera and iris in anterior staphyloma.

scleritis (sklĕ-ri′tis) inflammation of the sclera; it may involve the part adjoining the limbus of the cornea (*anterior s.*) or the underlying retina and choroid (*posterior s.*).

scleroblastema (skler″o-blas-te′mah) the embryonic tissue from which bone is formed. **scleroblastem′ic,** adj.

sclerochoroiditis (-kor″oi-di′tis) inflammation of the sclera and choroid.

sclerocornea (-kor′ne-ah) the sclera and choroid regarded as forming a single layer.

sclerodactyly (-dak′tĭ-le) localized scleroderma of the digits.

scleroderma (-der′mah) hardening and thickening of the skin, which may be a finding in several different diseases, occurring in localized and general forms. **circumscribed s.,** morphea. **systemic s.,** a systemic disorder of connective tissue characterized by induration and thickening of the skin, abnormalities of the blood vessels, and fibrotic degenerative changes in various body organs.

sclerogenous (sklĕ-roj′ĕ-nus) producing sclerosis or sclerous tissue.

scleroiritis (skler″o-i-ri′tis) inflammation of the sclera and iris.

sclerokeratitis (-ker″ah-ti′tis) inflammation of the sclera and cornea.

scleroma (sklĕ-ro′mah) a hardened patch or induration, especially of the nasal or laryngeal tissues. **respiratory s.,** rhinoscleroma.

scleromalacia (skler″o-mah-la′she-ah) degeneration and thinning (softening) of the sclera, occurring in rheumatoid arthritis.

scleromere (skler′o-mēr) 1. any segment or metamere of the skeletal system. 2. the caudal half of a sclerotome (2).

scleromyxedema (skler″o-mik″sĕ-de′mah) 1. lichen myxedematosus. 2. a term sometimes used to refer to lichen myxedematosus associated with scleroderma.

scleronyxis (-nik'sis) surgical puncture of the sclera.

sclero-oophoritis (-o''ah-fah-ri'tis) sclerosing inflammation of the ovary.

sclerophthalmia (sklēr''of-thal'me-ah) a condition, resulting from imperfect differentiation of the sclera and cornea, in which only the central part of the cornea remains clear.

sclerosant (sklē-ro'sant) a chemical irritant injected into a vein to produce inflammation and eventual fibrosis and obliteration of the lumen; used in the treatment of varicose veins.

sclerose (sklĕ-rōs') to become, or cause to become, hardened or sclerotic.

sclerosis (sklĕ-ro'sis) an induration or hardening, especially from inflammation and in diseases of the interstitial substance; applied chiefly to such hardening of the nervous system or to hardening of the blood vessels. **amyotrophic lateral s.,** progressive degeneration of the neurons that give rise to the corticospinal tract and of the motor cells of the brain stem and spinal cord, resulting in a deficit of upper and lower motor neurons; it usually has a fatal outcome within 2 to 3 years. **arterial s.,** arteriosclerosis. **arteriolar s.,** arteriolosclerosis. **disseminated s.,** multiple s. **familial centrolobar s.,** a progressive familial form of leukoencephalopathy, marked by nystagmus, ataxia, tremor, parkinsonian facies, dysarthria, and mental deterioration. **lateral s.,** degeneration of the lateral columns of the spinal cord; it may be primary, with spastic paraplegia, limb rigidity, increase of the tendon reflexes, and no sensory disturbances, or secondary to myelitis, with spastic paraplegia and sensory and other disturbances. **Mönckeberg's s.,** see under *arteriosclerosis.* **multiple s.,** demyelination occurring in patches throughout the white matter of the central nervous system, sometimes extending into the gray matter; symptoms of lesions of the white matter are weakness, incoordination, paresthesias, speech disturbances, and visual complaints. **progressive systemic s.,** systemic scleroderma. **tuberous s.,** an autosomal dominant disease characterized by hamartomas of the brain (tubers), retina, and viscera; mental retardation; seizures; and adenoma sebaceum.

sclerostenosis (sklēr''o-ste-no'sis) induration or hardening combined with contraction.

sclerostomy (sklē-ros'tah-me) surgical creation of an opening in the sclera; usually performed in treatment of glaucoma.

sclerotherapy (sklēr''o-ther'ah-pe) injection of sclerosing solutions in the treatment of hemorrhoids or other varicose veins.

sclerotic (sklē-rot'ik) 1. hard or hardening; affected with sclerosis. 2. sclera.

sclerotica (sklē-rot'ĭ-kah) [L.] sclera.

sclerotitis (sklēr''o-ti'tis) scleritis.

sclerotium (sklē-ro'she-um) a structure formed by fungi and certain protozoa in response to adverse environmental conditions, which will germinate under favorable conditions; in fungi, it is a hard mass of intertwined mycelia, usually with pigmented walls, and in protozoa it is a multinucleated hard cyst into which the plasmodium divides.

sclerotome (skle'ro-tōm) 1. an instrument used in the incision of the sclera. 2. the area of bone innervated from a single spinal segment. 3. one of the paired masses of mesenchymal tissue, separated from the ventromedial part of a somite, which develop into vertebrae and ribs.

sclerotomy (sklĕ-rot'o-me) incision of the sclera.

sclerous (sklēr'us) hard; indurated.

scolex (sko'leks), pl. *sco'lices* [Gr.] the attachment organ of a tapeworm, generally considered the anterior, or cephalic, end.

scoli(o)- word element [Gr.], *crooked; twisted.*

scoliokyphosis (sko''le-o-ki-fo'sis) combined lateral (scoliosis) and posterior (kyphosis) curvature of the spine.

scoliosiometry (-se-om'ĕ-tre) measurement of spinal curvature.

scoliosis (sko''le-o'sis) lateral curvature of vertebral column. **scoliot'ic,** adj.

scopolamine (sko-pol'ah-mēn) an anticholinergic alkaloid, $C_{17}H_{21}NO_4$, obtained from various solanaceous plants; the hydrobromide salt is used as a cerebral sedative, mydriatic, and cycloplegic.

scopophilia (sko-po-fil'e-ah) 1. voyeurism (*active s.*). 2. exhibitionism (*passive s.*).

scopophobia (sko''po-fo'be-ah) irrational fear of being seen.

-scopy word element [Gr.], *examination of.*

scorbutic (skor-bu'tik) pertaining to or affected with scurvy.

scorbutigenic (skor-bu''tĭ-jen'ik) causing scurvy.

scorbutus (skor-bu'tus) [L.] scurvy.

scordinema (skōr''dĭ-ne'mah) yawning and stretching with a feeling of lassitude, occurring as a preliminary symptom of some infectious disease.

score (skōr) a rating, usually expressed numerically, based on specific achievement or the degree to which certain qualities are manifest. **Apgar s.,** a numerical expression of an infant's condition, usually determined at 60 seconds after birth, based on heart rate, respiratory effort, muscle tone, reflex irritability, and color. **Bishop s.,** a score for estimating the prospects of induction of labor, arrived at by evaluating the extent of cervical dilatation, effacement, the station of the fetal head, consistency of the cervix, and the cervical position in relation to the vaginal axis.

scot(o)- word element [Gr.], *darkness.*

scotochromogen (sko''to-kro'mah-jen) a microorganism whose pigmentation develops in the dark as well as in the light. **scotochromogen'ic,** adj.

scotodinia (-din'e-ah) dizziness with blurring of vision and headache.

scotoma (sko-to'mah), pl. *scoto'mata.* an area of depressed vision in the visual field, surrounded by an area of less depressed or of normal vision. **scotom'atous,** adj. **annular s.,** a circular area of depressed vision surrounding the point of fixation. **central s.,** an area of depressed vision corresponding with the point of fixation and interfering with central vision. **centrocecal s.,** a horizontal oval defect in the field of vision situated between and embracing both the point of fixation and the blind spot. **color s.,** an isolated area of depressed or defective vision for color. **hemianopic s.,** depressed or lost vision affecting half of the central visual field. **mental s.,** in psychiatry, a figurative blind spot in a person's psychological awareness, the patient being unable to gain insight into and to understand his mental problems; lack of insight. **negative s.,** one which appears as a blank spot or hiatus in the visual field. **peripheral s.,** an area of depressed vision toward the periphery of the visual field. **physiologic s.,** that area of the visual field corresponding with the optic disk, in which the photosensitive receptors are absent. **positive s.,** one which appears as a dark spot in the visual field. **relative s.,** an area of the visual field in which perception of light is only diminished, or loss is restricted to light of certain wavelengths. **ring s.,** annular s. **scintillating s.,** teichopsia.

scotomagraph (sko-to′mah-graf) an instrument for recording a scotoma.

scotometry (sko-tom′ĕ-tre) the measurement of scotomas.

scotomization (sko″tah-mĭ-za′shun) the development of scotomata, especially mental scotomata, the patient attempting to deny existence of everything that conflicts with his ego.

scotophilia (sko″to-fil′e-ah) preference for night.

scotophobia (-fo′be-ah) irrational fear of darkness.

scotopia (sko-to′pe-ah) 1. night vision. 2. dark adaptation. **scotop′ic,** adj.

scotopsin (sko-top′sin) the protein moiety in the retinal rods that combines with 11-*cis* retinal to form rhodopsin; see *retinal* (2).

scours (skowrz) diarrhea in newborn animals.

scrapie (skra′pe) one of the transmissible spongiform encephalopathies occurring in sheep and goats, characterized by severe pruritus, debility, and muscular incoordination, and invariably ending fatally.

scratches (skrach′ez) eczematous inflammation of the feet of a horse.

screen (skrēn) 1. a structure resembling a curtain or partition, used as a protection or shield; such a structure used in fluoroscopy, or on which light rays are projected. 2. to examine by fluoroscopy (Great Britain). 3. protectant (2). 4. to separate well individuals in a population from those with an undiagnosed pathologic condition by means of tests, examinations, or other procedures.

screening (skrēn′ing) 1. examination of a group to separate well persons from those who have an undiagnosed pathologic condition or who are at high risk. 2. fluoroscopy (Great Britain).

screwworm (skroo′werm) the larva of *Cochliomyia hominivorax*.

scrobiculate (skro-bik′u-lāt) marked with pits.

scrobiculus (skro-bik′u-lus) [L.] pit. **s. cor′dis,** epigastric fossa.

scrofula (skrof′u-lah) primary tuberculosis of the cervical lymph nodes; the inflamed structures being subject to a cheesy degeneration.

scrofuloderma (skrof″u-lo-der′mah) a tuberculous or nontuberculous mycobacterial infection of the skin caused by direct extension of tuberculosis into the skin from underlying structures or by contact exposure to tuberculosis.

scrofulous (skrof′u-lus) pertaining to or characterized by scrofuloderma or scrofula.

scrotectomy (skro-tek′tah-me) partial or complete excision of the scrotum.

scrotitis (skro-ti′tis) inflammation of the scrotum.

scrotocele (skro′to-sēl) scrotal hernia.

scrotoplasty (-plas″te) plastic reconstruction of the scrotum.

scrotum (skro′tum) the pouch containing the testes and their accessory organs. **scro′tal,** adj. **lymph s.,** elephantiasis scroti.

scruple (skroo′p′l) 20 grains of the apothecaries' system, or 1.296 gm.

scurvy (sker′ve) a disease due to deficiency of ascorbic acid (vitamin C), marked by anemia, spongy gums, a tendency to mucocutaneous hemorrhages, and brawny induration of calf and leg muscles.

scute (skūt) any squama or scalelike structure, especially the bony plate separating the upper tympanic cavity and mastoid cells (*tympanic s.*).

scutiform (sku′tĭ-form) shaped like a shield.

scutulum (sku′tu-lum), pl. *scu′tula* [L.] one of the disk- or saucer-like crusts characteristic of favus.

scutum (sku′tum) 1. scute. 2. a hard chitinous plate on the anterior dorsal surface of hard-bodied ticks.

scybalum (sib′ah-lum), pl. *scyb′ala* [Gr.] a hard mass of fecal matter in the intestines. **scy′balous,** adj.

scyphoid (si′foid) shaped like a cup.

S.D. skin dose; standard deviation.

S.E. standard error.

Se chemical symbol, *selenium*.

searcher (serch′er) a sound used in examining the bladder for calculi.

seatworm (sēt′werm) any oxyurid, especially *Enterobius vermicularis*.

sebaceous (sĕ-ba′shus) pertaining to or secreting sebum.

sebiferous (sĕ-bif′er-us) sebiparous.

sebiparous (sĕ-bip′ah-rus) producing fatty secretion.

sebolith (seb′o-lith) calculus in a sebaceous gland.

seborrhea (seb″o-re′ah) 1. excessive secretion of sebum. 2. seborrheic dermatitis. **seborrhe′al, seborrhe′ic,** adj. **s. sic′ca,** dry, scaly seborrheic dermatitis.

sebotropic (seb″-o-trop′ik) having an affinity for or a stimulating effect on sebaceous glands; promoting the excretion of sebum.

sebum (se′bum) the oily secretion of the sebaceous glands, composed of fat and epithelial debris.

secobarbital (sek″o-bar′bĭ-tawl) a short- to intermediate-acting barbiturate, $C_{12}H_{18}N_2O_3$, used as a hypnotic; also used as the sodium salt.

secreta (se-kre′tah) [L., pl.] secretion products.

secretagogue (se-krēt′ah-gog) stimulating secretion; an agent that so acts.

secrete (sĭ-krēt′) to elaborate and release a secretion.

secretin (sĭ-kre′tin) a hormone secreted by the duodenal and jejunal mucosa when acid chyme enters the intestine; it stimulates secretion of pancreatic juice and, to a lesser extent, bile and intestinal secretion.

secretion (sĭ-kre′shun) 1. the cellular process of elaborating and releasing a specific product; this activity may range from separating a specific substance of the blood to the elaboration of a new chemical substance. 2. any substance so produced.

secretoinhibitory (sĭ-kre″to-in-hib′ĭ-tor″e) inhibiting secretion; antisecretory.

secretomotor, secretomotory (-mo′ter; -mo′ter-e) stimulating secretion; said of nerves.

secretor (sĭ-kre′ter) in genetics, one who secretes the ABH antigens of the ABO blood group in the saliva and other body fluids; also, the gene determining this trait.

secretory (sĭ-kre′tah-re) pertaining to secretion.

sectio (sek′she-o), pl. *sectio′nes* [L.] section.

section (sek′shun) 1. an act of cutting. 2. a cut surface. 3. a segment or subdivision of an organ. **abdominal s.**, laparotomy. **cesarean s.**, delivery of a fetus by incision through the abdominal wall and uterus. **frozen s.**, a specimen cut by microtome from tissue that has been frozen. **perineal s.**, external urethrotomy. **Saemisch's s.**, see under *operation*. **serial s's**, histologic sections made in consecutive order and so arranged for the purpose of microscopic examination.

secundigravida (sĭ-kun″dĭ-grav′ĭ-dah) a woman pregnant the second time; gravida II.

secundines (sĭ-kun′dĭnz, -dēnz) afterbirth.

secundipara (sek″un-, se″kun-dip′ah-rah) a woman who has had two pregnancies which resulted in viable offspring; para II.

S.E.D. skin erythema dose.

sedation (sĭ-da′shun) 1. the allaying of irritability or excitement, especially by administration of a sedative. 2. the state so induced.

sedative (sed′ah-tiv) 1. allaying irritability and excitement. 2. a drug that so acts.

sedentary (sed′en-tār″e) 1. sitting habitually; of inactive habits. 2. pertaining to a sitting posture.

sediment (sed′ĭ-ment) a precipitate, especially that formed spontaneously.

sedimentation (sed″ĭ-men-ta′shun) the settling out of sediment.

seed (sēd) 1. the mature ovule of a flowering plant. 2. semen. 3. a small cylindrical shield of gold or other suitable material, used in application of radiation therapy. 4. to inoculate a culture medium with microorganisms. **cardamom**

s., the dried ripe seed of *Elettaria cardamomum*, a plant of tropical Asia; used as a flavoring agent. **plantago s., psyllium s.**, cleaned, dried ripe seed of species of *Plantago*; used as a cathartic.

segment (seg′ment) a demarcated portion of a whole. **segmen′tal**, adj. **bronchopulmonary s's**, the smaller subdivisions of the lobes of the lungs, separated by connective tissue septa and supplied by branches of the respective lobar bronchi. **hepatic s's**, subdivisions of the hepatic lobes based on arterial and biliary supply and venous drainage. **uterine s.**, either of the portions into which the uterus differentiates in early labor; the upper contractile portion (corpus uteri) becomes thicker as labor advances, and the lower noncontractile portion (the isthmus) is expanded and thin-walled.

segmentation (seg″men-ta′shun) 1. division into similar parts. 2. cleavage.

segmentum (seg-men′tum), pl. *segmen′ta* [L.] segment.

segregation (seg″rah-ga′shun) 1. the separation of allelic genes during meiosis as homologous chromosomes begin to migrate toward opposite poles of the cell, so that eventually the members of each pair of allelic genes go to separate gametes. 2. the progressive restriction of potencies in the zygote to the various regions of the forming embryo.

segregator (seg′rah-ga″tor) an instrument for obtaining the urine from each kidney separately.

seizure (se′zhur) a sudden attack, as of disease or epilepsy. **absence s.**, an epileptic seizure marked by a momentary break in the stream of thought and activity, accompanied by a symmetrical 3-c.p.s. spike and wave activity on the electroencephalogram. **febrile s.**, convulsions associated with high fever.

selection (sĕ-lek′shun) the play of forces that determines the relative reproductive performance of the various genotypes in a population. **directional s.**, selection favoring individuals at one extreme of the distribution. **disruptive s., diversifying s.**, selection favoring the two extremes rather than the intermediate. **natural s.**, the survival in nature of those individuals and their progeny best equipped to adapt to environmental conditions. **sexual s.**, natural selection in which certain characteristics attract male or female members of a species, thus ensuring survival of those characteristics. **stabilizing s.**, selection favoring intermediate phenotypes rather than those at one or both extremes.

selectivity (sĕ-lek-tiv′ĭ-te) in pharmacology, the degree to which a dose of a drug produces the desired effect in relation to adverse effects. **selec′tive**, adj.

selenium (sĕ-le′ne-um) chemical element (see table), at. no. 34, symbol Se; it is an essential mineral nutrient, being a constituent of the enzyme glutathione peroxidase, but it occurs in toxic levels in plants growing in soil with high levels, causing disease in grazing animals. **s. sulfide**, SeS_2, an antiseborrheic, applied topically to the scalp.

self-antigen (self-an′tĭ-jen) autoantigen.

self-limited (-lim′it-ed) limited by its own peculiarities, and not by outside influence; said of a disease that runs a definite limited course.

self-tolerance (-tol′er-ans) immunological tolerance to self-antigens.

sella (sel′ah), pl. *sel′lae* [L.] a saddle-shaped depression. **sel′lar**, adj. **s. tur′cica,** a depression on the upper surface of the sphenoid bone, lodging the pituitary gland.

semeiography (se″mi-og′rah-fe) a description of the signs and symptoms of disease.

semeiotic (se″mi-ot′ik) 1. pertaining to signs or symptoms. 2. pathognomonic.

semeiotics (se″mi-ot′iks) symptomatology.

semelincident (sem″el-in′sĭ-dent) attacking only once, as an infectious disease which induces immunity thereafter.

semen (se′men) fluid discharged at ejaculation in the male, consisting of secretion of glands associated with the urogenital tract and containing spermatozoa. **sem′inal,** adj.

semi- word element [L.], *half.*

semicanal (sem″ĭ-kah-nal′) a channel open at one side.

semicoma (-ko′mah) a stupor from which the patient may be aroused. **semico′matose,** adj.

semiflexion (-flek′shun) position of a limb midway between flexion and extension; the act of bringing to such a position.

semilunar (-loo′nar) resembling a crescent or half-moon.

seminiferous (-nif′er-us) producing or carrying semen.

seminoma (se″mĭ-no′mah) a radiosensitive, malignant neoplasm of the testis, thought to be derived from primordial germ cells of the sexually undifferentiated embryonic gonad, and occuring as a gray to yellow-white nodule or mass; three histologic variants are recognized; *classical* (typical), the most common type; *anaplastic;* and *spermatocytic.*

seminuria (se″mĭ-nu′re-ah) discharge of semen in the urine.

semipermeable (sem″ĭ-per′me-ah-b'l) permitting passage only of certain molecules.

semiquantitative (-kwon′tĭ-ta′tiv) yielding an approximation of the quantity or amount of a substance; falling short of a quantitative result.

semis (se′mis) [L.] half; abbreviated ss.

semisulcus (sem″ĭ-sul′kus) a depression which, with an adjoining one, forms a sulcus.

semisupination (-soo″pĭ-na′shun) a position halfway toward supination.

semisynthetic (-sin-thet′ik) produced by chemical manipulation of naturally occurring substances.

senescence (sĕ-nes′ens) the process of growing old, especially the condition resulting from the transitions and accumulations of the deleterious aging processes.

senile (se′nīl) pertaining to old age.

senilism (se′nil-izm) premature old age.

senility (sĕ-nil′ĭ-te) the physical and mental deterioration associated with old age.

senna (sen′ah) the dried leaflets of *Cassia senna* or of *C. angustifolia;* used chiefly as a cathartic.

sennoside (sen′o-sīd) either of two anthraquinone glucosides, sennoside A and B, from senna; used as a cathartic.

senopia (se-no′pe-ah) second sight; improvement of vision, especially near vision, in the aged, a sign of incipient cataract.

sensation (sen-sa′shun) an impression produced by impulses conveyed by an afferent nerve to the sensorium. **girdle s.,** zonesthesia. **internal s.,** one perceptible only to the subject, and not associated with any object external to the body. **reflex s., referred s.,** one felt elsewhere than at the site of application of a stimulus. **subjective s.,** internal s.

sense (sens) a faculty by which the conditions or properties of things are perceived. **color s.,** the faculty by which colors are perceived and distinguished. **kinesthetic s.,** muscle s. **light s.,** the sense by which degrees of brilliancy are distinguished. **muscle s., muscular s.,** the sense by which muscular movements are perceived. **posture s.,** the muscular sense by which the position or attitude of the body or its parts is perceived. **pressure s.,** the sense by which pressure upon the surface of the body is perceived. **sixth s.,** cenesthesia. **space s.,** the sense by which relative positions and relations of objects in space are perceived. **special s.,** one of the five senses of seeing, feeling, hearing, taste, and smell. **stereognostic s.,** the sense by which form and solidity are perceived. **temperature s.,** the sense by which differences of temperature are appreciated.

sensibility (sen″sĭ-bil′ĭ-te) susceptibility of feeling; ability to feel or perceive. **deep s.,** the sensibility to pressure and movement that exists after the skin area is made completely anesthetic. **epicritic s.,** the sensibility to gentle stimulations permitting fine discriminations of touch and temperature, localized in the skin. **proprioceptive s.,** the sensibility afforded by receptors in muscles, joints, and other parts, by which one is made aware of their position and state. **protopathic s.,** sensibility to pain and temperature which is low in degree and poorly localized. **somesthetic s.,** proprioceptive s. **splanchnesthetic s.,** the sensibility to stimuli received by the splanchnic receptors.

sensible (sen′sĭ-b'l) capable of sensation; perceptible to the senses.

sensitive (sen′sĭ-tiv) 1. able to receive or respond to stimuli. 2. unusually responsive to stimulation, or responding quickly and acutely.

sensitivity (sen″sĭ-tiv′ĭ-te) 1. the state or quality of being sensitive. 2. the smallest concentration of a substance that can be reliably measured by a given analytical method. 3. the probability that a person having a disease will be correctly identified by a clinical test.

sensitization (sen″sĭ-tĭ-za′shun) 1. administration of an antigen to induce a primary immune response. 2. exposure to allergen that results in the development of hypersensitivity.

sensomobile (sen″so-mo′b'l) moving in response to a stimulus.

sensomotor (-mo′ter) sensorimotor.

sensorial (sen-sor′e-al) pertaining to the sensorium.

sensorimotor (sen″sor-e-mo′ter) both sensory and motor.

sensorineural (-nu′ral) of or pertaining to a sensory nerve or mechanism; see also under *deafness*.

sensorium (sen-sor′e-um) 1. a sensory nerve center. 2. the state of an individual as regards consciousness or mental awareness.

sensory (sen′ser-e) pertaining to sensation.

sentient (sen′she-ent) able to feel; sensitive.

Sephadex (sef′ah-deks) trademark for cross-linked dextran beads. Various forms are used in chromatography.

sepsis (sep′sis) the presence in the blood or other tissues of pathogenic microorganisms or their toxins; the condition associated with such presence. **catheter s.,** sepsis occurring as a complication of intravenous catheterization. **puerperal s.,** that occurring after childbirth, due to matter absorbed from the birth canal; see also *puerperal fever*.

septa (sep′tah) plural of *septum*.

septal (sep′tal) pertaining to a septum.

septate (sep′tāt) divided by a septum.

septectomy (sep-tek′tah-me) excision of part of the nasal septum.

septic (sep′tik) pertaining to sepsis.

septicemia (sep″tĭ-se′me-ah) blood poisoning; systemic disease associated with the presence and persistence of pathogenic microorganisms or their toxins in the blood. **septice′mic,** adj. **cryptogenic s.,** septicemia in which the focus of infection is not evident during life. **fowl s.,** a disease of fowl resembling fowl cholera, due to *Vibrio metchnikovii*, with diarrhea, hyperemia of the alimentary canal, and the presence of a blood-tinged, yellowish liquid in the small intestine. **hemorrhagic s.,** any of a group of animal diseases due to *Pasteurella multocida*, marked by hemorrhagic areas in various body organs and tissues. **puerperal s.,** see under *fever*.

septicopyemia (-pi-e′me-ah) septicemia and pyemia combined. **septicopye′mic,** adj.

septomarginal (sep″to-mar′jĭ-n'l) pertaining to the margin of a septum.

septonasal (-na′z'l) pertaining to the nasal septum.

septoplasty (-plas′te) surgical reconstruction of the nasal septum.

septostomy (sep-tos′to-me) surgical creation of an opening in a septum.

septotomy (sep-tot′ah-me) incision of the nasal septum.

Septra (sep′tra) trademark for a preparation of trimethoprim and sulfamethoxazole.

septulum (sep′tu-lum) pl. *sep′tula* [L.] a small separating wall or partition.

septum (sep′tum) pl. *sep′ta* [L.] a dividing wall or partition. **atrioventricular s.,** the part of the membranous portion of the interventricular septum between the left ventricle and the right atrium. **Bigelow's s.,** a layer of hard, bony tissue in the neck of the femur. **s. of Cloquet, crural s., femoral s.,** the thin fibrous membrane that helps close the femoral ring. **gingival s.,** the part of the gingiva interposed between adjoining teeth. **interalveolar s.,** one of the thin plates of bone separating the alveoli of the different teeth in the mandible and maxilla. **interatrial s.,** the partition separating the right and left atria of the heart. **interdental s.,** interalveolar s. **interventricular s.,** the partition separating the right and left ventricles of the heart. **s. lu′cidum,** pellucid s. **nasal s.,** the partition between the two nasal cavities. **s. pectinifor′me,** s. of penis. **pellucid s., s. pellu′cidum,** the triangular double membrane separating the anterior horns of the lateral ventricles of the brain. **s. of penis,** the fibrous sheet between the corpora cavernosa of the penis. **rectovaginal s.,** the membranous partition between the rectum and vagina. **rectovesical s.,** a membranous partition separating the rectum from the prostate and urinary bladder. **s. of scrotum, s. scro′ti,** the partition between the two chambers of the scrotum.

septuplet (sep′tu-plit, sep-tup′lit) one of seven offspring produced at one birth.

sequel (se′kwel) sequela.

sequela (sĭ-kwe′lah) pl. *seque′lae* [L.] a morbid condition following or occurring as a consequence of another condition or event.

sequester (sĭ-kwes′ter) to detach or separate abnormally a small portion from the whole. See *sequestration* and *sequestrum*.

sequestrant (sĭ-kwes′trant) a sequestering agent, as, for example, cholestyramine resin, which binds bile acids in the intestine, thus preventing their absorption.

sequestration (se″kwes-tra′shun) 1. the formation of a sequestrum. 2. the isolation of a patient. 3. a net increase in the quantity of blood within a limited vascular area, occurring physiologically, with forward flow persisting or not, or produced artificially by the application of tourniquets. **pulmonary s.,** loss of connection of lung tissue with the bronchial tree and the pulmonary veins.

sequestrectomy (-trek′tah-me) excision of a sequestrum.

sequestrum (sĭ-kwes′trum) pl. *seques′tra* [L.] a piece of dead bone separated from the sound bone in necrosis.

sequoiosis (se″kwoi-o′sis) a form of allergic alveolitis due to inhalation and tissue reaction to dust from moldy redwood bark.

sera (se′rah) plural of *serum*.

Ser-Ap-Es (ser′ap-es) trademark for a fixed combination preparation of hydralazine hydrochloride, reserpine, and hydrochlorothiazide.

Serax (ser′aks) trademark for a preparation of oxazepam.

series (se′rēz) a group or succession of events, objects, or substances arranged in regular order or forming a kind of chain; in electricity, parts of a circuit connected successively end to end to form a single path for the current. **se′rial,** adj. **erythrocytic s.,** the succession of developing cells which ultimately culminate in mature erythrocytes. **granulocytic s.,** the succession of developing cells that ultimately culminates in the mature granulocyte or granular leukocyte (*basophil, eosinophil,* or *neutrophil*). **lymphocytic s.,** the succession of developing cells that ultimately culminates in the lymphocyte. **monocytic s.,** the succession of developing cells that ultimately culminates in the monocyte. **thrombocytic s.,** the succession of developing cells that ultimately culminates in the blood platelets (thrombocytes).

serine (ser′ēn) a naturally occurring amino acid, $C_3H_7NO_3$, present in many proteins.

serocolitis (sēr′o-ko-li′tis) inflammation of the serous coat of the colon.

seroconversion (-con-ver′zhun) the change of a seronegative test from negative to positive, indicating the development of antibodies in response to immunization or infection.

serodiagnosis (-di″ag-no′sis) diagnosis of disease based on serologic tests. **serodiagnos′-tic,** adj.

seroenteritis (-en″tĕ-ri′tis) inflammation of the serous coat of the intestine.

serofibrinous (-fi′brĭ-nus) composed of serum and fibrin, as a serofibrinous exudate.

serogroup (sēr′o-grōōp″) an unofficial designation denoting a group of bacteria containing a common antigen, possibly including more than one serotype, species, or genus.

serology (se-rol′o-je) the study of antigen-antibody reactions *in vitro.* **serolog′ic,** adj.

seroma (se-ro′mah) a tumor-like collection of serum in the tissues.

seromembranous (sēr″o-mem′brah-nus) pertaining to or composed of serous membrane.

seromucous (-mu′kus) both serous and mucous.

seromuscular (-mus′ku-ler) pertaining to the serous and muscular coats of the intestine.

seronegative (-ne′gah-tiv) showing negative results on serological examination; showing a lack of antibody.

seropositive (-poz′ĭ-tiv) showing positive results or serological examination; showing a high level of antibody.

seropurulent (-pu′roo-lent) both serous and purulent.

seropus (-pus′) serum mingled with pus.

seroreaction (-re-ak′shun) a reaction occurring in serum or as a result of the action of a serum.

serosa (se-ro′sah, se-ro′zah) 1. any serous membrane (tunica serosa). 2. the chorion. **sero′sal,** adj.

serosanguineous (sēr″o-sang-gwin′e-us) composed of serum and blood.

seroserous (-se′rus) pertaining to two or more serous membranes.

serositis (-si′tis) inflammation of a serous membrane.

serosurvey (sēr″o-sur′va) a screening test of the serum of persons at risk to determine susceptibility to a particular disease.

serosynovitis (-sin″o-vi′tis) synovitis with effusion of serum.

serotherapy (-ther′ah-pe) treatment of infectious disease by injection of immune serum or antitoxin.

serotonin (-to′nin) a hormone and neurotransmitter, 5-hydroxytryptamine (5-HT), found in many tissues, including blood platelets, intestinal mucosa, pineal body, and central nervous system; it has many physiologic properties including inhibition of gastric secretion, stimulation of smooth muscles, and production of vasoconstriction.

serotoninergic (-to″nin-er′gik) 1. containing or activated by serotonin. 2. pertaining to neurons that secrete serotonin.

serotype (sēr′o-tīp) the type of a microorganism determined by its constituent antigens; a taxonomic subdivision based thereon.

serous (sēr′us) 1. pertaining to or resembling serum. 2. producing or containing serum.

serovaccination (sēr″o-vak″sĭ-na′shun) injection of serum combined with bacterial vaccination to produce passive immunity by the former and active immunity by the latter.

serpiginous (ser-pij′ĭ-nus) creeping; having a wavy or much indented border.

serrated (ser′āt-ed) having a sawlike edge.

Serratia (sĕ-ra′she-ah) a genus of bacteria (tribe *Serratieae*) made up of gram-negative rods which produce a red pigment. For the most part, they are free-living saprophytes, but they cause a variety of infections in immunocompromised patients.

serration (sĕ-ra′shun) 1. the state of being serrated. 2. a serrated structure or formation.

serum (sēr′um), pl. *se′ra, serums* [L.] 1. the clear portion of any liquid separated from its more solid elements; see *blood serum,* under B. 2. immune serum; blood serum from immunized animals used to produce passive immunity. **antilymphocyte s.,** serum from animals immunized with lymphocytes from a different species; a powerful immunosuppressive agent. **blood s.,** see under B. **foreign s.,** serum from an animal to be injected into one of another species. **immune s.,** antiserum. **muscle s.,** muscle plasma deprived of myosin. **polyvalent s.,** antiserum containing antibody to more than one kind of antigen. **pooled s.,** the mixed serum from a number of individuals.

serumal (se-roo′mal) pertaining to or formed from serum.

serum-fast (sēr′um-fast) resistant to the effects of serum.

sesamoid (ses′ah-moid) 1. denoting a small nodular bone embedded in a tendon or joint capsule. 2. a sesamoid bone.

sesamoiditis (ses″ah-moi-di′tis) inflammation of the sesamoid bones of a horse's foot.

sessile (ses′il) attached by a broad base, as opposed to being pedunculated or stalked.

setaceous (se-ta′shus) bristle-like.

Setaria (se-tār′e-ah) a genus of filarial nematodes.

sex (seks) 1. a distinctive character of most animals and plants, based on the type of gametes produced by the gonads, ova (macrogametes) being typical of the female, and sperm (microgametes) of the male, or the category in which the individual is placed on such basis. 2. to determine the sex of an organism. **chromosomal s.,** sex as determined by the presence of the XX (female) or the XY (male) genotype in somatic cells, without regard to phenotypic manifestations. **gonadal s.,** the sex as determined on the basis of gonadal tissue present (ovarian or testicular). **morphologic s.,** that determined on the basis of the external genital organs. **psychological s.,** the self-image of the gender role of an individual.

sexduction (seks-duk′shun) the process whereby part of the bacterial chromosome is attached to the autonomous F (sex) factor and thus is transferred from donor (male) bacterium to recipient (female).

sex-conditioned (-kon-dish′und) sex-influenced.

sex-influenced (-in′floo-enst) denoting an autosomal trait that is expressed differently, either in frequency or degree, in males and females, as for example, male-pattern baldness.

sex-limited (-lim′ĭ-ted) denoting a genetic trait exhibited by one sex only, although not determined by an X-linked gene.

sex-linked (seks′linkt) transmitted by a gene located on the X chromosome.

sexology (sek-sol′ah-je) the scientific study of sex and sexual relations.

sextuplet (seks′tu-plit, seks-tup′lit) any one of six offspring produced at the same birth.

sexual (sek′shoo-al) pertaining to sex.

sexuality (sek″shoo-al′ĭ-te) 1. the characteristic of the male and female reproductive elements. 2. the constitution of an individual in relation to sexual attitudes and behavior.

SGOT serum glutamic oxaloacetic transaminase; see *aspartate aminotransferase.*

SGPT serum glutamic pyruvic transaminase; see *alanine aminotransferase.*

shadow-casting (shad′o-kast″ing) application of a coating of gold, chromium, or other metal to ultramicroscopic structures to increase their visibility under the microscope.

shaft (shaft) a long slender part, such as the portion of a long bone between the wider ends or extremities.

shank (shangk) a leg, or leglike part.

shaping (shāp′ing) a technique in behavior therapy in which new behavior is produced by providing reinforcement for progressively closer approximations of the final desired behavior.

sheath (shēth) a tubular case or envelope. **arachnoid s.,** the delicate membrane between the pial and dural sheath of the optic nerve. **carotid s.,** a portion of the cervical fascia enclosing the carotid artery, the internal jugular vein, and the vagus nerve. **connective tissue s. of Key and Retzius,** the endoneurium, especially the delicate continuation around terminal branches of nerve fibers. **crural s.,** femoral s. **dentinal s.,** the layer of tissue forming the wall of a dentinal tubule. **dural s.,** the external investment of the optic nerve. **femoral s.,** the investing fascia of the proximal portion of the femoral vessels. **Henle's s.,** connective tissue s. of Key and Retzius. **Hertwig's s.,** root s. (1).

lamellar s., the perineurium. **Mauthner's s.,** axolemma. **medullary s., myelin s.,** the sheath surrounding the axon of myelinated nerve cells, consisting of concentric layers of myelin formed in the peripheral nervous system by the plasma membrane of Schwann cells, and in the central nervous system by oligodendrocytes. It is interrupted at intervals along the length of the axon by gaps known as *nodes of Ranvier.* Myelin is an electrical insulator that serves to speed the conduction of nerve impulses. **pial s.,** the innermost of the three sheaths of the optic nerve. **root s.,** 1. an investment of epithelial cells around the unerupted tooth and inside the dental follicle. 2. the epithelial portion of a hair follicle. **s. of Schwann,** neurilemma. **synovial s.,** synovial membrane lining the cavity of a bone through which a tendon moves.

sheep-pox (shēp-poks) a highly infectious, sometimes fatal, eruptive viral disease of sheep.

sheet (shēt) an oblong piece of cotton, linen, etc., for a bed covering. **draw s.,** one folded and placed under a patient's body so it may be removed with minimal disturbance of the patient.

shield (shēld) any protecting structure. **Buller's s.,** a watch glass fitted over the eye to guard it from infection. **embryonic s.,** the double-layered disk of the blastoderm from which the primary organ rudiments are formed. **nipple s.,** a device to protect the nipple of a nursing woman.

shift (shift) a change or deviation. **chloride s.,** the exchange of chloride (Cl) and bicarbonate (HCO_3^-) between plasma and the erythrocytes occurring whenever HCO_3^- is generated or decomposed within the erythrocytes. **Doppler s.,** the magnitude of frequency change due to the Doppler effect. **s. to the left,** an increase in the percentage of neutrophils having only one or a few lobes. **s. to the right,** an increase in the percentage of multilobed neutrophils.

Shigella (shĭ-gel′ah) a genus of gram-negative bacteria (family Enterobacteriaceae) which cause dysentery. They are separated into four species on the basis of biochemical reactions. (A) *S. dysente′riae,* (B) *S. flexne′ri,* (C) *S. boy′dii,* and (D) *S. son′nei.*

shigella (shĭ-gel′ah), pl. *shigel′lae.* An individual organism of the genus *Shigella.*

shigellosis (shĭ″gel-lo′sis) infection with *Shigella;* bacillary dysentery.

shin (shin) the prominent anterior edge of the tibia or the leg. **saber s.,** marked anterior convexity of the tibia, seen in congenital syphilis and in yaws.

shingles (shing′g′lz) herpes zoster.

shivering (-ing) 1. involuntary shaking of the body, as with cold. 2. a disease of horses, with trembling or quivering of various muscles.

shock (shok) 1. a sudden disturbance of mental equilibrium. 2. a profound hemodynamic and metabolic disturbance characterized by failure of the circulatory system to maintain adequate perfusion of vital organs. **anaphylactic s.,** a violent attack of symptoms produced by a second injection of serum or protein and due to anaphylaxis. **cardiogenic s.,** shock resulting from inadequate cardiac function, as from myocardial infarction or mechanical obstruction of the heart; manifestations include hypovolemia, hypotension, cold skin, weak pulse, mental confusion, and anxiety. **endotoxin s.,** septic shock due to release of endotoxins by gram-negative bacteria. **hypovolemic s.,** shock resulting from insufficient blood volume, either from hemorrhage or excessive fluid loss or from widespread vasodilation so that normal blood volume is inadequate to maintain tissue perfusion; manifestations are the same as for cardiogenic shock. **insulin s.,** a hypoglycemic reaction to overdosage of insulin, a skipped meal, or strenuous exercise in an insulin-dependent diabetic; early symptoms are tremor, irritability, dizziness, cool, moist skin, hunger, and tachycardia; if untreated it may progress to coma and convulsions. **septic s.,** shock associated with overwhelming infection, most commonly infection with gram-negative bacteria, thought to result from the actions of endotoxins and other products of the infectious agent that cause sequestration of blood in the capillaries and veins. **serum s.,** see *anaphylactic s.* and see under *sickness.*

shotty (shot′e) like shot; resembling the pellets used in shotgun cartridges.

shoulder (shōl′der) the junction of clavicle and scapula, where the arm joins the trunk. **frozen s.,** adhesive capsulitis.

shoulder-blade (-blād) scapula.

shoulder slip (-slip) inflammation and atrophy of the shoulder muscles and tendons in the horse.

show (sho) appearance of blood forerunning labor or menstruation.

shunt (shunt) 1. to turn to one side; to bypass. 2. a passage or anastomosis between two natural channels, especially between blood vessels, formed physiologically or anomalously. 3. a surgically created anastomosis; also, the operation of forming a shunt. **arteriovenous (A-V) s.,** the diversion of blood from an artery directly to a vein, bypassing the capillary network. **cardiovascular s.,** diversion of the blood flow through an anomalous opening from the left side of the heart to the right side or from the systemic to the pulmonary circulation (*left-to-right s.*), or from the right side to the left side or from the pulmonary to the systemic circulation (*right-to-left s.*). **left-to-right s.,** see *cardiovascular s.* **LeVeen peritoneovenous s.,** continuous shunting of ascites fluid from the peritoneal cavity to the jugular vein by means of a surgically implanted subcutaneous plastic tube. **portacaval s.,** surgical anastomosis of the portal vein and the vena cava. **right-to-left s.,** see *cardiovascular s.* **ventriculoatrial s.,** the surgical creation of a communication between a cerebral ventricle and a cardiac atrium by means of plastic tube, to permit drainage of cerebrospinal fluid for relief of hydrocephalus. **ventriculoperitoneal s.,** a communication between a cerebral ventricle and the peritoneum by means of plastic tubing; done for the relief of hydrocephalus.

SI Système International d'Unités, or International System of Units. See *SI unit,* under *unit.*

Si chemical symbol, *silicon.*

sial(o)- word element [Gr.], *saliva; salivary glands.*

sialadenitis (si″al-ad″in-īt′is) inflammation of a salivary gland.

sialadenosis (-ad″in-o′sis) sialadenitis.

sialagogue (si-al′ah-gog) an agent which stimulates the flow of saliva. **sialagog′ic,** adj.

sialectasia (si″al-ek-ta′ze-ah) dilatation of a salivary duct.

sialic acids (si-al′ik) a group of acetylated derivatives of neuraminic acid that occur in a number of mucopolysaccharides and glycolipids.

sialine (si′ah-līn″) pertaining to the saliva.

sialismus (si″ah-liz′mus) ptyalism.

sialitis (si″ah-li′tis) inflammation of a salivary gland or duct.

sialoadenectomy (si″ah-lo-ad″in-ek′tah-me) excision of a salivary gland.

sialoadenitis (-ad″in-īt′is) sialadenitis.

sialoadenotomy (-ad′in-ot′ah-me) incision and drainage of a salivary gland.

sialoaerophagia (-ār″o-fa′je-ah) the swallowing of saliva and air.

sialoangiectasis (-an″je-ek′tah-sis) sialectasia.

sialoangiitis (-an″je-i′tis) inflammation of a salivary duct.

sialoangiography (-an″je-og′rah-fe) radiography of the ducts of the salivary glands after injection of radiopaque material.

sialocele (si′ah-lo-sēl″) a salivary cyst.

sialodochitis (si″ah-lo-do-ki′tis) sialoangiitis.

sialodochoplasty (-do′ko-plas″te) plastic repair of a salivary duct.

sialoductitis (-duk-ti′tis) sialoangiitis.

sialogenous (si″ah-loj′ĕ-nus) producing saliva.

sialography (si″ah-log′rah-fe) sialoangiography.

sialolith (si-al′o-lith) a salivary calculus.

sialolithiasis (si″ah-lo-lĭ-thi′ah-sis) the formation of salivary calculi.

sialolithotomy (-lĭ-thot′ah-me) excision of a salivary calculus.

sialometaplasia (-met″ah-pla′ze-ah) metaplasia of the salivary glands. **necrotizing s.,** a benign inflammatory condition of the salivary glands, simulating mucoepidermoid and squamous cell carcinoma.

sialomucin (-mu′sin) mucin containing sialic acid, a component of airway secretions of the lungs.

sialorrhea (-re′ah) ptyalism.

sialoschesis (si″ah-los′kĕ-sis) suppression of secretion of saliva.

sialosis (si″ah-lo′sis) 1. the flow of saliva. 2. ptyalism. **sialot′ic,** adj.

sialostenosis (si″ah-lo-stĕ-no′sis) stenosis of a salivary duct.

sialosyrinx (sēr′inks) 1. salivary fistula. 2. a syringe for washing out the salivary ducts, or a drainage tube for the salivary ducts.

sib (sib) 1. a blood relative; one of a group of persons all descended from a common ancestor. 2. sibling.

sibilant (sib′ĭ-lant) whistling or hissing.

sibling (sib'ling) any of two or more offspring of the same parents; a brother or sister.

sibship (-ship) 1. relationship by blood. 2. a group of persons all descended from a common ancestor. 3. a group of siblings.

siccative (sik'ah-tiv) 1. drying; removing moisture. 2. an agent which produces drying.

siccus (sik'us) [L.] dry.

sick (sik) 1. not in good health; afflicted by disease; ill. 2. nauseous.

sicklemia (sik-le'me-ah) sickle cell anemia.

sickling (sik'ling) the development of sickle cells in the blood.

sickness (sik'nes) any condition or episode marked by pronounced deviation from the normal healthy state. **African sleeping s.**, African trypanosomiasis. **air s.**, 1. motion sickness due to travel by airplane. 2. high-altitude s. **altitude s.**, high-altitude s. **car s.**, motion sickness due to automobile or other vehicular travel. **decompression s.**, joint pain, respiratory manifestations, skin lesions, and neurologic signs, due to rapid reduction of air pressure in a person's environment. **falling s.**, epilepsy. **green tobacco s.**, a transient, recurrent occupational illness of tobacco harvesters, marked by headache, dizziness, vomiting, and prostration. **high-altitude s.**, the condition resulting from difficulty in adjusting to diminished oxygen pressure at high altitudes. It may take the form of mountain sickness, high-altitude pulmonary edema, or cerebral edema. **milk s.**, 1. an acute, often fatal disease due to ingestion of milk, milk products, or flesh of cattle or sheep affected with trembles (q.v.), marked by weakness, anorexia, vomiting, and sometimes muscular tremors. 2. trembles. **morning s.**, nausea of early pregnancy. **motion s.**, nausea and malaise due to unaccustomed motion, such as may be experienced in various modes of travel, as by airplane, automobile, ship, or train. **mountain s.**, oliguria, dyspnea, blood pressure and pulse rate changes, headache, and neurological disorders due to difficulty in adjusting to reduced oxygen pressure at high altitudes. **radiation s.**, a condition resulting from exposure to a whole-body dose of over 1 gray of ionizing radiation and characterized by the symptoms of the acute radiation syndrome. **serum s.**, a hypersensitivity reaction following the administration of foreign serum or serum proteins, marked by urticaria, arthralgia, edema, and lymphadenopathy. **sleeping s.**, increasing lethargy and drowsiness due to a protozoal infection, e.g., African trypanosomiasis, or by a viral infection, e.g., lethargic encephalitis.

side bone (sīd'bōn) a condition of horses marked by ossification of the lateral cartilages of the third phalanx of the foot.

side effect (ĭ-fekt') a consequence other than that for which an agent is used, especially an adverse effect on another organ system.

sider(o)- word element [Gr.], *iron.*

sideroblast (sid'er-o-blast″) a nucleated erythrocyte containing iron granules in its cytoplasm.

siderocyte (-sīt″) an erythrocyte containing nonhemoglobin iron.

sideroderma (sid″er-o-der'mah) bronzed coloration of the skin due to disordered iron metabolism.

siderofibrosis (-fi-bro'sis) fibrosis associated with deposits of iron, as in the spleen. **siderofibrot′ic**, adj.

sideromycin (sid″er-o-mi'sin) any of a class of antibiotics, synthesized by certain actinomycetes, that inhibit bacterial growth by interfering with iron uptake.

sideropenia (-pe′ne-ah) deficiency of iron in the body or blood. **sidērope′nic**, adj.

siderophil (sid′er-o-fil) 1. siderophilous. 2. a siderophilous cell or tissue.

siderophilous (sid″er-of′ĭ-lus) tending to absorb iron.

siderophore (sid′er-o-for″) a macrophage containing hemosiderin.

siderosis (sid″er-o′sis) 1. pneumoconiosis due to inhalation of iron particles. 2. excess of iron in the blood. 3. the deposit of iron in the tissues. **hepatic s.**, the deposit of an abnormal quantity of iron in the liver. **urinary s.**, the presence of hemosiderin granules in the urine.

siemens (se'menz) the SI unit of conductivity, measured by the quantity of electricity transferred across a unit area per unit potential gradient per unit time. Called also *mho.* Abbreviated S.

sight (sīt) 1. the act or faculty of vision. 2. a thing seen. **far s.**, hyperopia. **near s.**, myopia. **night s.**, hemeralopia; day blindness. **second s.**, senopia.

sigmatism (sig′mah-tizm) faulty enunciation or too frequent use of the s sound.

sigmoid (sig′moid) 1. shaped like the letter C or S. 2. the sigmoid colon.

sigmoidectomy (sig″moi-dek′tah-me) excision of part or all of the sigmoid colon.

sigmoiditis (sig″moi-di′tis) inflammation of the sigmoid colon.

sigmoidopexy (sig-moid′o-pek″se) fixation of the sigmoid colon, as for rectal prolapse.

sigmoidoproctostomy (sig-moid″o-prok-tos′-tah-me) surgical anastomosis of the sigmoid colon to the rectum.

sigmoidoscopy (sig″moi-dos′kah-pe) direct examination of the interior of the sigmoid colon.

sigmoidosigmoidostomy (sig-moid″o-sig″moi-dos′tah-me) surgical anastomosis of two portions of the sigmoid colon; the opening so created.

sigmoidostomy (sig″moi-dos′tah-me) creation of an artificial opening from the sigmoid colon to the body surface; the opening so created.

sigmoidotomy (sig″moi-dot′ah-me) incision of the sigmoid colon.

sigmoidovesical (sig-moid″o-ves′ĭ-k'l) pertaining to or communicating with the sigmoid colon and the urinary bladder.

sign (sīn) an indication of the existence of something; any objective evidence of a disease, i.e., such evidence as is perceptible to the examining physician, as opposed to the subjective sensations (symptoms) of the patient. **Abadie's s.,** 1. spasm of the levator muscle of the upper lid in Graves' disease. 2. insensibility of the Achilles tendon to pressure in tabes dorsalis. **Babinski's s's,** 1. loss or lessening of the triceps surae jerk in organic sciatica. 2. in organic hemiplegia, failure of the platysma muscle to contract on the affected side in opening the mouth, whistling, etc. 3. see under *reflex.* 4. in organic hemiplegia, flexion of the thigh and lifting of the heel from the ground when the patient tries to sit up from a supine position with arms crossed upon his chest; this is repeated when the patient resumes the lying posture. 5. in organic paralysis, when the affected forearm is placed in supination, it turns over to pronation. **Beevor's s.,** 1. in functional paralysis, inability to inhibit the antagonistic muscles. 2. in paralysis of the lower parts of the recti abdominis muscles, there is upward excursion of the umbilicus. **Bergman's s.,** in urologic radiography, (a) the ureter is dilated immediately below a neoplasm, rather than collapsed as below an obstructing stone and (b) the ureteral catheter tends to coil in this dilated portion of the ureter. **Biernacki's s.,** analgesia of the ulnar nerve in paralytic dementia and tabes dorsalis. **Blumberg's s.,** pain on abrupt release of steady pressure (rebound tenderness) over the site of a suspected abdominal lesion, indicative of peritonitis. **Branham's s.,** bradycardia produced by digital closure of an artery proximal to an arteriovenous fistula. **Braxton Hicks s.,** see under *contraction.* **Broadbent's s.,** retraction on the left side of the back, near the eleventh and twelfth ribs, related to pericardial adhesion. **Brudzinski's s.,** 1. in meningitis, flexion of the neck usually causes flexion of the hip and knee. 2. in meningitis, on passive flexion of one lower limb, the contralateral limb shows a similar movement. **Cardarelli's s.,** transverse pulsation in the laryngotracheal tube in aneurysms and dilatation of the aortic arch. **Chaddock's s.,** see under *reflex.* **Chvostek's s., Chvostek-Weiss s.,** spasm of the facial muscles elicited by tapping the facial nerve in the region of the parotid gland; seen in tetany. **Cullen's s.,** bluish discoloration around the umbilicus sometimes associated with intraperitoneal hemorrhage, especially after rupture of the uterine tube in ectopic pregnancy; similar discoloration occurs in acute hemorrhagic pancreatitis. **Dalrymple's s.,** abnormal wideness of the palpebral opening in Graves' disease. **Delbet's s.,** in aneurysm of a limb's main artery, if nutrition of the part distal to the aneurysm is maintained despite absence of the pulse, collateral circulation is sufficient. **de Musset's s.,** Musset's s. **Erb's s.,** 1. increased electric irritability of motor nerves in tetany. 2. dullness in percussion over the manubrium sterni in acromegaly. **Ewart's s.,** 1. undue prominence of the sternal end of the first rib in certain cases of pericardial effusion. 2. bronchial breathing and dullness on percussion at the lower angle of the left scapula in pericardial effusion. **fabere s.,** see *Patrick's test.* **Friedreich's s.,** 1. diastolic collapse of the cervical veins due to adhesion of the pericardium. 2. lowering of the pitch of the

percussion note over an area of cavitation during forced inspiration. **Goodell's s.,** softening of the cervix and vagina; a sign of pregnancy. **Graefe's s.,** tardy or jerky downward movement of the upper eyelids when the gaze is directed downward; noted in thyrotoxicosis. **halo s.,** a halo effect produced in the roentgenogram of the fetal head between the subcutaneous fat and the cranium; said to be indicative of intrauterine death of the fetus. **harlequin s.,** reddening of the lower half of the laterally recumbent body and blanching of the upper half, due to temporary vasomotor disturbance in newborn infants. **Hegar's s.,** softening of the lower uterine segment; indicative of pregnancy. **Hicks' s.,** Braxton Hicks contractions. **Hoffmann's s.,** 1. increased mechanical irritability of the sensory nerves in tetany; the ulnar nerve is usually tested. 2. a sudden nipping of the nail of the index, middle, or ring finger produces flexion of the terminal phalanx of the thumb and of the second and third phalanx of some other finger. **Homans' s.,** discomfort behind the knee on forced dorsiflexion of the foot, due to thrombosis in the calf veins. **Hoover's s.,** 1. in the normal state or in true paralysis, when the supine patient presses the leg against the surface on which he is lying, the other leg will lift. 2. movement of the costal margins toward the midline in inspiration, occurring bilaterally in pulmonary emphysema and unilaterally in conditions causing flattening of the diaphragm. **Joffroy's s.,** in Graves' disease, absence of forehead wrinkling when the gaze is suddenly directed upward. **Kernig's s.,** in meningitis, inability to completely extend the leg when sitting or lying with the thigh flexed upon the abdomen; when supine, the leg can be easily and completely extended. **Klippel-Feil s.,** in pyramidal tract disease, flexion and adduction of the thumb when the flexed fingers are quickly extended by the examiner. **Ladin's s.,** softening of the medial anterior surface of the body of the uterus just above the junction of the body and cervix; indicative of pregnancy. **Lasègue's s.,** in sciatica, flexion of the hip is painful when the knee is extended, but painless when the knee is flexed. **Leri's s.,** absence of normal flexion of the elbow on passive flexion of the hand at the wrist of the affected side in hemiplegia. **Lhermitte's s.,** electric-like shocks spreading down the body on flexing the head forward; seen mainly in multiple sclerosis but also in compression and other cervical cord disorders. **Macewen's s.,** a more than normal resonant note on percussion of the skull behind the junction of the frontal, temporal, and parietal bones in internal hydrocephalus and cerebral abscess. **McMurray's s.,** occurrence of a cartilage click on manipulation of the knee; indicative of meniscal injury. **Möbius' s.,** in Graves' disease, inability to keep the eyes converged due to insufficiency of the internal recti muscles. **Musset's s.,** rhythmical jerking of the head in aortic aneurysm and aortic insufficiency. **Nikolsky's s.,** in pemphigus vulgaris and some other bullous diseases, the outer epidermis separates easily from the basal layer on exertion of firm sliding manual pressure. **Oli-**

ver's s., tracheal tugging; see *tugging.* **Queck-enstedt's s.,** when the veins in the neck are compressed on one or both sides, there is a rapid rise in the pressure of the cerebrospinal fluid of healthy persons, and this rise quickly disappears when compression ceases. In obstruction of the vertebral canal, the pressure of the cerebrospinal fluid is little or not at all affected. **Romberg's s.,** swaying of the body or falling when the eyes are closed while standing with the feet close together; observed in tabes dorsalis. **Rossolimo's s.,** see under *reflex.* **setting-sun s.,** downward deviation of the eyes so that each iris appears to "set" beneath the lower lid, with white sclera exposed between it and the upper lid; indicative of intracranial pressure or irritation of the brain stem. **Stellwag's s.,** infrequent or incomplete blinking, a sign of Graves' disease. **Tinel's s.,** a tingling sensation in the distal end of a limb when percussion is made over the site of a divided nerve. It indicates a partial lesion or the beginning regeneration of the nerve. **Trousseau's s.,** 1. see under *phenomenon.* 2. tache cérébrale. **vital s's,** the pulse, respiration, and temperature.

signa (sig′nah) [L.] mark, or write; abbreviated S. or sig. in prescriptions.

signature (-chur) that part of a prescription which gives directions as to the taking of the medicine.

Silastic (sĭ-las′tik) trademark for polymeric silicone substances having the properties of rubber; it is biologically inert and used in surgical prostheses.

silica (sil′ĭ-kah) silicon dioxide, SiO_2, occurring in various allotropic forms, some of which are used in dental materials.

silicoanthracosis (sil″ĭ-ko-an″thrah-ko′sis) silicosis combined with pneumoconiosis of coal workers.

silicon (sil′ĭ-kon) chemical element (*see table*), at. no. 14, symbol Si. **s. carbide,** a compound of silicon and carbon used in dentistry as an abrasive agent. **s. dioxide,** silica.

silicone (sil′ĭ-kōn) any organic compound in which all or part of the carbon has been replaced by silicon.

silicosiderosis (sil″ĭ-ko-sid″er-o′sis) pneumoconiosis in which the inhaled dust is that of silica and iron.

silicosis (sil″ĭ-ko′sis) pneumoconiosis due to inhalation of the dust of stone, sand, or flint containing silica, with formation of generalized nodular fibrotic changes in both lungs. **silicot′ic,** adj.

siliquose (sil′ĭ-kwōs) pertaining to or resembling a pod or husk.

silver (sil′ver) chemical element (*see table*), at. no. 47, symbol Ag. **s. nitrate,** $AgNO_3$, used as a local anti-infective, as in the prophylaxis of ophthalmia neonatorum. **s. nitrate, toughened,** a compound of silver nitrate, hydrochloric acid, sodium chloride, or potassium nitrate; used as a caustic, applied topically after being dipped in water. **s. protein,** silver made colloidal by the presence of, or combination with,

protein; an active germicide with a local irritant and astringent effect. **s. sulfadiazine,** the silver derivative of sulfadiazine, $C_{10}H_9AgN_4$-O_2S, having bactericidal activity against many gram-positive and gram-negative organisms, as well as being effective against yeasts; used as a topical anti-infective for the prevention and treatment of wound sepsis in patients with second and third degree burns.

simethicone (sĭ-meth′ĭ-kōn) an antiflatulent substance consisting of a mixture of dimethyl polysiloxanes and silica gel.

simul (sim′ul) [L.] at the same time as.

simulator (sim′u-la″tor) something that stimulates, such as an apparatus that simulates conditions that will be encountered in real life. **electrocardiographic s.,** device that produces simulations of electrocardiographic wave forms.

Simulium (sĭ-mu′le-um) a genus of biting gnats; some species are intermediate hosts of *Onchocerca volvulus.*

simultanagnosia (si″mul-tān″ag-no′se-ah) the inability to comprehend more than one element of a visual scene at the same time or to integrate the parts as a whole.

sinciput (sin′sĭ-put) the upper and front part of the head. **sincip′ital,** adj.

Sinequan (sin′ĕ-kwan) trademark for a preparation of doxepin hydrochloride.

sinew (sin′u) a tendon of a muscle. **weeping s.,** an encysted ganglion, chiefly on the back of the hand, containing synovial fluid.

singultus (sing-gul′tus) [L.] hiccup.

sinister (sin′is-ter) [L.] left; on the left side.

sinistr(o)- word element [L.], *left; left side.*

sinistrad (sin′is-trad) to or toward the left.

sinistral (sin′is-tral) 1. pertaining to the left side. 2. a left-handed person.

sinistrality (sin″is-tral′ĭ-te) the preferential use, in voluntary motor acts, of the left member of the major paired organs of the body, as ear, eye, hand, and foot.

sinistraural (sin″is-traw′ral) hearing better with the left ear.

sinistrocerebral (-ser′ĕ-bral) pertaining to or situated in the left cerebral hemisphere.

sinistrocular (sin″is-trok′u-ler) having the left eye dominant.

sinistrogyration (sin″is-tro-ji-ra′shun) a turning to the left.

sinistromanual (-man′u-al) left-handed.

sinistropedal (sin″is-trop′ah-dal) using the left foot in preference to the right.

sinistrotorsion (sin″is-tro-tor′shun) a twisting toward the left, as of the eye.

sinoatrial (si″no-a′tre-al) pertaining to the sinus venosus and the atrium of the heart.

sinobronchitis (-brong-ki′tis) chronic paranasal sinusitis with recurrent episodes of bronchitis.

sinopulmonary (-pul′mo-nār″e) involving the paranasal sinuses and the lungs.

sinuous (sin′u-us) bending in and out; winding.

sinus (si′nus) 1. a recess, cavity, or channel, as (*a*) one in bone or (*b*) a dilated channel for venous blood. 2. an abnormal channel or fistula, permitting escape of pus. **si'nusal,** adj. **air s.,** an air-containing space within a bone. **anal s's,** furrows, with pouchlike openings at the distal end, separating the rectal columns. **aortic s.,** a dilatation between the aortic wall and each of the semilunar cusps of the aortic valve; from two of these sinuses the coronary arteries originate. **carotid s.,** a dilatation of the proximal portion of the internal carotid or distal portion of the common carotid artery, containing in its wall pressoreceptors which are stimulated by changes in blood pressure. **cavernous s.,** an irregularly shaped venous channel between the layers of dura mater of the brain, one on either side of the body of the sphenoid bone and communicating across the midline; it contains the internal carotid artery and abducent nerve. **cerebral s.,** one of the ventricles of the brain. **cervical s.,** a temporary depression caudal to the embryonic hyoid arch, containing the succeeding branchial arches; it is overgrown by the hyoid arch and closes off as the cervical vesicle. **circular s.,** the venous channel encircling the hypophysis, formed by the two cavernous sinuses and the anterior and posterior intercavernous sinuses. **coccygeal s.,** a sinus or fistula just over or close to the tip of the coccyx. **coronary s.,** the terminal portion of the great cardiac vein, lying in the coronary sulcus between the left atrium and ventricle, and emptying into the right atrium. **cortical s's,** lymph sinuses in the cortex of a lymph node, which arise from the marginal sinuses and continue into the medullary sinuses. **dermal s.,** a congenital sinus tract extending from the surface of the body, between the bodies of two adjacent lumbar vertebrae, to the spinal canal. **ethmoidal s.,** that paranasal sinus consisting of the ethmoidal cells collectively, and communicating with the nasal meatuses. See Plate XVI. **frontal s.,** one of the paired paranasal sinuses in the frontal bone, each communicating with the middle meatus of the ipsilateral nasal cavity. See Plate XVI. **intercavernous s's,** channels connecting the two cavernous sinuses, one passing anterior and the other posterior to the infundibulum of the hypophysis. **lacteal s's, lactiferous s's,** enlargements of the lactiferous ducts just before they open on the mammary papilla. **lymphatic s's,** irregular, tortuous spaces within lymphoid tissue (nodes) through which lymph passes, to enter efferent lymphatic vessels. **marginal s's,** 1. see under *lake.* 2. bowl-shaped lymph sinuses separating the capsule from the cortical parenchyma, and from which lymph flows into the cortical sinuses. **maxillary s.,** one of the paired paranasal sinuses in the body of the maxilla on either side, and opening into the middle meatus of the ipsilateral nasal cavity. See Plate XVI. **medullary s's,** lymph sinuses in the medulla of a lymph node, which divide the lymphoid tissue into a number of medullary cords. **occipital s.,** a venous sinus between the layers of dura mater, passing upward along the midline of the cerebellum. **oral s.,** stomodeum. **paranasal s's,** mucosa-lined air cavities in bones of the skull, communicating with the nasal cavity and including ethmoidal, frontal, maxillary, and

sphenoidal sinuses. See Plate XVI. **petrosal s., inferior,** a venous channel arising from the cavernous sinus and draining into the internal jugular vein. **petrosal s., superior,** one arising from the cavernous sinus and draining into the transverse sinus. **pilonidal s.,** a suppurating sinus containing hair, occurring chiefly in the coccygeal region. **s. pocula'ris,** prostatic utricle. **prostatic s.,** the posterolateral recess between the seminal colliculus and the wall of the urethra. **s's of pulmonary trunk,** slight dilatations in the wall of the pulmonary trunk just above the pulmonary valve. **renal s.,** a recess in the substance of the kidney, occupied by the renal pelvis, calices, vessels, nerves, and fat. **sagittal s., inferior,** a small venous sinus of the dura mater, opening into the straight sinus. **sagittal s., superior,** a venous sinus of the dura mater which ends in the confluence of sinuses. **sigmoid s.,** a venous sinus of the dura mater on either side, continuous with the transverse sinus and draining into the internal jugular vein of the same side. **sphenoidal s.,** one of the paired paranasal sinuses in the body of the sphenoid bone and opening into the highest meatus of the ipsilateral nasal cavity. See Plate XVI. **sphenoparietal s.,** a venous sinus of the dura mater, draining into the anterior part of the cavernous sinus. **s's of spleen,** dilated venous channels in the substance of the spleen. **straight s.,** a venous sinus of the dura mater formed by junction of the great cerebral vein and inferior sagittal sinus, commonly ending in the confluence of sinuses. **tarsal s.,** a space between the calcaneus and talus. **tentorial s.,** straight s. **terminal s.,** a vein which encircles the vascular area in the blastoderm. **transverse s.,** 1. either of two large venous sinuses of the dura mater. 2. a passage behind the aorta and pulmonary trunk and in front of the atria. **tympanic s.,** a deep recess on the medial wall of the tympanic cavity. **urogenital s.,** an elongated sac formed by division of the cloaca in the early embryo, forming the female vestibule, urethra, and vagina and some of the male urethra. **uterine s's,** venous channels in the wall of the uterus in pregnancy. **s. of venae cavae,** the portion of the right atrium into which the inferior and the superior vena cava open. **venous s., s. veno'sus,** 1. the common venous receptacle in the embryonic midheart, attached to the posterior wall of the primitive atrium. 2. s. of venae cavae. **venous s's of dura mater,** large channels for venous blood forming an anastomosing system between the layers of the dura mater of the brain, receiving blood from the brain and draining into the veins of the scalp or deep veins at the base of the skull. **venous s. of sclera,** a branching, circumferential vessel in the internal scleral sulcus, a major component of the drainage pathway for aqueous humor.

sinusitis (si″nu-si'tis) inflammation of a sinus.

sinusoid (si'nu-soid) 1. resembling a sinus. 2. a form of terminal blood channel consisting of a large, irregular anastomosing vessel having a lining of reticuloendothelium and found in the liver, heart, spleen, pancreas, and the adrenal, parathyroid, carotid, and hemolymph glands.

sinusotomy (si″nu-sot′ah-me) incision of a sinus.

siphon (si′fun) a bent tube with two arms of unequal length, used to transfer liquids from a higher to a lower level by the force of atmospheric pressure.

siphonage (si′fun-ij) the use of the siphon, as in gastric lavage or in draining the bladder.

sirenomelus (si″ren-om′ah-lus) a fetus with fused legs and no feet.

-sis word element [Gr.], *state; condition.*

SISI short increment sensitivity index.

sister (sis′ter) the nurse in charge of a hospital ward (Great Britain).

sit(o)- word element [Gr.], *food.*

site (sīt) a place, position, or locus. **allosteric s.,** a site on an enzyme that binds a nonsubstrate molecule (allosteric effector) and effects the catalytic activity. **antigen-binding s., antigen-combining s.,** the region of the antibody molecule that binds to antigens. **binding s's,** those portions of an enzyme molecule that contain chemical groups on amino acid residues in a geometric configuration bonding particular compounds with relatively high affinity. **operator s.,** a site adjacent to the structural genes in the operon, where repressor molecules are bound, thereby inhibiting the transcription of the genes in the adjacent operon. **restriction s.,** a base sequence in a DNA segment recognized by a particular restriction endonuclease.

sitology (sit″e-ol′o-je, si-tol′o-je) dietetics.

sitomania (si″to-ma′ne-ah) 1. excessive hunger, or morbid craving for food. 2. periodic bulimia.

sitosterol (si-tos′ter-ol) any of a group of closely related plant sterols; a preparation of β-sitosterol and related sterols of plant origin (called *sitosterols*) is used as an anticholesterolemic agent.

β-sitosterolemia (si-tos″ter-ol-e′me-ah) the presence of excessive levels of plant sterols, especially β-sitosterol, in the blood.

sitotherapy (si″to-ther′ah-pe) dietetic treatment.

sitotropism (si-tot′rah-pizm) response of living cells to the presence of nutritive elements.

situs (si′tus), pl. *si′tus* [L.] site or position. **s. inver′sus vis′cerum,** lateral transposition of the viscera of the thorax and abdomen. **s. transver′sus,** s. inversus viscerum.

skatole (skat′ōl) a strong-smelling crystalline amine from human feces, produced by protein decomposition in the intestine and directly from tryptophan by decarboxylation.

skelalgia (skēl-al′je-ah) pain in the leg.

skeletization (skel″ĭ-te-za′shun) 1. extreme emaciation. 2. removal of soft parts from the skeleton.

skeletogenous (skel″ĭ-toj′ĭ-nus) producing skeletal structures or tissues.

skeleton (skel′ĭ-tĭn) the hard framework of the animal body, especially that of higher vertebrates; the bones of the body collectively. See Plate II. **skel′etal,** adj. **appendicular s.,** the bones of the limbs and supporting thoracic (pectoral) and pelvic girdles. **axial s.,** the bones of the body axis, including the skull, vertebral column, ribs, and sternum.

skenitis (skēn-i′tis) inflammation of the paraurethral ducts (Skene's glands).

skin (skin) the outer protective covering of the body, consisting of the corium (or dermis) and the epidermis. **alligator s.,** ichthyosis sauroderma. **elastic s.,** Ehlers-Danlos syndrome. **farmer's s.,** actinic elastosis. **lax s., loose s.,** cutis laxa. **marble s.,** cutis marmorata. **sailor's s.,** actinic elastosis.

skull (skul) the cranium; the bony framework of the head, composed of the cranial and facial bones. See *Table of Bones.*

S.L.E. systemic lupus erythematosus.

sleep (slēp) a period of rest for the body and mind, during which volition and consciousness are in partial or complete abeyance and bodily functions are partially suspended; also described as a behavioral state, with characteristic immobile posture and diminished but readily reversible sensitivity to external stimuli. **NREM s.,** non-rapid eye movement sleep; the deep, dreamless period of sleep during which the brain waves are slow and of high voltage, and autonomic activities, such as heart rate and blood pressure, are low and regular. **REM s.,** the period of sleep during which the brain waves are fast and of low voltage, and autonomic activities, such as heart rate and respiration, are irregular. This type of sleep is associated with dreaming, mild involuntary muscle jerks, and rapid eye movements (REM). It usually occurs three to four times each night at intervals of 80 to 120 minutes, each occurrence lasting from 5 minutes to more than an hour.

sleepwalking (slēp′wok″ing) somnambulism (1).

slide (slīd) a glass plate on which objects are placed for microscopic examination.

sling (sling) a bandage or suspensory for supporting a part.

slough (sluf) 1. necrotic tissue in the process of separating from viable portions of the body. 2. to shed or cast off.

sludge (sluj) a suspension of solid or semisolid particles in a fluid which itself may or may not be a truly viscous fluid.

sludging (sluj′ing) settling out of solid particles from solution. **s. of blood,** intravascular agglutination.

Sm chemical symbol, *samarium.*

smallpox (smawl′poks) variola; an acute, highly contagious, often fatal infectious disease, now eradicated worldwide by vaccination programs, caused by an orthopoxvirus and marked by fever and distinctive progressive skin eruptions.

smear (smēr) a specimen for microscopic study prepared by spreading the material across the slide. **Pap s., Papanicolaou s.,** see under *tests.*

smegma (smeg′mah) the secretion of sebaceous glands, especially the cheesy secretion, consisting principally of desquamated epithelial cells, found chiefly beneath the prepuce. **smegmat′ic,** adj.

Sn chemical symbol, *tin* (L. *stannum*).

snap (snap) a short, sharp sound. **opening s.,** a short, sharp sound in early diastole caused by movement of the mitral leaflet into the ventricle at the start of ventricular filling.

snare (snār) a wire loop for removing polyps and tumors by encircling them at the base and closing the loop.

sneeze (snēz) 1. to expel air forcibly and spasmodically through the nose and mouth. 2. an involuntary, sudden, violent, and audible expulsion of air through the mouth and nose.

snore (snōr) 1. rough, noisy breathing during sleep, due to vibration of the uvula and soft palate. 2. to produce such sounds during sleep.

snow (sno) a freezing or frozen mixture consisting of discrete particles or crystals. **carbon dioxide s.,** solid carbon dioxide formed by rapid evaporation of liquid carbon dioxide; it gives a temperature of about −110° F. (−79° C.), and is used as an escharotic in various skin diseases.

snowblindness (sno'blīnd-nes) see under *blindness.*

snuffles (snuf'lz) catarrhal discharge from the nasal mucous membrane in infants, generally in congenital syphilis.

SOAP a device for conceptualizing the process of recording the progress notes in the *problem-oriented record* (see under *record*): S indicates subjective data obtained from the patient and others close to him; O designates objective data obtained by observation, physical examination, diagnostic studies, etc.; A refers to assessment of the patient's status through analysis of the problem, possible interaction of the problems, and changes in the status of the problems; P designates the plan for patient care.

soap (sōp) any compound of one or more fatty acids, or their equivalents, with an alkali. Soap is detergent and is much employed in liniments, enemas, and in making pills. It is also a mild aperient, antacid, and antiseptic.

socialization (so"shal-ĭ-za'shun) the process by which society integrates the individual and the individual learns to behave in socially acceptable ways.

sociobiology (so"se-o-bi-ol'ah-je) the branch of theoretical biology which proposes that all animal (including human) behavior has a biological basis, which is controlled by the genes. **sociobiolog'ic, sociobiolog'ical,** adj.

sociogenic (-jen'ik) arising from or imposed by society.

sociology (so"se-ol'ah-je) the scientific study of social relationships and phenomena.

sociometry (so"se-om'ĕ-tre) the branch of sociology concerned with the measurement of human social behavior.

sociopathy (so"se-op'ah-the) antisocial personality disorder. **sociopath'ic,** adj.

sociotherapy (so"se-o-ther'ah-pe) any treatment emphasizing modification of the environment and improvement in interpersonal relationships rather than intrapsychic factors.

socket (sok'it) a hollow into which a corresponding part fits. **dry s.,** a condition sometimes occurring after tooth extraction, with exposure of bone, inflammation of an alveolar crypt, and severe pain. **tooth s's,** the dental alveoli.

soda (so'dah) a term loosely applied to sodium bicarbonate, sodium hydroxide, or sodium carbonate. **baking s.,** sodium bicarbonate. **s. lime,** calcium hydroxide with sodium or potassium hydroxide, or both; used as adsorbent of carbon dioxide in equipment for metabolism tests, inhalant anesthesia, or oxygen therapy.

sodium (so'de-um) chemical element (*see table*), at. no. 11, symbol Na; the chief cation of extracellular body fluids. For sodium salts not listed here, see under the acid or the active ingredient. **s. acetate,** a systemic and urinary alkalizer. **s. alginate,** a product derived from brown seaweeds, used in formulating various pharmaceutical preparations. **s. ascorbate,** an antiscorbutic vitamin for parenteral administration. **s. benzoate,** a white, odorless granular or crystalline powder, used as an antifungal agent and as a test of liver function. **s. bicarbonate,** $NaHCO_3$, used as a gastric and systemic antacid and to alkalinize urine; also used, in solution, for washing the nose, mouth, and vagina, as a cleansing enema, and as a dressing for minor burns. **s. biphosphate,** the monohydrate salt of phosphoric acid, used as a urinary acidifier. **s. bisulfite,** salt, $NaHSO_3$, used as an antioxidant in pharmaceuticals. **s. borate,** $Na_2B_4O_7$, used as an alkalizing agent in pharmaceuticals. **s. carbonate,** $Na_2CO_3 \cdot H_2O$, used as an alkalizing agent in pharmaceuticals, and has been used as a lotion or bath in the treatment of scaly skin and as a detergent. **s. chloride,** common salt, a white crystalline compound, a necessary constituent of the body and therefore of the diet; sometimes used parenterally in solution to replenish electrolytes in the body. **s. citrate,** a crystalline compound, largely used as an anticoagulant in blood for transfusion. **s. fluoride,** NaF, used in the fluoridation of water or applied locally to the teeth, in 2% solution, to reduce the incidence of dental caries. **s. glutamate,** the monosodium salt of L-glutamic acid; used in treatment of encephalopathies associated with liver disease. Also used to enhance the flavor of foods. **s. hydrate, s. hydroxide,** a strongly alkaline and caustic compound, NaOH, used as an alkalinizing agent in pharmaceuticals. **s. iodide,** NaI, used as a source of iodine, and also as an expectorant. **s. lauryl sulfate,** a surface active agent, $CH_3(CH_2)_{10}CH_2$-$OSONa$, used as a wetting agent, emulsifying aid, and detergent in various dermatologic and cosmetic preparations, and as a toothpaste ingredient. **s. metabisulfite,** an antioxidant, $Na_2S_2O_5$. **s. monofluorophosphate,** a dental caries prophylactic, Na_2PFO_3. **s. nitrite,** a compound used as an antidote in cyanide poisoning. **s. nitroprusside,** sodium nitroferricyanide, an antihypertensive, $Na_2[Fe(CN)_5NO]$, used in the treatment of hypertensive crisis and to produce controlled hypotension during surgery; also used as a reagent. **s. peroxide,** a white water-soluble powder, Na_2O_2, which liberates oxygen. **s. phosphate,** a cathartic, Na_2HPO_4 $7H_2O$. **s. polystyrene sulfonate,** an ion-exchange resin used for treatment of hyperpotassemia. **s. propionate,** a compound used in fungal infections. **s. salicylate,** an analgesic compound. **s. sulfate,** a hydrogogue cathartic, $Na_2SO_4 \cdot 10H_2O$; also used as a diuretic and sometimes applied topically to wounds in solution to relieve edema and pain of infected wounds. **s. tetradecyl sulfate,** a sclerosing agent, $C_{14}H_{29}NaSO_4$, used in solution for varicose veins that are not prolapsed or thrombosed. **s. thiosulfate,** a compound, $NaS_2O_3 \cdot 5H_2O$, used as an antidote (with s. nitrite) for cyanide poisoning, in the prophylaxis of ringworm (added to foot baths), and as a topical application in solution in tinea versicolor.

sodoku (so'do-koo) the spirillary form of rat-bite fever, caused by *Spirillum minor.*

sodomy (sod'o-me) anal intercourse; also used to denote bestiality and fellatio.

softening (sof'en-ing) the process of becoming soft; any morbid process of becoming soft, as of the brain or spinal cord.

sol (sol) a liquid colloidal solution.

sol. solution.

solar (so'ler) denoting the great sympathetic plexus and its principal ganglia (especially the celiac); so called because of their radiating nerves.

solation (so-la'shun) the liquefaction of a gel.

sole (sōl) the bottom of the foot.

soluble (sol'u-b'l) susceptible of being dissolved.

solubility (sol"u-bil'ĭ-te) quality of being soluble; susceptibility of being dissolved.

solum (so'lum), pl. *so'la* [L.] the bottom or lowest part.

solute (sol'ūt) the substance dissolved in solvent to form a solution.

solution (sah-loo'shun) 1. a homogeneous mixture of one or more substances (solutes) dispersed in a sufficient quantity of dissolving medium (solvent). 2. the process of dissolving. 3. a loosening or separation. **aluminum acetate s.,** a preparation of aluminum subacetate solution, glacial acetic acid, and water; applied topically to the skin as an astringent, and also used as a topical antiseptic and antipruritic in various skin diseases. **aluminum subacetate s.,** a solution of aluminum sulfate, acetic acid, precipitated calcium carbonate, and water; applied topically to the skin as an astringent, and also as an antiseptic and a wet dressing. **ammonia s.,** a colorless, transparent liquid of alkaline reaction containing either 9–10 gm. of ammonia in each 100 ml. (*diluted ammonia s.*), or 20–30% of ammonia (*strong ammonia s.*); the former is a pharmaceutic necessity, the latter a solvent and source of ammonia. **anisotonic s.,** one having an osmotic pressure differing from that of the standard of reference. **antiseptic s.,** a preparation of boric acid, thymol, chlorothymol, menthol, eucalyptol, methyl salicylate, thyme oil, and alcohol in purified water; used as an antibacterial. **aqueous s.,** one in which water is the solvent. **Benedict's s.,** a sodium citrate, sodium carbonate, and copper sulfate water solution; used to determine presence of glucose in urine. **buffer s.,** one which resists appreciable change in its hydrogen ion concentration when acid or alkali is added to it. **colloid s., colloidal s.,** a preparation consisting of minute particles of matter suspended in a solvent. **Dakin's s.,** dilute sodium hypochlorite s. **formaldehyde s.,** an aqueous solution containing not less than 37% formaldehyde; used as a disinfectant. **hyperbaric s.,** one having a greater specific gravity than a standard of reference. **hypertonic s.,** one having an osmotic pressure greater than that of a standard of reference. **hypobaric s.,** one having a specific gravity less than that of a standard of reference. **hypotonic s.,** one having an osmotic pressure less than that of a standard of reference. **iodine s.,** a solution prepared with purified water, each 100 ml. containing 1.8–2.2 gm. of iodine and 2.1–2.6 gm. of sodium iodide; a local anti-infective. **iodine s., strong,** a solution containing, in each 100 ml., 4.5–5.5 gm. of iodine and 9.5–10.5 gm. of potassium iodide; a source of iodine. **isobaric s.,** a solution having the same specific gravity as a standard of reference. **isotonic s.,** one having an osmotic pressure the same as that of a standard of reference. **Lugol's s.,** iodine solution, strong. **magnesium citrate s.,** a preparation of magnesium carbonate, anhydrous citric acid, with syrup, talc, lemon oil, and potassium bicarbonate in purified water; used as a cathartic. **molar s.,** a solution each liter of which contains 1 mole of the dissolved substance; designated 1 M. The concentration of other solutions may be expressed in relation to that of molar solutions as tenth-molar (0.1 M), etc. **normal s.,** a solution each liter of which contains 1 chemical equivalent of the dissolved substance; designated 1 N. **ophthalmic s.,** a sterile solution, free from foreign particles, for instillation into the eye. **physiological salt s., physiological sodium chloride s.,** an aqueous solution of sodium chloride having an osmolality similar to that of blood serum. **Randall's s.,** a solution consisting of the acetate, bicarbonate, and citrate salts of potassium; used especially in the treatment of potassium deficiency. **Ringer's s.,** see under *irrigation.* **saline s., salt s.,** a solution of sodium chloride, or common salt, in purified water. **saturated s.,** one containing all of the solute which can be held in solution by the solvent. **sclerosing s.,** one containing an irritant substance which will cause obliteration of a space, as the lumen of a varicose vein or the cavity of a hernial sac. **Shohl's s.,** a solution containing 140 gm. citric acid and 98 gm. hydrated crystalline salt of sodium citrate in distilled water to make 1000 ml.; used to correct electrolyte imbalance in the treatment of renal tubular acidosis. **sodium hypochlorite s.,** a solution containing 4–6% by weight of sodium hypochlorite; used to disinfect various utensils. For wound disinfection, *dilute sodium hypochlorite s.* (Dakin's s., or fluid), containing 0.45–0.50% sodium hypochloride, is used. **standard s.,** one which contains in each liter a definitely stated amount of reagent; usually expressed in terms of normality (equivalent weights of solute per liter of solution) or molarity (g.mol.wts. of solute per liter of solution). **supersaturated s.,** an unstable solution containing more of the solute than it can permanently hold. **volumetric s.,** one which contains a specific quantity of solvent per stated unit of volume.

solvent (sol'vent) 1. dissolving; effecting a solution. 2. a liquid that dissolves or is capable of dissolving; the component of a solution present in greater amount.

soma (so'mah) 1. the body as distinguished from the mind. 2. the body tissue as distinguished from the germ cells. 3. the cell body.

somasthenia (so″mas-the′ne-ah) bodily weakness with poor appetite and poor sleep.

somat(o)- word element [Gr.], *body.*

somatalgia (so″mah-tal′je-ah) bodily pain.

somatesthesia (so″mat-es-the′ze-ah) body consciousness or awareness.

somatic (so-mat′ik) 1. pertaining to or characteristic of the soma or body. 2. pertaining to the body wall in contrast to the viscera.

somatization (so″mah-tĭ-za′shun) the conversion of mental experiences or states into bodily symptoms.

somatochrome (so-mat′o-krōm) any neuron which has a well marked cell body completely surrounding the nucleus, its colorable protoplasm having a distinct contour; used also adjectively.

somatoform (so-mat′o-form) denoting psychogenic symptoms that resemble those of physical disease.

somatogenic (so″mah-to-jen′ik) originating in the body.

somatology (so″mah-tol′ah-je) the sum of what is known about the body; the study of anatomy and physiology.

somatomedin (so″mah-to-me′din) any of a group of peptides found in the liver and in plasma which mediate the effect of growth hormone (somatotropin) on cartilage.

somatometry (so″mah-tom′ĕ-tre) measurement of the body.

somatopagus (so″mah-top′ah-gus) a double fetus with trunks more or less fused.

somatopathy (so″mah-top′ah-the) a bodily disorder as distinguished from a mental one. **somatopath′ic,** adj.

somatoplasm (so-mat′o-plazm) the protoplasm of the body cells exclusive of the germ cells.

somatopleure (-plōōr) the embryonic body wall, formed by ectoderm and somatic mesoderm. **somatopleur′al,** adj.

somatopsychic (so″mah-to-si′kik) pertaining to both mind and body; denoting a physical disorder which produces mental symptoms.

somatopsychosis (-si-ko′sis) a mental disorder associated with a physical disease.

somatoscopy (so″mah-tos′kah-pe) examination of the body.

somatosexual (so″mah-to-sek′shoo-al) pertaining to both physical and sex characteristics, or to physical manifestations of sexual development.

somatostatin (-stat′in) a polypeptide elaborated primarily by the median eminence of the hypothalamus and by the delta cells of the islets of Langerhans; it inhibits release of thyrotropin,

somatotropin, and corticotropin by the adenohypophysis, of insulin and glucagon by the pancreas, of gastrin by the gastric mucosa, of secretin by the intestinal mucosa, and of renin by the kidney.

somatotherapy (-ther′ah-pe) biological treatment of mental disorders.

somatotopic (so″mah-to-top′ik) related to particular areas of the body; describing organization of motor area of the brain, control of the movement of different parts of the body being centered in specific regions of the cortex.

somatotrope (so-mat′o-trōp) somatotroph.

somatotroph (so-mat′o-trōf″) any of the cells of the adenohypophysis that secrete growth hormone.

somatotrophic (so″mah-to-trof′ik) somatotropic.

somatotropic (so″mah-to-trop′ik) 1. having an affinity for or attacking the body cells. 2. having a stimulating effect on nutrition and growth. 3. having the properties of somatotrophin.

somatotrophin (so″mah-to-tro′fin) growth hormone.

somatotropin (-tro′pin) growth hormone.

somatotype (so-mat′o-tīp) a particular type of body build.

somesthesia (so″mes-the′ze-ah) somatesthesia. **somesthet′ic,** adj.

somite (so′mīt) one of the paired, blocklike masses of mesoderm, arranged segmentally alongside the neural tube of the embryo, forming the vertebral column and segmental musculature.

somnambulism (som-nam′bu-lizm) sleepwalking; rising out of bed and walking about during an apparent state of sleep.

somnifacient (som″nĭ-fa′shint) hypnotic (1).

somniferous (som-nif′er-us) producing sleep.

somniloquism (som-nil′o-kwizm) talking in one's sleep.

somnolence (som′no-lens) sleepiness; also, unnatural drowsiness.

somnolentia (som″no-len′she-ah) 1. drowsiness, or somnolence. 2. sleep drunkenness; a condition of incomplete sleep with disorientation and excited or violent behavior.

sonication (son″ĭ-ka′shun) exposure to sound waves; disruption of bacteria by exposure to high-frequency sound waves.

sonitus (son′ĭ-tus) tinnitus aurium.

sonography (sah-nog′rah-fe) ultrasonography. **sonograph′ic,** adj.

sonolucent (so″no-loo″sent) in ultrasonography, permitting the passage of ultrasound waves without reflecting them back to their source (without giving off echoes).

sopor (so′por) deep or profound sleep.

soporific (sop″ah-rif′ik, so″pah-rif′ik) producing deep sleep; an agent that so acts.

soporous (so′per-us) associated with coma or profound sleep.

sorb (sorb) to attract and retain substances by absorption or adsorption.

sorbefacient (sōr″bah-fa′shint) 1. promoting absorption. 2. a sorbefacient agent.

sorbent (sor'bent) an agent that sorbs.

sorbic acid (sor'bik) a fungistat, CH₃- CH=CHCH=CHCOOH, used as an antimicrobial inhibitor in pharmaceuticals.

sorbitan (sor'bĭ-tan) any of the anhydrides of sorbitol, the fatty acids of which are surfactants; see also *polysorbate 80*.

sorbitol (sor'bĭ-tol) a crystalline alcohol, C₆H₈- (OH)₆, found in various berries and fruits; a pharmaceutical preparation is used as a flavoring agent and as an osmotic diuretic.

Sorbitrate (sor'bĭ-trāt) trademark for a preparation of isosorbide dinitrate.

sordes (sor'dēz) debris, especially the encrustations of food, epithelial matter, and bacteria that collect on the lips and teeth during a prolonged fever. **s. gas'tricae,** undigested food, mucus, etc., in the stomach.

sore (sor) 1. popularly, almost any lesion of the skin or mucous membranes. 2. painful. **bed s.,** decubitus ulcer. **canker s.,** recurrent aphthous stomatitis. **cold s.,** see *herpes simplex*. **desert s.,** a form of tropical ulcer occurring in desert areas of Africa, Australia, and the Near East.

sore throat (sor thrōt) see *laryngitis, pharyngitis,* and *tonsillitis*. **septic s. t., streptococcal s. t.,** severe sore throat occurring in epidemics, usually due to *Streptococcus pyogenes,* with intense local hyperemia with or without a grayish exudate and enlargement of the cervical lymph glands.

sorption (sorp'shun) the process or state of being sorbed; absorption or adsorption.

S.O.S. [L.] *si o'pus sit* (if necessary).

souffle (soo'f'l) a soft, blowing auscultatory sound. **cardiac s.,** any cardiac or vascular murmur of a blowing quality. **fetal s.,** murmur sometimes heard over the pregnant uterus, supposed to be due to compression of the umbilical cord. **funic s., funicular s.,** hissing souffle synchronous with fetal heart sounds, probably from the umbilical cord. **placental s.,** the sound supposed to be produced by the blood current in the placenta. **uterine s.,** a sound made by the blood within the arteries of the gravid uterus.

sound (sownd) 1. the effect produced on the organ of hearing by vibrations of the air or other medium. 2. mechanical radiant energy, the motion of particles of the material medium through which it travels being along the line of transmission (longitudinal); such energy, having frequency of 20–20,000 Hz, provides the stimulus for the subjective sensation of hearing. 3. an instrument to be introduced into a cavity to detect a foreign body or to dilate a stricture. 4. a noise, normal or abnormal, heard within the body. **ejection s's,** high-pitched clicking sounds heard very shortly after the first heart sound, attributed to sudden distention of a dilated pulmonary artery or aorta or to forceful opening of the pulmonic or aortic cusps. **friction s.,** one produced by the rubbing of two surfaces. **heart s's,** the sounds heard over the cardiac region, which are produced by the functioning of the heart. The *first,* occurring at the beginning of ventricular systole, is dull, firm, and prolonged, and is heard as a "lubb" sound;

the *second,* produced essentially by closure of the semilunar valves, is shorter and sharper than the first, and is heard as a "dupp" sound; the *third,* produced by vibrations of the ventricular walls when they are suddenly distended by the rush of blood from the atria, is weak, low-pitched, and dull, and is usually audible only in children and young adults; and the *fourth,* produced by atrial contraction and ventricular filling, is low-pitched and short, and is rarely audible in the normal heart. **hippocratic s.,** the succussion sound heard in pyopneumothorax or seropneumothorax. **Korotkoff s's,** sounds heard during auscultatory determination of blood pressure. **percussion s.,** any sound obtained by percussion. **respiratory s.,** any sound heard on auscultation over the respiratory tract. **succussion s's,** splashing sounds heard on succussion over a distended stomach or in hydropneumothorax. **to-and-fro s.,** a friction sound or murmur heard with both systole and diastole. **urethral s.,** a long, slender instrument for exploring and dilating the urethra. **white s.,** that produced by a mixture of all frequencies of mechanical vibration perceptible as sound.

space (spās) 1. a delimited area. 2. an actual or potential cavity of the body. **spa'tial,** adj. **apical s.,** the region between the wall of the alveolus and the apex of the root of a tooth. **arachnoid s.,** see *subarachnoid s.* and *subdural s.* **axillary s.,** the axilla. **Bowman's s.,** capsular s. **bregmatic s.,** the anterior fontanel. **capsular s.,** a narrow chalice-shaped cavity between the glomerular and capsular epithelium of the glomerular capsule of the kidney. **cartilage s's,** the spaces in hyaline cartilage containing the cartilage cells. **corneal s's,** the spaces between the lamellae of the substantia propria of the cornea containing corneal cells and interstitial fluid. **cupular s.,** the part of the attic above the malleus. **dead s's,** 1. the space remaining after incomplete closure of surgical or other wounds, permitting accumulation of blood or serum and resultant delay in healing. 2. in the respiratory tract: (1) *anatomical dead s.,* those portions, from the nose and mouth to the terminal bronchioles, not participating in oxygen–carbon dioxide exchange, and (2) *physiologic dead s.,* which reflects nonuniformity of ventilation and perfusion in the lung, is the anatomical dead space plus the space in the alveoli occupied by air that does not participate in oxygen–carbon dioxide exchange. **epidural s.,** the space between the dura mater and the lining of the vertebral canal. **episcleral s.,** the space between the bulbar fascia and the eyeball. **haversian s.,** see under *canal*. **iliocostal s.,** the area between the twelfth rib and the crest of the ilium. **intercostal s.,** the space between two adjacent ribs. **interglobular s's,** small irregular spaces on the outer surface of the dentin in the tooth root. **interpeduncular s.,** see under *fossa*. **interpleural s.,** mediastinum. **interproximal s.,** the space between the proximal surfaces of adjoining teeth. **intervillous s.,** the space of the placenta into which the chorionic villi project and through which the maternal blood circulates. **Kiernan's s's,** the triangular spaces bounded by invaginated Glisson's capsule between the liver lobules, containing the larger interlobular branches of the portal vein, hepatic artery, and hepatic duct. **lymph s.,** any space in tissue occupied by lymph. **Meckel's s.,** a recess in the dura mater which lodges the gasserian ganglion. **mediastinal s.,** mediastinum. **medullary s.,** the central cavity and the intervals between the trabeculae of bone which contain the marrow. **palmar s.,** a large fascial space in the hand, divided by a fibrous septum into a midpalmar and a thenar space. **parasinoidal s's,** lateral lacunae in the dura mater, along the superior sagittal sinus, which receive meningeal and diploic veins. **perforated s.,** see under *substance*. **periaxial s.,** a fluid-filled cavity surrounding the nuclear bag and myotubule regions of a muscle spindle. **perilymphatic s.,** the fluid-filled space separating the membranous from the osseous labyrinth. **perineal s's,** spaces on either side of the inferior fascia of the urogenital diaphragm, the *deep* between it and the superior fascia, the *superficial* between it and the superficial perineal fascia. **periplasmic s.,** a zone between the plasma membrane and the outer membrane of the cell wall of gram-negative bacteria. **perivascular s.,** a lymph space within the walls of an artery. **pneumatic s.,** a portion of bone occupied by air-containing cells, especially the spaces constituting the paranasal sinuses. **Poiseuille's s.,** that part of the lumen of a tube, at its periphery, where no flow of liquid occurs. **retroperitoneal s.,** the space between the peritoneum and the posterior abdominal wall. **retropharyngeal s.,** the space behind the pharynx, containing areolar tissue. **retropubic s., Retzius s.,** the areolar space bounded by the reflection of peritoneum, symphysis pubis, and bladder. **subarachnoid s.,** the space between the arachnoid and the pia mater. **subdural s.,** the space between the dura mater and the arachnoid. **subgingival s.,** gingival crevice. **subphrenic s.,** the space between the diaphragm and subjacent organs. **subumbilical s.,** a somewhat triangular space in the body cavity beneath the umbilicus. **Tenon's s.,** episcleral s. **thenar s.,** the palmar space lying between the middle metacarpal bone and the tendon of the flexor pollicis longus. **zonular s's,** the lymph-filled spaces between the fibers of the ciliary zonule.

sparganosis (spar″gah-no′sis) infection with the larvae (spargana) of any of several species of tapeworms, which invade the subcutaneous tissues, causing inflammation and fibrosis.

sparganum (spar-ga′num), pl. *sparga′na* [Gr.] the larval stage of certain tapeworms, especially of the genera *Diphyllobothrium* and *Spirometra*; see also *sparganosis*. Also, a genus name applied to such larvae, usually when the adult stage is unknown.

spasm (spazm) 1. a sudden, violent, involuntary muscular contraction. 2. a sudden transitory constriction of a passage, canal, or orifice. **bronchial s.,** spasmodic contraction of the muscular coat of the bronchial tubes, as occurs in asthma. **carpopedal s.,** spasm of the hand or foot, or of the thumbs and great toes, seen in tetany. **clonic s.,** spasm with rigidity followed immediately by relaxation. **cynic s.,** risus sardonicus. **facial s.,** tonic spasm of the muscles supplied by the facial nerve, involving the entire side of the face or confined to a limited area about the eye. **habit s.,** tic. **intention s.,** muscular spasm on attempting voluntary movement. **myopathic s.,** spasm accompanying disease of the muscles. **nodding s.,** chronic spasm of the sternocleidomastoid muscles, causing a nodding motion of the head. **saltatory s.,** clonic spasm of the muscles of the legs, producing a peculiar jumping or springing motion when standing. **tetanic s., tonic s.,** tetanus (2). **toxic s.,** spasm caused by a toxin.

spasmodic (spaz-mod′ik) of the nature of a spasm; occurring in spasms.

spasmolysis (spaz-mol′ĭ-sis) the arrest of spasm. **spasmolyt′ic,** adj.

spasmophilia (spaz″mo-fil′e-ah) abnormal tendency to spasm or convulsions.

spasmus (spaz′mus) [L.] spasm. **s. nu′tans,** nodding spasm.

spastic (spas′tik) 1. of the nature of or characterized by spasms. 2. hypertonic, so that the muscles are stiff and movements awkward. 3. a person exhibiting spasticity, such as occurs in spastic paralysis or in cerebral palsy.

spasticity (spas-tis′ĭ-te) a state of increased muscle tone, with heightened deep tendon reflexes.

spatium (spa′she-um), pl. *spa′tia* [L.] space.

spatula (spach′ŭ-lah) a wide, flat, blunt, usually flexible instrument of little thickness, used for spreading material on a smooth surface.

spatulate (spach′ŭ-lāt) 1. having a flat blunt end. 2. to mix or manipulate with a spatula.

spavin (spav′in) in general, an exostosis, usually medial, of the tarsus of equines, distal to the tibiotarsal articulation and often involving the metatarsals.

spay (spa) to remove the ovaries.

SPCA serum prothrombin conversion accelerator (blood coagulation Factor VII).

specialist (spesh′ah-list) a physician whose practice is limited to a particular branch of medicine or surgery, especially one who, by virtue of advanced training, is certified by a specialty board as being qualified to so limit his practice. **clinical nurse s., nurse s.,** see under *nurse*.

specialty (spesh′ul-te) the field of practice of a specialist.

speciation (spe″se-a′shun) the evolutionary formation of new species.

species (spe′shēz) a taxonomic category subordinate to a genus (or subgenus) and superior to a subspecies or variety. **type s.,** the original species from which the description of the genus is formulated.

species-specific (-spe-sif′ik) characteristic of a particular species; having a characteristic effect on, or interaction with, cells or tissues of members of a particular species; said of an antigen, drug, or infective agent.

specific (spe-sif′ik) 1. pertaining to a species. 2. produced by a single kind of microorganism. 3.

restricted in application, effect, etc., to a particular structure, function, etc. 4. a remedy specially indicated for any particular disease. 5. in immunology, pertaining to the special affinity of antigen for the corresponding antibody.

specificity (spes″ĭ-fis′ĭ-te) 1. the quality or state of being specific. 2. the probability that a person who does not have a disease will be correctly identified by a clinical test.

specimen (spes′ĭ-men) a small sample or part taken to show the nature of the whole, as a small quantity of urine for analysis, or a small fragment of tissue for microscopic study.

spectacles (spek′tah-k′ls) a pair of lenses in a frame to assist vision.

spectinomycin (spek″tĭ-no-mi′sin) an antibiotic derived from *Streptomyces spectabilis,* used in treatment of gonorrhea.

spectra (spek′trah) plural of *spectrum.*

spectral (spek′tral) pertaining to a spectrum; performed by means of a spectrum.

spectrin (spek′trin) a contractile protein attached to glycophorin at the cytoplasmic surface of the cell membrane of erythrocytes, considered to be important in the determination of red cell shape.

spectrometry (spek-trom′ĕ-tre) determination of the place of lines in a spectrum.

spectrophotometer (spek″tro-fo-tom′ĕ-ter) 1. an apparatus for measuring light sense by means of a spectrum. 2. an apparatus for determining quantity of coloring matter in solution by measurement of transmitted light.

spectroscope (spek′tro-skōp) an instrument for developing and analyzing spectra.

spectrum (spek′trum) a charted band of wavelengths of electromagnetic radiation obtained by refraction or diffraction; by extension, a measurable range of activity, as the range of bacteria affected by an antibiotic (*antibacterial* s.) or the complete range of manifestations of a disease. **absorption s.,** one obtained by passing radiation with a continuous spectrum through a selectively absorbing medium, showing spaces or dark lines for wavelengths for which the spectrum of the medium itself would be bright. **broad-s.,** effective against a wide range of microorganisms. **electromagnetic s.,** the range of electromagnetic energy from cosmic rays to electric waves, including gamma, x- and ultraviolet rays, visible light, and infrared waves, and radio waves. **fortification s.,** scintillating scotoma. **visible s.,** that portion of the range of wavelengths of electromagnetic vibrations (from 7700 to 3900 Å) which is capable of stimulating specialized sense organs and is perceptible as light.

speculum (spek′u-lum) an instrument for opening or distending a body orifice or cavity to permit visual inspection.

speech (spēch) the expression of thoughts and ideas by vocal sounds. **esophageal s.,** that produced by vibration of the column of air in the esophagus against the contracting cricopharyngeal sphincter; used after laryngectomy. **explosive s.,** loud, sudden enunciation, seen in certain brain diseases. **mirror s.,** a speech abnormality in the order of syllables in a sentence is reversed. **pressured s.,** rapid, accelerated, frenzied speech, which may exceed the ability of the vocal musculature to articulate or may be incoherent to the listener. **scanning s., staccato s.,** speech in which syllables of words are separated by noticeable pauses; seen in multiple sclerosis.

sperm (sperm) 1. semen. 2. spermatozoon.

spermatic (sper-mat′ik) pertaining to the semen; seminal.

spermatid (sper′mah-tid) a cell derived from a secondary spermatocyte by fission, and developing into a spermatozoon.

spermatitis (sper″mah-ti′tis) deferentitis.

spermat(o)-, sperm(o)- word element [Gr.], *seed;* specifically, the male germinative element.

spermatoblast (sper-mat′o-blast) spermatid.

spermatocele (-sēl) cystic distention of the epididymis or rete testis, containing spermatozoa.

spermatocelectomy (sper″mah-to-se-lek′tah-me) excision of a spermatocele.

spermatocidal (-si′d′l) spermicidal.

spermatocyst (sper-mat′o-sist) 1. a seminal vesicle. 2. spermatocele.

spermatocystectomy (sper″mah-to-sis-tek′tah-me) excision of a seminal vesicle.

spermatocystitis (-sis-ti′tis) seminal vesiculitis.

spermatocystotomy (-sis-tot′ah-me) incision of a seminal vesicle.

spermatocyte (sper-mat′o-sīt) a cell developed from a spermatogonium in spermatogenesis. **primary s.,** the original large cell into which a spermatogonium develops. **secondary s.,** a cell produced by meiotic division of the primary spermatocyte and which gives rise to spermatids.

spermatocytogenesis (sper″mah-to-si″to-jen′ĕ-sis) the first stage of formation of spermatozoa in which the spermatogonia develop into spermatocytes and then into spermatids.

spermatogenesis (-jen′ĕ-sis) the process of the formation of spermatozoa, including spermatocytogenesis and spermiogenesis.

spermatogenic (-jen′ik) producing semen or spermatozoa.

spermatogonium (-go′ne-um), pl. *spermatogo′nia* [Gr.] an undifferentiated male germ cell, originating in a seminal tubule and dividing into two spermatocytes.

spermatoid (sper′mah-toid) resembling semen.

spermatolysis (sper″mah-tol′ĭ-sis) destruction or dissolution of spermatozoa. **spermatolyt′ic,** adj.

spermatopathia (sper″mah-to-path′e-ah) abnormality of the semen.

spermatorrhea (-re′ah) involuntary escape of semen, without orgasm.

spermatoschesis (sper″mah-tos′kĕ-sis) suppression of the secretion of semen.

spermatozoicide (sper″mah-to-zo′ĭ-sīd) spermicide.

spermatozoon (-zo′on), pl. *spermatozo′a* [Gr.] a mature male germ cell, which impregnates the ovum in sexual reproduction. Spermatozoa, formed in the seminiferous tubules, are derived from spermatogonia, which first develop into spermatocytes; these in turn produce spermatids by meiosis, which then differentiate into spermatozoa. **spermatozo′al,** adj.

spermaturia (sper″mah-tu′re-ah) seminuria.

spermectomy (sper-mek′tah-me) excision of a portion of the spermatic cord.

spermicide (sper′mĭ-sīd) an agent destructive to spermatozoa. **spermici′dal,** adj.

spermiduct (-dukt) the ejaculatory duct and vas deferens together.

spermiogenesis (sper″me-o-jen′ĕ-sis) the second stage in the formation of spermatozoa, in which the spermatids transform into spermatozoa.

spermolith (sper′mo-lith) a stone in the spermatic duct.

spermoneuralgia (sper″mo-nōōr-al′je-ah) neuralgic pain in the spermatic cord.

spermophlebectasia (-fleb″ek-ta′ze-ah) varicose state of the spermatic veins.

sp.gr. specific gravity.

sphacelate (sfas′ah-lāt) to become gangrenous.

sphacelation (sfas″ah-la′shun) the formation of a sphacelus; mortification.

sphacelism (sfas′ah-lizm) sphacelation or necrosis; sloughing.

sphaceloderma (sfas″ah-lo-der′mah) gangrene of the skin.

sphacelus (sfas′ah-lus) a slough; a mass of gangrenous tissue. **sphac′elous,** adj.

sphenion (sfe′ne-on) the point at the sphenoid angle of the parietal bone.

sphen(o)- word element [Gr.], *wedge-shaped; sphenoid bone.*

sphenoid (sfe′noid) 1. wedge-shaped. 2. see *Table of Bones.* **sphenoi′dal,** adj.

sphenoiditis (sfe″noi-di′tis) inflammation of the sphenoid sinus.

sphenoidotomy (sfe″noi-dot′ah-me) incision of a sphenoid sinus.

sphere (sfēr) a ball or globe. **attraction s.,** centrosome. **segmentation s.,** 1. morula. 2. a blastomere.

spher(o)- word element [Gr.], *round; a sphere.*

spherocyte (sfēr′o-sīt) a small, globular, completely hemoglobinated erythrocyte without the usual central pallor characteristically found in hereditary spherocytosis but also in acquired hemolytic anemia. **spherocyt′ic,** adj.

spherocytosis (sfēr″o-si-to′sis) the presence of spherocytes in the blood. **hereditary s.,** a congenital hereditary form of hemolytic anemia characterized by spherocytosis, abnormal fragility of erythrocytes, jaundice, and splenomegaly.

spheroid (sfēr′oid) a spherelike body.

spheroidal (sfēr-oi′d′l) resembling a sphere.

spheroma (sfēr-o′mah) a globular tumor.

sphincter (sfingk′ter) a ringlike muscle which closes a natural orifice or passage. **anal s., s. a′ni,** see *sphincter muscle of anus (external and internal)* in *Table of Muscles.* **cardiac s.,** muscle fibers about the opening of the esophagus into the stomach. **gastroesophageal s.,** the terminal few centimeters of the esophagus,

which prevents reflux of gastric contents into the esophagus. **O'Beirne's s.,** a band of muscle at the junction of the sigmoid colon and rectum. **Oddi's s.,** the sheath of muscle fibers investing the associated bile and pancreatic passages as they traverse the wall of the duodenum. **pharyngoesophageal s.,** a region of higher muscular tone at the junction of the pharynx and esophagus, which is involved in movements of swallowing. **precapillary s.,** a smooth muscle fiber encircling a true capillary where it originates from the arterial capillary, which can open and close the capillary entrance. **pyloric s.,** a thickening of the muscular wall of the stomach around the opening into the duodenum.

sphincteral, sphincteric (sfingk′ter-al; sfingkter′ik) pertaining to a sphincter.

sphincteralgia (sfingk″ter-al′je-ah) pain in a sphincter muscle.

sphincterectomy (-ek′tah-me) excision of a sphincter.

sphincterismus (-iz′mus) spasm of a sphincter.

sphincteritis (-i′tis) inflammation of a sphincter.

sphincterolysis (-ol′ĭ-sis) surgical separation of the iris from the cornea in anterior synechia.

sphincteroplasty (sfingk′ter-o-plas″te) plastic reconstruction of a sphincter.

sphincterotomy (sfingk″ter-ot′ah-me) incision of a sphincter.

sphingolipid (sfing″go-lip′id) a lipid containing sphingosine (e.g., ceramides, sphingomyelins, gangliosides, and cerebrosides), occurring in high concentrations in the brain and other nerve tissue.

sphingolipidosis (-lip″ĭ-do′sis), pl. *sphingolipido′ses* [Gr.] a general designation applied to diseases characterized by abnormal storage of sphingolipids, such as Gaucher's disease, Niemann-Pick disease, generalized gangliosidosis, and Tay-Sachs disease.

sphingolipodystrophy (-lip″o-dis′trah-fe) any of a group of disorders of sphingolipid metabolism.

sphingomyelin (-mi′ĕ-lin) a group of phospholipids which on hydrolysis yield phosphoric acid, choline, sphingosine, and a fatty acid.

sphingosine (sfing′go-sin) a long-chain, monounsaturated aliphatic amino alcohol found in sphingolipids.

sphygmic (sfig′mik) pertaining to the pulse.

sphygm(o)- word element [Gr.], *the pulse.*

sphygmodynamometer (-di″nah-mom′ĕ-ter) an instrument for measuring the force of the pulse.

sphygmogram (sfig′mo-gram) a record or tracing made by a sphygmograph.

sphygmograph (-graf) apparatus for registering the movements, form, and force of the arterial pulse. **sphygmograph′ic,** adj.

sphygmoid (sfig′moid) resembling the pulse.

sphygmomanometer (sfig″mo-mah-nom′ĕ-ter) an instrument for measuring arterial blood pressure.

sphygmometer (sfig-mom'ĕ-ter) an instrument for measuring the pulse.

sphygmoscope (sfig'mo-skōp) a device for rendering the pulse beat visible.

sphygmotonometer (sfig''mo-to-nom'ĕ-ter) an instrument for measuring elasticity of arterial walls.

sphyrectomy (sfi-rek'tah-me) excision of the malleus.

sphyrotomy (sfi-rot'ah-me) division of the malleus.

spica (spi'kah) a figure-of-8 bandage, with turns crossing each other.

spicule (spik'ūl) a sharp, needle-like body.

spiculum (spik'u-lum), pl. *spic'ula* [L.] spicule.

spider (spi'der) 1. an arthropod of the class Arachnida. 2. a spider-like nevus. **arterial s.**, vascular s. **black widow s.**, a spider, *Latrodectus mactans*, whose bite causes severe poisoning. **vascular s.**, a telangiectasis caused by dilatation and ramification of superficial cutaneous arteries, appearing as a bright red central area with branching rays somewhat resembling a spider; commonly associated with pregnancy and liver disease.

spike (spīk) a sharp upward deflection in a curve or tracing, as on the encephalogram.

spina (spi'nah), pl. *spi'nae* [L.] a spine; in anatomy, a thornlike process or projection. **s. bif'ida**, a developmental anomaly marked by defective closure of the bony encasement of the spinal cord, through which the meninges may (*s. bif'ida cys'tica*) or may not (*s. bif'ida occul'ta*) protrude. **s. vento'sa**, dactylitis affecting mostly infants and young children, with enlargement of digits, caseation, sequestration, and sinus formation.

spinal (spi'n'l) pertaining to a spine or to the vertebral column.

spinalgia (spi-nal'je-ah) pain in the spinal region.

spinate (spi'nāt) having thorns; thorn-shaped.

spindle (spin'd'l) 1. the fusiform figure occurring during metaphase of cell division, composed of microtubules radiating from the centrioles and connecting to the chromosomes at their centromeres. 2. see *brain waves*. 3. muscle s. **Krukenberg's s.**, a spindle-shaped, brownish-red opacity of the cornea. **mitotic s.**, spindle (1). **muscle s.**, one of the mechanoreceptors arranged in parallel between the fibers of skeletal muscle, being the receptor of impulses responsible for the stretch reflex. **nuclear s.**, spindle (1). **tendon s.**, Golgi tendon organ. **urine s's**, spindle-shaped, urine-filled segments of the ureter due to incomplete occlusion of the ureter during peristalsis.

spine (spīn) 1. a slender, thornlike process of bone. 2. the vertebral column. **alar s., angular s.**, s. of sphenoid. **bamboo s.**, the ankylosed spine produced by rheumatoid spondylitis, so called from its roentgenographic appearance. **cleft s.**, spina bifida. **ischial s.**, a bony process projecting backward and medialward from the posterior border of the ischium. **mental s.**, any of the small projections (usually four) on the inner surface of the mandible, near the lower end of the midline, serving for attachment of the genioglossal and geniohyoid muscles. **nasal s., anterior,** the sharp anterosuperior projection at the anterior extremity of the nasal crest of the maxilla. **nasal s., posterior,** a sharp, backward-projecting bony spine forming the medial posterior angle of the horizontal part of the palatine bone. **neural s.,** the spinous process of a vertebra. **palatine s's,** laterally placed ridges on the lower surface of the maxillary part of the hard palate, separating the palatine sulci. **poker s.,** the ankylosed spine produced by rheumatoid spondylitis. **rigid s.,** poker s. **s. of scapula,** a triangular bony plate attached by one end to the back of the scapula. **sciatic s.,** ischial s. **s. of sphenoid,** the posterior and downward projection from the lower aspect of the great wing of the sphenoid bone. **s. of tibia,** a longitudinally elongated, raised and roughened area on the anterior crest of the tibia. **trochlear s.,** a bony spicule on the anteromedial part of the orbital surface of the frontal bone for attachment of the trochlea of the superior oblique muscle.

spinipetal (spi-nip'ĭ-t'l) conducting or moving toward the spinal cord.

spinnbarkeit (spin'bahr-kīt) [Ger.] the formation of a thread by mucus from the cervix uteri when spread onto a glass slide and drawn out by a coverglass; the time at which it can be drawn to the maximum length usually precedes or coincides with the time of ovulation.

spinobulbar (spi''no-bul'ber) pertaining to the spinal cord and medulla oblongata.

spinocerebellar (-ser''ĕ-bel'er) pertaining to the spinal cord and cerebellum.

spinous (spi'nus) pertaining to or like a spine.

spir(o)- 1. word element [Gr.], *coil; spiral.* 2. word element [L.], *breath; breathing.*

spiradenoma (spīr''ad-ah-no'mah) syringocystadenoma.

spiral (spi'ral) 1. winding like the thread of a screw. 2. a structure curving around a central point or axis. **Curschmann's s's,** coiled mucinous fibrils sometimes found in the sputum in bronchial asthma.

spireme (spi'rēm) the threadlike continuous or segmented figure formed by the chromosome material during prophase.

spirilla (spi-ril'ah) plural of *spirillum.*

spirillicidal (spi-ril''ĭ-si'dal) destroying spirilla.

spirillosis (spi''rĭ-lo'sis) a disease caused by presence of spirilla.

Spirillum (spi-ril'um) a genus of gram-negative bacteria, including one species, *S. mi'nus,* which is pathogenic for guinea pigs, rats, mice, and monkeys and is the cause of rat-bite fever (sodoku) in man.

spirillum (spi-ril'um), pl. *spiril'la* [L.] an organism of the genus *Spirillum.*

Spirochaeta (spi''ro-ke'tah) a genus of bacteria found in fresh- or sea-water slime, especially when hydrogen sulfide is present. Most bacteria formerly assigned to this genus have been assigned to other genera.

spirochete (spi''ro-kēt) 1. a spiral bacterium; any microorganism of the order Spirochaetales. 2.

an organism of the genus *Spirochaeta*. **spiroche′tal**, adj.

spirocheticide (spi″ro-ke′tĭ-sīd) an agent which destroys spirochetes. **spirochetici′dal**, adj.

spirochetolysis (-ke-tol′ĭ-sis) the destruction of spirochetes by lysis. **spirochetolyt′ic**, adj.

spirochetosis (-ke-to′sis) infection with spirochetes. **avian s., fowl s.,** a septicemic disease of fowl caused by *Borrelia anserina* and transmitted by the tick *Argas persicus*.

spirogram (spi′ro-gram) a tracing or graph of respiratory movements.

spirograph (-graf) an instrument for registering respiratory movements.

spiroid (spi′roid) resembling a spiral.

spirolactone (spi″ro-lak′tōn) a group of compounds capable of opposing the action of sodium-retaining steroids on renal transport of sodium and potassium.

spirometer (spi-rom′ĕ-ter) an instrument for measuring the air taken into and exhaled by the lungs.

Spirometra (spi″ro-met′rah) a genus of tapeworms parasitic in fish-eating cats, dogs, and birds; larval infection (sparganosis) in man is caused by ingestion of inadequately cooked fish.

spirometry (spi-rom′ĕ-tre) the measurement of the breathing capacity of the lungs. **spiromet′ric**, adj.

spironolactone (spēr″o-no-lak′tōn) one of the spirolactones, $C_{24}H_{32}O_4S$, an aldosterone inhibitor highly effective when given orally; used as a diuretic.

spissated (spis′āt-ed) inspissated.

splanchn(o)- word element [Gr.], *viscus (viscera); splanchnic nerve.*

splanchnectopia (splangk″nek-to′pe-ah) displacement of one or more viscera.

splanchnesthesia (splangk″nes-the′ze-ah) visceral sensation. **splanchnesthet′ic**, adj.

splanchnic (splangk′nik) pertaining to the viscera.

splanchnicectomy (splangk″nĭ-sek′tah-me) excision of part of the splanchnic nerve.

splanchnicotomy (-kot′ah-me) transection of the splanchnic nerve.

splanchnocele (splangk′no-sēl) hernial protrusion of a viscus.

splanchnocoele (splangk′no-sēl) that portion of the coelom from which the visceral cavities are formed.

splanchnodiastasis (splangk″no-di-as′tah-sis) displacement of a viscus or viscera.

splanchnography (splangk-nog′rah-fe) descriptive anatomy of the viscera.

splanchnolith (splangk′no-lith) intestinal calculus.

splanchnology (splangk-nol′ah-je) the scientific study of the viscera of the body; applied also to the body of knowledge relating thereto.

splanchnomegaly (splangk″no-meg′ah-le) enlargement of the viscus; visceromegaly.

splanchnopathy (splangk-nop′ah-the) any disease of the viscera.

splanchnopleure (splangk′no-ploŏr) the layer

formed by union of the splanchnic mesoderm with entoderm; from it are developed the muscles and the connective tissue of the digestive tube.

splanchnoptosis (splangk″nop-to′sis) prolapse or downward displacement of the viscera.

splanchnosclerosis (splangk″no-sklĕ-ro′sis) hardening of the viscera.

splanchnoskeleton (-skel′ĭ-tĭn) skeletal structures connected with the viscera.

splanchnotomy (splangk-not′ah-me) anatomy or dissection of the viscera.

splanchnotribe (splangk′no-trīb) an instrument for crushing the intestine to obliterate its lumen.

splayfoot (spla′foot) flatfoot; talipes valgus.

spleen (splēn) a large, glandlike organ situated in the upper left part of the abdominal cavity, lateral to the cardiac end of the stomach. Among its functions are the disintegration of erythrocytes and the setting free of hemoglobin, which the liver converts into bilirubin; the genesis of new erythrocytes during fetal life and in the newborn; serving as a blood reservoir; and production of lymphocytes and plasma cells. **accessory s.,** a connected or detached outlying portion, or exclave, of the spleen. **diffuse waxy s.,** amyloid degeneration of the spleen involving especially the coats of the venous sinuses and the reticulum of the organ. **floating s., movable s.,** one displaced and preternaturally movable. **sago s.,** one with amyloid degeneration, the malpighian corpuscles looking like grains of sand. **wandering s.,** floating s. **waxy s.,** a spleen affected with amyloid degeneration.

splen (splen) [Gr.] spleen.

splen(o)- word element [Gr.], *spleen.*

splenadenoma (splēn″ad-ah-no′mah) hyperplasia of the spleen pulp.

splenalgia (sple-nal′je-ah) pain in the spleen.

splenectomy (sple-nek′tah-me) excision of the spleen.

splenectopia, splenectopy (sple″nek-to′pe-ah; sple-nek′tah-pe) displacement of the spleen; floating spleen.

splenic (splen′ik) pertaining to the spleen.

splenitis (sple-ni′tis) inflammation of the spleen.

splenium (sple′ne-um) a compress or bandage; a bandlike structure. **s. cor′poris callo′si,** the posterior, rounded end of the callosum.

splenization (splen″ĭ-za′shun) the conversion of a tissue, as of the lung, into tissue resembling that of the spleen, due to engorgement and condensation.

splenocele (sple′no-sēl) hernia of the spleen.

splenocolic (sple″no-kol′ik) pertaining to the spleen and colon.

splenocyte (splen′o-sīt) the monocyte characteristic of splenic tissue.

splenography (sple-nog′rah-fe) 1. roentgenography of the spleen. 2. a description of the spleen.

splenohepatomegaly (sple″no-hep″ah-to-meg′ah-le) enlargement of spleen and liver.

splenoid (sple'noid) resembling the spleen.

splenolysin (sple-nol'ĭ-sin) a lysin which destroys spleen tissue.

splenolysis (sple-nol'ĭ-sis) destruction of splenic tissue.

splenoma (sple-no'mah) a splenic tumor.

splenomalacia (sple''no-mah-la'she-ah) abnormal softness of the spleen.

splenomedullary (-med'u-lār''e) of or pertaining to the spleen and bone marrow.

splenomegaly (-meg'ah-le) enlargement of the spleen. **congestive s.,** splenomegaly secondary to portal hypertension. **hemolytic s.,** that associated with hemolytic anemia.

splenomyelogenous (-mi''ĕ-loj'ĕ-nus) formed in the spleen and bone marrow.

splenopancreatic (sple''no-pan''kre-at'ik) pertaining to the spleen and pancreas.

splenopathy (sple-nop'ah-the) any disease of the spleen.

splenopexy (sple'no-pek''se) surgical fixation of the spleen.

splenopneumonia (splen''o-noo-mōn'yah) pneumonia attended with splenization of the lung.

splenoptosis (sple''nop-to'sis) downward displacement of the spleen.

splenorrhagia (sple''no-ra'je-ah) hemorrhage from the spleen.

splenorrhaphy (sple-nor'ah-fe) surgical repair of the spleen.

splenotomy (sple-not'ah-me) incision of the spleen.

splint (splint) 1. a rigid or flexible appliance for fixation of displaced or movable parts. 2. the act of fastening or confining with such an appliance. **airplane s.,** one which holds the splinted limb suspended in the air. **anchor s.,** one for fracture of the jaw, with metal loops fitting over the teeth and held together by a rod. **Angle's s.,** one for fracture of the mandible. **Balkan s.,** see under *frame.* **coaptation s's,** small splints adjusted about a fractured limb for the purpose of producing coaptation of fragments. **Denis Browne s.,** a splint consisting of a pair of metal foot splints joined by a cross bar; used in talipes equinovarus. **dynamic s.,** a supportive or protective apparatus which aids in initiation and performance of motion by the supported or adjacent parts. **functional s.,** dynamic s. **shin s's,** strain of the flexor digitorum longus muscle occurring in athletes, marked by pain along the shin bone. **Thomas s.,** a leg splint consisting of two rigid rods attached to an ovoid ring that fits around the thigh; it can be combined with other apparatus to provide traction.

splinting (splint'ing) 1. application of a splint, or treatment by use of a splint. 2. in dentistry, the application of a fixed restoration to join two or more teeth into a single rigid unit. 3. rigidity of muscles occurring as a means of avoiding pain caused by movement of the part.

splints (splints) a condition characterized by the development of exostoses on the rudimentary second or fourth metacarpal or metatarsal bone in the horse.

spodogenous (spo-doj'ĕ-nus) caused by accumulation of waste material in an organ.

spondyl(o)- word element [Gr.], *vertebra; vertebral column.*

spondylalgia (spon''dil-al'je-ah) pain in the vertebrae.

spondylarthritis (spon''dil-ar-thri'tis) arthritis of the spine.

spondylitic (spon''dil-it'ik) pertaining to or marked by spondylitis.

spondylitis (spon''dil-i'tis) inflammation of vertebrae. **s. ankylopoiet'ica, ankylosing s., s. defor'mans,** rheumatoid s. **Kümmell's s.,** see under *disease.* **Marie-Strümpell s.,** rheumatoid s. **rheumatoid s.,** rheumatoid arthritis of the spine, affecting young males predominantly and producing pain and stiffness as a result of inflammation of the sacroiliac, intervertebral, and costovertebral joints; it may progress to cause complete spinal and thoracic rigidity. **s. tuberculo'sa,** tuberculosis of the spine. **s. typho'sa,** that following typhoid fever.

spondylizema (spon''dil-ĭ-ze'mah) downward displacement of a vertebra because of destruction or softening of the one below it.

spondylocace (spon''dil-ok'ah-se) tuberculosis of the vertebrae.

spondylodymus (spon''dil-od'ĭ-mus) twin fetuses united by the vertebrae.

spondylodynia (spon''dil-o-din'e-ah) spondylalgia.

spondylolisthesis (-lis'the-sis) forward displacement of a vertebra over a lower segment, usually of the fourth or fifth lumbar vertebra due to a developmental defect in the pars interarticularis. **spondylolisthet'ic,** adj.

spondylolysis (spon''dil-ol'ĭ-sis) the breaking down of a vertebra.

spondylopathy (spon''dil-op'ah-the) any disease of the vertebrae.

spondylopyosis (spon''dil-o-pi-o'sis) suppuration of a vertebra.

spondyloschisis (spon''dil-os'kĭ-sis) congenital fissure of a vertebral arch; spina bifida.

spondylosis (spon''dil-o'sis) vertebral ankylosis; also, any degenerative changes in the spine. **spondylot'ic,** adj. **rhizomelic s.,** rheumatoid spondylitis.

spondylosyndesis (spon''dil-o-sin'dĕ-sis) surgical creation of ankylosis between contiguous vertebrae; spinal fusion.

sponge (spunj) a porous, absorbent mass, as a pad of gauze or cotton surrounded by gauze, or the elastic fibrous skeleton of certain species of marine animals. **gelatin s., absorbable,** a sterile, absorbable, water-insoluble, gelatin-base material, used as a local hemostatic.

spongi(o)- word element [L., Gr.], *sponge; spongelike.*

spongiform (spun'jĭ-form) resembling a sponge.

spongioblast (spun'je-o-blast'') 1. any of the embryonic epithelial cells developed about the neural tube, which become transformed, some into neuroglial and some into ependymal cells. 2. amacrine cell.

spongioblastoma (spun''je-o-blas-to'mah) a tumor containing spongioblasts; glioblastoma or gliosarcoma.

spongiocyte (spun′je-o-sīt″) 1. a neuroglia cell. 2. one of the cells with spongy vacuolated protoplasm in the adrenal cortex.

spongioid (spun′je-oid) resembling a sponge.

spongioplasm (spun′je-o-plazm″) 1. a network of fibrils pervading the cell substance; seen in histological specimens following the use of certain fixatives. 2. the granular material of an axon.

spongiosa (spon″je-o′sah) spongy; sometimes used alone to mean the spongy substance of bone (substantia spongiosa ossium).

spongiosaplasty (spon″je-o′sah-plas″te) autoplasty of the substantia spongiosa ossium to potentiate formation of new bone or to cover bone defects.

spongiosis (spun″je-o′sis) intercellular edema within the epidermis.

spongiositis (spun″je-o-si′tis) inflammation of the corpus spongiosum of the penis.

sporadic (spo-rad′ic) occurring singly; widely scattered; not epidemic or endemic.

sporangium (spo-ran′je-um), pl. *sporan′gia* [Gr.] any encystment containing spores or sporelike bodies, as in certain fungi.

spore (spor) 1. a refractile, oval body formed within bacteria, especially *Bacillus* and *Clostridium*, which is regarded as a resting stage during the life history of the cell, and is characterized by its resistance to environmental changes. 2. the reproductive element, produced sexually or asexually, of one of the lower organisms, such as protozoa, fungi, algae, etc.

sporicide (spor′ĭ-sīd) an agent which kills spores. **sporici′dal**, adj.

sporoagglutination (spor″o-ah-gloo″tĭ-na′shun) agglutination of spores in the diagnosis of sporotrichosis.

sporoblast (spor′o-blast) one of the bodies formed in the oocyst of the malarial parasite in the mosquito and from which the sporozoite later develops; also, similar stages in certain other sporozoa.

sporocyst (spor′o-sist) 1. any cyst or sac containing spores or reproductive cells. 2. a germinal saclike stage in the life cycle of digenetic trematodes, produced by metamorphosis of a miracidium and giving rise to rediae. 3. a stage in the life cycle of certain coccidian protozoa, contained within the oocyst, produced by a sporoblast, and giving rise to sporozoites.

sporogenic (spor″o-jen′ik) producing spores.

sporogony (spo-rog′o-ne) sporulation involving multiple fission of a sporont, resulting in the formation of sporocysts and sporozoites. **sporogon′ic**, adj.

sporont (spor′ont) a zygote of coccidian protozoa enclosed in an oocyst, which undergoes sporogony to produce sporoblasts.

sporoplasm (spor′o-plazm″) 1. the protoplasm of spores. 2. in certain protozoa, the central mass of cytoplasm that leaves the spores as an amebula to infect the host.

Sporothrix (-thriks) a genus of fungi, including

S. schenck′ii (see *sporotrichosis*), and *S. car′nis*, which causes formation of white mold on meat in cold storage.

sporotrichosis (spor″o-trĭ-ko′sis) a chronic fungal disease caused by *Sporothrix schenckii*, occurring in three forms: a cutaneous lymphatic form, a disseminated form, and a pulmonary form.

sporozoan (-zo′an) 1. pertaining to sporozoa. 2. any protozoan of the phyla Apicocomplexa, Acetospora, Microspora, and Myxozoa. Organisms in the last three phyla form spores; many of the Apicocomplexa do not.

sporozoite (-zo′īt) the motile, infective stage of certain protozoa that results from sporogony.

sporozoon (-zo′on), pl. *sporozo′a* [Gr.] sporozoan (2).

sport (sport) a mutation.

sporulation (spor″u-la′shun) formation of spores.

sporule (spor′ūl) a small spore.

spot (spot) a circumscribed area; a small blemish; a macula. **Bitot's s's**, foamy gray, triangular spots of keratinized epithelium on the conjunctiva, associated with vitamin A deficiency. **blind s.**, the area marking the site of entrance of the optic nerve on the retina; it is not sensitive to light. **café au lait s's** (kah-fa′o-la′) [Fr.], macules, of a distinctive light brown color, occurring in neurofibromatosis and Albright's syndrome. **cherry-red s.**, the choroid appearing as a red circular area surrounded by gray-white retina, as viewed through the fovea centralis in Tay-Sachs disease. **cold s.**, see *temperature s's*. **cotton-wool s's**, white or gray soft-edged opacities in the retina composed of cytoid bodies; seen in hypertensive retinopathy, lupus erythematosus, and numerous other conditions. **Forschheimer s's**, a fleeting exanthem consisting of discrete rose spots on the soft palate sometimes seen in rubella just prior to the onset of the skin rash. **germinal s.**, the nucleolus of the fertilized ovum. **hot s.**, 1. see *temperature s's*. 2. the sensitive area of a neuroma. 3. an area of increased density on an x-ray or thermographic film. **Koplik's s's**, irregular, bright red spots on the buccal and lingual mucosa, with tiny bluish-white specks in the center of each; seen in the prodromal stage of measles. **liver s's**, a lay term for brownish spots on the face, neck, or backs of the hands in many older people. **Mariotte's s.**, blind s. **milky s's**, aggregations of macrophages in the subserous connective tissue of the pleura and peritoneum. **mongolian s.**, a smooth, brown to grayish blue nevus, consisting of an excess of melanocytes, typically found at birth in the sacral region in Orientals and dark-skinned races; it usually disappears during childhood. **pain s's**, spots on the skin where alone the sense of pain can be produced by a stimulus. **rose s's**, an eruption of rose-colored spots on the abdomen and thighs during the first seven days of typhoid fever. **Roth's s's**, round or oval white spots sometimes seen in the retina early in the course of subacute bacterial endocarditis. **Soemmering's s.**, macula lutea. **Tardieu's s's**, spots of ecchymosis under the pleura after death by suffocation. **temperature s's,** spots on the skin normally anesthetic to pain and pressure but sensitive respectively to heat and cold. **yellow s.,** macula retinae.

sprain (sprān) a joint injury in which some of the fibers of a supporting ligament are ruptured but the continuity of the ligament remains intact.

sprue (sproo) 1. a chronic form of malabsorption syndrome, occurring in both tropical and nontropical forms. 2. in dentistry, the hole through which metal or other material is poured or forced into a mold. **nontropical s.,** celiac disease; a malabsorption syndrome precipitated by ingestion of gluten-containing foods and marked by diarrhea with bulky, frothy, fatty fetid stools, abdominal distention, weight loss, asthenia, deficiency of vitamins B, D, and K, and electrolyte depletion. **tropical s.,** a malabsorption syndrome occurring in the tropics and subtropics, marked by stomatitis, diarrhea, and anemia.

spur (sper) 1. a projecting body, as from a bone. 2. in dentistry, a piece of metal projecting from a plate, band, or other dental appliance. **calcaneal s.,** a bone excrescence on the lower surface of the calcaneus which frequently causes pain on walking.

sputum (spu'tum) matter ejected from the trachea, bronchi, and lungs, through the mouth. **s. cruen'tum,** bloody sputum. **nummular s.,** sputum in rounded disks, shaped somewhat like coins. **rusty s.,** sputum stained with blood or blood pigments.

squama (squa'mah), pl. *squa'mae* [L.] a scale, or thin, platelike structure. **squa'mate,** adj.

squame (skwām) a scale or scalelike mass.

squamo-occipital (skwa"mo-ok-sip'ĭ-t'l) pertaining to the squamous portion of the occipital bone.

squamoparietal, squamosoparietal (skwa"-mo-pah-ri'ah-t'l, skwa-mo"so-pah-ri'ah-t'l) pertaining to the squamous portion of the temporal bone and the parietal bone.

squamous (skwa'mus) scaly or platelike.

squatting (skwot'ing) a position with hips and knees flexed, the buttocks resting on the heels; sometimes adopted by the parturient at delivery or by children with certain types of cardiac defects.

squill (skwil) the fleshy inner scales of the bulb of the white variety of *Urginea maritima;* it contains several cardioactive glycosides. The red variety is used as a rat poison.

squint (skwint) strabismus.

Sr chemical symbol, *strontium.*

SRH somatotropin releasing hormone; see *growth hormone releasing hormone.*

SRS-A slow-reacting substance of anaphylaxis; see under *substance.*

ss. [L.] *se'mis* (one half).

stabile (sta'b'l, -bīl) stable; stationary; resistant to change; opposed to *labile.*

stadium (sta'de-um), pl. *sta'dia* [L.] stage. **s. decremen'ti,** the period of decrease of severity in a disease; the defervescence of fever. **s. incremen'ti,** the period of increase in the

intensity of a disease; the stage of development of fever.

staff (staf) 1. a wooden rod or rodlike structure. 2. a grooved director used as a guide for the knife in lithotomy. 3. the professional personnel of a hospital. 4. see under *cell.* **s. of Aesculapius,** the rod or staff with entwining snake, symbolic of the god of healing, official insignia of the American Medical Association. See also *caduceus.* **attending s.,** the corps of attending physicians and surgeons of a hospital. **consulting s.,** specialists associated with a hospital and acting in an advisory capacity to the attending staff. **house s.,** the resident physicians and surgeons of a hospital.

stage (stāj) 1. a definite period or distinct phase, as of development of a disease or of an organism. 2. the platform of a microscope on which the slide containing the object to be studied is placed. **algid s.,** a period marked by flickering pulse, subnormal temperature, and varied nervous symptoms. **amphibolic s.,** the stage of an infectious disease between the acme and decline in which the diagnosis is uncertain. **anal s.,** in psychoanalysis, the second stage of psychosexual development, occurring between the ages of 1 and 3 years, during which the infant's activities, interests, and concerns are on the anal zone; preceded by the oral stage, followed by the phallic stage. **cold s.,** the period of chill or rigor in a malarial paraoxysm. **first s.** (of labor), see *labor.* **fourth s.** (of labor), a name sometimes applied to the immediate postpartum period. **genital s.,** in psychoanalysis, the final stage in psychosexual development, occurring during puberty, during which the person can receive sexual gratification from genital-to-genital contact and is capable of a mature relationship with a member of the opposite sex; preceded by the latency stage. **hot s.,** period of pyrexia in a malarial paroxysm. **latency s.,** 1. the incubation period of any infectious disorder. 2. the quiescent period following an active period in certain infectious diseases, during which the pathogen lies dormant before again initiating signs of active disease. 3. in psychoanalysis, the period of relative quiescence in psychosexual development, lasting from age 5 to 6 years to adolescence, during which interest in persons of the opposite sex ceases; preceded by the phallic stage, followed by the genital stage. **oral s.,** in psychoanalysis, the earliest stage of psychosexual development, from birth to about 18 months, during which the infant's needs, expression, and pleasurable experiences center on the oral zone; followed by the anal stage. **phallic s.,** in psychoanalysis, the third stage of psychosexual development, lasting from age 2 or 3 years to 5 or 6 years, during which sexual interest, curiosity, and pleasurable experiences center on the penis in boys and the clitoris in girls; preceded by the anal stage, followed by the latency stage. **second s.** (of labor), see *labor.* **third s.** (of labor), see *labor.*

staggers (stag'erz) 1. gid. 2. a form of vertigo occurring in decompression sickness.

staging (stāj'ing) 1. the determination of distinct phases or periods in the course of a disease, the life history of an organism, or any biological process. 2. the classification of neoplasms according to the extent of the tumor. **TNM s.,** staging of tumors according to three basic components: primary tumor (T), regional nodes (N), and metastasis (M). Adscripts are used to denote size and degree of involvement; for example, 0 indicates undetectable, and 1, 2, 3, and 4 a progressive increase in size or involvement. Thus, a tumor may be described as T1, N2, M0.

stain (stān) 1. a substance used to impart color to tissues or cells, to facilitate microscopic study and identification. 2. an area of discoloration of the skin. **differential s.,** one which facilitates differentiation of various elements in a specimen. **Giemsa s.,** a solution containing azure II-eosin, azure II, glycerin, and methanol; used for staining protozoan parasites, such as trypanosomes, *Leishmania*, etc., and *Leptospira, Borrelia*, viral inclusion bodies, and *Rickettsia*. **Gram's s.,** a staining procedure in which microorganisms are stained with crystal violet, treated with strong iodine solution, decolorized with ethanol or ethanol-acetone, and counterstained with a contrasting dye; those retaining the stain are *gram-positive*, and those losing the stain but staining with the counterstain are *gram-negative*. **hematoxylin-eosin s.,** a mixture of hematoxylin in distilled water and aqueous eosin solution, employed universally for routine tissue examination. **metachromatic s.,** one which produces in certain elements colors different from that of the stain itself. **portwine s.,** nevus flammeus. **supravital s.,** a stain introduced in living tissue or cells that have been removed from the body. **tumor s.,** an area of increased density in a radiograph, due to collection of contrast material in distorted and abnormal vessels, prominent in the capillary and venous phase of arteriography, and presumed to indicate neoplasm. **vital s.,** a stain introduced into the living organism, and taken up selectively by various tissue or cellular elements. **Wright's s.,** a mixture of eosin and methylene blue, used for demonstrating blood cells and malarial parasites.

staining (stān'ing) 1. artificial coloration of a substance to facilitate examination of tissues, microorganisms, or other cells under the microscope. For various techniques, see under *stain*. 2. in dentistry, the modification of the color of a tooth or denture base.

stalagmometer (stal″ag-mom'ĕ-ter) an instrument for measuring surface tension by determining the exact number of drops in a given quantity of a liquid.

stalk (stawk) an elongated anatomical structure resembling a plant stalk. **allantoic s.,** the more slender tube interposed in most mammals between the urogenital sinus and allantoic sac. It is the precursor of the umbilical cord. **yolk s.,** a narrow tube connecting the yolk sac (umbilical vesicle) with the midgut of the early embryo.

stammering (stam'er-ing) a disorder of speech behavior marked by involuntary pauses in speech; sometimes used synonymously with stuttering, especially in Great Britain.

standstill (stand'stil″) cessation of activity, as of the heart (*cardiac s.*) or chest (*respiratory s.*).

stannic acid (stan'ik) a vitreous acid of tin, H_2SnO_3, forming stannates.

stannous (stan'us) containing tin as a bivalent element.

stannum (stan'um) [L.] tin (symbol Sn).

stanozolol (stan'o-zo-lol″) an androgenic anabolic steroid, $C_{21}H_{32}N_2O$, used especially to increase hemoglobin levels in some patients with aplastic anemia.

stapedectomy (sta″pĭ-dek'tah-me) excision of the stapes.

stapedial (stah-pe'de-al) pertaining to the stapes.

stapediotenotomy (stah-pe″de-o-tĕ-not'o-me) cutting of the tendon of the stapedius muscle.

stapediovestibular (-ves-tib'u-ler) pertaining to the stapes and vestibule.

stapes (sta'pēz) [L.] see *Table of Bones* and Plate XII.

staphyl(o)- word element [Gr.], *uvula; resembling a bunch of grapes; staphylococci.*

staphyledema (staf″il-ĕ-de'mah) edema of the uvula.

staphyline (staf'ĭ-līn) 1. pertaining to the uvula. 2. shaped like a bunch of grapes.

staphylitis (staf″ĭ-li'tis) uvulitis.

staphylococcemia (staf″ĭ-lo-kok-se'me-ah) staphylococci in the blood.

Staphylococcus (-kok'us) a genus of gram-positive bacteria (family Micrococcaceae) that are potential pathogens, causing local lesions and serious opportunistic infections; it includes *S. au'reus*, a pathogenic species that causes serious suppurative infections and systemic disease and whose toxins cause food poisoning and toxic shock, *S. epider'midis*, which is commonly found on normal skin and includes many pathogenic strains, and *S. saprophyt'icus*, a usually nonpathogenic form that sometimes causes urinary tract infections.

staphylococcus (-kok'us), pl. *staphylococ'ci* [Gr.] any organism of the genus *Staphylococcus*. **staphylococ'cal, staphylococ'cic,** adj.

staphyloderma (-der'mah) pyogenic skin infection by staphylococci.

staphylodialysis (-di-al'ĭ-sis) relaxation of the uvula.

staphylolysin (staf″ĭ-lol'ĭ-sin) a hemolysin produced by staphylococci.

staphyloma (staf″ĭ-lo'mah) protrusion of the sclera or cornea, usually lined with uveal tissue, due to inflammation. **staphylom'atous,** adj. **anterior s.,** staphyloma in the anterior part of the eye. **corneal s.,** 1. bulging of the cornea with adherent uveal tissue. 2. one formed by protrusion of the iris through a corneal wound. **posterior s.,** backward bulging of the sclera at the posterior pole of the eye. **scleral s.,** protrusion of the contents of the eyeball where the sclera has become thinned.

staphyloncus (staf″ĭ-long'kus) a tumor or swelling of the uvula.

staphyloplasty (staf'ĭ-lo-plas″te) plastic repair of the soft palate and uvula.

staphyloptosia (staf″ĭ-lop-to-se-ah) elongation of the uvula.

staphylorrhaphy (staf″ĭ-lor′ah-fe) surgical correction of a midline cleft in the uvula and soft palate.

staphyloschisis (staf″ĭ-los′kĭ-sis) fissure of the uvula and soft palate.

staphylotomy (staf″ĭ-lot′ah-me) 1. incision of the uvula. 2. excision of a staphyloma.

starch (starch) 1. any of a group of polysaccharides of the general formula, $(C_6H_{10}O_5)_n$; it is the chief storage form of carbohydrates in plants. 2. granules separated from mature corn, wheat, or potatoes; used as a dusting powder and tablet disintegrant in pharmaceuticals.

stasis (sta′sis) 1. a stoppage or diminution of flow, as of blood or other body fluid. 2. a state of equilibrium among opposing forces. **intestinal s.**, impairment of the normal passage of intestinal contents, due to mechanical obstruction or to impaired intestinal motility. **urinary s.**, stoppage of the flow or discharge of urine, at any level of the urinary tract. **venous s.**, impairment or cessation of venous flow.

-stasis word element [Gr.], *maintenance of (or maintaining) a constant level; preventing increase or multiplication.* **-stat′ic**, adj.

stat. [L.] *sta′tim* (at once).

state (stāt) condition or situation. **alpha s.**, the state of relaxation and peaceful awakefulness, associated with prominent alpha brain wave activity. **persistent vegetative s.**, a condition of profound nonresponsiveness in the wakeful state caused by brain damage at any level and characterized by a nonfunctioning cerebral cortex, absence of response to the external environment, akinesia, mutism, and inability to signal. **refractory s.**, a condition of subnormal excitability of muscle and nerve following excitation. **resting s.**, the physiologic condition achieved by complete bed rest for at least one hour. **steady s.**, dynamic equilibrium.

statim (sta′tim) [L.] at once.

station (sta′shun) 1. the position assumed in standing; the manner of standing; in ataxic conditions it is sometimes pathognomonic. 2. the location of the presenting part of the fetus in the birth canal, designated as –5 to –1 according to the number of centimeters the part is above an imaginary plane passing through the ischial spines, 0 when at the plane, and +1 to +5 according to the number of centimeters the part is below the plane.

statistics (stah-tis′tiks) 1. a collection of numerical data. 2. a distinct scientific method that aims at solving real life problems by the use of the theory of probability. **vital s.**, the data collected by government bodies by the registration of all births, deaths, fetal deaths, marriages, and divorces.

statoacoustic (stat″o-ah-koo′stik) pertaining to balance and hearing.

statoconia (-ko′ne-ah), sing. *statoco′nium* [Gr.] minute calciferous granules within the gelatinous membrane surrounding the acoustic maculae.

statolith (stat′o-lith) 1. a granule of the statoco-

nia. 2. a solid or semisolid body occurring in the labyrinth of animals.

statometer (stah-tom′ĕ-ter) an apparatus for measuring the degree of exophthalmos.

stature (stach′ur) the height or tallness of a person standing. **stat′ural**, adj.

status (sta′tus) [L.] condition or state. **s. asthmat′icus**, a particularly severe asthmatic attack, usually requiring hospitalization, that does not respond adequately to ordinary therapeutic measures. **s. epilep′ticus**, rapid succession of epileptic spasms without intervening periods of consciousness. **s. lymphat′icus**, **s. thymicolymphat′icus**, lymphatism. **s. verruco′sus**, a wartlike appearance of the cerebral cortex, produced by disorderly arrangement of the neuroblasts so that the formation of fissures and sulci is irregular and unpredictable.

staxis (stak′sis) hemorrhage.

stear(o)- word element [Gr.], *fat.*

stearate (ste′ah-rāt) the ionic form of stearic acid; also, any compound of stearic acid.

stearic acid (ste′ah-rik) a saturated fatty acid, $C_{17}H_{35}COOH$, from animal and vegetable fats, used in pharmaceuticals, ointments, soaps, and suppositories.

steat(o)- word element [Gr.], *fat; oil.*

steatitis (ste″ah-ti′tis) inflammation of adipose tissue.

steatocystoma (ste″ah-to-sis-to′mah) an epithelial cyst. **s. mul′tiplex**, an autosomal dominant disorder, affecting men more often than women, characterized by the presence of multiple epidermal cysts containing an oily liquid, abortive hair follicles, lanugo hair, and sebaceous apocrine, or eccrine, glands.

steatogenous (ste″ah-toj′ĕ-nus) lipogenic.

steatolysis (ste″ah-tol′ĭ-sis) the emulsification of fats preparatory to absorption. **steatolyt′ic**, adj.

steatoma (ste″ah-to′mah), pl. *steatomata* or *steatomas.* 1. a lipoma. 2. a fatty mass retained within a sebaceous gland.

steatomatosis (ste″ah-to″mah-to′sis) 1. the presence of numerous sebaceous cysts. 2. steatocystoma multiplex.

steatonecrosis (-nĕ-kro′sis) fat necrosis.

steatopygia (ste″ah-to-pij′e-ah) excessive fatness of the buttocks. **steatop′ygous**, adj.

steatorrhea (-re′ah) excess fat in feces.

steatosis (ste″ah-to′sis) fatty degeneration.

stegnosis (steg-no′sis) constriction; stenosis. **stegnot′ic**, adj.

Stelazine (stel′ah-zēn) trademark for preparations of trifluoperazine hydrochloride.

stellate (stel′āt) star-shaped; arranged in rosettes.

stellectomy (stĕ-lek′tah-me) excision of a portion of the stellate ganglion.

stem (stem) a supporting structure comparable to the stalk of a plant. **brain s.**, see under *B.*

sten(o)- word element [Gr.], *narrow; contracted; constriction.*

stenochoria (-kor′e-ah) stenosis.

stenocoriasis (-kah-ri′ah-sis) contraction of the pupil.

stenopeic (-pe′ik) having a narrow opening or slit.

stenosed (stĕ-nōst′, stĕ-nōzd′) narrowed; constricted.

stenosis (stĕ-no′sis) narrowing or contraction of a body passage or opening. **aortic s.,** a narrowing of the aortic orifice of the heart or of the aorta itself. **idiopathic hypertrophic subaortic s.,** a cardiomyopathy of unknown cause, in which the left ventricle is hypertrophied and the cavity is small; it is marked by obstruction to left ventricular outflow. **mitral s.,** a narrowing of the left atrioventricular orifice. **pulmonary s.,** narrowing of the opening between the pulmonary artery and the right ventricle. **pyloric s.,** obstruction of the pyloric orifice of the stomach; it may be congenital or acquired. **tricuspid s.,** narrowing or stricture of the tricuspid orifice of the heart.

stenothermal, stenothermic (-ther′mal; -ther′mik) developing only within a narrow range of temperature; said of bacteria.

stenothorax (-thor′aks) abnormal narrowness of the chest.

stenotic (stĕ-not′ik) marked by stenosis; abnormally narrowed.

stent (stent) a device or mold of a suitable material, used to hold a skin graft in place or to support tubular structures that are being anastomosed.

stephanion (ste-fa′ne-on), pl. *stepha′nia* [Gr.] intersection of the superior temporal line and the coronal suture. **stepha′nial,** adj.

sterc(o)- word element [L.], *feces.*

stercobilin (ster′ko-bi′lin) a bile pigment derivative formed by air oxidation of stercobilinogen; it is a brown-orange-red pigmentation contributing to the color of feces and urine.

stercobilinogen (-bi-lin′o-jen) a bilirubin metabolite and precursor of stercobilin, formed by reduction of urobilinogen.

stercolith (ster′ko-lith) fecalith.

stercoraceous (ster′ko-ra′shus) consisting of feces.

stercoroma (-ro′mah) a tumor-like mass of fecal matter in the rectum.

stercus (ster′kus) [L.] dung or feces. **ster′coral, ster′corous,** adj.

stereo- word element [Gr.], *solid; three dimensional; firmly established.*

stereoarthrolysis (ster″e-o-ar-throl′ĭ-sis) operative formation of a movable new joint in cases of bony ankylosis.

stereoauscultation (-aus″kul-ta′shun) auscultation with two stethoscopes, on different parts of the chest.

stereocampimeter (-kam-pim′ĕ-ter) an instrument for studying unilateral central scotomas and central retinal defects.

stereochemistry (-kem′is-tre) the branch of chemistry treating of the space relations of atoms in molecules. **stereochem′ical,** adj.

stereocinefluorography (-sin″ĕ-floor‴-og′rah-fe) recording by motion picture camera of images observed by stereoscopic fluoroscopy.

stereoencephalotome (-en-sef′ah-lah-tōm″) a guiding instrument used in stereoencephalotomy.

stereoencephalotomy (-en-sef″ah-lot′ah-me) stereotaxic surgery.

stereognosis (ster″e-og-no′sis) 1. the faculty of perceiving and recognizing the form and nature of objects by the sense of touch. 2. perception by the senses of the solidity of objects. **stereognos′tic,** adj.

stereoisomer (ster″e-o-i′so-mer) one of a group of compounds having a stereoisomeric relationship.

stereoisomerism (-i-som′er-izm) isomerism in which the isomers have the same structure (same linkages between atoms) but different spatial arrangements of the atoms. **stereoisomer′ic,** adj.

Stereo-orthopter (-or-thop′ter) trademark for a mirror-reflecting instrument for correcting strabismus.

stereoscope (ster′e-o-skōp″) an instrument for producing the appearance of solidity and relief by combining the images of two similar pictures of an object.

stereoscopic (ster″e-o-skop′ik) having the effect of a stereoscope; giving objects a solid or three-dimensional appearance.

stereotaxic (-tak′sik) 1. pertaining to or characterized by precise positioning in space; said especially of discrete areas of the brain that control specific functions. 2. pertaining to or exhibiting stereotaxis.

stereotaxis (-tak′sis) taxis in response to contact with a solid or rigid surface.

stereotropism (ster″e-ot′rah-pizm) tropism in response to contact with a solid or rigid surface. **stereotrop′ic,** adj.

stereotypy (ster′e-o-ti″pe) persistent repetition of senseless acts or words.

steric (ster′ik) pertaining to the arrangement of atoms in space; pertaining to stereochemistry.

sterilant (ster′ĭ-lant) a sterilizing agent, i.e., an agent that destroys microorganisms.

sterile (ster′il) 1. not fertile; barren; not producing young. 2. aseptic; not producing microorganisms; free from living microorganisms.

sterilization (ster″ĭ-lĭ-za′shun) 1. the complete elimination or destruction of all living microorganisms. 2. any procedure by which an individual is made incapable of reproduction.

sterilizer (ster′ĭ-līz″er) an apparatus for the destruction of microorganisms.

stern(o)- word element [Gr.], *sternum.*

sternal (ster′n'l) of or relating to the sternum.

sternalgia (ster-nal′je-ah) pain in the sternum.

sternebra (ster′nĕ-brah), pl. *ster′nebrae* [L.] any of the segments of the sternum in early life, which later fuse to form the body of the sternum.

sternoclavicular (ster″no-klah-vik′u-ler) pertaining to the sternum and clavicle.

sternocleidomastoid (-kli″do-mas′toid) pertaining to the sternum, clavicle, and mastoid process.

sternocostal (-kos′t'l) pertaining to the sternum and ribs.

sternodymus (ster-nod′ĭ-mus) conjoined twins united at the anterior chest wall.

sternohyoid (ster″no-hi′oid) pertaining to the sternum and hyoid bone.

sternoid (ster′noid) resembling the sternum.

sternomastoid (ster″no-mas′toid) pertaining to the sternum and mastoid process.

sternopagus (ster-nop′ah-gus) sternodymus.

sternopericardial (ster″no-per″ĭ-kar′de-al) pertaining to the sternum and pericardium.

sternoschisis (ster-nos′kĭ-sis) congenital fissure of the sternum.

sternothyroid (ster″no-thy′roid) pertaining to the sternum and thyroid cartilage or gland.

sternotomy (ster-not′ah-me) the operation of cutting through the sternum.

sternum (ster′num) [L.] see *Table of Bones.*

sternutatory (ster-nu′tah-tor″e) 1. causing sneezing. 2. an agent that causes sneezing.

steroid (ster′oid, ste′roid) any of a group of polycyclic compounds having a 17-carbon-atom ring system as a nucleus, including progesterone, adrenocortical and gonadal hormones, bile acids, sterols, toad poisons, and some carcinogenic hydrocarbons. **anabolic s.,** any of a group of synthetic derivatives of testosterone, having pronounced anabolic properties and relatively weak androgenic properties, which are used clinically mainly to promote growth and repair of body tissues in senility, debilitating illness, and convalescence.

steroidogenesis (stĕ-roi″do-jen′ĕ-sis) production of steroids, as by the adrenal glands. **steroidogen′ic,** adj.

sterol (ster′ol, ste′rol) a steroid containing the 17-carbon-atom steroid nucleus, with an 8- to 10-carbon-atom side chain and at least one alcoholic group; sterols have lipid-like solubility. Examples are cholesterol and ergosterol.

stertor (ster′ter) the act of snoring; sonorous respiration. **ster′torous,** adj.

steth(o)- word element [Gr.], *chest.*

stethalgia (steth-al′je-ah) pain in the chest.

stethogoniometer (steth″o-go″ne-om′ĕ-ter) apparatus for measuring curvature of the chest.

stethometer (steth-om′ĕ-ter) an instrument for measuring the circular dimension or expansion of the chest.

stethoscope (steth′o-skōp) an instrument for performing mediate auscultation. **stethoscop′ic,** adj.

stethoscopy (steth-os′kah-pe) examination with the stethoscope.

stethospasm (steth′o-spazm) spasm of the chest muscles.

STH somatotropic hormone.

sthenia (sthe′ne-ah) a condition of strength and activity.

sthenic (sthen′ik) active; strong.

stibialism (stib′e-ah-lizm″) antimonial poisoning.

stibium (stib′e-um) [L.] antimony (symbol Sb).

stibocaptate (stib″o-kap′tāt) a trivalent antimony compound, $C_{12}H_6Na_6O_{12}Sb_2$, used as an antischistosomal.

stichochrome (stik′o-krōm) any neuron having the stainable substance arranged in more or less regular layers.

stigma (stig′mah), pl. *stig′mas, stig′mata* [Gr.] 1. any mental or physical mark or peculiarity that aids in identification or diagnosis of a condition. 2. [pl.] purpuric or hemorrhagic lesions of the hands and/or feet, resembling crucifixion wounds. **stigmat′ic,** adj. **malpighian stigmata,** the points where the smaller veins enter into the larger veins of the spleen.

stilet (sti′let) stylet.

stillbirth (stil′berth) delivery of a dead child.

stillborn (-born) born dead.

stimulant (stim′u-lant) 1. producing stimulation. 2. an agent which stimulates. **central s.,** a stimulant affecting the central nervous system. **diffusible s.,** one which acts promptly, but transiently. **general s.,** one which acts upon the whole body. **local s.,** one that affects only, or mainly, the part to which it is applied.

stimulate (stim′u-lāt) to excite functional activity.

stimulator (stim′u-la″tor) any agent that excites functional activity. **long-acting thyroid s. (LATS),** thyroid-stimulating antibody associated with Graves disease; it is an autoantibody reactive against thyroid cell receptors for thyroid stimulating hormone and thus mimics the effects of the hormone.

stimulus (stim′u-lus) any agent, act, or influence which produces functional or trophic reaction in a receptor or an irritable tissue. **adequate s.,** a stimulus of the specific form of energy to which a given receptor is sensitive. **aversive s.,** one which, when applied following the occurrence of a response, decreases the strength of that response on later occurrences. **conditioned s.,** a stimulus that acquires the capacity to evoke a particular response on repeated repairing with another stimulus naturally capable of eliciting the response. **discriminative s.,** a stimulus associated with reinforcement, which exerts control over a particular form of behavior; the subject discriminates between closely related stimuli and responds positively only in the presence of that stimulus. **eliciting s.,** any stimulus, conditioned or unconditioned, which elicits a response. **heterologous s.,** one that produces an effect or sensation when applied to any part of a nerve tract. **homologous s.,** adequate s. **threshold s.,** a stimulus that is just strong enough to elicit a response. **unconditioned s.,** any stimulus capable of eliciting an unconditioned response.

sting (sting) 1. injury due to a biotoxin introduced into an individual or with which he comes in contact, together with the mechanical trauma incident to its introduction. 2. the organ used to inflict such injury.

stippling (stip′ling) a spotted condition or appearance, as an appearance of the retina as if dotted with light and dark points, or the appearance of red blood cells in basophilia.

stirrup (stir′up) stapes.

stitch (stich) 1. a sudden, transient cutting pain. 2. a suture.

stoichiology   562

stoichiology (stoi″ke-ol′ah-je) the science of elements, especially the physiology of the cellular elements of tissues. **stoichiolog′ic,** adj.

stoichiometry (-om′ĕ-tre) the determination of the relative proportions of the compounds involved in a chemical reaction. **stoichiomet′ric,** adj.

stoke (stōk) a unit of kinematic viscosity, that of a fluid with a dynamic viscosity of 1 poise and a density of 1 gram per cubic centimeter. Abbreviated St.

stoma (sto′mah), pl. *sto′mas, sto′mata* [Gr.] a mouthlike opening, particularly an incised opening which is kept open for drainage or other purposes. **sto′mal,** adj.

stomach (stum′ak) the musculomembranous expansion of the alimentary canal between the esophagus and duodenum, consisting of a cardiac part, a fundus, a body, and a pyloric part. Its (gastric) glands secrete the gastric juice which, when mixed with food, forms chyme, a semifluid substance suitable for further digestion by the intestine. See Plates IV and V. **stom′achal, stomach′ic,** adj. **cascade s.,** an atypical form of hourglass stomach, characterized roentgenologically by a drawing up of the posterior wall; an opaque medium first fills the upper sac and then cascades into the lower sac. **hourglass s.,** one more or less completely divided into two parts, resembling an hourglass in shape; due to scarring which complicates chronic gastric ulcer. **leather bottle s.,** linitis plastica. **water-trap s.,** a stomach with an extremely high pylorus, so that it does not readily empty itself.

stomachalgia (stum″ah-kal′je-ah) pain in the stomach.

stomat(o)- word element [Gr.], *mouth.*

stomatalgia (sto″mah-tal′je-ah) pain in the mouth.

stomatitis (sto″mah-ti′tis) generalized inflammation of the oral mucosa. **angular s.,** perlèche. **aphthous s.,** recurrent aphthous s. **gangrenous s.,** see *noma.* **herpetic s.,** an acute infection of the oral mucosa with vesicle formation, due to the herpes simplex virus. **mycotic s.,** thrush. **recurrent aphthous s.,** a recurrent stomatitis of unknown etiology characterized by the appearance of small ulcers on the oral mucosa covered by a grayish exudate and surrounded by a bright red halo; they heal without scarring in 7 to 14 days. **ulcerative s.,** stomatitis with shallow ulcers on the cheeks, tongue, and lips. **Vincent's s.,** acute necrotizing ulcerative gingivostomatitis.

stomatodynia (sto″mah-to-din′e-ah) pain in the mouth.

stomatognathic (sto″mah-tog-nath′ik) denoting the mouth and jaws collectively.

stomatology (sto″mah-tol′ah-je) that branch of medicine which treats of the mouth and its diseases. **stomatolog′ic,** adj.

stomatomalacia (sto″mah-to-mah-la′she-ah) softening of the structures of the mouth.

stomatomenia (-me′ne-ah) bleeding from the mouth at the time of menstruation.

stomatomycosis (-mi-ko′sis) any fungal disease of the mouth.

stomatopathy (sto″mah-top′ah-the) any disorder of the mouth.

stomatoplasty (sto′mah-to-plas″te) plastic reconstruction of the mouth.

stomatorrhagia (sto″mah-to-ra′je-ah) hemorrhage from the mouth.

stomocephalus (sto″mo-sef′ah-lus) a fetus with rudimentary jaws and mouth.

stomodeum (-de′um) the ectodermal depression at the head end of the embryo, which becomes the front part of the mouth. **stomode′al,** adj.

-stomy word element [Gr.], *creation of an opening into* or *a communication between.*

stone (stōn) 1. a calculus. 2. a unit of weight, equivalent in the English system to 14 pounds avoirdupois.

stool (stōōl) the fecal discharge from the bowels. **rice water s.,** the watery evacuations of cholera. **silver s.,** stools having the color of aluminum or silver paint, due to a mixture of melena and white fatty stools; it occurs in tropical sprue, in children with diarrhea who are given sulfonamides, and with carcinoma of the ampulla of Vater.

storiform (stor′ĭ-form) denoting a matted, irregularly whorled pattern, somewhat resembling that of a straw mat; said of the microscopic appearance of fibrous histiocytomas.

storm (storm) a sudden and temporary increase in symptoms. **thyroid s., thyrotoxic s.,** a sudden and dangerous increase in the symptoms of thyrotoxicosis, especially after thyroidectomy.

strabismometer (strah-biz-mom′ĕ-ter) an apparatus for measuring strabismus.

strabismus (strah-biz′mus) squint; deviation of the eye which the patient cannot overcome; the visual axes assume a position relative to each other different from that required by the physiological conditions. **strabis′mic,** adj. **concomitant s.,** that due to faulty insertion of the eye muscles, resulting in the same amount of deviation in whatever direction the eyes are looking. **convergent s.,** esotropia. **divergent s.,** exotropia. **nonconcomitant s.,** that in which the amount of deviation of the squinting eye varies according to the direction of gaze. **vertical s.,** that in which the visual axis of the squinting eye deviates in the vertical plane (hypertropia or hypotropia).

strabotomy (strah-bot′ah-me) section of an ocular tendon in treatment of strabismus.

strain (strān) 1. to overexercise; to use to an extreme and harmful degree. 2. to filter or subject to colation. 3. an overstretching or overexertion of some part of the musculature. 4. excessive effort. 5. a group of organisms within a species or variety, characterized by some particular quality, as rough or smooth strains of bacteria.

strait (strāt) a narrow passage. **s's of pelvis,** the pelvic inlet (*superior pelvic s.*) and pelvic outlet (*inferior pelvic s.*).

straitjacket (strāt′jak″it) a contrivance for restraining the limbs, especially the arms, of a violently disturbed person.

strangles (strang′g′lz) 1. an infectious disease of

horses due to *Streptococcus equi*, with mucopurulent inflammation of the respiratory mucous membrane. 2. infection of the lymph nodes in swine, producing heavily encapsulated abscesses in the pharyngeal region.

strangulated (strang′gu-lāt″ed) congested by reason of constriction or hernial stricture.

strangulation (strang″gu-la′shun) 1. choking or throttling arrest of respiration by occlusion of the air passages. 2. arrest of circulation in a part due to compression.

strangury (strang′gu-re) slow and painful discharge of urine.

strap (strap) 1. a band or slip, as of adhesive plaster, used in attaching parts to each other. 2. to bind down tightly. **Montgomery's s's**, straps of adhesive tape used to secure dressings that must be changed frequently.

stratiform (strat′ĭ-form) occurring in layers.

stratigraphy (strah-tig′rah-fe) see *body-section roentgenography*. **stratigraph′ic**, adj.

stratum (stra′tum), pl. *stra′ta* [L.] a layer.

streak (strēk) a line or stripe. **angioid s's**, red to black irregular bands in the ocular fundus running outward from the optic disk. **fatty s.**, a small, flat, yellow-gray area, composed mainly of cholesterol, in an artery; possibly an early stage of atherosclerosis. **meningeal s.**, tache cérébrale. **primitive s.**, a faint white trace at the caudal end of the embryonic disk, formed by movement of cells at the onset of mesoderm formation, providing the first evidence of the embryonic axis.

strephosymbolia (stref″o-sim-bo′le-ah) 1. a perceptual disorder in which objects seem reversed as in a mirror. 2. a reading difficulty with confusion between similar but oppositely oriented letters (b-d, q-p) and a tendency to read backward.

strept(o)- word element [Gr.], *twisted.*

Streptobacillus (strep″to-bah-sil′lus) a genus of gram-negative bacteria of uncertain affiliation; organisms are highly pleomorphic. *S. monilifor′mis* is a cause of rat-bite fever.

streptobacillus (-bah-sil′us), pl. *streptobacil′li.* an organism of the genus *Streptobacillus.*

streptocerciasis (-ser-ki′ah-sis) infection with *Mansonella streptocerca*, whose microfilariae produce a pruritic rash resembling that in onchocerciasis; transmitted by midges of the genus *Culicoides*, it occurs in Central Africa.

Streptococcaceae (kah-ka′se-e) a family of gram-positive, facultative anaerobic cocci, which are usually nonmotile, and occur in pairs, chains, or tetrads.

streptococcemia (-kok-se′me-ah) occurrence of streptococci in the blood.

Streptococcus (-kok′us) a genus of gram-positive, facultatively anaerobic cocci (family Streptococcaceae) occurring in pairs or chains. The genus is separable into the *pyrogenic* group, the *viridans* group, the *enterococcus* group, and the *lactic* group. The first group includes the β-hemolytic human and animal pathogens, the second and third include α-hemolytic parasitic forms occurring as normal flora in the upper respiratory tract and the intestinal tract, respectively, and the fourth is made up of saprophytic forms associated with the souring of milk. Species include S. *mu′tans*, which has been implicated in the formation of dental caries; S. *pneumoniae*, an α-hemolytic species that is the most common cause of lobar pneumonia and also causes numerous other serious, acute pyogenic disorders, and S. *pyog′enes*, a β-hemolytic species that causes septic sore throat, scarlet fever, and rheumatic fever.

streptococcus (-kok′us), pl. *streptococ′ci* [Gr.] an organism of the genus *Streptococcus.* **streptococ′cal, streptococ′cic**, adj. **hemolytic s.**, any streptococcus capable of hemolyzing erythrocytes, classified as *α-hemolytic* or *viridans type*, producing a zone of greenish discoloration much smaller than the clear zone produced by the β type about the colony on blood agar; and the *β-hemolytic type*, producing a clear zone of hemolysis immediately around the colony on blood agar. The most virulent streptococci belong to the latter group. On immunological grounds, the β-hemolytic streptococci may be divided into groups A through T; most human pathogens belong to groups A through G.

streptodornase (-dor′nās) an enzyme produced by hemolytic streptococci which catalyzes the depolymerization of DNA.

streptokinase (-ki′nās) a proteolytic enzyme elaborated by hemolytic streptococci, which produces fibrinolysis by activating plasminogen to plasmin; it is used as a thrombolytic agent. **s.-streptodornase**, a mixture of enzymes elaborated by hemolytic streptococci; used as a proteolytic and fibrinolytic agent and as a skin test antigen in evaluating cell-mediated immunodeficiency.

streptolysin (strep-tol′ĭ-sin) the hemolysin of hemolytic streptococci.

Streptomyces (strep″to-mi′sēz) a genus of bacteria (order Actinomycetales), usually soil forms, but occasionally parasitic on plants and animals, and notable as the source of various antibiotics, e.g., the tetracyclines. S. *somalien′-sis* is a cause of mycetoma.

streptomycin (-mi′sin) an antibiotic produced by *Streptomyces griseus;* used chiefly in the treatment of tuberculosis.

streptosepticemia (-sep″tĭ-se′me-ah) septicemia due to streptococci.

streptozocin (-zo′sin) an antineoplastic antibiotic, $C_8H_{15}N_3O_7$, derived from *Streptomyces achromogenes;* used principally in the treatment of islet-cell tumors of the pancreas and also in the treatment of other endocrine tumors, e.g., gastrinomas associated with Zollinger-Ellison syndrome.

stress (stres) 1. forcibly exerted influence; pressure; in dentistry, the pressure of the upper teeth against the lower in mastication. 2. the sum of the biological reactions to any adverse stimulus, physical, mental, or emotional, internal or external, that tends to disturb an organism's homeostasis; also, the stimuli that elicit the reactions.

stretcher (strech′er) a contrivance for carrying the sick or wounded.

stria (stri'ah), pl. *stri'ae* [L.] 1. a streak or line. 2. a narrow bandlike structure; in anatomy, a general term for longitudinal collections of nerve fibers in the brain. **atrophic striae, stri'ae atroph'icae,** atrophic, pinkish or purplish, scarlike lesions, later becoming white (*lineae albicantes*), on the breasts, thighs, abdomen, and buttocks, due to weakening of elastic tissues, associated with pregnancy (*striae gravidarum*), overweight, rapid growth during puberty and adolescence, Cushing's syndrome, and topical or prolonged treatment with corticosteroids. **stri'ae gravida'rum,** see *atrophic striae.*

striate, striated (stri'āt; stri'āt-ed) having stripes or striae.

striation (stri-a'shun) 1. the quality of being marked by stripes or striae. 2. a streak or scratch, or a series of streaks.

striatum (stri-a'tum) corpus striatum. **stria'tal,** adj.

stricture (strik'chur) an abnormal narrowing of a duct or passage.

stricturization (strik''chur-ĭ-za'shun) the process of decreasing in caliber or of becoming constricted.

stridor (stri'der) a harsh, high-pitched respiratory sound. **strid'ulous,** adj. **laryngeal s.,** that due to laryngeal obstruction. A *congenital* form, marked by stridor and dyspnea, is due to an infolding of a congenitally flabby epiglottis and aryepiglottic folds during inspiration; it is usually outgrown by two years of age.

striocerebellar (stri''o-ser''ĕ-bel'er) pertaining to the corpus striatum and cerebellum.

strip (strip) 1. to press the contents from a canal, such as the urethra or a blood vessel, by running the finger along it. 2. to excise lengths of large veins and incompetent tributaries by subcutaneous dissection and the use of a stripper. 3. to remove tooth structure or restorative material from the mesial or distal surfaces of teeth utilizing abrasive strips; usually done to alleviate crowding.

strobila (stro-bi'lah), pl. *strobi'lae* [L., Gr.] the chain of proglottids constituting the bulk of the body of adult tapeworms.

stroke (strōk) a sudden and severe attack; see *stroke syndrome.* **apoplectic s.,** apoplexy (1). **heat s.,** a condition due to excessive exposure to heat, with dry skin, vertigo, headache, thirst, nausea, and muscular cramps; the body temperature may be dangerously elevated.

stroma (stro'mah), pl. *stro'mata* [Gr.] the supporting tissue or matrix of an organ. **stro'mal, stromat'ic,** adj.

stromuhr (strōm'oor) an instrument for measuring the velocity of blood flow.

Strongyloides (stron''jĭ-loi'dēz) a genus of widely distributed nematodes parasitic in the intestine of man and other mammals, including *S. stercora'lis,* found in the tropics and subtropics, where they cause diarrhea and intestinal ulceration.

strongyloidiasis (stron''jĭ-loi-di'ah-sis) infection with *Strongyloides stercoralis.*

strongyloidosis (-do'sis) strongyloidiasis.

strongylosis (stron''jĭ-lo'sis) infection with *Strongylus.*

Strongylus (stron'jĭ-lus) a genus of nematode parasites.

strontium (stron'she-um) chemical element (*see table*), at. no. 38, symbol Sr.

strophulus (strof'u-lus) papular urticaria.

struma (stroo'mah) goiter. **Hashimoto's s., s. lymphomato'sa,** a progressive disease of the thyroid gland with degeneration of its epithelial elements and replacement by lymphoid and fibrous tissue. **s. malig'na,** carcinoma of the thyroid gland. **s. ova'rii,** a teratoid ovarian tumor composed of thyroid tissue. **Riedel's s.,** a chronic, proliferating, fibrosing, inflammatory process involving usually one but sometimes both lobes of the thyroid gland, as well as the trachea and other adjacent structures.

strumectomy (stroo-mek'tah-me) excision of a goiter.

strumitis (stroo-mi'tis) thyroiditis.

strychnine (strik'nīn) a very poisonous alkaloid, $C_{21}H_{22}N_2O_2$, obtained chiefly from *Strychnos nux-vomica* and other species of *Strychnos.*

stump (stump) the distal end of a limb left after amputation.

stupe (stoōp) a hot, wet cloth or sponge, charged with a medication for external application.

stupefacient (stu''pah-fa'shent) 1. inducing stupor. 2. an agent that induces stupor.

stupor (stu'per) partial or nearly complete unconsciousness; in psychiatry, a disorder marked by reduced responsiveness.

stuttering (stut'er-ing) a speech problem characterized chiefly by spasmodic repetition of sounds, especially of initial consonants, and by prolongation of sounds and hesitation. Stuttering is usually distinguished from *stammering,* which is characterized by blocking or involuntary pauses in speech, sometimes with repetition of sounds.

sty, stye (sti), pl. *sties, styes.* Hordeolum.

styl(o)- word element [L., Gr.], *stake; pole; styloid process of the temporal bone.*

stylet (sti'lit) 1. a wire run through a catheter or cannula to render it stiff or to remove debris from its lumen. 2. a slender probe.

stylohyoid (sti''lo-hi'oid) pertaining to the styloid process and hyoid bone.

styloid (sti'loid) resembling a pillar; long and pointed; relating to the styloid process.

styloiditis (sti''loi-di'tis) inflammation of tissues around the styloid process.

stylomastoid (sti''lo-mas'toid) pertaining to the styloid and mastoid processes of the temporal bone.

stylomaxillary (-mak'sĭ-lār''e) pertaining to the styloid process of the temporal bone and the maxilla.

stylus (sti'lus) 1. stylet. 2. a pencil-shaped medicinal preparation, as of caustic.

stype (stīp) a tampon or pledget of cotton.

stypsis (stip'sis) 1. astringency; astringent action. 2. use of styptics.

styptic (stip'tik) 1. astringent; arresting hemorrhage by means of an astringent quality. 2. an astringent and hemostatic agent.

sub- word element [L.], *under; near; almost; moderately.*

subabdominal (sub″ab-dom′ĭ-n'l) below the abdomen.

subacromial (sub″ah-kro′me-al) below the acromion.

subacute (-ah-kūt) somewhat acute; between acute and chronic.

subalimentation (sub-al″′ĭ-men-ta′shun) insufficient nourishment.

subaponeurotic (-ap″o-noo-rot′ik) below an aponeurosis.

subarachnoid (sub″ah-rak′noid) between the arachnoid and the pia mater.

subareolar (-ah-re′o-ler) beneath the areola.

subastragalar (-as-trag′ah-ler) below the astragalus.

subatomic (-ah-tom′ik) of or pertaining to the constituent parts of an atom.

subaural (sub-aw′ral) below the ear.

subaurale (sub″aw-ra′le) the lowest point on the inferior border of the ear lobule when the subject is looking straight ahead.

subcapsular (sub-kap′su-ler) below a capsule, especially the capsule of the cerebrum.

subcartilaginous (-kar″tĭ-laj′ĭ-nus) 1. below a cartilage. 2. partly cartilaginous.

subclass (sub′klas) a taxonomic category subordinate to a class and superior to an order.

subclavian (sub-kla′ve-an) below the clavicle.

subclavicular (sub″klah-vik′u-ler) subclavian.

subclinical (sub-klin′ĭ-k'l) without clinical manifestations.

subclone (sub′klōn) the progeny of a mutant cell arising in a clone.

subconjunctival (sub″kon-jungk-ti′val) beneath the conjunctiva.

subconscious (sub-kon′shus) 1. imperfectly or partially conscious. 2. formerly, the preconscious and unconscious considered together.

subconsciousness (-kon′shus-nes) partial unconsciousness.

subcoracoid (-kor′ah-koid) situated under the coracoid process.

subcortex (-kor′teks) the brain substance underlying the cortex. **subcor′tical,** adj.

subcostal (-kos′t'l) below a rib or ribs.

subcranial (-kra′ne-al) below the cranium.

subcrepitant (-krep′ĭ-tint) somewhat crepitant in nature; said of a rale.

subculture (sub′kul-chur) a culture of bacteria derived from another culture.

subcutaneous (sub″ku-ta′ne-us) beneath the skin.

subcuticular (-ku-tik′u-ler) subepidermal.

subdelirium (-dĕ-lir′e-um) mild delirium.

subdiaphragmatic (sub-di″ah-frag-mat′ik) below the diaphragm.

subduct (-dukt′) to draw down.

subdural (-door′al) between the dura mater and the arachnoid.

subendocardial (sub″en-do-kar′de-al) beneath the endocardium.

subendothelial (-en-do-the′le-al) beneath the endothelium.

subepidermal (ep-ĭ-der′mal) beneath the epidermis.

subepithelial (-ep-ĭ-the′le-al) beneath the epithelium.

subfamily (sub′fam″ĭ-le) a taxonomic division between a family and a tribe.

subfascial (-fash′ul) beneath a fascia.

subgenus (sub′je″nus) a taxonomic category between a genus and a species.

subglenoid (sub-gle′noid) beneath the glenoid fossa.

subglossal (-glos′al) below the tongue.

subgrondation (sub″gron-da′shun) depression of one fragment of bone beneath another.

subhepatic (-hĕ-pat′ik) below the liver.

subhyoid (sub-hi′oid) below the hyoid bone.

subiculum (sŭ-bik′u-lum) an underlying or supporting structure.

subiliac (sub-il′e-ak) below the ilium.

subilium (-il′e-um) the lowest portion of the ilium.

subinvolution (sub″in-vah-loo′shun) incomplete involution.

subjacent (sub-ja′sent) located beneath.

subject (sub′jekt) 1. a person or animal subjected to treatment, observation, or experiment. 2. a body for dissection.

subjugal (-joo′gal) below the zygomatic bone.

sublatio retinae (-la′she-o ret″ĭ-ne) detachment of the retina.

sublethal (-le′thal) insufficient to cause death.

sublimate (sub′lĭ-māt) 1. a substance obtained by sublimation. 2. to accomplish sublimation.

sublimation (sub″′lĭ-ma″shun) 1. the conversion of a solid directly into the gaseous state. 2. an unconscious defense mechanism by which consciously unacceptable instinctual drives are expressed in personally and socially acceptable channels.

sublime (sub-līm′) to volatilize a solid body by heat and to collect it in a purified form as a solid or powder.

subliminal (-lim′ĭ-n'l) below the threshold of sensation or conscious awareness.

sublingual (-ling′gwal) beneath the tongue.

sublinguitis (sub″ling-gwi′tis) inflammation of the sublingual gland.

subluxation (sub″-luk-sa′shun) incomplete or partial dislocation.

submammary (sub-mam′ah-re) below the mammary gland.

submandibular (sub″man-dib′u-ler) below the mandible.

submaxilla (-mak-sil′ah) the mandible.

submaxillaritis (-mak-sĭ-ler-i′tis) inflammation of the submaxillary gland.

submaxillary (sub-mak′sĭ-lār″e) below the maxilla.

submental (-men′t'l) beneath the chin.

submetacentric (-met″ah-sen′trik) having the centromere almost, but not quite, at the metacentric position.

submicroscopic (-mi″kro-skop′ik) too small to be visible with the microscope.

submorphous (-mor′fus) neither amorphous nor perfectly crystalline.

submucosa (sub″mu-ko′sah) areolar tissue situated beneath a mucous membrane.

submucous (sub-mu′kus) beneath a mucous membrane.

subnarcotic (sub″nar-kot′ik) moderately narcotic.

subnasale (-na-sa′le) the point at which the nasal septum merges, in the midsagittal plane, with the upper lip.

subneural (sub-noor′al) beneath a nerve.

subnormal (-nor′m'l) below normal.

subnucleus (sub-noo′kle-us) a partial or secondary nucleus.

suboccipital (sub″ok-sip′ĭ-t'l) below the occiput.

suborbital (sub-or′bĭ-t'l) beneath the orbit.

suborder (sub′or″der) a taxonomic category between an order and a family.

subpapular (-pap′u-ler) indistinctly papular.

subpatellar (sub″pah-tel′er) below the patella.

subpericardial (-per-ĭ-kar′de-al) beneath the pericardium.

subperiosteal (-per-e-os′te-al) beneath the periosteum.

subperitoneal (-per-ĭ-to-ne′al) beneath or deep to the peritoneum.

subpharyngeal (-fah-rin′je-al) beneath the pharynx.

subphrenic (sub-fren′ik) beneath the diaphragm.

subphylum (sub′fi″lum) a taxonomic category between a phylum and a class.

subplacenta (sub″plah-sen′tah) the decidua basalis.

subpleural (sub-ploor′al) beneath the pleura.

subpreputial (sub″pre-pu′shal) beneath the prepuce.

subpubic (sub-pu′bik) beneath the pubic bone.

subpulmonary (-pul′mo-nār″e) beneath the lung.

subretinal (-ret′ĭ-n'l) beneath the retina.

subscapular (-skap′u-ler) below the scapula.

subscription (-skrip′shun) that part of a prescription giving the directions for compounding the ingredients.

subserous (sēr′us) beneath a serous membrane.

subspecies (sub′spe″sēz) a taxonomic category subordinate to a species, differing morphologically from others of the species but capable of interbreeding with them; a variety or race.

subspinale (sub″spi-na′le) point A.

substance (sub′stans) material constituting an organ or body. **black s.,** substantia nigra. **controlled s.,** any drug regulated under the Controlled Substances Act. **gray s.,** the gray nerve tissue composed of nerve cell bodies, unmyelinated nerve fibers, and supporting tissue. **ground s.,** the gel-like material in which connective tissue cells and fibers are embedded. **medullary s.,** 1. the white matter of the central nervous system, consisting of axons and their myelin sheaths. 2. the soft, marrow-like substance of the interior of an organ. **s. P,** an 11–amino acid peptide, present in nerve cells scattered throughout the body and in special endocrine cells in the gut. It increases the contraction of gastrointestinal smooth muscle and causes vasodilatation; it also seems to be a sensory neurotransmitter. **perforated s.,** 1. *anterior perforated s.,* an area anterolateral to each optic tract, pierced by branches of the anterior and middle cerebral arteries. 2. *posterior perforated s.,* an area between the cerebral peduncles, pierced by branches of the posterior cerebral arteries. **reticular s.,** the netlike mass of threads seen in red blood cells after vital staining. **Rolando's gelatinous s.,** substantia gelatinosa. **slow-reacting s. (SRS-A),** a substance released in the anaphylactic reaction that induces slow, prolonged contraction of certain smooth muscles. **threshold s's,** those substances (e.g., glucose) excreted into the urine only when their concentration in plasma exceeds a certain value. **transmitter s.,** neurotransmitter. **white s.,** the white nervous tissue, constituting the conducting portion of the brain and spinal cord, composed mostly of myelinated nerve fibers. **white s. of Schwann,** myelin (1).

substantia (sub-stan′she-ah), pl. *substan′tiae* [L.] substance. **s. al′ba,** white substance. **s. ferrugin′ea,** locus ceruleus. **s. gelatino′sa,** the gelatinous-appearing cap forming the dorsal part of the posterior horn of the spinal cord. **s. gris′ea,** gray substance. **s. ni′gra,** the layer of gray substance separating the tegmentum of the midbrain from the crus cerebri. **s. pro′pria,** 1. the tough, fibrous, transparent main part of the cornea, between Bowman's membrane and Descemet's membrane. 2. the main part of the sclera, between the episcleral lamina and the lamina fusca.

substernal (sub-ster′n'l) below the sternum.

substituent (sub-stich′u-ent) 1. a substitute; especially an atom, radical, or group substituted for another in a compound. 2. of or pertaining to such an atom, radical, or group.

substitution (sub″stĭ-too′shun) 1. the act of putting one thing in place of another, especially the chemical replacement of one atom or radical by another. 2. a defense mechanism, operating unconsciously, in which an unattainable or unacceptable goal, emotion, or object is replaced by one that is attainable or acceptable.

substrate (sub′strāt) a substance upon which an enzyme acts.

substructure (-struk″chur) the underlying or supporting portion of an organ or appliance; that portion of an implant denture embedded in the tissues of the jaw.

subsylvian (sub-sil′ve-an) situated deep in the lateral sulcus (sylvian fissure).

subtarsal (-tar′sal) below the tarsus.

subtentorial (sub″ten-to′re-al) beneath the tentorium of the cerebellum.

subthalamus (sub-thal′ah-mus) the ventral thalamus or subthalamic tegmental region: a transitional region of the diencephalon interposed between the (dorsal) thalamus, the hypothalamus, and the tegmentum of the mesencephalon (midbrain); it includes the subthalamic nucleus, Forel's fields, and the zona incerta. **subthalam′ic**, adj.

subtribe (sub′-trīb) a taxonomic category between a tribe and a genus.

subtrochanteric (sub″tro-kan-ter′ik) below the trochanter.

subungual (sub-ung′gwal) beneath a nail.

suburethral (sub″u-re′thral) beneath the urethra.

subvaginal (sub-vaj′ĭ-n′l) under a sheath, or below the vagina.

subvertebral (-ver′tĕ-bral) on the ventral side of the vertebrae.

subvirile (-vir′il) having deficient virility.

subvolution (sub″vo-loo′shun) the operation of turning over a flap to prevent adhesions.

succinate (suk′sĭ-nāt) any salt or ester of succinic acid.

succinic acid (suk-sin′ik) an intermediate in the tricarboxylic acid cycle, $HOOCCH_2CH_2COOH$.

succinylcholine (suk″sĭ-nil-ko′lēn) a skeletal muscle relaxant, $C_{14}H_{30}N_2O_4$, used as the chloride salt.

succinyl-CoA (suk′sĭ-nil) a high-energy intermediate formed in the tricarboxylic acid (Krebs) cycle by the oxidation of α-ketoglutaric acid.

succorrhea (suk″o-re′ah) excessive flow of a natural secretion.

succus (suk′us), pl. *suc′ci* [L.] any fluid derived from a living tissue; juice.

succussion (sŭ-kush′un) a procedure in which the body is shaken, a splashing sound being indicative of the presence of fluid and air in a body cavity.

sucrase (soo′krās) β-fructofuranosidase.

sucrose (soo′krōs) a disaccharide, $C_{12}H_{22}O_{11}$, from sugar cane, sugar beet, or other sources; used as a food and sweetening agent.

sucrosuria (soo″kro-su′re-ah) sucrose in the urine.

suction (suk′shun) aspiration of gas or fluid by mechanical means. **post-tussive s.,** a sucking sound heard over a lung cavity just after a cough.

Suctoria (suk-tor′e-ah) a class of protozoa (subphylum Ciliophora) whose members possess cilia only during the larval stage, the mature organism having suctorial tentacles that serve as locomotor and food-acquiring mechanisms; most are free-living, but some are parasites of other ciliates, of other protozoa, and of mammals.

suctorial (suk-tor′e-al) adapted for sucking.

suctorian (suk-tor′e-an) 1. any individual of the Suctoria. 2. of or pertaining to the Suctoria.

sudamen (soo-da′men), pl. *suda′mina* [L.] a whitish vesicle caused by retention of sweat in the horny layer of the skin.

Sudan (soo-dan′) a group of azo compounds used as biological stains for fats.

sudanophilia (soo-dan″o-fil′e-ah) affinity for Sudan stain. **sudanophil′ic**, adj.

sudation (soo-da′shun) the process of sweating.

sudomotor (soo″do-mo′ter) stimulating the sweat glands.

sudor (soo′dor) sweat; perspiration.

sudoresis (soo″do-re′sis) diaphoresis.

sudoriferous (-rif′er-us) 1. conveying sweat. 2. sudoriparous.

sudorific (-rif′ik) 1. promoting sweating; diaphoretic. 2. an agent that causes sweating.

sudoriparous (-rip′ah-rus) secreting or producing sweat.

suet (soo′et) the fat from the abdominal cavity of ruminants, especially the sheep or ox, used in preparing cerates and ointments and as an emollient; the pharmaceutical preparation (*prepared s.*) is obtained from sheep.

suffocation (suf″ŏ-ka′shun) asphyxiation; the stoppage of respiration, or the asphyxia that results from it.

suffusion (sŭ-fu′zhun) 1. the process of overspreading, or diffusion. 2. the condition of being moistened or of being permeated through, as by blood.

sugar (shoog′er) a sweet carbohydrate of both animal and vegetable origin, the two principal groups of which are the disaccharides and the monosaccharides.

suggestion (sug-jes′chun) 1. impartation of an idea to an individual from without. 2. an idea introduced from without. **posthypnotic s.,** implantation in the mind of a subject during hypnosis of a suggestion to be acted upon after recovery from the hypnotic state.

suggillation (sug″jĭ-la′shun) an ecchymosis.

sulcate (sul′kāt) furrowed; marked with sulci.

sulcus (sul′kus), pl. *sul′ci* [L.] a groove, trench, or furrow; in anatomy, a general term for such a depression, especially one on the brain surface, separating the gyri. **calcarine s.,** a sulcus of the medial surface of the occipital lobe, separating the cuneus from the lingual gyrus. **central s.,** one between the frontal and parietal lobes of the cerebral hemisphere. **cingulate s.,** one on the median surface of the hemisphere midway between the corpus callosum and the margin of the surface. **collateral s.,** one on the inferior surface of the cerebral hemisphere between the fusiform and parahippocampal gyri. **sul′ci cu′tis,** fine depressions of the skin between the ridges of the skin. **gingival s.,** the groove between the surface of the tooth and the epithelium lining the free gingiva. **hippocampal s.,** one extending from the splenium of the corpus callosum almost to the tip of the temporal lobe. **intraparietal s.,** one separating the parietal gyri. **lateral cerebral s.,** fissure of Sylvius. **s. of matrix of nail,** the skin fold in which the proximal part of the nail is embedded. **parieto-occipital s.,** one marking the boundary between the cuneus and precuneus, and also between the parietal and occipital lobes of the cerebral hemisphere. **posterior median s.,** 1. a shallow vertical groove in the closed part of the medulla oblongata, continuous with the posterior median sulcus of the spinal cord. 2. a shallow vertical groove dividing the spinal cord throughout its whole length in the midline posteriorly. **precentral s.,** one separating the pre-

sulfacetamide   568

central gyrus from the remainder of the frontal lobe. **scleral s.,** a slight groove on the outer surface of the eyeball, at the junction of the sclera and cornea.

sulfacetamide (sul″fah-set′ah-mīd) an antibacterial sulfonamide, $C_8H_{10}N_2O_3S$, used in urinary tract infections; the sodium salt is used topically in ophthalmic infections.

sulfacytine (-si′tēn) a rapidly excreted, oral sulfonamide used in treatment of acute urinary tract infections.

sulfadiazine (-di′ah-zēn) an antibacterial sulfonamide, $C_{10}H_{10}N_4O_2S$, often used in combination with other sulfonamides; the sodium salt is used in solution for intravenous administration.

sulfameter (sul′fah-me″ter) a long-acting sulfonamide, $C_{11}H_{12}N_4O_3S$, used in urinary tract infections.

sulfamethizole (sul″fah-meth′ĭ-zōl) an antibacterial sulfonamide, $C_9H_{10}N_4O_2S_2$, used mainly in urinary tract infections.

sulfamethoxazole (-meth-ok′sah-zōl) an antibacterial sulfonamide, $C_{10}H_{11}N_3O_3S$, especially useful in acute urinary tract infections and pyodermata and in infections of wounds and soft tissues.

sulfanilamide (-nil′ah-mīd) a potent antibacterial compound, the first of the sulfonamides discovered.

sulfasalazine (-sal′ah-zēn) a combination of sulfapyridine and salicylic acid used in the treatment and prophylaxis of ulcerative colitis.

sulfatase (sul′fah-tās) an enzyme which catalyzes the hydrolysis of sulfate esters.

sulfate (sul′fāt) a salt of sulfuric acid. **cupric s.,** a crystalline salt of copper used as an emetic, astringent, and fungicide.

sulfatide (sul′fah-tīd) any of a class of cerebroside sulfuric esters.

sulfhemoglobin (sulf″he′mo-glo″bin) sulfmethemoglobin.

sulfhemoglobinemia (-glo″bin-e′me-ah) sulfmethemoglobin in the blood.

sulfide (sul′fīd) any binary compound of sulfur; a compound of sulfur with another element or radical or base.

sulfinpyrazone (sul″fin-pi′rah-zōn) a uricosuric agent, $C_{23}H_{20}N_2O_3S$, used in the treatment of gout.

sulfisoxazole (sul″fĭ-sok′sah-zōl) an antibacterial sulfonamide, $C_{11}H_{13}N_3O_3S$, used in infections of the urinary and respiratory tracts and of soft tissues.

sulfite (sul′fīt) any salt of sulfurous acid. **s. oxidase,** an oxidoreductase that catalyzes the oxidation of sulfite (with O_2) to sulfate with release of H_2O_2; it is a mitochondrial hemoprotein containing molybdenum and is important in brain function.

sulfmethemoglobin (sulf″met-he′mo-glo″bin) a greenish substance formed by treating the blood with hydrogen sulfide or by absorption of this gas from the intestinal tract.

sulfobromophthalein (sul″fo-bro″mo-thal′e-in) a sulfur- and bromine-containing compound

used as the disodium salt in liver function tests.

sulfonamide (sul-fon′ah-mīd) a compound containing the $-SO_2NH_2$ group. The sulfonamides, or sulfa drugs, are derivatives of sulfanilamide, which competitively inhibits folic acid synthesis in microorganisms, and are bacteriostatic against a wide variety of bacteria. Sulfonamides have largely been supplanted by more effective and less toxic antibiotics.

sulfone (sul′fōn) a compound containing two hydrocarbon radicals attached to the $-SO_2-$ group, especially dapsone and its derivatives, which are potent antibacterials effective against many gram-positive and gram-negative organisms and are widely used as leprostatics.

sulfoxone (sul-fok′sōn) a dapsone derivative; its sodium salt is used as a leprostatic and dermatitis herpetiformis suppressant.

sulfur (sul′fer) chemical element (*see table*), at. no. 16, symbol S. **s. dioxide,** a colorless, noninflammable gas, SO_2, used as an antioxidant in pharmaceutical preparations; a dry form is used as an insecticide and rodenticide. **precipitated s.,** a fine, pale yellow powder used as a scabicide, antiparasitic, antifungal, and keratolytic. **sublimed s.,** a fine yellow crystalline powder; used as a scabicide and parasiticide.

sulfurated (sul′fu-rāt″ed) combined or charged with sulfur.

sulfuric acid (sul-fūr′ik) an oily, highly caustic, poisonous acid, H_2SO_4, widely used in chemistry, industry, and the arts.

sulfurous acid (sul′fūr-us) 1. a solution of sulfur dioxide in water, H_2SO_3; used as a reagent. 2. sulfur dioxide.

sulindac (sul-in′dak) an anti-inflammatory, analgesic, and antipyretic, $C_{20}H_{17}FO_3S$, used in the treatment of rheumatic disorders.

sulph- for words beginning thus, see those beginning *sulf-*.

sumac (soo′mak) name of various trees and shrubs of the genus *Rhus*. **poison s.,** a species, *Rhus vernix*, which causes an itching rash on contact with the skin.

summation (sŭ-ma′shun) the cumulative effect of a number of stimuli applied to a muscle, nerve, or reflex arc.

Sumycin (soo-mi′sin) trademark for preparations of tetracycline hydrochloride.

sunburn (sun′bern) injury to the skin, with erythema, tenderness, and sometimes blistering, after excessive exposure to sunlight, produced by unfiltered ultraviolet rays.

sunstroke (-strōk) a condition caused by excessive exposure to the sun, marked by high skin temperature, convulsions, and coma.

super- word element [L.], *above; excessive.*

superalimentation (soo″per-al″ĭ-men-ta′shun) treatment of wasting diseases by feeding beyond appetite requirements.

superalkalinity (-al″kah-lin′ĭ-te) excessive alkalinity.

supercilia (-sil′e-ah) [pl., L.] the hairs on the arching protrusion over either eye.

supercilium (-sil′e-um) [sing., L.] eyebrow; the

transverse elevation at the junction of the forehead and upper eyelid. **supercil′iary,** adj.

superclass (soo′per-klas″) a taxonomic category between a phylum and a class.

superego (soo″per-e′go) in psychoanalysis, the aspect of the personality that acts as a monitor and evaluator of ego functioning, comparing it with an ideal standard.

superexcitation (-ek″si-ta′shun) extreme or excessive excitement.

superfamily (soo″per-fam″ĭ-le) a taxonomic category between an order and a family.

superfecundation (soo″per-fe″kun-da′shun) fertilization of two or more ova during the same ovulatory cycle, by separate coital acts.

superfetation (-fe-ta′shun) fertilization and subsequent development of an ovum when a fetus is already present in the uterus, a result of fertilization of ova during different ovulatory cycles and yielding fetuses of different ages.

superficialis (-fish″e-a′lis) [L.] superficial.

superficies (-fish′e-ēz) [L.] an outer surface.

superinduce (in-do͞os′) to bring on in addition to an already existing condition.

superinfection (-in-fek′shun) a new infection complicating the course of antimicrobial therapy of an existing infection, due to invasion by bacteria or fungi resistant to the drug(s) in use.

superinvolution (-in″vo-lu′shun) prolonged involution of the uterus, after delivery, to a size much smaller than the normal, occurring in nursing mothers.

superior (soo-pēr′e-or) situated above, or directed upward.

superjacent (soo″per-ja′sent) located just above.

superlactation (-lak-ta′shun) hyperlactation.

supermotility (-mo-til′ĭ-te) excess of motility.

supernatant (-na′tant) the liquid lying above a layer of precipitated insoluble material.

supernumerary (-nu′mer-ār″e) in excess of the regular or normal number.

supernutrition (-noo-trish′un) excessive nutrition.

superolateral (-o-lat′er-al) above and to the side.

superoxide (-ok′sīd) any compound containing the highly reactive and extremely toxic oxygen radical O_2^-, a common intermediate in numerous biological oxidations.

supersaturate (-sach′er-āt) to add more of an ingredient than can be held in solution permanently.

superscription (-skrip′shun) the heading of a prescription, i.e., the symbol ℞ or the word Recipe, meaning "take."

superstructure (soo″per-struk″chur) the overlying or visible portion of an appliance.

supervascularization (soo″per-vas″ku-lar-ĭ-za′shun) in radiotherapy, the relative increase in vascularity that occurs when tumor cells are destroyed so that the remaining tumor cells are better supplied by the (uninjured) capillary stroma.

supervoltage (soo′per-vol″tij) very high voltage; in radiation therapy, a tube voltage between 500 and 1,000 kilovolts.

supinate (soo′pĭ-nāt) the act of turning the palm forward or upward, or of raising the medial margin of the foot.

supine (soo′pīn) lying with the face upward, or on the dorsal surface.

suppository (sŭ-poz′ĭ-tor″e) an easily fusible medicated mass to be introduced into a body orifice, as the rectum, urethra, or vagina.

suppressant (sŭ-pres′ant) 1. inducing suppression. 2. an agent that stops secretion, excretion, or normal discharge.

suppression (sŭ-presh′un) 1. sudden stoppage of a secretion, excretion, or normal discharge. 2. conscious inhibition as contrasted with repression, which is unconscious. 3. in genetics, a second mutation occurring at a site different from the first mutation site and masking the phenotypic expression of the first mutation.

suppurant (sup′u-rant) 1. promoting suppuration. 2. an agent that causes suppuration.

suppuration (sup″u-ra′shun) formation or discharge of pus. **sup′purative,** adj.

supra- word element [L.], *above; over.*

supra-acromial (soo″prah-ah-kro′me-al) above the acromion.

supra-auricular (-aw-rik′u-ler) above the auricle of the ear.

suprabulge (soo′prah-bulj″) the surface of the crown of a tooth sloping toward the occlusal surface from the height of contour.

suprachoroid (soo″prah-kor′oid) above or upon the choroid.

suprachoroidea (-ko-roi′de-ah) the outermost layer of the choroid.

supraclavicular (-klah-vik′u-ler) above the clavicle.

supraclusion (-kloo′zhun) projection of a tooth beyond the normal occlusal plane.

supracondylar (-kon′dĭ-ler) above a condyle.

supracostal (-kos′t'l) above or upon the ribs.

supracotyloid (-kot′ĭ-loid) above the acetabulum.

supradiaphragmatic (-di″ah-frag-mat′ik) above the diaphragm.

supraduction (soo″prah-duk′shun) upward rotation of an eye around its horizontal axis.

supraepicondylar (-ep″ĭ-kon′dĭ-ler) above an epicondyle.

suprahyoid (-hi′oid) above the hyoid bone.

supraliminal (-lim′ĭ-n'l) above the threshold of sensation.

supralumbar (-lum′ber) above the loin.

supramalleolar (-mah-le′o-ler) above a malleolus.

supramaxilla (-mak-sil′ah) maxilla.

supramaxillary (-mak′sĭ-lār″e) 1. pertaining to the upper jaw. 2. above the maxilla.

supramentale (-men-ta′le) point B.

supraocclusion (-ŏ-kloo′zhun) supraclusion.

supraorbital (-or′bĭ-t'l) above the orbit.

suprapelvic (-pel′vik) above the pelvis.

suprapharmacologic (-fahr″mah-ko-loj′ik) much greater than the usual therapeutic dose or pharmacologic concentration of a drug.

suprapontine (-pon'tĭn) above or in upper part of the pons.

suprapubic (-pu'bik) above the pubes.

suprarenal (-re'nal) 1. above a kidney. 2. pertaining to the suprarenal (adrenal) gland.

suprarenalectomy (-re"nal-ek'tah-me) adrenalectomy; excision of one or both adrenal glands.

suprarenalism (-re'nal-izm) adrenalism.

suprascapular (-skap'u-ler) above the scapula.

suprascleral (-skle'ral) on the outer surface of the sclera.

suprasellar (-sel'er) above the sella turcica.

supraspinal (-spi'n'l) above the spine.

suprasternal (-ster'n'l) above the sternum.

supratrochlear (-trok'le-ar) above the trochlea.

supravaginal (-vaj'ĭ-n'l) outside or above a sheath; specifically, above the vagina.

supraventricular (-ven-trik'u-ler) situated or occurring above the ventricles, especially in an atrium or atrioventricular node.

supravergence (soo"prah-ver'jens) disjunctive reciprocal movement of the eyes in which one eye rotates upward while the other one stays still.

supraversion (-ver'zhun) 1. abnormal elongation of a tooth from its socket. 2. sursumversion.

sura (su'rah) [L.] calf of the leg. **su'ral,** adj.

surfactant (ser-fak'tant) a surface-active agent, such as soap or a synthetic detergent. In pulmonary physiology, a mixture of phospholipids that reduces the surface tension of pulmonary fluids and thus contributes to the elastic properties of pulmonary tissue.

surgeon (ser'jun) 1. a physician who specializes in surgery. 2. the senior medical officer of a military unit.

surgery (ser'jer-e) 1. that branch of medicine which treats diseases, injuries, and deformities by manual or operative methods. 2. the place in a hospital, or doctor's or dentist's office, where surgery is performed. 3. in Great Britain, a room or office where a doctor sees and treats patients. 4. the work performed by a surgeon. **sur'gical,** adj. **antiseptic s., aseptic s.,** surgery according to antiseptic or aseptic methods. **bench s.,** surgery performed on an organ that has been removed from the body, after which it is reimplanted. **conservative s.,** surgery designed to preserve, or to remove with minimal risk, diseased or injured organs, tissues, or extremities. **dental s.,** operative dentistry. **general s.,** that which deals with surgical problems of all kinds, rather than those in a restricted area, as in a surgical specialty such as neurosurgery. **major s.,** surgery involving the more important, difficult, and hazardous operations. **minor s.,** surgery restricted to management of minor problems and injuries. **oral and maxillofacial s.,** the branch of dentistry that deals with the diagnosis and surgical and adjunct treatment of diseases and defects of the mouth and dental structures. **plastic s.,** surgery concerned with the restoration, reconstruction, correction, or improvement in the shape and appearance of body structures that are defective, damaged, or misshapened by injury, disease, or growth and development. **radical s.,** surgery designed to extirpate all areas of localized extensive disease and adjacent zones of lymphatic drainage. **stereotactic s., stereotaxic s.,** a technique for the production of sharply circumscribed lesions in specific groups of cells in deep-seated brain structures after locating the discrete structure by means of three-dimensional coordinates.

Surgicel (ser'jĭ-sel) trademark for an absorbable knitted fabric prepared by controlled oxidation of cellulose, used to control intraoperative hemorrhage when other conventional methods are impractical or ineffective.

surrogate (sur'o-git) a substitute; a thing or person that takes the place of something or someone else, as a drug used in place of another, or a person who takes the place of another in someone's affective existence.

sursumduction (sur"sum-duk'shun) supraduction.

sursumvergence (-ver'jens) supravergence.

sursumversion (-ver'zhun) the simultaneous and equal upward turning of the eyes.

susceptible (sŭ-sep'tĭ-b'l) 1. readily affected or acted upon. 2. lacking immunity or resistance and thus at risk of infection.

suscitate (sus'ĭ-tāt) to arouse to greater activity.

suscitation (sus"ĭ-ta'shun) arousal to greater activity.

suspension (sus-pen'shun) 1. a condition of temporary cessation, as of animation, of pain, or of any vital process. 2. a preparation of a finely divided drug intended to be incorporated (suspended) in some suitable liquid vehicle before it is used, or already incorporated in such a vehicle.

suspensoid (sus-pen'soid) a colloid system in which the disperse phase consists of particles of any insoluble substance, as a metal, in a solid, liquid, or gaseous dispersion medium.

suspensory (sus-pen'ser-e) 1. serving to hold up a part. 2. a ligament, bone, muscle, sling, or bandage that serves to hold up a part.

sustentaculum (sus"ten-tak'u-lum), pl. _susten-tac'ula_ [L.] a support. **sustentac'ular,** adj.

susurrus (sŭ-sur'us) [L.] murmur.

sutura (su-tu'rah), pl. _sutu'rae_ [L.] suture; in anatomy, a type of joint in which the apposed bony surfaces are united by fibrous tissue, permitting no movement; found only between bones of the skull. **s. denta'ta,** s. serrata. **s. no'tha,** a type formed by apposition of the roughened surfaces of the two participating bones. **s. pla'na,** a type in which there is simple apposition of the contiguous surfaces, with no interlocking of the edges of the participating bones. **s. serra'ta,** a type in which the participating bones are united by interlocking processes resembling the teeth of a saw. **s. squamo'sa,** a type formed by overlapping of the broad beveled edges of the participating bones. **s. ve'ra,** a true suture; see _sutura._

suture (su'cher) 1. sutura. 2. a stitch or series of stitches made to secure apposition of the edges of a surgical or traumatic wound. 3. to apply such stitches. 4. material used in closing a wound with stitches. **su'tural,** adj. **absorbable s.,** a strand of material used for closing wounds which is subsequently dissolved by the tissue fluids. **apposition s.,** a superficial suture used for exact approximation of the cutaneous edges of a wound. **approximation s.,** a deep suture for securing apposition of the deep tissue of a wound. **buried s.,** one placed deep in the tissues and concealed by the skin. **catgut s.,** see *catgut.* **coaptation s.,** apposition s. **cobblers' s.,** one made with suture material threaded through a needle at each end. **continuous s.,** one in which a continuous, uninterrupted length of material is used. **cranial s's,** the lines of junction between the bones of the skull. **Czerny's s.,** 1. an intestinal suture in which the thread is passed through the mucous membrane only. 2. union of a ruptured tendon by splitting one of the ends and suturing the other end into the slit. **false s.,** a line of junction between apposed surfaces without fibrous union of the bones. **figure-of-8 s.,** one in which the threads follow the contours of the figure 8. **Gély's s.,** a continuous stitch for wounds of the intestine, made with a thread having a needle at each end. **glovers' s.,** lock-stitch s. **Halsted s.,** a modification of the Lembert suture. **interrupted s.,** one in which each stitch is made with a separate piece of material. **Lembert s.,** an inverting suture used in gastrointestinal surgery. **lock-stitch s.,** a continuous hemostatic suture used in intestinal surgery, in which the needle is, after each stitch, passed through the loop of the preceding stitch. **loop s.,** interrupted s. **mattress s.,** a method in which the stitches are parallel with (*horizontal mattress s.*) or at right angles to (*vertical mattress s.*) the wound edges. **nonabsorbable s.,** suture material which is not absorbed in the body. **pursestring s.,** a continuous, circular inverting suture used to bury the stump of the appendix. **relaxation s.,** any suture so formed that it may be loosened to relieve tension as necessary. **subcuticular s.,** a method of skin closure involving placement of stitches in the subcuticular tissues parallel with the line of the wound. **uninterrupted s.,** continuous s.

svedberg (sfed'berg) Svedberg unit.

swab (swahb) a wad of cotton or other absorbent material attached to the end of a wire or stick, used for applying medication, removing material, collecting bacteriological material, etc.

swage (swāj) 1. to shape metal by hammering or by adapting it to a die. 2. to fuse, as suture material to the end of a suture needle.

sweat (swet) perspiration; the liquid secreted by the sweat glands.

sweeny (swe'ne) shoulder slip.

swelling (swel'ing) 1. transient abnormal enlargement of a body part or area not due to cell proliferation. 2. an eminence, or elevation. **cloudy s.,** an early stage of toxic degenerative changes, especially in protein constituents of organs in infectious diseases, in which the tissues appear swollen, parboiled, and opaque but revert to normal when the cause is removed.

sycosiform (si-ko'sĭ-form) resembling sycosis.

sycosis (si-ko'sis) papulopustular inflammation of hair follicles, especially of the beard. **s. bar'-** bae, bacterial folliculitis of the bearded region, usually caused by *Staphylococcus aureus.* **lupoid s.,** a chronic, scarring form of deep sycosis barbae. **s. vulga'ris, s.** barbae.

symballophone (sim-bal'o-fōn) a stethoscope with two chest pieces, making possible the comparison and localization of sounds.

symbiont (sim'bi-ont, sim'be-ont) an organism living in a state of symbiosis.

symbiosis (sim''bi-o'sis, -be-o'sis) 1. in parasitology, the close association of two dissimilar organisms, classified as mutualism, commensalism, parasitism, amensalism, or synnecrosis, depending on the advantage or disadvantage derived from the relationship. 2. in psychiatry, a mutually reinforcing relationship between persons who are dependent on each other; a normal characteristic of the relationship between mother and infant. 3. symbiotic psychosis. **symbiot'ic,** adj.

symbiote (sim'bi-ōt) symbiont.

symblepharon (sim-blef'ah-ron) adhesion of the eyelid(s) to the eyeball.

symblepharopterygium (-blef''ah-ro-ter-ij'e-um) symblepharon in which the adhesion is a cicatricial band resembling a pterygium.

symbolia (sim-bo'le-ah) ability to recognize the nature of objects by the sense of touch.

symbolism (sim'bo-lizm) 1. an abnormal mental condition in which every occurrence is conceived of as a symbol of the patient's own thoughts. 2. in psychoanalysis an unconscious mechanism whereby the real meaning of an object or idea becomes transformed so as not to be recognized as sexual by the superego.

symbolization (sim''bol-ĭ-za'shun) an unconscious defense mechanism in which one idea or object comes to represent another because of similarity or association between them.

symmelus (sim'ĕ-lus) a fetus with fused legs and one, two, or three feet, or no feet.

symmetry (sim'ĕ-tre) correspondence in size, form, and arrangement of parts on opposite sides of a plane or around an axis. **symmet'rical,** adj. **bilateral s.,** the configuration of an irregularly shaped body (as the human body or that of higher animals) which can be divided by a longitudinal plane into halves that are mirror images of each other. **inverse s.,** correspondence as between a part and its mirror image, wherein the right (or left) side of one part corresponds with the left (or right) side of the other. **radial s.,** that in which the body parts are arranged regularly around a central axis.

sympathectomy (-thek'tah-me) transection, resection, or other interruption of some portion of the sympathetic nervous pathway. **chemical s.,** that accomplished by means of a chemical agent.

sympathetic (sim''pah-thet'ik) 1. pertaining to, exhibiting, or caused by sympathy. 2. pertaining to the sympathetic nervous system.

sympathicoblast (sim-path'ĭ-ko-blast'') the primitive pluripotential undifferentiated cell that develops into a sympathetic nerve cell.

sympathicoblastoma (sim-path''ĭ-ko-blas-to'-

mah) a malignant tumor containing sympathicoblasts; see *neuroblastoma.*

sympathicotonia (-to′ne-ah) a stimulated condition of the sympathetic nervous system, marked by vascular spasm, heightened blood pressure, and gooseflesh. **sympathicoton′ic,** adj.

sympathicotripsy (-trip′se) the surgical crushing of a nerve, ganglion, or plexus of the sympathetic nervous system.

sympathicotropic (-trop′ik) 1. having an affinity for the sympathetic nervous system. 2. an agent having an affinity for or exerting its principal effect on the sympathetic nervous system.

sympathicus (sim-path′ĭ-kus) the sympathetic nervous system.

sympathin (sim′pah-thin) a neurohormonal mediator of nerve impulses at sympathetic nerve synapses; the term is used only when the nature of the mediator is unknown.

sympathoadrenal (sim″path-o-ah-dre′n'l) 1. pertaining to the sympathetic nervous system and the adrenal medulla. 2. involving the sympathetic nervous system and the adrenal glands, especially increased sympathetic activity that causes increased secretion of epinephrine and norepinephrine.

sympathogonia (-go′ne-ah) sing. *sympathogo′nium* [Gr.] undifferentiated embryonic cells which develop into sympathetic cells.

sympathogonioma (-go″ne-o′mah) sympathicoblastoma.

sympatholytic (-lit′ik) 1. antiadrenergic; blocking transmission of impulses from the postganglionic fibers to effector organs or tissues, inhibiting smooth muscle contraction and glandular secretion. 2. an agent that produces such an effect.

sympathomimetic (-mi-met′ik) 1. adrenergic; producing effects resembling those of impulses transmitted by the postganglionic fibers of the sympathetic nervous system. 2. an agent that produces such an effect.

sympathy (sim′pah-the) 1. an influence produced in any organ by disease or disorder in another part. 2. compassion for another's grief or loss. 3. the influence exerted by one individual upon another, or received by one from another, and the effects thus produced, as seen in hypnotism or in yawning.

symphalangia (sim″fah-lan′je-ah) congenital end-to-end fusion of contiguous phalanges of a digit.

symphyseal, symphysial (sim-fiz′e-al) pertaining to a symphysis.

symphysiorrhaphy (-fiz″e-or′ah-fe) suture of a divided symphysis.

symphysiotomy (-fiz″e-ot′ah-me) division of the symphysis pubis to facilitate delivery.

symphysis (sim′fĭ-sis), pl. *sym′physes* [Gr.] fibrocartilaginous joint; a type of joint in which the apposed bony surfaces are firmly united by a plate of fibrocartilage. **pubic s., s. pu′bica, s. pu′bis,** the line of union of the bodies of the pubic bones in the median plane.

sympodia (sim-po′de-ah) fusion of the lower extremities.

symport (sim′port) a structure that transports two compounds simultaneously across a cell membrane in the same direction, one compound being transported down a concentration gradient, the other against a gradient.

symptom (simp′tom) any subjective evidence of disease or of a patient's condition, i.e., such evidence as perceived by the patient; a change in a patient's condition indicative of some bodily or mental state. **objective s.,** one that is evident to the observer; see *sign.* **presenting s.,** the symptom or group of symptoms about which the patient complains or from which he seeks relief. **subjective s.,** one perceptible only to the patient. **withdrawal s's,** symptoms caused by sudden withholding of a drug to which a person is habituated or addicted.

symptomatic (simp″to-mat′ik) 1. pertaining to or of the nature of a symptom. 2. indicative (of a particular disease or disorder). 3. exhibiting the symptoms of a particular disease but having a different cause. 4. directed at the allaying of symptoms, as symptomatic treatment.

symptomatology (simp″to-mah-tol′ah-je) 1. the branch of medicine dealing with symptoms. 2. the combined symptoms of a disease.

symptomatolytic (simp″to-mat-o-lit′ik) causing the disappearance of symptoms.

symptosis (simp-to′sis) gradual wasting of the body or of an organ.

sympus (sim′pus) a fetus with fused legs.

syn- word element [Gr.], *union; association; together with.*

synapse (sin′aps) the junction between the processes of two neurons or between a neuron and an effector organ, where neural impulses are transmitted by electrical (see *ephapse*) or chemical means. In chemical transmission, the impulse causes the release of a neurotransmitter (e.g., acetylcholine or norepinephrine) from the presynaptic membrane of the axon terminal. The neurotransmitter molecules diffuse across the synaptic cleft and bind with specific receptors on the postsynaptic membrane causing depolarization or hyperpolarization of the postsynaptic cell.

synapsis (sĭ-nap′sis) the point-for-point pairing off of homologous chromosomes from male and female pronuclei during prophase of meiosis.

synaptic (sĭ-nap′tik) pertaining to a synapse or to synapsis.

synaptosome (sin-ap′to-sōm″) any of the membrane-bound sacs that break away from axon terminals at a synapse after brain tissue has been homogenized in sugar solution; it contains synaptic vessels and mitochondria.

synarthrodia (sin″ar-thro′de-ah) synarthrosis. **synarthro′dial,** adj.

synarthrophysis (-ar-thro-fi′sis) any ankylosing process.

synarthrosis (-ar-thro′sis), pl. *synarthro′ses* [Gr.] fibrous joint.

syncanthus (sin-kan′thus) adhesion of the eyeball to the orbital structures.

syncephalus (-sef′ah-lus) a twin fetus with heads fused into one, there being a single face, with four ears.

synchilia (-ki′le-ah) congenital adhesion of the lips.

synchiria (sin-ki′re-ah) a condition in which the sensation produced by a stimulus applied to one side of the body is referred to both sides.

synchondrosis (sin″kon-dro′sis), pl. *synchondro′ses* [Gr.] a type of cartilaginous joint in which the cartilage is usually converted into bone before adult life.

synchondrotomy (-kon-drot′ah-me) division of a synchondrosis.

synchronism (sin′kro-nizm) occurrence at the same time. **syn′chronous,** adj.

synchysis (-kĭ-sis) a softening or fluid condition of the vitreous body of the eye. **s. scintil′lans,** floating cholesterol crystals in the vitreous, developing as a secondary degenerative change.

synclitism (-klĭ-tizm) parallelism between the planes of the fetal head and those of the maternal pelvis. **synclit′ic,** adj.

synclonus (-klo-nus) muscular tremor or successive clonic contraction of various muscles together.

syncope (-ko-pe) a faint; temporary loss of consciousness due to generalized cerebral ischemia. **syn′copal, syncop′ic,** adj. **cardiac s.,** sudden loss of consciousness, with momentary premonitory symptoms or without warning, due to cerebral anemia caused by ventricular asystole, extreme bradycardia, or ventricular fibrillation. **carotid sinus s.,** see under *syndrome.* **laryngeal s.,** tussive s. **stretching s.,** syncope associated with stretching the arms upward with the spine extended. **swallow s.,** syncope associated with swallowing, a disorder of atrioventricular conduction mediated by the vagus nerve. **tussive s.,** brief loss of consciousness associated with paroxysms of coughing. **vasovagal s.,** see under *attack.*

syncytial (sin-sish′al) of or pertaining to a syncytium.

syncytioma (-sit″e-o′mah) syncytial endometritis. **s. malig′num,** choriocarcinoma.

syncytiotrophoblast (-sit″e-o-trof′o-blast) the outer syncytial layer of the trophoblast.

syncytium (-sish′e-um) a multinucleate mass of protoplasm produced by the merging of cells.

syndactyly (-dak′tĭ-le) persistence of webbing between adjacent digits of the hand or foot, so that they are more or less completely fused together. **syndac′tylous,** adj.

syndectomy (-dek′tah-me) peridectomy.

syndesis (sin′dĕ-sis) 1. arthrodesis. 2. synapsis.

syndesm(o)- word element [Gr.], *connective tissue; ligament.*

syndesmectomy (sin″dez-mek′tah-me) excision of a portion of ligament.

syndesmectopia (-mek-to′pe-ah) unusual situation of a ligament.

syndesmitis (-mi′tis) 1. inflammation of a ligament. 2. conjunctivitis.

syndesmography (-mog′rah-fe) a description of the ligaments.

syndesmology (-mol′ah-je) arthrology.

syndesmoma (-mo′mah) a tumor of connective tissue.

syndesmoplasty (sin-dez′mo-plas″te) plastic repair of a ligament.

syndesmosis (sin″dez-mo′sis), pl. *syndesmo′ses* [Gr.] a joint in which the bones are united by fibrous connective tissue forming an interosseous membrane or ligament.

syndesmotomy (-mot′o-me) incision of a ligament.

syndrome (sin′drōm) a set of symptoms occurring together; the sum of signs of any morbid state; a symptom complex. **Aarskog's s.,** a hereditary syndrome, transmitted as an X-linked trait, characterized by ocular hypertelorism, anteverted nostrils, broad upper lip, peculiar scrotal "shawl" above the penis, and small hands. **acquired immune deficiency s., acquired immunodeficiency s. (AIDS),** an epidemic, transmissible retroviral disease caused by infection with the human immunodeficiency virus, manifested in severe cases as profound depression of cell-mediated immunity, and affecting certain recognized risk groups. Diagnosis is by the presence of a disease indicative of a defect in cell-mediated immunity (e.g., life-threatening opportunistic infection) in the absence of any known causes of underlying immunodeficiency or of any other host defense defects reported to be associated with that disease (e.g., iatrogenic immunosuppression). **acute radiation s.,** a syndrome caused by exposure to a whole body dose of over 1 gray of ionizing radiation; symptoms, whose severity and time of onset depend on the size of the dose, include erythema, nausea and vomiting, fatigue, diarrhea, petechiae, bleeding from the mucous membranes, hematologic changes, gastrointestinal hemorrhage, epilation, hypotension, tachycardia, and dehydration; death may occur within hours or weeks of exposure. **Adams-Stokes s.,** see under *disease.* **Adie's s.,** tonic pupil associated with absence or diminution of certain tendon reflexes. **adrenogenital s.,** hyperfunction of the adrenal cortex, causing pseudohermaphroditism and virilism in the female, usually evident at birth, and precocious sexual development in the male, usually not evident until age three to four. **adult respiratory distress s. (ARDS),** fulminant pulmonary interstitial and alveolar edema, which usually develops a few days after the initiating trauma, thought to result from a massive sympathetic discharge due to brain injury or hypoxia and from increased capillary permeability. **afferent loop s.,** chronic partial obstruction of the proximal loop (duodenum and jejunum) after gastrojejunostomy, resulting in duodenal distention, pain, and nausea following ingestion of food. **Ahumada-Del Castillo s.,** a nonpuerperal triad consisting of galactorrhea, amenorrhea, and low gonadotropin secretion. **Albright's s.,** polyostotic fibrous dysplasia, patchy dermal pigmentation, and endocrine dysfunction. **Aldrich's s.,** Wiskott-Aldrich s. **Alport's s.,** a hereditary disorder marked by progressive nerve deafness, progressive pyelonephritis or glomerulonephritis, and occasionally ocular defects. **Alström's s.,** a hereditary syndrome of retinitis pigmentosa with nystagmus and early loss of central vision, deafness, obesity, and diabetes mellitus. **amnestic s.,** an organic mental disorder characterized by impairment of memory occurring in a normal state of consciousness; the most common cause is thiamine deficiency associated with alcohol abuse. **anorexia-cachexia s.,** a systemic response to cancer occurring as a result of a poorly understood relationship between anorexia and cachexia, manifested by malnutrition, weight loss, muscular weakness, acidosis, and toxemia. **anterior cord s.,** localized injury to the anterior portion of the spinal cord, characterized by complete paralysis and hypalgesia and hypesthesia to the level of the lesion, but with relative preservation of posterior column sensations of touch, position, and vibration. **Banti's s.,** congestive splenomegaly. **Barrett's s.,** peptic ulcer of the lower esophagus, often with stricture, due to the presence of columnar-lined epithelium, which may contain functional mucous cells, parietal cells, or chief cells, in the esophagus instead of normal squamous cell epithelium. **Bartter's s.,** hypertrophy and hyperplasia of the juxtaglomerular cells, producing hypokalemic alkalosis and hyperaldosteronism, characterized by absence of hypertension in the presence of markedly increased plasma renin concentration and by insensitivity to the pressor effects of angiotensin. It usually affects children and is perhaps hereditary. **basal cell nevus s.,** an autosomal dominant syndrome characterized by the development in early life of numerous basal cell carcinomas, in association with abnormalities of the skin, bone, nervous system, eyes, and reproductive tract. **Bassen-Kornzweig s.,** abetalipoproteinemia. **battered-child s.,** multiple traumatic lesions of the bones and soft tissues of young children, often accompanied by subdural hematomas, willfully inflicted by an adult. **Behçet's s.,** severe uveitis and retinal vasculitis, optic atrophy, and aphtha-like lesions of the mouth and genitalia, often with other signs and symptoms suggesting a diffuse vasculitis; it most often affects young males. **Bernard-Soulier s.,** a hereditary coagulation disorder marked by mild thrombocytopenia, giant and morphologically abnormal platelets, hemorrhagic tendency, prolonged bleeding time, and abnormal prothrombin consumption. **Boerhaave's s.,** spontaneous rupture of the esophagus. **Börjeson s., Börjeson-Forssman-Lehmann s.,** a hereditary syndrome, transmitted as an X-linked recessive trait, characterized by severe mental retardation, epilepsy, hypogonadism, hypometabolism, marked obesity, swelling of the subcutaneous tissues of the face, and large ears. **Brown-Séquard s.,** ipsilateral paralysis and loss of discriminatory and joint sensation, and contralateral loss of pain and temperature sensation; due to damage to one half of the spinal cord. **Budd-Chiari s.,** symptomatic obstruction or occlusion of the hepatic veins, causing hepatomegaly, abdominal pain and tenderness, intractable ascites, mild jaundice, and eventually portal hypertension and liver failure. **Caffey's s.,** infantile cortical hyperostosis. **Canada-Cronkhite s.,** familial polyposis of the gastroin-

testinal tract associated with alopecia, nail dystrophy, and hyperpigmentation of the skin. **carcinoid s.,** a symptom complex associated with carcinoid tumors (argentaffinomas), marked by attacks of severe cyanotic flushing of the skin lasting from minutes to days and by diarrheal watery stools, bronchoconstrictive attacks, sudden drops in blood pressure, edema, and ascites. Symptoms are caused by the secretion by the tumor of serotonin, prostaglandins, and other biologically active substances. **carotid sinus s.,** syncope sometimes associated with convulsions due to overactivity of the carotid sinus reflex when pressure is applied to one or both carotid sinuses. **carpal tunnel s.,** pain and burning or tingling paresthesias in the fingers and hand, sometimes extending to the elbow, due to compression of the median nerve in the carpal tunnel. **Carpenter's s.,** a hereditary disorder, transmitted as an autosomal recessive trait, characterized by acrocephalopolysyndactyly, brachydactyly, peculiar facies, obesity, mental retardation, hypogonadism, and other anomalies. **central cord s.,** injury to the central portion of the cervical spinal cord resulting in disproportionately more weakness or paralysis in the upper extremities than in the lower; pathological change is caused by hemorrhage or edema. **cerebrohepatorenal s.,** a hereditary disorder, transmitted as an autosomal recessive trait, characterized by craniofacial abnormalities, hypotonia, hepatomegaly, polycystic kidneys, jaundice, and death in early infancy. **cervical rib s.,** scalenus s. **Cestan's s., Cestan-Chenais s.,** an association of contralateral hemiplegia, contralateral hemianesthesia, ipsilateral lateropulsion and hemiasynergia, Horner's syndrome, and ipsilateral laryngoplegia, due to scattered lesions of the pyramid, sensory tract, inferior cerebellar peduncle, nucleus ambiguus, and oculopupillary center. **Charcot's s.,** 1. amyotrophic lateral sclerosis. 2. intermittent claudication. **Chédiak-Higashi s.,** a lethal, progressive, autosomal recessive, systemic disorder associated with oculocutaneous albinism, massive leukocyte inclusions (giant lysosomes), histiocytic infiltration of multiple body organs, development of pancytopenia, hepatosplenomegaly, recurrent or persistent bacterial infections, and a possible predisposition to development of malignant lymphoma. **Chinese restaurant s.,** transient arterial dilatation due to ingestion of monosodium glutamate, which is used liberally in seasoning Chinese food, marked by throbbing head, lightheadedness, tightness of the jaw, neck, and shoulders, and backache. **Chotzen's s.,** an autosomal dominant disorder characterized by acrocephalosyndactyly in which the syndactyly is mild and by hypertelorism, ptosis, and sometimes mental retardation. **compartmental s.,** a condition in which increased tissue pressure in a confined anatomic space causes decreased blood flow leading to ischemia and dysfunction of contained myoneural elements, marked by pain, muscle weakness, sensory loss, and palpable tenseness in the involved compartment; ischemia can lead to necrosis resulting in permanent impairment of function. **congenital**

rubella s., transplacental infection of the fetus with rubella, usually in the first trimester of pregnancy, as a consequence of maternal infection, resulting in various developmental anomalies in the newborn infant. **Conn's s.**, primary aldosteronism. **Costen's s.**, temporomandibular joint s. **couvade s.**, the occurrence in the mate of a pregnant woman of symptoms that are related to pregnancy, such as nausea, vomiting, and abdominal pain. **cri du chat s.**, a hereditary congenital syndrome characterized by hypertelorism, microcephaly, severe mental deficiency, and a plaintive catlike cry, due to deletion of the short arm of chromosome 5. **Crigler-Najjar s.**, an autosomal recessive form of nonhemolytic jaundice due to absence of the hepatic enzyme glucuronide transferase, marked by excessive amounts of unconjugated bilirubin in the blood, kernicterus, and severe central nervous system disorders. **s. of crocodile tears**, spontaneous lacrimation occurring parallel with the normal salivation of eating, and associated with facial paralysis; it seems to be due to straying of regenerating nerve fibers, some of those destined for the salivary glands going to the lacrimal glands. **crush s.**, the edema, oliguria, and other symptoms of renal failure that follow crushing of a part, especially a large muscle mass; see *lower nephron nephrosis.* **Cruveilhier-Baumgarten s.**, cirrhosis of the liver with portal hypertension associated with congenital patency of the umbilical and paraumbilical veins. **Cushing's s.**, a condition, more commonly seen in females, due to hyperadrenocorticism resulting from neoplasms of the adrenal cortex or anterior lobe of the pituitary; or to prolonged excessive intake of glucocorticoids for therapeutic purposes (*Cushing's s. medicamentosus*). The symptoms may include adiposity of the face, neck, and trunk, kyphosis caused by softening of the spine, amenorrhea, hypertrichosis (in females), impotence (in males), dusky complexion with purple markings, hypertension, polycythemia, pain in the abdomen and back, and muscular weakness. **Dandy-Walker s.**, congenital hydrocephalus due to obstruction of the foramina of Magendie and Luschka. **Down s.**, mongoloid features, short phalanges, widened space between the first and second toes and fingers, and moderate to severe mental retardation; associated with a chromosomal abnormality, usually trisomy of chromosome 21. **Dubin-Johnson s.**, hereditary chronic nonhemolytic jaundice thought to be due to defective excretion of conjugated bilirubin and certain other organic anions by the liver; a brown, coarsely granular pigment in hepatic cells is pathognomonic. **dumping s.**, nausea, weakness, sweating, palpitation, syncope, often a sensation of warmth, and sometimes diarrhea, occurring after ingestion of food in patients who have undergone partial gastrectomy. **Eaton-Lambert s.**, a myasthenia-like syndrome in which the weakness usually affects the limbs and ocular and bulbar muscles are spared; often associated with oat-cell carcinoma of the lung. **effort s.**, neurocirculatory asthenia. **Ehlers-Danlos s.**, a group of inherited disorders of connective tissue, varying in

clinical and biochemical evidence, in mode of inheritance, and in severity from mild to lethal; major manifestations include hyperextensible skin and joints, easy bruisability, friability of tissues, bleeding, poor wound healing, subcutaneous nodules, and cardiovascular, orthopedic, intestinal and ocular defects. **Eisenmenger's s.**, ventricular septal defect with pulmonary hypertension and cyanosis due to right-to-left (reversed) shunt of blood. Sometimes defined as pulmonary hypertension (pulmonary vascular disease) and cyanosis with the shunt being at the atrial, ventricular, or great vessel area. **EMG s.**, **exophthalmos-macroglossia-gigantism s.**, an autosomal dominant disorder characterized by exophthalmos, macroglossia, and gigantism, often associated with visceromegaly, adrenocortical cytomegaly, and dysplasia of the renal medulla. **extrapyramidal s.**, any of a group of clinical disorders marked by abnormal involuntary movements, including parkinsonism, athetosis, and chorea. **Faber's s.**, hypochromic anemia. **Fanconi's s.**, 1. a rare hereditary disorder, transmitted as an autosomal recessive trait, characterized by pancytopenia, hypoplasia of the bone marrow, and patchy brown discoloration of the skin due to the deposition of melanin, and associated with multiple congenital anomalies of the musculoskeletal and genitourinary systems. 2. a general term for a group of diseases marked by dysfunction of the proximal renal tubules, with generalized hyperaminoaciduria, renal glycosuria, hyperphosphaturia, and bicarbonate and water loss; the most common cause is cystinosis, but it is also associated with other genetic diseases and occurs in idiopathic and acquired forms. **Farber's s.**, **Farber-Uzman s.**, Farber's disease. **Felty's s.**, chronic (rheumatoid) arthritis, splenomegaly, leukopenia, pigmented spots on the skin of the legs, and other inconsistent evidence of hypersplenism, namely, anemia and thrombocytopenia. **fetal alcohol s.**, a syndrome of altered prenatal growth and morphogenesis, occurring in infants born of women who were chronically alcoholic during pregnancy; it includes maxillary hypoplasia, prominence of the forehead and mandible, short palpebral fissures, microophthalmia, epicanthal folds, severe growth retardation, mental retardation, and microcephaly. **fetal hydantoin s.**, poor growth and development with craniofacial and skeletal abnormalities, produced by prenatal exposure to hydantoin analogues, including phenytoin. **Ganser's s.**, amnesia, disturbance of consciousness, and hallucinations, associated with senseless answers to questions, and absurd acts. **Gardner's s.**, familial polyposis of the colon associated with osseous and soft tissue tumors. **gay bowel s.**, an assortment of sexually transmitted bowel and rectal diseases affecting homosexual males, caused by a wide variety of infectious agents. **general adaptation s.**, the total of all nonspecific reactions of the body to prolonged systemic stress. **Gilles de la Tourette's s.**, facial and vocal tics with onset in childhood, progressing to generalized jerking movements in any body part, with echolalia and coprolalia. **Goodpasture's s.**, glomerulonephritis associated with pulmonary hemorrhage and circulating antibodies against basement membranes, occurring most frequently in young men and usually having a course of rapidly progressing renal failure, with hemoptysis, pulmonary infiltrates, and dyspnea. **Gradenigo's s.**, sixth nerve palsy and unilateral headache in suppurative disease of the middle ear, due to involvement of the abducens and trigeminal nerves by direct spread of the infection. **gray s.**, a potentially fatal condition seen in neonates, particularly premature infants, due to a reaction to chloramphenicol, characterized by an ashen gray cyanosis, listlessness, weakness, and hypotension. **Guillain-Barré s.**, acute febrile polyneuritis. **Hallervorden-Spatz s.**, an autosomal recessive disorder involving marked reduction in the number of myelin sheaths of the globus pallidus and substantia nigra, with accumulations of iron pigment, progressive rigidity beginning in the legs, choreoathetoid movements, dysarthria, and progressive mental deterioration. **Hamman-Rich s.**, idiopathic pulmonary fibrosis. **Hand-Schüller-Christian s.**, see under *disease*. **Harada's s.**, bilateral diffuse exudative choroiditis and retinal detachment associated with headache, vomiting, an increase in lymphocytes in the cerebrospinal fluid, and temporary or permanent deafness; there may be transient vitiligo, alopecia, and poliosis. **Horner's s.**, sinking in of the eyeball, ptosis of the upper lid, slight elevation of the lower lid, miosis, narrowing of palpebral fissure, and anhidrosis and flushing of the affected side of the face; due to paralysis of the cervical sympathetic nerves. **Hurler's s.**, a mucopolysaccharidosis due to deficiency of the enzyme α-L-iduronidase, transmitted as an autosomal recessive trait, characterized by gargoyle-like facies, dwarfism, severe somatic and skeletal changes, severe mental retardation, cloudy corneas, deafness, cardiovascular defects, hepatosplenomegaly, and joint contractures. **hypereosinophilic s.**, a massive increase in the number of eosinophils in the blood, mimicking leukemia, and characterized by eosinophilic infiltration of the heart, brain, liver, and lungs and by a fatal course. **hyperkinetic s.**, attention-deficit hyperactivity disorder. **s. of inappropriate antidiuretic hormone (SIADH)**, persistent hyponatremia, inappropriately elevated urine osmolality, and no discernible stimulus for ADH release. **irritable bowel s.**, **irritable colon s.**, a chronic noninflammatory disease with a psychophysiologic basis, characterized by abdominal pain, diarrhea or constipation or both, and no detectable pathologic change; a variant form is marked by painless diarrhea. See *mucous colitis*. **Kartagener's s.**, a hereditary syndrome consisting of dextrocardia, bronchiectasis, and sinusitis. **Kimmelstiel-Wilson s.**, intercapillary glomerulosclerosis. **Klinefelter's s.**, a condition characterized by the presence of small testes, with fibrosis and hyalinization of seminiferous tubules, by variable degrees of masculinization, azoospermia, and infertility, and by increase in urinary gonadotropins. It is associated typically with an **XXY** chromosome complement although variants include XXYY, XXXY, XXXXY, and various mosaic patterns. **Klippel-Feil s.**, shortness of the neck due to reduction in the number of cervical vertebrae or the fusion of multiple hemivertebrae into one osseous mass, with limitation of neck motion and low hairline. **Korsakoff's s.**, amnestic syndrome; more narrowly, the amnestic component of Wernicke-Korsakoff s. **Laurence-Moon s.**, an autosomal recessive disorder characterized by mental retardation, pigmentary retinopathy, hypogonadism, and spastic paraplegia. **lazy leukocyte s.**, a syndrome occurring in children, marked by recurrent low-grade infections, associated with a defect in neutrophil chemotaxis and deficient random mobility of neutrophils. **Leriche's s.**, fatigue in the hips, thighs, or calves on exercising, absence of pulsation in femoral arteries, impotence, and often pallor and coldness of the legs, usually affecting males and due to obstruction of the terminal aorta. **Lesch-Nyhan s.**, an X-linked disorder of purine metabolism with physical and mental retardation, compulsive self-mutilation of fingers and lips by biting, choreoathetosis, spastic cerebral palsy, and impaired renal function, and by extremely excessive purine synthesis and consequently hyperuricemia and excessive urinary secretion of uric acid. **Libman-Sacks s.**, atypical verrucous endocarditis. **Lowe's s.**, oculocerebrorenal s. **Lown-Ganong-Levine s.**, an electrocardiographic abnormality characterized by a short P-R interval with a normal QRS complex, accompanied by atrial tachycardia. **Lutembacher's s.**, atrial septal defect with mitral stenosis (usually rheumatic). **lymphadenopathy s.**, unexplained lymphadenopathy for 3 or more months involving extrainguinal sites, which on biopsy reveal nonspecific lymphoid hyperplasia; seen in many male homosexuals and possibly a prodrome of acquired immune deficiency syndrome. **McArdle's s.**, see under *disease*. **Maffucci's s.**, enchondromatosis with multiple cutaneous or visceral hemangiomas. **malabsorption s.**, a group of disorders marked by subnormal absorption of dietary constituents, and thus excessive loss of nutrients in the stool, which may be due to a digestive defect, a mucosal abnormality, or lymphatic obstruction. **Marfan's s.**, a hereditary syndrome of abnormal length of the extremities, especially of fingers and toes, with subluxation of the lens, cardiovascular abnormalities, and other disorders. **Marie's s.**, hypertrophic pulmonary osteoarthropathy. **megacystis-megaureter s.**, chronic ureteral dilatation (megaureter) associated with hypotonia and dilatation of the bladder (megacystis) and gaping of the ureteral orifices, permitting vesicoureteral reflux of urine, and resulting in chronic pyelonephritis. **Menkes' s.**, a hereditary abnormality in copper absorption marked by severe cerebral degeneration and arterial changes resulting in death in infancy and by sparse, brittle scalp hair. It is transmitted as an X-linked recessive trait. **methionine malabsorption s.**, an inborn aminoacidopathy marked by white hair, mental retardation, convulsions, attacks of hyperpnea, and urine with an odor like an oasthouse (for drying hops) due to alpha-hydroxybutyric acid formed by bacterial action on the unabsorbed methionine. **middle lobe s.,** atelectasis of the middle lobe of the right lung, with chronic pneumonitis. **Mikulicz's s.,** chronic bilateral hypertrophy of the lacrimal, parotid, and salivary glands, associated with chronic lymphocytic infiltration; it may be associated with other diseases. **milk-alkali s.,** hypercalcemia without hypercalciuria or hypophosphatemia and with only mild alkalosis and other symptoms attributed to ingestion of milk and absorbable alkali for long periods. **Milkman's s.,** a generalized bone disease marked by multiple transparent stripes of absorption in the long and flat bones. **mitral valve prolapse s.,** prolapse of the mitral valve, often with regurgitation; a common, usually benign, often asymptomatic condition characterized by midsystolic clicks and late systolic murmurs on auscultation. **Möbius' s.,** agenesis or aplasia of the motor nuclei of the cranial nerves marked by congenital bilateral facial palsy, with unilateral or bilateral paralysis of the abductors of the eye, sometimes associated with cranial nerve involvement, and anomalies of the extremities. **Mohr s.,** oral-facial-digital s., type II. **Morquio's s.,** two biochemically distinct but clinically nearly indistinguishable forms of mucopolysaccharidosis, marked by genu valgum, pigeon breast, progressive flattening of the vertebral bodies, short neck and trunk, progressive deafness, and mild corneal clouding. **multiple glandular deficiency s.,** failure of any combination of endocrine glands, often accompanied by nonendocrine autoimmune abnormalities. **Munchausen s.,** habitual seeking of hospital treatment for apparent acute illness, the patient giving a plausible and dramatic history, all of which is false. **myeloproliferative s.,** a group of diseases related histogenetically and marked, at varying times in varying degrees, by medullary and extramedullary proliferation of one or more lines of bone marrow constituents, including myelocytic, erythroblastic, and megakaryocytic forms, in addition to various cells derived from the reticulum and mesenchymal elements. **Nelson's s.,** the development of an ACTH-producing pituitary tumor after bilateral adrenalectomy in Cushing's syndrome; it is characterized by aggressive growth of the tumor and hyperpigmentation of the skin. **nephrotic s.,** a condition marked by massive edema, heavy proteinuria, hypoalbuminemia, and peculiar susceptibility to intercurrent infections. **Noonan's s.,** webbed neck, ptosis, hypogonadism, and short stature, i.e., the phenotype of Turner's syndrome without the gonadal dysgenesis. **oculocerebrorenal s.,** an X-linked disorder marked by vitamin D–refractory rickets, hydrophthalmia, congenital glaucoma and cataracts, mental retardation, and renal tubule dysfunction as evidenced by hypophosphatemia, acidosis, and aminoaciduria. **oral-facial-digital s.,** any of a group of congenital syndromes characterized by a variety or oral, facial, and digital anomalies. *Type I,* a male-lethal X-linked dominant disorder, is associated

with mental retardation, familial trembling, alopecia, seborrhea, and milia; *type II,* an autosomal recessive disorder, is associated with episodic neuromuscular disturbances; *type III,* an autosomal recessive disorder, is associated with profound mental retardation. **organic affective s.,** a mental syndrome marked by manic or depressive mood disturbance caused by a specific organic factor and not associated with delirium. **organic anxiety s.,** a mental syndrome marked by prominent, recurrent panic attacks or generalized anxiety caused by a specific organic factor and not associated with delirium. **organic brain s.,** organic mental s. **organic delusional s.,** a mental syndrome marked by delusions caused by a specific organic factor and not associated with delirium. **organic personality s.,** a mental syndrome marked by a pronounced change in behavior or personality, e.g., emotional lability, caused by a specific organic factor and not associated with delirium. **organic mental s.,** a constellation of psychological or behavioral signs and symptoms associated with one or more organic causes. **ovarian vein s.,** obstruction of the ureter due to compression by an enlarged or varicose ovarian vein; typically the vein becomes enlarged during pregnancy. **Pancoast's s.,** 1. roentgenographic shadow at the apex of the lung, neuritic pain in the arm, atrophy of the muscles of the arm and hand, and Horner's syndrome, observed in tumor near the apex of the lung; due to involvement of the brachial plexus. 2. osteolysis in the posterior part of one or more ribs and sometimes involving also the corresponding vertebra. **paraneoplastic s.,** a symptom complex arising in a cancer-bearing patient that cannot be explained by local or distant spread of the tumor. **Parinaud's s.,** paralysis of conjugate upward movement of the eyes without paralysis of convergence; associated with tumors of the midbrain. **Parinaud's oculoglandular s.,** a general term applied to conjunctivitis, usually unilateral and of the follicular type, followed by tenderness and enlargement of the preauricular lymph nodes; often due to leptotrichosis but may be associated with other infections. **parkinsonian s.,** a form of parkinsonism due to idiopathic degeneration of the corpus striatum or substantia nigra; frequently a sequel of lethargic encephalitis, but other factors have also been implicated. **Peutz-Jeghers s.,** familial gastrointestinal polyposis, especially in the small bowel, associated with mucocutaneous pigmentation. **pickwickian s.,** obesity, somnolence, hypoventilation, and erythrocytosis. **Pierre Robin s.,** micrognathia occurring in association with cleft palate, glossoptosis, and absent gag reflex. **Plummer-Vinson s.,** dysphagia with glossitis, hypochromic anemia, splenomegaly, and atrophy in the mouth, pharynx, and upper end of the esophagus. **postcardiotomy s.,** anxiety, confusion, and perception disturbances occurring 2 to 5 days after an operation using cardiopulmonary bypass. **postcommissurotomy s.,** postpericardiotomy s. **postgastrectomy s.,** dumping s. **post-lumbar puncture s.,** headache in the erect posture, sometimes with nuchal pain, vomiting, diaphoresis, and malaise, all relieved by recumbency, occurring several hours after lumbar puncture; it is due to lowering of intracranial pressure by leakage of cerebrospinal fluid through the needle tract. **postpericardiotomy s.,** delayed pericardial or pleural reaction with fever, chest pains, and signs of pleural and/or pericardial inflammation, following opening of the pericardium. **preexcitation s.,** Wolff-Parkinson-White s. **premenstrual s.,** a syndrome of unknown cause sometimes marked by bloating, edema, emotional lability, headache, changes in appetite or craving for selected foods, breast swelling and tenderness, constipation, and decreased ability to concentrate. **Putnam-Dana s.,** subacute combined degeneration of the spinal cord. **Ramsay Hunt s.,** facial paralysis accompanied by otalgia and a vesicular eruption involving the external canal of the ear, sometimes extending to the auricle, due to herpes zoster virus infection of the geniculate ganglion. **Reiter's s.,** the triad of nongonococcal urethritis, conjunctivitis, and arthritis, frequently with mucocutaneous lesions. **respiratory distress s. of newborn,** a condition most often seen in premature infants, infants of diabetic mothers, and infants delivered by cesarean section, marked by dyspnea and cyanosis, and including two patterns: in *hyaline membrane disease,* affected infants often die of respiratory distress in the first few days of life and at autopsy have a hyaline-like membrane lining the terminal respiratory passages; in *idiopathic respiratory distress of newborn,* affected infants may live, but in those who die, only resorption atelectasis is seen. **Reye's s.,** a rare, acute and often fatal encephalopathy of childhood, marked by acute brain swelling associated with hypoglycemia, fatty infiltration of the liver, hepatomegaly, and disturbed consciousness and seizures. It most often occurs as a sequel of varicella or a viral infection of the upper respiratory tract. **Rh-null s.,** chronic hemolytic anemia affecting individuals who lack all Rh factors (Rh_{null}); it is marked by spherocytosis, stomatocytosis, and increased osmotic fragility. **Riley-Day s.,** dysautonomia. **salt-depletion s., salt-losing s.,** vomiting, dehydration, hypotension, and sudden death due to very large sodium losses from the body. It may be seen in abnormal losses of sodium into the urine (as in congenital adrenal hyperplasia, adrenocortical insufficiency, or one of the forms of salt-losing nephritis) or in large extrarenal sodium losses, usually from the gastrointestinal tract. **Sanfilippo's s.,** four biochemically distinct but clinically indistinguishable forms of mucopolysaccharidosis, characterized by urinary excretion of heparan sulfate and by mild Hurler-like symptoms, with death usually occurring before 20 years of age. **scalded skin s., staphylococcal,** an infectious disease, usually affecting infants and young children, following infection with certain strains of *Staphylococcus aureus,* varying in severity from a localized bullous skin eruption to exfoliation of large sheets of skin that leaves raw, denuded areas that make the skin look scalded. **scalenus s., scalenus anticus s.,** pain over the shoulder, often extending down the arm or radiating up the back, due to compression of the nerves and vessels between a cervical rib and the scalenus anticus muscle. **Schaumann's s.,** sarcoidosis. **Scheie's s.,** a relatively mild allelic variant of Hurler's syndrome, marked by corneal clouding, clawhand, aortic valve involvement, wide-mouthed facies, genu valgus, and pes cavus; stature, intelligence, and life span are normal. **Sertoli-cell–only s.,** congenital absence of the germinal epithelium of the testes, the seminiferous tubules containing only Sertoli cells, marked by testes slightly smaller than normal, azoospermia, and elevated titers of follicle-stimulating hormone and sometimes of luteinizing hormone. **Sézary s.,** a form of cutaneous T-cell lymphoma manifested by exfoliative erythroderma, intense pruritus, peripheral lymphadenopathy, and abnormal hyperchromatic mononuclear cells in the skin, lymph nodes, and peripheral blood. **Sheehan's s.,** postpartum pituitary necrosis. **short-bowel s., short-gut s.,** any of the malabsorption conditions resulting from massive resection of the small bowel, the degree and kind of malabsorption depending on the site and extent of the resection; it is characterized by diarrhea, steatorrhea, and malnutrition. **shoulder-hand s.,** a disorder of the upper extremity characterized by pain and stiffness in the shoulder, with puffy swelling and pain in the ipsilateral hand, sometimes occurring after myocardial infarction, but also produced by other causes. **Shwachman s., Shwachman-Diamond s.,** primary pancreatic insufficiency and bone marrow failure, characterized by normal sweat chloride values, pancreatic insufficiency, and neutropenia; it may be associated with dwarfism and metaphyseal dysostosis of the hips. **sick sinus s.,** a complex cardiac arrhythmia manifested as severe sinus bradycardia alone, sinus bradycardia alternating with tachycardia, or sinus bradycardia with atrioventricular block. **Sipple's s.,** a hereditary association of pheochromocytoma, medullary carcinoma of the thyroid, and a tendency to hyperparathyroidism due to hyperplasia or multiple parathyroid adenomas; it is transmitted as an autosomal dominant trait. **Sjögren's s.,** a symptom complex usually in middle-aged or older women, marked by keratoconjunctivitis sicca, xerostomia, and enlargement of the parotid glands; it is often associated with rheumatoid arthritis and sometimes with systemic lupus erythematosus, scleroderma, or polymyositis. **sleep apnea s.,** episodes of cessation of breathing occurring at the transition from NREM to REM sleep, with repeated waking and excessive daytime sleepiness; it occurs most frequently in middle-aged obese males. **Smith-Lemli-Opitz s.,** a hereditary syndrome, transmitted as an autosomal recessive trait, characterized by microcephaly, mental retardation, hypotonia, incomplete development of male genitalia, short nose with anteverted nostrils, and syndactyly of second and third toes. **social breakdown s.,** symptoms of a mental patient that are due to long-term institutionalization, rather than the primary illness, including excessive passivity, assumption of the sick role, and atrophy of work and social skills. **Steele-Richardson-Olszewski s.,** a progressive neurological disorder, having onset during the sixth decade, characterized by supranuclear ophthalmoplegia, especially paralysis of the downward gaze, pseudobulbar palsy, dysarthria, dystonic rigidity of the neck and trunk, and dementia. **Stein-Leventhal s.,** oligomenorrhea or amenorrhea, anovulation, and hirsutism associated with bilateral polycystic ovaries, but normal excretion of follicle-stimulating hormone and 17-ketosteroids. **Stevens-Johnson s.,** a sometimes fatal form of erythema multiforme presenting with a flulike prodrome and characterized by severe mucocutaneous lesions; pulmonary, gastrointestinal, cardiac, and renal involvement may occur. **Stewart-Treves s.,** lymphangiosarcoma occurring as a late complication of severe lymphedema of the arm after excision of the lymph nodes, usually in radical mastectomy. **stiff-man s.,** a condition of unknown etiology marked by progressive fluctuating rigidity of axial and limb muscles in the absence of signs of cerebral and spinal cord disease but with continuous electromyographic activity. **stroke s.,** stroke; a condition with sudden onset due to acute vascular lesions of the brain (hemorrhage, embolism, thrombosis, rupturing aneurysm), which may be marked by hemiplegia or hemiparesis, vertigo, numbness, aphasia, and dysarthria, and often followed by permanent neurologic damage. **Sturge-Kalischer-Weber s., Sturge-Weber s.,** a congenital syndrome of nevus flammeus of the face, angiomas of the leptomeninges and choroid, and late glaucoma, frequently associated with intracranial calcification, mental retardation, contralateral hemiplegia, and epilepsy. **subclavian steal s.,** cerebral or brain stem ischemia resulting from diversion of blood flow from the basilar artery to the subclavian artery, in the presence of occlusive disease of the proximal portion of the subclavian artery. **sudden infant death s.,** sudden and unexpected death of an infant who had previously been apparently well, and which is unexplained by careful postmortem examination. **Swyer-James s.,** acquired unilateral hyperlucent lung, with severe airway obstruction during expiration, oligemia, and a small hilum. **tarsal tunnel s.,** a complex of symptoms resulting from compression of the posterior tibial nerve or of the plantar nerves in the tarsal tunnel, with pain, numbness, and tingling paresthesia of the sole of the foot. **Taussig-Bing s.,** transposition of the great vessels of the heart and a ventricular septal defect straddled by a large pulmonary artery. **temporomandibular joint s.,** tinnitus, vertigo, discomfort in the ears, and other symptoms due to faulty articulation of the temporomandibular joint. **testicular feminization s.,** an extreme form of male pseudohermaphroditism, with external genitalia and secondary sex characters typical of the female, but with presence of testes and absence of uterus and uterine tubes; it is due to end-organ resistance to the action of testosterone. **thoracic outlet s.,** compression of the brachial plexus nerve trunks, with pain in arms, paresthesia of fingers, vasomotor symptoms, and weakness and wasting of small muscles of the hand; it may be caused by drooping shoulder girdle, a cervical rib or fibrous band, an abnormal first rib, continual hyperabduction of the arm (as during sleep), or compression of the edge of scalenus anterior muscle. **Tolosa-Hunt s.,** unilateral ophthalmoplegia associated with pain behind the orbit and in the area supplied by the first division of the trigeminal nerve; it is thought to be due to nonspecific inflammation and granulation tissue in the superior orbital fissure or cavernous sinus. **toxic shock s.,** a severe illness characterized by high fever of sudden onset, vomiting, diarrhea, and myalgia, followed by hypotension and, in severe cases, shock; a sunburn-like rash with peeling of the skin, especially of the palms and soles, occurs during the acute phase. The syndrome affects almost exclusively menstruating women using tampons, although a few women who do not use tampons and a few males have been affected. It is thought to be caused by infection with *Staphylococcus aureus.* **Treacher Collins s.,** see *mandibulofacial dysostosis.* **trisomy 8 s.,** a syndrome associated with an extra chromosome 8, usually mosaic (trisomy 8/normal), characterized by mild to severe mental retardation, prominent forehead, deep-set eyes, thick lips, prominent ears, and camptodactyly. **trisomy 13 s.,** holoprosencephaly due to an extra chromosome 13, in which central nervous system defects are associated with mental retardation, along with cleft lip and palate, polydactyly, and dermal pattern anomalies, and abnormalities of the heart, viscera, and genitalia. **trisomy 18 s.,** a condition characterized by neonatal hepatitis, mental retardation, scaphocephaly or other skull abnormality, micrognathia, blepharoptosis, low-set ears, corneal opacities, deafness, webbed neck, short digits, ventricular septal defects, Meckel's diverticulum, and other deformities. It is due to the presence of an extra chromosome 18. **trisomy 21 s.,** Down's s. **Trousseau's s.,** spontaneous venous thrombosis of upper and lower extremities occurring in association with visceral carcinoma. **tumor lysis s.,** severe hyperphosphatemia, hyperkalemia, hyperuricemia, and hypocalcemia occurring after effective induction chemotherapy of rapidly growing malignant neoplasms. **Turcot's s.,** familial polyposis of the colon associated with malignant tumors of the central nervous system. **Turner's s.,** a form of gonadal dysgenesis marked by short stature, undifferentiated (streak) gonads, and variable abnormalities that may include webbing of neck, low posterior hair line, increased carrying angle of elbow, cubitus valgus, and cardiac defects. The genotype is XO (45,X) or X/XX or X/XXX mosaic. The phenotype is female. **Turner's s., male,** Noonan's s. **urethral s.,** suprapubic arching and cramping, urinary frequency, and such bladder complaints as dysuria, urinary tenesmus, and low back pain, without evidence of urinary infection. **Vernet's s.,** paralysis of the glossopharyngeal, vagus, and spinal accessory nerves due to a lesion in the region of the jugular foramen. **Waardenburg's s.,** a hereditary disorder, transmitted as an autosomal dominant trait, characterized by wide bridge of the nose due to lateral displacement of the inner canthi and puncta, pigmentary disturbances, including white forelock, heterochromia iridis, white eyelashes, leukoderma, and sometimes cochlear deafness. **Waterhouse-Friderichsen s.,** the malignant or fulminating form of epidemic cerebrospinal meningitis, with sudden onset, short course, fever, collapse, coma, cyanosis, petechiae on the skin and mucous membranes, and bilateral adrenal hemorrhage. **s. of Weber,** paralysis of the oculomotor nerve on the same side as the lesion, causing ptosis, strabismus, and loss of light reflex and accommodation; also spastic hemiplegia on the side opposite the lesion with increased reflexes and loss of superficial reflexes. **Weil's s.,** a severe form of leptospirosis, marked by jaundice usually accompanied by azotemia, hemorrhage, anemia, disturbances of consciousness, and continued fever. **Werner's s.,** premature senility of an adult, with early graying and some hair loss, cataracts, hyperkeratinization, and scleroderma-like changes in the skin of the limbs, followed by chronic ulceration. **Wernicke-Korsakoff s.,** a neuropsychiatric disorder caused by thiamine deficiency, most often due to alcohol abuse, combining the features of Wernicke's encephalopathy and Korsakoff's syndrome. **whiplash shake s.,** subdural hematomas, retinal hemorrhage, and sometimes cerebral contusions caused by the stretching and tearing of cerebral vessels and brain substance that may occur when a child under 3 years of age (and usually less than 1 year of age) is shaken vigorously by the limbs or trunk with the head unsupported; paralysis, visual disturbances, blindness, convulsions, and death may result. **Wilson-Mikity s.,** a rare form of pulmonary insufficiency in low-birth-weight infants, marked by hyperpnea and cyanosis of insidious onset during the first month of life and often resulting in death. Radiographically, there are multiple cystlike foci of hyperaeration throughout the lung with coarse thickening of the interstitial supporting structures. **Wiskott-Aldrich s.,** a condition characterized by chronic eczema, chronic suppurative otitis media, anemia, and thrombocytopenic purpura; it is an immunodeficiency syndrome transmitted as an X-linked recessive trait, in which there is poor antibody response to polysaccharide antigens and dysfunction of cell-mediated immunity. **Wolf-Hirschhorn s.,** a syndrome associated with partial deletion of the short arm of chromosome 4, characterized by microcephaly, ocular hypertelorism, epicanthus, cleft palate, micrognathia, low-set ears simplified in form, cryptorchidism, and hypospadias. **Wolff-Parkinson-White s.,** the association of paroxysmal tachycardia (or atrial fibrillation) and preexcitation, in which the electrocardiogram displays a short P-R interval and a wide QRS complex which characteristically shows an early QRS vector (delta wave). **Zollinger-Ellison s.,** a triad comprising (1) intractable, sometimes fulminating, atypical peptic ulcers; (2) extreme gastric hyperacidity; and (3) benign or malignant gastrin-secreting islet cell tumors (gastrinomas) of the pancreas.

syndromic (sin-drom′ik) occurring as a syndrome.

syndromology (sin″drom-ol′ah-je) the field concerned with the taxonomy, etiology, and patterns of congenital malformations.

synechia (sĭ-nek′e-ah), pl. *synech′iae* [Gr.] adhesion, as of the iris to the cornea or lens. **s. vul′-vae,** a congenital condition in which the labia minora are sealed in the midline, with only a small opening below the clitoris through which urination and menstruation may occur.

synechotomy (sin″ĕ-kot′ah-me) incision of a synechia.

synencephalocele (-en-sef′ah-lo-sēl″) encephalocele with adhesions to adjoining parts.

syneresis (sĭ-ner′ĭ-sis) a drawing together of the particles of the dispersed phase of a gel, with separation of some of the disperse medium and shrinkage of the gel.

synergism (sin′er-jizm) the joint action of agents so that their combined effect is greater than the algebraic sum of their individual effects. **synergist′ic,** adj.

synergist (-er-jist) a muscle or agent which acts with another.

synergy (-er-je) correlated action or cooperation on the part of two or more structures or drugs. In neurology, the faculty by which movements are properly grouped for the performance of acts requiring special adjustments. **synerget′ic, syner′gic,** adj.

synesthesia (sin″es-the′ze-ah) a secondary sensation accompanying an actual perception; the experiencing of a sensation in one place, due to stimulation applied to another place; also, the condition in which a stimulus of one sense is perceived as sensation of a different sense, as when a sound produces a sensation of color.

synesthesialgia (-es-the″ze-al′je-ah) a condition in which a stimulus produces pain on the affected side but no sensation on the normal side.

syngamy (sing′gah-me) 1. sexual reproduction. 2. the union of two gametes to form a zygote in fertilization. **syn′gamous,** adj.

syngeneic (sin″jĕ-ne′ik) in transplantation biology, denoting individuals or tissues having identical genotypes, i.e., identical twins or animals of the same inbred strain, or their tissues.

syngenesis (sin-jen′ĕ-sis) 1. the origin of an individual from a germ derived from both parents and not from either one alone. 2. the state of having descended from a common ancestor.

synizesis (sin″ĭ-ze′sis) 1. occlusion. 2. a mitotic stage in which the nuclear chromatin is massed.

synkinesis (sin″ki-ne′sis) an associated movement; an involuntary movement accompanying a volitional movement. **synkinet′ic,** adj.

synnecrosis (-nĕ-kro′sis) symbiosis in which the relationship between populations (or individuals) is mutually detrimental.

synophthalmus (-of-thal′mus) cyclops.

synorchism (sin'or-kizm) congenital fusion of the testes into one mass.

synoscheos (sin-os'ke-us) adhesion between the penis and scrotum.

synosteotomy (sin''os-te-ot'ah-me) dissection of the joints.

synostosis (-os-to'sis), pl. *synosto'ses* [Gr.] 1. a union between adjacent bones or parts of a single bone formed by osseous material. 2. the osseous union of bones that are normally distinct. **synostot'ic,** adj.

synotia (sĭ-no'she-ah) persistence of the ears in their horizontal position beneath the mandible.

synovectomy (sin''o-vek'tah-me) excision of a synovial membrane.

synovia (sĭ-no've-ah) the transparent, viscid fluid secreted by the synovial membrane and found in joint cavities, bursae, and tendon sheaths. **syno'vial,** adj.

synovialis (sĭ-no''ve-a'lis) [L.] synovial.

synovioma (sĭ-no''ve-o'mah) a tumor of synovial membrane origin.

synoviorthesis (sin-o''ve-or-the'sis) irradiation of the synovium by intra-articular injection of radiocolloids to destroy inflamed synovial tissue.

synovitis (sin''o-vi'tis) inflammation of a synovial membrane, usually painful, particularly on motion, and characterized by fluctuating swelling, due to effusion in a synovial sac. **dry s., s. sic'ca,** that with little effusion. **simple s.,** that with clear or but slightly turbid effusion. **tendinous s.,** inflammation of a tendon sheath. **villonodular s.,** proliferation of synovial tissue, especially of the knee joint, composed of synovial villi and fibrous nodules infiltrated by giant cells and macrophages.

synovium (sĭ-no've-um) a synovial membrane.

synteny (sin'tĕ-ne) the presence together on the same chromosome of two or more gene loci whether or not in such proximity that they may be subject to linkage. **synten'ic,** adj.

synthase (sin'thās) lyase; an enzyme, which catalyzes a synthesis that does not involve the breakdown of a pyrophosphate bond.

synthesis (sin'thĕ-sis) 1. creation of a compound by union of elements composing it, done artificially or as a result of natural processes. 2. in psychiatry, the integration of the various elements of the personality. **synthet'ic,** adj.

synthetase (-thĕ-tās) ligase.

Synthroid (-throid) trademark for a preparation of levothyroxine sodium.

syntrophoblast (sin-trof'o-blast) syncytiotrophoblast.

syntropic (-trop'ik) 1. turning or pointing in the same direction. 2. denoting correlation of several factors, as the relation of one disease to the development or incidence of another.

syntropy (sin'trah-pe) the state of being syntropic.

syphilid (sif'ĭ-lid) any of the skin lesions of secondary syphilis.

syphilis (sif'ĭ-lis) a venereal disease caused by *Treponema pallidum,* leading to many structural and cutaneous lesions, transmitted by direct sexual contact or *in utero.* See *primary s., secondary s.,* and *tertiary s.* **syphilit'ic,** adj. **congenital s.,** syphilis acquired *in utero,* manifested by any of several characteristic malformations of teeth or bones and by active mucocutaneous syphilis at birth or shortly thereafter, and by ocular or neurologic changes. **endemic s., nonvenereal s.,** a chronic inflammatory infection caused by a treponema morphologically indistinguishable from *Treponema pallidum,* transmitted by direct nonsexual body contact and indirectly by the common use of table and drinking utensils; the early stage is marked by mucosis patches and by moist papules in the oxilla and skin folds; a latent stage and finally late complications, including gummata, follow. **primary s.,** syphilis in its first stage, the primary lesion being a chancre, which is infectious and painless; the nearby lymph nodes become hard and swollen. **secondary s.,** syphilis in the second of three stages, with fever, multiform skin eruptions (syphilids), iritis, alopecia, mucous patches, and severe pain in the head, joints, and periosteum. **tertiary s.,** late generalized syphilis, with involvement of many organs and tissues, including skin, bones, joints, and cardiovascular and central nervous systems; see also *tabes dorsalis.*

syphiloma (sif''ĭ-lo'mah) a tumor of syphilitic origin; a gumma.

syring(o)- word element [Gr.], *tube; fistula.*

syringe (sir'inj, sĭ-rinj') an instrument for injecting liquids into or withdrawing them from any vessel or cavity. **air s., chip s.,** a small, fine-nozzled syringe, used to direct an air current into a tooth cavity being excavated, to remove small fragments, or to dry the cavity. **dental s.,** a small syringe used in operative dentistry, containing an anesthetic solution. **hypodermic s.,** one for introduction of liquids through a hollow needle into subcutaneous tissues. **Luer's s., Luer-Lok s.,** a glass syringe for intravenous and hypodermic use.

syringectomy (sir''in-jek'tah-me) fistulectomy

syringitis (sir''in-ji'tis) inflammation of the auditory tube.

syringoadenoma (sĭ-ring''go-ad''ĕ-no'mah) syringocystadenoma.

syringobulbia (-bul'be-ah) the presence of cavities in the medulla oblongata.

syringocarcinoma (-kar''sĭ-no'mah) cancer of a sweat gland.

syringocele (sĭ-ring'go-sēl) a cavity-containing herniation of the spinal cord through the bony defect in spina bifida.

syringocoele (sĭ-ring'go-sēl) the central canal of the spinal cord.

syringocystadenoma (sĭ-ring''go-sist''ad-ĕ-no'-mah) adenoma of the sweat glands.

syringocystoma (-sis-to'mah) cystic tumor of a sweat gland.

syringoma (sir''ing-go'mah) syringocystadenoma.

syringomeningocele (sĭ-ring''go-mĕ-ning'go-sēl) meningocele resembling syringomyelocele.

syringomyelia (-mi-e'le-ah) a slowly progressive syndrome of varying etiology, in which cavitation occurs in the central segments of the spinal cord, generally in the cervical region, with resulting neurologic deficits; thoracic scoliosis is often present.

syringomyelitis (-mi″ah-li′tis) inflammation of the spinal cord with formation of cavities.

syringomyelocele (-mi′ah-lo-sēl″) hernial protrusion of the spinal cord through the bony defect in spina bifida.

syringotomy (sir″ing-got′o-me) fistulotomy.

syrinx (sir′inks) [Gr.] 1. a tube or pipe; a fistula. 2. in birds, the lower part of the trachea in which vocal sounds are produced.

syrup (sir′up) a concentrated solution of a sugar, such as sucrose, in water or other aqueous liquid, sometimes with a medicinal agent added; usually used as a flavored vehicle for drugs.

systaltic (sis-tal′tik) alternately contracting and dilating; pulsating.

system (sis′tim) 1. a set or series of interconnected or interdependent parts or entities (objects, organs, or organisms) that act together in a common purpose or produce results impossible by action of one alone. 2. a school or method of practice based on a specific set of principles. **alimentary s.,** digestive s. **cardiovascular s.,** the heart and blood vessels, by which blood is pumped and circulated through the body. See Plate VIII. **centimeter-gram-second s.,** see *C.G.S.* **centrencephalic s.,** the neurons in the central core of the brain stem from the thalamus down to the medulla oblongata, connecting the two hemispheres of the brain. **chromaffin s.,** the chromaffin cells of the body (which characteristically stain strongly with chromium salts) considered collectively; they occur along the sympathetic nerves, in the adrenal, carotid, and coccygeal glands, and in various other organs. **circulatory s.,** channels through which nutrient fluids of the body flow; often restricted to the vessels conveying blood. **conduction s., conductive s. (of heart),** the system comprising the sinoatrial and atrioventricular nodes, atrioventricular bundle, and Purkinje fibers. **digestive s.,** the organs concerned with ingestion, digestion, and absorption of food or nutritional elements; see Plate IV. **endocrine s.,** the system of glands and other structures that elaborate internal secretions (hormones) which are released directly into the circulatory system, influencing metabolism and other body processes; included are the pituitary, thyroid, parathyroid, and adrenal glands, pineal body, gonads, pancreas, and paraganglia. **extrapyramidal s.,** a functional, rather than anatomical, unit comprising the nuclei and fibers (excluding those of the pyramidal tract) involved in motor activities; they control and coordinate especially the postural, static, supporting, and locomotor mechanisms. It includes the corpus striatum, subthalamic nucleus, substantia nigra, and red nucleus, along with their interconnections with the reticular formation, cerebellum, and cerebrum; some authorities include the cerebellum and vestibular nuclei. **genitourinary s.,** urogenital s. **haversian s.,** a haversian canal and its concentrically arranged lamellae, constituting the basic unit of structure in compact bone (osteon). **hematopoietic s.,** the tissues concerned in the production of blood, including bone marrow and lymphatic tissue. **heterogeneous s.,** a system or structure made up of mechanically separable parts, as an emulsion or a suspension. **homogeneous s.,** a system or structure made up of parts which cannot be mechanically separated, as a solution. **hypophyseoportal s.,** the venules connecting the capillaries (gomitoli) in the median eminence of the hypothalamus with the sinusoidal capillaries of the anterior pituitary. **immune s.,** a complex system of cellular and molecular components having the primary functions of distinguishing self from not self and of defense against foreign organisms or substances. **International S. of Units,** see *SI unit,* under *unit.* **keratinizing s.,** the cells composing the bulk of the epithelium of the epidermis, which are of ectodermal origin and undergo keratinization and form the dead superficial layers of the skin. **limbic s.,** a group of brain structures common to all mammals, comprising the phylogenetically old cortex (archipallium and paleopallium) and its primarily related nuclei; it is associated with olfaction, autonomic functions, and certain aspects of emotion and behavior. **lymphatic s.,** the lymphatic vessels and lymphoid tissue, considered collectively. **lymphoid s.,** the lymphoid tissue of the body, collectively; it consists of (a) a central component, including the bone marrow, thymus, and an unidentified portion called bursal equivalent tissue; and (b) a peripheral component consisting of lymph nodes, spleen, and gut-associated lymphoid tissue (tonsils, Peyer's patches). **lymphoreticular s.,** the system consisting of the lymphoid tissues and the tissues of the reticuloendothelial system, i.e. reticular supporting cells, lymphoid cells, and the cells of the monocyte-macrophage series. **masticatory s.,** all bony and soft structures of the face and mouth involved in mastication, and the vessels and nerves supplying them. **metric s.,** a decimal system of weights and measures based on the meter; see *Table of Weights and Measures.* **mononuclear phagocyte s.,** the set of cells consisting of macrophages and their precursors (blood monocytes and their precursor cells in bone marrow). The term has been proposed to replace reticuloendothelial system, which does not include all macrophages and does include other unrelated cell types. **muscular s.,** the muscles of the body considered collectively; generally restricted to the voluntary, skeletal muscles. **nervous s.,** the organ system which, along with the endocrine system, correlates the adjustments and reactions of the organism to its internal and external environment, comprising the central and peripheral nervous systems. See Plates X and XI. **nervous s., autonomic,** the portion of the nervous system concerned with regulation of activity of cardiac muscle, smooth muscle, and glands. **nervous s., central,** the brain and spinal cord. **nervous s., parasympathetic,** the craniosacral portion of the autonomic nervous system, its preganglionic fibers traveling with cranial nerves III, VII, IX, X, and XI, and with the second to fourth sacral ventral roots; it innervates the heart, smooth muscle and glands of head and neck, and thoracic, abdominal, and pelvic viscera. **nervous s., peripheral,** all elements of the nervous system (nerves and ganglia) outside the brain and spinal cord. **nervous s., sympathetic,** the thoracolumbar part of the autonomic nervous system, the preganglionic fibers of which arise from cell bodies in the thoracic and first three lumbar segments of the spinal cord; postganglionic fibers are distributed to the heart, smooth muscle, and glands of the entire body. **portal s.,** an arrangement by which blood collected from one set of capillaries passes through a large vessel or vessels and another set of capillaries before returning to the systemic circulation, as in the pituitary gland and liver. **respiratory s.,** the tubular and cavernous organs that allow atmospheric air to reach the membranes across which gases are exchanged with the blood. See Plates VI and VII. **reticular activating s.,** the system of cells of the reticular formation of the medulla oblongata that receive collaterals from the ascending sensory pathways and project to higher centers; they control the overall degree of central nervous system activity, including wakefulness, attentiveness, and sleep; abbreviated RAS. **reticuloendothelial s., (RES),** a group of cells having the ability to take up and sequester inert particles and vital dyes, including macrophages and macrophage precursors, specialized endothelial cells lining the sinusoids of the liver, spleen, and bone marrow, and reticular cells of lymphatic tissue (macrophages) and bone marrow (fibroblasts). See also *lymphoreticular s.* and *mononuclear phagocyte s.* **stomatognathic s.,** structures of the mouth and jaws, considered collectively, as they subserve the functions of mastication, deglutition, respiration, and speech. **urogenital s.,** the organs concerned with production and excretion of urine, together with the organs of reproduction. **vascular s.,** the vessels of the body, especially the blood vessels. **vasomotor s.,** the part of the nervous system that controls the caliber of the blood vessels.

systema (sis-te′mah) [Gr.] system.

systemic (sis-tem′ik) pertaining to or affecting the body as a whole.

systole (sis′tah-le) the contraction, or period of contraction, of the heart, especially of the ventricles. **systol′ic,** adj. **aborted s.,** a systole, usually premature, not associated with pulsation of a peripheral artery. **atrial s.,** the contraction of the atria by which blood is propelled from them into the ventricles. **extra s.,** extrasystole. **ventricular s.,** the contraction of the cardiac ventricles by which blood is forced into the aorta and pulmonary artery.

systremma (sis-trem′ah) a cramp in the muscles of the calf of the leg.

syzygy (siz′ĭ-je) 1. the conjunction and fusion of organs without the loss of identity. 2. the temporary adherence of male and female gregarines prior to encystment and the production of gametes.

T

T symbol for *tesla, tera-, thymine* or *thymidine* (in nucleic acids), *thoracic vertebrae* (T-1–T-12), and *intraocular tension.* Normal intraocular tension is indicated by Tn, while T + 1, T + 2, etc., indicate increased tension, and T – 1, T – 2, etc., indicate decreased tension.

T symbol for *absolute temperature.*

T$_m$ tubular maximum (of the kidneys); used in reporting kidney function studies, with inferior letters representing the substance used in the test, as T$_{m_{PAH}}$ (tubular maximum for para-aminohippuric acid).

T$\frac{1}{2}$ symbol for half-life.

t$\frac{1}{2}$ symbol for half-life.

T$_3$ symbol for *triiodothyronine.*

T$_4$ symbol for *thyroxine.*

2,4,5-T a toxic chlorphenoxy herbicide (2,4,5-trichlorophenoxyacetic acid), a component of Agent Orange.

t in genetics, symbol for *translocation.*

T.A. toxin-antitoxin.

Ta chemical symbol, *tantalum.*

tabanid (tab′ah-nid) any gadfly of the family Tabanidae, including the horseflies and deerflies.

Tabanus (tah-ba′nus) a genus of bloodsucking biting flies (horseflies or gadflies) which transmit trypanosomes and anthrax to various animals.

tabes (ta′bēz) 1. any wasting of the body; progressive atrophy of the body or a part of it. 2. tabes dorsalis. **tabet′ic,** adj. **t. dorsa′lis,** parenchymatous neurosyphilis marked by degeneration of the posterior columns and posterior roots and ganglion of the spinal cord, with muscular incoordination, paroxysms of intense pain, visceral crises, disturbances of sensation, and various trophic disturbances, especially of bones and joints. **t. mesenter′ica,** tuberculosis of mesenteric glands in children.

tabescent (tah-bes′ent) growing emaciated; wasting away.

tabetiform (tah-bet′ĭ-form) resembling tabes.

tablature (tab′lah-chur) separation of the chief cranial bones into inner and outer tables, separated by a diploë.

table (ta′b′l) a flat layer or surface. **inner t.,** the inner compact layer of the bones covering the brain. **outer t.,** the outer compact layer of the bones covering the brain. **vitreous t.,** inner t.

tablet (tab′let) a solid dosage form containing a medicinal substance with or without a suitable diluent. **buccal t.,** one which dissolves when held between the cheek and gum, permitting direct absorption of the active ingredient through the oral mucosa. **enteric-coated t.,** one coated with material that delays release of the medication until after it leaves the stomach. **sublingual t.,** one that dissolves when held beneath the tongue, permitting direct absorption of the active ingredient by the oral mucosa.

taboparesis (ta″bo-pah-re′sis) dementia paralytica occurring concomitantly with tabes dorsalis.

tache (tahsh) [Fr.] a spot or blemish. **tachet′ic,** adj. **t. blanche** ("white spot"), a white spot on the liver in certain infectious diseases. **t's bleuâtres** ("bluish spots"), maculae caeruleae. **t. cérébrale** ("cerebral spot"), a congested streak produced by drawing the nail across the skin; a concomitant of various nervous or cerebral diseases. **t. motrice** ("motor spot"), a motor nerve ending in which the nerve fibril passes to a muscle cell, where it ends in a slight enlargement. **t. noire** ("black spot"), an ulcer covered with a black crust, a characteristic local reaction at the presumed site of the infective bite in certain tickborne rickettsioses.

tachography (tah-kog′rah-fe) the recording of the movement and speed of the blood current.

tachy- word element [Gr.], *rapid; swift.*

tachyarrhythmia (tak″e-ah-rith′me-ah) tachycardia associated with an irregularity in the normal heart rhythm.

tachycardia (-kar′de-ah) abnormally rapid heart rate. **tachycar′diac,** adj. **atrial t.,** a rapid cardiac rate, usually 160–190 per minute, originating from an atrial locus. **ectopic t.,** rapid heart action in response to impulses arising outside the sinoatrial node. **junctional t.,** that arising in response to impulses originating in the atrioventricular junction, i.e., in the atrioventricular node. **paroxysmal t.,** rapid heart action that starts and stops abruptly. **supraventricular t.,** a combination of junctional tachycardia and atrial tachycardia. **ventricular t.,** an abnormally rapid ventricular rhythm with aberrant ventricular excitation, usually above 150 per minute, generated within the ventricle, and most often associated with atrioventricular dissociation.

tachygastria (-gas′tre-ah) the occurrence of a sequence of electric potentials at abnormally high frequencies in the gastric antrum.

tachyphagia (-fa′je-ah) rapid eating.

tachyphylaxis (-fi-lak′sis) 1. rapid immunization against the effect of toxic doses of an extract by previous injection of small doses of it. 2. rapidly decreasing response to a drug or physiologically active agent after administration of a few doses. **tachyphylac′tic,** adj.

tachypnea (tak″ip-ne′ah) very rapid respiration.

tachyrhythmia (tak″e-rith′me-ah) tachycardia.

tachysterol (tak-is′ter-ol) an isomer of ergosterol produced by irradiation.

tactometer (tak-tom′ĕ-ter) an instrument for measuring tactile sensibility.

tactus (tak′tus) [L.] touch. **tac′tile, tac′tual,** adj.

Taenia (te′ne-ah) a genus of tapeworms. **T. echinococ′cus,** *Echinococcus granulosus.*

T. sagina′ta, a species 12–25 feet long, found in the adult form in the human intestine and in the larval state in muscles and other tissues of cattle and other ruminants; human infection usually results from eating inadequately cooked beef. **T. so′lium,** a species 3–6 feet long, found in the adult intestine; the larval form most often is found in muscle and other tissues of the pig; human infection results from eating inadequately cooked pork.

taenia (te′ne-ah) 1. a flat band or strip of soft tissue. 2. a tapeworm of the genus *Taenia.*

taeniacide (-sīd″) 1. lethal to tapeworms. 2, an agent lethal to tapeworms.

taeniafuge (-fūj″) teniafuge.

taeniasis (te-ni′ah-sis) infection with tapeworms of the genus *Taenia.*

Tagamet (tag′ah-met) trademark for preparations of cimetidine.

tail (tāl) 1. any slender appendage. 2. the appendage that extends from the posterior trunk of animals. **t. of spermatozoon,** the flagellum of a spermatozoon, which contains the axonema; it has four regions: the neck, middle piece, principal piece, and end piece.

talbutal (tal′bu-tal) a hypnotic and sedative, $C_{11}H_{16}N_2O_3$.

talc (talk) a native hydrous magnesium silicate, sometimes with a small amount of aluminum silicate; used as a dusting powder.

talcosis (tal-ko′sis) a condition due to inhalation or implantation in the body of talc.

talcum (tal′kum) talc.

talipes (tal′i-pēz) clubfoot; a congenital deformity of the foot, which is twisted out of shape or position; the foot may be in dorsiflexion (*t. calca′neus*) or plantar flexion (*t. equi′nus*), abducted, everted (*t. val′gus*), abducted, inverted (*t. va′rus*), or various combinations of these (*t. calcaneoval′gus, t. calcaneova′rus, t. equinoval′gus,* or *t. equinova′rus*).

talipomanus (tal″i-pom′ah-nus) clubhand.

talocalcaneal (ta″lo-kal-ka′ne-al) pertaining to the talus and calcaneus.

talocrural (-krōōr′al) pertaining to the talus and the leg bones.

talofibular (-fib′u-ler) pertaining to the talus and fibula.

talonavicular (-nah-vik′u-ler) pertaining to the talus and navicular bone.

talus (ta′lus), pl. *ta′li* [L.] see *Table of Bones.*

Talwin (tal′win) trademark for preparations of pentazocine.

tambour (tam-boor′) a drum-shaped appliance used in transmitting movements in a recording instrument.

tamoxifen (tah-moks′i-fen) a nonsteroidal oral antiestrogen, $C_{26}H_{29}NO$; used in the palliative treatment of breast cancer and to stimulate ovulation in infertility.

tampon (tam′pon) [Fr.] a pack, pad, or plug made of cotton, sponge, or other material, variously used in surgery to plug the nose, vagina, etc., for the control of hemorrhage or the absorption of secretions.

tamponade (tam″po-nād′) 1. surgical use of a

tampon. 2. pathologic compression of a part.
cardiac t., compression of the heart due to collection of blood in the pericardium.

Tandearil (tan-de′ah-ril) trademark for a preparation of oxyphenbutazone.

tannate (tan′āt) any of the salts of tannic acid, all of which are astringent.

tannic acid (tan′ik) a tannin, $C_{76}H_{52}O_{46}$, obtained from the bark and fruit of many plants, usually obtained from nutgalls; used as an astringent.

tannin (tan′in) tannic acid.

tantalum (tan′tah-lum) chemical element (*see table*), at. no. 73, symbol Ta; a noncorrosive and malleable metal that has been used for plates or disks to replace cranial defects, for wire sutures, and for making prosthetic appliances.

tanycyte (tan′ĭ-sīt) a modified cell of the ependyma of the infundibulum of the hypothalamus; its function is unknown, but it may transport hormones from the cerebrospinal fluid into the hypophyseal circulation or from the hypothalamic neurons to the cerebrospinal fluid.

tap (tap) 1. a quick, light blow. 2. to drain off fluid by paracentesis. **spinal t.,** lumbar puncture.

tape (tāp) a long, narrow strip of fabric or other flexible material. **adhesive t.,** a strip of fabric or other material evenly coated on one side with a pressure-sensitive adhesive material.

tapeinocephaly (tah-pi″no-sef′ah-le) flatness of the skull, with a vertical index below 72. **tapeinocephal′ic,** adj.

tapetum (tah-pe′tum), pl. *tape′ta* [L.] 1. a covering structure or layer of cells. 2. a stratum of fibers of the corpus callosum on the superolateral aspect of the occipital horn of the lateral ventricle. **t. lu′cidum,** the iridescent epithelium of the choroid of animals which gives their eyes the property of shining in the dark.

tapeworm (tāp′werm) a parasitic intestinal cestode worm having a flattened, bandlike form. **armed t.,** *Taenia solium.* **beef t.,** *Taenia saginata.* **broad t.,** *Dibothriocephalus latum.* **dog t.,** *Dipylidium caninum.* **fish t.,** *Diphyllobothrium latum.* **hydatid t.,** *Echinococcus granulosus.* **pork t.,** *Taenia solium.* **unarmed t.,** *Taenia saginata.*

tapotement (tah-pōt-maw′) [Fr.] a tapping manipulation in massage.

tar (tahr) a dark-brown or black, viscid liquid obtained from various species of pine or from bituminous coal. **coal t.,** a by-product obtained in destructive distillation of bituminous coal; used as a topical antieczematic and antipsoriatic. **juniper t.,** volatile oil obtained from wood of *Juniperus oxycedrus;* used as a topical antieczematic. **pine t.,** a product of destructive distillation of the wood of various pine trees; used as a local antieczematic and rubefacient.

tarantula (tah-ran′chu-lah) a venomous spider whose bite causes local inflammation and pain, usually not to a severe extent, including *Eurypelma hentzii* (American t.), *Sericopelma communis* (black t.) of Panama, and *Lycosa tarentula* (European wolf spider).

tardive (tahr′div) [Fr.] tardy; late.

tare (tār) 1. the weight of the vessel in which a

substance is weighed. 2. to weigh a vessel in order to allow for it when the vessel and a substance are weighed together.

target (tahr′gĭt) 1. an object or area toward which something is directed, such as the area of the anode of an x-ray tube where the electron beam collides, causing the emission of x-rays. 2. a cell or organ that is affected by a particular agent, e.g., a hormone or drug.

tarichatoxin (tar″ik-ah-tok′sin) a neurotoxin from the newt (*Taricha*), identical with tetrodotoxin.

tars(o)- word element [Gr.], *edge of eyelid; tarsus of the foot; instep.*

tarsadenitis (tahr″sad-ĕ-ni′tis) inflammation of the tarsus of the eyelid and the meibomian glands.

tarsal (tahr′s'l) pertaining to a tarsus.

tarsalgia (tahr-sal′je-ah) pain in a tarsus.

tarsalia (tahr-sa′le-ah) the bones of the tarsus.

tarsalis (tahr-sa′lis) [L.] tarsal.

tarsectomy (tahr-sek′tah-me) 1. excision of one or more bones of the tarsus. 2. excision of the cartilage of the eyelid.

tarsitis (tahr-si′tis) inflammation of the tarsus of the eyelid; blepharitis.

tarsoclasis (tahr-sok′lah-sis) surgical fracturing of the tarsus of the foot.

tarsomalacia (tahr″so-mah-la′she-ah) softening of the tarsus of an eyelid.

tarsometatarsal (-met″ah-tar′sal) pertaining to the tarsus and metatarsus.

tarsophyma (-fi′mah) any tumor of the tarsus.

tarsoplasty (tahr′so-plas″te) plastic surgery of the tarsus of the eyelid.

tarsoptosis (tahr″sop-to′sis) falling of the tarsus; flatfoot.

tarsorrhaphy (tahr-sor′ah-fe) suture of a portion of or the entire upper and lower eyelids together; done to shorten or entirely close the palpebral fissure.

tarsotomy (tahr-sot′ah-me) surgical incision of a tarsus, or an eyelid.

tarsus (tahr′sus) 1. the seven bones—talus, calcaneus, navicular, medial, intermediate and lateral cuneiform, and cuboid—composing the articulation between the foot and leg; the ankle or instep. 2. the cartilaginous plate forming the framework of either (upper or lower) eyelid.

tartar (tahr′ter) 1. potassium bitartrate. 2. dental calculus. **t. emetic,** antimony potassium tartrate.

tartaric acid (tar-tar′ik) $C_4H_6O_6$, obtained from the lees of wine and from various plants, used in baking and tanning, and as a chemical reagent.

tartrate (tahr′trāt) a salt of tartaric acid.

tastant (tās′tant) any substance, e.g., salt, capable of eliciting gustatory excitation, i.e., stimulating the sense of taste.

taste (tāst) the peculiar sensation caused by the contact of soluble substances with the tongue; the sense effected by the tongue, the gustatory and other nerves, and the gustation center. Four qualities are distinguished: sweet, sour, salty, and bitter.

taster (tās'ter) an individual capable of tasting a particular test substance (e.g., phenylthiocarbamide) used in genetic studies.

TAT thematic apperception test.

Tatlockia micda'dei (tat-lok'e-ah mik-da'de-i) Pittsburgh pneumonia agent; a waterborne legionella-like organism implicated as a cause of pneumonia.

tattooing (tah-too'ing) the introduction, by punctures, of permanent colors in the skin. **t. of cornea,** permanent coloring of the cornea, chiefly to conceal leukomatous spots.

taurine (taw'rēn) a crystallized acid, ethylamine sulfonic acid, from the bile; found also in small quantities in lung and muscle tissues.

taurocholate (taw''ro-ko'lāt) a salt of taurocholic acid.

taurocholic acid (taw''ro-ko'lik) a bile acid, C_{26}-$H_{45}NSO_7$; when hydrolyzed, it splits into taurine and cholic acid.

tautomer (taw'to-mer) a chemical compound exhibiting, or capable of exhibiting, tautomerism.

tautomeral (taw-tom'er-al) pertaining to the same part; said especially of neurons and neuroblasts sending processes to aid in formation of the white matter in the same side of the spinal cord.

tautomerase (-ās) an enzyme that catalyzes tautomeric reactions.

tautomerism (taw-tom'er-izm) the relationship that exists between two structural isomers that are in chemical equilibrium and freely change from one to the other. **tautomer'ic,** adj.

taxis (tak'sis) 1. an orientation movement of a motile organism in response to a stimulus; it may be either toward (positive) or away from (negative) the source of the stimulus; used also as a word ending, affixed to a stem denoting the nature of the stimulus. 2. exertion of force in manual replacement of a displaced organ or part.

taxon (tak'son), pl. *tax'a* [Gr.] 1. a particular taxonomic grouping, e.g., a species, genus, family, order, class, phylum, or kingdom. 2. the name applied to a taxonomic grouping.

taxonomy (tak-son'ah-me) the orderly classification of organisms into appropriate categories (taxa), with application of suitable and correct names. **taxonom'ic,** adj. **numerical t.,** a method of classifying organisms solely on the basis of the number of shared phenotypic characters, each character usually being given equal weight; used primarily in bacteriology.

Tb chemical symbol, *terbium.*

Tc chemical symbol, *technetium.*

TD₅₀ median toxic dose; a dose that produces a toxic effect in 50 per cent of a population.

Te chemical symbol, *tellurium.*

tears (tērz) the watery, slightly alkaline and saline secretion of the lacrimal glands, which moistens the conjunctiva.

tease (tēz) to pull apart gently with fine needles to permit microscopic examination.

teat (tēt) the nipple of the mammary gland.

tebutate (teb'u-tāt) USAN contraction for tertiary butyl acetate.

technetium (tek-ne'she-um) chemical element (*see table*), at. no. 43, symbol Tc. **t. 99m,** the most frequently used radioisotope in nuclear medicine, a gamma emitter having a half-life of 6.03 hours and a primary photon energy of 140 keV.

technic (tek'nik) technique.

technician (tek-nish'un) a person skilled in the performance of technical procedures.

technique (tek-nēk') the method of procedure and details of a mechanical process or surgical operation. **fluorescent antibody t.,** an immunofluorescence technique in which antigen in tissue sections is located by homologous antibody labeled with fluorochrome or by treating the antigen with unlabeled antibody followed by a second layer of labeled antiglobulin which is reactive with the unlabeled antibody. **Jerne plaque t.,** a hemolytic technique for detecting antibody-producing cells: a suspension of presensitized lymphocytes is mixed in an agar gel with erythrocytes; after a period of incubation, complement is added and a clear area of lysis of red cells can be seen around each of the antibody-producing cells.

tectorial (tek-tor'e-al) of the nature of a roof or covering.

tectorium (tek-tor'e-um) Corti's membrane.

tectospinal (tek''to-spi'n'l) extending from the tectum of the midbrain to the spinal cord.

tectum (tek'tum) a rooflike structure. **t. of mesencephalon, t. of midbrain,** the dorsal portion of the midbrain.

teething (tēth'ing) the entire process resulting in eruption of the teeth.

Teflon (tef'lon) trademark for preparations of polytef (polytetrafluoroethylene).

tegmen (teg'men), pl. *teg'mina* [L.] a covering structure or roof. **t. tym'pani,** 1. the thin layer of bone separating the tympanic antrum from the cranial cavity. 2. the roof of the tympanic cavity, related to part of the petrous portion of the temporal bone.

tegmentum (teg-men'tum), pl. *tegmen'ta* [L.] 1. a covering. 2. the part of the cerebral peduncle dorsal to the substantia nigra. **tegmen'tal,** adj.

Tegretol (teg'rĕ-tol) trademark for preparations of carbamazepine.

teichoic acids (ti-ko'ik) antigenic polymers of glycerol or ribitol phosphates found attached to the cell walls or in intracellular association with membranes of gram-positive bacteria; they determine group specificity of some species, e.g., the staphylococci.

teichopsia (ti-kop'se-ah) the sensation of a luminous appearance before the eyes, with a zigzag, wall-like outline.

tela (te'lah), pl. *te'lae* [L.] any weblike tissue. **t. conjuncti'va,** connective tissue. **t. elas'tica,** elastic tissue. **t. subcuta'nea,** subcutaneous tissue.

telalgia (tel-al'je-ah) referred pain.

telangiectasia (tel-an''je-ek-ta'ze-ah) a vascular lesion formed by dilation of a group of small blood vessels. **telangiectat'ic,** adj. **hereditary hemorrhagic t.,** a hereditary condition marked by multiple small telangiectases of the skin, mucous membranes, and other organs, associated with recurrent episodes of bleeding from attached sites and gross or occult melena.

telangiectasis (tel-an"je-ek-ta'sis), pl. *telangiec'-tases*. 1. the lesion produced by telangiectasia; which may present as a coarse or fine red line or as a punctum with radiating limbs (spider). **spider t.,** vascular spider.

telangiosis (-o'sis) any disease of the capillaries.

Teldrin (tel'drin) trademark for a preparation of chlorpheniramine maleate.

tele- word element [Gr.], *far away; operating at a distance; an end.*

telecanthus (tel"ah-kan'thus) abnormally increased distance between the medial canthi of the eyelids.

telecardiography (-kar"de-og'rah-fe) the recording of an electrocardiogram by transmission of impulses to a site at a distance from the patient.

telecardiophone (-kar'de-o-fōn") an apparatus for making heart sounds audible at a distance from the patient.

telediagnosis (-di"ag-no'sis) determination of the nature of a disease at a site remote from the patient on the basis of transmitted telemonitoring data or closed-circuit television consultation.

telefluoroscopy (-floor-os'ko-pe) television transmission of fluoroscopic images for study at a distant location.

telekinesis (-kǐ-ne'sis) 1. movement of an object produced without contact. 2. the ability to produce such movement. **telekinet'ic,** adj.

telemedicine (-med'ǐ-sin) the provision of consultant services by off-site physicians to health care professionals on the scene, as by means of closed-circuit television.

telemetry (tě-lem'ě-tre) the making of measurements at a distance from the subject, the measurable evidence of phenomena under investigation being transmitted by radio signals.

telencephalon (tel"en-sef'ah-lon) endbrain: 1. the paired brain vesicles, which are the anterolateral outpouchings of the forebrain, together with the median, unpaired portion, the terminal lamina of the hypothalamus; from it the cerebral hemispheres are derived. 2. the anterior of the two vesicles formed by specialization of the forebrain in embryonic development. **telencephal'ic,** adj.

teleneurite (tel"ah-noōr'īt) an end expansion of an axon.

teleneuron (-noōr'on) a nerve ending.

teleology (-ol'ah-je) the doctrine of final causes or of adaptation to a definite purpose.

teleomitosis (tel"e-o-mi-to'sis) completed mitosis.

teleopsia (tel"e-op'se-ah) a visual disturbance in which objects appear to be farther away than they actually are.

teleorganic (-or-gan'ik) necessary to life.

Telepaque (tel'ah-pāk) trademark for a preparation of iopanoic acid.

teleradiography (tel"ah-ra"de-og'rah-fe) teleroentgenography.

teleroentgenography (tel"ah-rent"gen-og'rah-fe) roentgenography with the x-ray tube $6\frac{1}{2}$ to 7 feet away from the plate in order more nearly to secure parallelism of the rays.

teletherapy (-ther'ah-pe) treatment in which the source of the therapeutic agent, e.g., radiation, is at a distance from the body.

telluric (tě-lu'rik) 1. pertaining to tellurium. 2. pertaining to or originating from the earth.

tellurium (tě-lu're-um) chemical element (*see table*), at. no. 52, symbol Te.

telo- word element [Gr.], *end.*

telodendron (tel"o-den'dron) any of the fine terminal branches of an axon.

telogen (tel'o-jen) the quiescent or resting phase of the hair cycle, following catagen, the hair having become a club hair and not growing further.

telognosis (tel"og-no'sis) diagnosis based on interpretation of roentgenograms transmitted by telephonic or radio communication.

telolecithal (tel"o-les'ǐ-thal) having a yolk concentrated at one of the poles.

telolemma (-lem'ah) the covering of a motor end-plate.

telomere (tel'o-mēr) an extremity of a chromosome, which has specific properties, one of which is a polarity that prevents reunion with any fragment after a chromosome has been broken.

telophase (-fāz) the last of the four stages of mitosis and of the two divisions of meiosis, in which the chromosomes arrive at the poles of the cell and the cytoplasm divides; in plants, the cell wall also forms.

temperature (tem'per-ah-chur) an expression of heat or coldness in terms of an arbitrary scale. See accompanying table. **absolute t.,** that reckoned from absolute zero (−273.15° C. or −459.67° F.). **critical t.,** that below which a gas may be converted to a liquid by pressure. **normal t.,** that of the human body in health, about 98.6° F or 37° C when measured orally.

template (tem'plit) 1. a pattern or mold. 2. in genetics, a strand of DNA or RNA (mRNA) that specifies the base sequence of a newly synthesized strand of DNA or RNA. 3. in dentistry, a curved or flat plate used as an aid in setting teeth in a denture.

temple (tem'p'l) the lateral region on either side of the head, above the zygomatic arch.

tempora (tem'po-rah) [L.] the temples.

temporal (-ral) 1. pertaining to the temple. 2. pertaining to time; limited as to time; temporary.

temporomandibular (tem"pah-ro-man-dib'u-ler) pertaining to the temporal bone and mandible.

temporomaxillary (-mak'sǐ-lar"e) pertaining to the temporal bone and maxilla.

temporo-occipital (-ok-sip'ǐ-t'l) pertaining to the temporal and occipital bones.

temporosphenoid (-sfe'noid) pertaining to the temporal and sphenoid bones.

tenaculum (tě-nak'u-lum) a hooklike surgical instrument for grasping and holding parts.

tenalgia (ten-al'je-ah) pain in a tendon.

TABLE OF TEMPERATURE EQUIVALENTS
CELSIUS (CENTIGRADE): FAHRENHEIT SCALE

CELSIUS:FAHRENHEIT $^\circ F = (^\circ C \times 9/5) + 32$				FAHRENHEIT:CELSIUS $^\circ C = (^\circ F - 32) \times 5/9$					
C°	F°	C°	F°	F°	C°	F°	C°	F°	C°
−50	−58.0	49	120.2	−50	−46.7	99	37.2	157	69.4
−40	−40.0	50	122.0	−40	−40.0	100	37.7	158	70.0
−35	−31.0	51	123.8	−35	−37.2	101	38.3	159	70.5
−30	−22.0	52	125.6	−30	−34.4	102	38.8	160	71.1
−25	−13.0	53	127.4	−25	−31.7	103	39.4	161	71.6
−20	−4.0	54	129.2	−20	−28.9	104	40.0	162	72.2
−15	−5.0	55	131.0	−15	−26.6	105	40.5	163	72.7
−10	14.0	56	132.8	−10	−23.3	106	41.1	164	73.3
−5	23.0	57	134.6	−5	−20.6	107	41.6	165	73.8
0	32.0	58	136.4	0	−17.7	108	42.2	166	74.4
+1	33.8	59	138.2	+1	−17.2	109	42.7	167	75.0
2	35.6	60	140.0	5	−15.0	110	43.3	168	75.5
3	37.4	61	141.8	10	−12.2	111	43.8	169	76.1
4	39.2	62	143.6	15	−9.4	112	44.4	170	76.6
5	41.0	63	145.4	20	−6.6	113	45.0	171	77.2
6	42.8	64	147.2	25	−3.8	114	45.5	172	77.7
7	44.6	65	149.0	30	−1.1	115	46.1	173	78.3
8	46.4	66	150.8	31	−0.5	116	46.6	174	78.8
9	48.2	67	152.6	32	0	117	47.2	175	79.4
10	50.0	68	154.4	33	+0.5	118	47.7	176	80.0
11	51.8	69	156.2	34	1.1	119	48.3	177	80.5
12	53.6	70	158.0	35	1.6	120	48.8	178	81.1
13	55.4	71	159.8	36	2.2	121	49.4	179	81.6
14	57.2	72	161.6	37	2.7	122	50.0	180	82.2
15	59.0	73	163.4	38	3.3	123	50.5	181	82.7
16	60.8	74	165.2	39	3.8	124	51.1	182	83.3
17	62.6	75	167.0	40	4.4	125	51.6	183	83.8
18	64.4	76	168.8	41	5.0	126	52.2	184	84.4
19	66.2	77	170.6	42	5.5	127	52.7	185	85.0
20	68.0	78	172.4	43	6.1	128	53.3	186	85.5
21	69.8	79	174.2	44	6.6	129	53.8	187	86.1
22	71.6	80	176.0	45	7.2	130	54.4	188	86.6
23	73.4	81	177.8	46	7.7	131	55.0	189	87.2
24	75.2	82	179.6	47	8.3	132	55.5	190	87.7
25	77.0	83	181.4	48	8.8	133	56.1	191	88.3
26	78.8	84	183.2	49	9.4	134	56.6	192	88.8
27	80.6	85	185.0	50	10.0	135	57.2	193	89.4
28	82.4	86	186.8	55	12.7	136	57.7	194	90.0
29	84.2	87	188.6	60	15.5	137	58.3	195	90.5
30	86.0	88	190.4	65	18.3	138	58.8	196	91.1
31	87.8	89	192.2	70	21.1	139	59.4	197	91.6
32	89.6	90	194.0	75	23.8	140	60.0	198	92.2
33	91.4	91	195.8	80	26.6	141	60.5	199	92.7
34	93.2	92	197.6	85	29.4	142	61.1	200	93.3
35	95.0	93	199.4	86	30.0	143	61.6	201	93.8
36	96.8	94	201.2	87	30.5	144	62.2	202	94.4
37	98.6	95	203.0	88	31.0	145	62.7	203	95.0
38	100.4	96	204.8	89	31.6	146	63.3	204	95.5
39	102.2	97	206.6	90	32.2	147	63.8	205	96.1
40	104.0	98	208.4	91	32.7	148	64.4	206	96.6
41	105.8	99	210.2	92	33.3	149	65.0	207	97.2
42	107.6	100	212.0	93	33.8	150	65.5	208	97.7
43	109.4	101	213.8	94	34.4	151	66.1	209	98.3
44	111.2	102	215.6	95	35.0	152	66.6	210	98.8
45	113.0	103	217.4	96	35.5	153	67.2	211	99.4
46	114.8	104	219.2	97	36.1	154	67.7	212	100.0
47	116.6	105	221.0	98	36.6	155	68.3	213	100.5
48	118.4	106	222.8	98.6	37.0	156	68.8	214	101.1

tenderness (ten′der-nes) a state of unusual sensitivity to touch or pressure. **rebound t.**, a state in which pain is felt on the release of pressure over a part.

tendinitis (ten″dĭ-ni′tis) inflammation of tendons and of tendon-muscle attachments. **calcific t.**, inflammation and calcification of the subacromial or subdeltoid bursa, resulting in pain, tenderness, and limitation of motion in the shoulder.

tendinoplasty (ten′dĭ-no-plas″te) tenoplasty.

tendinosuture (ten″dĭ-no-su′chur) tenorrhaphy.

tendinous (ten′dĭ-nus) pertaining to, resembling, or of the nature of a tendon.

tendo (ten′do), pl. *ten′dines* [L.] tendon. **t. Achil′lis, t. calca′neus,** Achilles tendon.

tendon (ten′don) a fibrous cord of connective tissue continuous with the fibers of a muscle and attaching the muscle to bone or cartilage. **Achilles t., calcaneal t.,** the powerful tendon at the back of the heel, attaching the triceps surae muscle to the calcaneus.

tendonitis (ten″do-ni′tis) tendinitis.

tendovaginal (-vaj′ĭ-n′l) pertaining to a tendon and its sheath.

tenectomy (tĕ-nek′tah-me) excision of a lesion of a tendon or of a tendon sheath.

tenesmus (tĕ-nez′mus) ineffectual and painful straining at stool or in urinating. **tenes′mic,** adj.

tenia (te′ne-ah), pl. *te′niae* [L.] 1. taenia (1). 2. a tapeworm of the genus *Taenia.*

teniacide (te′ne-ah-sīd″) 1. lethal to tapeworms. 2. an agent lethal to tapeworms.

teniafuge (-fūj″) an agent that expels tapeworms.

teniamyotomy (te″ne-ah-mi-ot′ah-me) an operation involving a series of transverse incisions of the teniae coli; done in diverticular disease.

teniasis (te-ni′ah-sis) taeniasis.

ten(o)- word element [Gr.], *tendon.*

tenodesis (ten-od′ĕ-sis) suture of the end of a tendon to a bone.

tenodynia (ten″o-din′e-ah) tenalgia.

tenolysis (ten-ol′ĭ-sis) the operation of freeing a tendon from adhesions.

tenomyoplasty (ten″o-mi′o-plas″te) plastic repair of a tendon and muscle.

tenomyotomy (-mi-ot′ah-me) excision of a portion of a tendon and muscle.

tenonectomy (-nek′tah-me) excision of part of a tendon to shorten it.

tenonitis (-ni′tis) 1. tendinitis. 2. inflammation of Tenon's capsule.

tenonometer (-nom′ĕ-ter) tonometer.

tenontitis (ten″on-ti′tis) tendinitis.

tenont(o)- word element [Gr.], *tendon.*

tenontodynia (ten″on-to-din′e-ah) tenalgia.

tenontography (ten″on-tog′rah-fe) a written description or delineation of the tendons.

tenontology (ten″on-tol′ah-je) sum of what is known about the tendons.

tenophyte (ten′o-fīt) a growth or concretion in a tendon.

tenoplasty (-plas″te) plastic repair of a tendon. **tenoplas′tic,** adj.

tenoreceptor (ten″o-re-sep′ter) a proprioreceptor in a tendon.

tenorrhaphy (tĕ-nor′ah-fe) suture of a tendon.

tenositis (ten″o-si′tis) tendinitis.

tenostosis (ten″os-to′sis) conversion of a tendon into bone.

tenosuture (ten″o-soo′chur) tenorrhaphy.

tenosynovectomy (-sin″o-vek′tah-me) excision or resection of a tendon sheath.

tenosynovitis (-sin″o-vi′tis) inflammation of a tendon sheath. **villonodular t.,** a condition marked by exaggerated proliferation of synovial membrane cells, producing a solid tumor-like mass, commonly occurring in periarticular soft tissues and less frequently in joints.

tenotomy (ten-ot′ah-me) transection of a tendon.

tenovaginitis (ten″o-vaj″ĭ-ni′tis) tenosynovitis.

tension (ten′shun) 1. the act of stretching or the condition of being stretched or strained. 2. the partial pressure of a component of a gas mixture. **arterial t.,** blood pressure within an artery. **intraocular t.,** see under *pressure.* **intravenous t.,** venous pressure. **premenstrual t.,** see under *syndrome.* **surface t.,** tension or resistance which acts to preserve the integrity of a surface. **tissue t.,** a state of equilibrium between tissues and cells which prevents overaction of any part.

tensor (ten′ser) any muscle that stretches or makes tense.

tent (tent) 1. a fabric covering designed to enclose an open space, especially such a covering over a patient's bed for administering oxygen or vaporized medication by inhalation. 2. a conical, expansible plug of soft material for dilating an orifice or for keeping a wound open, so as to prevent its healing except at the bottom. **sponge t.,** a conical plug made of compressed sponge used to dilate the os uteri.

tentorium (ten-tor′e-um), pl. *tento′ria* [L.] an anatomical part resembling a tent or covering. **tento′rial,** adj. **t. cerebel′li,** the process of the dura mater supporting the occipital lobes and covering the cerebellum.

Tenuate (ten′u-āt) trademark for preparations of diethylpropion hydrochloride.

tephromyelitis (tef″ro-mi″ĕ-li′tis) inflammation of the gray substance of the spinal cord.

tera- a word element ([Gr.] *monster*) used in naming units of measurement to designate a quantity 10^{12} (a trillion, or million million) times the unit specified by the root to which it is joined, as teracurie; symbol T.

teras (ter′as), pl. *ter′ata* [L., Gr.] a monster. **terat′ic,** adj.

teratism (ter′ah-tizm) an anomaly of formation or development; the condition of a monster.

terat(o)- word element [Gr.], *monster; monstrosity.*

teratoblastoma (ter″ah-to-blas-to′mah) a neoplasm containing embryonic elements, differing from a teratoma in that its tissue does not represent all germinal layers.

teratocarcinoma (-kar″sĭ-no′mah) a malignant neoplasm consisting of elements of teratoma with those of embryonal carcinoma or choriocarcinoma, or both; occurring most often in the testis.

teratogen (ter′ah-to-jen) an agent or influence that causes physical defects in the developing embryo. **teratogen′ic,** adj.

teratogenesis (ter″ah-to-jen′ĕ-sis) the production of deformity in the developing embryo, or of a monster. **teratogenet′ic,** adj.

teratogenous (ter″ah-toj′ĕ-nus) developed from fetal remains.

teratoid (ter′ah-toid) resembling a monster.

teratology (ter″ah-tol′ah-je) that division of embryology and pathology dealing with abnormal development and congenital deformations. **teratolog′ic,** adj.

teratoma (ter″ah-to′mah) a true neoplasm made up of different types of tissue, none of which is native to the area in which it occurs; usually found in the ovary or testis. **teratom′atous,** adj. **malignant t.,** a solid, malignant ovarian tumor resembling a dermoid cyst but composed of immature embryonal and/or extraembryonal elements derived from all three germ layers.

teratosis (ter″ah-to′sis) teratism.

terbium (ter′be-um) chemical element (see table), at. no. 65, symbol Tb.

terbutaline (ter-bu′tah-lēn) a β-adrenergic receptor antagonist, $(C_{12}H_{19}NO_3)_2$, used as a bronchodilator.

terebration (ter″ah-bra′shun) an act of boring or trephining; also, a boring pain.

teres (te′rēz) [L.] long and round.

ter in die (ter in de′a) [L.] three times a day.

term (term) a definite period, especially the period of gestation, or pregnancy.

terminatio (ter″mĭ-na′she-o), pl. *terminatio′nes* [L.] an ending; the site of discontinuation of a structure, as the free nerve endings (*termina′-tiones nervo′rum li′berae),* in which the peripheral fiber divides into fine branches that terminate freely in connective tissue or epithelium.

terminus (ter′mĭ-nus), pl. *ter′mini* [L.] an ending.

ternary (ter′nah-re) 1. third in order. 2. made up of three distinct chemical elements.

terpene (ter′pēn) any hydrocarbon of the formula $C_{10}H_{16}$.

terpin (ter′pin) a product obtained by the action of nitric acid on oil of turpentine and alcohol; used as an expectorant in the form of the hydrate.

tertian (ter′shun) recurring every three days (every second day); see under *malaria.*

tertiary (ter′she-ār″e) third in order.

tertigravida (ter″shĭ-grav′ĭ-dah) a woman pregnant for the third time; gravida III.

tertipara (ter-tip′ah-rah) a woman who has had three pregnancies which resulted in viable offspring; para III.

tesla (tes′lah) the SI unit of magnetic flux density, equal to one weber per square meter. Symbol T.

tessellated (tes′ah-lāt″ed) divided into squares, like a checker board.

test (test) 1. an examination or trial. 2. a significant chemical reaction. 3. a reagent. **abortus Bang ring t., abortus Bang ringprobe t.,** an agglutination test for brucellosis in cattle, performed by mixing a drop of stained brucellae with 1 ml of milk and incubating for 1 hour at 37°C; agglutinated bacteria rise to the surface to form a colored ring. Abbreviated ABR. **acid elution t.,** air-dried blood smears are fixed in 80 per cent methanol and immersed in a pH 3.3 buffer; all hemoglobins are eluted except fetal hemoglobin, which is seen in red cells after staining. **acidified serum t.,** incubation of red cells in acidified serum; after centrifugation, the supernatant is examined by colorimetry for hemolysis, which indicates paroxysmal nocturnal hemoglobinuria. **acoustic reflex t.,** measurement of the acoustic reflex threshold; used to differentiate between conductive and sensorineural deafness and to diagnose acoustic neuroma. **Adson's t.,** one for thoracic outlet syndrome; with the patient in a sitting position, his hands resting on thighs, the examiner palpates both radial pulses as the patient rapidly fills his lungs by deep inspiration and, holding his breath, hyperextends his neck and turns his head toward the affected side. If the radial pulse on that side is decidedly or completely obliterated, the result is positive. **alkali denaturation t.,** a spectrophotometric method for determining the concentration of fetal (F) hemoglobin. **Ames t.,** a strain of *Salmonella typhimurium* that lacks the enzyme necessary for histidine synthesis is cultured in the absence of histidine and in the presence of the suspected mutagen. If the substance causes DNA damage resulting in mutations (and is therefore carcinogenic), some of the bacteria will regain the ability to synthesize histidine and will proliferate to form colonies. **aptitude t.,** one designed to determine ability to undertake study or training in a particular field. **association t.,** one based on associative reaction, usually by mentioning words to a patient and noting what other words the patient will give as the ones called up in his mind. **Benedict's t.,** a qualitative or quantitative test for the determination of dextrose content of solutions. **Binet's t., Binet-Simon t.,** a method of ascertaining a child's or youth's mental age by asking a series of questions adapted to, and standardized on, the capacity of normal children at various ages. **Bing t.,** a vibrating tuning fork is held to the mastoid process and the auditory meatus is alternately occluded and left open; an increase and decrease in loudness (positive Bing) is perceived by the normal ear and in sensorineural hearing impairment, but in conductive hearing impairment no difference in loudness is perceived (negative Bing). **caloric t.,** Bárány's symptom (2). **cephalin-cholesterol flocculation t.,** one for liver disease based on the flocculation of a cephalin-cholesterol emulsion by the patient's serum. **chromatin t.,** determination of genetic sex of an individual by examination of body cells for the presence of sex chromatin.

cis-trans t., a test in microbial genetics to determine whether two mutations that have the phenotypic effect, in a haploid cell or a cell with single phage infection, are located in the same gene or in different genes; the test depends on the independent behavior of two alleles of a gene in a diploid cell or in a cell infected with two phages carrying different alleles. **complement fixation t.,** see under *fixation.* **conjunctival t.,** 1. see *ophthalmic reaction.* 2. the local reaction occurring after instillation of a pollen or pollen extract into the conjunctiva of a person sensitive to that pollen. **Coombs' t.,** one for detection of antibodies to red cells by means of antiglobulin. In the *direct* Coombs' test, used to detect cell-bound antibody, the red cells are washed free of serum and unbound antibody, and antiglobulin is added. Agglutination indicates the presence of antibody. This method is used to detect sensitized red cells in hemolytic disease of the newborn and autoimmune hemolytic anemia. In the *indirect* Coombs' test, used to detect circulating antibody, a sample of the subject's serum is incubated with donor red cells, the cells are washed, and the antiglobulin is added. If antibody has adsorbed to the cells, they will be agglutinated. **Denver Developmental Screening t.,** a test for identification of infants and preschool children with developmental delay. **Dick t.,** an intracutaneous test for determination of susceptibility to scarlet fever. **dilution t.,** a test for antibiotic sensitivity in bacteria; serial dilutions of an antibacterial agent in an agar or broth medium are inoculated with a suspension of a known concentration of a microorganism. Following incubation the lowest concentration at which there is no visible growth is referred to as the minimum inhibitory concentration for the specific antibiotic. **disk diffusion t.,** a test for antibiotic sensitivity in bacteria; agar plates are inoculated with a standardized suspension of a microorganism. Antibiotic-containing disks are applied to the agar surface. Following overnight incubation, the diameters of the zones of inhibition or clearing surrounding the disks are measured. Zone diameters are interpreted as sensitive (susceptible), indeterminate (or intermediate), or resistant. **early pregnancy t.,** a do-it-yourself immunological test for pregnancy, performed as early as 9 days after menstruation (missed period) was expected. Test materials consist of a mixture of human chorionic gonadotropin (HCG) antiserum and HCG-coated red blood cells in a glass test tube, a vial of water, and a medicine dropper. Three drops of urine are placed in the test tube and the vial of water is added. The tube is shaken for 10 seconds and placed in a holder for 2 hours. A brown ring of nonagglutinated red blood cells is positive (indicates pregnancy). **erythrocyte protoporphyrin t.,** determination of erythrocyte protoporphyrin levels as a screening test for lead toxicity; levels are increased in lead poisoning and iron deficiency. **exercise t's,** tests for detecting previously undetected coronary artery disease; they are graded tests of coronary fitness in which the subject performs exercise, as by walking a treadmill or pedaling a stationary bicycle, while under continuous electrocardiographic monitoring, usually by means of an oscilloscope, before, during, and after the exercise. **FE$_{Na}$ t.,** excreted fraction of filtered sodium test, a measure of renal tubular reabsorption of sodium, calculated as follows: (U/P)Na/(U/P)Cr $\times$ 100, where U and P represent concentrations of sodium and creatinine in urine and plasma, respectively. **finger-nose t.,** one for coordinated movements of the extremities; with the arm extended to one side the patient is asked to try to touch the end of his nose with the tip of his index finger. **Fishberg concentration t.,** determination of the ability of the kidneys to maintain excretion of solids under conditions of reduced water intake and a high protein diet, in which urine samples are collected and tested for specific gravity. **Frei t.,** intracutaneous injection of antigen derived from infected chick embryos, used in the diagnosis of lymphogranuloma venereum. **gel diffusion t.,** a precipitin test in which antigen and antibody are placed in a gel medium (e.g., agar) and one diffuses toward the other (single diffusion) or each diffuses toward the other (double diffusion) to form lines of precipitation. **glucose tolerance t.,** a test of the body's ability to utilize carbohydrates by measuring the blood sugar level at stated intervals after ingestion or intravenous injection of a large quantity of glucose. **glycosylated hemoglobin t.,** measurement of the percentage of hemoglobin A molecules that have formed a stable ketoamine linkage between their terminal amino acid position of the β-chains and a glucose group; in normal persons this amounts to about 7 per cent of the total, in diabetics about 14.5 per cent. **guaiac t.,** one for occult blood; glacial acetic acid and a solution of gum guaiac are mixed with the specimen; on addition of hydrogen peroxide, the presence of blood is indicated by a blue tint. **Ham t.,** acidified serum t. **Hanger's t.,** cephalin-cholesterol flocculation t. **histamine t.,** 1. subcutaneous injection of 0.1% solution of histamine to stimulate gastric secretion. 2. after rapid intravenous injection of histamine phosphate, normal persons experience a brief fall in blood pressure, but in those with pheochromocytoma, after the fall, there is a marked rise in blood pressure. **horse cell t.,** a modification of the Paul-Bunnell-Davidsohn test (q.v.) for antibodies associated with infectious mononucleosis, using horse erythrocytes instead of sheep erythrocytes. **Huhner t.,** determination of the number and condition of spermatozoa in mucus aspirated from the cervical canal within two hours after intercourse. **immobilization t.,** detection of antibody based on its ability to inhibit the motility of a bacterial cell or protozoon. **inkblot t.,** Rorschach t. **intradermal t.,** a skin test in which the antigen is injected intradermally. **Kveim t.,** an intracutaneous test for the diagnosis of sarcoidosis. **latex agglutination t., latex fixation t.,** a type of agglutination test using latex particles as passive carriers of adsorbed antigens. The particles agglutinate following the addition of specific antibody. Used for detection of rheumatoid factor and detection of urine human chorionic gonadotropin in pregnancy testing. **limulus t.,** an extract of blood cells from the horseshoe crab (*Limulus polyphemus*) is exposed to a blood sample from a patient; if gram-negative endotoxin is present in the sample, it will produce gelation of the extract of blood cells. **lupus band t.,** an immunofluorescence test to determine the presence and extent of immunoglobulin and complement deposits at the dermal-epidermal junction of skin specimens from patients with systemic lupus erythematosus. **McMurray's t.,** as the patient lies supine with one knee fully flexed, the examiner rotates the patient's foot fully outward and the knee is slowly extended; a painful "click" indicates a tear of the medial meniscus of the knee joint; if the click occurs when the foot is rotated inward, the tear is in the lateral meniscus. **Mantoux t.,** an intracutaneous tuberculin test. **Master "2-step" exercise t.,** a test of coronary circulation, electrocardiograms being recorded while and after the subject repeatedly ascends and descends two steps, each 9 inches high. **migration inhibitory factor t.,** an *in vitro* test for production of migration inhibitory factor by lymphocytes in response to specific antigens; used for evaluation of cell-mediated immunity. Production of migration inhibitory factor is absent in certain immunodeficiency diseases. **Moloney t.,** one for detection of delayed hypersensitivity to diphtheria toxoid. **multiple-puncture t.,** an intradermal test in which the material used (e.g., tuberculin) is introduced into the skin by pressure of several needles or pointed tines or prongs. **neutralization t.,** one for the bacterial neutralization power of a substance by testing its action on the pathogenic properties of the organism concerned. **Pap t., Papanicolaou t.,** an exfoliative cytological staining procedure for detection and diagnosis of various conditions, particularly malignant and premalignant conditions of the female genital tract; also used in evaluating endocrine function and in diagnosis of malignancies of other organs. **patch t.,** a test for hypersensitivity, performed by observing the reaction to application to the skin of filter paper or gauze saturated with the substance in question. **Patrick's t.,** thigh and knee of the supine patient are flexed, the external malleolus rests on the patella on the opposite leg, and the knee is depressed; production of pain indicates arthritis of the hip. Also known as *fabere sign*, from the initial letters of movements necessary to elicit it, i.e., *f*lexion, *ab*duction, *e*xternal *r*otation, and *e*xtension. **Paul-Bunnell t.,** determination of the highest dilution of the patients' serum that will agglutinate sheep erythrocytes; used to detect serum heterophile antibodies in the diagnosis of infectious mononucleosis. **Paul-Bunnell-Davidsohn t.,** a modification of the Paul-Bunnell test that differentiates among three types of heterophile sheep agglutinins: those associated with infectious mononucleosis and serum sickness, and natural antibodies against Forssman antigen. **precipitation t., precipitin t.,** any test in which the positive reaction consists in the formation and deposit of a precipitate in the fluid being tested.

prothrombin consumption t., a test to measure the formation of intrinsic thromboplastin by determining the residual serum prothrombin after blood coagulation is complete. **psychological t.,** any test to measure one's development, achievement, personality, intelligence, thought processes, etc. **psychomotor t.,** a test that assesses the subject's ability to perceive instructions and perform motor responses. **Queckenstedt's t.,** see under *sign*. **Quick's t.,** 1. a test for liver function based on excretion of hippuric acid after administration of sodium benzoate. 2. (*one-stage prothrombin time*) by adding an extrinsic thromboplastin to oxalated blood the integrity of the prothrombin complex, composed of Factors II, V, VII, X, may be defined; used to control administration of coumarin-type anticoagulants. **Quick tourniquet t.,** estimation of capillary fragility by counting the number of petechiae appearing in a limited area on the flexor surface of the forearm after obstruction to the circulation by a blood pressure cuff applied to the upper arm. **radioallergosorbent t. (RAST),** a radioimmunoassay test for the measurement of specific IgE antibody to a variety of allergens, using antigen fixed in a solid-phase matrix and radiolabeled anti-gamma globulin; used as an alternative to skin tests to determine sensitivity to specific antigens. **radioimmunosorbent t. (RIST),** a radioimmunoassay technique for measuring IgE immunoglobulins in serum, using radiolabeled IgE and anti-human IgE bound to an insoluble matrix. **rapid plasma reagin (RPR) t.,** a group of screening flocculation tests for syphilis, using a modified VDRL antigen. **Rinne t.,** a test of hearing made with tuning forks of 256, 512, and 1024 cycle frequency, comparing the duration of perception by bone and by air conduction. **Rorschach t.,** an association technique for personality testing based on the patient's response to a series of inkblot designs. **Rubin t.,** one for patency of the uterine tubes, made by transuterine inflation with carbon dioxide gas. **Schick t.,** an intracutaneous test for determination of susceptibility to diphtheria. **Schiller t.,** one for early squamous cell carcinoma of the cervix, performed by painting the uterine cervix with a solution of iodine and potassium iodide, diseased areas being revealed by a failure to take the stain. **Schilling t.,** a test for vitamin B_{12} absorption employing cyanocobalamin tagged with Co-57; used in the diagnosis of pernicious anemia. **Schirmer's t.,** a test of tear production in keratoconjunctivitis sicca, performed by measuring the area of moisture on a piece of filter paper inserted over the conjunctival sac of the lower lid, with the end of the paper hanging down on the outside. **Schwabach t.,** a hearing test made, with the opposite ear masked, with tuning forks of 256, 512, 1024, and 2048 cycles, alternately placing the stem of the vibrating fork on the mastoid process of the temporal bone of the patient and that of the examiner. The result is expressed as "Schwabach prolonged" if heard longer by the patient (indicative of conductive hearing impairment), as "Schwabach shortened or diminished" if heard longer by the examiner (indicative of sensorineural hearing impairment), and as "Schwabach normal" if heard for the same time by both. **scratch t.**, a skin test in which the antigen is applied to a superficial scratch. **sheep cell agglutination t. (SCAT)**, any agglutination test using sheep erythrocytes. **sickling t.**, one for demonstration of abnormal hemoglobin and the sickling phenomenon in erythrocytes. **skin t.**, any test in which an antigen is applied to the skin in order to observe the patient's reaction; used to determine immunity to infectious diseases, to identify allergens producing allergic reactions, and to assess ability to mount a cellular immune response. **stress t's**, exercise t's. **thematic apperception t. (TAT)**, a projective test in which the subject tells a story based on each of a series of standard ambiguous pictures, so that his responses reflect a projection of some aspect of his personality and his current psychological preoccupations and conflicts. **three-glass t.**, on arising in the morning, the patient urinates successively in three containers (I, II, III): in acute anterior urethritis, only the urine in I will be turbid from pus or will contain blood; in posterior urethritis the urine in all three will be turbid or contain blood; shreds in III point to chronic prostatitis. **thyroid suppression t.**, after administration of liothyronine for several days, radioactive iodine uptake is decreased in normal persons but not in those with hyperthyroidism. **tine t.**, four 2 mm.-long tines or prongs attached to a handle and coated with dip-dried Old tuberculin are pressed into the skin of the volar surface of the forearm; 48–72 hours later the skin is checked for palpable induration around the wounds. **tuberculin t.**, any of a large number of skin tests for tuberculosis using a variety of different types of tuberculin and methods of application. **unheated serum reagin t.**, a modification of the VDRL test using unheated serum; used primarily for screening. **VDRL t.**, a slide flocculation test for syphilis using VDRL antigen, which contains cardiolipin, cholesterol, and lecithin, to test heat-inactivated serum. **Weber's t.**, the stem of a vibrating tuning fork is placed on the vertex or midline of the forehead; if the sound is heard best in the affected ear, the impairment is probably of the conductive type; if heard best in the normal ear, the impairment is probably of the sensorineural type. **Widal's t.**, a test for the presence of agglutinins to O and H antigens of *Salmonella typhi* and *Salmonella paratyphi* in the serum of patients with suspected *Salmonella* infection.

testalgia (tes-tal'je-ah) testicular pain.

Tes-Tape (tes'tāp) trademark for a test strip impregnated with glucose oxidase, peroxidase, and orthotolidine; used for determining the approximate concentration of glucose in urine.

test card (test kard) a card printed with various letters or symbols, used in testing vision.

test type (test tīp) printed letters of varying size, used in the testing of visual acuity.

testectomy (tes-tek'tah-me) orchiectomy.

testicle (tes'tĭ-k'l) testis.

testicular (tes-tik'u-lar) pertaining to the testis.

testis (tes'tis), pl. *tes'tes* [L.] the male gonad; either of the paired egg-shaped glands normally situated in the scrotum, in which the spermatozoa develop. Specialized interstitial cells (Leydig cells) secrete testosterone. **Cooper's irritable t.**, a testis affected with neuralgia. **inverted t.**, one so positioned in the scrotum that the epididymis is attached anteriorly instead of posteriorly. **retained t**, **undescended t.**, one that has failed to descend into the scrotum, but remains within the abdomen or the inguinal canal.

testitis (tes-ti'tis) orchitis.

testolactone (tes″to-lak'tōn) an antineoplastic steroid, $C_{19}H_{24}O_3$, prepared from testosterone or progesterone by microbial synthesis; used in postmenopausal breast cancer.

testosterone (tes-tos'tah-rōn″) the principal androgenic hormone, $C_{19}H_{28}O_2$, produced by the interstitial cells of the testes (Leydig cells) in response to stimulation by the luteinizing hormone of the anterior pituitary gland; it is thought to be responsible for regulation of gonadotropic secretion, spermatogenesis, and wolffian duct differentiation. It is also responsible for other male characteristics after its conversion to dihydrotestosterone. In addition, testosterone possesses protein anabolic properties. It is used in the treatment of male hypogonadism, cryptorchism, and the symptoms of the male climacteric, and for palliative therapy of breast cancers.

tetanic (tĕ-tan'ik) pertaining to tetanus.

tetaniform (tĕ-tan'ĭ-form) resembling tetanus.

tetanigenous (tet″ah-nij'ĭ-nus) producing tetanic spasms.

tetanize (tet'ah-nīz) to induce tetanic convulsions or symptoms.

tetanode (tet'ah-nōd) the unexcited stage occurring between the tetanic contractions in tetanus.

tetanoid (tet'ah-noid) resembling tetanus.

tetanolysin (tet″ah-nol'ĭ-sin) the hemolytic fraction of the exotoxin formed by the tetanus bacillus (*Clostridium tetani*).

tetanospasmin (tet″ah-no-spaz'min) the neurotoxic component of the exotoxin (tetanus toxin) produced by *Clostridium tetani*, which causes the typical muscle spasms of tetanus.

tetanus (tet'ah-nus) an acute, often fatal, infectious disease caused by a neurotoxin (tetanospasmin) produced by *Clostridium tetani*, whose spores enter the body through wounds. There are two forms: generalized tetanus, marked by tetanic muscular contractions and hyperreflexia, resulting in trismus (lockjaw), glottal spasm, generalized muscle spasm, opisthotonus, respiratory spasm, seizures, and paralysis; and localized tetanus, marked by localized muscular twitching and spasm, which may progress to the generalized form. 2. a state of muscular contraction without periods of relaxation. **infantile t.**, **t. neonato'rum**, tetanus of very young infants, usually due to umbilical infection.

tetany (tet'ah-ne) 1. a syndrome manifested by sharp flexion of the wrist and ankle joints (carpopedal spasm), muscle twitchings, cramps, and convulsions, sometimes with attacks of stridor; due to hyperexcitability of nerves and muscles caused by a decrease in the concentration by extracellular ionized calcium; occurring in parathyroid hypofunction, vitamin D deficiency, and alkalosis, and as a result of ingestion of alkaline salts. 2. tetanus (2). **duration t.,** a continuous tetanic contraction in response to a strong continuous current, occurring especially in degenerated muscles. **gastric t.,** a severe form due to disease of the stomach, attended by difficult respiration and painful tonic spasms of the extremities. **hyperventilation t.,** tetany produced by forced inspiration and expiration continued for a considerable time. **latent t.,** tetany elicited by the application of electrical and mechanical stimulation. **neonatal t., t. of newborn,** hypocalcemic tetany occurring in the first few days of life, often marked by irritability, muscle twitchings, jitteriness, tremors, and convulsions, and less frequently by laryngospasm and carpopedal spasm. **parathyroid t., parathyroprival t.,** tetany due to removal or hypofunctioning of the parathyroids.

tetartanopia (tet″ar-tah-no′pe-ah) 1. quadrantanopia. 2. a rare dichromasy of doubtful existence, characterized by perception of red and green only, with blue and yellow perceived as an achromatic (gray) band.

tetartanopsia (-nop′se-ah) tetartanopia.

tetra- word element [Gr.], *four.*

tetrabrachius (tet″rah-bra′ke-us) a double fetus having four arms.

tetracaine (tet′rah-kān) a local and spinal anesthetic, $C_{15}H_{24}N_2O_2$, used in the form of the hydrochloride salt.

tetrachloroethylene (tet″rah-klōr″o-eth′ĭ-lēn) an anthelmintic, C_2Cl_4.

tetracrotic (-krot′ik) having four sphygmographic elevations to one beat of the pulse.

tetracycline (-si′klēn) an antibiotic, $C_{22}H_{24}N_2O_8$, isolated from elaboration products of certain species of *Streptomyces;* the base and the hydrochloride salt are used as an antiamebic, antibacterial, and antirickettsial.

tetrad (tet′rad) a group of four similar or related entities, as (1) any element or radical having a valence, or combining power, of four; (2) a group of four chromosomal elements formed in the pachytene stage of the first meiotic prophase; (3) a square of cells produced by division into two planes of certain cocci (*Sarcina*). **Fallot's t.,** tetralogy of Fallot.

tetradactyly (tet″rah-dak′tĭ-le) the presence of four digits on the hand or foot.

tetragonum (-go′num) [L.] a four-sided figure. **t. lumba′le,** the quadrangle bounded by the four lumbar muscles.

tetrahydrocannabinol (-hi″dro-kah-nab′ĭ-nol) the active principle of cannabis, occurring in two isomeric forms, both considered psychomimetically active. Abbreviated THC.

tetrahydrofolic acid (tĕ″trah-hi″dro-fo′lik) C_{19}-$H_{23}N_7O_6$, the coenzyme of folic acid, being a reduced folic acid with four hydrogen atoms attached; in dissociated form, called *tetrahydrofolate.*

tetrahydrozoline (-hi-drŏ′zah-lēn) an adrenergic, $C_{13}H_{16}N_2$, applied topically to the nasal mucosa and to the conjunctiva to produce vasoconstriction.

tetralogy (tĕ-tral′ah-je) a group or series of four. **t. of Fallot,** a complex of congenital heart defects consisting of pulmonary stenosis, interventricular septal defect, hypertrophy of right ventricle, and dextroposition of the aorta.

tetrameric (-mer′ik) having four parts.

tetranopsia (-nop′se-ah) quadrantanopia.

tetraparesis (-pah-re′sis) muscular weakness affecting all four extemities.

tetrapeptide (-pep′tid) a peptide which, on hydrolysis, yields four amino acids.

tetraplegia (-ple′je-ah) quadriplegia.

tetraploid (tet′rah-ploid) 1. characterized by tetraploidy. 2. an individual or cell having four sets of chromosomes.

tetrapus (-pus) a fetus with four feet.

tetrascelus (tĕ-tras′ah-lus) a fetus with four legs.

tetrasomy (tet′rah-so″me) the presence of two extra chromosomes of one type in an otherwise diploid cell. **tetraso′mic,** adj.

tetravalent (tet″rah-va′lent) having a valence of four.

tetrodotoxin (tet″ro-do-tok′sin) a highly lethal neurotoxin, $C_{11}H_{17}N_3O_3$, present in numerous species of puffer fish (suborder Tetraodontoidea) and in newts of the genus *Taricha* (tarichatoxin); ingestion results, within minutes, in malaise, dizziness, and tingling about the mouth, which may be followed by ataxia, convulsions, respiratory paralysis, and death.

textiform (teks′tĭ-form) formed like a network.

T-group training group; see *sensitivity group.*

Th chemical symbol, *thorium.*

thalamencephalon (thal″ah-men-sef′ah-lon) the part of the diencephalon comprising the thalamus, metathalamus, and epithalamus.

thalamocortical (thal″ah-mo-kor′tĭ-k'l) pertaining to the thalamus and cerebral cortex.

thalamolenticular (-len-tik′u-ler) pertaining to the thalamus and lenticular nucleus.

thalamotomy (thal″ah-mot′ah-me) a stereotaxic surgical technique for the discrete destruction of specific groups of cells within the thalamus, as for the relief of pain or for relief of tremor and rigidity in Parkinson's disease.

thalamus (thal′ah-mus), pl. *thal′ami* [L.] either of two large ovoid masses, consisting chiefly of gray substance, situated one on either side of and forming part of the lateral wall of the third ventricle. It is divided into dorsal and ventral parts; the term *thalamus* without a modifier usually refers to the dorsal thalamus, which functions as a relay center for sensory impulses to the cerebral cortex.

thalassemia (thal″ah-se′me-ah) a heterogeneous group of hereditary hemolytic anemias marked by a decreased rate of synthesis of one or more hemoglobin polypeptide chains, classified according to the chain involved (α, β, δ); the two major categories are α- and β-thalassemia. **α-t., alpha-t.,** that caused by diminished synthesis of alpha chains of hemoglobin. The *homozygous* form is incompatible with life, the stillborn infant displaying severe hydrops fetalis. The *heterozygous* form may be asymptomatic or marked by mild anemia. **β-t., beta-t.,** that caused by diminished synthesis of beta chains of hemoglobin. The *homozygous* form (Cooley's, Mediterranean, or erythroblastic anemia; t. major), in which hemoglobin A is completely absent, appears in the newborn period and is marked by hemolytic, hypochromic, microcytic anemia, hepatosplenomegaly, skeletal deformation, mongoloid facies, and cardiac enlargement. The *heterozygous* form (t. minor) is usually asymptomatic, but there is mild anemia. **t. major,** see *beta-t.* **t. minor,** see *beta-t.* **sickle cell–t.,** a hereditary anemia involving simultaneous heterozygosity for hemoglobin S and thalassemia.

thalidomide (thah-lid′o-mīd) a sedative and hypnotic, $C_{13}H_{10}N_2O$, commonly used in Europe in the early 1960's, and discovered to cause serious congenital anomalies in the fetus, notably amelia and phocomelia, when taken during early pregnancy.

thallium (thal′e-um) chemical element (*see table*), at. no. 81, symbol Tl. It may be absorbed from the gut and from the intact skin, causing a variety of neurologic and psychic symptoms and liver and kidney damage. **t.-201,** a radioactive isotope of thallium having a half-life of 73.5 hours. Used in cardiac imaging as thallous chloride Tl 201.

thanato- word element [Gr.], *death.*

thanatognomonic (than″ah-tog″no-mon′ik) indicating the approach of death.

thanatophidia (than″ah-to-fid′ě-ah) the venomous snakes, collectively.

thanatophoric (-for′ik) deadly; lethal.

THC tetrahydrocannabinol.

thebaine (the-ba′in) a crystalline, poisonous, and anodyne alkaloid from opium, having properties similar to those of strychnine.

theca (the′kah) pl. *the′cae* [L.] a case or sheath. **the′cal,** adj. **t. cor′dis,** pericardium. **t. follic′uli,** an envelope of condensed connective tissue surrounding a vesicular ovarian follicle, comprising an internal vascular layer (*t. interna*) and an external fibrous layer (*t. externa*).

thecitis (the-si′tis) tenosynovitis.

thecoma (the-ko′mah) theca cell tumor.

thecostegnosis (the″ko-steg-no′sis) contraction of a tendon sheath.

thelalgia (the-lal′je-ah) pain in the nipples.

thelarche (the-lar′ke) beginning of development of the breast at puberty.

Thelazia (the-la′ze-ah) a genus of nematode worms parasitic in the eyes of mammals, including, rarely, humans.

thelaziasis (the″la-zi′ah-sis) infection of the eye with *Thelazia.*

theleplasty (the′lě-plas″te) a plastic operation on the nipple.

thelerethism (thel-er′ě-thizm) erection of the nipple.

thelitis (the-li′tis) inflammation of a nipple.

thelium (the′le-um) 1. a papilla. 2. a nipple.

thelorrhagia (the″lo-ra′je-ah) hemorrhage from the nipple.

thenar (the′nar) 1. the fleshy part of the hand at the base of the thumb. 2. pertaining to the palm.

theobromine (the″o-bro′min) an alkaloid prepared from dried ripe seed of the tropical American tree *Theobroma cacao* or made synthetically from xanthine; it has properties similar to those of caffeine, and is used as a smooth muscle relaxant, as a diuretic, and as a myocardial stimulant and vasodilator.

theophylline (the-of′i-lin) a xanthine derivative, $C_7H_8N_4$; it is a smooth muscle relaxant, used chiefly for its bronchodilator effect; it may also be used for its myocardial stimulant and coronary vasodilator actions, diuretic action, and respiratory center stimulant effect. **t. cholinate,** oxtriphylline. **t. ethylenediamine,** aminophylline.

theory (the′o-re) 1. the doctrine or the principles underlying an art as distinguished from the practice of that particular art. 2. a formulated hypothesis or, loosely speaking, any hypothesis or opinion not based upon actual knowledge. **cell t.,** all organic matter consists of cells, and cell activity is the essential process of life. **clonal deletion t.,** a theory of immunologic self-tolerance according to which "forbidden clones" of immunocytes, those reactive with self antigens, are eliminated on contact with antigen during fetal life. **clonal-selection t.,** there are several million clones of antibody-producing cells in each adult, each programmed to make an antibody of a single specificity and carrying cell-surface receptors for specific antigens; exposure to antigen induces cells with receptors for that antigen to proliferate and produce large quantities of specific antibody. **information t.,** a system for analyzing, chiefly by statistical methods, the characteristics of communicated messages and the systems that encode, transmit, distort, receive, and decode them. **quantum t.,** radiation and absorption of energy occur in quantities (quanta) which vary in size with the frequency of the radiation. **recapitulation t.,** ontogeny recapitulates phylogeny, i.e., an organism in the course of its development goes through the same successive stages (in abbreviated form) as did the species in its evolutionary development. **Young-Helmholtz t.,** color vision depends on three sets of retinal receptors, corresponding to the colors red, green, and violet.

theque (těk) [Fr.] a round or oval collection, or nest, of melanin-containing nevus cells occurring at the dermoepidermal junction of the skin or in the dermis proper.

therapeutic (ther″ah-pu′tik) pertaining to therapeutics, or treatment of disease; curative.

therapeutics (-pu′tiks) 1. the science and art of healing. 2. a scientific account of the treatment of disease.

therapist (ther′ah-pist) a person skilled in the treatment of disease or other disorder. **physi-**

therapy

cal t., a person skilled in the techniques of physical therapy and qualified to administer treatment prescribed by a physician. **speech t.,** a person specially trained and qualified to assist patients in overcoming speech and language disorders.

therapy (ther′ah-pe) the treatment of disease; therapeutics. See also *treatment*. **aversion t.,** therapy directed at associating an undesirable behavior pattern with unpleasant stimulation. **behavior t.,** a therapeutic approach that focuses on modifying the patient's observable behavior, rather than on the conflicts and unconscious processes presumed to underlie the behavior. **collapse t.,** collapse and immobilization of the lung in treatment of pulmonary disease. **electroconvulsive t., electroshock t.,** a treatment for mental disorders, primarily depression, in which convulsions and loss of consciousness are induced by application of low-voltage alternating current to the brain via scalp electrodes for a fraction of a second; a muscle relaxant is used to prevent injury during the seizure. **group t.,** psychotherapy carried out with a group of patients under the guidance of a single therapist. **immunosuppressive t.,** treatment with agents, such as x-rays, corticosteroids, and cytotoxic chemicals, which suppress the immune response to antigen(s); used in various conditions, including organ transplantation, autoimmune disease, allergy, multiple myeloma, and chronic nephritis. **inhalation t.,** treatment of pathophysiologic alterations of gas exchange in the cardiopulmonary system by the use of respirators, aerosols, oxygen, and gas mixtures. **milieu t.,** treatment, usually in a psychiatric hospital, that emphasizes the provision of an environment and activities appropriate to the patient's emotional and interpersonal needs. **occupational t.,** the therapeutic use of self-care, work, and play activities to increase function, enhance development, and prevent disabilities. **photodynamic t.,** intravenous administration of hematoporphyrin derivative, which concentrates selectively in metabolically active tumor tissue, followed by exposure of the tumor tissue to red laser light to produce cytotoxic free radicals that destroy hematoporphyrin-containing tissue. **physical t.,** 1. treatment by physical means. 2. the health profession concerned with the promotion of health, the prevention of disability, and the evaluation and rehabilitation of patients disabled by pain, disease, or injury, and with treatment by physical therapeutic measures as opposed to medical, surgical, or radiologic measures. **replacement t.,** treatment to replace deficient formation or loss of body products by administration of the natural body products or synthetic substitutes. **substitution t.,** the administration of a hormone to compensate for glandular deficiency.

theriogenology (the″re-o-jen-ol′o-je) the branch of veterinary medicine that deals with reproduction in all its aspects. **theriogenolog′ic,** adj.

therm (therm) a unit of heat. The word has been used as equivalent to (a) large calorie; (b) small calorie; (c) 1000 large calories; (d) 100,000 British thermal units.

therm(o)- word element [Gr.], *heat.*

thermalgesia (ther″mal-je′ze-ah) painful sensation produced by heat.

thermalgia (ther-mal′je-ah) causalgia.

thermanalgesia (therm″an-al-je′ze-ah) absence of sensibility to heat.

thermanesthesia (-es-the′ze-ah) inability to recognize heat and cold.

thermesthesia (therm″es-the′ze-ah) ability to recognize heat and cold.

thermesthesiometer (-es-the″ze-om′ĕ-ter) an instrument for measuring sensibility to heat.

thermhyperesthesia (-hi″per-es-the′ze-ah) thermohyperesthesia.

thermhypesthesia (-hi-pes-the′ze-ah) thermohypesthesia.

thermic (ther′mik) pertaining to heat.

thermocautery (ther″mo-kaw′ter-e) cauterization by a heated wire or point.

thermochemistry (-kem′is-tre) the aspect of physical chemistry dealing with temperature changes that accompany chemical reactions.

thermocoagulation (-ko-ag″u-la′shun) tissue coagulation with high-frequency currents.

thermodiffusion (ther″mo-dĭ-fu′zhun) diffusion influenced by a temperature gradient.

thermodynamics (-di-nam′iks) the branch of science dealing with heat and energy, their interconversion, and problems related thereto.

thermoexcitory (-ek-si′ter-e) stimulating production of bodily heat.

thermogenesis (-jen′ĕ-sis) the production of heat, especially within the animal body. **thermogenet′ic, thermogen′ic,** adj.

thermogram (ther′mo-gram) 1. a graphic record of temperature variations. 2. the visual record obtained by thermography.

thermograph (-graf) 1. an instrument for recording temperature variations. 2. thermogram (2). 3. the apparatus used in thermography.

thermography (ther-mog′rah-fe) a technique wherein an infrared camera photographically portrays the body's surface temperature, based on self-emanating infrared radiation; sometimes used as a means of diagnosing underlying pathologic conditions, such as breast tumors.

thermohyperalgesia (ther″mo-hi″per-al-je′ze-ah) extreme thermalgesia.

thermohyperesthesia (-hi″per-es-the′ze-ah) increased sensibility to heat and cold.

thermohypesthesia (-hi″pes-the′ze-ah) decreased sensibility to heat and cold.

thermoinhibitory (ther″mo-in-hib′ĭ-tor″e) retarding generation of bodily heat.

thermolabile (-la′bĭl) easily affected by heat.

thermolysis (ther-mol′ĭ-sis) 1. chemical dissociation by means of heat. 2. dissipation of bodily heat by radiation, evaporation, etc. **thermolyt′ic,** adj.

thermomassage (ther″mo-mah-sahzh′) massage with heat.

thermometer (ther-mom′ĕ-ter) an instrument for determining temperatures, in principle making use of a substance with a physical property that varies with temperature and is susceptible of measurement on some defined scale. (see table accompanying temperature). **clinical t.**, one used to determine the temperature of the human body. **oral t.**, a clinical thermometer that is placed under the tongue. **recording t.**, a temperature-sensitive instrument by which the temperature to which it is exposed is continuously recorded. **rectal t.**, a clinical thermometer that is inserted into the rectum.

thermophile (ther′mo-fīl) an organism that grows best at elevated temperatures. **thermophil′ic**, adj.

thermophore (-for) 1. a device or apparatus for retaining heat. 2. an instrument for estimating heat sensibility.

thermoplacentography (ther″mo-plas″en-tog′rah-fe) use of thermography for determination of the site of placental attachment.

thermoplegia (-ple′je-ah) heatstroke or sunstroke.

thermopolypnea (-pol″ip-ne′ah) quickened breathing due to great heat.

thermoreceptor (-re-sep′ter) a nerve ending sensitive to stimulation by heat.

thermoregulation (-reg″u-la′shun) heat regulation.

thermostabile (-sta′b'l) not affected by heat.

thermosystaltic (-sis-tal′tik) contracting under the stimulus of heat.

thermotaxis (-tak′sis) 1. normal adjustment of bodily temperature. 2. movement of an organism in response to an increase in temperature. **thermotac′tic, thermotax′ic**, adj.

thermotherapy (-ther′ah-pe) therapeutic use of heat.

thermotonometer (ther″mo-to-nom′ĕ-ter) an instrument for measuring the amount of muscular contraction produced by heat.

thermotropism (ther-mot′rah-pizm) tropism in response to an increase in temperature. **thermotrop′ic**, adj.

thi(o)- a word element [Gr.], *sulfur.*

thiabendazole (thi″ah-ben′dah-zōl) a broad-spectrum anthelmintic, $C_{10}H_7N_3S$.

thiamine (thi′ah-min) vitamin B_1; a component of the B complex of vitamins, found in various foodstuffs and present in the free state in blood plasma and cerebrospinal fluid. Deficiency results in beriberi.

thiamylal (thi-am′ĭ-lal) an ultrashort-acting barbiturate; the sodium salt is used intravenously as a general anesthetic.

thiazide (thi′ah-zīd) any of a group of diuretics that act by inhibiting the reabsorption of sodium in the proximal renal tubule and stimulating chloride excretion, with resultant increase in excretion of water.

thiemia (thi-e′me-ah) sulfur in the blood.

thiethylperazine (thi-eth″il-per′ah-zēn) a phenothiazine derivative, $C_{22}H_{29}N_3S_2$, useful as an antiemetic and antinauseant.

thigh (thi) the portion of the leg above the knee; the femur.

thigmesthesia (thig″mes-the′ze-ah) tactile sensibility.

thigmotaxis (thig″mo-tak′sis) movement of an organism in response to contact. **thigmotac′tic, thigmotax′ic**, adj.

thigmotropism (thig-mot′rah-pizm) tropism of an organism elicited by touch or by contact with a solid or rigid surface. **thigmotrop′ic**, adj.

thimerosal (thi-mer′o-sal) a local anti-infective, $C_9H_9HgNaO_2S$.

thinking (thingk′ing) ideational mental activity (as opposed to emotional activity). **dereistic t.**, dereism.

thiobarbituric acid (thi″o-bar″bĭ-choor′ik) a condensation of malonic acid and thiourea, $C_8H_4N_2O_2S$, differing from barbituric acid only by the presence of a sulfur atom instead of an oxygen atom at the number 2 carbon. It is the parent compound of a class of drugs, the thiobarbiturates, which are analogous in their effects to barbiturates.

thioctic acid (thi-ok′tik) lipoic acid.

thiocyanate (thi″o-si′ah-nāt) a salt analogous in composition to a cyanate, but containing sulfur instead of oxygen.

thioguanine (-gwah′nēn) an antineoplastic derived from mercaptopurine; used in leukemia.

thiokinase (-ki′nās) any enzyme that catalyzes the joining of an acid and a thiol (—SH) group coupled with the release of inorganic phosphate from ATP or a similar triphosphate.

thionin (thi′o-nin) a dark-green powder, purple in solution, used as a metachromatic stain in microscopy.

thiopental (thi″o-pen′tal) an ultrashort-acting barbiturate, $C_{11}H_{17}N_2O_2S$; the sodium salt is used intravenously to induce general anesthesia, as an anticonvulsant, and for narcoanalysis and narcosynthesis.

thioridazine (-rid′ah-zēn) a tranquilizer, $C_{21}H_{26}N_2S_2$, used as the hydrochloride salt.

thiosulfate (thi″o-sul′fāt) the $SSO_3{}^{2-}$ anion, or a salt containing this ion; produced in cysteine metabolism.

thiotepa (-te′pah) a cytotoxic alkylating agent, $C_6H_{12}N_3PS$, used as an antineoplastic.

thiothixene (-thik′sēn) a tranquilizer, $C_{23}H_{29}N_3O_2S_2$.

thioxanthene (-zan′thēn) any of a class of structurally related neuroleptic drugs, including chlorprothixene and thiothixene.

thiphenamil (thi-fen′ah-mil) an anticholinergic, $C_{20}H_{26}ClNOS$, having potent antispasmodic and smooth muscle relaxant properties.

thirst (therst) a sensation, often referred to the mouth and throat, associated with a craving for drink; ordinarily interpreted as a desire for water.

thixotropism (thik-sot′rah-pizm) thixotropy.

thixotropy (thik-sot′rah-pe) the property of certain gels of becoming fluid when shaken and then becoming semisolid again. **thixotrop′ic**, adj.

thlipsencephalus (thlip″sen-sef′ah-lus) a fetus with a defective skull.

thorac(o)- word element [Gr.], *chest.*

thoracalgia (thor″ah-kal′je-ah) pain in the chest wall.

thoracectomy (-sek′to-me) thoracotomy with resection of part of a rib.

thoracentesis (-sen-te′sis) surgical puncture of the chest wall into the parietal cavity for aspiration of fluids.

thoracic (thah-ras′ik) pertaining to the chest.

thoracoacromial (thor″ah-ko-ah-kro′me-al) pertaining to the chest and acromion.

thoracoceloschisis (-se-los′ki-sis) congenital fissure of the thorax and abdomen.

thoracocyllosis (-si-lo′sis) deformity of the thorax.

thoracocyrtosis (-sir-to′sis) abnormal curvature of the thorax or unusual prominence of the chest.

thoracodelphus (-del′fus) a double fetus with one head, two arms, and four legs, the bodies being joined above the navel.

thoracodidymus (-did′ĭ-mus) thoracopagus.

thoracodynia (-din′e-ah) pain in the thorax.

thoracogastroschisis (-gas-tros′ki-sis) congenital fissure of the thorax and abdomen.

thoracolumbar (-lum′bar) pertaining to thoracic and lumbar vertebrae.

thoracolysis (thor″ah-kol′ĭ-sis) the freeing of adhesions of the chest wall.

thoracomelus (-kom′ah-lus) a fetus with a supernumerary limb attached to the thorax.

thoracometer (-kom′ah-ter) stethometer.

thoracomyodynia (-ko-mi″o-din′e-ah) pain in the muscles of the chest.

thoracopagus (-kop′ah-gus) conjoined twins united at the thorax.

thoracopathy (-kop′ah-the) any disease of the thoracic organs or tissues.

thoracoplasty (thor′ah-ko-plas″te) surgical removal of ribs, allowing the chest wall to collapse a diseased lung.

thoracoschisis (thor″ah-kos′ki-sis) congenital fissure of the chest wall.

thoracoscope (tho-ra′ko-skōp) an endoscope for examining the pleural cavity through an intercostal space.

thoracostenosis (ko-stĕ-no′sis) abnormal contraction of the thorax.

thoracostomy (-kos′tah-me) incision of the chest wall, with maintenance of the opening for drainage.

thoracotomy (-kot′ah-me) incision of the chest wall.

thorax (thor′aks) the chest; the part of the body between the neck and the respiratory diaphragm, encased by the ribs. **Peyrot's t.,** an obliquely oval thorax associated with massive pleural effusions.

Thorazine (thor′ah-zēn) trademark for preparations of chlorpromazine.

thorium (thor′e-um) chemical element (*see table*), at. no. 90, symbol Th.

thoroughpin (thur′o-pin) distention of the synovial sheaths at the upper portion and back of the hock joint of a horse.

thought broadcasting (thawt brawd′kas-ting) the feeling that one's thoughts are being broadcast to the environment.

thought insertion (thawt in-ser′shun) the delusion that thoughts that are not one's own are being inserted into one's mind.

thought withdrawal (thawt with-draw′al) the delusion that someone or something is removing thoughts from one's mind.

threadworm (thred′werm) any long slender nematode, especially *Enterobius vermicularis.*

threonine (thre′o-nin) a naturally occurring amino acid essential for human metabolism.

threshold (thresh′old) the level that must be reached for an effect to be produced, as the degree of intensity of a stimulus that just produces a sensation, or the concentration that must be present in the blood before certain substances are excreted by the kidney (*renal t.*).

thrill (thril) a vibration felt by the examiner on palpation. **diastolic t.,** one felt over the precordium during diastole in advanced aortic insufficiency. **hydatid t.,** one sometimes felt on percussing over a hydatid cyst. **presystolic t.,** one felt just before the systole over the apex of the heart. **systolic t.,** one felt over the precordium during systole in aortic stenosis, pulmonary stenosis, and ventricular septal defect.

thrix (thriks) [Gr.] hair.

-thrix word element [Gr.], *hair.*

throat (thrōt) 1. pharynx. 2. fauces. 3. anterior aspect of the neck. **sore t.,** see under S.

thromb(o)- word element [Gr.], *clot; thrombus.*

thrombasthenia (throm″bas-the′ne-ah) a platelet abnormality characterized by defective clot retraction and defective ADP-induced platelet aggregation; clinically manifested by epistaxis, inappropriate bruising, and excessive posttraumatic bleeding. **Glanzmann's t.,** thrombasthenia.

thrombectomy (throm-bek′tah-me) surgical removal of a clot from a blood vessel.

thrombi (throm′bi) plural of *thrombus.*

thrombin (throm′bin) an enzyme resulting from activation of prothrombin, which catalyzes the conversion of fibrinogen to fibrin.

thromboangiitis (throm″bo-an″je-i′tis) inflammation of a blood vessel, with thrombosis. **t. oblit′erans,** Buerger's disease; an inflammatory and obliterative disease of the blood vessels of the limbs, primarily the legs, leading to ischemia and gangrene.

thromboarteritis (-ar″ter-i′tis) thrombosis associated with arteritis.

thromboclasis (throm-bok′lah-sis) the dissolution of a thrombus. **thromboclas′tic,** adj.

thrombocyst, thrombocystis (throm′bo-sist; throm″bo-sis′tis) a chronic sac formed around a thrombus in a hematoma.

thrombocytapheresis (throm″bo-sīt″ah-fĕ-re′-sis) the selective separation and removal of thrombocytes (platelets) from withdrawn blood, the remainder of the blood then being retransfused into the donor.

thrombocyte (throm′bo-sīt) a blood platelet. **thrombocyt′ic,** adj.

thrombocythemia (throm″bo-si-the′me-ah) a

fixed increase in the number of circulating blood platelets. **essential t., hemorrhagic t.,** a clinical syndrome with repeated spontaneous hemorrhages, either external or into the tissues, and greatly increased number of circulating platelets.

thrombocytocrit (-si′to-krit) the volume of packed blood platelets in a given quantity of blood; also, the instrument used to measure platelet volume.

thrombocytolysis (-si-tol′ĭ-sis) destruction of blood platelets.

thrombocytopathy (-si-top′ah-the) any qualitative disorder of blood platelets.

thrombocytopenia (-si″to-pe′ne-ah) decrease in number of platelets in circulating blood. **immune t.,** that associated with the presence of anti-platelet antibodies (IgG).

thrombocytopoiesis (-si″to-poi-e′sis) the production of blood platelets. **thrombocytopoiet′ic,** adj.

thrombocytosis (-si-to′sis) an increased number of platelets in circulating blood.

thromboembolism (-em′bo-lizm) obstruction of a blood vessel with thrombotic material carried by the blood from the site of origin to plug another vessel.

thromboendarterectomy (-end″ar-ter-ek′tah-me) excision of an obstructing thrombus together with a portion of the inner lining of the obstructed artery.

thromboendarteritis (-end″ar-ter-i′tis) inflammation of the innermost coat of an artery, with thrombus formation.

thromboendocarditis (-en″do-kar-di′tis) 1. formation of a thrombus on a heart valve which has previously been eroded. 2. an infectious disease of rabbits.

thrombogenesis (-jen′ĕ-sis) clot formation. **thrombogen′ic,** adj.

thromboid (throm′boid) resembling a thrombus.

thrombokinase (throm″bo-ki′nās) activated coagulation Factor X.

thrombokinetics (-ki-net′iks) the dynamics of blood coagulation.

thrombolymphangitis (-lim″fan-ji′tis) inflammation of a lymph vessel due to a thrombus.

thrombolysis (throm-bol′ĭ-sis) dissolution of a thrombus. **thrombolyt′ic,** adj.

thrombophilia (-fil′e-ah) a tendency to the occurrence of thrombosis.

thrombophlebitis (-flĕ-bi′tis) inflammation of a vein associated with thrombus formation. **t. mi′grans,** a recurring thrombophlebitis involving different vessels simultaneously or at intervals. **postpartum iliofemoral t.,** thrombophlebitis of the iliofemoral vein following childbirth.

thromboplastic (-plas′tik) causing or accelerating clot formation in the blood.

thromboplastin (-plas′tin) a substance in blood and tissues which, in the presence of ionized calcium, aids in the conversion of prothrombin to thrombin. **tissue t.,** coagulation Factor III.

thrombopoiesis (-poi-e′sis) 1. thrombogenesis. 2. thrombocytopoiesis. **thrombopoiet′ic,** adj.

thrombosed (throm′bōzd) affected with thrombosis.

thrombosis (throm-bo′sis) the formation or presence of a thrombus. **thrombot′ic,** adj. **cerebral t.,** thrombosis of a cerebral vessel, which may result in cerebral infarction. **coronary t.,** thrombosis of a coronary artery, often leading to myocardial infarction.

thrombostasis (throm-bos′tah-sis) stasis of blood in a part with formation of a thrombus.

thromboxane (throm-bok′sān) either of two compounds, one designated A_2 and the other B_2. Thromboxane A_2 is synthesized by platelets and is an inducer of platelet aggregation and platelet release functions and is a vasoconstrictor; it is very unstable and is hydrolyzed to thromboxane B_2.

thrombus (throm′bus), pl. *throm′bi.* An aggregation of blood factors, primarily platelets and fibrin with entrapment of cellular elements, frequently causing vascular obstruction at the point of its formation. **mural t.,** one attached to the wall of the endocardium in a diseased area. **occluding t.,** one that occupies the entire lumen of a vessel and obstructs blood flow. **parietal t.,** one attached to a vessel or heart wall.

thrush (thrush) candidiasis of the oral mucous membranes, usually affecting sick, weak infants or elderly adults in poor health, with formation of whitish spots (aphthae), which are followed by shallow ulcers; it is caused by *Candida albicans.*

thrypsis (thrip′sis) a comminuted fracture.

thulium (thoo′le-um) chemical element (*see table*), at. no. 69, symbol Tm.

thumb (thum) the radial or first digit of the hand. **tennis t.,** tendinitis of the tendon of the long flexor muscle of the thumb, with calcification.

thumbprinting (thum′print-ing) a roentgenographic sign appearing as smooth indentations on the barium-filled colon, as though made by depression with the thumb.

thym(o)- word element [Gr.], *thymus; mind, soul, or emotions.*

thymectomize (thi-mek′tah-mīz) to excise the thymus.

thymectomy (thi-mek′tah-me) excision of the thymus.

thymelcosis (thi″mel-ko′sis) ulceration of the thymus.

-thymia word element [Gr.], *condition of mind.* **-thy′mic,** adj.

thymic (thi′mik) pertaining to the thymus.

thymicolymphatic (thi″mĭ-ko-lim-fat′ik) pertaining to the thymus and lymphatic nodes.

thymidine (thi′mĭ-dēn) 1. deoxy thymidine, a nucleoside of DNA. 2. a rarely occurring base in rRNA and tRNA.

thymin (thi′min) thymopoietin.

thymine (thi′mēn) a pyrimidine base, $C_5H_6N_2O$, in DNA.

thymitis (thi-mi′tis) inflammation of the thymus.

thymocyte (thi′mo-sīt) a lymphocyte arising in the thymus.

thymokinetic (-kĭ-net′ik) tending to stimulate the thymus.

thymol (thi′mol) a phenol, $C_{10}H_{14}O$, obtained from thyme oil and other volatile oils or produced synthetically; used as a stabilizer in pharmaceutical preparations.

thymoleptic (thi″mo-lep′tik) any drug that favorably modifies mood in serious affective disorders such as depression or mania; the main categories of thymoleptics include the tricyclic antidepressants, monoamine oxidase inhibitors, and lithium compounds.

thymoma (thi-mo′mah) a tumor derived from the epithelial or lymphoid elements of the thymus.

thymopathy (thi-mop′ah-the) any disease of the thymus. **thymopath′ic,** adj.

thymopoietin (thi″mo-poi′ĕ-tin) a polypeptide hormone secreted by thymic epithelial cells that induces differentiation of precursor lymphocytes into thymocytes.

thymoprivic, thymoprivous (thi″mo-priv′ik; thi-mop′rĭ-vus) pertaining to or resulting from removal or atrophy of the thymus.

thymosin (thi′mo-sin) a humoral factor secreted by the thymus, which promotes the maturation of T lymphocytes.

thymus (thi′mus) a bilaterally symmetrical lymphoid organ consisting of two pyramidal lobules situated in the anterior superior mediastinum, each lobule consisting of an outer cortex, rich in lymphocytes (thymocytes) and an inner medulla, rich in epithelial cells. The thymus is the site of production of T lymphocytes: precursor cells migrate to the outer cortex, where they proliferate, then move through the inner cortex, where T-cell surface markers are acquired, and finally into the medulla, where they become mature T cells; maturation is controlled by hormones produced by the thymus, including thymopoietin and thymosin. The thymus reaches maximal development at about puberty and then undergoes gradual involution.

thyr(o)- word element [Gr.], *thyroid.*

thyroadenitis (thi″ro-ad″ĕ-ni′tis) inflammation of the thyroid.

thyroaplasia (-ah-pla′ze-ah) defective development of the thyroid with deficient activity of its secretion.

thyroarytenoid (-ar″ĭ-te′noid) pertaining to the thyroid and arytenoid cartilages.

thyrocardiac (-kar′de-ak) pertaining to the thyroid and heart.

thyrocele (thi′ro-sēl) tumor of the thyroid gland; goiter.

thyrochondrotomy (thi″ro-kon-drot′ah-me) surgical incision of the thyroid cartilage.

thyrocricotomy (-kri-kot′o-me) incision of the cricothyroid membrane.

thyroepiglottic (-ep″ĭ-glot′ik) pertaining to the thyroid and epiglottis.

thyrogenic, thyrogenous (thi″ro-jen′ik; thi-roj′ĕ-nus) originating in the thyroid.

thyroglobulin (thi″ro-glob′u-lin) 1. an iodine-containing glycoprotein of high molecular weight, occurring in the colloid of the follicles of the thyroid gland; the iodinated tyrosine moieties of thyroglobulin form the active hormones thyroxine and triiodothyronine. 2. a substance obtained by fractionation of thyroid glands from the hog; administered orally as a thyroid supplement in the treatment of hypothyroidism.

thyroglossal (-glos′al) pertaining to the thyroid and tongue.

thyrohyal (-hi′al) pertaining to the thyroid cartilage and the hyoid bone.

thyrohyoid (-hi′oid) pertaining to the thyroid gland or cartilage and the hyoid bone.

thyroid (thi′roid) 1. resembling a shield. 2. the thyroid gland; see under *gland.* 3. a pharmaceutical preparation of cleaned, dried, powdered thyroid gland, obtained from those domesticated animals used for food by man.

thyroidectomize (thi″roi-dek′tah-mīz) to excise the thyroid.

thyroidectomy (thi″roi-dek′tah-me) excision of the thyroid.

thyroiditis (thi″roi-di′tis) inflammation of the thyroid. **Hashimoto's t.,** struma lymphomatosa.

thyroidotomy (thi″roi-dot′ah-me) incision of the thyroid.

thyromegaly (thi″ro-meg′ah-le) goiter.

thyromimetic (-mi-met′ik) producing effects similar to those of thyroid hormones or the thyroid gland.

thyroparathyroidectomy (-par″ah-thi″roi-dek′tah-me) excision of thyroid and parathyroids.

thyroprival, thyroprivic (-pri′v'l; -priv′ik) pertaining to, marked by, or due to deprivation or loss of thyroid function.

thyroptosis (thi″rop-to′sis) downward displacement of the thyroid gland into the thorax.

thyrotherapy (thi″ro-ther′ah-pe) treatment with preparations of thyroid.

thyrotomy (thi-rot′ah-me) 1. surgical division of the thyroid cartilage. 2. the operation of cutting the thyroid gland. 3. biopsy of the thyroid gland.

thyrotoxic (thi″ro-tok′sik) 1. marked by the effects of presentation of excessive quantities of thyroid hormones to the tissues. 2. describing a patient suffering from thyrotoxicosis.

thyrotoxicosis (-tok″sĭ-ko′sis) a morbid condition due to overactivity of the thyroid gland; see *Graves' disease.*

thyrotrope, thyrotroph (thi′ro-trōp; thi′ro-trōf) one of the basophils (beta cells) of the adenohypophysis, the granules of which secrete thyrotropin.

thyrotrophic (thi″ro-trōf′ik) thyrotropic.

thyrotrophin (-trōf′in) thyrotropin.

thyrotropic (-trop′ik) 1. pertaining to or marked by thyrotropism. 2. having an influence on the thyroid gland.

thyrotropin (-trop′in) a hormone of the anterior pituitary gland having an affinity for and specifically stimulating the thyroid gland.

thyroxine (thi-rok′sin) an iodine-containing hormone secreted by the thyroid gland; its chief function is to increase the rate of cell metabolism. Thyroxine is deiodinated in peripheral tissues to form triiodothyronine, which has a greater biological activity. A synthetic preparation is used in treating hypothyroidism. Symbol T$_4$.

Ti chemical symbol, *titanium.*

tibia (tib′e-ah) see *Table of Bones.* **tib′ial,** adj. **t. val′ga,** bowing of the leg in which the angulation is away from the midline. **t. va′ra,** medial angulation of the tibia in the metaphyseal region, due to a growth disturbance of the medial aspect of the proximal tibial epiphysis.

tibialis (tib″e-a′lis) [L.] tibial.

tibiofemoral (tib″e-o-fem′o-ral) pertaining to the tibia and femur.

tibiofibular (-fib′u-ler) pertaining to the tibia and fibula.

tibiotarsal (-tar′s'l) pertaining to the tibia and tarsus.

tic (tik) an involuntary, compulsive, repetitive, stereotyped movement, usually involving the face and shoulders. **t. douloureux** (doo-loo-roo′), trigeminal neuralgia. **facial t.,** spasm of the facial muscles.

ticarcillin (ti″kar-sil′in) a semisynthetic penicillin, $C_{15}H_{16}N_2O_6S_2$, bactericidal against both gram-negative and gram-positive organisms.

tick (tik) a bloodsucking acarid parasite of the superfamily Ixodoidea, divided into *soft-bodied ticks* and *hard-bodied ticks.* Some ticks are vectors and reservoirs of disease-causing agents.

t.i.d. [L.] *ter in di′e* (three times a day).

tide (tīd) a physiological variation or increase of a certain constituent in body fluids. **acid t.,** temporary increase in the acidity of the urine which sometimes follows fasting. **alkaline t.,** temporary increase in the alkalinity of the urine during gastric digestion. **fat t.,** the increase of fat in the lymph and blood after a meal.

Tigan (ti′gan) trademark for a preparation of trimethobenzamide.

timbre (tim′ber, tam′br) [Fr.] musical quality of a tone or sound.

time (tīm) a measure of duration. **bleeding t.,** the duration of bleeding after controlled, standardized puncture of the earlobe or forearm; a relatively inconsistent measure of capillary and platelet function. **circulation t.,** the time required for blood to flow between two given points. **clotting t., coagulation t.,** the time required for blood to clot in a glass tube. **inertia t.,** the time required to overcome the inertia of a muscle after reception of a stimulus from a nerve. **prothrombin t.,** the time required for clot formation after thromboplastin (brain extract) and calcium have been added to blood plasma. **reaction t.,** the time elapsing between the application of a stimulus and the resulting reaction.

timolol (ti′mo-lol) a beta-adrenergic blocking agent, $C_{13}H_{24}N_4O_3$, with antihypertensive and antiarrhythmic properties; timolol maleate is used topically to lower intraocular pressure in glaucoma.

tin (tin) chemical element (*see table*), at. no. 50, symbol Sn.

tinct. tincture.

tinctorial (tingk-tor′e-al) pertaining to dyeing or staining.

tincture (tingk′chur) an alcoholic or hydroalcoholic solution prepared from an animal or vegetable drug or a chemical substance. **benzoin t., compound,** a mixture of benzoin, aloes, storax, and tolu balsam in alcohol; used as a topical protectant. **iodine t.,** a mixture of iodine and sodium iodide in a menstruum of alcohol and water; an anti-infective for the skin. **sweet orange peel t.,** a flavoring agent prepared by maceration of the outer rind of natural colored fresh ripe fruit of *Citrus sinensis* in alcohol.

tinea (tin′e-ah) ringworm; a name applied to many different superficial fungal infections of the skin, the specific type (depending on appearance, etiology, or site) usually designated by a modifying term. **t. bar′bae,** infection of the bearded parts of the face and neck caused by species of *Trichophyton.* **t. cap′itis,** fungal infection of the scalp, due to species of *Trichophyton* and *Microsporum.* **t. circina′ta,** tinea corporis. **t. cor′poris,** fungal infection of glabrous skin, usually due to species of *Trichophyton* or *Microsporum.* **t. cru′ris,** fungal infection involving the groin, perineum, and perineal regions and sometimes spreading to the contiguous areas; it most often accompanies tinea pedis, so that the causative organism is the same for both infections. **t. facia′le, t. facie′i,** tinea of the face, other than the bearded area. **t. imbrica′ta,** a form of tinea corporis seen in the tropics, due to *Trichophyton concentricum;* the early lesion is annular with a circle of scales at the periphery. **t. pe′dis,** athlete's foot; a chronic superficial fungal infection of the skin of the foot, especially between the toes and on the soles, due to species of *Trichophyton* or to *Epidermophyton floccosum.* **t. profun′da,** trichophytic granuloma. **t. syco′sis,** an inflammatory, deep type of tinea barbae, due to *Trichophyton violaceum* or *T. rubrum.* **t. unguium,** tinea involving the nails; the surface and lateral and distal edges are involved at first, followed by establishment of infection beneath the nail plate. **t. versico′lor,** a chronic, noninflammatory, usually asymptomatic disorder due to *Pityrosporon orbiculare,* marked only by multiple macular patches.

tingible (tin′jĭ-b'l) stainable.

tinnitus (tĭ-ni′tus) a noise in the ears, which may at times be heard by others than the patient. **t. au′rium,** a subjective sensation of noise in the ears.

tissue (tish′u) an aggregation of similarly specialized cells which together perform certain special functions. **adenoid t.,** lymphoid t. **adipose t.,** connective tissue made of fat cells in meshwork of areolar tissue. **adipose t., brown,** a thermogenic type of adipose tissue containing a dark pigment, and arising during embryonic life in certain special areas in many mammals, including man; it is prominent in the newborn. **adipose t., white, adipose t., yellow,** the adipose tissue comprising the bulk of the body fat.

areolar t., connective tissue made up largely of interlacing fibers. **bony t.**, bone. **bursa-equivalent t.**, a hypothesized tissue in nonavian vertebrates equivalent to the bursa of Fabricius in birds; the site of B-lymphocyte maturation. It now appears that B-cell maturation occurs primarily in the bone marrow. **cancellous t.**, the spongy tissue of bone. **cartilaginous t.**, the substance of cartilage. **chromaffin t.**, a tissue composed largely of chromaffin cells, well supplied with nerves and vessels; it occurs in the adrenal medulla and also forms the paraganglia of the body. **cicatricial t.**, the dense fibrous tissue forming a cicatrix, derived directly from granulation tissue. **connective t.**, the stromatous or nonparenchymatous tissues of the body; that which binds together and is the ground substance of the various parts and organs of the body. **elastic t.**, elastic t., **yellow,** connective tissue made up of yellow elastic fibers, frequently massed into sheets. **endothelial t.**, endothelium. **epithelial t.**, epithelium. **erectile t.**, spongy tissue that expands and becomes hard when filled with blood. **extracellular t.**, the total of tissues and body fluids outside the cells. **fatty t.**, adipose t. **fibrous t.**, the common connective tissue of the body, composed of yellow or white parallel fibers. **gelatinous t.**, mucous t. **glandular t.**, an aggregation of epithelial cells that elaborate secretions. **granulation t.**, the newly formed vascular tissue normally produced in healing of wounds of soft tissue, ultimately forming the cicatrix. **gut-associated lymphoid t. (GALT)**, lymphoid tissue associated with the gut, including the tonsils, Peyer's patches, lamina propria of the gastrointestinal tract, and appendix. **indifferent t.**, undifferentiated embryonic tissue. **interstitial t.**, connective tissue between the cellular elements of a structure. **lymph- adenoid t.**, tissue resembling that of lymph nodes, found in the spleen, bone marrow, tonsils, and other organs. **lymphoid t.**, a lattice work of reticular tissue, the interspaces of which contain lymphocytes. **mesenchymal t.**, mesenchyma. **mucous t.**, a jelly-like connective tissue, as occurs in the umbilical cord. **muscular t.**, the substance of muscle. **myeloid t.**, red bone marrow. **nerve t., nervous t.**, the substance of which the nerve centers are composed. **osseous t.**, the specialized tissue forming the bones. **reticular t., reticulated t.**, connective tissue consisting of reticular cells and fibers. **scar t.**, cicatricial t. **sclerous t's,** the cartilaginous, fibrous, and osseous tissue. **skeletal t.**, the bony, ligamentous, fibrous, and cartilaginous tissue forming the skeleton and its attachments. **subcutaneous t.**, the layer of loose connective tissue directly under the skin.

titanium (ti-ta′ne-um) chemical element (*see table*), at. no. 22, symbol Ti; used for fixation of fractures. **t. dioxide**, TiO_2, used as a topical protectant in ointment or lotion.

titer (ti′ter) the quantity of a substance required to react with or to correspond to a given amount of another substance. **agglutination t.**, the highest dilution of a serum which causes clumping of microorganisms or other particulate antigens.

titration (ti-tra′shun) determination of a given component in solution by addition of a liquid reagent of known strength until the endpoint is reached when the component has been consumed by reaction with the reagent.

titubation (tit″u-ba′shun) the act of staggering or reeling; a staggering gait with shaking of the trunk and head, commonly seen in cerebellar disease.

Tl chemical symbol, *thallium.*

TLC total lung capacity.

Tm chemical symbol, *thulium.*

TNM see under *staging.*

TNT trinitrotoluene.

tobacco (tah-bak′o) the dried prepared leaves of the plant *Nicotiana tabacum,* the source of various alkaloids, the principal one being nicotine.

tobramycin (to″brah-mi′sin) a purified fraction of an aminoglycoside antibiotic produced by *Streptomyces tenebrarius,* $C_{18}H_{37}N_5O_9$, bactericidal against many gram-negative and some gram-positive organisms; also used as the sulfate salt.

toc(o)- word element [Gr.], *childbirth; labor.* See also words beginning *tok(o)-.*

tocology (to-kol′ah-je) obstetrics.

tocometer (to-kom′ĕ-ter) tokodynamometer.

tocopherol (to-kof′er-ol) an alcohol having the properties of vitamin E; it is isolated from wheat germ oil or produced synthetically. **alpha t.**, vitamin E.

toe (to) a digit of the foot. **hammer t.**, deformity of a toe, most often the second, in which the proximal phalanx is extended and the second and distal phalanges are flexed, giving a clawlike appearance. **Morton's t.**, a form of metatarsalgia due to compression on a branch of the plantar nerve by the metatarsal heads; chronic compression may lead to formation of a neuroma. **pigeon t.**, permanent toeing-in position of the feet. **tennis t.**, painful great toe associated with subungual hematoma; so called because it develops usually after vigorous tennis playing. **webbed t's,** toes abnormally joined by strands of tissue at their base.

toenail (to′nāl) the nail on any of the digits of the foot. **ingrown t.**, aberrant growth of a toenail, with one (usually the outer) margin growing deeply into the nail groove and surrounding tissues.

Tofranil (to-fra′nil) trademark for preparations of imipramine.

togavirus (to″gah-vi′rus) a subgroup of arboviruses, including mosquito-borne and tickborne viruses that cause hemorrhagic fever; they are RNA viruses with envelopes (or "togas").

toilet (toi′lit) the cleansing and dressing of a wound.

tok(o)- word element [Gr.], *childbirth; labor.* See also words beginning *toc(o)-.*

tokodynagraph (to″ko-di′nah-graf) a tracing obtained by the tokodynamometer.

tokodynamometer (-di″nah-mom′ĕ-ter) an instrument for measuring and recording the expulsive force of uterine contractions.

tolazamide (tol-az'ah-mīd) a hypoglycemic, $C_{14}H_{21}N_3O_3S$.

tolazoline (tol-az'o-lēn) a smooth muscle relaxant and peripheral vasodilator, $C_{10}H_{12}N_2$, used as the hydrochloride salt.

tolbutamide (tol-bu'tah-mīd) an oral hypoglycemic agent, $C_{12}H_{18}N_2O_3S$, used also as the monosodium salt.

Tolectin (tol'ek-tin) trademark for a preparation of tolmetin sodium.

tolerance (tol'er-ans) the ability to endure without effect or injury. **tol'erant,** adj. **drug t.,** decrease in susceptibility to the effects of a drug due to its continued administration. **immunologic t.,** specific nonreactivity of lymphoid tissues to a particular antigen capable under other conditions of inducing immunity.

tolerogen (tol'er-o-jen) an antigen that induces a state of specific immunological unresponsiveness to subsequent challenging doses of the antigen.

Tolinase (tōl'in-ās) trademark for a preparation of tolazamide.

tolmetin (tol'met-in) an anti-inflammatory, analgesic, and antipyretic $C_{15}H_{15}NO_3$, used in the treatment of certain cases of rheumatoid arthritis.

tolnaftate (tol-naf'tāt) a topical antifungal, $C_{19}H_{17}NOS$, used in the treatment of tinea.

toluene (tol'u-ēn) the hydrocarbon C_7H_8.

-tome word element [Gr.], *an instrument for cutting; a segment.*

tom(o)- word element [Gr.], *a section; a cutting.*

tomogram (to'mo-gram) an image of a tissue section produced by tomography.

tomograph (-graf) an apparatus for moving an x-ray source in one direction as the film is moved in the opposite direction, thus showing in detail a predetermined plane of tissue while blurring or eliminating detail in other planes.

tomography (to-mog'rah-fe) any imaging method that produces images of cross-sections of the body. **tomograph'ic,** adj. **computed t. (CT), computerized axial t. (CAT),** an imaging method in which a cross-sectional image of the structures in a body plane is reconstructed by a computer program from the x-ray absorption of beams projected through the body in the image plane. **positron emission t. (PET),** a nuclear medicine imaging method similar to computed tomography, except that the image shows the tissue concentration of a positron-emitting radioisotope. **ultrasonic t.,** the ultrasonographic visualization of a cross-section of a predetermined plane of the body; see *B-mode ultrasonography.*

-tomy word element [Gr.], *incision; cutting.*

tone (tōn) 1. normal degree of vigor and tension; in muscle, the resistance to passive elongation or stretch. 2. a healthy state of a part; tonus. 3. a particular quality of sound or of voice.

tongue (tung) the movable muscular organ on the floor of the mouth; it is the chief organ of taste, and aids in mastication, swallowing, and speech. **bifid t.,** one with an anterior length-

wise cleft. **black t.,** the presence of a brown furlike patch on the dorsum of the tongue, composed of hypertrophied filiform papillae with microorganisms and some pigment. **cleft t.,** bifid t. **coated t.,** one covered with a whitish or yellowish layer consisting of desquamated epithelium, debris, bacteria, fungi, etc. **fissured t., furrowed t.,** a tongue with numerous furrows or grooves on the dorsal surface, often radiating from a groove on the midline. **geographic t.,** a tongue with denuded patches surrounded by thickened epithelium. **hairy t.,** one with the papillae elongated and hairlike. **raspberry t.,** a red, uncoated tongue, with elevated papillae, as seen a few days after the onset of the rash in scarlet fever. **scrotal t.,** fissured t. **strawberry t., red,** raspberry tongue. **strawberry t., white,** the white-coated tongue with prominent red papillae characteristic of the early stage of scarlet fever.

tongue-tie (tung'ti) abnormal shortness of the frenum of the tongue, interfering with its motion; ankyloglossia.

tonic (ton'ik) 1. producing and restoring normal tone. 2. characterized by continuous tension.

tonicity (to-nis'ĭ-te) the state of tissue tone or tension; in body fluid physiology, the effective osmotic pressure equivalent.

ton(o)- word element [Gr.], *tone; tension.*

tonoclonic (ton″o-klon'ik) both tonic and clonic; said of muscular spasms.

tonofibril (ton'o-fi″bril) a bundle of fine filaments (tonofilaments) in certain cells, especially epithelial cells, the individual strands of which traverse the cytoplasm in all directions and extend into the cell processes to converge and insert on the desmosomes.

tonography (to-nog'rah-fe) recording of changes in intraocular pressure due to sustained pressure on the eyeball. **carotid compression t.,** a test for occlusion of the carotid artery by measuring ocular pressure and pulse before, during, and after the proximal portion of the carotid artery is compressed by the fingers.

tonometry (to-nom'ĕ-tre) measurement of tension or pressure, e.g., intraocular pressure. **digital t.,** estimation of the degree of intraocular pressure by pressure exerted on the eyeball by the examiner's finger.

tonoplast (ton'o-plast) the limiting membrane of an intracellular vacuole.

tonsil (ton'sil) a small, rounded mass of tissue, especially of lymphoid tissue; generally used alone to designate the palatine tonsil. **ton'sillar,** adj. **t. of cerebellum,** a rounded mass of tissue forming part of the caudal lobe of the hemisphere of the cerebellum. **faucial t.,** palatine t. **lingual t.,** an aggregation of lymph follicles at the root of the tongue. **Luschka's t.,** pharyngeal t. **palatine t.,** a small mass of lymphoid tissue between the pillars of the fauces on either side of the pharynx. **pharyngeal t.,** the diffuse lymphoid tissue and follicles in the roof and posterior wall of the nasopharynx.

tonsilla (ton-sil'ah), pl. *tonsil'lae* [L.] tonsil.

tonsillectomy (ton"sĭ-lek'tah-me) excision of a tonsil.

tonsillitis (ton"sĭ-li'tis) inflammation of the tonsils, especially the palatine tonsils. **follicular t.,** tonsillitis especially affecting the crypts. **parenchymatous t., acute,** that affecting the whole substance of the tonsil.

tonsillolith (ton-sil'o-lith) a calculus in a tonsil.

tonsillotomy (ton"sĭ-lot'ah-me) incision of a tonsil.

tonus (to'nus) tone or tonicity; the slight, continuous contraction of a muscle, which in skeletal muscles aids in the maintenance of posture and in the return of blood to the heart.

tooth (tooth), pl. *teeth.* One of the hard, calcified structures set in the alveolar processes of the jaws for the biting and mastication of food. **accessional teeth,** those having no deciduous predecessors: the permanent molars. **artificial t.,** one made of porcelain or other synthetic compound in imitation of a natural tooth. **auditory teeth,** toothlike projections in the cochlea. **bicuspid t.,** one of the premolar teeth. **canine t., cuspid t.,** the third tooth on either side from the midline in each jaw. **deciduous teeth,** the 20 teeth of the first dentition in man which are supplanted by the permanent teeth. **eye t.,** a canine tooth of the upper jaw. **Hutchinson teeth,** notched, narrow-edged permanent incisors; regarded as a sign of congenital syphilis, but not always of such origin. **impacted t.,** one prevented from erupting by a physical barrier. **incisor teeth,** the four front teeth, two on each side of the midline, in each jaw. **milk teeth,** deciduous teeth. **molar teeth,** the three (in the permanent dentition, two in the deciduous) posterior teeth on either side in each jaw; see Plate XV. **peg t.,** a tooth whose sides converge or taper together incisally. **permanent teeth,** the 32 teeth of the second dentition. **premolar teeth,** the two permanent teeth on either side in each jaw, between the canine and the molar teeth. **primary teeth,** deciduous teeth. **stomach t.,** a canine tooth of the lower jaw. **succedaneous teeth, succesional teeth,** the permanent teeth that have deciduous predecessors. **temporary teeth,** deciduous teeth. **wisdom teeth,** the last molar tooth on either side in each jaw.

top(o)- word element [Gr.], *particular place* or *area.*

topagnosia (top"ag-no'ze-ah) 1. loss of touch localization. 2. loss of ability to recognize familiar surroundings.

topalgia (tah-pal'je-ah) fixed or localized pain.

topectomy (tah-pek'tah-me) ablation of a small and specific area of the frontal cortex in the treatment of mental illness.

topesthesia (top"es-the'ze-ah) ability to recognize the location of a tactile stimulus.

tophaceous (tah-fa'shus) gritty or sandy; pertaining to tophi.

tophus (to'fus), pl. *to'phi.* a deposit of sodium urate in the tissues about the joints in gout, producing a chronic, foreign-body inflammatory response.

topical (top'ĭ-k'l) pertaining to a particular area,

as a topical anti-infective applied to a certain area of the skin and affecting only the area to which it is applied.

topoanesthesia (top"o-an"es-the'ze-ah) inability to recognize the location of tactile stimuli.

topography (tah-pog'rah-fe) the description of an anatomic region or a special part.

torpor (tor'per) [L.] sluggishness. **tor'pid,** adj. **t. ret'inae,** sluggish response of the retina to the stimulus of light.

torque (tork) a rotary force; in dentistry, the rotation of a tooth on its long axis, especially the movement of the apical portions of the teeth by use of orthodontic appliances.

torsion (tor'shun) 1. act of twisting; state of being twisted; in dentistry, the condition of a tooth when it is turned on its long axis. 2. in ophthalmology, any rotation of the vertical corneal meridians. **tor'sive,** adj.

torsiversion (tor"sĭ-ver'zhun) turning of a tooth on its long axis out of normal position.

torso (tor'so) the body, exclusive of the head and limbs.

torticollis (tor"tĭ-kol'is) wryneck; a contracted state of the cervical muscles, with torsion of the neck.

tortipelvis (-pel'vis) dystonia musculorum deformans.

torulus (tor'u-lus), pl. *tor'uli* [L.] a small elevation; a papilla. **t. tac'tilis,** a tactile elevation in the skin of the palms and soles.

torus (to'rus), pl. *to'ri* [L.] a swelling or bulging projection.

totipotential (to"tĭ-po-ten'shul) exhibiting totipotency; characterized by the ability to develop in any direction; said of cells that can give rise to cells of all types. **totip'otent,** adj.

touch (tuch) 1. the sense by which contact of an object with the skin is recognized. 2. palpation with the finger.

tourniquet (toor'nĭ-kit) a band to be drawn tightly around a limb for the temporary arrest of circulation in the distal area.

tox(o)- word element [Gr.; L.], *toxin; poison.*

Toxascaris (tok-sas'kah-ris) a genus of nematode parasites, including *T. leoni'na,* found in lions, tigers, and other large Felidae, as well as dogs and cats.

toxemia (tok-se'me-ah) 1. the condition resulting from the spread of bacterial products (toxins) by the bloodstream. 2. a condition resulting from metabolic disturbances, e.g., toxemia of pregnancy. **toxe'mic,** adj. **alimentary t.,** toxemia due to absorption from the alimentary canal of chemical poisons generated therein; a form of autointoxication. **t. of pregnancy,** a group of pathologic conditions, essentially metabolic disturbances, occurring in pregnant women, manifested by preeclampsia and fully developed eclampsia.

toxic (tok'sik) poisonous; pertaining to poisoning manifesting the symptoms of severe infection.

toxic(o)- word element [Gr.], *poison; poisonous.*

toxicant (tok'sĭ-kant) 1. poisonous. 2. a poison.

toxicity (tok-sis'ĭ-te) the quality of being poisonous, especially the degree of virulence of a toxic microbe or of a poison. **O₂ t., oxygen t.,** serious, sometimes irreversible, damage to the pulmonary capillary endothelium associated with breathing high partial pressures of oxygen for prolonged periods.

toxicogenic (-jen′ik) producing or elaborating toxins.

toxicology (tok″sĭ-kol′ah-je) the science or study of poisons. **toxicolog′ic,** adj.

toxicopathy (tok″sĭ-kop′ah-the) toxicosis. **toxicopath′ic,** adj.

toxicopexis (tok″sĭ-ko-pek′sis) the fixation or neutralization of a poison in the body. **toxicopec′tic, toxicopex′ic,** adj.

toxicophobia (-fo′be-ah) irrational fear of being poisoned.

toxicosis (tok″sĭ-ko′sis) any diseased condition due to poisoning.

toxiferous (tok-sif′er-us) conveying or producing a poison.

toxigenicity (-jĕ-nis′ĭ-te) the property of producing toxins.

toxin (tok′sin) a poison, especially a protein or conjugated protein produced by some higher plants, certain animals, and pathogenic bacteria, that is highly poisonous for other living organisms. **bacterial t's,** toxins produced by bacteria, including exotoxins, endotoxins, and toxic enzymes. **botulinus t.,** an exotoxin produced by *Clostridium botulinum* that produces paralysis by blocking the release of acetylcholine in the central nervous system; there are seven immunologically distinct types (A–G). **clostridial t.,** one produced by species of *Clostridium,* including those causing botulinus, gas gangrene, and tetanus. **Dick t.,** erythrogenic t. **diphtheria t.,** a protein exotoxin produced by *Corynebacterium diphtheriae* that is primarily responsible for the pathogenesis of diphtheritic infection; it is an enzyme that activates transferase II of the mammalian protein synthesizing system. **diphtheria t. for Schick test,** a sterile solution of the diluted, standardized toxic products of *Corynebacterium diphtheriae;* used as a dermal reactivity indicator. **erythrogenic t.,** an exotoxin produced by many strains of *Streptococcus pyogenes,* which produces an erythematous reaction on intradermal inoculation in man, and is responsible for the scarlatiniform rash of scarlet fever. **extracellular t.,** exotoxin. **gas gangrene t.,** an exotoxin produced by *Clostridium perfringens* that causes gas gangrene; at least 10 types have been identified. **intracellular t.,** endotoxin. **tetanus t.,** the potent exotoxin produced by *Clostridium tetani,* consisting of two components, one a neurotoxin (*tetanospasmin*) and the other a hemolysin (*tetanolysin*).

toxin-antitoxin (tok″sin-an′tĭ-tok″sin) a nearly neutral mixture of diphtheria toxin with its antitoxin; used for diphtheria immunization.

toxinology (tok″sin-ol′ah-je) the science dealing with the toxins produced by certain higher plants and animals and by pathogenic bacteria.

toxipathy (tok-sip′ah-the) toxicosis.

Toxocara (tok″so-kār′ah) a genus of nematode parasites found in the dog (*T. ca′nis*) and cat (*T.*

ca′ti); both species are sometimes found in man.

toxocariasis (-kah-ri′ah-sis) infection by worms of the genus *Toxocara.*

toxoid (tok′soid) a modified or inactivated exotoxin that has lost toxicity but retains the ability to combine with, or stimulate the production of, antitoxin. **diphtheria t.,** a sterile preparation of formaldehyde-treated toxin of *Corynebacterium diphtheriae,* used as an active immunizing agent. **tetanus t.,** a sterile preparation of formaldehyde-treated toxin of *Clostridium tetani,* used as an active immunizing agent.

toxophilic (tok″so-fil′ik) easily susceptible to poison; having affinity for toxins.

toxophore (tok′so-for) the group of atoms in a toxin molecule which produces the toxic effect. **toxoph′orous,** adj.

Toxoplasma (tok″so-plaz′mah) a genus of sporozoa that are intracellular parasites of many organs and tissues of birds and mammals, including man. *T. gon′dii* is the etiologic agent of toxoplasmosis.

toxoplasmosis (-plaz-mo′sis) an acute or chronic, widespread disease of animals and humans caused by *Toxoplasma gondii* and transmitted by oocysts in the feces of cats. Most human infections are asymptomatic; when symptoms occur, they range from a mild, self-limited disease resembling mononucleosis to a disseminated, fulminating disease that may damage the brain, eyes, muscles, liver, and lungs. Severe manifestations are seen principally in immunocompromised patients and in fetuses infected transplacentally as a result of maternal infection. Chorioretinitis may be associated with all forms, but it is usually a late sequel of congenital disease.

TPN total parenteral nutrition; see *parenteral hyperalimentation.*

trabecula (trah-bek′u-lah), pl. *trabec′ulae* [L.] a little beam; in anatomy, a general term for a supporting or anchoring strand of connective tissue, e.g., a strand extending from a capsule into the substance of the enclosed organ. **trabec′ular,** adj. **trabeculae of bone,** anastomosing bony spicules in cancellous bone which form a meshwork of intercommunicating spaces that are filled with bone marrow.

trabeculate (trah-bek′u-lāt) marked with transverse or radiating bars or trabeculae.

trabeculoplasty (trah-bek″u-lo-plas′te) plastic surgery of a trabecula. **laser t.,** the placing of surface burns in the trabecular network of the eye to lower intraocular pressure in open-angle glaucoma.

tracer (trās′er) a means by which something may be followed, as (*a*) a mechanical device by which the outline or movements of an object can be graphically recorded, or (*b*) a material by which the progress of a compound through the body may be observed. **radioactive t.,** a radioactive isotope replacing a stable chemical element in a compound introduced into the body, enabling its metabolism, distribution, and elimination to be followed.

trachea (tra′ke-ah) windpipe; the cartilaginous and membranous tube descending from the larynx and branching into the left and right main bronchi. **tra′cheal,** adj.

trachealgia (tra″ke-al′je-ah) pain in the trachea.

tracheitis (-i′tis) inflammation of the trachea.

trachel(o)- word element [Gr.], *neck; necklike structure,* especially the uterine cervix.

trachelagra (tra″kah-lag′rah) gout in the neck.

trachelectomy (-lek′tah-me) cervicectomy.

trachelematoma (-lem″ah-to′mah) a hematoma on the sternocleidomastoid muscle.

trachelism, trachelismus (tra′kah-lizm; tra″-kah-liz′mus) spasm of the neck muscles; spasmodic retraction of the head in epilepsy.

trachelitis (tra″kah-li′tis) cervicitis.

trachelocystitis (tra″kah-lo-sis-ti′tis) inflammation of the neck of the bladder.

trachelodynia (-din′e-ah) pain in the neck.

trachelomyitis (-mi-i′tis) inflammation of the muscles of the neck.

trachelopexy (tra′ke-lo-pek″se) fixation of the uterine cervix.

tracheloplasty (-plas″te) plastic repair of the uterine cervix.

trachelorrhaphy (tra″kah-lor′ah-fe) suture of the uterine cervix.

trachelotomy (-lot′ah-me) incision of the uterine cervix.

trache(o)- word element [Gr.], *trachea.*

tracheoaerocele (tra″ke-o-ār′-o-sēl″) a tracheal hernia containing air.

tracheobronchial (-brong′ke-al) pertaining to the trachea and bronchi.

tracheobronchitis (-brong-ki′tis) inflammation of the trachea and bronchi.

tracheobronchoscopy (-brong-kos′kah-pe) inspection of the interior of the trachea and bronchi.

tracheocele (tra′ke-o-sēl″) hernial protrusion of tracheal mucous membrane.

tracheoesophageal (tra″ke-o-e-sof″ah-je′al) pertaining to the trachea and esophagus.

tracheolaryngeal (-lah-rin′je-al) pertaining to the trachea and larynx.

tracheomalacia (-mah-la′she-ah) softening of the tracheal cartilages.

tracheopathy (tra″ke-op′ah-the) disease of the trachea.

tracheopharyngeal (tra″ke-o-fah-rin′je-al) pertaining to the trachea and pharynx.

tracheophony (tra″ke-of′o-ne) sound heard in auscultation over the trachea.

tracheoplasty (tra′ke-o-plas″te) plastic repair of the trachea.

tracheopyosis (tra″ke-o-pi-o′sis) purulent tracheitis.

tracheorrhagia (-ra′je-ah) hemorrhage from the trachea.

tracheoschisis (tra″ke-os′kĭ-sis) fissure of the trachea.

tracheoscopy (-os′kah-pe) inspection of interior of the trachea. **tracheoscop′ic,** adj.

tracheostenosis (tra″ke-o-stĕ-no′sis) constriction of the trachea.

tracheostomy (-os′tah-me) creation of an opening into the trachea through the neck, with the tracheal mucosa being brought into continuity with the skin; also, the opening so created.

tracheotomy (tra″ke-ot′ah-me) incision of the trachea through the skin and muscles of the neck. **inferior t.,** performed below, and **superior t.,** above, the isthmus of the thyroid.

trachoma (trah-ko′mah) a contagious disease of the conjunctiva and cornea, producing photophobia, pain, and lacrimation, caused by a strain of *Chlamydia trachomatis.* Clinically, it progresses from a mild infection with tiny follicles on the eyelid conjunctiva to invasion of the cornea, with scarring and contraction which may result in blindness. **tracho′matous,** adj.

trachyphonia (tra″ke-fo′ne-ah) roughness of the voice.

tract (trakt) a longitudinal assemblage of tissues or organs, especially a bundle of nerve fibers having a common origin, function, and termination, or a number of anatomic structures arranged in series and serving a common function. **alimentary t.,** see under *canal.* **biliary t.,** the organs, ducts, etc., participating in secretion (the liver), storage (the gallbladder), and delivery (hepatic and bile ducts) of bile into the duodenum. **digestive t.,** alimentary canal. **dorsolateral t.,** a group of nerve fibers in the lateral funiculus of the spinal cord dorsal to the posterior column. **extrapyramidal t′s,** see under *system.* **Flechsig's t.,** spinocerebellar t., posterior. **gastrointestinal t.,** the stomach and intestine in continuity. **Gowers' t.,** spinocerebellar t., anterior. **iliotibial t.,** a thickened longitudinal band of fascia lata extending from the tensor muscle downward to the lateral condyle of the tibia. **intestinal t.,** the small and large intestines in continuity. **optic t.,** the nerve tract proceeding backward from the optic chiasm, around the cerebral peduncle, and dividing into a lateral and medial root, which end in the superior colliculus and lateral geniculate body, respectively. **pyramidal t′s,** collections of nerve fibers arising in the brain and passing down through the spinal cord to motor cells in the anterior horns. **respiratory t.,** the organs which allow entrance of air into the lungs and exchange of gases with the blood, from air passages in the nose to the pulmonary alveoli. See Plate VI. **spinocerebellar t., dorsal,** a group of nerve fibers in the lateral funiculus of the spinal cord, arising mostly from the nucleus thoracicus, and ascending to the cerebellum through the inferior cerebellar peduncle. **spinocerebellar t., ventral,** a group of nerve fibers in the lateral funiculus of the spinal cord, arising mostly in the gray matter of the opposite side, and ascending to the cerebellum through the superior cerebellar peduncle. **urinary t.,** the organs concerned with the elaboration and excretion of urine: kidneys, ureters, bladder, and urethra. **uveal t.,** the vascular tunic of the eye, comprising the choroid, ciliary body, and iris.

traction (trak′shun) the act of drawing or pulling. **axis t.,** traction along an axis, as of the pelvis in obstetrics. **elastic t.,** traction by an elastic force or by means of an elastic appliance.

skeletal t., traction applied directly upon long bones by means of pins, wires, etc., **skin t.,** traction on a body part maintained by an apparatus affixed by dressings to the body surface.

tractotomy (trak-tot′ah-me) transection of a nerve tract in the central nervous system.

tractus (trak′tus), pl. *trac′tus* [L.] tract.

tragus (tra′gus), pl. *tra′gi* [L.] the cartilaginous projection anterior to the external opening of the ear; used also in the plural to designate hairs growing on the pinna of the external ear, especially on the tragus. **tra′gal,** adj.

trainable (tra′nah-b′l) capable of being trained; the term is used with special reference to persons with moderate mental retardation (I.Q. approximately 36–51) who are capable of achieving self-care, social adjustment at home, and economic usefulness under close supervision.

training (trān′ing) a system of instruction or teaching; preparation by instruction and practice. **assertiveness t.,** a form of behavior therapy in which individuals are taught appropriate interpersonal responses, involving expression of their feelings, both negative and positive.

trait (trāt) 1. any genetically determined characteristic; also, the condition prevailing in the heterozygous state of a recessive disorder, as the sickle cell trait. 2. a distinctive behavior pattern. **sickle cell t.,** the condition, usually asymptomatic, due to heterozygosity for hemoglobin S.

trance (trans) a sleeplike state of altered consciousness marked by heightened focal awareness and reduced peripheral awareness.

tranquilizer (tran′kwĭ-li″zer) a drug with a calming, soothing effect. **major t.,** antipsychotic agent; see *antipsychotic.* **minor t.,** antianxiety agent; see under *antianxiety.*

trans (tranz) 1. in organic chemistry, having certain atoms or radicals on opposite sides of a nonrotatable parent structure. 2. in genetics, having one of the two mutant genes on each homologous chromosome.

trans- word element [L.], *through; across; beyond.*

transabdominal (trans″ab-dom′ĭ-nal) across the abdominal wall or through the abdominal cavity.

transacetylation (trans-as″ĕ-til-a′shun) a chemical reaction involving the transfer of the acetyl radical.

transacylase (-as′ĭ-lās) an enzyme that catalyzes transacylation.

transacylation (-as″ĭ-la′shun) a chemical reaction involving the transfer of an acyl radical.

transaminase (-am′ĭ-nās) aminotransferase.

transamination (-am″ĭ-na′shun) the reversible exchange of amino groups between different amino acids.

transaortic (trans″a-or′tik) performed through the aorta.

transaudient (trans-aw′de-ent) penetrable by sound waves.

transaxial (-ak′se-al) directed at right angles to the long axis of the body or a part.

transbasal (-ba′s′l) through the base, as a surgical approach through the base of the skull.

transcalvarial (trans″kal-vār′e-al) through or across the calvaria.

transcatheter (trans-kath′ĕ-ter) performed through the lumen of a catheter.

transcobalamin (trans″ko-bal′ah-min) either of two plasma proteins (transcobalamin I and II) that bind and transport cobalamins (vitamin B_{12}).

transcortical (trans-kor′tĭ-k′l) connecting two parts of the cerebral cortex.

transcortin (-kor′tin) an α-globulin that binds and transports biologically active, unconjugated cortisol in plasma.

transcriptase (-krip′tās) RNA polymerase; an enzyme that catalyzes the synthesis (polymerization) of RNA from ribonucleoside triphosphates, with DNA serving as a template. **reverse t.,** RNA-directed DNA polymerase; an enzyme of RNA viruses that catalyzes the transcription of RNA to DNA, which is then incorporated into the genome of the host cell.

transcription (-krip′shun) the synthesis of RNA using a DNA template catalyzed by RNA polymerase; the base sequences of the RNA and DNA are complementary.

transducer (-doo′ser) a device that translates one form of energy to another, e.g., the pressure, temperature, or pulse to an electrical signal. **neuroendocrine t.,** a neuron, such as a neurohypophyseal neuron, that on stimulation secretes a hormone, thereby translating neural information into hormonal information.

transduction (-duk′shun) the transfer of a genetic fragment from one bacterium to another by bacteriophage.

transdural (-dōōr′al) through or across the dura mater.

transection (tran-sek′shun) a cross section; division by cutting transversely.

transepithelial (trans-ep″ĭ-thēl′e-al) occurring through or across an epithelium.

transferase (trans′fer-ās) a class of enzymes that transfer a chemical group from one compound to another.

transference (trans-fer′ens) 1. the passage of a symptom or disorder from one part of the body to another. 2. in psychotherapy, the unconscious tendency to assign to others in one's present environment feelings and attitudes associated with significance in one's early life, especially the patient's transfer to the therapist of feelings and attitudes associated with a parent.

transferrin (-fer′in) a serum globulin that binds and transports iron.

transfixion (-fik′shun) a cutting through from within outward, as in amputation.

transformation (-for-ma′shun) change of form or structure; conversion from one form to another. In oncology, the change that a normal cell undergoes as it becomes malignant. **bacterial t.,** the exchange of genetic material between strains of bacteria by the transfer of a fragment of naked DNA from a donor cell to a recipient cell, followed by recombination in the recipient chromosome.

transfusion (trans-fu'zhun) the introduction of whole blood or blood components directly into the blood stream. **direct t.,** immediate t. **exchange t.,** repetitive withdrawal of small amounts of blood and replacement with donor blood, until a large proportion of the original volume has been replaced. **immediate t.,** transfer of blood directly from a vessel of the donor to a vessel of the recipient. **indirect t., mediate t.,** introduction of blood which has been stored in a suitable container after withdrawal from the donor. **placental t.,** return to an infant after birth, through the intact umbilical cord, of the blood contained in the placenta. **replacement t., substitution t.,** exchange t.

transglutaminase (trans"gloo-tam'in-ās) the activated form of protransglutaminase, which forms stabilizing covalent bonds within fibrin strands.

transiliac (trans-il'e-ak) across the two ilia.

transillumination (trans"ĭ-lu"mĭ-na'shun) the passage of strong light through a body structure, to permit inspection by an observer on the opposite side.

translation (trans-la'shun) in genetics, the process by which polypeptide chains are synthesized, the sequence of amino acids being determined by the sequence of bases in a messenger RNA, which in turn is determined by the sequence of bases in the DNA of the gene from which it was transcribed.

translocation (trans"lo-ka'shun) the attachment of a fragment of one chromosome to a nonhomologous chromosome. **reciprocal t.,** the complete exchange of fragments between two broken chromosomes, one part of one uniting with part of the other, with no fragments left over. **robertsonian t.,** translocation involving two acrocentric chromosomes, which fuse at the centromere region and lose their short arms.

transmethylation (trans"meth-ĭ-la'shun) the transfer of a methyl group (CH_3—) from the molecules of one compound to those of another.

transmission (trans-mish'un) the transfer, as of a disease, from one person to another.

transmural (-mu'ral) through the wall of an organ; extending through or affecting the entire thickness of the wall of an organ or cavity.

transmutation (trans"mu-ta'shun) 1. evolutionary change of one species into another. 2. the change of one chemical element into another.

transphosphorylation (-fos"for-ĭ-la'shun) the exchange of phosphate groups between organic phosphates, without their going through the stage of inorganic phosphates.

transpiration (tran"spĭ-ra'shun) discharge of air, vapor, or sweat through the skin.

transplacental (-plah-sen'tal) through the placenta.

transplant 1. (trans'plant) tissue used in grafting or transplanting. 2. (trans-plant') to transfer tissue from one part to another.

transport (trans'port) movement of materials in biological systems, particularly into and out of cells and across epithelial layers. **active t.,** movement of materials in biological systems resulting directly from expenditure of metabolic energy. **bulk t.,** the uptake by or extrusion from a cell of fluid or particles, accomplished by invagination and vacuole formation (uptake) or by evagination (extrusion); it includes endocytosis, phagocytosis, pinocytosis, and exocytosis.

transposition (trans"po-zish'un) 1. displacement of a viscus to the opposite side. 2. the operation of carrying a tissue flap from one situation to another without severing its connection entirely until it is united at its new location. 3. the exchange of position of two atoms within a molecule. **t. of great vessels,** a congenital cardiovascular malformation in which the position of the chief blood vessels of the heart is reversed. Life then depends on a crossflow of blood between the right and left sides of the heart, as through a ventricular septal defect.

transposon (trans-po'zon) a discrete DNA sequence that transposes flocks of genetic material back and forth within a bacterial cell or from the chromosome to plastids or bacteriophages, by which the material may be transferred to another cell.

transpubic (trans-pu'bik) performed through the pubic bone after removal of a segment of the bone.

transsegmental (trans"seg-men'tal) extending across segments.

transseptal (trans-sep'tal) extending or performed through or across a septum.

transsexualism (-sek"shoo-al-izm") a disturbance of gender identity in which the affected person has an overwhelming desire to change anatomic sex, stemming from the fixed conviction that he or she is a member of the opposite sex; such persons often seek hormonal and surgical treatment to bring their anatomy into conformity with their belief.

transthalamic (trans"thah-lam'ik) across the thalamus.

transthoracic (-thah-ras'ik) through the thoracic cavity or across the chest wall.

transtympanic (-tim-pan'ik) across the tympanic membrane or cavity.

transudate (tran'su-dāt) a fluid substance that has passed through a membrane or has been extruded from a tissue; in contrast to an exudate, it is of high fluidity and has a low content of protein, cells, or solid materials derived from cells.

transurethral (trans"u-re'thral) performed through the urethra.

transvaginal (trans-vaj'ĭ-nal) through the vagina.

transversalis (trans"ver-sa'lis) [L.] transverse.

transverse (trans-vers') extending from side to side; at right angles to the long axis.

transversectomy (trans"ver-sek'tah-me) excision of a transverse process of a vertebra.

transversus (trans-ver'sus) [L.] transverse.

transvesical (-ves'ĭ-kal) through the bladder.

transvestism (-ves'tizm) the practice of wearing articles of clothing of the opposite sex.

Tranxene (tran'zēn) trademark for a preparation of clorazepate dipotassium.

tranylcypromine (tran"il-si'pro-mēn) a monoamine oxidase inhibitor, $(C_9H_{11}N)_2$; the sulfate salt is used as an antidepressant.

trapezium (trah-pe'ze-um) an irregular, four-sided figure; see *Table of Bones*.

trauma (traw'mah) a wound or injury, whether physical or psychic. **traumat'ic**, adj. **birth t.**, an injury to the infant during the process of being born. In some psychiatric theories, the psychic shock produced in an infant by the experience of being born. **psychic t.**, an emotional shock that produces an emotional or mental disorder.

traumat(o)- word element [Gr.], *trauma*.

traumatism (traw'mah-tizm) 1. the physical or psychic state resulting from an injury or wound. 2. a wound.

traumatology (traw"mah-tol'o-je) the branch of surgery dealing with wounds and disability from injuries.

traumatopnea (traw"mah-top-ne'ah) partial asphyxia with collapse caused by traumatic opening of the pleural space.

travail (trah-vāl') childbirth; see *labor*.

tray (tra) a flat-surfaced utensil for the conveyance of various objects or material. **impression t.**, a contoured container to hold the material for making an impression of the teeth and associated structures.

treatment (trēt'ment) management and care of a patient or the combating of disease or disorder. **active t.**, that directed immediately to the cure of the disease or injury. **causal t.**, treatment directed against the cause of a disease. **conservative t.**, that designed to avoid radical medical therapeutic measures or operative procedures. **dietetic t.**, treatment of disease by regulation of the diet. **empiric t.**, treatment by means which experience has proved to be beneficial. **expectant t.**, treatment directed toward relief of untoward symptoms, leaving cure of the disease to natural forces. **palliative t.**, treatment designed to relieve pain and distress with no attempt to cure. **preventive t., prophylactic t.**, that in which the aim is to prevent the occurrence of the disease; prophylaxis. **rational t.**, that based upon knowledge of disease and the action of the remedies given. **shock t.**, electroconvulsive therapy. **specific t.**, treatment particularly adapted to the disease being treated. **supporting t.**, that which is mainly directed to sustaining the strength of the patient. **symptomatic t.**, expectant t.

tree (tre) an anatomic structure with branches resembling a tree. **bronchial t.**, the bronchi and their branching structures. **tracheobronchial t.**, the trachea, bronchi, and their branching structures.

Trematoda (trem"ah-to'dah) a class of Platyhelminthes, including the flukes; they are parasitic in man and animals, infection usually resulting from ingestion of inadequately cooked fish, crustaceans, or vegetation containing their larvae.

trematode (trem'ah-tōd) an individual of the class Trematoda.

trembles (trem'b'lz) poisoning in cattle and sheep feeding on the white snakeroot (*Eupato-*

rium rugosum), in which the animal has muscular tremors and becomes weak and may suddenly stumble and fall; see also *milk sickness* (1).

tremor (trem'er, tre'mer) an involuntary trembling or quivering. **action t.**, rhythmic, oscillatory, involuntary movements of the outstretched upper limb; it may also affect the voice and other parts. **coarse t.**, one in which the vibrations are slow. **fibrillary t.**, rapidly alternating contraction of small bundles of muscle fibers. **fine t.**, one in which the vibrations are rapid. **flapping t.**, asterixis. **Hunt's t.**, the tremor attending every voluntary movement, characteristic of cerebellar lesions. **intention t.**, that occurring when the patient attempts voluntary movement. **rest t.**, tremor occurring in a relaxed and supported limb, as in parkinsonism. **senile t.**, that due to the infirmities of old age. **volitional t.**, trembling of entire body during voluntary effort; seen in multiple sclerosis.

tremulous (trem'u-lus) shaking, trembling, or quivering.

trendscriber (trend'skīb-er) the apparatus used in trendscription.

trendscription (-skrip'shun) a programmed method of continuous electrocardiographic monitoring, wherein the tracing is condensed on a rotating drum recorder and the program permits selective sampling of rhythm data.

trepan (trah-pan') to trephine.

trephination (tref"ĭ-na'shun) the operation of trephining.

trephine (trah-fīn', trah-fēn') 1. a crown saw for removing a circular disk of bone, chiefly from the skull. 2. an instrument for removing a circular area of cornea. 3. to remove with a trephine.

trepidation (trep"ĭ-da'shun) 1. a trembling or oscillatory movement. 2. nervous anxiety and fear. **trep'idant**, adj.

Treponema (trep"o-ne'mah) a genus of bacteria (family Spirochaetaceae), some of them pathogenic and parasitic for man and other animals, including the etiologic agents of pinta (*T. cara'teum*), syphilis (*T. pal'lidum*), and yaws (*T. per'ten'ue*).

treponema (-ne'mah) an organism of the genus *Treponema*. **trepone'mal**, adj.

treponematosis (-ne"mah-to'sis) infection with organisms of the genus *Treponema*.

treponemicidal (-ne"mĭ-si'dal) destroying treponemas.

trepopnea (tre"pop-ne'ah) more comfortable respiration with the patient turned in a definite recumbent position.

treppe (trep'ĕ) [Ger.] the gradual increase in muscular contraction following rapidly repeated stimulation.

tresis (tre'sis) perforation.

tretinoin (tret'ĭ-noin) the *all-trans* stereoisomer of retinoic acid, $C_{20}H_{28}O_2$, used as a topical keratolytic, especially in the treatment of certain cases of acne vulgaris.

TRH thyrotropin releasing hormone.

tri- 610

tri- word element [Gr., L.], *three.*

triacetin (tri-as′ĕ-tin) an antifungal agent, $C_9H_{14}O_6$, used topically.

triad (tri′ad) 1. any trivalent element. 2. a group of three associated entities or objects. **Beck's t.,** rising venous pressure, falling arterial pressure, and small quiet heart; characteristic of cardiac compression. **Hutchinson's t.,** diffuse interstitial keratitis, labyrinthine disease, and Hutchinson's teeth, seen in congenital syphilis. **Saint's t.,** hiatus hernia, colonic diverticula, and cholelithiasis.

triage (tre-ahzh′) [Fr.] the sorting out and classification of casualties of war or other disaster to determine priority of need and proper place of treatment.

trial (tri′al, trīl) a test or experiment. **clinical t.,** an experiment performed on human beings in order to evaluate the comparative efficacy of two or more therapies.

triamcinolone (tri″am-sin′o-lōn) an anti-inflammatory glucocorticoid, $C_{21}H_{27}FO_6$.

triamterene (tri-am′ter-ēn) a diuretic, $C_{12}H_{11}N_7$, which increases sodium and chloride excretion, but not potassium excretion.

triangle (tri′ang-g'l) a three-cornered object, figure, or area, as such an area on the surface of the body capable of fairly precise definition. **carotid t., inferior,** the part of the carotid trigone medial to the omohyoid muscle. **carotid t., superior,** the part of the carotid trigone lateral to the omohyoid muscle. **cephalic t.,** one on the anteroposterior plane of skull, between lines from the occiput to the forehead and to the chin, and from the chin to the forehead. **Codman's t.,** a triangular area visible roentgenographically where the periosteum, elevated by a bone tumor, rejoins the cortex of normal bone. **digastric t.,** submandibular t. **t. of elbow,** in front, the supinator longus on the outside and pronator teres inside, the base toward the humerus. **facial t.,** a triangle whose points are the basion, and alveolar and nasal points. **Farabeuf's t.,** one in the upper part of the neck bound by the internal jugular vein, the facial nerve, and the hypoglossal nerve. **femoral t.,** the area formed superiorly by the inguinal ligament, laterally by the sartorius muscle, and medially by the adductor longus muscle. **frontal t.,** one bounded by the maximum frontal diameter and the lines to the glabella. **Hesselbach's t.,** inguinal t. (1). **iliofemoral t.,** one formed by Nélaton's line, another line through the superior iliac spine, and a third from this to the greater trochanter. **infraclavicular t.,** one formed by the clavicle above, upper border of the pectoralis major on the inside, and the anterior border of the deltoid on the outside. **inguinal t.,** 1. the area on the inferoanterior abdominal wall bounded by the rectus abdominis muscle, the inguinal ligament, and inferior epigastric vessels. 2. femoral t. **Langenbeck's t.,** one whose apex is the anterior superior iliac spine, its base the anatomic neck of the femur, and its external side the external base of the greater trochanter. **Lesser's t.,** one formed by the hypoglossal nerve above, and the two bellies of the digastricus on the two sides. **lumbocostoab-**

dominal t., one between the obliquus externus, the serratus posterior inferior, the erector spinae, and the obliquus internus. **Macewen's t.,** mastoid fossa. **occipital t.,** one having the sternomastoid in front, the trapezius behind, and the omohyoid below. **occipital t., inferior,** one having a line between the two mastoid processes as its base and the inion its apex. **Pawlik's t.,** an area on the anterior vaginal wall corresponding to the trigone of the bladder. **Petit's t.,** the inferolateral margin of the latissimus dorsi and the external oblique muscle of the abdomen. **Scarpa's t.,** femoral t. **subclavian t.,** a deep region of the neck: the triangular area bounded by the clavicle, sternocleidomastoid, and omohyoid. **submandibular t., submaxillary t.,** the triangular region of the neck bounded by the mandible, the stylohyoid muscle and posterior belly of the digastric muscle, and the anterior belly of the digastric muscle. **suboccipital t.,** one between the rectus capitis posterior major and superior and inferior oblique muscles. **suprameatal t.,** mastoid fossa.

triangularis (-ang″gu-la′ris) [L.] triangular.

Triatoma (tri″ah-to′mah) a genus of bugs (order Hemiptera), the cone-nosed bugs, important in medicine as vectors of *Trypanosoma cruzi.*

triatomic (-ah-tom′ik) containing three atoms.

tribe (trīb) a taxonomic category subordinate to a family (or subfamily) and superior to a genus (or subtribe).

tribrachius (tri-bra′ke-us) a fetus with three arms.

TRIC *tr*achoma *i*nclusion *c*onjunctivitis (group of organisms); see *Chlamydia trachomatis.*

tricephalus (tri-sef′ah-lus) a fetus with three heads.

triceps (tri′seps) three-headed, as a triceps muscle. **t. su′rae,** see *Table of Muscles.*

trich(o)- word element [Gr.], *hair.*

trichiasis (trĭ-ki′ah-sis) 1. a condition of ingrowing hairs about an orifice, or ingrowing eyelashes. 2. appearance of hairlike filaments in the urine.

trichilemmoma (trik″ĭ-lem-o′mah) a benign neoplasm of the lower outer root sheath of the hair.

trichina (trĭ-ki′nah), pl. *trichi′nae* [Gr.] an individual organism of the genus *Trichinella.*

Trichinella (trik″ĭ-nel′ah) a genus of nematode parasites, including *T. spira′lis,* the etiologic agent of trichinosis, found in the muscles of the rat, pig, and man.

trichinosis (-no′sis) a disease due to eating inadequately cooked meat infected with *Trichinella spiralis,* attended by diarrhea, nausea, colic, and fever, and later by stiffness, pain, muscle swelling, fever, sweating, eosinophilia, circumorbital edema, and splinter hemorrhages.

trichlormethiazide (tri-klor″mĕ-thi′ah-zīd) a diuretic and antihypertensive, $C_8H_8ClN_3O_4S_2$.

trichloroacetic acid (tri-klor″o-ah-sēt′ik) an extremely caustic acid, CCl_3COOH, used in medicine as a topical caustic for local destruction of lesions and in clinical chemistry as a protein precipitating agent.

trichloroethylene (-klor″o-eth′ĭ-lēn) a clear,

mobile liquid used as an industrial solvent; formerly used as an inhalant anesthetic.

trichoanesthesia (trik″o-an″es-the′ze-ah) loss of hair sensibility.

trichobezoar (-be′zor) hairball; a bezoar composed of hair.

trichoepithelioma (-ep″ĭ-the″le-o′mah) a benign skin tumor originating in the follicles of the lanugo; it may occur as an inherited condition marked by multiple tumors (*t. papillo′sum mul′tiplex*).

trichoesthesia (-es-the′ze-ah) sensibility of the hair to touch.

trichoglossia (-glos′e-ah) hairy tongue.

trichome (tri′kōm) a filamentous or hairlike structure.

trichomegaly (trik″o-meg′ah-le) a congenital syndrome consisting of excessive growth of the eyelashes and brow hair associated with dwarfism, mental retardation, and pigmentary degeneration of the retina.

trichomonacide (-mo′nah-sīd) an agent destructive to trichomonads.

trichomonad (-mo′nad) a parasite of the genus *Trichomonas.*

Trichomonas (-mo′nas) a genus of flagellate protozoa parasitic in various invertebrates and vertebrates, including humans; it includes *T. homi′nis,* a common intestinal parasite of man, *T. te′nax,* a nonpathogenic species found in the human mouth, and *T. vagina′lis,* found in the vagina and the male genital tract, which produces a refractory vaginal discharge and pruritus. **trichomo′nal,** adj.

trichomoniasis (-mo-ni′ah-sis) infection by organisms of the genus *Trichomonas.*

trichomycosis (-mi-ko′sis) any disease of the hair caused by fungi. **t. axilla′ris,** infection of the axillary and sometimes of the pubic hair, due to *Corynebacterium tenuis* (not a fungus), with development of clumps of bacteria on the hairs, appearing as red, yellow, or black nodules.

trichonodosis (-no-do′sis) a condition characterized by apparent or actual knotting of the hair.

trichopathy (trĭ-kop′ah-the) disease of the hair.

trichophytid (trĭ-kof′ĭ-tid) a dermophytid associated with trichophytosis; applied especially to the allergic manifestations of ringworm.

trichophytin (trĭ-kof′ĭ-tin) a filtrate from cultures of *Trichophyton;* used in testing for trichophytosis.

trichophytobezoar (trik″o-fi″to-be′zor) a bezoar composed of animal hair and vegetable fiber.

Trichophyton (trĭ-kof′ĭ-ton) a genus of fungi, species of which attack skin, hair, and nails.

trichophytosis (trik″o-fi-to′sis) infection with fungi of the genus *Trichophyton.* **trichophyt′ic,** adj.

trichoptilosis (-tĭ-lo′sis) splitting of hairs at the end.

trichorrhexis (-rek′sis) the condition in which the hairs break. **t. nodo′sa,** a condition marked by fracture and splitting of the cortex of a hair

into strands, giving the appearance of white nodes at which the hair is easily broken.

trichoschisis (trĭ-kos′kĭ-sis) trichoptilosis.

trichoscopy (trĭ-kos′kah-pe) examination of the hair.

trichosis (trĭ-ko′sis) any disease or abnormal growth of the hair.

Trichosporon (trĭ-kos′po-ron) a genus of fungi that are normal flora of the respiratory and digestive tracts of man and animals, and may infect the hair.

trichosporosis (trik″o-spo-ro′sis) infection with *Trichosporon;* see *piedra.*

trichostasis spinulosa (trĭ-kos′tah-sis spin″u-lo′sah) a condition in which the hair follicles contain a dark, horny plug that contains a bundle of vellus hair.

trichostrongyliasis (trik″o-stron″jĭ-li′ah-sis) infection with *Trichostrongylus.*

Trichostrongylus (-stron′jĭ-lus) a genus of nematodes parasitic in animals and man.

trichotillomania (-til″o-ma′ne-ah) compulsive pulling out of one's hair.

trichotomous (trĭ-kot′ah-mus) divided into three parts.

trichroism (tri′kro-izm) the exhibition of three different colors in three different aspects. **trichro′ic,** adj.

trichromasy (tri-kro′mah-se) 1. the ability to distinguish the three primary colors and mixtures thereof. 2. normal color vision. **anomalous t.,** defective color vision in which the patient has all three cone pigments but one is deficient.

trichromatopsia (tri″kro-mah-top′se-ah) trichromasy.

trichromic (tri-kro′mik) 1. pertaining to or exhibiting three colors. 2. able to distinguish only three of the seven colors of the spectrum.

trichuriasis (trik″u-ri′ah-sis) infection with *Trichuris.*

Trichuris (trik-u′ris) a genus of intestinal nematode parasites, including *T. trichiu′ra* (whipworm), the species principally infecting man.

tricipital (tri-sip′ĭ-tal) 1. three-headed. 2. relating to the triceps muscle.

triclofos (tri′klo-fōs) a hypnotic and sedative, $C_2H_3Cl_3NaO_4P$, used as the sodium salt.

tricornute (tri-kor′nūt) having three horns, cornua, or processes.

tricrotism (tri′krot-izm) quality of having three sphygmographic waves or elevations to one beat of the pulse. **tricrot′ic,** adj.

tricuspid (tri-kus′pid) having three points or cusps, as a valve of the heart.

tricyclic (-sik′lik) containing three fused rings in the molecular structure; see also under *antidepressant.*

tridactylism (-dak′tĭ-lizm) presence of only three digits on the hand or foot.

tridentate (-den′tāt) having three prongs.

tridermic (-der′mik) derived from the ectoderm, endoderm, and mesoderm.

tridihexethyl chloride (tri″di-heks-eth′il) a quaternary ammonium anticholinergic, C_{21}-

$H_{36}ClNO$, used in the treatment of peptic ulcer and irritable bowel syndrome.

trifid (tri′fid) split into three parts.

trifluoperazine (tri″floo-o-per′ah-zēn) a phenothiazine derivative, $C_{21}H_{24}F_3N_3S$; its hydrochloride salt is used as a major tranquilizer.

triflupromazine (-pro′mah-zēn) a phenothiazine derivative, $C_{18}H_{19}F_3N_2S$; its hydrochloride salt is used as a major tranquilizer.

trifurcation (tri″fer-ka′shun) division, or the site of separation, into three branches.

trigeminy (tri-jem′ĭ-ne) the condition of occurring in threes, especially the occurrence of three pulse beats in rapid succession.

triglyceride (-glis′er-īd) a compound consisting of three molecules of fatty acid esterified to glycerol; a neutral fat that is the usual storage form of lipids in animals.

trigonal (tri′go-nal) 1. triangular. 2. pertaining to a trigone.

trigone (tri′gōn) 1. a triangular area. 2. the first three cusps of an upper molar tooth. **t. of bladder,** vesical t. **carotid t.,** the triangular area bounded by the posterior belly of the digastric muscle, the sternocleidomastoid muscle, and the anterior midline of the neck. **olfactory t.,** the triangular area of gray matter between the roots of the olfactory tract. **vesical t.,** the smooth triangular portion of the mucosa at the base of the bladder, bounded behind by the interureteric fold, ending in front in the uvula of the bladder.

trigonectomy (tri″gon-ek′tah-me) excision of the vesical trigone.

trigonitis (tri″go-ni′tis) inflammation or localized hyperemia of the vesical trigone.

trigonocephalus (trig″o-no-sef′ah-lus) an individual exhibiting trigonocephaly.

trigonocephaly (-sef′ah-le) triangular shape of the head due to sharp forward angulation at the midline of the frontal bone. **trigonocephal′ic,** adj.

trigonum (tri-go′num), pl. *trigo′na* [L.] a three-cornered area; triangle or trigone.

trihexyphenidyl (tri-hek″sĭ-fen′ĭ-dil) an anticholinergic, $C_{20}H_{31}NO$, used as the hydrochloride salt in parkinsonism.

triiodothyronine (tri″i-o″do-thi′ro-nēn) one of the thyroid hormones, an organic iodine-containing compound liberated from thyroglobulin by hydrolysis. It has several times the biological activity of thyroxine. Symbol T_3.

trilaminar (tri-lam′ĭ-ner) three-layered.

trilobate (tri-lo′bāt) having three lobes.

trilocular (-lok′u-ler) having three compartments or cells.

trilogy (tril′o-je) a group or series of three. **t. of Fallot,** a term sometimes applied to concurrent pulmonic stenosis, atrial septal defect, and right ventricular hypertrophy.

trimeprazine (-mep′rah-zēn) a drug, $(C_{18}H_{22}N_2S)_2$, with mild central nervous depressant, moderate antiemetic and anticonvulsant, and powerful antihistaminic action; used as an antipruritic in the form of the tartrate salt.

trimester (-mes′ter) a period of three months.

trimethadione (tri″meth-ah-di′ōn) an anticonvulsant, $C_6H_9NO_3$.

trimethaphan camsylate (tri-meth′ah-fan) a short-acting ganglionic blocking agent, $C_{32}H_{40}$-$N_2O_5S_2$, used as an antihypertensive to produce controlled hypotension during surgery and for the emergency treatment of hypertensive crises.

trimethobenzamide (-meth″o-ben′zah-mīd) an antiemetic, $C_{21}H_{28}N_2O_5$, used as the hydrochloride salt.

trimethoprim (-meth′o-prim) an antibacterial, $C_{14}H_{18}N_4O_3$, closely related to pyrimethamine; administered in combination with a sulfonamide because these drugs blockade two consecutive steps in the synthesis of tetrahydrofolate by microorganisms; used primarily for the treatment of urinary tract infections.

trimorphous (tri-mor′fus) existing in three different forms.

trinitrophenol (-ni″tro-fe′nol) a substance, C_6-$H_2(NO_2)_3OH$, used as dye, tissue fixative, antiseptic, astringent, and stimulant of epithelialization; it can be detonated on percussion or by heating above 300° C.

trinitrotoluene (-tol′u-ēn) TNT: a high explosive, $C_6H_2(NO_2)_3CH_3$, derived from toluene; it sometimes causes poisoning in those who work with it, marked by dermatitis, gastritis, abdominal pain, vomiting, constipation, and flatulence.

triocephalus (tri″o-sef′ah-lus) a fetus with no organs of sight, hearing, or smell.

triorchidism (tri-or′kĭ-dizm) the presence of three testes.

triose (tri′ōs) a monosaccharide containing three carbon atoms in a molecule.

trioxsalen (tri-ok′sah-len) a psoralen, $C_{14}H_{12}O_3$, used in conjunction with ultraviolet exposure in treatment of vitiligo and psoriasis.

tripelennamine (tri″pĕ-len′ah-min) an antihistaminic, $C_{16}H_{21}N_3$, used as the citrate and monohydrochloride salts in the symptomatic treatment of various allergic disorders.

tripeptide (tri-pep′tīd) a peptide that on hydrolysis yields three amino acids.

triphalangism (-fal′an-jizm) three phalanges in a digit normally having only two.

triphasic (-fa′zik) having three phases.

triphenylmethane (-fen″il-meth′ān) a substance from coal tar, the basis of various dyes and stains, including aurin, rosaniline, basic fuchsin, and gentian violet.

triple blind (trip′'l blind) pertaining to a clinical trial in which neither the subject nor the person administering the treatment nor the person evaluating the response to treatment knows which treatment any particular subject is receiving.

triplegia (-ple′je-ah) paralysis of three extremities.

triplet (trip′lit) 1. one of three offspring produced at one birth. 2. a combination of three objects or entities acting together, as three lenses or three nucleotides.

triplex (tri′pleks) triple or threefold.

triploid (trip'loid) having triple the haploid number of chromosomes (3n).

triplopia (trĭ-plo'pe-ah) the perception of three images of a single object.

triprolidine (tri-pro'lĭ-dēn) an antihistaminic, $C_{19}H_{22}N_2$, used as the hydrochloride salt.

-tripsy word element [Gr.], *crushing;* used to designate a surgical procedure in which a structure is intentionally crushed.

tripus (tri'pus) a conjoined twin monster having three feet.

trismus (triz'mus) motor disturbance of the trigeminal nerve, especially spasm of the masticatory muscles, with difficulty in opening the mouth (lockjaw); a characteristic early symptom of tetanus.

trisomy (tri'so-me) the presence of an additional (third) chromosome of one type in an otherwise diploid cell (2n + 1). See also under *syndrome.* **triso'mic,** adj.

trisplanchnic (tri-splangk'nik) pertaining to the three great visceral cavities.

trisulcate (tri-sul'kāt) having three furrows.

trisulfapyrimidines (-sul″fah-pi-rim'ĭ-dēnz) preparations containing a mixture of the sulfonamides sulfadiazine, sulfamerazine, and sulfamethazine.

trisulfide (-sul'fīd) a sulfur compound containing three atoms of sulfur to one of the base.

tritanomaly (tri″tah-nom'ah-le) tritanomalopia.

tritanope (trit'ah-nōp″) a person exhibiting tritanopia.

tritanopia (tri″tah-no'pe-ah) a rare dichromasy marked by retention of the sensory mechanism for two hues only (red and green), with blue and yellow being absent. **tritanop'ic,** adj.

tritium (trit'e-um, trish'e-um) see *hydrogen.*

trituration (trich″ĕ-ra'shun) 1. reduction to powder by friction or grinding. 2. a finely powdered substance. 3. the creation of a homogeneous whole by mixing, as the combining of particles of an alloy with mercury to form dental amalgam.

trivalent (tri-va'lent) having a valence of three.

tRNA transfer RNA; see *ribonucleic acid.*

trocar (tro'kar) a sharp-pointed instrument equipped with a cannula, used to puncture the wall of a body cavity and withdraw fluid.

trochanter (tro-kan'ter) a broad, flat process on the femur, at the upper end of its lateral surface (*greater t.*), or a short conical process on the posterior border of the base of its neck (*lesser t.*). **trochanter'ic, trochanter'ian,** adj.

troche (tro'ke) a medicinal preparation for solution in the mouth, consisting of an active ingredient incorporated in a mass made of sugar and mucilage or fruit base.

trochlea (trok'le-ah), pl. *troch'leae* [L.] a pulley-shaped part or structure; used in anatomic nomenclature to designate various bony or fibrous structures through or over which tendons pass or with which other structures articulate. **troch'lear,** adj.

trochocephaly (tro″ko-sef'ah-le) a rounded appearance of the head due to synostosis of the frontal and parietal bones.

trochoid (tro'koid) pivot-like, or pulley-shaped.

trochoides (tro-koi'dēz) a pivot joint.

Troglotrema (trog″lo-tre'mah) a genus of flukes, including *T. salmin'cola* (salmon fluke), a parasite of various fish, especially salmon and trout, which is a vector of *Neorickettsia helminthoeca.*

Trombicula (trom-bik'u-lah) a genus of acarine mites (family Trombiculidae), including *T. akamu'shi, T. delien'sis, T. fletch'eri, T. interme'dia, T. pal'lida,* and *T. scutella'ris,* whose larvae (chiggers) are vectors of *Rickettsia tsutsugamushi,* the cause of scrub typhus.

trombiculiasis (trom-bik″u-li'ah-sis) infestation with mites of the genus *Trombicula.*

Trombiculidae (trom-bik″u-li'de) a family of mites cosmopolitan in distribution, whose parasitic larvae (chiggers) infest vertebrates.

tromethamine (tro-meth'ah-mēn) an alkalizing agent, $C_4H_{11}NO_3$, used intravenously in metabolic acidosis.

troph(o)- word element [Gr.], *food; nourishment.*

trophedema (trof″ĕ-de'mah) a chronic disease with permanent edema of the feet or legs.

trophic (trof'ik) pertaining to nutrition.

-trophic, -trophin word element [Gr.], *nourishing; stimulating.*

trophoblast (trof″o-blast) the peripheral cells of the blastocyst, which attach the fertilized ovum to the uterine wall become the placenta and the membranes that nourish and protect the developing organisms. **trophoblas'tic,** adj.

trophoblastoma (trof″o-blas-to'mah) choriocarcinoma.

trophodermatoneurosis (-der″mah-to-nu-ro'-sis) acrodynia.

trophoneurosis (trof″o-nu-ro'sis) any tɪ hic disorder of a part due to deficiency of its ɪ rve supply. **trophoneurot'ic,** adj.

trophonosis (-no'sis) any disease due to nu ritional causes.

trophont (tro'font) the active, motile, feediɪg stage in the life cycle of certain ciliate protozoa.

trophopathy (tro-fop'ah-the) any derangement of nutrition.

trophoplast (trof″o-plast) a granular protoplasmic body.

trophotaxis (trof″o-tak'sis) taxis in response to nutritive materials.

trophotherapy (-ther'ah-pe) treatment of disease by dietary measures.

trophozoite (-zo'īt) the active, motile feeding stage of a sporozoan parasite.

tropia (tro'pe-ah) strabismus.

-tropic word element [Gr.], *turning toward; changing; tending to turn or change.*

tropine (tro'pēn) a crystalline alkaloid from atropine and from various plants.

tropism (tro'pizm) the turning, bending, movement, or growth of an organism or part of an organism elicited by an external stimulus, either toward (*positive t.*) or away from (*negative t.*) the stimulus; used as a word element combined with a stem indicating the nature of the stimulus (e.g., phototropism) or material or entity for which an organism (or substance) shows a special affinity (e.g., neurotropism). Usually applied to nonmotile organisms.

tropocollagen (tro″po-kol′ah-jen) the molecular unit of all forms of collagen; it is a helical structure of three polypeptides.

tropomysin (-mi′o-sin) a muscle protein of the I band that inhibits contraction by blocking the interaction of actin and myosin, except when influenced by troponin.

troponin (tro′po-nin) a complex of muscle proteins which, when combined with Ca^{++}, influence tropomyosin to initiate contraction.

truncate (trung′kāt) 1. to amputate; to deprive of limbs. 2. having the end cut squarely off.

truncus (trung′kus), pl. *trun′ci* [L.] trunk.

trunk (trungk) the main part, as the part of the body to which the head and limbs are attached, or a larger structure (e.g., vessel or nerve) from which smaller divisions or branches arise, or which is created by their union. **trun′cal**, adj. **brachiocephalic t.**, a vessel arising from the arch of the aorta and giving rise to the right common carotid and right subclavian arteries. **celiac t.**, the arterial trunk arising from the abdominal aorta and giving origin to the left gastric, common hepatic, and splenic arteries. **encephalic t.**, brain stem. **lumbosacral t.**, a trunk formed by union of the lower part of the ventral branch of the fourth lumbar nerve with the ventral branch of the fifth lumbar nerve. **lymphatic t's**, the lymphatic vessels that drain lymph from the various regions of the body into the right lymphatic or the thoracic duct. **pulmonary t.**, a vessel arising from the conus arteriosus of the right ventricle and bifurcating into the right and left pulmonary arteries. **sympathetic t.**, two long ganglionated nerve strands, one on each side of the vertebral column, extending from the base of the skull to the coccyx.

truss (trus) an elastic, canvas, or metallic device for retaining a reduced hernia within the abdominal cavity.

trypanocidal (tri-pan″o-si′dal) destructive to trypanosomes.

trypanolysis (tri″pan-ol′ĭ-sis) the destruction of trypanosomes. **trypanolyt′ic**, adj.

Trypanosoma (tri″pan-o-so′mah) a multispecies genus of protozoa parasitic in the blood and lymph of invertebrates and vertebrates, including man. Trypanosomal infections of man include Gambian and Rhodesian forms of African trypanosomiasis (caused by *T. gambien′se* and *T. rhodesien′se*, respectively) and Chagas' disease (caused by *T. cru′zi*). Other species cause serious diseases of domestic animals, including *T. bru′cei, T. congolen′se, T. evan′si*, etc.

trypanosome (tri-pan′o-sōm) an individual of the genus *Trypanosoma*. **trypanoso′mal**, adj.

trypanosomiasis (tri-pan″o-so-mi′ah-sis) infection with trypanosomes. **African t.**, human trypanosomiasis endemic in tsetse fly–infested areas of tropical Africa, due to infection with *Trypanosoma gambiense* (Gambian t.) or *T. rhodesiense* (Rhodesian t.); it is transmitted by the bite of various species of *Glossina*, and in the ad-

vanced stage involves the central nervous system, resulting in meningoencephalitis that leads to lethargy, tremors, convulsions, and eventually coma and death. **South American t.**, Chagas' disease.

trypanosomicide (-so′mĭ-sīd) 1. lethal to trypanosomes. 2. an agent lethal to trypanosomes.

trypanosomid (-so′mid) a skin eruption occurring in trypanosomiasis.

trypsin (trip′sin) an enzyme of the hydrolase class, secreted as trypsinogen by the pancreas and converted to the active form in the small intestine, that catalyzes the cleavage of peptide linkages involving the carboxyl group of either lysine or arginine; a purified preparation derived from ox pancreas is used for its proteolytic effect in débridement and in the treatment of empyema. **tryp′tic**, adj.

trypsinogen (trip-sin′o-jen) the inactive precursor of trypsin, secreted by the pancreas.

tryptophan (trip′to-fan) a naturally occurring amino acid, existing in proteins and essential for human metabolism.

tryptophanuria (trip″to-fan-ūr′e-ah) excessive urinary excretion of trytophan.

tsetse (tset′se) an African fly of the genus *Glossina*, which transmits trypanosomiasis.

TSH thyroid-stimulating hormone.

TU tuberculin unit.

tuaminoheptane (too″ah-me″no-hep′tān) an adrenergic, $C_7H_{17}N$, used as a nasal decongestant in the form of the base (for inhalation) and sulfate salt (topical solution).

tuba (too′bah), pl. *tu′bae* [L.] tube.

Tubadil (too′bah-dil) trademark for a preparation of tubocurarine.

Tubarine (-rin) trademark for a preparation of tubocurarine.

tube (tūb) a hollow cylindrical organ or instrument. **tu′bal**, adj. **auditory t.**, eustachian tube; the narrow channel connecting the middle ear and the nasopharynx. **drainage t.**, a tube used in surgery to facilitate escape of fluids. **Durham's t.**, a jointed tracheotomy tube. **endobronchial t.**, a double-lumen tube inserted into the bronchus of one lung, permitting complete deflation of the other lung; used in anesthesia and thoracic surgery. **endotracheal t.**, an airway catheter inserted in the trachea in endotracheal intubation. **eustachian t.**, auditory t. **fallopian t.**, uterine t. **feeding t.**, one for introducing high-caloric fluids into the stomach. **Levin t.**, a gastroduodenal catheter of sufficiently small caliber to permit transnasal passage. **Miller-Abbott t.**, a double-channel intestinal tube with an inflatable balloon at its distal end, for use in treatment of obstruction of the small intestine, and occasionally as a diagnostic aid. **nasogastric t.**, a soft tube to be inserted through a nostril and into the stomach, for instilling liquids or other substances, or for withdrawing gastric contents. **neural t.**, the epithelial tube produced by folding of the neural plate in the early embryo. **otopharyngeal t.**, auditory t. **Ryle's t.**, a thin rubber tube for giving a test meal. **Sengstaken-Blakemore t.**, a multilumen tube used for tamponade of bleeding esophageal varices. **stomach t.**, one which is passed through the esophagus to the stomach, for introduction of nutrients or for gastric lavage. **test t.**, a tube of thin glass, closed at one end; used in chemical tests and other laboratory procedures. **tracheotomy t.**, a curved tube that is inserted into the trachea through the opening made in the neck at tracheotomy. **uterine t.**, a slender tube extending laterally from the uterus toward the ovary on the same side, conveying ova to the cavity of the uterus and permitting passage of spermatozoa in the opposite direction. **vacuum t.**, a glass tube from which gaseous contents have been evacuated. **Wangensteen t.**, a small nasogastric tube connected with a special suction apparatus to maintain gastric and duodenal decompression. **x-ray t.**, a vacuum tube used for the production of x-rays; when a suitable current is applied, high-speed electrons travel from the cathode to the anode, where they are suddenly arrested, giving rise to x-rays.

tubectomy (too-bek′tah-me) excision of a portion of the uterine tube.

tuber (too′ber), pl. *tubers* or *tu′bera* [L.] a swelling or protuberance. **t. cine′reum**, a layer of gray matter forming part of the floor of the third ventricle, to which the infundibulum of the hypothalamus is attached.

tubercle (too′ber-k'l) 1. any small, rounded mass produced by infection with *Mycobacterium tuberculosis*. 2. a nodule or small eminence, especially one on a bone, for attachment of a tendon. **tuber′cular**, adj. **anatomic t.**, tuberculosis verrucosa cutis. **auricular t.**, **darwinian t.**, a small projection sometimes found on the edge of the helix; conjectured by some to be a relic of simioid ancestry. **Farre's t's**, masses beneath the capsule of the liver in certain cases of hepatic cancer. **fibrous t.**, one of bacillary origin which contains connective-tissue elements. **genial t.**, mental t. **Ghon's t.**, see under *focus*. **gracile t.**, an enlargement of the fasciculus gracilis in the medulla oblongata, produced by the underlying nucleus gracilis. **intervenous t.**, a ridge across the inner surface of the right atrium between the openings of the venae cavae. **Lisfranc's t.**, an eminence on the first rib, for attachment of the anterior scalene muscle. **Lower's t.**, intervenous t. **mental t.**, a prominence on the inner border of either side of the mental protuberance of the mandible. **miliary t.**, one of the many minute tubercles formed in many organs in acute miliary tuberculosis. **pubic t.**, a prominent tubercle at the lateral end of the pubic crest. **scalene t.**, Lisfranc's t. **supraglenoid t.**, one on the scapula for attachment of the long head of the biceps.

tuberculate, tuberculated (too-ber′ku-lāt″; too-ber′ku-lāt″ed) covered or affected with tubercles.

tuberculid (too-ber′ku-lid) recurrent eruptions of the skin usually characterized by spontaneous involution; considered by some authorities to be hyperergic reactions to mycobacteria or their antigens. **papulonecrotic t.**, a grouped, symmetric eruption of symptomless papules,

appearing in successive crops and healing spontaneously with superficially depressed scars.

tuberculigenous (too-ber″ku-lij′ĭ-nus) causing tuberculosis.

tuberculin (too-ber′ku-lin) a sterile liquid containing the growth products of, or specific substances extracted from, the tubercle bacillus; used in various forms in the diagnosis of tuberculosis; see also under *test*. **New t.**, a suspension of the fragments of tubercle bacilli, freed from all soluble materials and with glycerin added. **Old t.**, a heat-concentrated filtrate of tubercle bacillus culture grown on a special medium; used for tuberculin tests. **purified protein derivative (PPD) t.**, a soluble purified protein fraction precipitated from filtrate of tubercle bacillus grown on a special medium; used in tuberculin tests.

tuberculitis (too-ber″ku-li′tis) inflammation of or near a tubercle.

tuberculocele (too-ber′ku-lo-sēl″) tuberculous disease of a testis.

tuberculofibroid (too-ber″ku-lo-fi′broid) characterized by a tubercle that has undergone fibroid degeneration.

tuberculoid (too-ber′ku-loid) resembling a tubercle or tuberculosis.

tuberculoma (too-ber″ku-lo′mah) a tumor-like mass resulting from enlargement of a caseous tubercle.

tuberculosis (too-ber″ku-lo′sis) any of the infectious diseases of man and other animals due to species of *Mycobacterium* and marked by formation of tubercles and caseous necrosis in tissues of any organ; in man, the lung is the major seat of infection and the usual portal through which infection reaches other organs. **avian t.**, a form affecting various birds, due to *Mycobacterium avium*, which may be communicated to man and other animals. **bovine t.**, an infection of cattle due to *Mycobacterium bovis*, transmissible to man and other animals. **disseminated t.**, acute miliary t. **genital t.**, tuberculosis of the genital tract, e.g., tuberculous endometritis. **t. of lungs**, pulmonary tuberculosis; infection of the lungs due to *Mycobacterium tuberculosis*, marked by tuberculous pneumonia, formation of tuberculous granulation tissue, caseous necrosis, calcification, and cavity formation. Symptoms include weight loss, fatigue, night sweats, purulent sputum, hemoptysis, and chest pain. **miliary t., acute**, an acute form in which minute tubercles are formed in a number of organs, due to dissemination of the bacilli through the body by the blood stream. **open t.**, 1. that in which there are lesions from which tubercle bacilli are being discharged out of the body. 2. tuberculosis of the lungs with cavitation. **pulmonary t.**, t. of lungs. **t. of spine**, Pott's disease. **t. verruco′sa, warty t.**, a condition usually resulting from external inoculation of the tubercle bacilli into the skin, with wartlike papules coalescing to form distinctly verrucous patches with an inflammatory, erythematous border.

tuberculostatic (too-ber″ku-lo-stat′ik) 1. inhibiting the growth of *Mycobacterium tuberculosis*. 2. a tuberculostatic agent.

tuberculotic (too-ber″ku-lot′ik) pertaining to or affected with tuberculosis.

tuberculous (too-ber′ku-lus) pertaining to or affected with tuberculosis; caused by *Mycobacterium tuberculosis.*

tuberculum (too-ber′ku-lum), pl. *tuber′cula* [L.] a tubercle, nodule, or small eminence; in anatomy, used principally to designate a small eminence on a bone. **t. arthrit′icum,** a gouty concretion in a joint. **t. doloro′sum,** a painful nodule or tubercle.

tuberosis (too-ber-o′sis) a condition characterized by the presence of nodules.

tuberositas (too″ber-os′ĭ-tas), pl. *tuberosita′tes* [L.] tuberosity; in anatomy, an elevation on a bone to which a muscle is attached.

tuberosity (too″bĕ-ros′ĭ-te) an elevation or protuberance.

tuberous (too″ber-us) covered with tubers; knobby. See also under *sclerosis.*

tubo- word element [L.], *tube.*

tubocurarine (too″bo-kūr-ar′ēn) an alkaloid from the bark and stems of *Chondrodendron tomentosum;* it is the active principle of curare, used as a skeletal muscle relaxant.

tuboligamentous (-lig″ah-men′tus) pertaining to the uterine tube and broad ligament.

tubo-ovarian (-o-vār′e-an) pertaining to the uterine tube and ovary.

tuboperitoneal (-per″ĭ-tah-ne′al) pertaining to the uterine tube and the peritoneum.

tuboplasty (too′bo-plas″te) plastic repair of a tube, such as the uterine tube or auditory tube.

tubotympanum (too″bo-tim′pah-num) the auditory tube and tympanic cavity considered together.

tubouterine (-u′ter-in) pertaining to the uterine tube and uterus.

tubule (too′būl) a small tube. **tu′bular,** adj. **collecting t's,** the terminal channels of the nephrons which open on the summits of the renal pyramids in the renal papillae. **dentinal t's,** dental canaliculi. **Henle's t's,** the straight ascending and descending portions of a renal tubule forming Henle's loop. **mesonephric t's,** the tubules composing the mesonephros, or temporary kidney, of amniotes. **metanephric t's,** the tubules composing the permanent kidney of amniotes. **renal t's,** the minute reabsorptive canals made up of basement membrane and lined with epithelium, composing the substance of the kidney and secreting, collecting, and conducting the urine; see also *nephron.* **seminiferous t's,** the tubules of the testis in which the spermatozoa develop and through which they leave the gland. **T t's,** the transverse intracellular tubules invaginating from the cell membrane and surrounding the myofibrils of the T system of skeletal and cardiac muscle, serving as a pathway for the spread of electrical excitation within a muscle cell. **uriniferous t's,** renal t's.

tubulin (too′bu-lin) the constituent protein of microtubules.

tubulorrhexis (too″bu-lo-rek′sis) rupture of the renal tubules.

tubulus (too′bu-lus), pl. *tu′buli* [L.] tubule; a minute canal.

tuft (tuft) a small clump or cluster; a coil. **malpighian t.,** renal glomerulus.

tuftsin (tuft′sin) a tetrapeptide cleaved from IgG that stimulates phagocytosis by neutrophils.

tugging (tug′ing) a pulling sensation, as a pulling sensation in the trachea (*tracheal t.*), due to aneurysm of the arch of the aorta.

tularemia (too″lah-re′me-ah) a plaguelike disease of rodents, caused by *Francisella (Pasteurella) tularensis,* which is transmissible to man. **oculoglandular** tularemia in which the primary site of entry of the pathogen is the conjunctival sac, marked by conjunctivitis, itching, lacrimation, pain, corneal lesions, and enlargement of preauricular lymph nodes. **pulmonary t., pulmonic t.,** tularemia associated with involvement of the lungs by spread of a primary infection or by inhalation of the pathogen, marked by cough, headache, fever, substernal pain, and bloody mucoid sputum. **typhoidal t.,** the most serious form of tularemia, caused by swallowing an inoculum of the pathogen, marked by symptoms similar to those of typhoid. **ulceroglandular t.,** the most common form of human tularemia, beginning with a painful, swollen, erythematus papule at the point of inoculation, which ruptures to form a shallow ulcer; lymphadenopathy, hepatosplenomegaly, and pneumonia may also occur.

tumefacient (too″mah-fa′shent) producing tumefaction.

tumefaction (-fak′shun) a swelling; the state of being swollen, or the act of swelling; puffiness; edema.

tumescence (too-mes′ens) 1. the condition of being swollen. 2. a swelling.

tumid (too′mid) swollen; edematous.

tumor (too′mer) 1. swelling, one of the cardinal signs of inflammation; morbid enlargement. 2. neoplasm; a new growth of tissue in which cell multiplication is uncontrolled and progressive. **benign t.,** one lacking the properties of invasion and metastasis and showing a lesser degree of anaplasia than do malignant tumors; it is usually surrounded by a fibrous capsule. **Brenner t.,** a benign fibroepithelioma of the ovary. **brown t.,** a giant-cell granuloma produced in and replacing bone, occurring in osteitis fibrosa cystica and due to hyperparathyroidism. **Buschke-Löwenstein t.,** a large cauliflower-like mass of warts occurring on the prepuce, especially in uncircumcised males, and also in the perianal region. **carotid body t.,** a firm, round mass at the bifurcation of the common carotid artery. **desmoid t.,** desmoid (1). **erectile t.,** cavernous hemangioma. **Ewing's t.,** a malignant tumor of bone, arising in medullary tissue and more often in cylindrical bones. **false t.,** structural enlargement due to extravasation, exudation, echinococcus, or retained sebaceous matter. **giant cell t.,** 1. a bone tumor, ranging from benign to frankly malignant, composed of cellular spindle cell stroma containing multinucleated giant cells resembling osteoclasts. 2. a benign, small, yellow, tumor-like nodule of tendon sheath origin, most often of the wrist and fingers or ankle and toes, laden with lipophages and containing multinucleated giant cells. **glomus t.**, a blue-red, painful chemodectoma involving a glomeriform arteriovenous anastomosis (glomus body). **glomus jugulare t.**, a chemodectoma involving the tympanic body (glomus jugulare). **granular cell t.**, a usually benign, circumscribed, tumor-like lesion of soft tissue, particularly of the tongue, composed of large cells with prominent granular cytoplasm; the histiogenesis is uncertain, but Schwann cell derivation is favored. **granulosa t., granulosa cell t.**, an ovarian tumor originating in the cells of the membrana granulosa. **granulosa-theca cell t.**, an ovarian tumor composed of granulosa (follicular) cells and theca cells; either form may predominate. **heterologous t., heterotypic t.**, one made up of tissue differing from that in which it grows. **homoiotypic t., homologous t.**, one resembling the surrounding parts in its structure. **Hürthle cell t.**, a new growth of the thyroid gland, usually benign but sometimes malignant, composed wholly or predominantly of large cells (Hürthle cells) having abundant granular, eosinophilic cytoplasm. **islet cell t.**, a tumor of the islands of Langerhans, which may result in hyperinsulinism. **Krukenberg's t.**, carcinoma of the ovary, usually metastatic from gastrointestinal cancer, marked by areas of mucoid degeneration and by the presence of signet-ring–like cells. **Leydig cell t.**, a tumor of the Leydig cells of the testis. **lipoid cell t. of ovary**, a usually benign ovarian tumor composed of eosinophilic cells or cells with lipoid vacuoles; it causes masculinization. **malignant t.**, one having the properties of invasion and metastasis and showing a high degree of anaplasia. **mast cell t.**, mastocytosis. **melanotic neuroectodermal t.**, a benign, rapidly growing, dark tumor of the jaw and occasionally of other sites; seen almost exclusively in infants. **mixed t.**, one composed of more than one type of neoplastic tissue. **papillary t.**, papilloma. **pearl t.**, cholesteatoma. **sand t.**, psammoma. **teratoid t.**, teratoma. **theca cell t.**, a fibroid-like ovarian tumor containing yellow areas of lipoid material derived from theca cells. **true t.**, a neoplasm. **turban t's**, a term used to describe the gross appearance of multiple cutaneous cylindromas of the scalp. **Warthin's t.**, papillary adenocystoma lymphomatosum. **Wilms' t.**, a rapidly developing malignant mixed tumor of the kidneys, made up of embryonal elements, usually affecting children before the fifth year.

tumoricidal (too″mer-ĭ-si′dal) destructive to cancer cells.

tumorigenesis (-jen′ĕ-sis) the production of tumors. **tumorigen′ic**, adj.

Tunga (tun′gah) a genus of fleas, including *T. pen'etrans*, the chigoe (q.v.).

tungsten (tung′sten) chemical element (*see table*), at. no. 74, symbol W.

tunica (too′nĭ-kah), pl. *tu'nicae* [L.] a tunic; in anatomy, a general term for a membrane or other structure covering or lining a body part or organ. **t. adventi′tia**, the outer coat of various tubular structures. **t. albugin′ea**, a dense, white, fibrous sheath enclosing a part or organ. **t. conjuncti′va**, the conjunctiva. **t. dar′tos**, the thin layer of subcutaneous tissue underlying the skin of the scrotum. **t. exter′na**, an outer coat, especially the fibroelastic coat of a blood vessel. **t. fibro′sa**, fibrous coat; an enveloping fibrous membrane. **t. in′tima**, the innermost coat of blood vessels. **t. me′dia**, the middle coat of blood vessels. **t. muco′sa**, mucous membrane. **t. muscula′ris**, the muscular coat or layer surrounding the tela submucosa in most portions of the digestive, respiratory, urinary, and genital tracts. **t. pro′pria**, a proper coat or layer of a part, as distinguished from an investing membrane. **t. sero′sa**, the membrane lining the external walls of body cavities and reflected over the surfaces of protruding organs; it secretes a watery exudate. **t. vagina′lis**, the serous membrane covering the front and sides of the testis and epididymis. **t. vasculo′sa**, a vascular coat, or a layer well supplied with blood vessels.

tunnel (tun′el) a passageway of varying length through a solid body, completely enclosed except for the open ends, permitting entrance and exit. **carpal t.**, the osseofibrous passage for the median nerve and the flexor tendons, formed by the flexor retinaculum and the carpal bones. **Corti's t.**, inner t. **flexor t.**, carpal t. **inner t.**, a canal extending the length of the cochlea, formed by the pillar cells of the organ of Corti. **tarsal t.**, the osseofibrous passage for the posterior tibial vessels, tibial nerve, and flexor tendons, formed by the flexor retinaculum and the tarsal bones.

turbidimeter (ter″bĭ-dim′ĕ-ter) an apparatus for measuring turbidity of a solution.

turbidity (ter-bid′ĭ-te) cloudiness; disturbance of solids (sediment) in a solution, so that it is not clear. **tur′bid**, adj.

turbinal (ter′bĭ-n'l) turbinate.

turbinate (-nāt) 1. shaped like a top. 2. a turbinate bone (nasal concha).

turbinectomy (-nek′tah-me) excision of a turbinate bone (nasal concha).

turbinotomy (-not′ah-me) incision of a turbinate bone.

turgescence (ter-jes′ens) distention or swelling of a part.

turgid (ter′jid) swollen and congested.

turgor (ter′ger) condition of being turgid; normal, or other fullness.

turista (too-rēs′tah) Mexican name for traveler's diarrhea.

turmschädel (toorm′sha-del) a developmental anomaly in which the head is high and rounded, due to early synostosis of the three major sutures of the skull.

turnover (tern′o-ver) the movement of something into, through, and out of a place; the rate at which a thing is depleted and replaced. **erythrocyte iron t.**, the rate at which iron moves from the bone marrow into circulating red cells. **plasma iron t.**, the rate at which iron moves from the blood plasma to the bone marrow or other tissues.

turricephaly (tur″ĭ-sef′ah-le) oxycephaly.

tussigenic (tus″ĭ-jen′ik) causing cough.

tussis (tus′is) [L.] cough. **tus′sal, tus′sive,** adj.

tutamen (too-ta′men), pl. *tuta′mina* [L.] a protective covering or structure. **tuta′mina oc′uli,** the protecting appendages of the eye, as the lids, lashes, etc.

twig (twig) a final ramification, as of branches of a nerve or blood vessel.

twin (twin) one of two offspring produced in one pregnancy. **allantoidoangiopagous t's,** twins united by the umbilical vessels only. **conjoined t's,** monozygotic twins whose bodies are joined to a varying extent. **dizygotic t's,** twins developed from two separate ova fertilized at the same time. **enzygotic t's,** monozygotic t's. **fraternal t's, heterologous t's,** dizygotic t's. **identical t's,** monozygotic t's. **impacted t's,** twins so situated during delivery that pressure of one against the other produces incomplete simultaneous engagement of both. **monoamniotic t's,** twins developing within a single amniotic cavity; they are always monozygotic. **monozygotic t's,** two individuals developed from one fertilized ovum. **omphaloangiopagous t's,** allantoidoangiopagous t's. **Siamese t's,** conjoined t's. **similar t's,** monozygotic t's. **uniovular t's,** monozygotic t's.

twinning (twin′ing) 1. the production of symmetrical structures or parts by division. 2. the simultaneous intrauterine production of two or more embryos.

twitch (twich) a brief, contractile response of a skeletal muscle elicited by a single maximal volley of impulses in the neurons supplying it.

tybamate (ti′bah-māt) a minor tranquilizer, C₁₃-H₂₆N₂O₄.

tylectomy (ti-lek′tah-me) lumpectomy.

Tylenol (ti′lĕ-nol) trademark for preparations of acetaminophen.

tylion (til′e-on) a point on anterior edge of the optic groove in the median line.

tyloma (ti-lo′ma) a callus or callosity.

tylosis (ti-lo′sis) formation of callosities. **tylot′ic,** adj.

tyloxapol (ti-loks′ah-pol) a nonionic liquid polymer used as a surfactant to aid liquefaction and removal of mucopurulent bronchopulmonary secretions, administered by inhalation.

tympan(o)- word element [Gr.], *tympanic cavity; tympanic membrane.*

tympanal (tim′pah-n′l) pertaining to the tympanum or to the tympanic membrane.

tympanectomy (tim″pah-nek′tah-me) excision of the tympanic membrane.

tympanic (tim-pan′ik) 1. of or pertaining to the tympanum. 2. bell-like; resonant.

tympanism (tim′pah-nizm) tympanites.

tympanites (tim″pah-ni′tēz) abnormal distention due to the presence of gas or air in the intestine or the peritoneal cavity.

tympanitic (tim″pah-nit′ik) 1. pertaining to or affected with tympanites. 2. bell-like; tympanic.

tympanitis (tim″pah-ni′tis) otitis media.

tympanocentesis (tim″pah-no-sen-te′sis) surgical puncture of the tympanic membrane or tympanum.

tympanogenic (-jen′ik) arising from the tympanum or middle ear.

tympanogram (-gram″) a graphic representation of the relative compliance and impedance of the tympanic membrane and ossicles of the middle ear obtained by tympanometry.

tympanomastoiditis (tim″pah-no-mas″toi-di′tis) inflammation of the middle ear and the pneumatic cells of the mastoid process.

tympanometry (tim″pah-nom′ĕ-tre) indirect measurement of the compliance (mobility) and impedance of the tympanic membrane and ossicles of the middle ear.

tympanoplasty (tim′pah-no-plas″te) surgical reconstruction of the tympanic membrane and establishment of ossicular continuity from the tympanic membrane to the oval window. **tympanoplas′tic,** adj.

tympanosclerosis (tim″pah-no-sklĕ-ro′sis) a condition characterized by the presence of masses of hard, dense connective tissue around the auditory ossicles in the tympanic cavity.

tympanotomy (tim″pah-not′ah-me) myringotomy.

tympanous (tim′pah-nus) distended with gas.

tympanum (tim′pah-num) 1. loosely, the tympanic membrane. 2. tympanic cavity.

tympany (tim′pah-ne) 1. tympanites. 2. a tympanic, or bell-like, percussion note. **t. of stomach,** a kind of indigestion in cattle and sheep, marked by abnormal collection of gas in the first stomach.

type (tīp) the general or prevailing character of any particular case of disease, person, substance, etc. **blood t's,** see *blood group.* **constitutional t.,** a constellation of traits related to body build. **mating t.,** in ciliate protozoa, certain bacteria, and certain fungi, the equivalent of a sex. **phage t.,** an intraspecies type of bacterium demonstrated by phage typing.

typhl(o)- word element [Gr.], *cecum; blindness.*

typhlectasis (tif-lek′tah-sis) distention of the cecum.

typhlitis (tif-li′tis) inflammation of the cecum.

typhlodicliditis (tif″lo-dik″lĭ-di′tis) inflammation of the ileocecal valve.

typhlolexia (-lek′se-ah) alexia.

typhlolithiasis (-lĭ-thi′ah-sis) calculi in the cecum.

typhlosis (tif-lo′sis) blindness.

typhlotomy (tif-lot′o-me) cecotomy.

typhoid (ti′foid) 1. resembling typhus. 2. typhoid fever. 3. typhoidal.

typhoidal (ti-foi′dal) resembling typhoid fever.

typhus (ti′fus) a group of closely related, acute, arthropod-borne rickettsial diseases that differ in the intensity of certain signs and symptoms, severity, and fatality rate; all are characterized by headache, chills, fever, stupor, and a macular, maculopapular, petechial, or papulovesicular eruption. Often used alone in English-speaking countries to refer to epidemic typhus, and in several European languages to refer to typhoid fever. **ty′phous,** adj. **endemic t.,** murine t. **epidemic t.,** the classic form, due to *Rickettsia prowazekii* and transmitted from man to man by body lice. **Kenya t.,** see *boutonneuse fever,* under *fever.* **murine t.,** an infectious disease, clinically similar to epidemic typhus but milder, due to *Rickettsia typhi,* transmitted from man to man by the rat flea and rat louse. **recrudescent t.,** Brill's disease. **scrub t.,** an acute, typhus-like infectious disease caused by *Rickettsia tsutsugamushi* and transmitted by chiggers, characterized by a primary skin lesion at the site of inoculation and development of a rash, regional lymphadenopathy, and fever. **tropical t.,** scrub typhus.

typology (ti-pol′ah-je) the study of types; the science of classifying, as bacteria according to type.

tyroma (ti-ro′mah) a caseous tumor.

tyromatosis (ti″ro-mah-to′sis) a condition characterized by caseous degeneration.

tyropanoate (-pah-no′āt) a radiopaque medium used as the sodium salt in oral cholecystography, $C_{15}H_{18}I_3NO_3$.

tyrosine (ti′ro-sēn) a naturally occurring amino acid present in most proteins; it is a product of phenylalanine metabolism and a precursor of thyroid hormones, catecholamines, and melanin.

tyrosinemia (ti″ro-sĭ-ne′me-ah) a hereditary disorder of tyrosine metabolism occurring in several types. *Type I* shows an excess of tyrosine, with inhibition of some liver enzymes and renal tubular function; the acute form leads to death from liver failure 6–8 months after birth, while the chronic form has similar but milder features. *Type II* is marked by crystallization of the accumulated tyrosine in the epidermis and cornea and is frequently accompanied by mental retardation. *Neonatal tyrosinemia* is asymptomatic and quickly cured by dietary restriction of protein, with few, if any, long-term effects.

tyrosinosis (-sĭ-no′sis) a condition characterized by faulty metabolism of tyrosine in which an intermediate product, para-hydroxyphenyl pyruvic acid, appears in the urine and gives it an abnormal reducing power.

tyrosinuria (-sĭ-nu′re-ah) presence of tyrosine in the urine.

tyrosyluria (ti″ro-sil-u′re-ah) increased urinary secretion of para-hydroxyphenyl compounds derived from tyrosine, as in tyrosinemia.

tyvelose (ti′vel-ōs) an unusual sugar that is a polysaccharide somatic antigen of certain *Salmonella* serotypes.

tzetze (tset′se) tsetse.

U

U chemical symbol, *uranium;* symbol for *uracil* or *uridine* (in nucleic acids) and for International Unit (of enzyme activity).

ubiquinol (u-bik′wĭ-nol) the reduced form of ubiquinone.

ubiquinone (u-bik′wĭ-nōn) a group of quinones occurring in the lipid core of inner mitochondrial membranes and functioning in electron transfer reactions.

UDP uridine diphosphate.

ul(o)- word element [Gr.], (1) *scar;* (2) *gingiva.*

ulcer (ul′ser) a local defect, or excavation of the surface, of an organ or tissue, produced by sloughing of necrotic inflammatory tissue. **Curling's u.,** acute ulceration of the stomach or duodenum following severe burns of the body. **decubital u., decubitus u.,** bedsore; an ulceration due to prolonged pressure from lying too still in bed for too long a time. **dental u.,** a lesion on the oral mucosa due to trauma inflicted by the teeth. **duodenal u.,** a peptic ulcer situated in the duodenum. **gastric u.,** an ulcer of the gastric mucosa. **Hunner's u.,** one involving all layers of the bladder wall, occurring in chronic interstitial cystitis. **jejunal u.,** an ulcer of the jejunum; such an ulcer following surgery is called a *secondary jejunal u.* **marginal u.,** a gastric ulcer in the jejunal mucosa near the site of a gastrojejunostomy. **peptic u.,** an ulceration of the mucous membrane of the esophagus, stomach, or duodenum, due to action of the acid gastric juice. **perforating u.,** one involving the entire thickness of an organ or of the wall of an organ creating an opening on both surfaces. **phagedenic u.,** a necrotic lesion associated with prominent tissue destruction, due to secondary bacterial invasion of an existing cutaneous lesion or of intact skin in a person with impaired resistance as the result of systemic disease. **rodent u.,** ulcerating basal cell carcinoma of the skin. **stercoraceous u., stercoral u.,** one caused by pressure of impacted feces; also, a fistulous ulcer through which fecal matter escapes. **stress u.,** peptic ulcer, usually gastric, resulting from stress. **trophic u.,** one due to imperfect nutrition of the part. **tropical u.,** 1. a lesion of cutaneous leishmaniasis. 2. tropical phagedenic u. **tropical phagedenic u.,** a chronic, painful, phagedenic ulcer of unknown cause, occurring usually on the lower extremities of malnourished children in the tropics. **varicose u.,** an ulcer due to varicose veins. **venereal u.,** a condition marked by formation of ulcers resembling chancre or chancroid about the vulvae of women not exposed to venereal disease.

ulcerate (ul′ser-āt) to undergo ulceration.

ulceration (ul″ser-a′shun) 1. the formation or development of an ulcer. 2. an ulcer. **ul′cerative,** adj.

ulcerogenic (-jen′ik) causing ulceration; leading to the production of ulcers.

ulceromembranous (-mem′brah-nus) characterized by ulceration and a membranous exudation.

ulcerous (ul′ser-us) 1. of the nature of an ulcer. 2. affected with ulceration.

ulcus (ul′kus), pl. *ul′cera* [L.] ulcer.

ulectomy (u-lek′to-me) 1. excision of scar tissue. 2. gingivectomy.

ulerythema (u″ler-ĭ-the′mah) an erythematous skin disease with formation of cicatrices and atrophy. **u. ophryog′enes**, a hereditary form in which keratosis pilaris involves the hair follicles of the eyebrows.

ulna (ul′nah), pl. *ul′nae* [L.] the inner and larger bone of the forearm; see *Table of Bones*.

ulnad (ul′nad) toward the ulna.

ulnar (ul′ner) pertaining to the ulna or to the ulnar (medial) aspect of the arm as compared to the radial (lateral) aspect.

ulnaris (ul-na′ris) [L.] ulnar.

ulnocarpal (ul″no-kar′p'l) pertaining to the ulna and carpus.

ulnoradial (-ra′de-al) pertaining to the ulna and radius.

ulocarcinoma (u″lo-kar″sĭ-no′mah) carcinoma of the gums.

ulorrhagia (u″lo-ra′je-ah) a sudden or free discharge of blood from the gums.

ulotomy (u-lot′ah-me) 1. incision of scar tissue. 2. incision of the gums.

ultra- word element [L.], *beyond; excess.*

ultracentrifugation (ul″trah-sen-trif″u-ga′-shun) subjection of material to an exceedingly high centrifugal force, which will separate and sediment the molecules of a substance.

ultradian (ul-tra′de-an) pertaining to a period of less than 24 hours; applied to the rhythmic repetition of certain phenomena in living organisms occurring in cycles of less than a day (*ultradian rhythm*).

ultrafiltration (-fil-tra′shun) filtration through a filter capable of removing very minute (ultramicroscopic) particles.

ultramicroscope (-mi′kro-skōp″) a special darkfield microscope for the examination of particles of colloidal size. **ultramicroscop′ic**, adj.

ultrasonic (-son′ik) beyond the upper limit of perception by the human ear; relating to sound waves having a frequency of more than 20,000 Hz.

ultrasonics (-son′iks) the science dealing with ultrasonic sound waves.

ultrasonography (-son-og′rah-fe) the imaging of deep structures of the body by recording the echoes of pulses of 1–10 megahertz ultrasound reflected by tissue planes where there is a change in density. **ultrasonograph′ic**, adj. **A-mode u.**, that in which one axis on the cathode-ray tube (CRT) display represents the time required for the return of the echo and the other corresponds to the strength of the echo, as in echoencephalography. **B-mode u.**, that in which the position of a spot on the CRT display corresponds to the time elapsed (and thus to the position of the echogenic surface) and the brightness of the spot to the strength of the echo; movement of the transducer produces a sweep of the ultrasound beam and a tomographic scan of a cross section of the body.

Doppler u., that in which measurement and a visual record are made of the shift in frequency of a continuous ultrasonic wave proportional to the blood flow velocity in underlying vessels; used in diagnosis of extracranial occlusive vascular disease. It is also used in detection of the fetal heart beat or of the velocity of movement of a structure such as the beating heart. **gray-scale u.**, B-mode ultrasonography in which the strength of echoes is indicated by a proportional brightness of the displayed dots. **real-time u.**, B-mode ultrasonography using an array of detectors so that scans can be made electronically at a rate of 30 frames a second.

ultrasound (ul′trah-sownd) mechanical radiant energy of a frequency greater than 20,000 Hz.

ultrastructure (-struk″chur) the structure beyond the resolution power of the light microscope, i.e., visible only under the ultramicroscope and electron microscope.

ultraviolet (ul″trah-vi′o-let) denoting electromagnetic radiation between violet light and roentgen rays, having wavelengths of 4–400 nanometers.

umbilical (um-bil″ĭ-k'l) pertaining to the umbilicus.

umbilication (um-bil″ĭ-ka′shun) a depression resembling the umbilicus.

umbilicus (um-bil″ĭ-kus, um″bĭ-li′kus) the navel; the scar marking the site of attachment of the umbilical cord in the fetus.

umbo (um′bo), pl. *umbo′nes* [L.] 1. a rounded elevation. 2. the slight projection at the center of the outer surface of the tympanic membrane.

UMP uridine monophosphate.

uncal (un′kal) of or pertaining to the uncus.

unciform (un′sĭ-form) hook shaped.

uncinate (un′sĭ-nāt) 1. unciform. 2. relating to or affecting the uncinate gyrus.

uncipressure (-presh″ur) pressure with a hook to stop hemorrhage.

unconscious (un-kon′shus) 1. insensible; incapable of responding to sensory stimuli and of having subjective experiences. 2. the part of the mind not readily accessible to conscious awareness but whose existence may be manifested in symptom formation, in dreams, or under the influence of drugs. **collective u.**, the portion of the unconscious which is theoretically common to mankind.

uncovertebral (un″ko-ver′tah-bral) pertaining to the uncinate processes of a vertebra.

unction (ungk′shun) 1. an ointment. 2. application of an ointment or salve; inunction.

uncus (ung′kus) the medially curved anterior end of the parahippocampal gyrus. **un′cal**, adj.

undecylenic acid (un-des″ĭ-len′ik) an unsaturated fatty acid, $C_{11}H_{20}O_2$, present in sweat; used as an antifungal agent.

undine (un′dēn) a small glass flask for irrigating the eye; a vibration.

ung. [L.] *unguen′tum* (ointment).

ungual (ung′gwal) pertaining to the nails.

unguent (ung′gwent) an ointment.

unguiculate (ung-gwik′u-lāt) having claws or nails; clawlike.

unguis (ung′gwis), pl. *un′gues* [L.] nail (2).

uni- word element [L.], *one.*

uniaxial (u″ne-ak′se-al) 1. having only one axis. 2. developing in an axial direction only.

unicameral (u″nĭ-kam′er-al) having only one cavity or compartment.

unicellular (-sel′u-ler) made up of a single cell, as the bacteria.

unicornous (-kor′nus) having only one cornu.

uniglandular (-glan′du-ler) affecting only one gland.

unilateral (-lat′er-al) affecting only one side.

unilocular (-lok′u-ler) monolocular.

uninucleated (-noo′kle-āt″ed) mononuclear (1).

uniocular (u″ne-ok′u-ler) monocular.

union (ūn′yun) the renewal of continuity in a broken bone or between the edges of a wound.

uniovular (u″ne-ov′u-ler) monozygotic, monovular.

uniparous (u-nip′ah-rus) 1. producing only one ovum or offspring at a time. 2. primiparous.

unipolar (u″nĭ-po′ler) 1. having a single pole or process, as a nerve cell. 2. pertaining to mood disorders in which only depressive episodes occur.

unipotent (u-nip′o-tent) unipotential.

unipotential (u″nĭ-po-ten′shul) having only one power, as giving rise to cells of one type only.

unit (u′nit) 1. a single thing; one segment of a whole that is made up of identical or similar segments. 2. a specifically defined amount of anything subject to measurement, as of activity, dimension, velocity, volume, or the like. **Ångström u.,** angstrom. **atomic mass u.,** the unit mass equal to $\frac{1}{12}$ the mass of the nuclide of carbon-12. Called also *dalton.* **Bethesda u.,** a measure of the level of inhibitor to Factor VIII; equal to the amount of inhibitor in patient plasma that will inactivate 50 per cent of inhibitor in patient plasma following a 2-hour incubation period. **Bodansky u.,** the quantity of phosphatase in 100 ml of serum that will liberate 1 mg of phosphorus as phosphate ion from sodium β-glycerophosphate in 1 hour under standard conditions. **British thermal u.,** a unit of heat, being the amount necessary to raise the temperature of 1 lb. of water from 39° to 40° F; abbreviated B.T.U. **C.G.S. u.,** any unit in the centimeter-gram-second system. **coronary care u.,** a specially designed and equipped hospital area containing a small number of private rooms, with all facilities necessary for constant observation and possible emergency treatment of patients with severe heart disease. **intensive care u.,** a hospital unit in which are concentrated special equipment and skilled personnel for the care of seriously ill patients requiring immediate and continuous attention; abbreviated ICU. **International u.,** a unit of biological material, as of enzymes, hormones, vitamins, etc., established by the International Conference for the Unification of Formulas. **motor u.,** the unit of motor activity formed by a motor nerve cell and its many innervated muscle fibers. **SI u.,** any of the units of the Système International d′Unités (International System of Units) adopted in 1960 at the Eleventh General Conference of Weights and Measures. See accompanying tables. **Somogyi u.,** that amount of amylase which will liberate reducing equivalents equal to 1 mg of glucose per 30 minutes under defined conditions. **Svedberg u.,** a unit equal to 10^{-13} second used for expressing sedimentation coefficients of macromolecules. **toxic u., toxin u.,** the smallest dose of a toxin which will kill a guinea pig weighing about 250 gm in three to four days. **U.S.P. u.,** one used in the United States Pharmacopeia in expressing potency of drugs and other preparations.

United States Pharmacopeia see *U.S.P.*

univalent (u″nĭ-va′lent) having a valence of one.

unmyelinated (un-mi′ĕ-lĭ-na″ted) not having a myelin sheath.

unphysiologic (un″fiz-e-o-loj′ik) not in harmony with the laws of physiology.

unsaturated (un-sach′ur-āt″ed) 1. not holding all of a solute which can be held in solution by the solvent. 2. denoting compounds in which two or more atoms are united by double or triple bonds.

unstriated (-stri′āt-ed) having no striations, as smooth muscle.

uptake (up′tāk) absorption and incorporation of a substance by living tissue.

urachus (ūr′ah-kus) a fetal canal connecting the bladder with the allantois, persisting throughout life as a cord (median umbilical ligament). **u′rachal,** adj.

uracrasia (ūr″ah-kra′ze-ah) disordered state of urine.

uragogue (ūr′ah-gog) diuretic.

uran(o)- word element [Gr.], *palate.*

uraniscus (ūr″ah-nis′kus) the palate.

uranium (u-ra′ne-um) chemical element (*see table*), at. no. 92, symbol U.

uranorrhaphy (ūr″ah-nor′ah-fe) staphylorrhaphy.

uranoschisis (ūr″ah-nos′kĭ-sis) cleft palate.

uranostaphyloschisis (ūr″ah-no-staf″ĭ-los′kĭ-sis) fissure of the soft and hard palates.

urarthritis (ūr″ah-thri′tis) gouty arthritis.

uratoma (ūr″ah-to′mah) a concretion made up of urates; tophus.

uraturia (-tu′re-ah) urates in the urine.

urceiform (er-se′ĭ-form) pitcher-shaped.

urea (u-re′ah) 1. the chief nitrogenous end-product of protein metabolism, formed in the liver from amino acids and from ammonia compounds; found in urine, blood, and lymph. 2. a pharmaceutical preparation of urea occasionally used to lower intracranial or intraocular pressure. **ure′al,** adj. **u. nitrogen,** the urea concentration of serum or plasma, conventionally specified in terms of nitrogen content and called *blood urea nitrogen (BUN);* an important indicator of renal function.

Ureaplasma (u-re′ah-plaz″ma) a genus of nonmotile pleomorphic, gram-negative bacteria, (family Mycoplasmataceae), lacking a cell wall and hydrolyzing urea; *U. urealyt′icum* is associated with nonspecific urethritis in males and genital tract infections in females.

QUANTITY	UNIT	SYMBOL	PRONUNCIATION	DERIVATION
Base Units				
length	meter	m	me'ter	
mass	kilogram	kg	kil'o-gram	
time	second	s	sek'und	
electric current	ampere	A	am'pêr	
temperature	kelvin	K	kel'vin	
luminous intensity	candela	cd	kan-del'ah	
amount of substance	mole	mol	mōl	
Supplementary Units				
plane angle	radian	rad	ra'de-an	
solid angle	steradian	sr	stĕ-ra'de-an	
Derived Units				
force	newton	N	noo'ton	$kg \cdot m/s^2$
pressure	pascal	Pa	pas'kal	N/m^2
energy, work	joule	J	jōōl	$N \cdot m$
power	watt	W	waht	J/s
electric charge	coulomb	C	koo'lom	$A \cdot s$
electric potential	volt	V	volt	J/C
electric capacitance	farad	F	far'ad	C/V
electric resistance	ohm	Ω	ōm	V/A
electric conductance	siemens	S	se'menz	Ω^{-1}
magnetic flux	weber	Wb	web'er	$V \cdot s$
magnetic flux density	tesla	T	tes'la	Wb/m^2
inductance	henry	H	hen're	Wb/A
frequency	hertz	Hz	herts	s^{-1}
luminous flux	lumen	lm	loo'men	$cd \cdot sr$
illumination	lux	lx	luks	lm/m^2
temperature	degree celsius	°C	sel'ze-us	$K - 273.15$
radioactivity	becquerel	Bq	bek-rel'	s^{-1}
absorbed dose	gray	Gy	gra	J/kg
absorbed dose equivalent	sievert	Sv	se'vert	J/kg

PREFIXES FOR SI UNITS

MULTIPLICATION	PREFIX	SYMBOL	PRONUNCIATION
$1\ 000\ 000\ 000\ 000\ 000\ 000\ =\ 10^{18}$	exa	E	ek'sah
$1\ 000\ 000\ 000\ 000\ 000\ =\ 10^{15}$	peta	P	pet'ah
$1\ 000\ 000\ 000\ 000\ =\ 10^{12}$	tera	T	ter'ah
$1\ 000\ 000\ 000\ =\ 10^{9}$	giga	G	jig'ah
$1\ 000\ 000\ =\ 10^{6}$	mega	M	meg'ah
$1\ 000\ =\ 10^{3}$	kilo	k	kil'o
$100\ =\ 10^{2}$	hecto	h	hek'to
$10\ =\ 10$	deka	dk	dek'ah
$0.1\ =\ 10^{-1}$	deci	d	des'ĭ
$0.01\ =\ 10^{-2}$	centi	c	sen'tĭ
$0.001\ =\ 10^{-3}$	milli	m	mil'ĭ
$0.000\ 001\ =\ 10^{-6}$	micro	μ	mi'kro
$0.000\ 000\ 001\ =\ 10^{-9}$	nano	n	na'no
$0.000\ 000\ 000\ 001\ =\ 10^{-12}$	pico	p	pe'ko
$0.000\ 000\ 000\ 000\ 001\ =\ 10^{-15}$	femto	f	fem'to
$0.000\ 000\ 000\ 000\ 000\ 001\ =\ 10^{-18}$	atto	a	at'o

ureapoiesis (u-re″ah-poi-e′sis) formation of urea. **ureapoiet′ic,** adj.

urease (ur′e-ās) an enzyme which catalyzes the decomposition of urea to ammonia and carbon dioxide.

urecchysis (u-rek′ĭ-sis) an effusion of urine into cellular tissue.

uredema (ūr-ĕ-de′mah) swelling from extravasated urine.

urelcosis (ūr″el-ko′sis) ulceration in the urinary tract.

uremia (u-re′me-ah) 1. azotemia; an excess of the nitrogenous end products of protein and amino acid metabolism in the blood. 2. the entire constellation of signs and symptoms of chronic renal failure. **ure′mic,** adj.

uremigenic (u-re″mĭ-jen′ik) 1. caused by uremia. 2. causing uremia.

ureotelic (ūr″e-o-tel′ik) having urea as the chief excretory product of nitrogen metabolism.

uresiesthesis (u-re″se-es-the′sis) the normal impulse to pass the urine.

uresis (u-re′sis) the passage of urine; urination.

-uresis word element [Gr.], *urinary excretion of.* **-uret′ic,** adj.

ureter (u-re′ter) the fibromuscular tube through which urine passes from kidney to bladder. **ure′teral, ureter′ic,** adj.

ureter(o)- word element [Gr.], *ureter.*

ureteralgia (u-re″ter-al′je-ah) pain in the ureter.

ureterectasis (-ek′tah-sis) distention of the ureter.

ureterectomy (-ek′tah-me) excision of a ureter.

ureteritis (-i′tis) inflammation of a ureter.

ureterocele (u-re′ter-o-sēl″) intravesical ballooning of the lower end of the ureter.

ureterocelectomy (u-re″ter-o-se-lek′tah-me) excision of a ureterocele.

ureterocolostomy (-ko-los′tah-me) anastomosis of a ureter to the colon.

ureterocystoscope (-sis′to-skōp) a cystoscope with a catheter for insertion into the ureter.

ureterocystostomy (-sis-tos′tah-me) ureteroneocystostomy.

ureterodialysis (-di-al′ĭ-sis) rupture of a ureter.

ureteroenterostomy (-en″ter-os′tah-me) anastomosis of one or both ureters to the wall of the intestine.

ureterography (u-re″ter-og′rah-fe) roentgenography of the ureter after injection of a contrast medium.

ureteroileostomy (-il″e-os′tah-me) anastomosis of the ureters to an isolated loop of the ileum drained through a stoma on the abdominal wall.

ureterolith (u-re′ter-o-lith″) a calculus in the ureter.

ureterolithiasis (u-re″ter-o-lĭ-thi′ah-sis) formation of a calculus in the ureter.

ureterolithotomy (-lĭ-thot′ah-me) incision of ureter for removal of calculus.

ureterolysis (u-re″ter-ol′ĭ-sis) 1. rupture of the ureter. 2. paralysis of the ureter. 3. the operation of freeing the ureter from adhesions.

ureteroneocystostomy (u-re″ter-o-ne″o-sis-tos′tah-me) surgical transplantation of a ureter to a different site in the bladder.

ureteroneopyelostomy (-pi″ĕ-los′tah-me) ureteropyeloneostomy.

ureteronephrectomy (u-re″ter-o-nĕ-frek′to-me) excision of a kidney and ureter.

ureteropathy (u-re″ter-op′ah-the) any disease of the ureter.

ureteropelvioplasty (u-re″ter-o-pel′ve-o-plas″-te) surgical reconstruction of the junction of the ureter and renal pelvis.

ureteroplasty (u-re′ter-o-plas″te) plastic repair of a ureter.

ureteropyelitis (u-re″ter-o-pi″ĕ-li′tis) inflammation of a ureter and renal pelvis.

ureteropyelography (-pi-ĕ-log′rah-fe) roentgenography of the ureter and renal pelvis.

ureteropyeloneostomy (-pi″ĕ-lo-ne-os′tah-me) surgical creation of a new communication between a ureter and the renal pelvis.

ureteropyelonephritis (-pi″ĕ-lo-nĕ-fri′tis) inflammation of the ureter, renal pelvis, and kidney.

ureteropyeloplasty (-pi′ĕ-lo-plas″te) plastic repair of a ureter and renal pelvis.

ureteropyelostomy (-pi″ĕ-los′tah-me) ureteropyeloneostomy.

ureteropyosis (-pi-o′sis) suppurative inflammation of a ureter.

ureterorenoscope (-re′no-skōp) a fiberoptic endoscope used in ureterorenoscopy.

ureterorenoscopy (-re-nos′ko-pe) visual inspection of the interior of the ureter and kidney by means of a fiberoptic endoscope for such purposes as biopsy or removal or crushing of stones.

ureterorrhagia (-ra′je-ah) discharge of blood from a ureter.

ureterorrhaphy (u-re″ter-or′ah-fe) suture of the ureter.

ureterosigmoidostomy (u-re″ter-o-sig″moid-os′to-me) anastomosis of a ureter to the sigmoid colon.

ureterostomy (u-re″ter-os′tah-me) creation of a new outlet for a ureter.

ureterotomy (-ot′ah-me) incision of a ureter.

ureteroureterostomy (u-re″ter-o-u-re″ter-os′-tah-me) end-to-end anastomosis of the two portions of a transected ureter.

ureterovaginal (-vaj′ĭ-n'l) pertaining to or communicating with a ureter and the vagina.

ureterovesical (-ves′ĭ-k'l) pertaining to a ureter and the bladder.

urethr(o)- word element [Gr.], *urethra.*

urethra (u-re′thrah) the membranous canal through which urine is discharged from the bladder to the exterior of the body. **ure′thral,** adj.

urethralgia (ūr″e-thral′je-ah) pain in the urethra.

urethratresia (u-re″thrah-tre′ze-ah) imperforation of the urethra.

urethrectomy (ūr″e-threk′tah-me) excision of the urethra or a part of it.

urethremphraxis (ūr″e-threm-frak′sis) obstruction of the urethra.

urethrism (u-re′thrizm) irritability or chronic spasm of the urethra.

urethritis (ūr″e-thri′tis) inflammation of the urethra. **u. cys′tica,** inflammation of the urethra with formation of multiple submucosal cysts. **nongonococcal u., nonspecific u.,** urethritis without evidence of gonococcal infection. **u. petrif′icans,** urethritis with formation of calcareous matter in the urethral wall. **simple u.,** nongonococcal u. **specific u.,** that due to gonorrheal infection of the urethra.

urethrobulbar (u-re″thro-bul′ber) pertaining to the urethra and the bulb of the penis.

urethrocele (u-re′thro-sēl) prolapse of the female urethra.

urethrocystitis (u-re″thro-sis-ti′tis) inflammation of the urethra and bladder.

urethrodynia (-din′e-ah) urethralgia.

urethrography (ūr″e-throg′rah-fe) radiography of the urethra.

urethrometry (ūr″e-throm′ĕ-tre) 1. determination of the resistance of various segments of the urethra to retrograde flow of fluid. 2. measurement of the urethra.

urethropenile (u-re″thro-pe′nīl) pertaining to the urethra and penis.

urethroperineal (-per″ĭ-ne′al) pertaining to the urethra and perineum.

urethroperineoscrotal (-per″ĭ-ne″o-skro′t′l) pertaining to the urethra, perineum, and scrotum.

urethropexy (-pek′se) surgical fixation of the urethra to the overlying symphysis pubis and fascia of the rectus abdominis muscle; done to correct stress incontinence in the female.

urethrophraxis (-frak′sis) obstruction of the urethra.

urethrophyma (-fi′mah) a tumor or growth in the urethra.

urethroplasty (u-re′thro-plas″te) plastic repair of the urethra.

urethroprostatic (u-re″thro-pros-tat′ik) pertaining to the urethra and prostate.

urethrorectal (-rek′t′l) pertaining to the urethra and rectum.

urethrorrhagia (-ra′je-ah) flow of blood from the urethra.

urethrorrhaphy (ūr″e-thror′ah-fe) suture of a urethral fistula.

urethrorrhea (u-re″thro-re′ah) abnormal discharge from the urethra.

urethroscope (u-re′thro-skōp) an instrument for viewing the interior of the urethra.

urethroscopy (ūr″e-thros′ko-pe) visual inspection of the urethra. **urethroscop′ic,** adj.

urethrospasm (u-re′thro-spazm) spasm of the urethral muscular tissue.

urethrostaxis (u-re″thro-stak′sis) oozing of blood from the urethra.

urethrostenosis (-stĕ-no′sis) constriction of the urethra.

urethrostomy (ūr″e-thros′tah-me) surgical formation of a permanent opening of the urethra at the perineal surface.

urethrotome (u-re′thro-tōm) an instrument for cutting a urethral stricture.

urethrotomy (ūr″e-throt′ah-me) incision of the urethra.

urethrotrigonitis (u-re″thro-tri″go-ni′tis) inflammation of the urethra and the trigone of the bladder.

urethrovaginal (-vaj′ĭ-n′l) pertaining to the urethra and vagina.

urethrovesical (-ves′ĭ-k′l) pertaining to the urethra and bladder.

urgency (ur′jen-se) the sudden compelling desire to urinate.

urhidrosis (ur″hĭ-dro′sis) the presence in the sweat of urinous materials, chiefly uric acid and urea.

-uria word element [Gr.], *characteristic or constituent of the urine.* **-u′ric,** adj.

uric acid (ūr′ik) the end product of purine metabolism, 2,6,8-trioxypurine. Deposition of urate crystals in the joints and kidneys causes gout.

uricacidemia (ūr″ik-as″ĭ-de′me-ah) hyperuricemia.

uricaciduria (-as″ĭ-du′re-ah) hyperaciduria.

uricemia (ūr″ĭ-se′me-ah) hyperuricemia.

uricometer (ūr″ĭ-kom′ĕ-ter) an instrument for measuring uric acid in the urine.

uricosuria (ūr″ĭ-ko-su′re-ah) excretion of uric acid in the urine.

uricosuric (-su′rik) 1. pertaining to, characterized by, or promoting uricosuria. 2. an agent that promotes uricosuria.

uridine (ūr′ĭ-dēn) a nucleoside containing uracil and ribose. **u. diphosphate (UDP),** a nucleotide that participates in glycogen metabolism and in some processes of nucleic acid synthesis. **u. monophosphate (UMP),** a nucleotide, uridine 5′-phosphate. Called also *uridylic acid.* **u. triphosphate (UTP),** a nucleotide involved in RNA synthesis.

uridylic acid (ūr″i-dil′ik) uridine monophosphate.

uriesthesis (ūr″e-es-the′sis) uresiesthesis.

urin(o)- word element [Gr., L.], *urine.*

urina (u-ri′nah) [L.] urine.

urinal (ūr′ĭ-n′l) a receptacle for urine.

urinalysis (ūr″ĭ-nal′ĭ-sis) analysis of the urine.

urinate (ūr′ĭ-nāt) to void urine.

urination (ūr″ĭ-na′shun) the discharge of urine from the bladder.

urine (ūr′in) the fluid excreted by the kidneys, stored in the bladder, and discharged through the urethra. **u′rinary,** adj. **residual u.,** urine remaining in the bladder after urination.

uriniferous (ūr″ĭ-nif′er-us) transporting or conveying urine.

uriniparous (ūr″ĭ-nip′ah-rus) excreting urine.

urinogenous (ūr″ĭ-noj′ĕ-nus) of urinary origin.

urinoma (ūr″ĭ-no′mah) a cyst containing urine.

urinometer (ūr″ĭ-nom′ĕ-ter) an instrument for determining the specific gravity of urine.

urinometry (ūr″ĭ-nom′ĕ-tre) determination of the specific gravity of urine.

urinous (ūr′ĭ-nus) pertaining to or of the nature of urine.

uro- word element [Gr.], *urine* (urinary tract, urination).

urobilin (ūr″o-bi′lin) a brownish pigment formed by oxidation of urobilinogen.

urobilinemia (-bi″lĭ-ne′me-ah) urobilin in the blood.

urobilinogen (-bi-lin′o-jen) a colorless compound formed in the intestines by reduction of bilirubin.

urocanic acid (ūr″o-kan′ik) an intermediate metabolite of histamine, $C_6H_8N_2O_2$, convertible normally to glutamic acid.

urocele (ūr′o-sēl) distention of the scrotum with extravasated urine.

urochezia (ūr″o-ke′ze-ah) the discharge of urine in the feces.

urochrome (ūr′o-krōm) a breakdown product of hemoglobin related to the bile pigments, found in the urine and responsible for its yellow color.

urocyst (ūr′o-sist) the urinary bladder. **urocys′tic,** adj.

urocystitis (ūr″o-sis-ti′tis) inflammation of the urinary bladder.

urodynamics (-di-nam′iks) the dynamics of the propulsion and flow of urine in the urinary tract. **urodynam′ic,** adj.

urodynia (-din′e-ah) pain on urination.

uroedema (-ĕ-de′mah) edema due to infiltration of urine.

urogastrone (-gas′trōn) a polypeptide secreted by the salivary glands and by Brunner's glands, which is a potent inhibitor of gastric acid secretion.

urogenital (-jen′ĭ-tal) pertaining to the urinary apparatus and genitalia.

urogenous (u-roj′ĕ-nus) 1. producing urine. 2. produced from or in the urine.

urogram (ūr′o-gram) a film obtained by urography.

urography (u-rog′rah-fe) radiography of any part of the urinary tract. **ascending u., cystoscopic u.,** retrograde u. **descending u., excretion u., excretory u., intravenous u.,** urography after intravenous injection of an opaque medium which is rapidly excreted in the urine. **retrograde u.,** urography after injection of a contrast medium into the bladder through the urethra.

urokinase (ūr″o-ki′nās) an enzyme in the urine of man and other mammals; it is elaborated by the parenchymal cells of the human kidney and functions as a plasminogen activator. It is used as a thrombolytic (fibrinolytic) agent.

urolith (ūr′o-lith) a calculus in the urine or the urinary tract. **urolith′ic** adj.

urolithiasis (ūr″o-lĭ-thi′ah-sis) the formation of urinary calculi, or the condition associated with urinary calculi.

urology (u-rol′o-je) the branch of medicine dealing with the urinary system in the female and genitourinary tract in the male. **urolog′ic,** adj.

urometry (u-rom′ĕ-tre) the measurement and recording of pressure changes caused by contraction of the ureter during ureteral peristalsis. **uromet′ric,** adj.

uroncus (u-rong′kus) a swelling caused by retention or extravasation of urine.

uronephrosis (ūr″o-nĕ-fro′sis) distention of the renal pelvis and tubules with urine.

uropathy (u-rop′ah-the) any disease of the urinary tract.

urophanic (ūr″o-fan′ik) appearing in the urine.

uropoiesis (-poi-e′sis) the formation of urine. **uropoiet′ic,** adj.

uroporphyria (-por-fir′e-ah) porphyria with excessive excretion of uroporphyrin.

uroporphyrin (-por′fĭ-rin) one of a group of porphyrins produced during biosynthesis of natural porphyrins and excreted in urine.

uroporphyrinogen (-por″fĭ-rin′o-jen) a precursor of uroporphyrin and coproporphyrinogen.

uropsammus (-sam′us) urinary gravel.

uroradiology (-ra″de-ol′ah-je) radiology of the urinary tract.

urorrhagia (-ra′je-ah) excessive secretion of urine.

urorrhea (-re′ah) involuntary flow of urine.

uroscopy (u-ros′ko-pe) diagnostic examination of the urine. **uroscop′ic,** adj.

urosepsis (ur″o-sep′sis) septic poisoning from retained and absorbed urinary substances. **urosep′tic,** adj.

uroureter (-u-re′ter) distention of the ureter with urine.

urticant (er′tĭ-kant) producing urticaria.

urticaria (er″tĭ-kār′e-ah) hives; a vascular reaction of the upper dermis marked by transient appearance of slightly elevated patches (wheals) which are redder or paler than the surrounding skin and often attended by severe itching; the exciting cause may be certain foods or drugs, infection, or emotional stress. **urticar′ial,** adj. **u. bullo′sa, bullous u.,** that in which bullae are superimposed on the wheals. **cold u.,** urticaria precipitated by cold air, water, or objects, occurring in a hereditary and an acquired form. **giant u., u. gigan′tea,** angioedema. **u. medicamento′sa,** that due to use of a drug. **papular u.,** a hypersensitivity reaction to insect bites, manifested by crops of small papules and wheals, which may become infected or lichenified because of rubbing and excoriation. **u. pigmento′sa,** the most common form of mastocytosis, characterized by small, reddish brown macules or papules that occur mainly on the trunk and tend to urtication upon mild mechanical trauma or chemical irritation.

urtication (er″tĭ-ka′shun) 1. the development or formation of urticaria. 2. a burning sensation as of stinging with nettles.

urushiol (u-roo′she-ol) the toxic irritant principle of poison ivy and various related plants.

USAN United States Adopted Names, non-proprietary designations for compounds used as drugs, established by negotiation between their manufacturers and a council sponsored jointly by the American Medical Association, American Pharmaceutical Association, and United States Pharmacopeial Convention.

U.S.P. United States Pharmacopeia, a legally recognized compendium of standards for drugs, published by the United States Pharmacopeial Convention, Inc., and revised periodically; it also includes assays and tests for determination of strength, quality, and purity.

U.S.P.H.S. United States Public Health Service.

ustilaginism (us′tĭ-laj′ĭ-nizm) a condition resembling ergotism due to ingestion of maize containing *Ustilago maydis*, the corn smut fungus.

uter(o)- word element [L.], *uterus*.

uteralgia (u″ter-al′je-ah) pain in the uterus.

uterine (u′ter-in, u′ter-īn) pertaining to the uterus.

uteroabdominal (u″ter-o-ab-dom′ĭ-n′l) pertaining to the uterus and abdomen.

uterocervical (-ser′vĭ-k′l) pertaining to the uterus and cervix uteri.

uterogestation (-jes-ta′shun) uterine gestation; normal pregnancy.

uterolith (u′ter-o-lith″) hysterolith.

uterometer (u″ter-om′ĕ-ter) hysterometer.

utero-ovarian (u″ter-o-o-va′re-an) pertaining to the uterus and ovary.

uteroplacental (u″ter-o-plah-sen′tal) pertaining to the placenta and uterus.

uteroplasty (u′ter-o-plas″te) any plastic operation on the uterus.

uterorectal (u″ter-o-rek′t′l) pertaining to or communicating with the uterus and rectum.

uterosacral (-sa′kr′l) pertaining to the uterus and sacrum.

uterosclerosis (-sklĕ-ro′sis) sclerosis of the uterus.

uterotonic (u″ter-o-ton′ik) 1. increasing the tone of uterine muscle. 2. a uterotonic agent.

uterotubal (-too′b′l) pertaining to the uterus and oviducts.

uterovaginal (-vaj′ĭ-n′l) pertaining to the uterus and vagina.

uterovesical (-ves′ĭ-k′l) pertaining to the uterus and bladder.

uterus (u′ter-us) the hollow muscular organ in female mammals in which the fertilized ovum normally becomes embedded and in which the developing embryo and fetus is nourished. Its

cavity opens into the vagina below and into a uterine tube on either side. **u. bicor′nis,** one with two cornua. **u. cordifor′mis,** a heart-shaped uterus. **u. du′plex,** a double uterus, normal in marsupials but rarely seen in humans. **gravid u.,** one containing a developing fetus. **u. masculi′nus,** prostatic utricle. **u. unicor′nis,** one with a single cornu.

UTP uridine triphosphate.

utricle (u′tri-k′l) 1. any small sac. 2. the larger of the two divisions of the membranous labyrinth of the internal ear. **prostatic u., urethral u.,** a small blind pouch in the substance of the prostate.

utricular (u-trik′u-ler) 1. pertaining to the utricle. 2. bladderlike.

utriculitis (u-trik″u-li′tis) inflammation of the prostatic utricle or the utricle of the ear.

utriculosaccular (u-trik″u-lo-sak′u-ler) pertaining to utricle and saccule of the labyrinth.

utriculus (u-trik′u-lus) utricle. **u. masculi′nus, u. prostat′icus,** prostatic utricle.

uve(o)- word element, *uvea*.

uvea (u′ve-ah) the iris, ciliary body, and choroid together. **u′veal,** adj.

uveitis (u″ve-i′tis) inflammation of all or part of the uvea. **uveit′ic,** adj. **heterochromic u.,** see under *iridocyclitis*. **sympathetic u.,** see under *ophthalmia*.

uveoscleritis (-skle-ri′tis) scleritis due to extension of uveitis.

uviform (u′vĭ-form) shaped like a grape.

uvula (u′vu-lah), pl. *u′vulae* [L.] a pendant, fleshy mass, specifically the palatine uvula. **u′vular,** adj. **u. of bladder,** u. vesicae. **u. cerebel′li, u. of cerebellum,** u. vermis. **u. palati′na, palatine u.,** the small, fleshy mass hanging from the soft palate above the root of the tongue. **u. ver′mis,** the part of the vermis of the cerebellum between the pyramid and nodule. **u. vesi′cae,** a rounded elevation at the neck of the bladder, formed by convergence of muscle fibers terminating in the urethra.

uvulectomy (u″vu-lek′tah-me) excision of the uvula.

uvulitis (u″vu-li′tis) inflammation of the uvula.

uvuloptosis (u″vu-lop-to′sis) a relaxed, pendulous state of the uvula.

uvulotomy (u″vu-lot′ah-me) the cutting off of the uvula or a part of it.

V

V chemical symbol, *vanadium*.

v. *vein*, or [L.] *vena*; volt.

VAC a regimen of vincristine, dactinomycin, and cyclophosphamide, used in cancer therapy.

vaccigenous (vak-sij′ĕ-nus) producing vaccine.

vaccinal (vak′sĭ-n′l) 1. pertaining to vaccinia, to vaccine, or to vaccination. 2. having protective qualities when used by way of inoculation.

vaccination (vak″sĭ-na′shun) the introduction of vaccine into the body to produce immunity.

vaccine (vak′sēn) a suspension of attenuated or killed microorganisms (viruses, bacteria, or rickettsiae), administered for prevention, amelioration, or treatment of infectious diseases. **attenuated v.,** a vaccine prepared from live microorganisms or viruses cultured under adverse conditions leading to loss of their virulence but retention of their ability to induce protective immunity. **autogenous v.,** a bacterial vaccine prepared from cultures of material derived from a lesion of the patient to be treated. **BCG v.,** a preparation used as an active immunizing agent against tuberculosis and in cancer immunotherapy, especially against malignant melanoma, consisting of a dried, living, avirulent culture of the Calmette-Guérin strain of *Mycobacterium bovis.* **cholera v.,** a preparation of killed *vibrio cholerae,* used in immunization against cholera. **heterologous v.,** a vaccine that confers protective immunity against a pathogen that shares cross-reacting antigens with the microorganisms in the vaccine, e.g., vaccinia virus protects against smallpox. **influenza virus v.,** a killed virus vaccine used in immunization against influenza; usually bivalent or trivalent, containing one or two influenza A virus strains and one influenza B virus strain. **live v.,** a vaccine prepared from live microorganisms or viruses that have been attenuated but that retain their immunogenic properties. **measles, mumps, and rubella virus v. live,** a combination of the live measles, mumps, and rubella vaccines. **measles and rubella virus v. live,** a combination of live measles and rubella vaccines. **measles virus v. live,** a live attenuated virus vaccine used for immunization against measles; children are usually immunized with measles-mumps-rubella (MMR) combination vaccine. **mumps virus v. live,** a live attenuated virus vaccine used in immunization against mumps; children are usually immunized with measles-mumps-rubella (MMR) combination vaccine. **mixed v.,** polyvalent v. **pertussis v.,** a preparation of killed *Bordetella pertussis* bacilli, used to immunize against whooping cough; generally used in combination with diphtheria and tetanus toxoids (DTP). **plague v.,** a preparation of killed *Yersinia pestis* bacilli, used as an active immunizing agent. **poliovirus v., attenuated,** a suspension of formalin-inactivated polioviruses (*Salk v.*) used for immunization against poliomyelitis. **poliovirus v. live oral,** a preparation of one or a combination of the three types of live, attenuated polioviruses (*Sabin oral v.*) used as an active immunizing agent. **polyvalent v.,** a vaccine prepared from more than one strain or species of microorganisms. **rabies v.,** a killed virus vaccine used for preexposure immunization against rabies and, together with rabies immune globulin, for postexposure prophylaxis. **replicative v.,** any vaccine containing organisms that are able to reproduce, including live and attenuated viruses and bacteria. **rubella and mumps v., live,** a combination of live rubella and mumps vaccines. **rubella virus v., live,** a live attenuated virus vaccine used for immunization against rubella; children are usually immunized with measles-mumps-rubella (MMR) combination vaccine. **Sabin oral v.,** see *poliovirus v., live oral.* **Salk v.,** see *poliovirus v., attenuated.* **smallpox v.,** a live vaccinia virus vaccine, grown by various methods, used to produce immunity to smallpox. **subunit v.,** a vaccine produced from specific protein subunits of a virus and thus having less risk of adverse reactions than whole virus vaccines. **tuberculosis v.,** BCG v. **typhoid v.,** a killed bacteria vaccine used for immunization against typhoid fever. **yellow fever v.,** a preparation of attenuated yellow fever virus, used to immunize against yellow fever.

vaccinia (vak-sin′e-ah) the cutaneous and sometimes systemic reactions associated with vaccination with smallpox vaccine (cf. *cowpox*). **vaccin′ial,** adj. **v. gangreno′sa,** progressive v. **generalized v.,** a usually self-limited skin eruption resembling smallpox, sometimes occurring after primary smallpox vaccination, caused by transient viremia. **progressive v.,** a rare but often fatal complication of smallpox vaccination in those with deficient immune mechanisms or receiving immunosuppressive therapy, marked by tissue necrosis that spreads from the inoculation site, which may result in vaccinial metastasis to the skin, bones, and viscera.

vacciniform (vak-sin′ĭ-form) resembling vaccinia.

vacuolar (vak′u-o″lar) containing, or of the nature of, vacuoles.

vacuolated (vak′u-ah-lāt″ed) containing vacuoles.

vacuolation (vak″u-ah-la′shun) the process of forming vacuoles; the condition of being vacuolated.

vacuole (vak′u-ōl) a space or cavity in the protoplasm of a cell.

vagal (va′gal) pertaining to the vagus nerve.

vagina (vah-ji′nah) 1. a sheath or sheathlike structure. 2. the canal in the female, from the vulva to the cervix uteri, that receives the penis in copulation. **vag′inal,** adj.

vaginitis (vaj″ĭ-nah-li′tis) inflammation of the tunica vaginalis testis.

vaginate (vaj′ĭ-nāt) enclosed in a sheath.

vaginectomy (vaj″ĭ-nek′to-me) excision of the vagina.

vaginismus (vaj″ĭ-niz′mus) painful spasm of the vagina due to involuntary muscular contraction severe enough to prevent intercourse; the cause may be organic or psychogenic.

vaginitis (vaj″ĭ-ni′tis) 1. inflammation of the vagina. 2. inflammation of a sheath. **adhesive v.,** see *atrophic v.* **atrophic v.,** vaginitis with tissue atrophy occurring in postmenopausal women and associated with estrogen deficiency. **desquamative inflammatory v.,** a form resembling atrophic vaginitis but affecting women with normal estrogen levels. **emphysematous v.,** inflammation of the vagina and adjacent cervix, characterized by numerous, asymptomatic, gas-filled cystlike lesions. **senile v.,** atrophic v.

vaginoabdominal (vaj″ĭ-no-ab-dom′ĭ-nal) pertaining to the vagina and abdomen.

vaginocele (vaj′ĭ-no-sēl″) 1. hernia into the vagina. 2. prolapse of the vagina.

vaginodynia (vaj″ĭ-no-din′e-ah) colpodynia.

vaginofixation (-fik-sa′shun) suture of the vagina to the abdominal wall.

vaginolabial (-la′be-al) pertaining to the vagina and labia.

vaginomycosis (-mi-ko′sis) any fungal disease of the vagina.

vaginopathy (vaj″ĭ-nop′ah-the) any disease of the vagina.

vaginoperineal (vaj″ĭ-no-per″ĭ-ne′al) pertaining to the vagina and perineum.

vaginoperineorrhaphy (-per″ĭ-ne-or′ah-fe) suture repair of the vagina and perineum.

vaginoperineotomy (-per″ĭ-ne-ot′o-me) paravaginal incision.

vaginoperitoneal (-per″ĭ-to-ne′al) pertaining to the vagina and peritoneum.

vaginopexy (vah-ji′no-pek″se) vaginofixation.

vaginoplasty (-plas″te) colpoplasty.

vaginoscopy (vaj″ĭ-nos′ko-pe) colposcopy.

vaginotomy (vaj″ĭ-not′ah-me) colpotomy.

vaginovesical (vaj″ĭ-no-ves′ĭ-k'l) pertaining to the vagina and bladder.

vagitus (vah-ji′tus) [L.] the cry of an infant. **v. uteri′nus,** the cry of an infant in the uterus.

vagolysis (va-gol′ĭ-sis) surgical destruction of the vagus nerve.

vagolytic (va″go-lit′ik) having an effect resembling that produced by interruption of impulses transmitted by the vagus nerve.

vagomimetic (-mi-met′ik) having an effect resembling that produced by stimulation of the vagus nerve.

vagotomy (va-got′o-me) interruption of the impulses carried by the vagus nerve or nerves. **highly selective v.,** division of only those vagal fibers supplying the acid-secreting glands of the stomach, with preservation of those supplying the antrum as well as the hepatic and celiac branches. **medical v.,** that accomplished by administration of suitable drugs. **parietal cell v.,** selective severing of the vagus nerve fibers supplying the proximal two-thirds (parietal area) of the stomach; done for duodenal ulcer. **selec-**

tive v., division of the vagal fibers to the stomach with preservation of the hepatic and celiac branches. **surgical v.,** transection of the vagus nerve by surgical means. **truncal v.,** surgical division of the two main trunks of the abdominal vagus nerve.

vagotonia (va″go-to′ne-ah) hyperexcitability of the vagus nerve, characterized by vasomotor instability, sweating, constipation, and involuntary motor spasms with pain. **vagoton′ic,** adj.

vagotropic (va″go-trop′ik) having an effect on the vagus nerve.

vagovagal (-va′gal) arising as a result of afferent and efferent impulses mediated through the vagus nerve.

vagus (va′gus), pl. *va′gi* [L.] the vagus nerve; see *Table of Nerves.*

valence (va′lens) 1. a positive number that represents the number of bonds that each atom of an element makes in a chemical compound; now replaced the concept "oxidation number." 2. in immunology, the number of antigen binding sites possessed by an antibody molecule.

valgus (val′gus) [L.] bent out, twisted; denoting a deformity in which the angulation is away from the midline of the body, as in talipes valgus. The meanings of valgus and varus are often reversed.

valine (va′lēn) a naturally occurring amino acid, essential for human metabolism.

valinemia (val″ĭ-ne′me-ah) hypervalinemia.

Valisone (val′ĭ-sōn) trademark for preparations of betamethasone valerate.

Valium (val′e-um) trademark for a preparation of diazepam.

vallate (val′āt) having a wall or rim; cup-shaped.

vallecula (vah-lek′u-lah), pl. *vallec′ulae* [L.] a depression or furrow. **vallec′ular,** adj. **v. cerebel′li,** the longitudinal fissure on the inferior cerebellum, in which the medulla oblongata rests. **v. syl′vii,** a depression made by the fissure of Sylvius at base of the brain. **v. un′guis,** the sulcus of the matrix of the nail.

valproic acid (val-pro′ik) an anticonvulsant, 2-propylpentanoic acid, used for the control of absence seizures.

value (val′u) a measure of worth or efficiency; a quantitative measurement of the activity, concentration, etc., of specific substances. **normal v's,** the range in concentration of specific substances found in normal healthy tissues, secretions, etc. **reference v's,** a set of values of a quantity measured in the clinical laboratory that characterize a specified population in a defined state of health.

valva (val′vah), pl. *val′vae* [L.] a valve.

valve (valv) a membranous fold in a canal or passage that prevents backward flow of material passing through it. **aortic v.,** that guarding the entrance to the aorta from the left ventricle. **atrioventricular v's,** the valves between the right atrium and right ventricle (tricuspid v.) and the left atrium and left ventricle (mitral v.). **Béraud's v.,** a fold at the beginning of the nasolacrimal duct. **bicuspid v.,** mitral v. **caged-ball v.,** a heart valve prosthesis consisting of a sewing ring attached to a cage composed of struts that contains a free-floating ball. **cardiac v's,** those controlling the flow of blood through and from the heart. **cardiac v., artificial,** a substitute, mechanical or composed of tissue, for a cardiac valve. **coronary v.,** that at the entrance of the coronary sinus into the right atrium. **flair v.,** a cardiac valve having a cusp that has lost its normal support (as in ruptured chordae tendineae) and flutters in the blood stream. **Houston's v.,** the middle one of three transverse folds of the rectum. **ileocecal v., ileocolic v.,** that guarding the opening between the ileum and cecum. **mitral v.,** that between the left atrium and left ventricle, usually having two cusps (anterior and posterior). **pulmonary v.,** that at the entrance of the pulmonary trunk from the right ventricle. **pyloric v.,** a prominent fold of mucous membrane at the pyloric orifice of the stomach. **semilunar v.,** one having semilunar cusps, i.e., the aortic and pulmonary valves; sometimes used to designate the semilunar cusps composing these valves. **thebesian v.,** coronary v. **tilting disk v.,** a heart valve prosthesis consisting of a sewing ring and a valve housing containing a suspended disk that swings between open and closed positions. **tricuspid v.,** that guarding the opening between the right atrium and right ventricle. **ureteral v.,** a congenital transverse fold across the lumen of the ureter, composed of redundant mucosa made prominent by circular muscle fibers; it usually disappears in time but may rarely cause urinary obstruction.

valvotomy (val-vot′ah-me) incision of a valve.

valvula (val′vu-lah), pl. *vul′vulae* [L.] a small valve.

valvular (val′vu-ler) pertaining to, affecting, or of the nature of a valve.

valvulitis (val-vu-li′tis) inflammation of a valve, especially a heart valve.

valvuloplasty (val′vu-lo-plas″te) plastic repair of a valve, especially a heart valve.

valvulotome (-tōm) an instrument for cutting a valve.

vanadium (vah-na′de-um) chemical element (*see table*), at. no. 23, symbol V. Its salts have been used in treating various diseases. Absorption of its compounds, usually via the lungs, causes chronic intoxication, the symptoms of which include respiratory tract irritation, pneumonitis, conjunctivitis, and anemia.

vancomycin (van″ko-mi′sin) an antibiotic produced by *Streptomyces orientalis,* highly effective against gram-positive bacteria, especially against staphylococci; used as the hydrochloride salt.

vanillism (vah-nil′izm) dermatitis, coryza, and malaise seen in raw vanilla handlers, due to the mite *Acarus siro.*

vanillylmandelic acid (vah-nil″il-man-del′ik) an excretory product of the catecholamines, used as a test for epinephrine metabolism.

vaporization (va″por-ĭ-za′shun) 1. the conversion of a solid or liquid into a vapor without chemical change; distillation. 2. treatment by vapors; vapotherapy.

vapotherapy (va″po-ther′ah-pe) therapeutic use of vapor, steam, or spray.

variation (var″e-a′shun) the act or process of changing; in genetics, deviation in characters in an individual from the group to which it belongs or deviation in characters of the offspring from those of its parents. **antigenic v.,** a mechanism by which parasites can escape the immune surveillance of a host by modifying or completely altering their surface antigens. **microbial v.,** the range of characteristics within a species used in identification and differentiation. **phenotypic v.,** the total variation, for whatever cause, observed in one character.

varic(o)- word element [L.], *varix; swollen.*

varication (var″ĭ-ka′shun) 1. the formation of a varix. 2. a varicose condition; a varicosity.

variceal (var″ĭ-se′al) of or pertaining to a varix.

varicella (var″ĭ-sel′ah) chickenpox.

varicelliform (var″i-sel′ĭ-form) resembling varicella.

varices (văr′ĭ-sēz) [L.] plural of *varix.*

variciform (vah-ris′ĭ-form) resembling a varix; varicose.

varicoblepharon (var″ĭ-ko-blef′ah-ron) a varicose swelling of the eyelid.

varicocele (var′ĭ-ko-sēl) varicosity of the pampiniform plexus of the spermatic cord, forming a scrotal swelling that feels like a "bag of worms."

varicocelectomy (var″ĭ-ko-se-lek′tah-me) ligation and excision of the enlarged veins for varicocele.

varicography (var″ĭ-kog′rah-fe) x-ray visualization of varicose veins.

varicomphalus (var″ĭ-kom′fah-lus) a varicose tumor of the umbilicus.

varicophlebitis (var″ĭ-ko-flĕ-bi′tis) varicose veins with inflammation.

varicose (var′ĭ-kōs) of the nature of or pertaining to a varix; unnaturally and permanently distended (said of a vein); variciform.

varicosity (var″ĭ-kos′ĭ-te) 1. a varicose condition; the quality or fact of being varicose. 2. a varix, or varicose vein.

varicotomy (var″ĭ-kot′ah-me) excision of a varix or of a varicose vein.

varicula (vah-rik′u-lah) a varix of the conjunctiva.

variety (vah-ri′ĕ-te) in taxonomy, a subcategory of a species.

variola (vah-ri′o-lah) smallpox. **vari′olar, vari′olous,** adj.

variolate (var′e-o-lāt) 1. having the nature or appearance of smallpox. 2. to inoculate with smallpox virus.

varioliform (va″re-o′lĭ-form) resembling smallpox.

varix (văr′iks), pl. *var′ices* [L.] an enlarged tortuous vein, artery, or lymphatic vessel. **aneurysmal v.,** a markedly dilated tortuous vessel. **arterial v.,** a racemose aneurysm or varicose artery. **esophageal varices,** varicosities of branches of the azygos vein which anastomose with tributaries of the portal vein in the lower esophagus, due to portal hypertension in cirrhosis of the liver. **lymph v., v. lymphat'icus,** a soft, lobulated swelling of a lymph node, due to obstruction of lymphatic vessels.

varolian (vah-ro'le-an) pertaining to the pons varolii.

varus (var'us) [L.] bent inward; denoting a deformity in which the angulation of the part is toward the midline of the body, as in talipes varus. The meanings of *varus* and *valgus* are often reversed.

vas (vas), pl. *va'sa* [L.] a vessel. **va'sal,** adj. **v. aber'rans,** 1. a blind tubule sometimes connected with the epididymus; a vestigial mesonephric tubule. 2. any anomalous or unusual vessel. **va'sa afferen'tia,** vessels that convey fluid to a structure or part. **va'sa bre'via,** short gastric arteries. **v. capilla're,** a capillary. **v. def'erens,** ductus deferens. **va'sa efferen'tia,** vessels that convey fluid away from a structure or part. **v. lymphat'icum,** lymphatic vessels. **va'sa prae'via,** presentation, in front of the fetal head during labor, of the blood vessels of the umbilical cord where they enter the placenta. **va'sa rec'ta,** long U-shaped vessels arising from the efferent glomerular arterioles of juxtamedullary nephrons and supplying the renal medulla. **va'sa vaso'rum,** the small nutrient arteries and veins in the walls of the larger blood vessels. **va'sa vortico'sa,** vorticose veins.

vas(o)- word element [L.], *vessel; duct.*

vascular (vas'ku-ler) pertaining to blood vessels or indicative of a copious blood supply.

vascularization (vas''ku-ler-ĭ-za'shun) the formation of new blood vessels in tissues.

vasculature (vas'ku-lah-chur) the vascular system of the body, or any part of it.

vasculitis (vas''ku-li'tis) inflammation of a vessel; angiitis. **vasculit'ic,** adj.

vasculogenic (vas''ku-lo-jen'ik) inducing vascularization.

vasculopathy (vas''ku-lop'ah-the) any disorder of blood vessels.

vasectomy (vah-sek'tah-me) excision of the vas (ductus) deferens, or a portion of it.

vasiform (vas'ĭ-form) resembling a vessel.

vasitis (vah-si'tis) inflammation of the vas (ductus) deferens.

vasoactive (vas''o-ak'tiv) exerting an effect on the caliber of blood vessels.

vasoconstriction (-kon-strik'shun) decrease in the caliber of blood vessels. **vasoconstric'tive,** adj.

vasodepression (-de-presh'un) decrease in vascular resistance with hypotension.

vasodepressor (-de-pres'sor) 1. having the effect of lowering the blood pressure through reduction in peripheral resistance. 2. an agent that causes vasodepression.

Vasodilan (-di'lan) trademark for a preparation of isoxsuprine.

vasodilatation (-dil''ah-ta'shun) a state of increased caliber of the blood vessels. **vasodi'lative,** adj.

vasodilation (-di-la'shun) increase in the caliber of blood vessels.

vasodilator (-di-la'ter) 1. causing dilatation of blood vessels. 2. a nerve or agent which causes dilatation of blood vessels.

vasoepididymography (-ep''ĭ-did''ĭ-mog'rah-fe) radiography of the vas deferens and epididymis after injection of a contrast medium.

vasoepididymostomy (-ep''ĭ-did''ĭ-mos'tah-me) anastomosis of the vas (ductus) deferens and the epididymis.

vasoformative (-for'mah-tive) pertaining to or promoting the formation of blood vessels.

vasoganglion (-gang'gle-on) a vascular ganglion or rete.

vasography (vas-og''rah-fe) radiography of the blood vessels.

vasohypertonic (vas''o-hi''per-ton'ik) vasoconstrictor.

vasohypotonic (-hi''po-ton'ik) vasodilator.

vasoinhibitor (-in-hib'ĭ-ter) an agent which inhibits vasomotor nerves. **vasoinhib'itory,** adj.

vasoligation (-li-ga'shun) ligation of the vas (ductus) deferens.

vasomotor (-mo'tor) 1. affecting the caliber of blood vessels. 2. a vasomotor agent or nerve.

vasoneuropathy (-noo-rop'ah-the) a condition caused by combined vascular and neurologic defect.

vasoneurosis (-noo-ro'sis) angioneuropathy.

vaso-orchidostomy (-or''kĭ-dos'tah-me) anastomosis of the epididymis to the severed end of the vas (ductus) deferens.

vasoparesis (-pah-re'sis) partial paralysis of vasomotor nerves.

vasopermeability (-per''me-ah-bil'ĭ-te) the extent to which a blood vessel is permeable.

vasopressin (-pres'in) a hormone secreted by cells of the hypothalamic nuclei and stored in the posterior pituitary for release as necessary; it constricts blood vessels, raising the blood pressure, and increases peristalsis, exerts some influence on the uterus, and influences resorption of water by the kidney tubules, resulting in concentration of urine. Also prepared synthetically or obtained from the posterior pituitary of domestic animals; used as an antidiuretic.

vasopressor (-pres'er) 1. stimulating contraction of the muscular tissue of the capillaries and arteries. 2. a vasopressor agent.

vasopuncture (-pungk'chur) puncture of the vas (ductus) deferens.

vasoreflex (-re'fleks) a reflex of blood vessels.

vasorelaxation (-re''lak-sa'shun) decrease of vascular pressure.

vasorrhaphy (vah-sor'ah-fe) suture of the vas (ductus) deferens.

vasosection (vas''o-sek'shun) resection of the ductus (vas) deferens.

vasosensory (-sen'sor-e) supplying sensory filaments to the vessels.

vasospasm (vas'o-spazm) spasm of blood vessels, decreasing their caliber. **vasospas'tic,** adj.

vasostimulant (vas''o-stim'u-lant) stimulating vasomotor action.

vasostomy (vah-sos'tah-me) surgical formation of an opening into the ductus (vas) deferens.

vasotomy (vah-sot′ah-me) incision of the vas (ductus) deferens.

vasotonia (vas″o-to′ne-ah) tone or tension of the vessels. **vasoton′ic,** adj.

vasotrophic (-trof′ik) affecting nutrition through alteration of blood vessel caliber.

vasotropic (-trop′ik) tending to act on blood vessels.

vasovagal (-va′gal) vascular and vagal; see also under *attack.*

vasovasostomy (vas″o-vah-sos′tah-me) anastomosis of the ends of the severed vas (ductus) deferens.

vasovesiculectomy (-vĕ-sik″u-lek′to-me) excision of the vas (ductus) deferens and seminal vesicles.

vastus (vas′tus) [L.] great; describes muscles.

VC vital capacity.

VCG vector cardiogram.

V-Cillin (ve-sil′in) trademark for a preparation of penicillin V.

V.D. venereal disease.

V.D.H. valvular disease of the heart.

V.D.R.L. Venereal Disease Research Laboratory.

vection (vek′shun) the carrying of disease germs from an infected person to a well person.

vectis (vek′tis) a curved lever for making traction on the fetal head in labor.

vector (vek′ter) 1. a carrier, especially the animal (usually an arthropod) that transfers an infective agent from one host to another. 2. a plasmid or viral chromosome into whose genome a fragment of foreign DNA is inserted; used to introduce foreign DNA into a host cell in the cloning of DNA. 3. a quantity possessing magnitude, direction, and sense (positivity or negativity). **vecto′rial,** adj. **biological v.,** an arthropod vector in whose body the infecting organism develops or multiplies before becoming infective to the recipient individual. **mechanical v.,** an arthropod vector which transmits an infective organism from one host to another but which is not essential to the life cycle of the parasite.

vectorcardiogram (vek″ter-kar′de-o-gram″) the record, usually a photograph, of the loop formed on the oscilloscope in vectorcardiography.

vectorcardiography (-kar″de-og′rah-fe) the registration, usually by formation of a loop display on an oscilloscope, of the direction and magnitude (vector) of the moment-to-moment electromotive forces of the heart during one complete cycle. **vectorcardiograph′ic,** adj.

vectorscope (vek′ter-skōp) a device utilized in viewing vectorcardiograms.

vegan (vej′an, ve′gan) a vegetarian who excludes from the diet all protein of animal origin.

vegetarian (vej″ĕ-tar′e-an) one who eats only foods of vegetable origin.

vegetation (vej″ĕ-ta′shun) any plantlike fungoid neoplasm or growth; a luxuriant fungus-like growth of pathologic tissue.

vegetative (vej″ĕ-ta″tiv) 1. concerned with growth and nutrition. 2. functioning involun-

tarily or unconsciously. 3. resting; denoting the portion of a cell cycle during which the cell is not replicating. 4. of, pertaining to, or characteristic of plants. 5. of or pertaining to asexual reproduction, as by budding or fission.

vehicle (ve′ĭ-k′l) 1. an excipient. 2. any medium through which an impulse is propagated.

veil (vāl) 1. a covering structure. 2. a caul or piece of amniotic sac occasionally covering the face of a newborn child. 3. slight huskiness of the voice.

Veillonella (va″yon-el′ah) a genus of gram-negative bacteria (family Veillonellaceae), found as nonpathogenic parasites in the mouth, intestines, and urogenital and respiratory tracts of man and other animals.

vein (vān) a vessel in which blood flows toward the heart, in the systemic circulation carrying blood that has given up most of its oxygen. For names of veins of the body, *see the table,* and see Plates VIII and IX. **accompanying v.,** a vein that closely follows the artery of the same name, occurring especially in the extremities. **afferent v's,** veins that carry blood to an organ. **allantoic v's,** paired vessels that accompany the allantois, growing out from the primitive hindgut and entering the body stalk of the early embryo. **cardinal v's,** embryonic vessels that include the precardinal and postcardinal veins and the ducts of Cuvier (*common cardinal v's*). **emissary v.,** one passing through a foramen of the skull and draining blood from a cerebral sinus into a vessel outside the skull. **postcardinal v's,** paired vessels in the early embryo caudal to the heart. **precardinal v's,** paired venous trunks in the embryo cranial to the heart. **pulp v's,** vessels draining the venous sinuses of the spleen. **subcardinal v's,** paired vessels in the embryo, replacing the postcardinal veins and persisting to some degree as definitive vessels. **sublobular v's,** tributaries of the hepatic veins that receive the central veins of hepatic lobules. **supracardinal v's,** paired vessels in the embryo, developing later than the subcardinal veins and persisting chiefly as the lower segment of the inferior vena cava. **trabecular v's,** vessels coursing in splenic trabeculae, formed by tributary pulp veins. **varicose v.,** a dilated, tortuous vein, usually in the subcutaneous tissues of the leg; incompetency of the venous valve is associated. **vesalian v.,** an emissary vein connecting the cavernous sinus with the pterygoid venous plexus. **vitelline v's,** veins that return the blood from the yolk sac to the primitive heart of the early embryo.

velamen (ve-la′men), pl. *velam′ina* [L.] a membrane, meninx, or velum.

velamentous (vel″ah-men′tus) membranous and pendent; like a veil.

vellus (vel′us) the fine hair that succeeds the lanugo over most of the body.

velopharyngeal (vel″o-fah-rin′je-al) pertaining to the soft palate and pharynx.

velum (ve′lum), pl. *ve′la* [L.] a covering structure or veil. **ve′lar,** adj. **v. interpos′itum,** membranous roof of the third ventricle. **medullary v.,** one of the two portions (*rostral medullary v.* and *caudal medullary v.*) of the white substance

COMMON NAME*	NA TERM†	REGION*	RECEIVES BLOOD FROM*	DRAINS INTO*
accompanying v. of hypoglossal nerve	v. comitans nervi hypoglossi	accompanies hypoglossal nerve	formed by union of profunda linguae v. and sublingual v.	facial, lingual, or internal jugular v's
adrenal v's. See suprarenal v., left and right.				
anastomotic v., inferior	v. anastomotica inferior	interconnects superficial middle cerebral v. and transverse sinus		
anastomotic v., superior	v. anastomotica superior	interconnects superficial middle cerebral v. and superior sagittal sinus		
angular v.	v. angularis	between eye and root of nose	formed by union of supratrochlear v. and supraorbital v.	continues inferiorly as facial v.
antebrachial v., median	v. intermedia antebrachii	forearm between cephalic v. and basilic v.		cephalic v. and/or basilic v., or median cubital v.
appendicular v.	v. appendicularis	accompanies appendicular artery	a palmar venous plexus	joins anterior and posterior cecal v's to form ileocolic v.
v. of aqueduct of cochlea	v. aqueductus cochleae	along aqueduct of cochlea	cochlea	superior bulb of internal jugular v.
v. of aqueduct of vestibule	v. aqueductus vestibuli	passes through aqueduct of vestibule	internal ear	superior petrosal sinus
arcuate v's of kidney	vv. arcuatae renis	a series of complete arches across the bases of the renal pyramids, formed by union of interlobular v's and straight venules of kidney		interlobar v's
articular v's	vv. articulares		plexus around temporomandibular joint	retromandibular v.
atrial v., lateral	v. lateralis atrii	passes through lateral wall of lateral ventricle	temporal and parietal lobes	superior thalamostriate v.
atrial v., medial	v. medialis atrii	passes through medial wall of lateral ventricle	parietal and occipital lobes	internal cerebral or great cerebral v.
auditory v's, internal. See labyrinthine v's				
auricular v's, anterior	vv. auriculares anteriores	anterior part of auricle		superficial temporal v.
auricular v., posterior	v. auricularis posterior	passes down behind auricle	a plexus on side of head	joins retromandibular v. to form external jugular v.
axillary v.	v. axillaris	the upper limb	formed at lower border of teres major muscle by junction of basilic v. and brachial v.	continuous with subclavian v. at lateral border of first rib

azygos v.	v. azygos	intercepting trunk for right intercostal v's as well as connecting branch between superior and inferior venae cavae; ascends in front of and on right side of vertebrae	ascending lumbar v.	superior vena cava
azygos v., left. See hemiazygos v.				
azygos v., lesser superior. See hemiazygos v., accessory.				
basal v.	v. basalis	passes from anterior perforated substance backward and around cerebral peduncle	anterior perforated substance	internal cerebral v.
basilic v.	v. basilica	forearm, superficially	ulnar side of dorsal rete of hand	joins brachial v's to form axillary v.
basilic v., median	v. intermedia basilica	sometimes present as medial branch of a bifurcation of median antebrachial v.		basilic v.
basivertebral v's	vv. basivertebrales		venous sinuses in cancellous tissue of bodies of vertebrae, which communicate with venous plexus on anterior surface of vertebrae and with external and internal vertebral plexuses	
brachial v's	vv. brachiales	accompany brachial artery		joins basilic v. to form axillary v.
brachiocephalic v's	vv. brachiocephalicae (dextra/sinistra)	thorax	head, neck, and upper limbs; formed at root of neck by union of ipsilateral internal jugular and subclavian v's	unite to form superior vena cava
bronchial v's	vv. bronchiales		larger subdivisions of bronchii	azygos v. on left; hemiazygos or superior intercostal v. on right
v of bulb of penis	v. bulbi penis		bulb of penis	internal pudendal v.
v. of bulb of vestibule	v. bulbi vestibuli		bulb of vestibule of vagina	internal pudendal v.
cardiac v's, anterior	vv. cardiacae anteriores		anterior wall of right ventricle	right atrium of heart or lesser cardiac v.
cardiac v., great	v. cardiaca magna		anterior surface of ventricles	coronary sinus
cardiac v., middle	v. cardiaca media		diaphragmatic surface of ventricles	coronary sinus
cardiac v., small	v. cardiaca parva		right atrium and ventricle	coronary sinus

*v. = vein; v's = (pl.) veins.
†v. = vena; vv. = [L.(pl.)] venae.

COMMON NAME*	NA TERM†	REGION*	RECEIVES BLOOD FROM*	DRAINS INTO*
cardiac v's, smallest	vv. cardiacae minimae	numerous small veins arising in myocardium, draining independently into cavities of heart and most readily seen in the atria		
carotid v., external. See retromandibular v.				
cavernous v's of penis	vv. cavernosae penis		corpora cavernosa	deep v's and dorsal v. of penis
central v's of liver	vv. centrales hepatis	in middle of hepatic lobules	liver substance	hepatic v.
central v. of retina	v. centralis retinae	eyeball	retinal v's	superior ophthalmic v.
central v. of suprarenal gland	v. centralis glandulae suprarenalis	the large single vein into which the various veins within the substance of the gland empty, and which continues at the hilum as the suprarenal v.		
cephalic v.	v. cephalica	winds anteriorly to pass along anterior border of brachioradial muscle; above elbow, ascends along lateral border of biceps of deltoid muscle	radial side of dorsal rete of hand	axillary v.
cephalic v., accessory	v. cephalica accessoria	forearm	dorsal rete of hand	joins cephalic v. just above elbow
cephalic v., median	v. intermedia cephalica	sometimes present as lateral branch formed by bifurcation of median antebrachial v.		cephalic v.
cerebellar v's, inferior	vv. cerebelli		inferior surface of cerebellum	transverse, sigmoid, and inferior petrosal sinuses, or occipital sinus
cerebellar v's, superior			superior surface of cerebellum	straight sinus and great cerebral v., or transverse and superior petrosal sinuses
v's of cerebellar hemisphere, inferior	vv. inferirores hemispherii cerebelli		inferior surface of cerebellum	transverse, sigmoid, superior petrosal sinuses, or into occipital sinus
v's of cerebellar hemisphere, superior	vv. superiores hemispherii cerebelli		superior surfaces of cerebellum	transverse or superior petrosal sinuses
cerebral v's, anterior	vv. anteriores cerebri	accompany anterior cerebral artery		basal v.
cerebral v., great	v. magna cerebri	curves around splenium of corpus callosum	formed by union of the 2 internal cerebral veins	continues as or drains into straight sinus
cerebral v's, inferior	vv. inferiores cerebri	veins that ramify on base and inferolateral surface of frontal lobe draining into inferior sagittal sinus and cavenous sinus; those on temporal lobe into superior petrosal sinus and transverse sinus; and those on occipital lobe into straight sinus		

cerebral v's, internal (2)	vv. internae cerebri	pass backward from interventricular foramen through tela choroidea	formed by union of thalamostriate v. and choroid v.; collect blood from basal nuclei	unite at splenium or corpus callosum to form great cerebral v.
cerebral v., middle, deep	v. media profunda cerebri	accompanies middle cerebral artery in floor of lateral sulcus	lateral surface of cerebrum	basal v.
cerebral v's, middle, superficial	vv. cerebri superficiales mediae	follow lateral cerebral fissure		cavernous sinus
cerebral v's, superior	vv. superiores cerebri	8–12 veins draining superolateral and medial surfaces of cerebrum toward longitudinal fissure		superior sagittal sinus
cervical v., deep	v. cervicalis profunda	accompanies deep cervical artery down neck	a plexus in suboccipital triangle	vertebral v. of brachiocephalic v.
cervical v's, transverse	vv. transversae cervicis	accompanies transverse cervical artery		subclavian v.
choroid v., inferior	v. choroidea inferior	runs whole length of choroid plexus	inferior choroid plexus	basal v.
choroid v., superior	v. choroidea superior		choroid plexus, hippocampus, fornix, corpus callosum	joins superior thalamostriate v. to form internal cerebral v.
ciliary v's	vv. ciliares	anterior vessels follow anterior ciliary arteries; posterior follow posterior ciliary arteries	arise in eyeball by branches from ciliary muscle; anterior ciliary v's also receive branches from sinus venosus, sclerae, episcleral v's and conjunctiva of eyeball	superior ophthalmic v.; posterior ciliary v's empty also into inferior ophthalmic v.
circumflex femoral v's, lateral	vv. circumflexae laterales femoris	accompany lateral circumflex femoral artery		femoral v. or profunda femoris v.
circumflex femoral v's, medial	vv. circumflexae mediales femoris	accompany medial circumflex femoral artery		femoral v. or profunda femoris v.
circumflex iliac v., deep	v. circumflexa ilium profunda	a common trunk formed by veins accompanying deep circumflex iliac artery		external iliac v.
circumflex iliac v., superficial	v. circumflexa superficialis ilium	accompanies superficial circumflex iliac artery		great saphenous v.
v. of cochlear canal. See v. of aqueduct of cochlea.				
colic v., left	v. colica sinistra	accompanies left colic artery		inferior mesenteric v.
colic v., middle	v. colica media	accompanies middle colic artery		superior mesenteric v.
colic v., right	v. colica dextra	accompanies right colic artery		superior mesenteric v.
conjunctival v's	vv. conjunctivales		conjunctiva	superior ophthalmic v.

635

TABLE OF VEINS

COMMON NAME*	NA TERM†	REGION*	RECEIVES BLOOD FROM*	DRAINS INTO*
coronary v's. *See* entries under cardiac v's.				
v. of corpus callosum, posterior	v. posterior corporis callosi		posterior surface of corpus callosum	great cerebral v.
cubital v., median	v. intermedia cubiti	passes obliquely upward across cubital fossa	cephalic v., below elbow	basilic v.
cutaneous v.	v. cutanea	one of the small veins that begin in papillae of skin, form subpapillary plexuses, and open into the subcutaneous veins		
cystic v.	v. cystica	within substance of liver	gallbladder	right branch of portal v.
deep v's of clitoris	vv. profundae clitoridis		clitoris	vesical venous plexus
deep v's of penis	vv. profundae penis	accompany deep artery of penis	penis	dorsal v. of penis
digital v's of foot, dorsal	vv. digitales dorsales pedis	dorsal surfaces of toes		unite at clefts to form dorsal metatarsal v's
digital v's, palmar	vv. digitales palmares	accompany proper and common palmar digital arteries		superficial palmar venous arch
digital v's, plantar	vv. digitales plantares	plantar surfaces of toes		unite at clefts to form plantar metatarsal v's
diploic v., frontal	v. diploica frontalis		frontal bone	supraorbital v. externally, or superior sagittal sinus internally
diploic v., occipital	v. diploica occipitalis		occipital bone	occipital v. of transverse sinus
diploic v., temporal, anterior	v. diploica temporalis anterior		lateral portion of frontal bone, anterior part of parietal bone	sphenoparietal sinus internally, or a deep temporal v. externally
diploic v., temporal, posterior	v. diploica temporalis posterior		parietal bone	transverse sinus
direct v's, lateral	vv. directae laterales		lateral ventricle	great cerebral v.
dorsal v. of clitoris, deep	v. dorsalis profunda clitoridis			vesical plexus
dorsal v's of clitoris, superficial	vv. dorsales superficiales clitoridis	accompanies dorsal artery of clitoris	clitoris, subcutaneously	external pudendal v.
dorsal v. of corpus callosum	v. dorsalis corporis callosi		superior surface of corpus callosum	great cerebral vein
dorsal v. of penis, deep	v. dorsalis profunda penis	the single median vein lying subfascially in penis between the dorsal arteries; it begins in small veins around corona of glans, is joined by deep veins of penis as it passes proximally, and passes between arcuate pubic and transverse perineal ligaments, where it divides into a left and a right vein to join prostatic plexus		
dorsal v's of penis, superficial	vv. dorsales superficiales penis		penis, subcutaneously	external pudendal v.

636

dorsal v's, of tongue. *See* lingual v's, dorsal		
emissary v., condylar v. emissaria condyloidea	a small vein running through condylar canal of skull connecting sigmoid sinus with vertebral v. or internal jugular v.	
emissary v., mastoid v. emissaria mastoidea	a small vein passing through mastoid foramen of skull, connecting sigmoid sinus with occipital v. or posterior auricular v.	
emissary v., occipital v. emissaria occipitalis	an occasional small vein running through a minute foramen in occipital protuberance of skull, connecting confluence of sinuses with occipital v.	
emissary v., parietal v. emissaria parietalis	a small vein passing through parietal foramen of skull, connecting superior sagittal sinus with superficial temporal v's	
epigastric v., inferior v. epigastrica inferior	accompanies inferior epigastric artery	external iliac v.
epigastric v., superficial v. epigastrica superficialis	accompanies superficial epigastric artery	great saphenous v. or femoral v.
epigastric v's, superior vv. epigastricae superiores	accompany superior epigastric artery	internal thoracic v.
episcleral v's vv. episclerales	around cornea	vorticose v's and ciliary v's
esophageal v's vv. oesophageales	esophagus	hemiazygos v. and azygos v., or left brachiocephalic v.
ethmoidal v's vv. ethmoidales	accompany anterior and posterior ethmoidal arteries and emerge from ethmoidal foramina	superior ophthalmic v.
facial v. v. facialis	the vein beginning at medial angle of eye as angular v., descending behind facial artery, and usually ending in internal jugular v.; sometimes joins retromandibular v. to form a common trunk	
facial v., deep v. profunda faciei	pterygoid plexus	facial v.
facial v., posterior. *See* retromandibular v.		
facial v., transverse v. transversa faciei	passes backward with transverse facial artery just below zygomatic arch	retromandibular v.
femoral v. v. femoralis	follows course of femoral artery in proximal two thirds of thigh	at inguinal ligament becomes external iliac v.
femoral v., deep v. profunda femoris	accompanies deep femoral artery	femoral v.
fibular v's. *See* peroneal v's		
gastric v., left v. gastrica sinistra	accompanies left gastric artery	portal v.

637

TABLE OF VEINS

COMMON NAME*	NA TERM†	REGION*	RECEIVES BLOOD FROM*	DRAINS INTO*
gastric v., right	v. gastrica dextra	accompanies right gastric artery		portal v.
gastric v's, short	vv. gastricae breves		left portion of greater curvature of stomach	splenic v.
gastroepiploic v., left. See gastro-omental v., left.				
gastroepiploic v., right. See gastro-omental v., right.				
gastro-omental v., left	v. gastro-omentalis sinistra	accompanies left gastro-omental artery		splenic v.
gastro-omental v., right	v. gastro-omentalis dextra	accompanies right gastro-omental artery		superior mesenteric v.
genicular v's	vv. geniculares	accompany genicular arteries		popliteal v.
gluteal v's, inferior	vv. gluteae inferiores	accompany inferior gluteal artery; unite into a single vessel after passing through greater sciatic foramen	subcutaneous tissue of back of thigh, muscles of buttock	internal iliac v.
gluteal v's, superior	vv. gluteae superiores	accompany superior gluteal artery and pass through greater sciatic foramen	muscles of buttock	internal iliac v.
hemiazygos v.	v. hemiazygos	an intercepting trunk for lower left posterior intercostal v's; ascends on left side of vertebrae to eighth thoracic vertebra, where it may receive accessory branch, and crosses vertebral column	ascending lumbar v.	azygos v.
hemiazygos v., accessory	v. hemiazygos accessoria	the descending intercepting trunk for upper, often fourth through eighth, left posterior intercostal v's; it lies on left side and at eighth thoracic vertebra joins hemiazygos v. or crosses to right side to join azygos v. directly; above, it may communicate with left superior intercostal v.		
hemorrhoidal v's. See entries under rectal v's				
hepatic v's	vv. hepaticae	2 or 3 large veins in an upper group and 6 to 20 small veins in a lower group, forming successively larger vessels	central v's of liver	inferior vena cava on posterior aspect of liver
hypogastric v. See iliac v., internal.				

638

ileal v's		
ileocolic v.	accompanies ileocolic artery	ileum
iliac v., common	ascends to right side of fifth lumbar vertebra	superior mesenteric v.
		superior mesenteric v.
		unites with fellow of opposite side to form inferior vena cava
	arises at sacroiliac joint by union of external and internal iliac v's	
iliac v., external	extends from inguinal ligament to sacroiliac joint	joins internal iliac v. to form common iliac v.
	continuation of femoral v.	
iliac v. internal	extends from greater sciatic notch to brim of pelvis	joins external iliac v. to form common iliac v.
iliolumbar v.	accompanies iliolumbar artery	formed by union of parietal branches
		internal iliac v. and/or common iliac v.
innominate v's. See brachiocephalic v's		
insular v's		
vv. insulares	veins at clefts of fingers that pass between metacarpal bones and establish communication between dorsal and palmar venous systems of hand	insula
intercapitular v's		deep middle cerebral v.
vv. intercapitulares manus		
intercostal v's, anterior (12 pairs)	accompany anterior thoracic arteries	
vv. intercostales anteriores		
intercostal v., highest	first posterior intercostal veins of either side, which passes over apex of lung	internal thoracic v's
v. intercostalis suprema		brachiocephalic, vertebral, or superior intercostal v.
intercostal v's, posterior	accompany posterior intercostal arteries	
vv. intercostales posteriores		brachiocephalic or vertebral v., superior intercostal v., azygos v. on right; hemiazygos or accessory hemiazygos v. on left
intercostal v., superior, left	crosses arch of aorta	intercostal spaces
v. intercostalis superior sinistra		left brachiocephalic v.
intercostal v., superior, right		formed by union of second, third, and sometimes fourth posterior intercostal v's
v. intercostalis superior dextra		azygos v.
		formed by union of second, third, and sometimes fourth posterior intercostal v's
interlobar v's of kidney	pass down between renal pyramids	
vv. interlobares renis		unite to form renal v.
interlobular v's of kidney		venous arcades of kidney
vv. interlobulares renis	venous arcades of kidney	
interlobular v's of liver	arise between hepatic lobules	capillary network of renal cortex
vv. interlobulares hepatis		venous arcades of kidney
		liver
		portal v.
interosseous v's of foot, dorsal. See metatarsal v's, dorsal.		

COMMON NAME*	NA TERM†	REGION*	RECEIVES BLOOD FROM*	DRAINS INTO*
intervertebral v.	v. intervertebralis	vertebral column	vertebral venous plexuses	in neck, vertebral v.; in thorax, intercostal v's; in abdomen, lumbar v's; in pelvis, lateral sacral v's
jejunal v's	vv. jejunales		jejunum	superior mesenteric v.
jugular v., anterior	v. jugularis anterior	arises under chin and passes down neck		external jugular v. or subclavian v., or jugular venous arch
jugular v., external	v. jugularis externa	begins in parotid gland behind angle of jaw and passes down neck	formed by union of retromandibular v. and posterior auricular v.	subclavian v., internal jugular v., or brachiocephalic v.
jugular v., internal	v. jugularis interna	from jugular fossa, descends in neck with internal carotid artery and then with common carotid artery	begins as superior bulb, draining much of head and neck	joins subclavian v. to form brachiocephalic v.
labial v's, anterior	vv. labiales anteriores		anterior aspect of labia in female	external pudendal v.
labial v's, inferior	vv. labiales inferiores		region of lower lip	facial v.
labial v's, posterior	vv. labiales posteriores		labia in female	vesical venous plexus
labial v., superior	v. labialis superior		region of upper lip	facial v.
labyrinthine v's	vv. labyrinthi	pass through internal acoustic meatus	cochlea	inferior petrosal sinus or transverse sinus
lacrimal v.	lacrimalis		lacrimal gland	superior ophthalmic v.
laryngeal v., inferior	v. laryngea inferior		larynx	inferior thyroid v.
laryngeal v., superior	v. laryngea superior		larynx	superior thyroid v.
lingual v.	v. lingualis			internal jugular v.
lingual v., deep	v. profunda linguae	a deep vein following distribution of lingual artery	deep aspect of tongue	joins sublingual v. to form accompnaying v. of hypoglossal nerve
lingual v's, dorsal	vv. dorsales linguae	veins that unite with a small vein accompanying lingual artery and join main lingual trunk		
lumbar v's	vv. lumbales	4 or 5 v's on each side accompanying corresponding lumbar arteries and draining posterior wall of abdomen, vertebral canal, spinal cord, and meninges; first four usually end in inferior vena cava, although first may end in ascending lumbar v.; fifth is generally a tributary of common iliac v.		
lumbar v., ascending	v. lumbalis ascendens	an ascending intercepting vein for lumbar v's on either side; it begins in lateral sacral region and ascends to first lumbar vertebra, where by union with subcostal v. it becomes on right side the azygos v. and on left the hemiazygos v.		

maxillary v's	vv. maxillares	usually form a single short trunk with pterygoid plexus		join superficial temporal v. in parotid gland to form retromandibular v.
mediastinal v's	vv. mediastinales		anterior mediastinum	brachiocephalic v's, azygos v., or superior vena cava
v's of medulla oblongata	vv. medullae oblongatae		medulla oblongata	v's of spinal cord, dura venous sinuses, inferior petrosal sinus, superior bulb of jugular v.
meningeal v's	vv. meningeae	accompanying meningeal arteries	dura mater (also communicate with lateral lacunae)	regional sinuses and veins
meningeal v's, middle	vv. meningeae mediae	accompany middle meningeal artery		pterygoid venous plexus
mesenteric v., inferior	v. mesenterica inferior	follows distribution of inferior mesenteric artery		splenic v.
mesenteric v., superior	v. mesenterica superior	follows distribution of superior mesenteric artery		joins splenic v. to form portal v.
metacarpal v's dorsal	vv. metacarpales dorsales	veins arising from union of dorsal veins of adjacent fingers and passing proximally to join in forming dorsal venous network of hand		
metacarpal v's, palmar	vv. metacarpales palmares	accompany palmar metacarpal arteries		deep palmar venous arch
metatarsal v's, dorsal	vv. metatarsales dorsales		arise from dorsal digital v's of toes at clefts of toes	dorsal venous arch
metatarsal v's, plantar	vv. metatarsales plantares	deep veins of foot	arise from plantar digital v's at clefts of toes	plantar venous arch
musculophrenic v's	vv. musculophrenicae	accompany musculophrenic artery	parts of diaphragm and wall of thorax and abdomen	internal thoracic v's
nasal v's, external	vv. nasales externae	small ascending branches from nose		angular v., facial v.
nasofrontal v.	v. nasofrontalis		supraorbital v.	superior ophthalmic v.
oblique v. of left atrium	v. obliqua atrii sinistri	left atrium of heart		coronary sinus
obturator v's	vv. obturatoriae	enter pelvis through obturator canal	hip joint and regional muscles	internal iliac v. and/or inferior epigastric v.
occipital v.	v. occipitalis	scalp; follows distribution of occipital artery		opens under trapezius muscle into suboccipital venous plexus, or accompanies occipital artery to end in internal jugular v.

COMMON NAME*	NA TERM†	REGION*	RECEIVES BLOOD FROM*	DRAINS INTO*
ophthalmic v., inferior	v. ophthalmica inferior	a vein formed by confluence of muscular and ciliary branches, and running backward either to join superior ophthalmic v. or to open directly into cavernous sinus; it sends a communicating branch through inferior orbital fissure to joint pterygoid venous plexus		
ophthalmic v., superior	v. ophthalmica superior	a vein beginning at medial angle of eye, where it communicates with frontal, supraorbital, and angular v's; it follows distribution of ophthalmic artery, and may be joined by inferior ophthalmic v. at superior orbital fissure before opening into cavernous sinus		
ovarian v., left	v. ovarica sinistra		pampiniform plexus of broad ligament on the left	left renal v.
ovarian v., right	v. ovarica dextra		pampiniform plexus of broad ligament on the right	inferior vena cava
palatine v., external	v. palatina externa		tonsils and soft palate	facial v.
palpebral v's, inferior	vv. palpebrales inferiores	small branches from eyelids	lower eyelid	superior ophthalmic v.; facial v.
palpebral v's, superior	vv. palpebrales superiores		upper eyelid	angular v.
pancreatic v's	vv. pancreaticae		pancreas	splenic v., superior mesenteric v.
pancreaticoduodenal v's	vv. pancreaticoduodenales	4 veins that drain blood from pancreas and duodenum, closely following pancreaticoduodenal arteries, a superior and an inferior vein originating from an anterior and a posterior venous arcade; anterior superior v. joins right gastro-omental v., and posterior superior v. joins portal v.; anterior and posterior inferior v's join, sometimes as one trunk, uppermost jejunal v. or superior mesenteric v.		
paraumbilical v's	vv. paraumbilicales	veins that communicate with portal v. above and descend to anterior abdominal wall to anastomose with superior and inferior epigastric and superior vesical v's in region of umbilicus; they form a significant part of collateral circulation of portal v. in event of hepatic obstruction		
parotid v's	vv. parotideae		parotid gland	superficial temporal v.
perforating v's	vv. perforantes	empty into deep femoral v. and establish anastomosis between deep femoral v. and popliteal v. (below) and inferior gluteal v. (above)		
pericardiac v's	vv. pericardiales		pericardium	brachiocephalic, inferior thyroid, and azygos v's, superior vena cava
pericardiacophrenic v's	vv. pericardiacophrenicae		pericardium and diaphragm	left brachiocephalic v.

peroneal v's	vv. fibulares	accompany peroneal artery	posterior tibial v.
petrosal v.	v. petrosa	a short trunk arising from union of 4 or 5 cerebellar and pontine v's opposite middle cerebellar peduncle	superior petrosal sinuses
pharyngeal v's	vv. pharyngeales	pharyngeal plexus	internal jugular v.
phrenic v's, inferior	vv. phrenicae inferiores	accompany inferior phrenic arteries	on right, enters inferior vena cava; on left, enters left suprarenal or renal v., or inferior vena cava
phrenic v's, superior. *See* pericardiacophrenic v's.			
pontine v's	vv. pontis	pons	basal v., cerebellar v's, petrosal or venous sinuses, or venous plexus of foramen ovale
pontomesencephalic v., anterior	v. pontomesencephalica anterior	lies on superior and anterior aspects of pons in midline of interpeduncular fossa; interconnects basal v. and petrosal v.	
popliteal v.	v. poplitea	follows popliteal artery; formed by union of anterior and posterior tibial v's	at adductor hiatus becomes femoral v.
portal v.	v. portae hepatis	a short, thick trunk formed by union of superior mesenteric and splenic v's behind neck of pancreas; it ascends to right end of porta hepatis, where it divides into successively smaller branches, following branches of hepatic artery, until it forms a capillary-like system of sinusoids that permeates entire substance of liver	
posterior v. of left ventricle	v. posterior ventriculi sinistri cordis	posterior surface of left ventricle	coronary sinus
precentral v. of cerebellum	v. precentralis cerebelli	arises in precentral cerebellar fissure and passes anterior and superior to culmen	great cerebral v.
prepyloric v.	v. prepylorica	accompanies prepyloric artery, passing upward over anterior surface of junction between pylorus and duodenum	right gastric v.
profunda femoris v. *See* femoral v., deep.			
profunda linguae v. *See* lingual v., deep.			
v. of pterygoid canal	v. canalis pterygoidei	passes through pterygoid canal	pterygoid plexus
pudendal v's, external	vv. pudendae externae	follow distribution of external pudendal artery	great saphenous v.
pudendal v., internal	v. pudenda interna	follows course of internal pudendal artery	internal iliac v.

COMMON NAME*	NA TERM†	REGION*	RECEIVES BLOOD FROM*	DRAINS INTO*
pulmonary v., inferior, left	v. pulmonalis sinistra inferior		lower lobe of left lung	left atrium of heart
pulmonary v., inferior, right	v. pulmonalis dextra inferior		lower lobe of right lung	left atrium of heart
pulmonary v., superior, left	v. pulmonalis sinistra superior		upper lobe of left lung	left atrium of heart
pulmonary v., superior, right	v. pulmonalis dextra superior		upper and middle lobes of right lung	left atrium of heart
pyloric v. *See* gastric v., right. radial v's		accompany radial artery		brachial v's
ranine v. *See* sublingual v. rectal v's, inferior	vv. rectales inferiores		rectal plexus	internal pudendal v.
rectal v's, middle	vv. rectales mediae		rectal plexus	internal iliac and superior rectal v's
rectal v., superior	v. rectalis superior	establishes connection between portal and systemic systems	upper part of rectal plexus	inferior mesenteric v.
retromandibular v.	v. retromandibularis	the vein formed in upper part of parotid gland behind neck of mandible by union of maxillary and superficial temporal v's; it passes downward through the gland, communicates with facial v. and, emerging from the gland, joins with posterior auricular v. to form external jugular v.		
sacral v's, lateral	vv. sacrales laterales	follow lateral sacral arteries		help form lateral sacral plexus; empty into internal iliac v. or superior gluteal v's
sacral v., median	v. sacralis mediana	follows median sacral artery		common iliac v.
saphenous v., accessory	v. saphena accessoria		when present, medial and posterior superficial parts of thigh	great saphenous v.
saphenous v., great	v. saphena magna	extends from dorsum of foot to just below inguinal ligament		femoral v.
saphenous v., small	v. saphena parva	from behind ankle passes up back of leg to knee		popliteal v.
scleral v's	vv. sclerales		sclera	anterior ciliary v's
scrotal v's, anterior	vv. scrotales anteriores		anterior aspect of scrotum	external pudendal v.
scrotal v's, posterior	vv. scrotales posteriores		scrotum	vesical venous plexus
v. of septum pellucidum, anterior	v. anterior septi pellucidi		anterior septum pellucidum	superior thalamostriate v.
v. of septum pellucidum, posterior	v. posterior septi pellucidi		septum pellucidum	superior thalamostriate v.
sigmoid v's	vv. sigmoideae		sigmoid colon	inferior mesenteric v.

644

English name	NA term (Latin)	Description / course	Drains into / continues
spinal v's, anterior and posterior	vv. spinales anteriores/posteriores	anastomosing networks of small veins that drain blood from spinal cord and its pia mater into internal vertebral venous plexuses	
spiral v. of modiolus	v. spiralis modioli	modiolus	labyrinthine v's
splenic v.	v. splenica	passes from left to right of neck of pancreas; formed by union of several branches at hilus of spleen	joins superior mesenteric v. to form portal v.
stellate v's of kidney	venulae stellatae renis	superficial parts of renal cortex	interlobular v's of kidney
sternocleidomastoid v.	v. sternocleidomastoidea	follows course of sternocleidomastoid artery	internal jugular v.
striate v's	vv. striatae		
stylomastoid v.	v. stylomastoidea	follows stylomastoid artery	retromandibular v.
subclavian v.	v. subclavia	follows subclavian artery; continues axillary v. as main venous channel of upper limb	joins internal jugular v. to form brachiocephalic v.
subcostal v.	v. subcostalis	accompanies subcostal artery	joins ascending lumbar v. to form azygos v. on right, hemiazygos v. on left
subcutaneous v's of abdomen	vv. subcutaneae abdominis	superficial layers of abdominal wall	
sublingual v.	v. sublingualis	follows sublingual artery	lingual v.
submental v.	v. submentalis	follows submental artery	facial v.
supraorbital v.	v. supraorbitalis	passes down forehead lateral to supratrochlear v.	joins supratrocheal v. at root of nose to form angular v.
suprarenal v., left	v. suprarenalis sinistra	left adrenal gland	left renal v.
suprarenal v., right	v. suprarenalis dextra	right adrenal gland	inferior vena cava
suprascapular v.	v. suprascapularis	accompanies suprascapular artery (sometimes as 2 veins that unite)	usually into external jugular v., occasionally into subclavian v.
supratrochlear v's (2)	vv. supratrochleares	venous plexuses high up on forehead	joins supraorbital v. at root of nose to form angular v.
temporal v's, deep	vv. temporales profundae	deep portions of temporal muscle	pterygoid plexus
temporal v., middle	v. temporalis media	arises in substance of temporal muscle; descends deep to fascia to zygoma	joins superficial temporal v.
temporal v's, superficial	vv. temporales superficiales	veins that drain lateral part of scalp in frontal and parietal regions, the branches forming a single superficial temporal v. in front of ear, just above zygoma; this descending vein receives middle temporal and transverse facial v's and, entering parotid gland, unites with maxillary v. deep to neck of mandible to form retromandibular v.	
testicular v., left	v. testicularis sinistra	left pampiniform plexus	left renal v.
testicular v., right	v. testicularis dextra	right pampiniform plexus	inferior vena cava

TABLE OF VEINS

COMMON NAME*	NA TERM†	REGION*	RECEIVES BLOOD FROM*	DRAINS INTO*
thalamostriate v's, inferior	vv. thalamostriatae inferiores		anterior perforated substance of brain	joins deep middle cerebral and anterior cerebral v's to form basal v.
thalamostriate v., superior	v. thalamostriata superior		corpus striatum and thalamus	joins choroid v. to form internal cerebral v.
thoracic v's, internal	vv. thoracicae internae	2 veins formed by junction of the veins accompanying internal thoracic artery of either side; each continues along the artery to open into brachiocephalic v.		
thoracic v., lateral	v. thoracica lateralis	accompanies lateral thoracic artery		axillary v.
thoracoacromial v.	v. thoracoacromialis	follows thoracoacromial artery		subclavian v.
thoracoepigastric v's	vv. thoracoepigastricae	long, longitudinal, superficial veins in anterolateral subcutaneous tissue of trunk		superiorly into lateral thoracic v.; inferiorly into femoral v.
thymic v's	vv. thymicae		thymus	left brachiocephalic v.
thyroid v., inferior	v. thyroidea inferior	either of 2 veins, left and right, that drain thyroid plexus into left and right brachiocephalic v's; occasionally they may unite into a common trunk to empty, usually into left brachiocephalic v.		
thyroid v's, middle	vv. thyroideae mediae	arises from side of upper part of thyroid gland	thyroid gland	internal jugular v.
thyroid v., superior	v. thyroidea superior		thyroid gland	internal jugular v., occasionally in common with facial v.
tibial v's, anterior	vv. tibiales anteriores	accompany anterior tibial artery		join posterior tibial v's to form popliteal v.
tibial v's, posterior	vv. tibiales posteriores	accompany posterior tibial artery		join anterior tibial v's to form popliteal v.
tracheal v's	vv. tracheales		trachea	brachiocephalic v.
tympanic v's	vv. tympanicae	small veins from midde ear that pass through petrotympanic fissure and open into the plexus around temporomandibular joint		retromandibular v.
ulnar v's	vv. ulnares	accompany ulnar artery		join radial v's at elbow to form brachial v's
umbilical v.	v. umbilicalis (formerly)	in the early embryo, either of the paired veins that carry blood from chorion to sinus venosus and heart; they later fuse and become left umbilical v. of fetus		
umbilical v. of fetus, left	v. umbilicalis sinistra	the vein formed by fusion of atrophied right umbilical v. with the left umbilical v., which carries all the blood from placenta to ductus venosus		
v. of uncus	v. unci		uncus	ipilateral inferior cerebral v.
uterine v's	vv. uterinae		uterine plexus	internal iliac v.

646

vena cava, inferior	vena cava inferior	the venous trunk for the lower limbs and for pelvic and abdominal viscera; it begins at level of fifth lumbar vertebra by union of common iliac v's and ascends on right of aorta	right atrium of heart
vena cava, superior	vena cava superior	the venous trunk draining blood from head, neck, upper limbs, and thorax; it begins by union of 2 brachiocephalic v's and passes directly downward	right atrium of heart
ventricular v., inferior	v. ventricularis inferior	temporal lobe	basal v.
v. of vermis, inferior	v. inferior vermis	runs backward on inferior vermis	straight sinus or one of the sigmoid sinuses
v. of vermis, superior	v. superior vermis	runs forward and medially across superior vermis	great cerebral v.
vertebral v.	v. vertebralis	passes with vertebral artery through foramina of transverse processes of upper 6 cervical vertebrae	suboccipital venous plexus
vertebral v., accessory	v. vertebralis accessoria	when present, a plexus formed by vertebral v. around vertebral artery	brachiocephalic v.
vertebral v., anterior	v. vertebralis anterior	a v. that descends with vertebral v., emerging through transverse foramen of seventh cervical vertebra	brachiocephalic v.
vorticose veins (4)	vv. vorticosae	accompanies ascending cervical artery	vertebral v.
		venous plexus adjacent to more cranial cervical transverse processes	superior ophthalmic v.
		pierce sclera	choroid

that form the roof of the fourth ventricle. **v. palati'num,** soft palate.

vena (ve'nah), pl. *ve'nae* [L.] vein. **v. ca'va,** see *Table of Veins.*

venacavogram (ve''nah-ka'vo-gram) a film obtained by venacavography.

venacavography (ve''nah-ka-vog'rah-fe) radiography of a vena cava, usually the inferior vena cava.

vene-, veni-, ven(o)- word element [L.], *vein.*

venectasia (ve''nek-ta'ze-ah) phlebectasia.

venectomy (ve-nek'to-me) phlebectomy.

venereal (vĕ-nēr'e-al) due to or propagated by sexual intercourse.

venereologist (vĕ-nēr''e-ol'o-jist) a specialist in venereology.

venereology (vĕ-nēr''e-ol'o-je) the study and treatment of venereal diseases.

venesection (ven''ĕ-sek'shun) phlebotomy.

venipuncture (ven''ĭ-pungk'chur) surgical puncture of a vein.

venisuture (-su'chur) phleborrhaphy.

venography (ve-nog'rah-fe) phlebography.

venom (ven'om) poison, especially a toxic substance normally secreted by a serpent, insect, or other animal.

venomotor (ve''no-mo'ter) controlling dilation of constriction of the veins.

veno-occlusive (ve''no-ŏ-kloo'siv) characterized by obstruction of the veins.

venoperitoneostomy (-per''ĭ-to''ne-os'tah-me) anastomosis of the saphenous vein with the peritoneum for drainage of ascites.

venopressor (-pres'er) 1. pertaining to venous blood pressure. 2. an agent that causes venous constriction.

venosclerosis (-sklĕ-ro'sis) phlebosclerosis.

venosity (ve-nos'ĭ-te) 1. excess of venous blood in a part. 2. a plentiful supply of blood vessels or of venous blood.

venostasis (ve''no-sta'sis) retardation of the venous outflow in a part; see *phlebostasis.*

venotomy (ve-not'ah-me) phlebotomy.

venous (ve'nus) pertaining to the veins.

venovenostomy (ve''no-ve-nos'tah-me) phlebophlebostomy.

vent (vent) an opening or outlet, such as an opening that discharges pus, or the anus.

venter (ven'ter), pl. *ven'tres* [L.] 1. any belly-shaped part; a fleshy contractile part of a muscle. 2. the abdomen or stomach. 3. a hollowed part or cavity.

ventilation (ven''tĭ-la'shun) 1. the process or act of supplying a house or room continuously with fresh air. 2. the process of exchange of air between the lungs and the ambient air. 3. in psychiatry, verbalization of one's emotional problems. **alveolar v.,** the amount of gas expelled from the alveoli to the outside of the body per minute. **mechanical v.,** ventilation accomplished by extrinsic means. **minute v.,** the total amount of gas (in liters) expelled from the lungs per minute.

ventilator (ven'tĭ-la-tor) an apparatus designed to qualify the air breathed through it or to assist or control pulmonary ventilation, either intermittently or continuously.

ventrad (ven'trad) toward a belly, venter, or ventral aspect.

ventral (ven'tral) 1. pertaining to the abdomen or to any venter. 2. directed toward or situated on the belly surface; opposite of dorsal.

ventralis (ven-tra'lis) [L.] ventral.

ventri-, ventr(o)- word element [L.], *belly; front (anterior) aspect of the body; ventral aspect.*

ventricle (ven'trĭ-k'l) a small cavity or chamber, as in the brain or heart. **ventric'ular,** adj.

v. of Arantius, 1. the rhomboid fossa, especially its lower end. 2. fifth v. **fifth v.,** the median cleft between the two laminae of the septum pellucidum. **fourth v.,** a median cavity in the hindbrain, containing cerebrospinal fluid. **v. of larynx,** the space between the true and false vocal cords. **lateral v.,** the cavity in each cerebral hemisphere, derived from the cavity of the embryonic tube, containing cerebrospinal fluid. **left v.,** the lower chamber of the left side of the heart, which pumps oxygenated blood out through the aorta to all the tissues of the body. **Morgagni's v.,** v. of larynx. **pineal v.,** an extension of the third ventricle into the stalk of the pineal body. **right v.,** the lower chamber of the right side of the heart, which pumps venous blood through the pulmonary trunk and arteries to the capillaries of the lung. **third v.,** a narrow cleft below the corpus callosum, within the diencephalon between the two thalami. **Verga's v.,** an occasional space between the corpus callosum and fornix.

ventricornu (ven''trĭ-kor'nu) the anterior horn of gray matter in the spinal cord. **ventricor'nual,** adj.

ventricul(o)- word element [L.], *ventricle (of heart or brain).*

ventriculitis (ven-trik''u-li'tis) inflammation of a ventricle, especially a cerebral ventricle.

ventriculoatriostomy (ven-trik''u-lo-a''tre-os'-tah-me) ventriculoatrial shunt.

ventriculocisternostomy (-sis''ter-nos'tah-me) surgical creation of a communication between the third ventricle and the interpeduncular cistern, for drainage of cerebrospinal fluid.

ventriculography (ven-trik''u-log'rah-fe) 1. radiography of the cerebral ventricles after introduction of air or other contrast medium. 2. radiography of a ventricle of the heart after injection of a contrast medium.

ventriculometry (ven-trik''u-lom'ĕ-tre) measurement of intracranial pressure.

ventriculopuncture (ven-trik''u-lo-pungk'-chur) surgical puncture of a lateral ventricle of the brain.

ventriculoscopy (ven-trik''u-los'kah-pe) endoscopic or cystoscopic examination of cerebral ventricles.

ventriculostomy (ven-trik''u-los'tah-me) surgical creation of a free communication between the third ventricle and the interpeduncular cistern for relief of hydrocephalus.

ventriculosubarachnoid (ven-trik''u-lo-sub''-ah-rak'noid) pertaining to the cerebral ventricles and subarachnoid space.

ventriculotomy (ven-trik″u-lot′ah-me) incision of a ventricle of the brain or heart.

ventriculus (ven-trik′u-lus), pl. *ventric′uli* [L.] 1. a ventricle. 2. the stomach.

ventriduct (ven′trĭ-dukt) to bring or carry ventrad.

ventrofixation (ven″tro-fik-sa′shun) fixation of a viscus, e.g., the uterus, to the abdominal wall.

ventrohysteropexy (-his′ter-o-pek″se) ventrofixation of the uterus.

ventrolateral (-lat′er-al) both ventral and lateral.

ventromedian (-me′de-an) both ventral and median.

ventroposterior (-pos-tēr′e-or) both ventral and posterior (caudal).

ventroscopy (ven-tros′ko-pe) peritoneoscopy.

ventrose (ven′trōs) having a belly-like expansion.

ventrosuspension (ven″tro-sus-pen′shun) ventrofixation.

ventrotomy (ven-trot′ah-me) celiotomy.

venula (ven′u-lah), pl. *ven′ulae* [L.] venule.

venule (ven′ūl) any of the small vessels that collect blood from the capillary plexuses and join to form veins. **ven′ular**, adj. **postcapillary v's**, venous capillaries. **stellate v's of kidney**, see *Table of Veins.*

verbigeration (ver-bij″er-a′shun) stereotyped and meaningless repetition of words and phrases.

verge (verj) a circumference or ring. **anal v.**, the opening of the anus on the surface of the body.

vergence (ver′jens) a disjunctive reciprocal rotation of both eyes so that the axes of fixation are not parallel; the kind of vergence is indicated by a prefix, e.g., convergence, divergence.

vermicide (ver′mĭ-sīd) an agent lethal to intestinal animal parasites.

vermicular (ver-mik′u-ler) wormlike in shape or appearance.

vermiculation (ver-mik″u-la′shun) peristaltic motion; peristalsis.

vermiculous (ver-mik′u-lus) 1. wormlike. 2. infested with worms.

vermiform (ver′mĭ-form) worm-shaped.

vermifuge (ver′mĭ-fūj) an agent that expels worms or intestinal animal parasites; an anthelmintic. **vermifu′gal**, adj.

vermilionectomy (ver-mil″yon-ek′tah-me) excision of the vermilion border of the lip.

vermin (ver′min) an external animal parasite; such parasites collectively. **ver′minous**, adj.

vermis (ver′mis) [L.] 1. a worm, or wormlike structure. 2. v. cerebelli. **v. cerebel′li**, the median part of the cerebellum, between the two hemispheres.

vernix (ver′niks) [L.] varnish. **v. caseo′sa**, an unctuous substance composed of sebum and desquamated epithelial cells.

verruca (vě-roo′kah), pl. *verru′cae* [L.] 1. common wart; a lobulated hyperplastic epidermal lesion with a horny surface, caused by a human papillomavirus, transmitted by contact or autoinoculation, and usually occurring on the dorsa

of the hands and fingers. 2. any of various nonviral, wartlike epidermal proliferations. **ver′rucose, verru′cous**, adj. **v. acumina′ta**, condyloma acuminatum. **v. necrogen′ica**, tuberculosis verrucosa cutis. **v. perua′na, v. peruvia′na**, verruga peruana. **v. pla′na**, a small, smooth, usually skin-colored or light brown, slightly raised wart sometimes occurring in great numbers; seen most often in children. **v. planta′ris**, a viral epidermal tumor on the sole of the foot.

verruciform (vě-roo′sĭ-form) wartlike.

verruga (vě-roo′gah) [Sp.] wart. **v. perua′na**, a hemangioma-like tumor or nodule occurring in Carrión's disease.

version (ver′zhun) 1. the act or process of turning or changing direction. 2. the situation of an organ or part in relation to an established normal position. 3. in gynecology, misalignment or tilting of the uterus. 4. in obstetrics, the manual turning of the fetus. 5. in opthalmology, rotation of the eyes in the same direction. **bimanual v.**, version by combined external and internal manipulation. **bipolar v.**, turning effected by acting upon both poles of the fetus, either by external or combined version. **cephalic v.**, turning of the fetus so that the head presents. **combined v.**, bimanual v. **external v.**, turning effected by outside manipulation. **internal v.**, turning effected by the hand or fingers inserted through the dilated cervix. **pelvic v.**, version by manipulation of the breech. **podalic v.**, conversion of a more unfavorable presentation into a footling presentation. **spontaneous v.**, one which occurs without aid from any extraneous force.

vertebr(o)- word element [L.], *vertebra; spine.*

vertebra (ver′tĕ-brah), pl. *ver′tebrae* [L.] any of the 33 bones of the vertebral (spinal) column, comprising 7 *cervical,* 12 *thoracic,* 5 *lumbar,* 5 *sacral,* and 4 *coccygeal* vertebrae. See *Table of Bones.* **ver′tebral**, adj. **basilar v.**, the lowest lumbar vertebra. **cervical vertebrae**, the seven vertebrae closest to the skull, constituting the skeleton of the neck. **coccygeal vertebrae**, the three to five segments of the vertebral column most distant from the skull, which fuse to form the coccyx. **cranial v.**, the segments of the skull and facial bones regarded by some as modified vertebrae. **v. denta′ta**, the second cervical vertebra, or axis. **dorsal vertebrae**, thoracic vertebrae. **false vertebrae**, those vertebrae which normally fuse with adjoining segments: the sacral and coccygeal vertebrae. **lumbar vertebrae**, the five segments of the vertebral column between the twelfth thoracic vertebra and the sacrum. **v. mag′num**, the sacrum. **odontoid v.**, the second cervical vertebra, or axis. **v. pla′na**, a condition of spondylitis in which the body of the vertebra is reduced to a sclerotic disk. **sacral vertebrae**, the segments (usually five) below the lumbar vertebrae, which normally fuse to form the sacrum. **sternal v.**, sternebra. **thoracic vertebrae**, the 12 segments of the vertebral column between the cervical and the lumbar vertebrae, giving attachment to the ribs and forming part of the posterior wall of the thorax. **true vertebrae,**

those segments of the vertebral column that normally remain unfused throughout life: the cervical, thoracic, and lumbar vertebrae.

Vertebrata (ver″tĕ-bra′tah) a subphylum of the Chordata, comprising all animals having a vertebral column, including mammals, birds, reptiles, amphibians, and fishes.

vertebrate (ver′tĕ-brāt) 1. having a spinal column (vertebrae). 2. an animal with a vertebral column; any member of the Vertebrata.

vertebrectomy (ver″tĕ-brek′tah-me) excision of a vertebra.

vertebrobasilar (ver″tĕ-bro-bas′ĭ-ler) pertaining to or affecting the vertebral and basilar arteries.

vertebrochondral (-kon′dral) pertaining to a vertebra and a costal cartilage.

vertebrocostal (-kos′t'l) pertaining to a vertebra and a rib.

vertebrogenic (-jen′ik) arising in a vertebra or in the vertebral column.

vertebrosternal (-ster′n'l) pertaining to a vertebra and the sternum.

vertex (ver′teks) the summit or top, especially the top of the head (v. cra′nii). **ver′tical**, adj.

verticalis (ver″tĭ-ka′lis) [L.] vertical.

verticillate (ver-tis′ĭ-lāt) arranged in whorls.

vertigo (ver′tĭ-go) a sensation of rotation or movement of one's self (subjective v.) or of one's surroundings (objective v.) in any plane; sometimes used erroneously to mean any form of dizziness. **vertig′inous**, adj. **alternobaric v.,** a transient, true, whirling vertigo sometimes affecting those subjected to large, rapid variations in barometric pressure. **auditory v., aural v.,** Meniere's disease. **benign paroxysmal positional (or postural) v.,** recurrent vertigo and nystagmus occurring when the head is placed in certain positions, usually not associated with lesions of the central nervous system. **disabling positional v.,** constant vertigo and dysequilibrium and nausea with the head in the upright position, without hearing disturbance or loss of vestibular function. **labyrinthine v.,** a form associated with disease of the labyrinth of the ear. **objective v.,** see vertigo. **ocular v.,** a form due to eye disease. **organic v.,** that due to vestibular brain disease or to tabes dorsalis. **postural v.,** that associated with a specific position of the head in space or with changes in position of the head in space or head. **subjective v.,** see vertigo. **vestibular v.,** vertigo due to disturbances of the vestibular centers or pathways in the central nervous system.

verumontanum (ver″u-mon-ta′num) colliculus seminalis.

vesalianum (vĕ-sa″le-a′num) a sesamoid bone in the tendon of origin of the gastrocnemius muscle, or in the angle between the cuboid and fifth metatarsal.

vesic(o)- word element [L.], blister; bladder.

vesica (vĕ-si′kah), pl. vesi′cae [L.] bladder. **v. bilia′ris, v. fel′leae,** gallbladder. **v. urina′ria,** urinary bladder.

vesical (ves′ĭ-k'l) pertaining to the urinary bladder.

vesicant (ves′ĭ-kant) 1. producing blisters. 2. an agent that produces blisters.

vesication (ves″ĭ-ka′shun) 1. the process of blistering. 2. a blistered spot or surface.

vesicle (ves′ĭ-k'l) 1. a small bladder or sac containing liquid. 2. a small circumscribed elevation of the epidermis containing a serous fluid; a small blister. **acrosomal v.,** a membrane-bounded vacuole-like structure which spreads over the upper two thirds of the head of a spermatozoon to form the head cap. **allantoic v.,** internal hollow portion of allantois; see under diverticulum. **auditory v.,** a detached ovoid sac formed by closure of the auditory pit in the early embryo, in embryonic development of the inner ear. **blastodermic v.,** blastocyst. **brain v's,** the five divisions of the closed neural tube in the developing embryo, including the telencephalon, diencephalon, mesencephalon, metencephalon, and myelencephalon. **brain v's, primary,** the three earlier subdivisions of the embryonic neural tube, including the forebrain, midbrain, and hindbrain. **brain v's, secondary,** the four brain vesicles formed by specialization of the forebrain and of the hindbrain in later embryonic development. **cerebral v's,** brain v's. **chorionic v.,** the developing ovum at the time of its invasion of the endometrium of the uterus. **compound v.,** multilocular v. **encephalic v's,** brain v's. **germinal v.,** the fluid-filled nucleus of an oocyte toward the end of prophase of its meiotic division. **lens v.,** a vesicle formed from the lens pit of the embryo, developing into the crystalline lens. **matrix v's,** small membrane-limited structures at sites of calcification of the cartilage matrix. **olfactory v.,** 1. the vesicle in the embryo which later develops into the olfactory bulb and tract. 2. a bulbous expansion at the distal end of an olfactory cell, from which the olfactory hairs project. **optic v.,** an evagination on either side of the forebrain of the early embryo, from which the percipient parts of the eye develop. **otic v.,** auditory v. **seminal v's,** paired sacculated pouches attached to the posterior urinary bladder; the duct of each joins the ipsilateral ductus deferens to form the ejaculatory duct. **umbilical v.,** the pear-shaped expansion of the yolk sac growing out into the cavity of the chorion, joined to the midgut by the yolk stalk.

vesicocele (ves′ĭ-ko-sēl″) hernia of bladder.

vesicocervical (ves″ĭ-ko-ser′vĭ-k'l) pertaining to the bladder and cervix uteri, or communicating with the bladder and cervical canal.

vesicoclysis (ves″ĭ-kok′lĭ-sis) introduction of fluid into the bladder.

vesicoenteric (-en-ter′ik) vesicointestinal.

vesicointestinal (-in-tes′tĭ-n'l) pertaining to or communicating with the urinary bladder and intestine.

vesicoprostatic (-pros-tat′ik) pertaining to the bladder and prostate.

vesicopubic (-pu′bik) pertaining to the bladder and pubes.

vesicosigmoidostomy (-sig″moi-dos′to-me) creation of a permanent communication between the urinary bladder and the sigmoid flexure.

vesicospinal (-spi′nal) pertaining to the bladder and spine.

vesicostomy (ves″ĭ-kos′tah-me) the formation of an opening into the bladder; cystostomy. **cutaneous v.**, surgical anastomosis of the bladder mucosa to an opening in the skin below the umbilicus, creating a stoma for bladder drainage.

vesicotomy (ves″ĭ-kot′ah-me) cystotomy.

vesicoureteral, vesicoureteric (ves″ĭ-ko-u-re′ter-al, -u-re′ter-ik) pertaining to the bladder and ureter.

vesicouterine (-u′ter-in) pertaining to the bladder and uterus.

vesicovaginal (-vaj′ĭ-n′l) pertaining to the bladder and vagina.

vesicula (vĕ-sik′u-lah), pl. *vesic′ulae* [L.] vesicle.

vesicular (vĕ-sik′u-ler) 1. composed of or relating to small, saclike bodies. 2. pertaining to or made up of vesicles on the skin.

vesiculectomy (vĕ-sik″u-lek′tah-me) excision of a vesicle, especially the seminal vesicles.

vesiculiform (vĕ-sik′u-lĭ-form″) shaped like a vesicle.

vesiculitis (vĕ-sik″u-li′tis) inflammation of a vesicle, especially a seminal vesicle (*seminal v.*).

vesiculocavernous (vĕ-sik″u-lo-kav′er-nus) both vesicular and cavernous.

vesiculography (vĕ-sik″u-log′rah-fe) radiography of the seminal vesicles.

vesiculopapular (vĕ-sik″u-lo-pap′u-ler) marked by or having characteristics of vesicles and papules.

vesiculopustular (-pus′tu-ler) marked by or having characteristics of vesicles and pustules.

vesiculotomy (vĕ-sik″u-lot′ah-me) incision into a vesicle, especially the seminal vesicles.

vessel (ves′′l) any channel for carrying a fluid, such as blood or lymph. **absorbent v′s**, lymphatic v′s. **blood v.**, one of the vessels conveying the blood, comprising arteries, capillaries, and veins. **chyliferous v′s**, lacteal v′s. **collateral v′s**, 1. a vessel that parallels another vessel, nerve, or other structure. 2. a vessel important in establishing and maintaining a collateral circulation. **great v′s**, the large vessels entering the heart, including the aorta, the pulmonary arteries and veins, and the venae cavae. **lacteal v′s**, those that take up chyle from the intestinal wall during digestion. **lymph v′s, lymphatic v′s**, the capillaries, collecting vessels, and trunks that collect lymph from the tissues and carry it to the blood stream. **nutrient v′s**, vessels supplying nutritive elements to special tissues, as arteries entering the substance of bone or the walls of large blood vessels.

vestibule (ves′tĭ-būl) a space or cavity at the entrance to a canal. **vestib′ular**, adj. **v. of aorta**, a small space at root of the aorta. **v. of ear**, an oval cavity in the middle of the bony labyrinth. **v. of mouth**, the portion of the oral cavity bounded on the one side by teeth and gingivae, or residual alveolar ridges, and on the other by the lips (*labial v.*) and cheeks (*buccal v.*). **v. of nose**, the anterior part of the nasal cavity. **v. of pharynx**, 1. fauces. 2. oropharynx. **v. of**

vagina, the space between the labia minora into which the urethra and vagina open.

vestibulogenic (ves-tib″u-lo-jen′ik) arising in a vestibule, as that of the ear.

vestibulo-ocular (-ok′u-ler) pertaining to the vestibular and oculomotor nerves; or to the maintenance of visual stability during head movements.

vestibuloplasty (ves-tib″u-lo-plas″te) surgical modification of gingival–mucous membrane relationships in the vestibule of the mouth.

vestibulotomy (ves-tib″u-lot′ah-me) surgical opening of the vestibule of the ear.

vestibulourethral (ves-tib″u-lo-u-re′thral) pertaining to the vestibule of the vagina and the urethra.

vestibulum (ves-tib′u-lum), pl. *vestib′ula* [L.] vestibule.

vestige (ves′tij) the remnant of a structure that functioned in a previous stage of species or individual development. **vestig′ial,** adj.

vestigium (ves-tij′e-um), pl. *vestig′ia* [L.] vestige.

veterinarian (vet″er-ĭ-nār′e-an) a person trained and authorized to practice veterinary medicine and surgery; a doctor of veterinary medicine.

veterinary (vet′er-ĭ-nār″e) 1. pertaining to domestic animals and their diseases. 2. veterinarian.

V.F. vocal fremitus.

v.f. visual field.

viable (vi′ah-b′l) able to maintain an independent existence; able to live after birth.

vibesate (vi′bĕ-sāt) a modified polyvinyl plastic applied topically as a spray to form an occlusive dressing for surgical wounds and other surface lesions.

vibex (vi′beks), pl. *vib′ices* [L.] a narrow linear mark or streak; a linear subcutaneous effusion of blood.

Vibramycin (vi″brah-mi′sin) trademark for preparations of doxycycline.

vibratile (vi′brah-til) swaying or moving to and fro; vibratory.

vibration (vi-bra′shun) 1. a rapid movement to and fro; oscillation. 2. the shaking of the body as a therapeutic measure. 3. a form of massage.

vibrator (vi′bra-tor) an instrument for producing vibrations used in the mechanical treatment of disease.

Vibrio (vib′re-o) a genus of gram-negative bacteria (family Spirillaceae). *V. chol′erae* (*V. com′ma*), or cholera vibrio, is the cause of Asiatic cholera; *V. metschnikov′ii* causes gastroenteritis; *V. parahaemoly′ticus* causes gastroenteritis due to consumption of raw or undercooked seafood; and *V. vulni′ficus* causes septicemia and cellulitis in persons who have consumed raw seafood.

vibrio (vib′re-o) an organism of the genus *Vibrio* or other spiral motile organism. **cholera v.,** *Vibrio cholerae.* **El Tor v.,** a biotype of *Vibrio cholerae.*

vibriocidal (vib″re-o-si′dal) destructive to *Vibrio*, especially *V. cholerae.*

vibrissa (vi-bris′ah), pl. *vibris′sae* [L.] one of the

hairs growing in the vestibule of the nose in man or about the muzzle of an animal.

vibrocardiography (-kar″de-og′rah-fe) graphic recording of chest wall vibrations produced by action of the heart.

Vicia (vish′e-ah) a genus of herbs, including V. fa′ba (V. fa′va), the fava or broad bean, whose beans or pollen contain a component capable of causing favism in susceptible persons.

vidarabine (vi-dār′ah-bēn) a purine analogue, adenine arabinoside (ara-A), $C_{10}H_{13}N_5O_4$, that inhibits DNA synthesis; used as an antiviral agent to treat herpes simplex keratitis and encephalitis.

vigilambulism (vij″il-am′bu-lizm) an ambulatory automatism resembling somnambulism, but occurring in the waking state.

villi (vil′i) plural of villus.

villoma (vĭ-lo′mah) papilloma.

villose (vil′ōs) shaggy with soft hairs; covered with villi.

villositis (vil″o-si′tis) a bacterial disease with alterations in the villi of the placenta.

villosity (vĭ-los′ĭ-te) 1. condition of being covered with villi. 2. a villus.

villus (vil′us), pl. vil′li [L.] a small vascular process or protrusion, as from the free surface of a membrane. **arachnoid villi,** microscopic projections of the arachnoid into some of the venous sinuses; see arachnoid granulations. **chorionic villi,** threadlike projections growing in tufts on the external surface of the chorion. **intestinal villi,** multitudinous threadlike projections covering the surface of the mucous membrane lining the small intestine, serving as the sites of absorption of fluids and nutrients. See Plates V and XV. **synovial villi,** slender projections from the surface of the synovial membrane into the cavity of a joint.

villusectomy (vil″ŭ-sek′tah-me) synovectomy.

vinblastine (vin-blas′tēn) an antineoplastic alkaloid, $C_{46}H_{58}N_4O_9$, extracted from Vinca rosea; used as the sulfate salt in palliative treatment of a variety of malignancies.

vincristine (vin-kris′tēn) an antineoplastic alkaloid, $C_{46}H_{56}N_4O_{10}$, extracted from Vinca rosea; used as the sulfate salt primarily as a component in combination chemotherapy, especially for Hodgkin disease, acute lymphocytic leukemia, and non-Hodgkin lymphoma.

vinculum (ving′ku-lum), pl. vin′cula [L.] a band or bandlike structure. **vin′cula ten′dinum,** filaments which connect the phalanges with the flexor tendons.

Vioform (vi′o-form) trademark for preparations of iodochlorhydroxyquin.

violet (vi′ah-let) the reddish-blue color produced by the shortest rays of the visible spectrum. **crystal v., gentian v., methyl v.,** see under G.

viper (vi′per) any venomous snake especially any member of the families Viperidae (true vipers) and Crotalidae (pit vipers).

vipoma (vĭ-po′mah) an endocrine tumor, usually arising in the pancreas, that produces vasoactive polypeptide, which is the mediator of a syndrome of watery diarrhea, hypokalemia, and

hypochlorhydria, leading to renal failure and death.

viral (vi′ral) pertaining to or caused by a virus.

viremia (vi-re′me-ah) the presence of viruses in the blood.

virgin (ver′jin) a female who has not had coitus.

virile (vir′il) 1. peculiar to men or the male sex. 2. possessing masculine traits, especially copulative power.

virilescence (vir″ĭ-les′ens) the development of male secondary sex characters in the female.

virilism (vir′ĭ-lizm) the presence of male characteristics in women.

virility (vĭ-ril′ĭ-te) possession of normal primary sex characters in a male.

virilization (vir″ĭ-lĭ-za′shun) induction or development of male secondary sex characters, especially appearance of such changes in the female.

virion (vi′re-on) the complete viral particle, found extracellularly and capable of surviving in crystalline form and infecting a living cell; it comprises the nucleoid (genetic material) and the capsid.

virolactia (vi″ro-lak′she-ah) secretion of viruses in the milk.

virology (vi-rol′o-je) the study of viruses and virus diseases.

virucide (vi′rŭ-sīd) an agent which neutralizes or destroys a virus. **viruci′dal,** adj.

virulence (vir′u-lens) the degree of pathogenicity of a microorganism as indicated by the severity of disease produced and the ability to invade the tissues of the host; by extension, the competence of any infectious agent to produce pathologic effects. **vir′ulent,** adj.

viruliferous (vir″u-lif′er-us) conveying or producing a virus or other noxious agent.

viruria (vi-roo′re-ah) the presence of viruses in the urine.

virus (vi′rus) a minute infectious agent which, with certain exceptions, is not resolved by the light microscope, lacks independent metabolism and is able to replicate only within a living host cell; the individual particle (virion) consists of nucleic acid (nucleoid)—DNA or RNA (but not both)—and a protein shell (capsid), which contains and protects the nucleic acid and which may be multilayered. **arbor** (arthropod-borne) **v.,** arbovirus. **attenuated v.,** one whose pathogenicity has been reduced by serial passage or other means. **Coxsackie v.,** coxsackievirus. **defective v.,** one that cannot be completely replicated or cannot form a protein coat; in some cases replication can proceed if missing gene functions are supplied by other viruses; see helper v. **dengue v.,** a flavivirus existing as four distinct types (designated 1,2,3, and 4) that causes dengue. **Ebola v.,** an RNA virus almost identical to the Marburg virus but serologically distinct; it causes a similar disease. **ECHO** (enteric cytopathogenic human orphan) **v.,** echovirus. **encephalomyocarditis v.,** an enterovirus that causes mild aseptic meningitis and encephalomyocarditis. **enteric v.,** enterovirus. **enteric orphan v's,** orphan viruses isolated from the intestinal tract of man and various other animals; they include such viruses isolated from cattle (ecboviruses), dogs (ecdoviruses), man (echoviruses), monkeys (ecmoviruses), and swine (ecsoviruses). **Epstein-Barr v. (EB v., EBV),** a herpeslike virus that causes infectious mononucleosis and is associated with Burkitt's lymphoma and nasopharyngeal carcinoma. **equine encephalomyelitis v.,** a group of arboviruses that cause encephalomyelitis in horses, mules, and humans, transmitted by mosquitoes; there are three strains: *eastern, western,* and *Venezuelan.* **filterable v., filtrable v.,** a pathogenic agent capable of passing through fine filters of diatomite or unglazed porcelain; ultravirus. **v. fixé, fixed v.,** rabies virus whose virulence and incubation period have been stabilized by serial passage and remained fixed during further transmission; used for inoculating animals from which rabies vaccine is prepared. **helper v.,** one that aids in the development of a defective virus by supplying or restoring the activity of the viral gene or enabling it to form a protein coat. **hepatitis v.,** the etiologic agent of viral hepatitis. Four types are recognized: *hepatitis A virus,* the agent causing infectious hepatitis, acquired by parenteral inoculation or by ingestion; *hepatitis B virus,* the agent causing serum hepatitis, transmitted by inadequately sterilized syringes and needles, or through infectious blood plasma, or certain blood products; *hepatitis C virus,* which causes non-A, non-B hepatitis; and *hepatitis delta virus,* a defective RNA viral agent that can replicate only in the presence of hepatitis B virus and is transmitted with it and causes hepatitis delta. **herpes v.,** herpesvirus. **human immunodeficiency v. (HIV),** a human T-cell leukemia/lymphoma virus with a selective affinity for helper T cells that is the agent of acquired immune deficiency syndrome. **human T-cell leukemia/lymphoma v., human T-cell lymphotrophic v. (HTLV),** a family of retroviruses that have a selective affinity for helper/inducer T lymphocytes and have been isolated from unusual and epidemiologically distinct T-cell leukemias and lymphomas; see also *human immunodeficiency v.* **influenza v.,** any of a group of myxoviruses that causes influenza, including at least three serotypes (A, B, and C). Serotype A viruses are subject to major antigenic changes (antigenic shifts) as well as minor gradual antigenic changes (antigenic drift) and cause the major pandemics. **lytic v.,** one that is replicated in the host cell and causes death and lysis of the cell. **Marburg v.,** an RNA virus occurring in Africa, transmitted by insect bite and causing Marburg disease. **measles v.,** a paramyxovirus that is the cause of measles. **monkeypox v.,** an orthopoxvirus that produces mild exanthematous disease in monkeys and a smallpox-like disease in humans. **Norwalk v.,** a common agent of epidemics of acute gastroenteritis. **orphan v's,** viruses isolated in tissue culture but not found specifically associated with any illness. **papilloma v.,** papillomavirus. **parainfluenza v.,** one of a group of viruses, classified in four types, isolated from patients with upper respiratory tract disease of varying severity. **pox v.,** poxvirus.

rabies v., an RNA virus of the rhabdovirus group that causes rabies. **respiratory syncytial v.,** a virus isolated from children with bronchopneumonia and bronchitis, which causes syncytium formation in tissue culture. **Rous-associated v. (RAV),** a helper virus in whose presence a defective Rous sarcoma virus is able to form a protein coat. **Rous sarcoma v.,** see *Rous sarcoma.* **satellite v.,** a strain of virus unable to replicate except in the presence of helper virus; considered to be deficient in coding for capsid formation. **street v.,** rabies virus from a naturally infected animal, as opposed to a laboratory-adapted strain of the virus. **tickborne v.,** one transmitted by ticks.

vis (vis), pl. *vi'res* [L.] force, energy. **v. a ter'go,** the factor of pressure transmitted through the capillaries to the veins by the blood pumped into the arteries by the heart.

viscer(o)- word element [L.], *viscera.*

viscera (vis'er-ah) plural of *viscus.*

viscerad (vis'er-ad) toward the viscera.

visceral (vis'er-al) pertaining to a viscus.

visceralgia (vis"er-al'je-ah) pain in any viscera.

visceromegaly (-meg'ah-le) splanchnomegaly.

visceromotor (-mo'tor) concerned in the essential movements of the viscera.

visceroparietal (-pah-ri'ah-tal) pertaining to the viscera and the abdominal wall.

visceroperitoneal (-per"ĭ-to-ne'al) pertaining to the viscera and peritoneum.

visceropleural (-ploo'ral) pertaining to the viscera and the pleura.

visceroskeletal (-skel'ah-tal) pertaining to the visceral skeleton.

viscerotropic (-trop'ik) primarily acting on the viscera; having a predilection for the abdominal or thoracic viscera.

viscid (vis'id) glutinous or sticky.

viscosity (vis-kos'ĭ-te) resistance to flow; a physical property of a substance that is dependent on the friction of its component molecules as they slide by one another.

viscous (vis'kus) sticky or gummy; having a high degree of viscosity.

viscus (vis'kus), pl. *vis'cera* [L.] any large interior organ in any of the three great body cavities, especially those in the abdomen.

vision (vizh'un) faculty of seeing; sight. **vis'ual,** adj. **achromatic v.,** monochromatism. **binocular v.,** the use of both eyes together without diplopia. **central v.,** that produced by stimuli impinging directly on the macula retinae. **chromatic v., color v. color v.,** 1. perception of the different colors making up the spectrum of visible light. 2. chromatopsia. **day v.,** visual perception in the daylight or under conditions of bright illumination. **dichromatic v.,** dichromasy. **direct v.,** central v. **double v.,** diplopia. **indirect v.,** peripheral v. **low v.,** impairment of vision such that there is significant visual handicap but also significant usable residual vision. **monocular v.,** vision with one eye. **multiple v.,** polyopia. **night v.,** visual perception in the darkness of night or under conditions of reduced illumination. **oscillating v.,** oscillopsia. **peripheral v.,** that produced by stimuli falling on areas of the retina distant from the macula. **solid v., stereoscopic v.,** perception of the relief of objects or of their depth; vision in which objects are perceived as having three dimensions. **tunnel v.,** that in which the visual fields are severely constricted to about 10 degrees from the fixation point.

Vistaril (vis′tah-ril) trademark for preparations of hydroxyzine.

visualization (vizh″u-al-ĭ-za′shun) the act of viewing or of achieving a complete visual impression of an object.

visuoauditory (vizh″u-o-aw′dĭ-tor″e) audiovisual.

visuosensory (-sen′sor-e) pertaining to perception of stimuli giving rise to visual impressions.

Vitallium (vi-tal′e-um) trademark for a cobalt-chromium alloy used for cast dentures and surgical appliances.

vitamin (vi′tah-min) any of a group of unrelated organic substances occurring in many foods in small amounts and necessary in trace amounts for the normal metabolic functioning of the body; they may be water- or fat-soluble. **antihemorrhagic v.,** see *v. K.* **antineuritic v.,** thiamine. **antipellagra v.,** niacin. **antiscorbutic v.,** ascorbic acid. **fat-soluble v's,** those (vitamins A, D, E, and K) that are soluble in fat solvents and are absorbed along with dietary fats; they are not normally excreted in the urine and tend to be stored in the body in moderate amounts. **permeability v.,** a substance necessary to ensure integrity of the capillary walls. **water-soluble v's,** the vitamins soluble in water (i.e., all but vitamins A, D, E, and K); they are excreted in the urine and are not stored in the body in appreciable quantities.

v. A, a fat-soluble vitamin occurring in nature in two forms: *retinol* and *dehydroretinol.* It is found in fish liver oils, liver, butter, egg yolk, cheese, and many vegetables, in most of which it exists as its precursor, carotene; deficiency in the diet causes (*a*) inadequate production and regeneration of rhodopsin with resultant nightblindness, and (*b*) epithelial tissue disturbances resulting in keratomalacia, xerophthalmia, and lessened resistance to infection through epithelial surfaces. It is toxic when taken in excess; see *hypervitaminosis A.*

v. A₁, retinol.

v. A₂, dehydroretinol.

v. B, any member of the *vitamin B complex,* a group of water-soluble substances including thiamine, riboflavin, niacin, niacinamide, the vitamin B₆ group, biotin, pantothenic acid, folic acid, possibly para-aminobenzoic acid, inositol, cyanocobalamine (vitamin B₁₂), and possibly choline.

v. B₁, thiamine.

v. B₂, riboflavin.

v. B₆, a group of water-soluble substances (including pyridoxine, pyridoxal, and pyridoxamine) widely distributed in animal and plant tissues, concerned in amino acid metabolism, in degradation of tryptophan, and in breakdown of glycogen to glucose-1-phosphate.

v. B₁₂, cyanocobalamine.

v. Bc, folic acid.

v. C, ascorbic acid.

v. D, any of several fat-soluble compounds, including cholecalciferol and ergocalciferol; they are present in fish liver oils and in butter and egg yolk and produced in the body on exposure to sunlight, and may be produced artificially by irradiation of ergosterol and a few related sterols. Deficiency tends to cause rickets in children and osteomalacia and osteoporosis in adults. Known collectively as *calciferol.*

v. D₂, ergocalciferol.

v. D₃, cholecalciferol.

v. E, a fat-soluble vitamin necessary in the diet of many species for normal reproduction, normal muscular development, normal resistance of erythrocytes to hemolysis, and various other biochemical functions; chemically, it is α-tocopherol (q.v.), found in wheat germ oil, cereals, egg yolk, and beef liver, or produced synthetically.

v. G, riboflavin.

v. H, biotin.

v. K, a group of fat-soluble compounds found in alfalfa, spinach, cabbage, putrefied fish meal, hog-liver fat, egg yolk, and hempseed, which promote clotting of blood by increasing the synthesis of prothrombin by the liver.

v. K₁, phytonadione.

v. K₂, menaquinone.

v. K₃, menadione.

v. L, a factor necessary for lactation in rats; L₁ is found in beef-liver extract, L₂ in yeast.

v. M, folic acid.

vitellus (vi-tel′us) the yolk of egg. **vitel′line,** adj.

vitiligines (vit″ĭ-lij′ĭ-nēz) depigmented areas of the skin.

vitiligo (vit″ĭ-li′go) a usually progressive, chronic pigmentary anomaly of the skin manifested by depigmented white patches that may be surrounded by a hyperpigmented border. **vitilig′inous,** adj.

vitrectomy (vĭ-trek′tah-me) surgical extraction, usually via the pars plana, of the contents of the vitreous chamber of the eye.

vitreoretinal (-ret′ĭ-n'l) of or pertaining to the vitreous and retina.

vitreous (vit′re-us) 1. glasslike or hyaline. 2. vitreous body. **primary persistent hyperplastic v.,** a congenital anomaly, usually unilateral, due to persistence of embryonic remnants of the fibromuscular tunic of the eye and part of the hyaloid vascular system. Clinically, there is a white bright, elongated ciliary processes, and often microphthalmia; the lens, although clear initially, may become completely opaque.

vivi- word element [L.], *alive; life.*

vividialysis (viv″ĭ-di-al′ĭ-sis) dialysis through a living membrane (the peritoneum).

vividiffusion (-dĭ-fu′zhun) circulation of the blood through a closed apparatus in which it is passed through a membrane for removal of substances ordinarily removed by the kidneys.

vivification (-fĭ-ka′shun) conversion of lifeless into living protein matter by assimilation.

viviparous (vi-vip′ah-rus) giving birth to living young which develop within the maternal body.

vivisection (viv″ĭ-sek′shun) surgical procedures

performed upon a living animal for purpose of physiologic or pathologic investigation.

VLDL very low-density lipoprotein.

V.M.D. Doctor of Veterinary Medicine.

voice (vois) sound produced by the speech organs and uttered by the mouth. **vo′cal,** adj.

void (void) to cast out as waste matter, especially the urine.

vola (vo′lah) a concave or hollow surface. **v. ma′nus,** the palm. **v. pe′dis,** the sole.

volar (vo′lar) pertaining to sole or palm; indicating the flexor surface of the forearm, wrist, or hand.

volaris (vo-la′ris) palmar.

volatile (vol′ah-til) evaporating rapidly.

volatilization (vol″ah-til-ĭ-za′shun) conversion into a vapor or gas without chemical change.

volley (vol′e) a rhythmical succession of muscular twitches artificially induced; the aggregate of nerve impulses set up by a single stimulus.

volsella (vol-sel′ah) vulsella.

volt (volt) the SI unit of the electromotive force or electric potential, equal to 1 joule per coulomb or 1 ampere-ohm. **electron v. (eV),** a unit of energy equal to the energy acquired by an electron in being accelerated through a potential difference of 1 volt; equal to 1.602×10^{-19} joule.

volume (vol′ūm) the space occupied by a substance or a three-dimensional region; the capacity of such a region or of a container. **expiratory reserve v.,** the maximal amount of gas that can be expired from the resting end-expiratory level. **inspiratory reserve v.,** the maximal amount of gas that can be inspired from the end-inspiratory position. **mean corpuscular v.,** see *MCV.* **minute v.,** the volume of air expelled from the lungs per minute. **packed-cell v.,** the volume of packed red cells in milliliters per 100 ml. of centrifuged blood. **residual v.,** the amount of gas remaining in the lung at the end of a maximal expiration. **stroke v.,** the volume of blood ejected from a ventricle at each beat of the heart. **tidal v.,** the volume of gas inspired and expired during one respiratory cycle.

volumetric (vol″u-met′rik) pertaining to or accompanied by measurement in volumes.

volute (vo-lūt′) rolled up.

volvulosis (vol″vu-lo′sis) onchocerciasis due to *Onchocerca volvulus.*

volvulus (vol′vu-lus) [L.] torsion of a loop of intestine, causing obstruction.

vomer (vo′mer) [L.] see *Table of Bones.* **vo′merine,** adj.

vomeronasal (vo″mer-o-na′z'l) pertaining to the vomer and the nasal bone.

vomica (vom′ĭ-kah), pl. *vom′icae* [L.] 1. the profuse and sudden expectoration of pus and putrescent matter. 2. an abnormal cavity in an organ, especially in the lung, caused by suppuration and the breaking down of tissue.

vomit (vom′it) 1. matter expelled from the stomach by the mouth. 2. to eject stomach contents through the mouth. **black v.,** vomit consisting of blood which has been acted upon by the gastric juice, seen in yellow fever and other conditions in which blood collects in the stomach. **coffee-ground v.,** vomit consisting of dark altered blood mixed with stomach contents.

vomiting (-ing) forcible ejection of contents of stomach through the mouth. **cyclic v.,** recurring attacks of vomiting. **dry v.,** attempts at vomiting, with the ejection of nothing but gas. **pernicious v.,** vomiting in pregnancy so severe as to threaten life. **v. of pregnancy,** that occurring in pregnancy, especially early morning vomiting (morning sickness). **projectile v.,** vomiting with the material ejected with great force. **stercoraceous v.,** vomiting of fecal matter.

vomitory (vom′ĭ-to″re) an emetic.

vomiturition (vom″ĭ-chur-ish′un) repeated ineffectual attempts to vomit; retching.

vomitus (vom′ĭ-tus) [L.] 1. vomiting. 2. matter vomited.

vortex (vor′teks), pl. *vor′tices* [L.] a whorled or spiral arrangement or pattern, as of muscle fibers, or of the ridges or hairs of the skin.

vox (voks) [L.] voice. **v. choler′ica,** the peculiar suppressed voice of true cholera.

voyeurism (voi′yer-izm) a paraphilia characterized by recurrent, intense sexual urges or sexually arousing fantasies involving watching unsuspecting people who are naked, disrobing, or engaging in sexual activity.

V.R. vocal resonance.

V.S. volumetric solution.

v.s. vibration seconds (the unit of measurement of sound waves).

vuerometer (vu″er-om′ĕ-ter) an instrument for measuring distance between the pupils.

vulgaris (vul-ga′ris) [L.] ordinary; common.

vulnus (vul′nus), pl. *vul′nera* [L.] a wound.

vulsella, vulsellum (vul-sel′ah; vul-sel′um) a forceps with clawlike hooks at the end of each blade.

vulva (vul′vah) [L.] the external genital organs of the female, including the mons pubis, labia majora and minora, clitoris, and vestibule of the vagina. **vul′val, vul′var,** adj. **fused v.,** synechia vulvae.

vulvectomy (vul-vek′tah-me) excision of the vulva.

vulvitis (vul-vi′tis) inflammation of the vulva.

vulvouterine (-u′ter-in) pertaining to the vulva and uterus.

vulvovaginal (-vaj″ĭ-n'l) pertaining to the vulva and vagina.

vulvovaginitis (-vaj″ĭ-ni′tis) inflammation of the vulva and vagina.

vv. venae (L. pl.); veins.

v/v volume (of solute) per volume (of solvent).

W

W chemical symbol, *tungsten (wolfram)*; symbol for *watt*.

waist (wāst) the portion of the body between the thorax and the hips.

wall (wawl) a structure bounding or limiting a space or a definitive mass of material. **cell w.,** a rigid structure that lies just outside of and is joined to the plasma membrane of plant cells and most prokaryotic cells, which protects the cell and maintains its shape. **nail w.,** a fold of skin overlapping the sides and proximal end of a fingernail or toenail. **parietal w.,** somatopleure. **splanchnic w.,** splanchnopleure.

walleye (wawl′i) 1. leukoma of the cornea. 2. exotropia.

ward (ward) a large room in a hospital, with beds for the accommodation of many patients.

warfarin (war′ah-rin) an anticoagulant, $C_{19}H_{16}$-O_4, usually used as the sodium salt.

wart (wort) verruca; a hyperplastic epidermal lesion with a horny surface, caused by a human papillomavirus; also loosely applied to any of various wartlike, epidermal proliferations of nonviral origin. **anatomic w.,** the wart in tuberculosis verrucosa. **moist w.,** condyloma latum. **mosaic w.,** an irregularly shaped lesion on the sole, with a granular surface, formed by an aggregation of contiguous plantar warts. **necrogenic w.,** tuberculosis verrucosa cutis. **Peruvian w.,** verruga peruana; see *Carrión's, disease,* under *disease.* **pitch w's,** precancerous, keratotic, epidermal tumors occurring in those working with pitch and coal tar derivatives. **plantar w.,** verruca plantaris. **pointed w.,** condyloma acuminatum. **postmortem w., prosector's w.,** tuberculosis verrucosa cutis. **soot w.,** chimney-sweeps' cancer. **tuberculous w.,** tuberculosis verrucosa cutis. **venereal w.,** condyloma acuminatum.

wash (wosh) a solution used for cleansing or bathing a part, as an eye or the mouth.

water (wot′er) 1. clear, colorless, odorless, tasteless liquid, H_2O. 2. an aqueous solution of a medicinal substance. 3. purified w. **w. of crystallization,** that which is an ingredient of many salts, forming a structural part of a crystal. **distilled w.,** water purified by distillation. **w. for injection,** water that has been purified by distillation and contains no added substance. **w. for injection, bacteriostatic,** sterile water for injection, containing one or more suitable antimicrobial agents. **w. for injection, sterile,** water for injection that has been sterilized. **purified w.,** water obtained by either distillation or ion-exchange treatment; used when mineral-free water is required.

waters (wot′erz) popular name for *amniotic fluid.*

watt (wot) a unit of electric power, being the work done at the rate of 1 joule per second. It is equivalent to 1 ampere under pressure of 1 volt.

wave (wāv) a uniformly advancing disturbance in which the parts moved undergo a double oscillation; any wavelike pattern. **alpha w's,** see under *rhythm.* **beta w's,** see under *rhythm.* **brain w's,** the fluctuations of electric potential in the brain, as recorded by electroencephalography. **delta w's,** 1. an early QRS vector in the electrocardiogram in Wolff-Parkinson-White syndrome. 2. see under *rhythm* (1). **electromagnetic w's,** the spectrum of waves propagated by an electromagnetic field, having a velocity of 3×10^8 m/s in a vacuum and including, in order of decreasing wavelength, radio waves, microwaves, infrared, visible, and ultraviolet light, x-rays, gamma rays, and cosmic rays. **P w.,** a deflection in the electrocardiogram produced by excitation of the atria. **pulse w.,** the elevation of the pulse felt by the finger or shown graphically in a recording of pulse pressure. **Q w.,** in the QRS complex, the initial downward (negative) deflection, related to the initial phase of depolarization. **R w.,** the initial upward deflection of the QRS complex, following the Q wave in the normal electrocardiogram. **S w.,** a downward deflection of the QRS complex following the R wave in the normal electrocardiogram. **T w.,** the second major deflection of the normal electrocardiogram, reflecting the potential variations occurring with repolarization of the ventricles. **theta w's,** see under *rhythm.* **U w.,** a potential undulation of unknown origin immediately following the T wave, seen in the normal electrocardiogram and accentuated in hypokalemia.

wavelength (wāv′length) the distance between the top of one wave and the identical phase of the succeeding one.

wax (waks) a plastic substance deposited by insects or obtained from plants. **wax′y,** adj. **dental w.,** a mixture of two or more natural and synthetic waxes, resins, coloring agents, and other additives; used in dentistry for casting, constructing nonmetallic denture bases, registering jaw relations, and as an aid in laboratory work. **ear w.,** cerumen. **grave w.,** adipocere. **white w.,** bleached, purified wax from the honeycomb of the bee, *Apis mellifera;* used as an ingredient of several ointments. **yellow w.,** beeswax; purified wax from the honeycomb of the bee, *Apis mellifera;* used as a stiffening agent, and as an ingredient of yellow ointment.

waxing (wak′sing) the shaping of a wax pattern or the wax base of a trial denture into the contours desired.

Wb weber.

W.B.C. white blood cell; white blood (cell) count.

wean (wēn) to discontinue breast feeding and substitute other feeding habits.

web (web) a tissue or membrane. **laryngeal w.,** a web spread between the vocal folds near the anterior commissure; the most common congenital malformation of the larynx. **terminal w.,** a feltwork of fine filaments in the cytoplasm immediately beneath the free surface of certain epithelial cells; it is thought to have a supportive or cytoskeletal function.

weber (web′er) the SI unit of magnetic flux which, linking a circuit of one turn, produces in it an electromotive force of one volt as it is reduced to zero at a uniform rate in one second.

wedge (wej) a piece of material thick at one end and tapering to a thin edge at the other. **step w.**, a block of absorber, usually aluminum, machined in steps of increasing thickness, used to measure the penetrating power of roentgen rays.

weight (wāt) heaviness; the degree to which a body is drawn toward the earth by gravity. See *Table of Weights and Measures*. **apothecaries′ w.**, a system of weights used in compounding prescriptions based on the grain (equivalent 64.8 mg). Its units are the scruple (20 grains), dram (3 scruples), ounce (8 drams), and pound (12 ounces). **atomic w.**, the weight of an atom of a substance as compared with the weight of an atom of carbon-12, which is taken as 12.00000. Abbreviated at. wt. **avoirdupois w.**, the system of weight commonly used for ordinary commodities in English-speaking countries; its units are the dram (27.344 grains), ounce (16 drams), and pound (16 ounces). **molecular w.**, the weight of a molecule of a substance as compared with that of an atom of carbon-12; it is equal to the sum of the atomic weights of its constituent atoms. Abbreviated mol. wt.

wen (wen) 1. a sebaceous or epidermal inclusion cyst. 2. pilar cyst.

wheal (hwēl) a localized area of edema on the body surface, often attended with severe itching and usually evanescent; it is the typical lesion of urticaria.

wheeze (hwēz) a whistling respiratory sound.

whiplash (hwip′lash) a popular term for an acute cervical sprain.

whipworm (-werm) *Trichuris trichiura.*

whitlow (hwit′lo) felon. **herpetic w.**, primary herpes simplex infection of the terminal segment of a finger, with extensive tissue destruction, sometimes accompanied by systemic symptoms. **melanotic w.**, acral lentiginous melanoma.

W.H.O. World Health Organization, an international agency associated with the United Nations and based in Geneva.

whoop (hōōp) the sonorous and convulsive inspiration of whooping cough.

whooping cough (hōōp′ing kawf) pertussis.

window (win′do) a circumscribed opening in a plane surface. **aortic w.**, a transparent region below the aortic arch, formed by the bifurcation of the trachea, visible in the left anterior oblique radiograph of the heart and great vessels. **oval w.**, fenestra vestibuli. **round w.**, fenestra cochleae.

windpipe (wind′pīp) the trachea.

winking (wingk′ing) quick opening and closing of the eyelids. **jaw w.**, involuntary closing of the eyelid occasionally associated with jaw movements.

wire (wīr) a slender, elongated, flexible structure of metal. **Kirschner w.**, a steel wire for skeletal transfixion of fractured bones and for obtaining skeletal traction in fractures.

withdrawal (with-drawl′) 1. pathological retreat from interpersonal contact and social involvement. 2. a specific organic brain syndrome that follows cessation of use or reduction of intake of a psychoactive substance that had been regularly used to induce intoxication.

Wohlfahrtia (vōl-fahr′te-ah) a genus of flies. The larvae of *W. magnif′ica* produce wound myiasis; those of *W. o′paca* and *W. vig′il* cause cutaneous myiasis.

wolfram (wool′fram) tungsten (symbol W).

work-up (werk′up) the procedures done to arrive at a diagnosis, including history taking, laboratory tests, x-rays, and so on.

worm (werm) 1. any of the soft-bodied, naked, elongated invertebrates of the phyla Annelida, Acanthocephala, Aschelminthes, and Platyhelminthes. 2. The spiral tube of a distilling apparatus. **flat w.**, any of the Platyhelminthes. **spiny-headed w., thorny-headed w.**, any of the Acanthocephala.

wound (wōōnd) a bodily injury caused by physical means, with disruption of the normal continuity of structures. **contused w.**, one in which the skin is unbroken. **incised w.**, one caused by a cutting instrument. **lacerated w.**, one in which the tissues are torn. **open w.**, one having a free outward opening. **penetrating w.**, one caused by a sharp, usually slender object, which passes through the skin into the underlying tissues. **perforating w.**, a penetrating wound that extends into a viscus or body cavity. **puncture w.**, penetrating w.

wrist (rist) the region of the joint between the forearm and hand; the carpus. Also, the corresponding forelimb joint in quadrupeds.

wristdrop (rist′drop) a condition resulting from paralysis of the extensor muscles of the hand and fingers.

wryneck (ri′nek) torticollis.

wt. weight.

Wuchereria (voo″ker-e′re-ah) a genus of filarial nematodes indigenous to the warmer regions of the world, including *W. bancrof′ti*, which causes elephantiasis, lymphangitis, and chyluria by interfering with the lymphatic circulation.

wuchereriasis (voo″ker-ĕ-ri′ah-sis) infestation with worms of the genus *Wuchereria.*

w./v. weight (of solute) per volume (of solvent).

TABLES OF WEIGHTS AND MEASURES

MEASURES OF MASS

Avoirdupois Weight

GRAINS	DRAMS	OUNCES	POUNDS	METRIC EQUIVALENTS (grams)
1	0.0366	0.0023	0.00014	0.0647989
27.34	1	0.0625	0.0039	1.772
437.5	16	1	0.0625	28.350
7000	256	16	1	453.5924277

Apothecaries' Weight

GRAINS	SCRUPLES (℈)	DRAMS (ʒ)	OUNCES (℥)	POUNDS (℔)	METRIC EQUIVALENTS (grams)
1	0.05	0.0167	0.0021	0.00017	0.0647989
20	1	0.333	0.042	0.0035	1.296
60	3	1	0.125	0.0104	3.888
480	24	8	1	0.0833	31.103
5760	288	96	12	1	373.24177

Metric Weight

MICRO-GRAM	MILLI-GRAM	CENTI-GRAM	DECI-GRAM	GRAM	DECA-GRAM	HECTO-GRAM	KILO-GRAM	METRIC TON	EQUIVALENTS Avoirdupois	EQUIVALENTS Apothecaries'
1									0.000015 gr	0.000015 gr
10^3	1								0.015432 gr	0.015432 gr
10^4	10	1							0.154323 gr	0.154323 gr
10^5	100	10	1						1.543235 gr	1.543235 gr
10^6	1000	100	10	1					15.432356 gr	15.432356 gr
10^7	10^4	1000	100	10	1				5.6438 dr	7.7162 scr
10^8	10^5	10^4	1000	100	10	1			3.527 oz	3.215 oz
10^9	10^6	10^5	10^4	1000	100	10	1		2.2046 lb	2.6792 lb
10^{12}	10^9	10^8	10^7	10^6	10^5	10^4	1000	1	2204.6223 lb	2679.2285 lb

Troy Weight

GRAINS	PENNYWEIGHTS	OUNCES	POUNDS	METRIC EQUIVALENTS (grams)
1	0.042	0.002	0.00017	0.0647989
24	1	0.05	0.0042	1.555
480	20			

APOTHECARIES' (WINE) MEASURE

								EQUIVALENTS	
MINIMS	FLUID DRAMS	FLUID OUNCES	GILLS	PINTS	QUARTS	GALLONS	Cubic Inches	Milliliters	Cubic Centimeters
1	0.0166	0.002	0.0005	0.00013	—	—	0.00376	0.06161	0.06161
60	1	0.125	0.0312	0.0078	0.0039	—	0.22558	3.6967	3.6967
480	8	1	0.25	0.0625	0.0312	0.0078	1.80468	29.5737	29.5737
1920	32	4	1	0.25	0.125	0.0312	7.21875	118.2948	118.2948
7680	128	16	4	1	0.5	0.125	28.875	473.179	473.179
15360	256	32	8	2	1	0.25	57.75	946.358	946.358
61440	1024	128	32	8	4	1	231	3785.434	3785.434

METRIC MEASURE

MICRO-LITER	MILLI-LITER	CENTI-LITER	DECI-LITER	LITER	DEKA-LITER	HECTO-LITER	KILO-LITER	MEGA-LITER	EQUIVALENTS (Apothecaries' Fluid)
1	—	—	—	—	—	—	—	—	0.01623108 min
10^3	1	—	—	—	—	—	—	—	16.23 min
10^4	10	1	—	—	—	—	—	—	2.7 fl dr
10^5	100	10	1	—	—	—	—	—	3.38 fl oz
10^6	10^3	100	10	1	—	—	—	—	2.11 pts
10^7	10^4	10^3	100	10	1	—	—	—	2.64 gal
10^8	10^5	10^4	10^3	100	10	1	—	—	26.418 gals
10^9	10^6	10^5	10^4	10^3	100	10	1	—	264.18 gals
10^{12}	10^9	10^8	10^7	10^6	10^5	10^4	10^3	1	26418 gals

1 liter = 2.113363738 pints (Apothecaries')

MEASURES OF LENGTH

METRIC MEASURE

MICRO-METER	MILLI-METER	CENTI-METER	DECI-METER	METER	DEKA-METER	HECTO-METER	KILO-METER	MEGA-METER	EQUIVALENTS
1	0.001	10^{-4}	—	—	—	—	—	—	0.000039 inch
10^3	1	10^{-1}	—	—	—	—	—	—	0.03937 inch
10^4	10	1	—	—	—	—	—	—	0.3937 inch
10^5	100	10	1	—	—	—	—	—	3.937 inches
10^6	1000	100	10	1	—	—	—	—	39.37 inches
10^7	10^4	1000	100	10	1	—	—	—	10.9361 yards
10^8	10^5	10^4	1000	100	10	1	—	—	109.3612 yards
10^9	10^6	10^5	10^4	1000	100	10	1	—	1093.6121 yards
10^{10}	10^7	10^6	10^5	10^4	1000	100	10	—	6.2137 miles
10^{12}	10^9	10^8	10^7	10^6	10^5	10^4	1000	1	621.370 miles

CONVERSION TABLES

AVOIRDUPOIS—METRIC WEIGHTS

OUNCES	GRAMS	OUNCES	GRAMS	POUNDS	GRAMS	KILOGRAMS
1/16	1.772	7	198.447	1 (16 oz)	453.59	
1/8	3.544	8	226.796	2	907.18	
1/4	7.088	9	255.146	3	1360.78	1.36
1/2	14.175	10	283.495	4	1814.37	1.81
1	28.350	11	311.845	5	2267.96	2.27
2	56.699	12	340.194	6	2721.55	2.72
3	85.049	13	368.544	7	3175.15	3.18
4	113.398	14	396.893	8	3628.74	3.63
5	141.748	15	425.243	9	4082.33	4.08
6	170.097	16 (1 lb)	453.59	10	4535.92	4.54

METRIC—AVOIRDUPOIS WEIGHT

GRAMS	OUNCES	GRAMS	OUNCES	GRAMS	POUNDS
0.001 (1 mg)	0.000035274	1	0.035274	1000 (1 kg)	2.2046

APOTHECARIES'—METRIC WEIGHT

GRAINS	GRAMS	GRAINS	GRAMS	SCRUPLES	GRAMS
1/150	0.0004	2/5	0.03	1	1.296(1.3)
1/120	0.0005	1/2	0.032	2	2.592(2.6)
1/100	0.0006	3/5	0.04	3 (1 ℈)	3.888(3.9)
1/90	0.0007	2/3	0.043	**DRAMS**	**GRAMS**
1/80	0.0008	3/4	0.05	1	3.888
1/64	0.001	7/8	0.057	2	7.776
1/60	0.0011	1	0.065	3	11.664
1/50	0.0013	1 1/2	0.097(0.1)	4	15.552
1/48	0.0014	2	0.12	5	19.440
1/40	0.0016	3	0.20	6	23.328
1/36	0.0018	4	0.24	7	27.216
1/32	0.002	5	0.30	8 (1 ℥)	31.103
1/30	0.0022	6	0.40		
1/25	0.0026	7	0.45	**OUNCES**	**GRAMS**
1/20	0.003	8	0.50	1	31.103
1/16	0.004	9	0.60	2	62.207
1/12	0.005	10	0.65	3	93.310
1/10	0.006	15	1.00	4	124.414
1/9	0.007	20 (1 ℈)	1.30	5	155.517
1/8	0.008	30	2.00	6	186.621
1/7	0.009			7	217.724
1/6	0.01			8	248.828
1/5	0.013			9	279.931
1/4	0.016			10	311.035
1/3	0.02			11	342.138
				12 (1 ℔)	373.242

METRIC—APOTHECARIES' WEIGHT

MILLIGRAMS	GRAINS	GRAMS	GRAINS	GRAMS	EQUIVALENTS
1	0.015432	0.1	1.5432	10	2.572 drams
2	0.030864	0.2	3.0864	15	3.858 "
3	0.046296	0.3	4.6296	20	5.144 "
4	0.061728	0.4	6.1728	25	6.430 "
5	0.077160	0.5	7.7160	30	7.716 "
6	0.092592	0.6	9.2592	40	1.286 oz
7	0.108024	0.7	10.8024	45	1.447 "
8	0.123456	0.8	12.3456	50	1.607 "
9	0.138888	0.9	13.8888	100	3.215 "
10	0.154320	1.0	15.4320	200	6.430 "
15	0.231480	1.5	23.1480	300	9.644 "
20	0.308640	2.0	30.8640	400	12.859 "
25	0.385800	2.5	38.5800	500	1.34 lb
30	0.462960	3.0	46.2960	600	1.61 "
35	0.540120	3.5	54.0120	700	1.88 "
40	0.617280	4.0	61.728	800	2.14 "
45	0.694440	4.5	69.444	900	2.41 "
50	0.771600	5.0	77.162	1000	2.68 "
100	1.543240	10.0	154.324		

APOTHECARIES'—METRIC LIQUID MEASURE

MINIMS	MILLILITERS	FLUID DRAMS	MILLILITERS	FLUID OUNCES	MILLILITERS
1	0.06	1	3.70	1	29.57
2	0.12	2	7.39	2	59.15
3	0.19	3	11.09	3	88.72
4	0.25	4	14.79	4	118.29
5	0.31	5	18.48	5	147.87
10	0.62	6	22.18	6	177.44
15	0.92	7	25.88	7	207.01
20	1.23	8 (1 fl oz)	29.57	8	236.58
25	1.54			9	266.16
30	1.85			10	295.73
35	2.16			11	325.30
40	2.46			12	354.88
45	2.77			13	384.45
50	3.08			14	414.02
55	3.39			15	443.59
60 (1 fl dr)	3.70			16 (1 pt)	473.17
				32 (1 qt)	946.33
				128 (1 gal)	3785.32

METRIC—APOTHECARIES' LIQUID MEASURE

MILLILITERS	MINIMS	MILLILITERS	FLUID DRAMS	MILLILITERS	FLUID OUNCES
1	16.231	5	1.35	30	1.01
2	32.5	10	2.71	40	1.35
3	48.7	15	4.06	50	1.69
4	64.9	20	5.4	500	16.91
5	81.1	25	6.76	1000 (1 L)	33.815
		30	7.1		

U.S. AND BRITISH—METRIC LENGTH

INCHES	MILLIMETERS	CENTIMETERS	METERS
1/25	1.00	0.1	0.001
1/8	3.18	0.318	0.00318
1/4	6.35	0.635	0.00635
1/2	12.70	1.27	0.00127
1	25.40	2.54	0.0254
12 (1 foot)	304.80	30.48	0.3048

These *approximate* dose equivalents represent the quantities usually prescribed, under identical conditions, by physicians using, respectively, the metric system or the apothecary system of weights and measures. In labeling dosage forms in both the metric and the apothecary systems, if one is the approximate equivalent of the other, the approximate figure shall be enclosed in parentheses.

When prepared dosage forms such as tablets, capsules, pills, etc., are prescribed in the metric system, the pharmacist may dispense the corresponding *approximate* equivalent in the apothecary system, and vice versa, as indicated in the following table.

For the conversion of specific quantities in converting pharmaceutical formulas, equivalents must be used. In the compounding of prescriptions, the exact equivalents, rounded to three significant figures, should be used.

Note—A milliliter (ml) is the *approximate* equivalent of a cubic centimeter (cc).

LIQUID MEASURE

METRIC	APPROXIMATE APOTHECARY EQUIVALENTS		METRIC	APPROXIMATE APOTHECARY EQUIVALENTS	
1000 ml	1	quart	3 ml	45	minims
750 ml	1 1/2	pints	2 ml	30	minims
500 ml	1	pint	1 ml	15	minims
250 ml	8	fluid ounces	0.75 ml	12	minims
200 ml	7	fluid ounces	0.6 ml	10	minims
100 ml	3 1/2	fluid ounces	0.5 ml	8	minims
50 ml	1 3/4	fluid ounces	0.3 ml	5	minims
30 ml	1	fluid ounce	0.25 ml	4	minims
15 ml	4	fluid drams	0.2 ml	3	minims
10 ml	2 1/2	fluid drams	0.1 ml	1 1/2	minims
8 ml	2	fluid drams	0.06 ml	1	minims
5 ml	1 1/4	fluid drams	0.05 ml		3/4 minim
4 ml	1	fluid dram	0.03 ml		1/2 minim

METRIC	APPROXIMATE APOTHECARY EQUIVALENTS	METRIC	APPROXIMATE APOTHECARY EQUIVALENTS
30 g	1 ounce	30 mg	1/2 grain
15 g	4 drams	25 mg	3/8 grain
10 g	2 1/2 drams	20 mg	1/3 grain
7.5 g	2 drams	15 mg	1/4 grain
6 g	90 grains	12 mg	1/5 grain
5 g	75 grains	10 mg	1/6 grain
4 g	60 grains (1 dram)	8 mg	1/8 grain
3 g	45 grains	6 mg	1/10 grain
2 g	30 grains (1/2 dram)	5 mg	1/12 grain
1.5 g	22 grains	4 mg	1/15 grain
1 g	15 grains	3 mg	1/20 grain
750 mg	12 grains	2 mg	1/30 grain
600 mg	10 grains	1.5 mg	1/40 grain
500 mg	7 1/2 grains	1.2 mg	1/50 grain
400 mg	6 grains	1 mg	1/60 grain
300 mg	5 grains	800 μg	1/80 grain
250 mg	4 grains	600 μg	1/100 grain
200 mg	3 grains	500 μg	1/120 grain
150 mg	2 1/2 grains	400 μg	1/150 grain
125 mg	2 grains	300 μg	1/200 grain
100 mg	1 1/2 grains	250 μg	1/250 grain
75 mg	1 1/4 grains	200 μg	1/300 grain
60 mg	1 grain	150 μg	1/400 grain
50 mg	3/4 grain	120 μg	1/500 grain
40 mg	2/3 grain	100 μg	1/600 grain

The above *approximate* dose equivalents have been adopted by the *United States Pharmacopeia* and the *National Formulary*, and these dose equivalents have the approval of the federal Food and Drug Administration.

X

xanth(o)- word element [Gr.], *yellow.*

xanthelasma (zan″thah-laz′mah) xanthoma affecting the eyelids; see *planar xanthoma.*

xanthemia (zan-the′me-ah) carotenemia.

xanthic (zan′thik) 1. yellow. 2. pertaining to xanthine.

xanthine (zan′thēn) a compound, $C_5H_4N_4O_2$, found in most bodily tissues and fluids; it is a precursor of uric acid.

xanthinuria (zan″thin-ūr′e-ah) a rare hereditary disorder of purine metabolism due to a deficiency of the enzyme xanthine oxidase, which causes excessive urinary secretion of xanthine.

xanthochromatic (zan″thah-kro-mat′ik) yellow-colored.

xanthochromia (-kro′me-ah) yellowish discoloration, as of the skin or spinal fluid.

xanthochromic (-kro′mik) yellow-colored; applied almost exclusively to cerebrospinal fluid.

xanthocyanopsia (-si″ah-nop′se-ah) ability to discern yellow and blue tints, but not red or green.

xanthoderma (-der′mah) any yellowish discoloration of the skin.

xanthogranuloma (-gran″u-lo′mah) a tumor having histologic characteristics of both granuloma and xanthoma. **juvenile x.,** a benign, self-limited disorder of infants and children, manifested by single or multiple yellow, pink, orange, or reddish brown papules or nodules on the scalp, face, proximal extremities, or trunk, with possible involvement of the mucous membranes, viscera, eye, and other organs.

xanthoma (zan-tho′mah) a tumor composed of lipid-laden foam cells, which are histiocytes containing cytoplasmic lipid material. **diabetic x., x. diabetico′rum,** eruptive x. **disseminated x., x. dissemina′tum,** a rare, normolipoproteinemic form manifested by the development of reddish yellow to brown papules and nodules that may coalesce to form plaques, chiefly involving flexural ureases, the mucous membranes of the mouth and respiratory tract, cornea, sclera, and central nervous system. **eruptive x., x. erupti′va, x. multiplex,** a form marked by sudden eruption of crops of small, yellow or yellowish brown papules encircled by an erythematous halo, especially on the buttocks, posterior thighs, and elbows, and caused by high concentrations of plasma triglycerides, especially that associated with uncontrolled diabetes mellitus. **planar x., plane x., x. pla′num,** xanthomatosis marked by yellowish to orange, flat macules or slightly elevated plaques, sometimes having a central white area, which may be localized or generalized, often occurring in association with other xanthomas and certain hyperlipoproteinemias. **tendinous x., x. tendinosum,** a form manifested by free movable papules or nodules in the tendons, ligaments, fascia, and periosteum, especially on the backs of the hands, fingers, elbows, knees, and heels, in association with some hyperlipoproteinemias and certain other xanthomas. **x. tubero′sum, tuberous x.,** a form manifested by groups of flat, or elevated and rounded, yellowish or orangish nodules on the skin over joints, especially the elbows and knees; it may be associated with certain types of hyperlipoproteinemia, biliary cirrhosis, and myxedema.

xanthomatosis (zan″thah-mah-to′sis) a condition marked by the presence of xanthomas. **x. bul′bi,** fatty degeneration of the cornea.

xanthomatous (zan-tho′mah-tus) pertaining to xanthoma.

xanthophose (zan′thah-fōz) a yellow phose.

xanthopsia (zan-thop′se-ah) chromatopsia in which objects are seen as yellow.

xanthopsin (zan-thop′sin) all-*trans* retinal; see *retinal* (2).

xanthosine (zan′thah-sēn) a nucleoside composed of xanthine and ribose.

xanthosis (zan-tho′sis) yellowish discoloration; degeneration with yellowish pigmentation.

xanthurenic acid (zanth″u-rēn′ik) $C_9H_5N(OH)_2COOH$, a metabolite of L-tryptophan, present in normal urine and in increased amounts in vitamin B_6 deficiency.

Xe chemical symbol, *xenon.*

xen(o)- word element [Gr.], *strange; foreign.*

xenoantigen (zen″o-an′tĭ-jen) an antigen occurring in organisms of more than one species.

xenodiagnosis (zen″o-di″ag-no′sis) a method of animal inoculation using laboratory-bred bugs and animals in the diagnosis of certain parasitic infections when the infecting organism cannot be demonstrated in blood films; used in Chagas' disease (examination of the feces of clean bugs fed on the patient's blood) and trichinosis (examination of rats to which the patient's muscle tissue has been fed). **xenodiagnos′tic,** adj.

xenogeneic (-jen-a′ik) in transplantation biology, denoting individuals or tissues from individuals of different species and hence of disparate cell type.

xenogenesis (-jen′ĕ-sis) 1. heterogenesis (1). 2. the hypothetical production of offspring unlike either parent.

xenogenous (ze-noj′ĕ-nus) caused by a foreign body, or originating outside the organism.

xenograft (zen′o-graft) a graft of tissue transplanted between animals of different species.

xenon (ze′non) chemical element (*see table*), at. no. 54, symbol Xe.

xenoparasite (zen″o-par′ah-sīt) an organism not usually parasitic on a particular species, but which becomes so because of a weakened condition of the host.

xenophobia (-fo′be-ah) irrational fear of strangers.

xenophonia (-fo′ne-ah) alteration in the quality of the voice.

xenophthalmia (zen″of-thal′me-ah) ophthalmia caused by a foreign body in the eye.

Xenopsylla (zen″op-sil′ah) a genus of fleas, many species of which transmit pathogens; *X. che′opis*, the rat flea, transmits plague and murine typhus.

xer(o)- word element [Gr.], *dry; dryness.*

xeroderma (zēr″o-der′mah) a mild form of ichthyosis, marked by a dry, rough, discolored state of the skin. **x. pigmento′sum,** a rare pigmentary and atrophic autosomal recessive disease in which extreme cutaneous sensitivity to ultraviolet light results from an enzyme deficiency in the repair of DNA damaged by ultraviolet light. It begins in childhood, with early development of excessive freckling, telangiectases, keratomas, papillomas, and malignancies in sun-exposed skin, severe opthalmologic abnormalities, and, in some cases, neurological disorders. **xerodermat′ic,** adj.

xerography (zĭ-rog′rah-fe) xeroradiography.

xeroma (zĭ-ro′mah) abnormal dryness of the conjunctiva; xerophthalmia.

xeromammography (zēr″o-mă-mog′rah-fe) xeroradiography of the breast.

xeromenia (-me′ne-ah) the appearance of constitutional symptoms at the menstrual period without any flow of blood.

xerophthalmia (zēr″of-thal′me-ah) abnormal dryness and thickening of the conjunctiva and cornea due to vitamin A deficiency.

xeroradiography (zēr-o-ra″de-og′rah-fe) the making of radiographs by a dry, direct photoelectric process, using metal plates coated with a semiconductor, such as selenium.

xerosialography (-si″ah-log′rah-fe) sialography in which the images are recorded by xerography.

xerosis (ze-ro′sis) abnormal dryness, as of the eye, skin, or mouth. **xerot′ic,** adj.

xerostomia (zēr″o-sto′me-ah) dryness of the mouth due to salivary gland dysfunction.

xerotomography (-to-mog′rah-fe) tomography in which the images are recorded by xeroradiography.

xiph(o)- word element [Gr.], *xiphoid process.*

xiphisternum (zif″ĭ-ster′num) xiphoid process. **xiphister′nal,** adj.

xiphocostal (zif″ah-kos′tal) pertaining to the xiphoid process and ribs.

xiphoid (zif′oid, zi′foid) 1. sword-shaped; ensiform. 2. xiphoid process.

xiphoiditis (zif″oi-di′tis) inflammation of the xiphoid process.

xiphopagus (zĭ-fop′ah-gus) symmetrical conjoined twins united in the region of the xiphoid process.

X-linked (eks′linkt) transmitted by genes on the X chromosome; sex-linked.

x-ray (eks′ra) roentgen ray; see under *ray.*

xylene (zi′lēn) dimethylbenzene, C_8H_{10}; used as a solvent in microscopy.

Xylocaine (zi′lo-kān) trademark for preparations of lidocaine.

xylometazoline (zi″lo-met″ah-zo′lēn) an adrenergic, $C_{16}H_{24}N_2$, used as a topical nasal decongestant in the form of the hydrochloride salt.

xylose (zi′lōs) a pentose occurring in mucopolysaccharides of connective tissue and sometimes in the urine; also obtained from vegetable gum, beechwood, and jute. D-xylose is used in a diagnostic test of intestinal absorption.

xylulose (zi′lu-lōs) a pentose sugar occurring as L-xylulose, one of the few L sugars found in nature and sometimes excreted in the urine (see *pentosuria*), and D-xylulose.

xysma (zis′mah) material resembling bits of membrane in stools of diarrhea.

xyster (zis′ter) a file-like instrument used in surgery.

Y

Y chemical symbol, *yttrium.*

yaw (yaw) a lesion of yaws. **mother y.,** the initial cutaneous lesions of yaws.

yaws (yawz) an endemic infectious tropical disease caused by *Treponema pertenue*, usually affecting persons under 15 years of age, spread by direct contact with skin lesions or by contaminated fomites. It is initially manifested by the appearance of a papilloma at the site of inoculation; this heals, leaving a scar, and is followed by crops of generalized granulomatous lesions that may relapse repeatedly. There may be bone and joint involvement.

Yb chemical symbol, *ytterbium.*

yeast (yēst) a general term including single-celled, usually rounded fungi that produce by budding; some yeasts transform to a mycelial stage under certain environmental conditions, while others remain single-celled. They are fer-

menters of carbohydrates, and a few are pathogenic for humans. **brewer's y.,** *Saccharomyces cerevisiae*, used in brewing beer, making alcoholic liquors, and baking bread. **dried y.,** dried cells of any suitable strain of *Saccharomyces cerevisiae*, usually a by-product of the brewing industry; used as a natural source of protein and B-complex vitamins.

yellow (yel′o) 1. the primary color of wavelength of 571.5–578.5 mμ. 2. a dye or stain which produces a yellow color. **visual y.,** all-*trans* retinal; see *retinal* (2).

Yersinia (yer-sin′e-ah) a genus of nonmotile, ovoid or rod-shaped, nonencapsulated, gram-negative bacteria (family Enterobacteriaceae); *Y. enterocolitica* is a ubiquitous species that causes acute gastroenteritis and mesenteric lymphadenitis in children and arthritis, septicemia, and erythema nodosum in adults; *Y. pes-*

tis causes plague in humans and rodents, transmitted from rat to rat and from rats to humans by the rat flea, and from person to person by the human body louse; *Y. pseudotuberculosis* caused pseudotuberculosis in rodents and mesenteric lymphadenitis in humans.

yoke (yōk) a connecting structure; a depression or ridge connecting two structures.

yolk (yōk) the stored nutrient of the ovum.

ytterbium (ĭ-ter′be-um) chemical element (*see table*), at. no. 70, symbol Yb.

yttrium (ĭ′tre-um) chemical element (*see table*), at. no. 39, symbol Y.

Z

Z symbol, *atomic number*.

Zarontin (zah-ron′tin) trademark for a preparation of ethosuximide.

Zaroxolyn (zah-rok′so-lin) trademark for a preparation of metolazone.

zero (zēr′o) the point on a thermometer scale at which the graduation begins; zero of the Celsius (centigrade) scale is the ice point, and that of the Fahrenheit scale is 32 degrees below the ice point. **absolute z.,** the lowest possible temperature, designated as 0 on the Kelvin or Rankine scale, the equivalent of −273.15° C. or −459.67° F.

zidovudine (zi-do′vu-dēn) a synthetic thymidine analog that inhibits the human immunodeficiency virus.

zigzagplasty (zig″zag-plas″te) the surgical technique of minimizing the visual impact of a long linear scar by breaking it up into short irregular segments at right or acute angles to each another.

zinc (zingk) chemical element (*see table*), at. no. 30, symbol Zn; it is an essential micronutrient present in many enzymes. Its salts are both poisonous when absorbed by the system, producing a chronic poisoning. **z. acetate,** $Zn(C_2-H_3O_2)2\cdot 2H_2O$, an astringent and styptic. **z. chloride,** a salt used topically as an astringent, desensitizer for dentin, caustic antiseptic, and deodorant. **z. oxide,** ZnO, a topical astringent and protectant. **z. stearate,** a compound of zinc with stearic and palmitic acids, used as a water-repellent protective powder in dermatoses. **z. sulfate,** $ZnSO_4$, an ophthalmic astringent. **z. undecylenate,** $C_{22}H_{38}O_4Zn$, used topically in a 20% ointment as an antifungal.

zirconium (zir-ko′ne-um) chemical element (*see table*), at. no. 40, symbol Zr.

Zn chemical symbol, *zinc*.

zo(o)- word element [Gr.], *animal.*

zoacanthosis (zo″ak-an-tho′sis) dermatitis caused by animal structures, such as bristles, sting, or hairs.

zoanthropy (zo-an′thro-pe) delusion that one has become an animal. **zoanthrop′ic,** adj.

zona (zo′nah), pl. *zo′nae* [L.] 1. zone. 2. herpes zoster. **zo′nal,** adj. **z. arcua′ta,** canal of Corti. **z. cartilagin′ea,** limbus laminae spiralis osseae. **z. cilia′ris,** ciliary zone. **z. denticula′ta,** the inner zone of the lamina basilaris of the cochlear duct within the limbus of the osseous spiral lamina. **z. fascicula′ta,** the thick middle layer of the adrenal gland. **z. glomerulo′sa,** the outermost layer of the adrenal cortex. **z. hemorrhoida′lis,** that part of the anal canal extending from the anal valves to the anus and containing the rectal venous plexus. **z. incer′ta,** a narrow band of gray matter between the subthalamic nucleus and thalamic fasciculus. **z. ophthal′mica,** herpetic infection of the cornea. **z. orbicula′ris,** a ring around the neck of the femur formed by circular fibers of the articular capsule of the hip joint. **z. pectina′ta,** the outer part of the lamina basilaris of the cochlear duct running from the rods of Corti to the spiral ligament. **z. pellu′cida,** 1. the transparent, noncellular secreted layer surrounding an oocyte. 2. area pellucida. **z. perfora′ta,** the inner portion of the lamina basilaris of the cochlear duct. **z. radia′ta,** a zona pellucida, def. 1. **z. reticula′ris,** the innermost layer of the adrenal cortex. **z. stria′ta,** a zona pellucida exhibiting conspicuous striations. **z. tec′ta,** canal of Corti. **z. vasculo′sa,** a region in the supramastoid fossa containing many foramina for the passage of blood vessels.

zone (zōn) an encircling region or area; by extension, any area with specific characteristics or boundary. **ciliary z.,** the outer of the two regions into which the anterior surface of the iris is divided by the angular line. **comfort z.,** an environmental temperature between 13° and 21° C. (55°–70° F.) with a humidity of 30 to 55 per cent. **epileptogenic z.,** an area which when stimulated may bring on an epileptic attack. **erogenous z's, erotogenic z's,** areas of the body whose stimulation produces erotic desire. **Lissauer's marginal z.,** a bridge of white substance between the apex of the posterior horn and the periphery of the spinal cord. **transitional z.,** any anatomical region that marks the point at which the constituents of a structure change from one type to another.

zonesthesia (zo″nes-the′zhah) a sensation of constriction, as by a girdle.

zonifugal (zo-nif′u-g′l) passing outward from a zone or region.

zonipetal (zo-nip′ah-t′l) passing toward a zone or region.

zonula (zōn′u-lah), pl. *zon′ulae* [L.] zonule.

zonule (zōn′ūl) a small zone. **zon′ular,** adj. **ciliary z., z. of Zinn,** a series of fibers connecting the ciliary body and lens of the eye.

zonulitis (zōn″u-li′tis) inflammation of the ciliary zonule.

zonulolysis (zōn″u-lol′ĭ-sis) dissolution of the

ciliary zonule by use of enzymes to permit surgical removal of the lens.

zonulotomy (zōn″u-lot′o-me) incision of the ciliary zonule.

zoodermic (-der′mik) performed with the skin of an animal, as in skin grafting.

zoogenous (zo-oj′ĕ-nus) 1. acquired from animals. 2. viviparous.

zooglea (zo″o-gle′ah) a colony of bacteria embedded in a gelatinous matrix.

zoogony (zo-og′ah-ne) the production of living young from within the body. **zoog′onous,** adj.

zoografting (zo′o-graf″ting) the grafting of animal tissue.

zooid (zo′oid) 1. animal-like. 2. an animal-like object or form. 3. an individual in a united colony of animals.

zoolagnia (zo″o-lag′ne-ah) sexual attraction toward animals.

zoology (zo-ol′o-je) the biology of animals.

Zoomastigophorea (zo″o-mas″tĭ-go-for′e-ah) a class of protozoa (subphylum Mastigophora), including all the animal-like, as opposed to plant-like, protozoa.

zoonosis (-no′sis, zo-on′ah-sis), pl. *zoono′ses, zoon′oses.* Disease of animals transmissible to man. **zoonot′ic,** adj.

zooparasite (zo″o-par′ah-sīt) any parasitic animal organism or species. **zooparasit′ic,** adj.

zoopathology (-pah-thol′ah-je) the science of the diseases of animals.

zoophagous (zo-of′ah-gus) carnivorous.

zoophilia (zo″o-fil′e-ah) 1. abnormal fondness for animals. 2. a paraphilia in which intercourse or other sexual activity with animals is the preferred method of achieving sexual excitement.

zoophobia (-fo′be-ah) irrational fear of animals.

zooplasty (zo′o-plas″te) zoografting.

zoospore (zo′o-spor) a motile, flagellated, sexual or asexual spore, as produced by certain algae, fungi, and protozoa.

zootomy (zo-ot′ah-me) the dissection or anatomy of animals.

zootoxin (zo″o-tok′sin) a toxic substance of animal origin, e.g., venom of snakes, spiders, and scorpions.

zoster (zos″ter) herpes zoster.

zosteriform (zos-ter′ĭ-form) resembling herpes zoster.

zosteroid (zos′ter-oid) zosteriform.

Z-plasty (ze′plas-te) repair of a skin defect by the transposition of two triangular flaps, for relaxation of scar contractures.

Zr chemical symbol, *zirconium.*

zwitterion (tsvit′er-i″on) an ion that has both positive and negative regions of charge.

zyg(o)- word element [Gr.], *yoked; joined; a junction.*

zygal (zi′g′l) shaped like a yoke.

zygapophysis (zi″gah-pof′ĭ-sis) the articular process of a vertebra.

zygion (zij′e-on), pl. *zyg′ia.* The most lateral point on the zygomatic arch.

zygodactyly (zi″go-dak′tĭ-le) union of digits by soft tissues (skin), without bony fusion of the phalanges.

zygoma (zi-go′mah) 1. the zygomatic process of the temporal bone. 2. zygomatic arch. 3. a term sometimes applied to the zygomatic bone. **zygomat′ic,** adj.

zygomaticofacial (zi″go-mat″ĭ-ko-fa′shul) pertaining to the zygoma and face.

zygomaticotemporal (-tem′pah-rul) pertaining to the zygoma and temporal bone.

zygon (zi′gon) the stem connecting the two branches of a zygal fissure.

zygosity (zi-gos′ĭ-te) the condition relating to conjugation, or to the zygote, as (a) the state of a cell or individual in regard to the alleles determining a specific character, whether identical (homozygosity) or different (heterozygosity); or (b) in the case of twins, whether developing from one zygote (monozygosity) or two (dizygosity).

zygote (zi′gōt) the cell resulting from union of a male and a female gamete; the fertilized ovum. More precisely, the cell after synapsis at the completion of fertilization until first cleavage. **zygot′ic,** adj.

zygotene (zi′go-tēn) the synaptic stage of the first meiotic prophase in which the two leptotene chromosomes undergo pairing by the formation of synaptonemal complexes to form a bivalent structure.

Zyloprim (zi′lo-prim) trademark for preparations of allopurinol.

zym(o)- word element [Gr.], *enzyme; fermentation.*

zymase (zi′mās) enzyme.

zymogen (zi′mo-jen) proenzyme. **zymogen′ic,** adj.